Textbook of
CRITICAL CARE NURSING
Diagnosis and Management

LYNNE ANN THELAN, MN, RN

Critical Care Consultant and Lecturer
formerly Critical Care Instructor
Grossmont College
San Diego, California

JOSEPH KEVIN DAVIE, MSN, RN

Director, Department of Nursing
Associate Professor of Perioperative and Critical Care Nursing
Grossmont College
Administrative Coordinator, Alvarado Hospital Medical Center
San Diego, California

LINDA DIANN URDEN, DNSc, RN, CNA

Director, Staff/Program Development
Children's Hospital
San Diego, California

Foreword by

Phyllis B. Kritek, PhD, RN, FAAN

Professor and Dean
Marquette University College of Nursing
Milwaukee, Wisconsin

with 415 illustrations

The C. V. Mosby Company

ST. LOUIS • BALTIMORE • PHILADELPHIA • TORONTO   1990

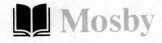

Editor: Don Ladig
Developmental editors: Jane Kinney, Sally Adkisson, Jeanne Rowland
Project manager: Suzanne Seeley
Production editor: Catherine M. Vale
Book and cover design: Gail Morey Hudson

Printed in the United States of America

The C.V. Mosby Company
11830 Westline Industrial Drive, St. Louis, Missouri 63146

Library of Congress Cataloging-in-Publication Data

Thelan, Lynne A.
    Textbook of critical care nursing.

    1. Intensive care nursing.   2.   Emergency nursing.
I.   Davie, Joseph Kevin.   II.   Urden, Linda Diann.
III.   Title.   [DNLM: 1.   Critical Care—nurses' instruction.
WY 154 T379t]
RT120.I5T48   1990   610.73'61   89-14020
ISBN 0-8016-5003-8

GW/VH/VH 9 8 7 6 5 4 3 2

To my husband **John**
confidant, consultant, baby-sitter, and
steadfast supporter throughout this project

L.A.T.

To my **Dad**
for teaching me to love work
To my **Mom**
for teaching me to love words

J.K.D.

To my **Mother**
for her faith in me

L.D.U.

From all of us to **Scout**—whose perpetual "tail wagging"
and playfulness have made many moments bearable

Contributors

CAROL ARCHIBALD, MPH, RN

Clinical Specialist/Research Associate-Pulmonary
University of California-San Diego Medical Center
San Diego, California

Chapter 17

JENNIFER BLOOMQUIST, MN, RN

Cardiothoracic Clinical Nurse Specialist
San Diego VA Medical Center
La Jolla, California

Chapters 12 and 13

JOY BOARINI, MSN, RN, CETN

Professional Education Manager, Hollister, Inc.
Libertyville, Illinois

Chapters 35, 36, and 37

KAREN BRASFIELD, MSN, RN, CNN

Instructor of Nursing, Point Loma Nazarene College
San Diego, California

Chapters 29, 30, 31, 32, 33, and 34

DOROTHY J. BRUNDAGE, PhD, RN, FAAN

Associate Professor of Nursing
Duke University School of Nursing
Durham, North Carolina

Chapter 47

RUTH BRYANT, MS, RN, CETN

Director, ET Nursing Education Program; Manager,
ET Nursing Services
Abbott-Northwest Hospital
Minneapolis, Minnesota

Chapters 35, 36, and 37

JOANN CLARK, MSN, RN

Professor of Nursing
Grossmont College
San Diego, California

Chapters 39, 40, 41, and 42

KATHLEEN S. CROCKER, MSN, RN, CNSN

Director of Nursing, New England Critical Care
Nutritional Support Clinical Specialist
Westboro, Massachusetts

Chapter 38

JOSEPH K. DAVIE, MSN, RN

Associate Professor of Perioperative and Critical Care Nursing
Grossmont College
San Diego, California

Chapters 1, 16, 22, 28, 34, 38, 42, and 47

KATHERINE M. FORTINASH, MSN, RN, CS

Professor of Psychiatric-Mental Health Nursing
Grossmont College
San Diego, California

Chapters 28, 48, and 49

JANE FREIN, MN, RN

Education Services Manager, Marian Medical Center
Santa Maria, California

Chapter 5

SHEANA WHELAN FUNKHOUSER, MN, RN

Doctoral Student, UCLA School of Nursing
Los Angeles, California

Chapter 11

JUDITH R. HEGGIE, MS, RN, CCRN

Clinical Nurse Specialist MICU/CCU
San Diego VA Medical Center
La Jolla, California

Chapter 16

BONNIE JENNINGS, DNSc, RN, LTC, AN

Nurse Researcher, Health Care Studies Division
US Army Health Services Command
Houston, Texas

Chapter 50

JACQUELINE L. KARTMAN, MS, RNC, CCRN

Cardiovascular Clinical Nurse Specialist
LaCrosse, Wisconsin

Chapters 6, 7, and 8

CHRISTINE KENNEDY-CALDWELL, MSN, RNC, CNSN

Doctoral Student
Brown University
Providence, Rhode Island

Chapters 35, 36, and 37

GERE HARRIS LANE, MSN, MEd, RN, GNP

Director, Medical-Surgical Services
Cheshire Medical Center
Keene, New Hampshire

Chapters 18, 19, 20, and 21

GAIL B. LEWIS, MSN, RN, CCRN

Instructor, Barnes Hospital School of Nursing
St. Louis, Missouri

Chapter 43

MARY E. LOUGH, MS, RN, CCRN

Assistant Clinical Professor
University of California-San Francisco
San Francisco, California
Critical Care Educator, Sequoia Hospital
Redwood City, California

Chapter 13

MARTHA LOVE, MN, RN

Cardiovascular Clinical Nurse Specialist
VA Medical Center
Asheville, North Carolina

Chapter 13

MARY COURTNEY MOORE, MSN, RN, RD

Doctoral Student, Vanderbilt University
Nashville, Tennessee

Chapters 9 and 10

CYNTHIA E. NORTHROP, MS, JD, RN

Nurse Attorney
New York, New York

Chapter 3 and Legal Reviews

MADELINE M. O'DONNELL, MS, RN, CCRN

Cardiovascular Clinical Nurse Specialist
Massachusetts General Hospital
Boston, Massachusetts

Chapter 14

THOMAS W. OERTEL, MSN, RN

Instructor of Nursing
Grossmont College
San Diego, California

Chapters 45 and 46

ANGELA S. PALOMO, MN, RN

Clinical Nurse Specialist-Cardiovascular Surgery
University of Colorado Health Sciences Center
Denver, Colorado

Chapter 15

JEANNE RAIMOND, MSN, RN, CCRN

Neuroscience Clinical Nurse Specialist
Alvarado Hospital Medical Center
San Diego Rehabilitation Institute at Alvarado
San Diego, California

Chapter 28

JUDITH HARTMAN RUEKBERG, MSN, RN

Coordinator-Pulmonary Rehabilitation
Pulmonary Clnical Nurse Specialist
Alvarado Hospital Medical Center
San Diego Rehabilitation Institute at Alvarado
San Diego, California

Chapter 21

PENNY SCHOENMEHL, MN, RN, CS

Clinical Nurse Specialist
San Diego VA Medical Center
La Jolla, California

Appendix D

LYNNE A. THELAN, MN, RN

Critical Care Consultant and Lecturer
San Diego, California

Chapters 16, 17, 19, 20, 22, 28, 34, 38, and 42

SONDRA THIEDERMAN, PhD

President, Cross-Cultural Communications
San Diego, California

Chapter 4

LAURA TOLEDO, MS, RN

Consultant in Post-Anesthesia and Critical Care
San Diego, California

Chapter 18

DAVID UNKLE, MSN, RN, CCRN, CEN

Clinical Research Coordinator
Division of Trauma and Emergency Services
Robert Wood Johnson Medical School at Camden
Camden, New Jersey

Chapter 44

LINDA D. URDEN, DNSc, RN, CNA

Director, Staff/Program Development
Children's Hospital and Health Center
San Diego, California

Chapter 2, Research Abstracts

HELEN VOS, MS, RN, CNRN, CCRN

Director of Clinical Projects
University of California-San Diego Medical Center
San Diego, California

Chapters 23, 24, 25, 26, and 27

EVELYN WASSLI, DNSc, RN

Unit Coordinator, Community Mental Health Services
Washington, DC

Chapter 48

Consultants

TOM AHRENS, DNS, RN, CCRN

Barnes Hospital
St. Louis, Missouri

MARTHA BAKER, MEd

Baylor University
Dallas, Texas

DIANE BILLINGS, EdD, RN

Indiana University
Indianapolis, Indiana

SARA BRENNER, MS, RN

State University of New York at Brockport
Brockport, New York

SHARON BROSCIOUS, MSN, RN, CCRN

Norfolk State University
Norfolk, Virginia

PAMELA BUTLER, MS, JD, RN

University of Tulsa
Tulsa, Oklahoma

FRANCESCA P. CARIELLO, MSN, RN, CCRN

University of California-San Diego Medical Center
San Diego, California

MICHAEL J. DAVIE, Esq.

Jacksonville, Florida

DARE DOMICO, MN, RN

Medical College of Georgia
Athens, Georgia

SARA DOUGLAS, MSN, CCRN

Illinois State University
Normal, Illinois

SALLY DUCHIN, PhD, RN

University of Texas
Houston, Texas

SARA FRY, PhD, RN

University of Maryland
Baltimore, Maryland

TONI GALVAN, MSN, RN, CCRN

University of Texas at Tyler
Tyler, Texas

GAYLING GEE, MS, RN

San Francisco General Hospital
San Francisco, California

ROBERT W. GILLESPIE, MD

Burn Surgery
Lincoln, Nebraska

RENEE HOLLERAN, MSN, RN, CEN, CCRN

University Air Care
Cincinnati, Ohio

CHERI HOWARD, MSN, RN

Indiana University Hospital
Indianapolis, Indiana

DEBBIE KLEIN, MSN, RN, CCRN, CS

Case Western Reserve University
Cleveland, Ohio

SISTER KATHLEEN KREKELER, PhD, MSN, BSN

St. Louis University
St. Louis, Missouri

GENELLE LEE, MSN, RN

UCLA Medical Center
Los Angeles, California

GAIL LEWIS, MSN, RN

St. Louis University
St. Louis, Missouri

HELEN MIRAMENTES, MS, BS, BA, CCRN

California Nurses Association
San Francisco, California

LEONA MOURAD, MSN, RN

Ohio State University
Columbus, Ohio

KELLY HAMPTON NADEAU, MN, RN, CCRN

DeKalb Medical Center
Atlanta, Georgia

AMY PERRIN ROSS, MSN, RN, CNRN

Loyola University Medical Center
Maywood, Illinois

KAREN RUSSELL, RRT, RCP

Division of Pulmonary Medicine
Grossmont District Hospital
San Diego, California

BARBARA SOULE, BS, RN, CIC

St. Peter's Hospital
Olympia, Washington

DEBORAH SPRITZ, MS, RN, CCRN

University of Maryland
Baltimore, Maryland

JULIE STANIK, MA, MS, RN, CCRN

Old Dominion University
Norfolk, Virginia

ROBERTA M. STEWART, MSN, RN

Neurosurgical Associates
Norfolk, Virginia

MARY ALICE SUSCA, CCC-SP

San Diego, Rehabilitation Institute at Alvarado
San Diego, California

LAURA TALBOT, MSN, RN

Texas Christian University
Fort Worth, Texas

GAYLE A. TRAVER, MSN, RN

University of Arizona
Tucson, Arizona

LINDA YACONE, BS, RN, CCRN

Halifax Medical Center
Daytona Beach, Florida

Foreword

In 1973 I stood on the edges of the first National Conference, which had convened to struggle toward a collective exploration of the concept of nursing diagnosis. A good deal of energy was directed at confronting the concept itself: soul-searching questions about acceptability, imitation of medical science, political repercussions. I wondered then what made these such central issues. We seemed brilliantly able to identify problems, stymied with the call for solutions.

As the process of creating a national organization and a consensus model of decision making progressed, I noted how we nurses seemed caught in a web of self-doubt, uncertain of our vision, nervously struggling for status, power, and control of our fate. Among ourselves, we danced the dance of the chronically oppressed and longed for freedom. Our discourse seemed driven by the desire to prove our worth by denigrating the worth of others. We could spar better than we could create.

During those years we also intensified our drift toward specialization and found ourselves fragmented by the experience. We moved further and further *from* a common language. In my reflective moments, when I surveyed the effects of this fragmentation on myself and others, I saw us as clumsy in our effort at self-definition. Like my clients, depressed women without identities, we found that even when we let go of our overidentification with others, there was still the enormous challenge of finding our own voice and of speaking clearly to one another. Letting go of a borrowed identity from medicine was difficult; assuming a nursing identity often seemed impossible. We suddenly discovered ours was the more complex, more diffuse, more multifaceted, more mysterious identity. We had not planned on this.

Slowly, the idea of nursing diagnosis took center stage, and the marginal status of those who had nurtured the idea from inception found themselves somewhat nervously embroiled in the new dynamic of an emerging discipline, with a growing fixation on power, control, recognition, status, and victory in a traditionally zero sum game. Granted the mantle of victory in a struggle over ideas, we wore it awkwardly. For many of us, the struggle had never been the intent or motivation. We had worried about the quality and nature of nursing care: the work undone because it was

unknown, the self-defeat of staff nurses that overflowed in ways that hurt patients, the systematic silencing of the creative impulse in nursing practice.

During these years, I found that these experiences usually evoked ambivalence: we were making progress, I thought, but at what price? I was sustained in these moments of discomfort by moments of healing light. I would serendipitously discover what I called pockets of hope: dedicated groups of nurses struggling to create, to make a difference in the quality of patient care, to bring us to a collective intellectual and emotional maturity simply because they shared with me a passion for nursing, a conviction about its nature and potential, its import for humans.

That is why I am writing this Foreword. This book is a manifestation for me of one such pocket of hope, a gift from other nurses who keep me both energized and committed to our common dreams. It is my way of saying thank you to the authors for their gift of hope.

And what does it give you, the reader? An opportunity to participate in the process of creation. The authors respect you, value you, and have written a book designed to bring together a complex matrix of facts, insights, beliefs, intuitions, and convictions to enhance the care you give. Critical care nurses, from the most experienced to the purest neophyte, will find here a new window on their world, one that emerges from a conviction that what we do for a living is a great deal more than we have yet to understand. Herein you will meet three nurses who not only value and respect all that critical care has been, but have both the courage and insight to sketch for you all that it can become.

Once we thought of critical care nursing as the elitist practitioner corps in acute care environments. It was a mixed perception: admiration mixed with envy of the recognition, the expertise, the capacity to deal with complexity; irritation at the blurring of nursing's identity with that of medicine coupled with a hunger for a comparably collaborative model of practice. This book can put that ambivalence to rest. It gives critical care nurses an opportunity to both continue their proud history of expertise and competence and also make manifest and clear the *nursing* character of that expertise and competence. In that world of nursing where we can most easily be misperceived as mechanistic super-technicians, this book provides a corrective: we are nurses here, and it is extraordinary because we *synthesize the whole*.

Yes, technology is a piece. But here, too, find me struggling with sleep interventions, with altered sexuality, with enormous dilemmas of morality, with the infinite potential of the human spirit, both mine and that of every patient. Yes, I am busy grasping a complex array of physiological indicators and its meaning for my patient. But notice, my contribution is one of enabling wholeness, of integration, of putting it all together for someone's health and well-being. The courage of critical care nurses is a given; the complexity of their intellectual, intuitive, and ethical competence is herein given recognition.

Increasingly, I find the metaphor of a quilt useful in understanding nursing. Each individual piece of fabric, each painstakingly made stitch, all the fibers of filling, and a backdrop of whole cloth: every component, unique in itself, is necessary to create the whole. It is useful in experiencing a quilt to study each component. It intensifies one's appreciation of the whole. And it is imperative to do so in that state of tension in which studying one component is done focusing intensely on its individual realities, and concurrently focusing on the whole. The tension of the paradox is obvious: we only understand a piece by knowing it as a unique entity; we only understand a piece by seeing it as always within a given context which shapes it uniquely.

You have in your hands a book developed by three nurses committed to quilt making. If you read it and study it in the spirit in which it was written, it will enable you to fashion your own critical care nursing quilt. That in itself is a wonderful opportunity, and I believe you will grow and be enriched by the experience. If you do, write to the authors and tell them. They are the kind of nurses who would like to receive the letter. Sometimes, as you read, you will develop new insights, ones that the authors did not have or record. If you do, write to them and tell them. They are the kind of nurses who would like to receive the letter. And somewhere in this book you may find something that bothers you, with which you disagree. If you do, write to the authors and tell them. They are the kind of nurses who would like to receive the letter. Quilt makers are that way.

Which brings me full circle to how I started this Foreword. You have before you an opportunity to look at critical care through a new set of lenses. I invite you to enjoy, even become anxious, looking through these lenses. Perhaps you could think of yourself as a participant in a dialogue. When you want to talk back, do so. The spirit of the authors is that way. And we need the dialogue in nursing. When you suddenly sense that critical care nursing, as envisioned by these authors, is a lot more than you have said out loud to yourself, enjoy the moment. We need the enjoyment in nursing. And when you sense that there is a good deal more to both nursing diagnosis and critical care than you noticed before, take pride in the moment. We need that pride in nursing.

There are moments in nursing in which pockets of hope make a difference. In a world increasingly willing to reduce the human spirit to a chronic state of despair and cynicism, hope is a precious creature. I invite you to share in the spirit of hope this book evokes in me. And I wish for you, along with the learning and quilting, an equal measure of hope.

Phyllis B. Kritek, PhD, RN, FAAN
Professor and Dean
Marquette University College of Nursing

Preface

Our intent was to create a critical care nursing text that captured and proclaimed the outstanding contributions of critical care nurses. We wanted to depict the practice of critical care nursing as being bordered only by the limits of a nurse's imagination and as vast in scope and complexity as one's creativity in posing research questions. We believe we have been successful in this.

A dominant theme of this book is nursing diagnosis and management, hence the title, *Textbook of Critical Care Nursing: Diagnosis and Management*. The book is organized around alterations in dimensions of human functioning that span biopsychosocial realms. We've gone beyond the traditional physiological focus of critical care texts and incorporated chapters on the following:

- Nursing process
- Ethical issues
- Legal issues
- Cultural issues
- Health promotion and patient education
- Sleep alterations
- Nutritional alterations
- Self-concept alterations
- Coping alterations
- Sexuality alterations
- The stress of critical care

We have treated nursing diagnosis as a prime focus for the critical care practitioner. Each nursing diagnosis is accompanied by a *Theoretical Basis* section, which examines the theoretical background of the phenomenon, its etiological influences, clinical manifestations, and sources of variance. Diagnostic phenomena are presented in a concept analysis fashion, enabling the learner to fully know the disorder she or he diagnoses. The power of a research-based critical care practice has been incorporated into nursing interventions. To foster critical thinking and decision making, a boxed "menu" of nursing diagnoses complete with specific etiological/related factors accompanies each medical disorder discussion and directs the learner to the section in the book where appropriate nursing management is detailed.

Research abstracts are integrated throughout the book to encourage incorporation of research findings into clinical practice. The abstracts are derived from published research in critical care and specialty journals of 1988 and 1989 and are distinguished by having at least one nurse as a principal investigator.

Reviews of medical malpractice case law pertinent to critical care are highlighted throughout the text to focus on the importance of safe delivery of patient care and to illustrate actions for which the nurse may be liable.

Organizationally, the book is composed of 12 major units. The chapter content of Unit I, *Foundations of Critical Care Nursing Practice*, forms the basis of practice regardless of the physiological alterations of the critically ill patient. The book may be studied in any sequence; however, it is recommended that Chapter 1, *The Nursing Process*, be studied first because it clarifies the major assumptions on which the entirety of the book is based.

Unit II, *Sleep Alterations*, examines a perennial problem in critical care and is divided into three chapters: *Sleep Physiology and Assessment, Sleep Disorders,* and *Sleep Care Plans*. Unit III, *Nutritional Alterations*, is an in-depth analysis of nutritional assessment, support, and management. This unique approach covers key nutritional aspects of body systems, as well as disorders specific to each body system.

Unit IV, *Cardiovascular Alterations*; Unit V, *Pulmonary Alterations*; Unit VI, *Neurological Alterations*; and Unit VII, *Renal and Fluids Alterations*, are each structured with the following chapters:

- Anatomy and Physiology
- Clinical Assessment
- Laboratory Assessment and Diagnostic Procedures
- Disorders
- Therapeutic Management
- Care Plans: Theoretical Basis and Management

This organization permits easy retrieval of information and provides flexibility for the instructor to individualize teaching methods by assigning chapters which best suit student needs. Unit VIII, *Gastrointestinal Alterations*, and Unit IX, *Endocrine Alterations*, are organized similarly. However, the assessment parameters, such as clinical, laboratory, and diagnostic procedures, are discussed in one chapter. In addition, disorders and therapeutic management are combined into one chapter.

Unit X, *Multisystem Alterations*, covers disorders that affect multiple body systems and necessitate discussion as a separate category. Unit X includes four chapters: *Burns, Trauma, Anaphylaxis*, and *Disseminated Intravascular Coagulation (DIC)*.

The interrelationship of human biopsychosocial dimensions is explored and applied to practice in this book to a genuine degree. Unit XI, *Psychosocial Alterations*, consists of three chapters that examine the theoretical basis and nursing process for alterations in self-concept, coping, and sexuality as consequences of critical illness and care.

Unit XII, *Stress in the Critical Care Unit*, addresses the impact of the critical care environment on the nurse and presents excellent strategies for management of this stress.

Finally, five appendixes have been included that contain extremely useful information for all students and practitioners of critical care. Appendix A, *North American Nursing Diagnosis Association's (NANDA) Taxonomy I Revised*, contains all diagnostic categories approved at the Eighth Conference on the Classification of Nursing Diagnoses. These categories are organized into the nine human response patterns of the profession's official taxonomic structure. A glossary of terms for Taxonomy I Revised is also included in this appendix. Appendix B, *Advanced Cardiac Life Support (ACLS) Guidelines*, presents the American Heart Association's decision trees for use in treating life-threatening dysrhythmias, administering emergency drugs and defibrillation during cardiopulmonary resuscitation. Appendix C, *Physiological Formulas for Critical Care*, features ten com-

monly encountered hemodynamic and oxygenation calculations presented in easily understood formulas. Recommendations for fluid replacement based on body surface area (BSA) calculation are also included. Appendix D, *Therapeutic Touch in a High-Tech Environment*, is an excellent discussion of nursing's premier "independent therapy." The discussion details the conceptual and scientific basis for therapeutic touch and includes a step-by-step guide for learning to perform the technique. Appendix E, *Universal Precautions*, is the official updated guide for prevention of infection transmission in acute care settings developed by the Centers for Disease Control.

Textbook of Critical Care Nursing: Diagnosis and Management represents a commitment on *our* part to bring you the best and the brightest in all things a textbook can offer: the best and the brightest in contributing and consulting authors from around the United States, the latest in scientific research befitting the brink of the 1990s, outstanding original artwork by one of this country's most prominent medical illustrators, George J. Wassilchenko, and an organizational format that exercises diagnostic reasoning skills and is logical and consistent. A commitment on *your* part to develop a comprehensive research-based critical care specialty practice is not a simple one, nor one casually made. This is precisely, however, our challenge to you now.

Lynne Ann Thelan
Joseph Kevin Davie
Linda Diann Urden

Acknowledgments

A project of this book's magnitude is never merely the work of its authors. The concerted talent, hard work, and inspiration of a multitude of people have produced *Textbook of Critical Care Nursing: Diagnosis and Management*, and helped to make it the state-of-the-science text we affirm it to be. A "tradition of publishing excellence" has been evident throughout our partnership with The C.V. Mosby Company. We deeply appreciate the assistance of our Executive Editor, Don Ladig, and Developmental Editors, Jane Kinney, Sally Adkisson, and Jeanne Rowland who have helped us document and refine our ideas and transform our book into a reality. Their creativity, expertise, availability, and generosity of time and resources have been invaluable to us throughout this endeavor. We are also grateful to Catherine Vale, manuscript editor, for her scrupulous attention to detail. Kathie Schmit, typist for the final manuscript, is commended for her excellent work. We are indebted to artists George J. Wassilchenko and Donald O'Connor for their extraordinary talent. Their detailed work appears throughout the text and its beauty is in itself an inspiration to learning.

Contents

Detailed Contents

FOUNDATIONS OF CRITICAL CARE NURSING PRACTICE

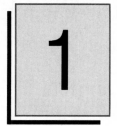

The Nursing Process

Very early in your critical care education and practice you will doubtless be impressed, perhaps even intimidated, by the magnitude and complexity of clinical decisions made by critical care nurses. This reaction is reasonable because, in actuality, critical care is critical nursing care—of highly unstable, highly at-risk patients whose health conditions change not day by day, but minute by minute.

To the casual observer, critical care in the 1990s might appear to be characterized by the application of highly sophisticated technology, but as you shall very soon see, when used alone, technology is abysmally inadequate. Its application in health care is adjunct to nursing and medical decision making. The core of critical care nursing—clinical decision making—is the focus of this chapter and of most of this book.

THE NURSING PROCESS

The nursing process is a method for making clinical decisions. It is a way of thinking and acting in relation to the clinical phenomena of concern to nurses. Classically, the nursing process comprises five phases or dimensions: data collection, nursing diagnosis, planning, implementation, and evaluation. The nursing process is a systematic decision making model that is cyclical, not linear (see Fig. 1-1). By virtue of its evaluation phase, the nursing process incorporates a feedback loop that maintains quality control of its decision-making outputs.

The nursing process is indeed a method for solving clinical problems, but it is not merely a problem-solving method. Similar to a problem-solving method, it offers an organized, systematic approach to clinical problems. Unlike a problem-solving method, the nursing process is continuous, not episodic. The nursing process doesn't become activated only in the face of an identified problem, and then deactivated when the problem is resolved. The five phases constitute a continuous cycle throughout the nurse's moment-to-moment data interpretation and management of patient care. Kritek[18] describes the phases of the nursing process as being not only continuous but "interactive"; in other words, all phases operate and influence each other and the patient simultaneously. Fig. 1-2 illustrates this interactive nature of the nursing process, wherein each phase is represented by a line that intersects with the others and converging at a point in time to which the nurse attends.[18]

Why a nursing process? Why a systematic method for approaching, analyzing, and managing clinical problems? Because it yields sound decisions. And it grooms the novice critical care practitioner for expert practice by necessitating organized thinking and maximizing the nurse's analytical skills.

The nursing process, then, serves as a template for clinical practice reasoning: data collection and analysis, the nursing conclusion about the data's collective meaning, the approach to planning and implementation of treatment, and evaluation. Two important elements strongly influence the nursing process: (1) intuition, and (2) breadth of clinical practice experience.

Intuition, or intuitive reasoning, may be defined as a person's insight into a situation without his or her conscious analysis. An intuitive insight can be likened to a "strong hunch." Intuition has been described as an individual's capacity to solve problems with relatively few data.[32]

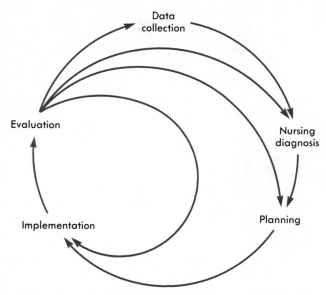

Fig. 1-1   The cyclical nature of the nursing process.

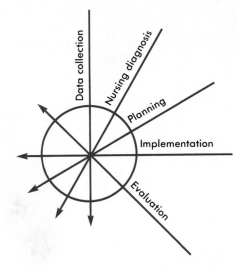

Fig. 1-2   The interactive nature of the nursing process.

The status of intuitive problem solving in nursing has had an interesting history. At one time, long before clinical decision making formally became an object of interest to the profession, it was acknowledged and accepted that nurses relied heavily on intuitive hunches or "gut feelings" to guide their clinical assessments and direct their nursing actions. Then, with the development of nursing as a science, came a scrutiny of nurses' clinical processes and methods of "knowing." Intuition as a method or ingredient of clinical problem solving was seen as "embarrassing" to the profession because of its historical association with gender and things unscientific.[23] Consequently, nursing endeavored to divest itself of intuitive processes and any lingering associations thereof. And so it was buried. What emerged in its place, as if by reaction formation, were some very narrow, stark paradigms of clinical reasoning, which eradicated all elements of subjectivity and intuition from the process. The vast complexity of nurses' decision making was reduced to what amounted to a linear equation: $a + b + c = d$.

In recent years, the nature of intuition and the complexity of clinical reasoning has begun to surface in the scientific literature. The usefulness, indeed the advantage, of intuitive reasoning as an influence on the assessment and management of clinical problems is now given considerable attention in the literature.[5,10,12,25,28]

Patricia Benner's landmark work *From Novice to Expert: Excellence and Power in Clinical Nursing Practice*[5] analyzed the reasoning processes used by expert nurse clinicians. It was found that many of these nurses were not consciously aware of the mental processes that they employed in the assessment and management of patient care problems, but that the sense on which they operated yielded remarkably superior insights.

Smith[28] analyzed the phenomenon of deterioration in critically ill adults. It was found that critical care nurses consistently sensed or felt a patient's impending crisis before any discernible physiological changes had actually taken place.[28]

Intuition can influence the nursing process in any of its five phases. It has been reported, however, as being more commonly associated with data collection and implementation of nursing interventions.[25] The usefulness of intuition and the process of intuitive reasoning will likely occupy a priority position on nursing's research agenda well into the twenty-first century.

Expertise, which is developed through clinical experience, is a second important element influencing the nursing process and has much to do with the first, intuition. In fact, the empirical limitation of intuitive problem solving is that it cannot be taught and, other than through clinical experience, cannot be learned. Clinical practice experience, beyond all other variables, is what consistently characterizes the nurse expert.[5]

Expertise in the specialty practice of clinical care nursing might seem to the beginning specialist to be dishearteningly far off, and intuition, a domain of the expert, even farther. This is an understandable perception, but one that will gradually be replaced with a more realistic perception that, given time and experience, these qualities are attainable.

Expertise: a feature of time, yes, but also of high-quality experiences, exemplary role modeling, a passionate sense of inquiry on your part, and a strong start. This chapter provides you with the latter.

Data Collection: Organizational Frameworks

By virtue of nursing's unique orientation and commitment to holism, nurses collect an enormous amount of data about a patient's biopsychosocial health status. By virtue of a vast array of technophysiological monitoring devices, critical care nurses process an additional layer of data in the form of physiological parameter measurements. Consequently, in the process of assembling this data base, the critical care nurse needs some place to file the information as it is collected. Ideally, this storage system would contain compartments, which could keep the data separated and organized. Such a system is called an *organizational framework*. Organizational frameworks also serve as guides for assessment, and their compartments consist of headings corresponding to the attributes the nurse accepts as constituting the nature of humans, health, illness, and nursing. In this way, the framework helps guide the identification of diagnoses that are within the domain of nursing.

Organizational frameworks are neither new nor unique to nursing. Traditionally, nursing used medicine's organizational framework for the collection and organization of data, but as nursing's knowledge base and conceptual orientation became increasingly differentiated and complex, the biological mechanistic scheme of medicine was found to be insufficiently comprehensive for its use by nurses as a tool for holistic assessment. The organizational framework for generalist medical practice, and two frameworks for nursing practice are shown in Table 1-1.

Functional health pattern typology. Developed by Marjory Gordon, functional health patterns are categories of human biological, psychological, developmental, cultural, social, and spiritual assessments. Health patterns, or sequences of health behavior across time, are identified and interpreted by the nurse and determined to be either functional or dysfunctional. Functional health patterns are the patient's strengths; dysfunctional health patterns form the basis for the patient's nursing diagnoses.[14] The functional health pattern typology has gained wide acceptance in nursing service and education systems as an organizational framework.

Unitary person assessment tool. In 1986, at the Seventh Conference of the North American Nursing Diagnosis Association (NANDA), a classification system for nursing diagnoses was endorsed. Named Taxonomy I Revised (see Appendix A), this classification system is based on unitary person framework (NANDA's conceptual framework) and replaces the alphabetized listing of diagnoses used previously. A taxonomy organizes known phenomena into a hierarchical structure and helps direct the discovery of new phenomena. An example of a taxonomic system from zoology is the familiar division: Kingdom, Phylum, Class, Order, Family, Genus, and Species. Strictly speaking, the alphabetized list of approved nursing diagnoses (discussed later in this chapter) constitutes a nomenclature, or system of names. The specification of a nomenclature and its successor, a taxonomy, are important preliminary steps in building nursing theory and science.

Developed by Guzzetta and associates,[15] the Unitary Person Assessment Tool is an organizational framework for use in cardiovascular critical care, though adaptable to other critical care specialties. The major categories of the tool are those of Taxonomy I Revised, the nine human response patterns (see Table 1-2).

Organizational frameworks are necessary to process the volume of information nurses accrue in the assessment of a patient. Frameworks facilitate diagnostic reasoning (discussed later in this chapter) by guiding data collection and organizing it into manageable parts. Organizing incoming information in this way increases its availability for retrieval and facilitates subsequent identification of relationships among the data.

The selection of any one framework over another, as long as it is designed to organize nursing data, is an individual choice.

Nursing Diagnosis

The concept of nursing diagnosis, a process whereby nurses interpret assessment data and apply standardized labels to health problems they identify and anticipate treating, is rapidly evolving in clinical and educational settings. Not coincidentally, this evolution is taking place parallel to the

Table 1-1 Comparison of selected organizational frameworks

Medicine	Nursing	
BODY SYSTEMS	**NANDA TAXONOMY I REVISED**	**FUNCTIONAL HEALTH PATTERNS**
Cardiovascular	Exchanging	Health perception–health management
Respiratory	Communication	
Neurological	Relating	Nutritional-metabolic
Endocrine	Valuing	
Metabolic	Choosing	Elimination
Hematopoietic	Moving	Activity-exercise
Integumentary	Perceiving	Sleep-rest
Gastrointestinal	Feeling	Cognitive-perceptual
Genitourinary	Knowing	
Reproductive		Self-perception–self-concept
Psychiatric		Role-relationship
		Sexuality-reproductive
		Coping–stress tolerance
		Value-belief

Table 1-2 Nine human response patterns of unitary person

1. Exchanging	A human response pattern involving mutual giving and receiving
2. Communicating	A human response pattern involving sending messages
3. Relating	A human response pattern involving establishing bonds
4. Valuing	A human response pattern involving the assigning of relative worth
5. Choosing	A human response pattern involving the selection of alternatives
6. Moving	A human response pattern involving activity
7. Perceiving	A human response pattern involving the reception of information
8. Knowing	A human response pattern involving the meaning associated with information
9. Feeling	A human response pattern involving the subjective awareness of information

overall process of professionalization of nursing. Critical attention is currently being focused on aspects of nursing practice and education that either foster or inhibit the establishment of the discipline of nursing as a profession.

A traditional reliance on the language and therapeutics of other sciences is inhibiting the establishment of nursing as a free-standing profession. Efforts to identify and name the conditions that nurses study and treat, on the other hand, fosters nursing's professional identity by clarifying its distinct services to society and providing a vehicle for the building of its science.

Historical development of nursing diagnosis

Pre–North American Nursing Diagnosis Association (NANDA) era. Diagnosis by nurses of health problems amenable to their treatment is not new. There is evidence that this activity spans nursing's history. During the Crimean War, Florence Nightingale identified and treated such health problems as alterations in comfort and nutrition, fear, anxiety, and potential for injury.[14] In fact, Nightingale, by her writings, teachings, and example, set the precedent for the scrupulous data collection and goal-directed planning of care that today characterizes the practice of nursing.

The term *nursing diagnosis* first appeared in the literature in the 1950s. Gordon points out that along with the genesis of this term, a fundamental change in the process whereby nurses moved from data collection to care planning began to occur: a pause in which the data collected are analyzed and grouped, the signs and symptoms of a suspected health problem identified, a possible cause uncovered, and the diagnostic conclusion stated. Only *then* was care planning begun.[14]

Historically, nursing interventions tended to be disjointed and episodic. The nurse often looked on each piece of assessment data as separate, discrete entities, neither seeking nor perceiving relationships among groups of symptoms. Intervention strategies were planned and carried out in relation to what were considered to be series of independent findings. For example, if soft tissue swelling, frequent infections, and delayed healing were observed in a patient, it is likely these would be interpreted and managed separately, that is, interventions slated to reduce swelling, some to avoid or control infection, and others to promote healing. Consider the gains if the nurse instead considers the possibility of a relationship among these symptoms, uncovers a cause, and organizes a treatment plan corresponding to the diagnosis, Altered Nutrition: Less Than Body Protein Requirements.

With nursing diagnosis as a component of our decision-making methods, we necessarily become more systematic in the collection and interpretation of data and accomplish a change in the substance of our clinical operations, from symptom management to problem solving.

NANDA era. Prompted initially by a need to clarify the nurse's role and to distinguish it from that of other health professionals in their own practice setting, two faculty members at St. Louis University, Kristine Gebbie and Mary Ann Lavin, called together the First National Conference on the Classification of Nursing Diagnoses in 1973.[13] The group organized around the task of identifying, standardizing, and classifying health problems treated by nurses. This confer-

ence has heralded a now-international professional movement. The organization, now known as the *North American Nursing Diagnosis Association (NANDA),* consists of nurse theorists, nurse researchers, nurse educators, and advanced and grass roots clinicians.

The impetus for the work of NANDA and its scientific sessions derives from the necessity of establishing a vocabulary that specifically reflects the treatment domain of nursing practice. In addition to its being requisite to nursing's status as a profession, such a vocabulary serves to coordinate communication among nurses in relation to the health problems they are observing and treating, and is as much for purposes of social policy as it is, says Carpenito, for "clarifying nursing for nurses."[9]

Approved nursing diagnoses are listed on the endpaper of this book. Though not included in the table, accompanying each diagnosis are possible causative factors (etiological/related factors) and the signs and symptoms of the health problem (defining characteristics). These are used by the nurse to help formulate the diagnostic statement and tailor it to the individual patient characteristics and circumstance.

An "approved" nursing diagnosis is one accepted by NANDA as having been refined to the point of clinical usefulness and approved for beginning clinical validation through formal research methods. Practitioners using approved nursing diagnoses, their etiologies, and defining characteristics are in fact participating in the preliminary testing of the diagnoses as they relate to the health problems described by the diagnostic labels. NANDA actively seeks input from practicing nurses regarding the development and refinement of nursing diagnoses. The Association publishes guidelines for submitting new diagnoses to its Diagnosis Review Committee, and direct input into the proceedings of the biennial conferences is possible through membership and participation in NANDA and any of its regional associations.

The immediate goals of NANDA include (1) further validation and refinement of existing diagnoses and their etiologies and defining characteristics, (2) the generation of new diagnoses, (3) the incorporation of a category of wellness diagnoses, which describe patients' strengths and potential for growth, (4) the refinement of NANDA's Taxonomy I Revised, and (5) the incorporation of approved diagnoses into the tenth revision of the World Health Organization's *International Classification of Diseases.*

Definitions of nursing diagnosis. No single definition of nursing diagnosis is sufficiently comprehensive to convey its identity as a concept, a skill, and an international professional movement. Basic to any definition is the recognition that nursing diagnosis exists both as part of a process—the nursing process—and is a process unto itself—the diagnostic reasoning process.

Several of the most enduring definitions of nursing diagnosis are found in the box on p. 5. Key terms emerging from these definitions are *conclusion, judgment, inference, person's response,* and *actual* or *potential health problem.*

A nursing diagnosis is a conclusion the nurse reaches after collecting and analyzing data relative to the patient's biopsychosocial health status. It is a professional judgment in that, in addition to the collection and analysis of data, interpretations are made by the nurse about the meaning and significance of these findings both individually and collectively. This conclusion, this judgment, forms the basis for nursing action: intervention.

The term *inference* is useful in defining nursing diagnosis because it emphasizes the tentative and assumptive nature of diagnoses. Webster's Collegiate Dictionary defines inference as the "process of arriving at a conclusion by reasoning from evidence" and warns that "if the evidence is slight the term comes close to *surmise*.[31] In recognizing that elements of both judgment and inference are part of nursing diagnosis, one can appreciate the need to limit or control the influence of bias on the part of the diagnostician and in the act of diagnosing so that the diagnostic conclusion reached is as logical and factually based as possible. Inference in the context of diagnostic reasoning is discussed in greater detail later in this chapter.

The person's response to health and illness situations constitutes the focus, or phenomenon, of concern to nurses, and it is the object of nurses' diagnostic activities. In 1980, the American Nurses' Association (ANA) issued *Nursing: A Social Policy Statement,* which defined the nature and scope of the profession as follows: "Nursing is the diagnosis and treatment of human responses to actual or potential health problems."[2] Actual or potential health problems to which nurses direct their diagnosis and treatment, then, are human responses—human responses to the health challenges encountered in birth, illness, wellness, growth and development, and death.

The most essential and distinguishing feature of any nursing diagnosis is that it describe a health condition *primarily resolved by nursing interventions or therapies*. There is, however, some difficulty in applying this criterion to the broad spectrum of health problems that nurses have historically, do currently, and will in the future identify and treat. The boundaries of nursing and those, particularly, that it shares with other health professions, are dynamic and not at once easily delineated.[2]

To assist in clarifying the boundaries of nursing and provide a framework for the development and classification of nursing diagnoses, the ANA outlines the following categories of health problems, the treatment of which lies within the profession's domain[9]:

1. Self-care limitations
2. Impaired functioning in areas such as rest, sleep, ventilation, circulation, activity, nutrition, elimination, skin, sexuality, and the like
3. Pain and discomfort
4. Emotional problems related to illness and treatment; life-threatening events; or daily life experiences, such as anxiety, loss, loneliness, and grief
5. Distortion of symbolic functions, reflected in interpersonal and intellectual processes, such as hallucinations
6. Deficiencies in decision making and ability to make personal choices
7. Self-image changes required by health status
8. Dysfunctional perceptual orientations to health
9. Strains related to processes that occur during life such

> # DEFINITIONS OF NURSING DIAGNOSIS
>
> *Gebbie and Lavin:* The judgment or conclusion that occurs as a result of nursing assessment.[13]
>
> *Mundinger:* A statement of a person's response to a situation or illness which is actually or potentially unhealthful and which nursing intervention can change in the direction of health.[22]
>
> *Aspinall:* A process of clinical inference from observed changes in the patient's physical or psychological condition.[3]
>
> *Gordon:* Actual or potential health problems which nurses, by virtue of their education and experience, are capable and licensed to treat.[14]
>
> *Shoemaker:* A clinical judgment about an individual, family or community which is derived through a deliberate, systematic process of data collection and analysis. It provides the basis for prescriptions for definitive therapy for which the nurse is accountable. It is expressed concisely and it includes the etiology of the condition when known.[27]

---

as birth, growth and development, and death
10. Problematic affiliative relationships

Although the above categories are not in themselves nursing diagnoses, standardization of diagnostic labels developed from within this framework helps to ensure a discipline-specific perspective for the intervention activities of professional nurses.

Nursing diagnosis in critical care. Currently there is controversy regarding the application of nursing diagnosis in critical care.[11,17,26,29] The appropriateness of critical care nurses contending that they diagnose and treat phenomena such as decreased cardiac output, impaired pulmonary gas exchange, and altered tissue perfusion is disputed, although some of the strongest reservations appear to have come from nurses outside the critical care specialty.

In addition to the scientific and general assembly sessions of the biennial NANDA Conference, the American Association of Critical-Care Nurses (AACN) and Marquette University have cosponsored national conferences addressing nursing diagnosis in critical care and the professional issues from which it is inseparable. The basic elements of the controversy follow.

The physiological diagnosis controversy. Since the inception of an organized nursing diagnosis movement, controversy has surrounded the question of what is and is not the domain of nursing diagnosis. On one side of this issue, it is held that the term nursing diagnosis should refer only to health states that professional nurses manage independent of other health care professionals. Health problems for which nurses do not assume exclusive responsibility, it is argued, do not meet the criteria for a nursing diagnosis. Out of this argument has come a persistent focus on "the physiological diagnoses" (for example, Decreased Cardiac Output and Dysreflexia) as being the outliers from mainstream nursing diagnoses.

On the other side of the issue, however, it is not the physiological diagnoses alone that necessitate or profit from interdisciplinary collaboration. Body Image Disturbance, Rape-Trauma Syndrome, Impaired Verbal Communication, Dysfunctional Grieving, and others are diagnoses not uniformly managed independently by nurses—independent, that is, of the perspective of such allied disciplines as psychiatry, psychology, speech pathology, social work, and thanatology. So, the argument goes, what is the actual distinction between the domain of "physiological" and "nonphysiological" diagnoses?

Moreover, Roberts[26] points out that since the original formulations on the application of nursing diagnosis "times have changed and critical care nursing has become a highly technical and advanced area of practice in which most nursing diagnoses are primarily physiologic." Critical care nurses work intimately with physiological phenomena and, through a research-based practice, may independently and successfully manipulate variables such as left ventricular afterload, ventilation-perfusion ratios and intracranial pressure. The deliberate, substantive, and research-based contribution of any health discipline to a therapeutic regimen constitutes the practice domain of that discipline.[11] That which nurses treat should be described with nursing diagnoses.

For clarity, the position taken in this book is one of inclusion versus exclusion: all phenomena—physiological, psychological, and social—of concern to critical care nurses and the object of their treatment are represented by nursing diagnoses throughout this text. The factors contributing to their development (their etiological factors) are modifiable by nursing intervention.

Kritek[18] asserts that the categorization of nursing diagnoses as *independent* or *collaborative* constitutes a political distinction, not a conceptual one. If this designation is desired, however, it can be easily superimposed by the practitioner.

Formulating nursing diagnosis statements. *PES format.* There are three distinct components to a nursing diagnosis statement. The format for documenting these components is called the PES format, where:

P = *Problem.* This is a concise statement of the patient's actual or potential human response to the health state and is also called a *diagnostic label* or *category label.* Problem statements come from the list of approved nursing diagnoses (see end paper). An example is Impaired Skin Integrity.

E = *Etiology.* This is a specification of the source(s) from which the health problem is thought to arise, also called *related* or *contributing factors.* The etiology of a problem is its cause (to the extent that cause and effect can be known or shown). A nursing diagnosis may be, and often is, based on several etiological factors. These factors, whether they are psychological, biological, environmental, circumstantial, or interpersonal, interact to produce the health problem. Each diagnostic label has accompanying listings of possible causative factors. Examples of etiological factors for the diagnosis Impaired Skin Integrity are *shearing forces, physical immobilization,* and *nutritional deficit.*

S = *Signs and symptoms.* These are observed, reported, or measured biopsychosocial findings that serve as supporting evidence of the diagnosis, also called the *defining characteristics* or *manifestations.* Defining characteristics are listed for each diagnostic label. Examples of defining characteristics for the diagnostic label Impaired Skin Integrity are *disruption of skin surface* and *destruction of skin layers.*

When communicating nursing diagnoses, either verbally or in writing, nurses customarily link the PES components with words that indicate the direction of the relationship between the problem, its etiologic factors, and defining characteristics. The problem and etiology are linked with the indicator *related to* and the defining characteristics are linked by the indicator *as evidenced by.* To illustrate documenting diagnostic statements in this way, a diagnosis of Pain would be written:

Pain *related to muscle spasm as evidenced by (patient statements) "8/10," "sharp knifelike pain,"* and *(nurse observations) guarding behaviors, tightened brow, tachycardia.*

Additionally, it is common practice to abbreviate *related to* and *as evidenced by* as *R/T* and *AEB,* respectively. A diagnosis of Constipation would be written:

Constipation *R/T immobility, fluid volume deficit, AEB no BM × 5 days, hypoactive bowel sounds, straining at stool.*

Guidelines for use of the list of approved nursing diagnoses. It is important to recognize that classification of the phenomena to which a profession addresses itself is a sizable and ongoing task. The development and refinement of nursing's nomenclature of health problems is in its earliest stages and subject to much revision based on the research and clinical reports presented and reviewed at each of NANDA's conferences and by the Diagnosis Review Committee. Work on existing diagnoses is also incomplete. Several have etiologies and defining characteristics yet to be developed, making clinical use difficult and frustrating. Other diagnoses may be deleted from the approved list from conference to conference. Such changes are both necessary and usual in the process of taxonomy development. One has only to look at the system of names describing health problems treated by physicians not many years ago (for example, chilblains, consumption, dropsy) to appreciate nursing's progress to date.

Guidelines for PROBLEMS (P)

DEFINITIONS OF HEALTH PROBLEMS. Many diagnoses have accompanying definitions to better explain the health problem. These definitions are important for the student of nursing diagnosis to consider, because they clarify more about the problem than is apparent from the label alone. For example, the definitions accompanying the diagnoses Fear and Anxiety draw a particularly useful distinction between the two problems: Fear is an emotion that has an identifiable source or object that the patient validates, whereas Anxiety is an emotion whose source is nonspecific or unknown to the patient. Other good examples of such definitions accompany the diagnoses Social Isolation, Powerlessness, Altered Parenting, and Ineffective Family Coping.

Until definitions accompany all approved diagnoses, it will be important for nurses collaborating in care to establish consensus about the meaning and scope of the health problems stated.

MAKING DIAGNOSTIC LABELS SPECIFIC. Some nursing diagnoses need accompanying qualifiers or specifiers based on the characteristics of the health problem as it manifests itself in a particular patient. For example, the diagnosis Fear needs specification as to the object of the patient's particular fear, such as death, pain, disfigurement, or malignancy. Similarly, the diagnosis Knowledge Deficit needs specification about the content of the deficiency, such as use of incentive spirometer, counting the pulse rate, or respiratory muscle strengthening exercise. Below is a list of nursing diagnoses needing specification, each with an example of a particular patient circumstance so specified:

Fear: *Postoperative Pain*
Knowledge Deficit: *Self-Monitoring of Oral Anticoagulation Therapy*
Altered *Peripheral* Tissue Perfusion
Altered Nutrition: Less than Body *Potassium* Requirements
Altered Nutrition: More Than Body *Calorie* Requirements
Self-Care Deficit: *Bathing and Feeding*
(Note: this diagnosis needs even further specification as to the functional level classification.)
Noncompliance: *Prescribed Activity Restrictions*

Guidelines for ETIOLOGIES (E)

MAKING ETIOLOGIES SPECIFIC. In many instances, etiologies are broad categories or examples needing to be made specific based on characteristics of the problem and the patient being treated. For example, one of several possible etiologies for the diagnosis Fluid Volume Excess is *compromised regulatory mechanism*. Considering this the cause of the fluid excess in a particular patient, the nurse would need to specify which regulatory mechanism and in what way compromised (for example, inappropriate ADH secretion by the neurohypophysis) before the diagnosis could be formally stated (leaving aside the question as to whether this problem is treatable by nurses or would need referral).

Several etiologies needing to be made specific are listed below, along with examples of such specification in parentheses:

Situational crisis (recent diagnosis of terminal illness)
Psychological injuring agent (hurtful relationship, verbal abuse)
Developmental factors (developmental arrest, extremes of age)

NURSING DIAGNOSES AS ETIOLOGIES. Nursing diagnostic labels may rightfully serve as etiologies for other diagnoses. Examples are Anxiety R/T knowledge deficit, and Activity Intolerance R/T decreased cardiac output.

ETIOLOGIES AS THE FOCUS OF TREATMENT. The treatment plan formulated for a given diagnosis must include interventions aimed at resolution or management of the etiologic factors as well as the health problem. In fact, in some instances nursing treatment will be directed exclusively at the etiology of a problem, with the logical expectation that, if the causative factors are reduced in influence, the problem should begin to be resolved. This will be especially true in instances where a nursing diagnosis has as its etiology another nursing diagnosis. Consider treatment approaches to the diagnosis Ineffective Breathing Pattern R/T high abdominal incision pain. Predictably little effectiveness would be shown were the interventions to be focused solely on reviewing the rationale for slow, deep, symmetrical breathing; demonstrating the technique; and encouraging the patient in its performance without some plan for manipulation of the pain variable.

MEDICAL DIAGNOSES AS ETIOLOGIES. Because, as previously mentioned, the etiology of a nursing diagnosis becomes a focus of intervention in the treatment of the overall problem, citing a medical condition or diagnosis as the etiology is conceptually inadvisable if the problem statement is to retain its identity as a health problem primarily resolved by nursing therapies. And yet many problems of concern to critical care nurses and amenable to their treatment *are* consequent to medical conditions. Examples are the Ineffective Airway Clearance that results from chronic obstructive pulmonary disease (COPD), and Sensory-Perceptual Alterations resulting from coronary artery bypass graft surgery. In these instances, the nurse should isolate those aspects of the contributing pathological state that are modifiable by nursing intervention, and cite these factors as etiological; for instance, Ineffective Airway Clearance R/T thick tracheobronchial secretions, respiratory muscle weakness, and knowledge deficit: effective cough and hydration techniques; and Sensory-Perceptual Alterations R/T sensory overload, sensory deprivation, and sleep pattern disturbance. These problem statements are more clearly worded and provide a much sharper focus for nursing intervention.

Guidelines for DEFINING CHARACTERISTICS [*signs and symptoms*] (S)

MAKING DEFINING CHARACTERISTICS SPECIFIC. As with problem statements and statements of etiology, defining characteristics cited for diagnoses are in nonspecific form and often need to be modified to reflect the particular situation presented by the patient being diagnosed. For example, the diagnosis Impaired Gas Exchange has as one of its possible defining characteristics *abnormal blood gases*. In the nurse's formulation of this diagnostic statement for clinical use, the specific blood gas value used to diagnose the problem should be cited in the statement (for example, PO_2: 54 mm Hg and/or PCO_2: 50 mm Hg) versus the nonspecific symptom category, abnormal blood gases.

Several defining characteristics are cited below in nonspecific form, with accompanying examples of proper specification:

Respiratory depth changes (hypoventilation)
Blood pressure changes (hypotension)
Autonomic responses (dilated pupils, tachycardia)
Altered electrolytes (hypokalemia)

Change in mental state (confusion, obtundation, apprehension)

MAJOR OR CRITICAL DEFINING CHARACTERISTICS. Major or critical defining characteristics are designated signs and/or symptoms that *must be present for the health problem to be considered present.* Major defining characteristics, when applicable, must be present in the nurse's assessment profile to diagnose the corresponding health problem with any degree of certainty. For example, the diagnosis Unilateral Neglect has as its major defining characteristic *consistent inattention to stimuli on affected side.* It is essential, then, that this characteristic be present in the patient's situation (in addition, perhaps, to several other noncritical signs) for the diagnosis of this problem. The assignment of major or critical status to a defining characteristic is based on research or extensive clinical experience in which the signs and symptoms of a health problem are tested for their ability to most reliably predict the presence of the diagnosis and can therefore be used with confidence by the nurse diagnostician.

Guidelines for diagnosing high-risk states and potential health problems

DETERMINING A RISK-STATE FOR DIAGNOSIS. Predicting a potential health problem in a given patient involves an estimation of probability. The potential for an event, or pattern of response, to occur can truly be said to exist in almost any situation. Consider the potential health problems facing the postoperative patient. This risk state includes Potential Noncompliance with the rehabilitative regime, Potential Body Image Disturbance, Potential Sleep Pattern Disturbance, Potential Ineffective Airway Clearance, Potential Constipation, and Potential for Aspiration to name only a few. To state each of these diagnoses on a treatment plan without regard for probabilities and develop desired patient outcomes and interventions for each is pointless.

What needs to occur is an appraisal of the patient's health status and the identification of risk factors that place him or her at higher risk for the health problem than the general population. For example, all persons recovering from abdominal surgery have Potential for Constipation because of the effects of general anesthesia and narcotic analgesics, manipulation of abdominal viscera, and postoperative immobility. All nurses have a tacit undertanding of this risk, and monitoring and intervention are carried out to avert the problem as part of routine nursing care, hence no need to state the problem.* A patient is at higher risk than the general population of postoperative patients if there is, for example, a history of dependence on laxatives, fluid volume deficit, prolonged immobility, or noncompliance with nursing prescription for ambulation. The diagnosis indicating this potential and its risk factors would be stated so that additional and/or more intensified interventions, over those that are routine, can be planned.

STATING POTENTIAL DIAGNOSES. Several of the approved diagnoses address potential dysfunctional states and cite defining characteristics as risk factors. Examples of such diagnoses are:

Altered Nutrition: Potential for More Than Body Requirements
Potential For Aspiration
Potential For Disuse Syndrome
Potential For Infection
Potential for Impaired Skin Integrity
Potential For Injury
Potential for Poisoning
Potential for Suffocation
Potential for Trauma
Potential for Violence

In addition to those diagnoses formally listed as potential, any diagnosis from the approved list can be stated as a potential problem by simply adding the modifier *potential* to the label. For example, Self-Esteem Disturbance can be written Potential Self-Esteem Disturbance by virtue of there being risk factors present but not yet the actual health problem.

Potential nursing diagnoses have only two parts to the statement: the *health problem at risk* and the *risk factors.*[14] An example is Potential Ineffective Individual Coping, risk factors: malignant biopsy results, absence of interpersonal support system, and history of alcohol abuse.

DIAGNOSING THE POTENTIAL FOR A MEDICAL PROBLEM. Nurses were speaking the language of prevention long before it became economically imperative to do so. Many activities that make up the professional nursing role in general, and the critical care nursing role specifically, relate to the promotion of health and prevention of illness and complications. Hence the prevention of some medical conditions is justifiably well within the nursing domain. Potential for Atelectasis, Potential for Joint Contractures, and Potential for Thrombophlebitis, though not so designated within NANDA's list of approved diagnoses, are examples of health problems primarily resolved by nursing interventions or therapies—problems that nurses "by virtue of their education and experience are capable and licensed to treat."[14]

Scrutiny of the entire scope and context of situations in which these and other potentials for a medical condition are diagnosed is necessary, however, to determine that the problem can and will respond *primarily* to nursing intervention. Certainly there are medical conditions that are not directly preventable by nursing therapies, such as potential for asthma and potential for breast cancer. Additionally, once the potential for a medical condition becomes an *actual* problem, it loses its designation as a nursing diagnosis and is referred to a physician.

Diagnostic reasoning. Diagnostic reasoning is the process through which the nurse moves to arrive at a nursing diagnosis. Like any process, it is often orderly and systematic. However, unlike a process, not all of its factors and operations exist in our conscious awareness. The challenge of refining one's diagnostic reasoning is to bring into awareness the factors and operations that influence the process and are necessary in arriving at an accurate "answer," or diagnosis. Four key components of diagnostic reasoning are collecting and organizing the data base, cues, inferences, and validating inferences.

---

* No need to state the problem on an individualized nursing care plan; however, this potential problem should be on record in a standards of care manual or standardized care plan.

Components

COLLECTING AND ORGANIZING THE DATA BASE. Collecting and organizing a data base was discussed earlier in this chapter, under Data Collection.

CUES. A *cue* is a piece of information, a raw fact. Nurses notice and seek cues regarding patients' health status and functioning. Sweaty palms, restlessness, and a heart rate of 102 beats/min are cues. In the process of diagnostic reasoning, cues are the units of information that are collected and recorded for later analysis.

INFERENCES. An *inference* is the assignment of meaning to cues. A nursing diagnosis is an example of an inference. When individual cues are clustered and interpreted collectively, they begin to assume an identity either the same as or different from what each represented individually. Sweaty palms, restlessness, and a heart rate of 102 beats/min, when interpreted as a cluster, can now mean anxiety, shock, fear, or pain.

Inferences are created, whereas cues exist. The process of creating inferences from cues, therefore, carries with it the risk of error in logic. If the cues sweaty palms, restlessness, and a heart rate of 102 beats/min were grouped and interpreted in a patient who also manifested gurgling respiratory sounds and a rapid, shallow breathing pattern—and these additional cues were overlooked or ignored by the person assigning meaning to the cluster—the inference might be erroneous, the more probable inference now being ineffective airway clearance. Nursing diagnoses are inferences, and the defining characteristics are the cues that lead to these inferences.

VALIDATING INFERENCES. Once a diagnostic inference is formulated, the nurse will develop and implement a treatment plan designed to resolve or reduce the problem represented by that inference. Erroneous inferences carry an obvious implication in terms of potential patient harm resulting from treatment of a nonexistent health problem or from treatment withheld for a missed diagnosis: nursing malpractice. Consequently, it is essential to seek validation of diagnostic inferences before implementing treatment.

Four approaches to the validation of inferences are recommended. The first is to consult with an authoritative source. This may be a clinical nurse specialist, nurse educator, a textbook, or published research, for example. Seek confirmation of the logical and scientific integrity of your diagnostic statement. Second, reexamine the cues: Could the ones in this diagnostic statement support any other diagnosis or only the one chosen? Could the cues from the data base felt *not* to be a part of the cluster supporting this diagnosis belong to some other cluster, or could several of them, together with cues supporting this diagnosis, suggest an altogether different diagnosis? Third, nurses should validate inferences with the patient. Nurses may share with the patient the cluster of cues identified and what is represented. Patients often have remarkable insight into what underlies their patterns of response and can be of great resource in validating the nurse's conclusions. Additionally, people benefit significantly from having their situations reflected back to them. Indeed, collaborating with the patient in this way may be all the intervention that is necessary. Fourth is to seek evidence of the reliability of the diagnostic inference from within the appropriate reference group. Do most professional peers conclude the same explanation for the available cues?

These approaches are workable strategies for seeking validation of diagnostic inferences before the institution of treatment; however, the only way to achieve or confirm validation of a diagnosis is to treat the problem and evaluate the outcome. If favorable and predicted outcomes result, strong evidence exists that the problem and its etiology and defining characteristics were accurately inferred.

Sources of diagnostic error. Currently there is much scientific curiosity within the nursing profession regarding the diagnostic reasoning process, strategies effective in increasing diagnostic accuracy, and sources of diagnostic error. Many of the principles identified through research thus far have come from studying differences in the diagnostic strategies employed by experts and those used by novices.[5,6,8,30] The following discussion will focus only on the most common type of diagnostic error, *the inferential leap*, and several of its sources. For more in-depth examinations of the skills of clinical problem solving and decision making, the reader is referred to Gordon, Carnevali, Tanner, and Benner.

INFERENTIAL LEAP. As the term implies, the inferential leap involves a jump to a conclusion based on premature termination of the data gathering/data analysis phase of the nursing process. Numerous studies have shown that this jump to an erroneous conclusion is most frequently made because not all of the variables were known or examined at the time the inference was formulated.[5,8,30] Interestingly, the novice often closes the *search* for cues prematurely, whereas the expert will more often prematurely terminate the *analysis* of cues.

The novice may close the search for cues prematurely because of a lack of understanding of the scope of the problem to be diagnosed. Diagnoses such as Disturbance in Self-Concept and Ineffective Individual Coping are reported to be at the highest level of abstraction among nursing diagnoses and are therefore more difficult to fully grasp, let alone discriminate from other diagnostic possibilities.[21] The expert has an advantage in this regard by virtue of a greater breadth of experience, both with the label and the clinical presentation of patients demonstrating the problem.

Additionally, the novice will often halt the collection of data and conclude a diagnosis prematurely because of a discomfiture with uncertainty. The erring expert will, however, occasionally rely too heavily on knowledge from previous experience, which can foster a tendency to stereotype patients and their health alterations, thereby obscuring vital relationships among assessment data.[8]

Professional advantages of nursing diagnosis. Baer has assembled from the literature the following statements in advocacy of nursing diagnosis. They are presented here to highlight the advantages nursing diagnosis brings to the profession.

Nursing diagnosis

■ Assists in organizing, defining, and developing nursing knowledge

■ Aids in identifying and describing the domain and scope of nursing practice

- Focuses nursing care on the patient's response to problems
- Prescribes diagnosis-specific nursing interventions that should increase the effectiveness of nursing care
- Facilitates the evaluation of nursing practice
- Provides a framework for testing the validity of nursing interventions
- Provides a standardized vocabulary to enhance intra-professional and interprofessional communication
- Prescribes the content of nursing curricula
- Provides a framework for developing a system to direct third-party reimbursements for nursing services
- Indicates specific rationales for patient care based on nursing assessment
- Leads to more comprehensive and individualized patient care[4]

In summary, nursing diagnoses are standardized labels that represent clinical judgments made by professional nurses and describe health problems resolved primarily by nursing therapies. Nursing diagnosis focuses nursing assessment and intervention on the human response to altered health states, thus constituting a unique, distinct, and imperative component to critical health care. Nursing diagnosis is mandated as part of competent registered nurse criteria by many state Nurse Practice Acts, as well as constituting the core of the ANA's formal definition of nursing.

Planning

Two things are accomplished in the planning phase of the nursing process: (1) patient *outcome criteria* are established and (2) *nursing interventions* are selected.

Outcome criteria. Outcome statements consist of highly specific indicators that will be used by the nurse in the evaluation phase as criteria that either (1) the actual problem has been resolved or reduced, or (2) the potential problem has not occurred. An outcome statement is a projection of the expected influence that the nursing intervention will have on the patient in relation to the identified problem. Though often confused, statements of expected patient outcome are *not* patient goals or nursing goals, nor should they describe nursing interventions.

As shown in Fig. 1-3, outcome criteria for an *actual* problem are developed from the signs and symptoms of the nursing diagnosis. In other words, the assessment findings that were used to certify the existence of a diagnosis should also be used to establish its resolution or improvement. For example:

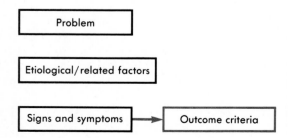

Fig. 1-3 Developing outcome criteria for an actual problem.

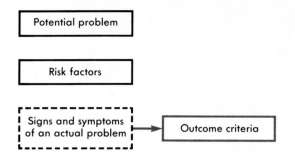

Fig. 1-4 Developing outcome criteria for a potential problem.

Nursing diagnosis	Outcome criteria
Ineffective Breathing Pattern R/T respiratory muscle fatigue AEB-P_{CO_2} = 52 -RR = 28	$P_{CO_2} \leq 45$ RR ≤ 20 at rest

Outcome criteria for *potential* problems differ only in that, being a two-part statement, signs and symptoms will be absent from the diagnostic statement. Fig. 1-4 illustrates how the outcome criteria are developed from what would be the signs and symptoms of the potential problem *were it to become actual*. For example:

Nursing diagnosis	Outcome criteria
Potential for Aspiration	Lungs clear to auscultation
RISK FACTORS:	Absence of blue tinge to
Endotracheal tube	tracheal aspirate
Continuous intraenteral feedings	Afebrile
Decreased level of consciousness	$SvO_2 \geq 94\%$

Outcome criteria should be measurable, desirable, and, given full consideration to the resources of the patient and those of the nurse, attainable.

Measurable outcome criteria consist of patient behaviors, statements, and/or physiological parameters that are recognizable on their occurrence. Many of the phenomena critical care nurses diagnose and treat are readily measurable, such as adequacy of ventilation, cardiac output, and tissue perfusion. Many, however, are not readily measurable and thus present a challenging task to care planning in general and outcome criteria development specifically. Phenomena such as anxiety, powerlessness, body image, and coping involve the patient's subjective perception and, as such, elude the nurse's quantification. Outcome statements such as "less anxiety," "perceives personal power," or "copes effectively" represent favorable goals for nursing interventions but offer little in the way of criteria against which successful patient attainment can be measured. Again, here it is helpful to consider the signs and symptoms of the problem being treated and to modify them to reflect a situation in which the problem is absent or reduced. Several examples are:

Signs and symptoms	Outcome criteria
"Why is it I have no say in any of this?"	Patient makes five decisions regarding his or her care
Distracted, preoccupied	Maintains eye contact throughout interactions
Looks away during stoma care	Visually regards stoma

Table 1-3   Correct and incorrect outcome criteria statements

Nursing diagnosis	Incorrect outcome	Correct outcome
Fluid volume deficit	Improved hydration	Systolic blood pressure ≥100 mm Hg
	Patient will be offered 100 cc fluid q 2 hr	24 hr fluid intake ≥body surface area fluid requirements
		Skin turgor ≤3 seconds
Decreased cardiac output	Hemodynamic stability	Cardiac index 2.5-4.0
Potential for thrombophlebitis	Patient will be taught active leg exercises	No calf tenderness
	Patient will perform active leg exercises 10 x q 1 hr	No ankle swelling
Pain	Patient will have a reduction in pain	Pain ≤"4/10" 10 minutes after IV narcotic
Powerlessness	Patient will perceive greater control over situation	Patient will make five decisions regarding his or her care

Outcome statements are made further measurable by indicating the date and time of anticipated attainment. Projecting outcome attainment seems in some situations to be an arbitrary exercise, such as predicting the date or hour for the return of clear lung fields. The importance of this aspect of outcome criteria development lies however in the fact that a specific deadline for evaluation of outcome attainment has been designated. Evaluating attainment of the outcome at designated intervals ensures that certain problems do not persist beyond acceptable time periods (such as Altered Peripheral Tissue Perfusion, Urinary Retention, and Pain) and that modification of the treatment approach occurs regularly. The outcome criteria applied throughout this text purposefully do not include date and time projection for attainment as this should be a reflection of actual, not hypothetical, patient characteristics.

The desirability and attainability of patient outcome criteria is another important aspect of planning nursing management. Individual patient baseline, patterns, and nurse and patient resources are the dominant considerations given to a projection of desired outcome, versus normative values. An example of an undesirable outcome is "RR <16 at rest" for a patient with an unmodifiable chest wall restriction. "Absence of pain" in a patient with a sternotomy incision is also an undesirable target for early postoperative intervention. Examples of outcome criteria that are unattainable (and therefore undesirable) are "P_{CO_2} <40" in a patient who chronically retains carbon dioxide and "no anxiety" preoperatively for open heart surgery (see Table 1-3 for examples of correct and incorrect outcome criteria statements for assorted nursing diagnoses).

Developing outcome criteria statements has particular relevance to critical care nursing, because they describe, in measurable terms, the effects or results of critical care nursing. And they communicate the influence nursing intervention has in preventing, resolving, or improving various health states and provide a basis for justifying the allocation and reimbursement of professional nursing resources.

Nursing intervention

THE POWER OF NURSING INTERVENTION. Interventions are the power of nursing and a distinct strength of this text.

Also known as *nursing orders* or *nursing prescriptions,* interventions constitute the treatment approach to an identified problem. Interventions are selected to satisfy the outcome criteria and prevent or resolve the nursing diagnosis.

A common shortcoming of nursing interventions, as much in the literature as in individual practice, is the prescription of very vague, weak, nonsubstantive nursing actions. By definition, a nursing diagnosis is a health problem that nurses treat. *Treatment* implies producing a change in a situation, not merely maintaining equilibrium. And *prescribe* connotes recommending a course of action, not simply supporting an existing regimen. Intervention strategies that consist solely of monitoring, measuring, checking, obtaining physician orders, documenting, reporting, and notifying do not fulfill criteria for the treatment of a problem. Nursing intervention for nursing diagnoses should designate therapeutic activity that assists the patient in moving from one state of health to another. The growing body of research-based independent nursing therapies should be liberally applied to treatment plans for nursing diagnoses in critical care. Exciting advances in nurse management of such phenomena as ventilation-perfusion inequalities, excessive preload and afterload, increased intracranial pressure, and sensory-perceptual alterations associated with critical illness afford the critical care nurse the opportunity to incorporate potency into treatment plans.

FOCUS FOR INTERVENTIONS. As discussed earlier in this chapter, interventions have the greatest impact when they are directed at the etiological/related factors of the diagnosis (see Fig. 1-5) or, in the case of a potential problem, the risk factors (see Fig. 1-6). This stipulates that the etiological factors of a problem be modifiable by nursing. To achieve the most favorable patient outcome, the multiple etiological factors of a problem should be studied carefully and interventions selected to modify each.

SPECIFICITY OF INTERVENTIONS. Planned interventions should provide clarity, specificity, and direction to the spectrum of nurses implementing care for a patient. Statements such as "check vital signs" and "measure I and O" provide no real direction to nursing care and are therefore quite useless. Instead, "monitor for heart rate elevations 30 beats/

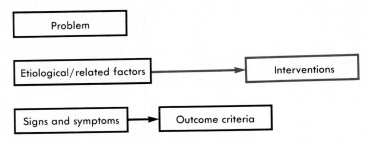

Fig. 1-5 Developing interventions for an actual problem.

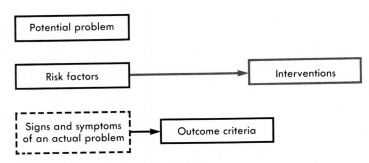

Fig. 1-6 Developing interventions for a potential problem.

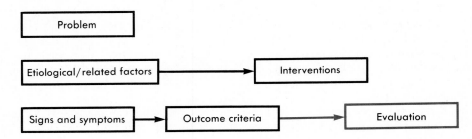

Fig. 1-7 Evaluating an actual problem.

min over baseline" and "look for 24 hr positive fluid balances" are preferable.

Include a brief rationale as part of intervention statement where this would enhance understanding of the treatment maneuver. For example, "change position dynamically q2hr, *to best match ventilation with perfusion*." Rationales are *italicized* throughout the care planning sections of this book.

Medically delegated actions, such as administering medications and initiating ventilator setting changes, should be included in the interventions but with the emphasis placed clearly on the assessments and judgments the nurse makes in evaluating their effectiveness, patient tolerance, safety, dosage, titration, and discontinuance. In critical care there is no such thing, for example, as "administer nitroprusside as ordered." Adequate specificity of nursing orders has been achieved when one is reasonably certain that a nurse unfamiliar with the patient can review the treatment plan and

implement the kind of care intended by the primary nurse or case manager.

Implementation

Implementation is the action component of planning. It is the phase of the nursing process in which the nursing treatment plan is carried out. Data collection and evaluation are continuous throughout this phase.

Evaluation

Evaluation of attainment of the expected patient outcomes occurs formally at intervals designated in the outcome criteria. Informal evaluation occurs continuously. Fig. 1-7 and Fig. 1-8 illustrate how evaluation is conducted in relation to the outcome criteria for actual and potential problems, respectively. There are two components to the evaluation phase of the nursing process. First, the nurse should compare the patient's current state with that described by the outcome

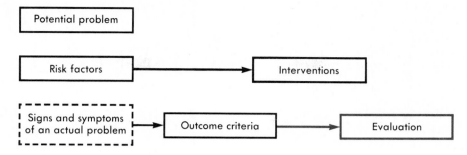

Fig. 1-8   Evaluating a potential problem.

criteria: Are his breath sounds clear and equal bilaterally? Is the tidal volume of his spontaneous respirations >500 cc, as they were projected to be by this point in time? An evaluation of nursing effectiveness is done by commenting on the extent to which a predicted outcome has been attained.

Second, the nurse should query: If not, why not? Is it too soon to evaluate? Should implementation of the plan be continued for 24 hours longer and then reevaluated? Should the interventions be intensified; perhaps increase the frequency of respiratory muscle strengthening exercises? Are the outcome criteria impractical for this patient? Is the validity of the nursing diagnosis questionable? Are more data needed? Specific recommendations are then proposed which include either continuing implementation as outlined or returning to the data collection, nursing diagnosis, planning, or implementation phase of the process.

The evaluation phase and the activities that take place within it is perhaps the most important dimension of the nursing process (see Fig. 1-1). Evaluation of patient progress against a standard of nursing care incorporates accountability into the process—accountability to the standard of care. Lack of progress in outcome attainment or lack of progress in problem solving is readily identified and kept in check, and alternate solutions can then be proposed.

REFERENCES

1. American Association of Critical-Care Nurses: Demonstration project, Newport Beach, Calif, 1988, The Association.
2. American Nurses' Association: Nursing: a social policy statement, Kansas City, Mo, 1980, The Association.
3. Aspinall NJ: Nursing diagnosis: the weak link, Nurs Outlook 24:433, 1976.
4. Baer CL: Nursing diagnosis, Top Clin Nurs 5:89, 1984.
5. Benner P: From novice to expert: excellence and power in clinical nursing practice, Menlo Park, Calif, 1984, Addison-Wesley.
6. Benner P and Tanner C: How expert nurses use intuition, Am J Nurs 87:23, 1987.
7. Carnevali DL: Nursing care planning: diagnosis and management, Philadelphia, 1983, JB Lippincott Co.
8. Carnevali DL, and others: Diagnostic reasoning in nursing, Philadelphia, 1984, JP Lippincott Co.
9. Carpenito LJ: Nursing diagnosis: application to clinical practice, Philadelphia, 1989, JB Lippincott Co.
10. Cosier RA and Alpin JC: Intuition and decision-making: some empirical evidence, Psychol Rep 51:275, 1982.
11. Davie JK: Independent and interdependent/collaborative nursing practice, Newsletter of the Southern California Nursing Diagnosis Association 5:3, 1988.
12. Dreyfus H and Dreyfus S: Mind over machine: the power of human intuition and expertise in the era of the computer, New York, 1985, Free Press.
13. Gebbie KM and Lavin MA: Classification of nursing diagnoses: proceedings of the first national conference, St Louis, 1975, The CV Mosby Co.
14. Gordon M: Nursing diagnosis: process and application, New York, 1987, McGraw-Hill Book Co.
15. Guzzetta CE, and others: Clinical assessment tools for use with nursing diagnoses, St Louis, 1989, The CV Mosby Co.
16. Guzzetta CE, and others: Unitary person assessment tool: easing problems with nursing diagnoses, Focus Crit Care 15:12, 1988.
17. Kim M: The dilemma of physiological problems: without collaboration, what's left?, Am J Nurs 85:281, 1985.
18. Kritek PB: Generation and classification of nursing diagnoses: toward a theory of nursing, Image J Nurs Sch 10:33, 1978.
19. Kritek PB: Nursing diagnosis in perspective: response to a critique, Image J Nurs Sch 17:3, 1985.
20. Kritek PB: Development of a taxonomic structure for nursing diagnoses: a review and an update. In Hurley, ME, editor: Classification of nursing diagnoses: proceedings of the sixth conference, St Louis, 1986, The CV Mosby Co.
21. Kritek PB: Advantages and limitations of using nursing diagnostic categories as a framework for nursing practice research. Audiotape transcription: Debate at the National Teaching Institute of American Association of Critical-Care Nurses, Anaheim, Calif, May 1986.
22. Mundinger MO: Nursing diagnoses for cancer patients, Cancer Nurs 1:122, 1978.
23. Munhall PL and Oiler CJ: Nursing research, Norwalk, Conn, 1986, Appleton-Century-Crofts.
24. Prescott PA, Dennis KE, and Jacox AK: Clinical decision-making of staff nurses, Image J Nurs Sch 19:56, 1987.
25. Rew L: Intuition in decision-making, Image J Nurs Sch 20:150, 1988.
26. Roberts SL: Physiologic nursing diagnoses are necessary and appropriate for critical care, Focus Crit Care 15:42, 1988.
27. Shoemaker J: Essential features of a nursing diagnosis. In Kim MJ, McFarland G, and McLane A, editors: Classification of nursing diagnoses: proceedings of the fifth national conference, St Louis, 1984, The CV Mosby Co.
28. Smith SK: An analysis of the phenomenon of deterioration in the critically ill, Image J Nurs Sch 20:12, 1988.
29. Tanner C: Overview. Symposium on nursing diagnosis in critical care, Heart Lung 14:423, 1985.
30. Tanner C, and others: Diagnostic reasoning strategies of nurses and nursing students, Nurs Res 36:358, 1987.
31. Webster's New Collegiate Dictionary, ed 9, Springfield, Mass, 1986, Merriam-Webster, Inc.
32. Wescott MR: Antecedents and consequences of intuitive thinking. Final report to US Department of Health, Education & Welfare, Poughkeepsie, New York, 1968, Vassar College.

CHAPTER

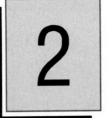

2

Ethical Issues

CHAPTER OBJECTIVES

- *Differentiate between morals and ethics.*
- *Relate the ethical theories of consequentialism and formalism to decision making in critical care.*
- *Discuss ethical principles as they relate to the critical care patient.*
- *Delineate ways in which resources are allocated in critical care.*
- *Describe landmark court cases that have impacted the management of critical care patients.*
- *Describe what constitutes an ethical dilemma.*
- *List steps for making ethical decisions.*
- *Delineate strategies for ethical decision making in critical care.*

There has been a revolution in health care in the last 50 years as the result of new technologies and treatments that were used during World War II. Issues that require ethical decisions about treatments, therapies, and life support are found in all health care settings and are most evident in technologically advanced critical care units. A multiplicity of factors surrounds ethical decisions and has an impact on both the health care recipient and the health care provider: autonomy, philosophical views of health and life, moral and ethical beliefs, societal trends, cultural background, legal directives, health care costs, and bureaucratic constraints.

The most common ethical issues that occur in critical care units are those of foregoing treatment and allocating the scarce critical care unit resource. Historically, the critical care professionals believed that life had to be maintained at all costs and that death signified the failure of medicine and technology. More recently, long-term prognosis in terms of quality of life has replaced the earlier emphasis on sanctity of life as a major factor in ethical decision making. Dracup described the conflict that is prevalent in critical care today[22]:

There are no easy answers for the myriad of ethical dilemmas that arise each day in an intensive care unit. Although knowledge of ethical principles and legal guidelines are critical to appropriate decisions, every case has its specific and often unique aspects. Each clinical situation requires open and respectful discussion

among all the concerned parties—physicians, nurses, patients (when able), and family members.

The critical care nurse is confronted with moral and ethical conflicts on a frequent, sometimes daily, basis and is the health care professional who is most involved with all persons affected by the decision.[62] It is essential that the critical care nurse has an understanding of professional nursing ethics and ethical theories and principles and that she or he is able to use a decision-making model to guide nursing actions. The purpose of this chapter is to provide the reader with an overview of moral development, ethical theories and principles, and professional nursing ethics. An ethical decision-making model will be described and illustrated. Landmark court cases will be discussed with emphasis on implications for the critical care nurse. Finally, recommendations will be given about methods to discuss ethical issues in the critical care setting.

MORALS AND ETHICS
Morals Defined

The word *moral* is derived from the Latin *moralis,* which is defined as "good or right in conduct or character . . . making the distinction between right and wrong . . . principles of right and wrong based on custom."[33] Morals are the "shoulds," "should nots," "oughts," and "ought nots" of actions and behaviors and have been related closely to sexual mores and behaviors in Western society. Religious and cultural values and beliefs largely mold one's moral thoughts and actions. Morals form the basis for action and provide a framework for evaluation of behavior.

Ethics Defined

The word *ethics* is derived from the Greek *ethos,* which is defined as "the system or code of morals of a particular person, religion, group, or profession . . . the study of standards of conduct and moral judgment."[33] The term ethics is sometimes used interchangeably with the word morals. However, ethics is more concerned with the "why" of the action rather than with whether the action is right or wrong, good or bad.[58] Ethics implies that an evaluation is being made that is theoretically based on or derived from a set of standards. *Normative ethics* is the division of ethics that focuses on "norms or standards of behavior and value and their ultimate application to daily life"[29] with an emphasis on evaluation for purposes of guiding moral action. *Bioethics* incorporates all aspects of life but most frequently refers to health care ethics and the application of ethical principles to individual cases.

MORAL DEVELOPMENT

The variables that affect moral thinking and behavior have been studied primarily in the fields of psychology and education.[29] An understanding of moral development forms the basis for the facilitation of moral reasoning in personal and professional practice. The cognitive developmental model of moral development proposed by Kohlberg[39] and modified by Gilligan[52] will be discussed as a basis for moral reasoning.

Cognitive developmental models convert certain inherent attitudes and beliefs into a complete model of moral standards from which behaviors and actions are derived. The process depends on the cognitive level of the individual and follows a series of thought patterns that are qualitatively different from each other. The stages are theorized to follow the same sequence for all persons in all cultures and to integrate life experiences.[52] Kohlberg formulated a three-level model with two stages at each level based on work done earlier by Piaget.

Kohlberg focused on a social perspective, or the view of one's relationship to society, as the basic structural element in moral development. Kohlberg's six stages of moral development are delineated in the box at right. From this view, a preconventional person in level A views rules and various adult social expectations as external to himself or herself. In stage one of level A, physical consequences of action determine whether an action is "good" or "bad." In stage 2, the right action consists of that which satisfies one's own needs and occasionally the needs of others. Children up to age 10 are usually in the preconventional level and persons in this stage are "pragmatically opportunistic" and have converted the Golden Rule into "Do unto others as others have done unto you." An individual in stage 2 functions by using others as a means to an end.[58]

A level B conventional person is one who has internalized the expectations of society and authority and uses appropriate guidelines for conduct. Inherent is an attitude of conformity and loyalty along with support and justification of moral guidelines. Stages 3 and 4 are classified in level B. In stage 3, the person now operates by the Golden Rule "Do unto others as you would have them do unto you." Mutual relations are important and peer pressure influences one's behaviors and actions. Behavior is frequently judged by intention; that is, the motivation behind a behavior is a very important consideration. Stage 4 is the law and order stage. There is an orientation toward authority, fixed rules, and the maintenance of social order. Doing one's duty in society is important.

A level C postconventional person is one who has differentiated himself or herself from others' expectations and

---

KOHLBERG'S SIX STAGES OF MORAL DEVELOPMENT

LEVEL A

Preconventional level

Stage 1

The stage of punishment and obedience

Stage 2

The stage of individual instrumental purpose and exchange

LEVEL B

Conventional level

Stage 3

The stage of mutual interpersonal expectations, relationships, and conformity

Stage 4

The stage of social system and conscience maintenance

LEVEL B/C

Transitional level

LEVEL C

Postconventional and principled level

Stage 5

The stage of prior rights and social contract or utility

Stage 6

The stage of universal ethical principles

Modified with permission from Kohlberg L: The philosophy of moral development, San Francisco, 1981, Harper & Row Publishers.

---

rules and has adopted self-chosen principles instead. Self-chosen principles may coincide with those of society, but morality is an individual choice and commitment rather than an internalization of others' expectations. Stages 5 and 6 are categorized in level C. In stage 5, individual differences are recognized and standards and laws are structures that demonstrate personal values and opinions. Law is a rational consideration that is open to change for social utility and fairness to all.[58] Stage 6 is based on self-chosen ethical principles that are abstract and universal: justice, equality of human rights, and respect for the dignity of human beings as individuals.

Kohlberg estimated that approximately 25% of society reaches the postconventional level. Progression through the stages of moral development takes about 5 years to move from one stage to the next. Most high school students reason at stages 2 and 3, and teachers reason at stages 3 and 4. High school and college graduates tend to remain at the same stage they were in at the time of graduation. Kohlberg has demonstrated that "persons understand the next higher stage from their predominant one, but cannot understand two stages higher."[58] From these findings, it can be seen that decisions regarding moral dilemmas will be made differently depending on the level of moral development of the various decision makers involved in the situation.

Kohlberg's research has demonstrated that female moral develoment is arrested at stage 3, which is reflective of her social world. He felt that women would continue to operate at this stage as long as they felt that they were successfully resolving their moral dilemmas.[58] It was at this point that Gilligan disagreed with Kohlberg regarding moral development. Kohlberg had studied only male subjects and had formulated a model of moral development that used male subjects as the standard for comparison. Gilligan contended that females were not arrested at any certain stage of development but instead developed differently than males. She purported that female moral development was based on caring and relationships rather than on a male hierarchy of values.[52] She proposed a model with three levels and two transitional stages, which is illustrated in the box below for comparison to the Kohlberg model.[52]

In Gilligan's model, the moral development of women begins with an early concern of not causing hurt to others. This concern evolves into a "more mature concern and responsibility for self and others"[34] in which she will always consider the context of the problem when faced with moral decisions. Women do not deal with absolutes and are thus more holistic in their approach to problem solving and always consider the context and relationships. Gilligan's view of moral maturity is clearly in conflict with Kohlberg's model in which context-free rules govern in the postconventional stage. Although application of the models will demonstrate different ethical practices, one view is not superior to the other.[34]

Kohlberg stressed the importance of education as a mechanism in assisting individuals to reach a higher level of moral development. Through his own research, he has validated that this education can be carried out through exposure to the thought processes of persons who function at higher levels of moral development. It is by engaging in open discussions, offering various options, and examining reasons for approaches and decisions that nurses and other health care professionals can facilitate their own moral development and that of their patients.

ETHICAL THEORIES

Philosophers have described ethical theories to be the combination of thinking processes, related principles, and rationales. The approach is normative, because it attempts to provide a basis for action. There are two traditional ethical theories that will be briefly discussed in this chapter: teleological and deontological.

Teleological Theory (Consequentialism)

The focus of this theoretical approach is on the consequence of an action. There is an obligation for individuals to provide the greatest amount of happiness for the greatest number or the least amount of harm to the greatest number. The underlying assumption is that harm and benefit can be weighed and measured and that the outcome will demonstrate a good over evil for most people.[20] According to Fowler, utilitarian ethics is the most important teleological theory for use in health care today.[29] Two common aphorisms summarize the utilitarianism approach: "the greatest good for the greatest number" and "the end justifies the means."[58]

Philosophers Jeremy Bentham and John Stuart Mill professed the utilitarian theory and presented arguments for the approach with what has been described as "calculus morality." The outcomes of all alternative actions on the welfare of present and future generations are calculated. Based on these possibilities, a decision is made as to which alternative best benefits the greatest number.[20] Rather than determining utility of an action on a single situation or act (act utilitarianism), rule utilitarians judge actions on moral rules, which leads to the greatest good for the greatest number.[29]

The effect of consequences on present and future conditions of persons and groups takes precedence in utilitar-

---

GILLIGAN'S COGNITIVE-DEVELOPMENTAL MODEL

LEVEL I: ORIENTATION TO INDIVIDUAL SURVIVAL

Morality comprises sanctions imposed by society. Being moral is surviving by being submissive to authority. This perspective is egocentric.

Transition from selfishness to responsibility

Responsibility for and to others is more important than surviving through submission.

LEVEL II: GOODNESS AS SELF-SACRIFICE

Goodness is viewed as relying on shared norms or expectations. Being moral is above all not hurting others, with no thought of the hurt that might be done to self.

Transition from goodness to truth

Responsibility for not hurting others shifts to include not only others, but self.

LEVEL III: MORALITY OF NONVIOLENCE

The injunction against hurting becomes the moral principle governing all moral judgments. This injunction inlcudes an equality of self and others. Care, instead of individual rights, becomes the universal obligation.

Reprinted from *Ethical Issues in Nursing* by P.L. Chinn (Ed.), p. 42, with permission of Aspen Publishers, Inc., © 1986.

ianism.[40,64] Given the scarce resources of health care dollars, this approach for ethical decision making may be increasingly important. Future productivity of patients may serve to determine the types and amount of treatment or health care services that they receive.[40,64] Emergency situations may require a standard to be violated, such as omitting a sterile procedure to save a life or safely triage patients. According to utilitarian theory, truth telling may not be upheld if it is determined to not be in the best interest of the patient.[35,40]

Deontological Theory (Formalism)

The focus of the deontological approach to ethical problems is on the rules that determine the rightness or wrongness of the action.[29,64] Immanuel Kant, a German philosopher, has been credited with the formulation of this approach. Democratic principles or laws are stressed and universality is the basis for decisions.[64] Past moral or ethical judgments are considered, and value is assigned to significant relationships, commitments, and promises. Actions are independently assessed for their own value, and the consequences are not part of the decision.[40]

Kant espoused the belief that moral actions would supercede all other reasons for action and issued a "categorical imperative" that only actions that should become universal law be demonstrated.[35] Categorical imperatives are unconditional commands that are morally necessary and required under any circumstances. One has a duty to obey categorical imperatives with no exceptions and under all circumstances. The aphorism inherent in formalism is "the end does not justify the means." Decisions based on formalism are normally congruent with one's moral convictions and serve to validate one's strong sense of duty when acting out of principle regardless of consequences.[40,42] Strict adherence to rules, policies, and standards may stifle creativity and examination of alternatives in the fast-paced health care environment of today.

ETHICAL PRINCIPLES

There are certain ethical principles that were derived from classic ethical theories that are used in health care decision making.[40] Principles are general guidelines that govern conduct, provide a basis for reasoning, and direct actions.[20] The six ethical principles that will be discussed in this chapter are autonomy, beneficence, nonmaleficence, veracity, fidelity, and justice.

LEGAL REVIEW

Informed consent: use of experimental drugs in critical care

HUMAN SUBJECTS RESEARCH SOURCE: 46 C.F.R. 46.116 (a)
Elements of informed consent.

Physicians may prescribe experimental drugs for critically ill patients. When nurses are asked to administer these drugs, they should do so only after knowing the legal implications of such an act. Experimental drugs are those that have not been fully approved by the Food and Drug Administration (FDA), the federal agency that must approve all drugs for use in health care. The FDA grants trial approval for the use of new and experimental drugs. Before giving experimental drugs, nurses should:

- Know the drug's approval status (by the FDA and the hospital).
- Be assured by the physician that proper informed consent has been obtained from the patient or surrogate, if indicated.
- If part of a research study, be assured by the principal investigator that the study has been approved by the committee within the facility that reviews research projects and that patients have given an informed consent to participate in the research project.

The principal investigator, the person responsible for the study, must obtain prior approval of an institutional review board (IRB). Among many responsibilities of the IRB is the responsibility that human subjects are protected. For federally funded research projects, it is mandated that each human subject be provided the following:

- A statement that the study involves research, an explanation of the purposes of the research, the expected duration of the subject's participation, a description of the procedures to be followed, and identification of any procedures that are experimental.
- A description of any reasonably foreseeable risks or discomforts to the subject.
- A description of any benefits to the subjects or to others that may reasonably be expected from the research.
- A disclosure of appropriate alternative procedures or courses of treatment, if any might be advantageous to the subject.
- A statement describing the extent, if any, to which confidentiality of records identifying the subject will be maintained.
- For research involving more than minimal risk, an explanation of whether compensation or medical treatments are available if injury occurs and, if so, what they consist of or where further information may be obtained.
- An explanation of whom to contact for answers to pertinent questions about the research and research subjects' rights and whom to contact in the event of a research-related injury.
- A statement that participation is voluntary and that refusal to participate or a discontinuation of participation at any time will involve no penalty or loss of benefits to which the subject is otherwise entitled.

Autonomy

The concept of autonomy appears in all ancient writings and early Greek philosophy. Immanueal Kant described an ethical person as one who is guided and motivated in response to one's own inward obedience, free from coercion, desire, or fear of future consequences.[35] Persons are not to be treated as a means to an end but rather as an end themselves.[31] In health care, autonomy can be viewed as the freedom to make decisions about one's own body without the coercion or interference of others. Autonomy is a freedom of choice or a self-determination that is a basic human right. It can be experienced in all human life events.

The obligation for health care professionals is to respect the values, thoughts, and actions of patients and not to let their own values or morals influence treatment decisions.[44] Fry described this as a respect for the "unconditional worth of the individual."[31] Often there is a conflict between the values of the patient and the health care professionals when dealing with life-sustaining matters in critical care. Miller suggested that any conflict can be "resolved by taking a firm line on autonomy: any autonomous decision of a patient must be respected."[44]

The critical care nurse is often "caught in the middle" in ethical situations and promoting autonomous decision making is one of those situations. As the nurse works closely with patients and families to promote autonomous decision making, another crucial element becomes clear. Patients and families must have all of the information about a certain situation to make a decision that is best for them. Not only should they be given all of the information and facts, but they must also have a clear understanding of what was presented. This is where the nurse is a most important member of the health care team—that is, providing more information, clarifying points, reinforcing information, and providing support during the process. The legal implications of informed consent are discussed in Chapter 3.

Beneficence

The concept of doing good and preventing harm to patients is a *sine qua non* for the nursing profession. However, the ethical principle of beneficence, which requires that one promote the well-being of patients, points to the importance of this duty for the health care professional. According to Davis and Aroskar, the principle of beneficence presupposes that harms and benefits are balanced, leading to positive or beneficial outcomes.[20]

Murphy described the ethical mandate of the nurse as being different from that of the physician in some aspects of care. Because nurses diagnose and treat human responses to health problems, it is they who deal most closely with quality of life issues.[45] In these situations, the nurse is obligated to act different from the physician, whose duty is to preserve life at all means.

In approaching issues related to beneficence, there is frequently conflict with another principle, that of autonomy. *Paternalism* exists when the nurse or physician makes a decision for the patient without consulting or including the patient in the decision process. *Paternalism* is "making people do what is good for them" and "preventing people from doing what is bad for them."[35] Jameton[35] described two types of paternalists: strong paternalists who make decisions for obviously competent persons and weak paternalists who make decisions for persons who are mentally or physically unable to make their own decision.

Traditional health care has been based on a paternalistic approach to patients. Many patients are still more comfortable in deferring all decisions about care and treatment to their health care provider. Active involvement by various organizations and agencies regarding health care has demonstrated a trend toward the public's need and desire for more information about health care and alternative treatments and providers. Paternalism, or maternalism in the case of female providers, may always be a possibility in the health care setting, but enlightened consumers are changing this practice of health care professionals.

In the critical care setting, there are many instances and possibilities for paternalistic actions by the nurse. Postoperative care, which is designed to assist the patient with a quick recovery, is a good example of paternalistic action by the nurse. Encouraging the patient to turn, cough, and deep breathe and increasing activity in the form of dangling, sitting in a chair, and ambulating are all paternalistic when the patient is in pain, sleep deprived, and wanting to be left alone. However, there are times when the priorities of benefits and harms must be balanced. In this instance, the duty to do no harm, which is the next principle to be discussed, takes precedence over paternalistic actions. When there are conflicts in ethical principles, one must weigh all of the benefits and choose the best one.[20]

Nonmaleficence

The ethical principle of nonmaleficence, which dictates that one prevent harm and remove harmful situations is a *prima facie* duty for the nurse.[20] Thoughtfulness and care is necessary, as is balancing risks and benefits, which was discussed earlier with beneficence. Beneficence and nonmaleficence are on two ends of a continuum and are often carried out differently, depending on the views of the practitioner. A practitioner using a utilitarian approach will consider long-term consequences and the good to society as a whole. The practitioner operating from a deontological basis will consider the principle and its effect on the single individual in the situation.

Such complex situations as quality of life versus sanctity of life are always difficult to analyze in the critical care setting as well as in non–critical care settings. Flynn described such decisions as withholding and withdrawing treatments as being based on not one ethical principle alone, but rather on a balance of all ethical principles so that the most appropriate moral decision can be made.[27] Nonmaleficence should serve as the guide for practice of health care professionals.[40]

Veracity

Veracity or truth-telling is an important ethical principle that underlies the nurse-patient relationship. In 1860 Florence Nightingale described veracity with patients: "Far more now than formerly does the medical attendant tell the truth to the sick who are really desirous to hear it about their own state."[48] Nightingale's philosophy was not agreed on by

RESEARCH ABSTRACT

The clinical nurse's role in informed consent

Davis A: Prof Nursing 4(2):88, 1988.

PURPOSE

The purpose of this study was to clarify elements that nurses thought were necessary for consent to be considered informed and to identify roles that nurses assumed in obtaining consent from patients.

FRAMEWORK

The framework for this study was the recognition of respect for autonomy of patients' right to know and make choices about their own care. The role that nurses play in situations in which patients are asked to give consent to research and treatments by other health professionals had not been clearly identified in the literature and served as the focus of this study.

METHODS

Four treatment vignettes and four research vignettes were formulated in which both beneficial and non-beneficial benefits were possible. The vignettes were discussed in semistructured interviews with 27 Masters-prepared staff nurses, clinical nurse specialists, and head nurses. This sample of nurses worked in two settings: a large medical center and a city hospital, both of which served as clinical, teaching, and research facilities.

RESULTS

Respondents viewed informed consent as a process that occurs over time, and they judged consent as more informed when patients had prior preparation. They also indicated that the most acutely ill patients did not have as much idea of their rights as those patients with chronic illness or those who had been previously hospitalized. Five roles were identified in which nurses had assumed active involvement: (1) watchdog to monitor informed consent situations, (2) resource person to provide information on alternatives, (3) advocate to mediate on behalf of patients, (4) coordinator to preserve an open, friendly atmosphere for discussion, and (5) facilitator to clarify misconceptions or misunderstandings.

IMPLICATIONS

Nurses need to become involved in the consent process as early as possible, whether it be preoperatively for scheduled treatments or surgeries or on admission to the hospital or unit. Nurses should be included in research protocols, and they should have input into patient care issues and reinforce information given by other health care professionals and researchers. The timing of explanations and consent is essential for the patient, and the nurse can have input into the appropriate time and context for informed consent to occur. The advocacy role of the nurse for the patient is essential to promote autonomy and informed consent.

other health care providers of the time (that is, physicians), but she was sensitive to the needs of patients who sought information about their own conditions.

Veracity is important in soliciting informed consent, so that the patient is aware of all potential risks and benefits from specific treatments or their alternatives. Once again, the critical care nurse can be in the middle of a situation where all of the facts and information about a particular treatment option are not disclosed. Sometimes information has been given accurately but has been delivered with bias or in a way that is misleading. In this case and other instances with veracity, the ethical principle of autonomy has been violated.[6]

Are there ever any situations in which nurses should lie to patients? This subject was discussed in depth by Schmelzer and Anema[56] who posed that nurses make many value judgments in their daily practice, some of which are made after careful consideration and some of which are made quickly with minimal thought. Veracity is also related closely to the principle of beneficence in which the nurse must consider whether the lie will benefit the patient and if so, how. They stressed the importance of designating lies as negative benefits when comparing them with the positive benefits of the truth.

When faced with a veracity dilemma, one should analyze the personal abilities, values, and beliefs of the patient. All possible options and truthful alternatives should be examined. The long-term effects of a lie may be the loss of credibility of the nurse with the patient, the need for additional "cover-up" lies, and stress to the nurse who told the lie. Schmelzer and Anema concluded that "nurses should be committed to telling the truth and, when faced with situations where they are tempted to lie, should instead seek alternative actions based on honesty."[56] This principle should guide all areas of practice for the nurse, that is, colleague relationships, employee relationships, as well as the nurse-patient relationship.

Fidelity

Another ethical principle that is closely related to autonomy and veracity is fidelity. Fidelity, or faithfulness and promise-keeping to patients, is also a *sine qua non* for nursing. It forms a bond between individuals and is the basis of all relationships, both professional and personal. Regardless of the amount of autonomy that patients have in the critical care areas, they are still quite dependent on the nurse for a multitude of types of physical care and emotional support. A trusting relationship that establishes and maintains an open atmosphere is one that is very positive for all involved.

Aroskar[6] pointed out that making a promise to a patient is voluntary for the nurse, whereas respect for a patient's making decisions is a moral obligation. She described the critical care nurse as experiencing a great deal of moral conflict. "Fidelity to patients in high-tech care units may require that nurses question the use of specific technologies for a specific patient or even the admission of a hopelessly ill patient . . . to such a unit."[6]

As do all the other principles, fidelity extends to the family of the critical care patient. When a promise is made to the family that they will be called if an emergency arises or that they will be informed of other special events, the nurse should make every effort to follow through on the promise. Not only will fidelity be upheld for the nurse-family relationship, but there will also be a positive reflection on the nursing profession as a whole and on the institution in which the nurse is employed.

Confidentiality is one element of fidelity that is based on traditional health care professional ethics. According to Veatch and Fry,[60] the nursing and medical professions have established ethical codes that allow no patient-centered reasons for breaking the principle of confidentiality. Confidentiality is described as a right whereby patient information can only be shared with those involved in the care of the patient. An exception to this guideline might be when the welfare of others is at risk by keeping patient information confidential. Again in this situation, the nurse must balance ethical principles and weigh risks with benefits. Special circumstances, such as mandatory reporting laws, will guide the nurse in certain situations.

Privacy has also been described as inherent in the principle of fidelity. It may be closely aligned with confidentiality of patient information and a patient's right to privacy of his or her person, such as maintaining privacy for the patient by pulling the curtains around the bed or making sure that he or she is adequately covered.

Justice/Allocation of Resources

The principle of justice is often used synonymously with the concept of allocation of scarce resources. According to Krekeler, "Justice necessitates giving to persons what they are entitled to deserve or can legitimately claim."[40] Contrary to the belief of many people, health care is not a right guaranteed by the Constitution of the United States. Rather, *access* to health care should be provided to all people. With escalating health care costs, expanded technologies, an aging population with its own special health care needs, and (in some instances) a scarcity of health care personnel, the question of health care allocation becomes even more complex.

The application of the justice principle in health care is concerned primarily with allocation of goods and services, which is termed *distributive justice*. According to Jameton, distributive justice appears at three levels of health care: national policies and budget, state or local distribution of resources, and distribution in the individual health care settings.[35] Traditionally, six criteria for making decisions about allocation of resources have been used.[35,41] Distribution has been based on:

- Equality for all persons
- Individual merit
- Societal contributions
- Availability in an open market
- Individual need
- Similar treatment for similar cases

Equality for all persons. Equality for all persons has been a traditional stance of health care and has been evidenced in ethical codes and in the practices of professionals. With equality, all persons are given equal treatments and resources, such as access to health care, technologies, specialists, personnel to perform necessary care and treatment, and support for physical and emotional needs during the process. This clearly is not the case in current health care. Is a rural or small community health care agency equal to larger urban centers or medical centers in the ability to provide such comprehensive services described? Is there equality in care across the health care continuum, that is, access to treatment and home, community, or follow-up care for all persons? The answer to both questions is "no" for a myriad of reasons and circumstances.

Escalating health care costs and technological advances of expensive treatments have resulted in the inability to provide equality in health care services to all.[26] Elderly retired persons on Medicare, the unemployed with no insurance, and the middle-class working family with moderate insurance coverage receive differing types and amounts of services. Most persons do not receive health care along the entire continuum, that is, from health care *promotion* to health care *illness*. The quality of care provided has traditionally been the same. But might this also be changing in the future, or has it already changed to varying degrees in some instances?

Veatch[59] delineated three objections to the egalitarian interpretation of justice. First, he raised the question of whether equality should be applied to health status, that is, specific illness or condition, or to equality of health welfare in general, that is, overall health care services across the continuum. Second, he posited that the egalitarian approach does not allow for any consideration of other ethical principles. And lastly, he raised concern that there might be infinite patient demands for services and that the individual patient-centered principle of autonomy would take precedence over societal needs.

Individual merit. Distribution of services based on individual merit has not been a traditional practice of health care professionals and is an area that may be subtle to observe. Individual merit might be based on that which has already been achieved or that which is expected to occur in the future, such as in the case of an infant or child or a person who may have potential for success in some endeavor. Basically, the issue at hand is whether this type of person deserves a particular treatment. The decision is based on values that are subjective and not driven by a set of rules or principles.

Greater merit may be given to those who are rich and famous, have a particular profession or type of work, or lead a certain lifestyle. Thus a person who smokes, drinks excessively, or uses recreational drugs may have a lower priority for treatments, surgery, and care. Health care professionals may judge that persons have abused themselves, such as in the case of the alcoholic or drug abuser, or have neglected themselves, such as in the case of one who has not sought necessary health care. Such persons may receive varying levels of care or might be denied care altogether.

Societal contribution. Decisions based on the societal contribution of the individual examine the worth of that individual in society and are subjective and value based. Using this as a framework for making decisions causes the elderly, the young, persons who have conditions that are socially undesirable such as alcoholism or mental diseases, and those who are handicapped to a degree that makes them very dependent to be considered to not have worth to society.

Societal worth has not been a factor traditionally espoused by health care professionals as a basis for decisions. However, in the early days of renal transplantation, criteria such as age and personal demographics were considered in the decision to transplant, which resulted in public discomfort with the decision method.[11,41]

Free market acquisition. Justice determined by free market acquisition is guided by money and what individuals can acquire with their money. Persons both in the past and in the present who have unlimited money are able to receive the ultimate in services and are able to quickly search for and find services to meet their needs and desires. They are usually limited only by the technologies and services available. However, when time is not crucial, money will pay for technologies or services that can be developed if there is money to support such efforts.

Differences can be noted through private rooms; many nurses or attendants; the best, world-renowned specialist being brought to the patient; or the patient being taken anywhere in the world to obtain treatment. Money and the free market open up lines of communication that do not exist for others. Through free market, those with money and necessary resources may be the first in line for a treatment and take priority over others.

Individual need. Jameton described individual need as most applicable to health care in deciding allocation of resources.[35] The dilemma arises when one considers one individual's need for heart transplantation or other technologies versus the possibility of using those resource dollars for early education on preventing heart disease for many people. In delineating problematic areas in the determination of individual needs, Levine-Ariff asserted that level and type of need should be identified.[41] If harm would come to the individual were the need not met, then the need takes precedence and should be met.

Similar treatment for similar cases. The concept of similar treatment for similar cases expands on the concept of equality and applies the same basic principle at the societal level. However, consideration of contribution to society is also inherent in this method of decision. For instance, criteria may be established that designate that all who have a certain conditon and who are under a certain age will be given the treatment, surgery, or service. This allows equal access of all who meet those criteria but disallows others who do not meet the criteria. Decisions based on this standard cover groups of people, whereas decisions based on individual need hold only for that one person.

ALLOCATION OF SCARCE RESOURCES IN CRITICAL CARE

According to Englelhardt and Rie[24]:

It is impossible to discover a concrete view of a just system of health care allocation. . . . At best, moral arguments will be able to establish a range of acceptable models. As a result, moral justifiable concrete system for providing health care is secured through common agreement, rather than through rational arguments alone.

They described critical care units as providing optimal care to all who require it, yet those responsible for the costs of critical care can no longer afford to pay for the advanced treatments and technologies that have been developed and refined and made available.

There have been reductions in federally funded health care programs and a leveling off of monies for health care research funds from previous years. Resources available for health needs are no longer unlimited, as they previously appeared to be. It has become evident that both resource allocation and allocation decisions will become inevitable and may appear in forms of public policies and guidelines.[25] Allocation will be discussed in two areas: allocation of technologies and treatments and allocation of health care energy.

Allocation of Technologies and Treatments

Limitations of resources force society and the critical care health professionals to reexamine the goals of critical care for patients. Once considered experimental, heart transplantation is now widely accepted and funded by payers. Survival rates for 1 year are 70% to 80% and for greater than 5 years are 50%. In 1987 it was stated that potential candidates for transplants must prove in advance their ability to pay the estimated $95,000 average cost of a heart transplant. Postoperative care and life-long medications were not described but are additional costs that are difficult to estimate.[55]

According to Murray, "Human bodies have value, and not just to the persons whose bodies they are. Organs can be transplanted; tissues used for research and product development. One way of looking at these body parts is as property to be bought and sold . . . another way . . . is to see them as gifts."[46] Because the possibilities and number of organ transplants are increasing, there are not enough available organs. To increase the availability of donated organs, most states have enacted "required request" laws, which mandate that families must be approached about donation of organs on the death of their loved ones. Procurement of organs has posed new ethical dilemmas for health care professionals who must now act in accordance with state laws. Implications for critical care nurses regarding organ procurement are posited in Chapter 3.

Marsden[43] described health care professionals as dealing with the needs of their current patients and families, not as anticipating future patients' needs. Health care providers may be required to act based on rules and regulations that are in conflict with their code of ethics or ethical principles. Discussions of the moral and ethical dilemmas inherent in organ procurement and transplantation are liberally demonstrated in the literature.[9,12,13,23,43,46]

Other technologies found in critical care that were considered experimental only a few years ago are the intraaortic balloon pump (IABP),[8] the left ventricular assist device (LVAD), and the artificial heart.[50] Essential in the use of all technologies and critical care treatments are veracity, autonomy, and informed consent,[8] which have been discussed earlier in this chapter. Legal implications about informed consent are discussed in Chapter 3. In cases in which research protocols are used with patients in the critical care units, all ethical principles apply.[21]

Quality of life is an issue that should be considered when examining the use of technologies. It is an area that is very personal and value laden and one that will be different for all involved and dependent on the content. O'Mara[50] described quality of life having dual dimensions of both objectivity and subjectivity. Objectivity examines the person's functionability, whereas subjectivity analyzes his or her psychosocial state. He stated that an evaluation of quality of life issues can only take place after one has received the technology and "lived" that "new" life.

Allocation of Health Care Energy

In 1986, 6% to 10% of all hospital beds in the United States were designated as critical care, which reflects a higher proportion than in any other country.[38] Knaus stated that "access to an expensive and complex resource like intensive care can never be absolute."[38] Critical care nurses are faced with rationing of critical care beds and nursing staff on a daily basis. Strengths and weaknesses of the staff must be balanced with the needs of the patient. Orientation and other special circumstances, such as designation for charge nurse, trauma nurse, and code nurse, must be taken into consideration when scheduling staff and making out assignments. Any inexperienced staff, float staff, or registry staff must be given appropriate orientation and backup during the shift.

There is frequently a triage system for critical care units that is called on when there are more admissions than available beds. The critical care nurse is instrumental in assisting the medical director to determine patient selection for transfer, if appropriate. Some hospitals use a set of standards, criteria, or guidelines for determining patient admission and transfer to and from critical care areas.

Pinch described allocation of scarce resources in terms of three theories: goal-based theory, duty-based theory, and rights-based theory.[54] Use of the *goal-based theory* results in the most happiness or good for the majority. Utilitarian theory is applied, which seeks the best solution to benefit the most. Weighing benefits and establishing criteria for patient selection into critical care areas is an example of this theoretical application.

By analyzing the dilemma with a *duty-based theory*, one acts according to obligations. The basic principle of nonmaleficence governs actions, and all individuals would be treated alike. No priority is assigned to any one individual, and all would be cared for equally. In the event that there were no beds for admission, the nurse's first and prime consideration would be the patients already in the unit under her care. Other alternatives would be explored, such as admitting the patient elsewhere in the hospital with a critical care nurse in attendance or transporting the patient to another institution that had adequate resources.

The last theory to be discussed is that of the *rights-based theory*. The focus here is on the benefits that the individual deserves or is entitled to receive from that individual's point of view and value system. Individual autonomy is the major ethical principle in this theory. In the critical care setting, all patients would appear to be voluntary patients in need of critical care. If there were any cases in which individual patients were questioning treatments or not wanting certain procedures done, they would be self-selecting a transfer out of the unit. In other cases in which all patients were medically competitive for the critical care bed, random selection would be the recommended method of decision making.

The final decision in any of the three theoretically based decision models would involve examining several ethical principles and many factors related to each case. No easy answers can be given, and there are no set rules or standards for these difficult issues. Pinch suggested the application of sound management principles and the adherence to legal guidelines as essential to decision situations.[54]

WITHHOLDING AND WITHDRAWING TREATMENT

The technological support of life at all costs has recently come to be questioned by both health care professionals and health care consumers. Physicians and nurses who are closest to the issues have debated the moral and ethical implications and have looked to ethicists for guidance and legal opinion. Both medical and nursing associations have developed guidelines for their practitioners about withholding and withdrawing treatments. The American Medical Association formulated a *Statement on Withholding or Withdrawing Life Prolonging Medical Treatment* in 1986. The statement delineated that life-prolonging treatments and technological support of respiration, nutrition, and hydration could be withheld when a patient is in an irreversible coma, regardless of whether death is imminent.[32]

The American Nurses' Association's *Guidelines on Withdrawing or Withholding Food and Fluid* are found in the box on p. 23 and will not be discussed in depth in this chapter. The decision not to employ aggressive measures or to discontinue treatments that have been in place is always difficult and stressful for all involved in the decision, particularly those who continue to care for the patient on a daily basis.[51] Legal implcations for withholding or withdrawing treatments and orders not to resuscitate the patient are delineated in Chapter 3.

There appears to be more reluctance to withdraw treatments, which is reflective of ethical and moral conflicts within each of the practitioners. Withholding usually means

GUIDELINES ON WITHDRAWING OR WITHHOLDING FOOD AND FLUID

Is it morally permissible to withhold or withdraw food or fluid from sick patients—and should nurses ever be involved in doing so? The answers to these two related questions are no, under most circumstances, and yes, in a few instances. The focus of these guidelines, therefore, is upon the *circumstances* under which it is morally permissible to withhold food and fluid.

The starting point for our understanding of what nurses ought to do is based on the general moral consensus of civilized societies, religions, and generations regarding the usual obligation to provide food and fluid to the needy, sick, and dependent who can be helped by it. Such an obligation is central to the common understanding of a nurse's professional and moral duties.

An aspect of nursing care, as carried out regularly and routinely by all bedside nurses, is the provision of some form of food and fluid. Patients need food and fluid in order to feel better physically and emotionally. The benefits of life and health from receiving food and fluid are so clear that, especially for those in the health professions (and perhaps most especially for nurses), there is a generally unambiguous moral duty to provide them. Thus under most circumstances, it is *not* morally permissible for nurses to withhold or withdraw food or fluid from persons in their care, and nurses should not do so.

The most frequent instance when it is morally permissible, indeed obligatory, for nurses to withhold feedings are those occasions when patients would clearly be more harmed by receiving than by doing without feeding. Clinical examples include patients preparing for or just recovering from surgery, infants with such conditions as tracheoesophageal fistula or anal atresia, and certain overeating disorders. These circumstances are temporary and usually involve substitute provision of specified nutrients. The goal is to provide proper nutrition later, when it is safe and beneficial.

Harm, as used in this moral reasoning, is not simply synonymous with hurt, pain, or discomfort, though it may involve each. It refers rather to serious damage, often irreparable, and involving the loss of valued capacities or pleasures. There are occasions when the provision of food and fluid is both painful and beneficial and there is justification for the temporary imposition of some short-term discomfort from hunger and thirst.

Thus far, we have identified the two instances that are ethically the most common and clear-cut. First, the nurse should almost always provide food and fluid because their provision is almost always an essential, life-preserving, health-giving benefit. Second, the nurse should temporarily withhold food and fluid when their very provision clearly causes harm.

Ethical difficulties arise when it is unclear whether food and fluid are more beneficial or harmful. Since they are essential for life, this uncertainty ultimately leads to questions about whether life, under certain conditions, might be a greater harm than death. Determination of benefit and harm should be decisive. Should the evaluation by the patient, the family, the professional care giver, a religious advisor, or that of society, through the court, predominate? There are also questions about whether possible harms and benefits to others, in addition to the patient, should be considered.

Since competent, reflective adults are generally in the best position to evaluate various harms and benefits to themselves in the context of their own values, life projects, and tolerance of pain, their acceptance or refusal of food and fluid should usually be respected. This ethical judgment is now well established legally through various cases affirming the right of competent patients to refuse treatment, including food and fluid. It is morally as well as legally permissible for nurses to honor the refusal of food and fluid by competent patients in their care. The Code for Nurses, the historical evolution of nurses' professional responsibilities as patient advocates, and the general moral principle of respect for persons, sometimes referred to as the principle of autonomy, support this view.

It is important, however, to guard against the possibility that respect for a competent patient's right to refuse food and fluid could lead to indifference or a misplaced respect for patient autonomy. The danger, in this instance, results in nurses' failure to interest themselves in a patient's reason for exercising his or her presumed right. It is the patient's *reasons* that establish the right and are, therefore, pivotal in determining what the nurse should do. Moreover, because such serious harms to the patient are associated with the refusal of food and fluid (initial discomfort from hunger and thirst, illness, physical wasting, and ultimately death), it is not enough simply to fulfill the obligation to respect the wishes of competent persons. Obligations to prevent harm and bring benefit also require that nurses seek to understand the patient's reasons for refusal.

First, it is important to establish clearly the patient's ability to understand her or his situation, the alternatives, and the associated harms and benefits. The refusal of food and fluid, however, is not itself evidence of incompetence. Patients who refuse based on their evaluation of life with severe physical constraints, or with intractable pain, or as a choice about the way and time to die in the face of an eventually fatal illness, or as a last resort to draw attention to important social causes* will usually have weighed carefully the harms and benefits associated with refusal, in the light of their own values and capacities. Such reasoned reflection should be respected by nurses. Thus in the case of competent patients with good reasons, "the patient" is the answer to questions about whose evaluation of benefit and harm should be decisive.

From the American Nurses' Association Committee on Ethics, Kansas City, Mo, June 1988, The Association.
*A suicide attempt as a prima facie refusal of life itself should not be taken as unquestionably entailing a refusal of food and fluid. Intervention to halt or reverse suicide rightly includes the emergency provision of food and fluid until the patient's reasons for the suicide attempt can be ascertained.

Continued.

GUIDELINES ON WITHDRAWING OR WITHHOLDING FOOD AND FLUID—cont'd

This answer should not, however, be taken automatically to apply to all circumstances of competent refusal. Competent patients can refuse for incongruous reasons. They may not have an accurate picture of the facts or they may despair for reasons that are reversible, though they may not think this is true. These patients should receive special, sympathetic attention from nurses. Nurses should make every effort to correct inaccurate views, to modify superficially held beliefs and overly dramatic gestures, and to restore hope where there is reason to hope.

In certain instances, when a patient is no longer competent but it is possible to establish with certainty the patient's projected refusal, the same respect for a patient's values is indicated. Documents such as a living will, other written or well-established verbal advance directives, or the legal assignment of a durable power of attorney† for health care can be taken as aids in discerning the patient's view. The application of a previously stated refusal will, of necessity, require the judgment—both clinical and moral—of nurses and other care givers as to whether the current situation is one to which the patient intended her or his refusal to apply. In general, advance directives, even those involving the withholding or withdrawing of food and fluid, should carry great weight in care givers' discussions with the patient's family or surrogate. It is imperative in this process for nurses not to substitute their own views about which lives are worth saving and living for the views of their competent or formerly competent patients.

In circumstances in which the patient has never been competent (including infants, children, many mentally retarded persons, and the never competent mentally ill), nurses along with others have the moral and professional responsibility to decide whether provision of food and fluid is in the patient's best interest. The same moral and professional responsibility falls to care givers in the situation of the patient who is not now competent and whose views when he or she was competent cannot be discovered. Patients who are incompetent make an *exceedingly vulnerable* population dependent upon care givers for careful thought and compassionate action, including the provision of nutrition.

The withholding of food and fluid might be indicated only when feeding is futile because of underlying, incorrectable absorption problems or when feeding is severely burdensome to the patient or sustains life only long enough for the patient to die of other more painful causes. Only under very special circumstances is it morally permissible to withhold feeding or give less than adequate feeding to those who cannot speak for themselves. In such circumstances, the nurse's responsibility for care continues and special attention should be given to mouth and skin care, and other forms of compassionate touch.

If withholding food and fluid appears more harmful than expected or if the patient's condition changes and hydration or nutrition appears potentially beneficial, the giving of food and fluid should be reinstituted. The views and moral sensibilities of care-giving family members should be influential in decisions for such patients unless there is clear indication that family members do not wish to be involved in decision making, are not themselves competent, or substitute their own interests for those of the patient.

In almost all cases the provision of food and fluid is in the patient's best interest. For some, it is one of life's central pleasures. Rarely is feeding more burdensome than beneficial. In addition, the nurse's obligation to fulfill the duties of the profession and remain faithful to patients includes the general role promise that the nurse will engage in activities that are nurturing, even when such care is not clearly beneficial so long as it is not harmful.

Central to the benefit of life itself is the benefit of nourishment that sustains physical being and provides psychological or emotional comfort. Thus, even in circumstances where food and fluid do not provide adequate nourishment, food and fluid should continue to be given if they provide comfort. For example, infants with irreversible absorption problems still enjoy sucking and mouthing food, and older adults who have refused further renal dialysis may still derive pleasure from sips of fluid or bits of food despite their impending death. Feeding should not be continued or forced, however, when it is futile and when it inflicts suffering or harm that is not outweighed by an important long-term benefit.

The nursing profession believes that the social and economic responsibilities that result from this position should be shared by all citizens, not solely those with a family member in need of nursing. We further believe that the good conscience, security, and sense of well-being among citizens rests in part on the knowledge that the vulnerable will be nourished and that carefully considered refusals of food and fluid will be respected.

REFERENCES

1. Nelson LJ: The law, professional responsibility and decisions to forego treatment, QRB p. 8, January 1986.
2. Grant ER and Forsythe C: A plight of the last friend: legal issues for physicians and nurses in providing nutrition and hydration, Issues Law Med 2(4):279, 1987.
3. American Nurses' Association: Code for nurses with interpretive statements, Kansas City, Mo, 1985, The Association.
4. Hastings Center: Guidelines on the termination of life-sustaining treatment and the care of the dying, New York, 1987, Hastings Center.

—Interpretation issued by
ANA Committee on Ethics
January 1988

---

†A durable power of attorney is an individual's written designation of another person to act on his or her behalf, when the designation is authorized by a state's durable power of attorney statute. Under state law, a power of attorney terminates when the designating individual loses decision-making capacity, whereas a durable power of attorney does not.

that there is no hope for success from the onset, whereas withdrawing means surrendering hope. There are also difficult discussions that must take place between the health care professionals and the family. The nurse must be sure to examine the treatment with regard for the patient's best interests and wishes and to act accordingly.[16,44,45,49]

LANDMARK COURT DECISIONS

There have been several cases with ethical dilemmas that were decided by the courts and have now become landmark cases on which to base treatment decisions. Fear of litigation has formed the basis of many ethical health care decisions in the past and even in the present. Legal issues in critical care and implications for nurses are discussed in Chapter 3. Five cases will be briefly discussed in this chapter: Quinlan, Von Stetina, Herbert, Bartling, and Brophy.

Quinlan Case

Karen Ann Quinlan was a New Jersey teenager who was left in a persistent vegetative state following a cardiac arrest in 1975. When it appeared that Karen would not recover and would remain in a vegetative state, her parents requested that the ventilator be removed. Physicians were unable to honor their request, because this would set a precedent and would conflict with their moral responsibility to maintain life at all costs.

Karen's father petitioned the court to name him Karen's guardian, thereby granting him permission to have the ventilator removed and to forego all future extraordinary procedures. The trial judge refused to appoint Mr. Quinlan as guardian, but a 1976 appeal to the New Jersey Supreme Court reversed this decision. The appellate court decided that Karen had a right to privacy and to refuse treatments and that those rights outweighed the right of the state to preserve life at all costs. It also acknowledged that decisions of this type should be made between patients and family, and the courts were not the appropriate place for health care decisions to be made. This case removed legal ramifications for health care professionals in discontinuing ventilators in cases such as Karen Quinlan.[27]

Von Stetina Case

Susan Von Stetina was a 27-year-old woman who was taken to a trauma center emergency room after being injured in an automobile accident in 1982. She had surgery for abdominal injuries and was transferred to the critical care unit, where she was showing steady improvement. Two days after her admission, she was found severely bradycardic and nonresponsive for an unknown period of time. She was successfully resuscitated and was intubated and placed on mechanical ventilation. She never regained consciousness and was eventually transferred to a nursing home with a tracheostomy and a gastrostomy.

A subsequent lawsuit demonstrated that Susan had been disconnected from her ventilator for an undetermined amount of time and that alarm systems failed to alert the staff. Furthermore, at the time of the arrest, the unit was understaffed by nurses, and safe care was not delivered as the result of the inadequate staffing. In addition to the inadequate staffing situation, patients continued to be admitted to the unit despite the availability of beds in other nearby hospitals and available safe transport to these hospitals. Expert testimony was given concerning the one-to-one care that Susan should have received. The court decision was in favor of the plaintiff, and the family was awarded $12,470,000.[24]

The Von Stetina case demonstrates the court's concern for rationing of resources in health care—in this case, in the critical care unit. Despite the constraints that the unit or hospital might be operating under in any given situation, steps and assurances must be taken to protect the rights and lives of those who are receiving care in the current situation. In other words, although there is an obligation of health care institutions and providers to care for society to the best of their abilities, the most pressing obligation is to those who are already hospitalized. Some sort of triage, procedure, guidelines, or lottery system that provides direction for decisions must be in place before those on staff are actually faced with making the decision.

Herbert Case

Clarence Herbert suffered a respiratory arrest with a subsequent coma after a noneventful elective surgery procedure in 1983. He was transferred to the critical care unit where he remained comatose on ventilatory support with intravenous and nasogastric feeding. After his wife requested that "no heroics" be done, the physician removed the ventilator and ordered that no treatments be instituted other than supportive care. Mr. Herbert continued breathing on his own and his vital signs remained stable. The physician discontinued intravenous and nasogastric feedings 3 days later and transferred Mr. Herbert to the surgical floor, where he died 6 days later.[60]

The nursing supervisor of the critical care unit persisted in her efforts to have written guidelines for "heroic" and "supportive" care. Her requests were denied, and she was warned against discussing the case. She subsequently resigned and filed a complaint about the medical management with the health department. After a year of investigation, murder charges were filed against physicians Barber and Nejdl.[60] The murder charges were dismissed by the lower court but were reinstated on request by the district attorney. The higher court of appeal once again reversed the charges and asserted that the physicians were not obligated to continue treatment that had been demonstrated to be ineffective.[27]

By the ruling, no differences were seen to exist between nutritional procedures and life support technologies. Instead of examining specific treatments as central to a decision, the court analyzed life support in general.[27] Also of importance in the case is that the nursing supervisor refused to allow the nurses in the critical care unit to practice illegally and unethically—that is, without any written guidelines or policies to direct management and care of patients in the critical care unit. Clearly written and published criteria must be available to assist health care professionals who care for the critically ill in all situations.

Bartling Case

Mr. William Bartling had multisystem disease involvement with emphysema, arteriosclerosis, abdominal aneurysm, and lung cancer. During a lung biopsy in 1984, he sustained a pneumothorax and had a tracheostomy and was placed on a ventilator. Previous to this time and immediately following the events, he was alert and competent to make decisions. He had both a living will and durable power of attorney, which stated that he did not wish to have extraordinary measures such as a ventilator and that he understood the consequences of removal of the ventilator. The physicians and hospital did not comply with his wishes and took the case to court.

The court's decision was not to remove the ventilator. Mr. Bartling died 6 months after the decision was made, and on the day following his death, the decision was overturned. The court found that the patient's right to refuse treatment and exercise autonomy in decisions about his or her care was essential.[27]

Brophy Case

Paul Brophy was a 37-year-old Massachusetts resident who had a brain aneurysm resulting in an irreversible coma. His wife was appointed as legal guardian and requested that nasogastric tube feedings and fluids be discontinued. Both she and other members of the family stated that Paul had voiced desires such as this in discussions before the event. The medical staff and administrators of the hospital refused to comply with the request, because they felt that their medical code of ethics and moral values would be compromised. Thus the courts were approached for a legal decision.

The court decision required that the physicians assist the family in transferring Paul to another institution or to his home where others could be responsible for the care that the family requested. This court decision reflected the desire of the court that decisions should not be forced on colleagues and patients who disagree.[10] This case also acknowledged the concept of *substitutive judgment,* which is a decision based on what another person would have wanted done in the situation.[4] In this case, Paul Brophy had verbalized his wishes for treatment before the event.

Court Decisions Versus Clinical Decisions

According to Armstrong, there has been a remarkable transition in the legal view of ethical/moral issues in a relatively short time. The legal principles are now clear, but the implementation of the principles is not consistent among hospital counsel and physicians. Armstrong listed six points that are clear from a legal standpoint[4]:

1. Competent patients have the right to refuse treatment.
2. Incompetent patients have the same right, which can be exercised by a surrogate, that is, a family member or attorney.
3. Courts should not be involved in treatment decisions except in cases where there is no family or guardian or when there is disagreement among them.
4. There is no difference in the eyes of the law between withholding treatments and withdrawing treatments.
5. Artificial nutritional support, such as nasogastric or gastrostomy tubes and intravenous lines, can be withheld or withdrawn if no benefits are given to the patient by these forms of treatment.
6. Hospitals and physicians who withhold or withdraw

treatments will be protected from lawsuits if they act in good faith on desires that have been articulated in some manner by the patient and no harm comes to the patient.

ETHICS AS A FOUNDATION FOR NURSING PRACTICE

Traditional theories of professions have included a code of ethics as the basis for the practice of professionals. The moral foundation of nursing has been discussed in the literature by various authors who describe the unique relationship of the professional nurse with the patient, which establishes a caring, trusting approach.[15,19,53,63] It is by adherence to a code of ethics that the professional fulfills an obligation for quality practice to society.

According to Curtin,[18] nursing ethics is concerned with duties that are assumed by nurses and with the consequences

---

CODE OF ETHICS FOR NURSES

1. The nurse provides services with respect for human dignity and the uniqueness of the client, unrestricted by considerations of social or economic status, personal attributes, or the nature of health problems.
2. The nurse safeguards the client's right to privacy by judiciously protecting information of a confidential nature.
3. The nurse acts to safeguard the client and the public when health care and safety are affected by the incompetent, unethical, or illegal practice of any person.
4. The nurse assumes responsibility and accountability for individual nursing judgments and actions.
5. The nurse maintains competence in nursing.
6. The nurse exercises informed judgment and uses individual competence and qualifications as criteria in seeking consultation, accepting responsibilities, and delegating nursing activities to others.
7. The nurse participates in activities that contribute to the ongoing development of the profession's body of knowledge.
8. The nurse participates in the profession's efforts to implement and improve standards of nursing.
9. The nurse participates in the profession's efforts to establish and maintain conditions of employment conducive to high quality nursing care.
10. The nurse participates in the profession's effort to protect the public from misinformation and misrepresentation and to maintain the integrity of nursing.
11. The nurse collaborates with members of the health professions and other citizens in promoting community and national efforts to meet the health needs of the public.

Used with permission from American Nurses' Association: Code for nurses with interpretive statements, Kansas City, Mo, 1985, The Association.

of decisions that affect patients, colleagues, society, and the nursing profession. A professional ethic is based on three elements: the profesional code of ethics, the purpose of the profession, and the standards of practice of the profession. The need for the profession and its inherent promise to provide certain duties form a contract between nursing and society. The code of ethics developed by the professionals is the delineation of its values and relationships with and among members of the profession and society. The professional standards describe specifics of practice in a variety of settings and subspecialties. Each element is dynamic, and ongoing evaluations are necessary as societal expectations change, technologies increase, and the profession evolves.

Nursing Code of Ethics

The American Nurses' Association (ANA) provides the major source of ethical guidance for the nursing profession. According to the preamble of the *Code for Nurses,* "When individuals become nurses, they make a moral commitment to uphold the values and special moral obligations expressed in their code."[1] The 11 statements of the Code are found in the box on p. 26. They are based on the underlying assumption that nursing is concerned with protection, promotion, and restoration of health; prevention of illness; and the alleviation of suffering of patients.[1]

The *Code for Nurses* was adopted by the ANA in 1950 and has undergone revisions over the years. It provides a framework for the nurse in ethical decision making and provides society with a set of expectations of the profession. The Code is "not open to negotiation in employment settings, nor is it permissible for individuals or groups of nurses to adapt or change the language of this code."[1] The ANA also suggests that the requirements of the Code may not be in concert with the law and that it is the nurse's obligation to uphold the Code because of the societal commitment inherent in nursing.

The Nurse as Patient Advocate

Winslow[61] described the evolution of nursing ethics from traditional loyalty to physicians to contemporary advocacy of patient rights. The loyalty ethic was based on a military model; advocacy is based on a legal model. He further dicussed areas of concern for the nurse when serving in an advocacy role. Patients and their families are sometimes not ready or willing to accept the nurse as an advocate. Advocacy is frequently associated with controversy, and the nurse may experience conflict between interests and loyalties.[47,61] Advocacy "involves an act of free will and a studied choice to view ourselves in a particular way in our relationship to others."[47] Active advocacy reflects the nurse's responsibility and obligation to the patient and incorporates both personal and professional values and standards.[7]

Curtin[17] delineated four major conditions that cause patients and families to be more vulnerable: loss of independence, loss of freedom of action, interference with the ability to make choices, and the power of health care professionals. If these issues are not addressed, "patients' values are ignored, or replaced with others' values, [and] patients cease to exist as unique human beings."

PATIENT RIGHTS

1. Informed participation in health care decisions.
2. Information about research and experimental protocols and alternatives available elsewhere.
3. Respect and privacy regarding source of payment for treatment.
4. Complete and accurate information concerning all care and procedures.
5. Prompt attention, especially in emergencies.
6. Clear, concise, and understandable explanation of procedures, including risks, potential sequelae, and probability of their success.
7. Clear, thorough, and accurate evaluation of one's condition and prognosis without treatment before consenting to treatment.
8. Knowledge of identity and professional status of caregivers.
9. Access to an interpreter as needed.
10. Access to one's medical records.
11. Access to a consultant specialist to discuss one's condition.
12. Tests or procedures performed for only personal benefit.
13. Personal and informational privacy.
14. Opportunity to refuse any drug, test, procedure, or treatment.
15. Access to persons and support outside the health care facility.
16. Opportunity to discharge oneself from the institution, regardless of physical condition or economic status.
17. Notification of discharge at least 24 hours in advance and notification of person of choice.
18. Access to a complete copy of one's medical record on discharge.
19. Access to a patient rights advocate 24 hours a day.

Modified from Annas GJ: Supervisor Nurse 5:21, 1974.

Rights protection model. The legal model of nursing advocacy espoused by Winslow is reflective of the nurse as the protector of patient rights.[31,61] The underlying assumption is that one's rights are violated in the patient role and that assistance is needed in the form of an advocate. Ethicist George Annas has delineated the rights of patients that are illustrated in the box above.

Values-based decision model. Inherent in this model is the nurse's respect for the individual's own values and beliefs. It is the responsibility of the nurse to provide information and to clarify it as necessary so that the patient can make informed decisions. Personal values and decisions of the nurse are not imposed on the patient and family.[31] Supporting the patient and family during this process does not necessarily mean agreement with the decision, but rather support of the patient and family to make their own decision.

ASSESSING THE RISKS IN THE ADVOCATE ROLE

- Are channels of communication between health care professionals open and clear regarding client needs and choices?
- Once channels of communication are open and clear, are these channels being maintained?
- Are members of the health care team clear regarding the obligations and responsibilities of the nurse in the nurse-patient relationship?
- Has trust been established and maintained in the nurse-patient relationship.
- What role in the decision-making process does the patient have (i.e., degree of autonomy)?
- What influence do significant others have in health care decisions regarding the patient?
- What role expectations do the patient and family have of the nurse and other members of the health care team?
- What information and knowledge must the nurse have to support and teach the patient?
- What are the legal and ethical implications involved in assuming the advocate role in this situation?

Reprinted from *Holistic Nursing Practice,* Vol. 1, No. 1, p. 60, with permission of Aspen Publishers, Inc., © November 1986.

Respect-for-persons model. Respect for the individual as an autonomous decision maker whose human dignity and privacy is to be protected forms the basis for this model. In cases in which patients are unable to determine their own choices, the nurse defers to a surrogate decision maker or advocates in these patients' best interests.[31]

The Risks of Advocacy

As discussed previously, there are occasions in which conflicts exist between professional loyalties. Becker[7] asserted that assessing risks in an advocate situation will serve to minimize risks to both nurse and patient. The box above delineates questions that should be asked when assessing advocacy risks. She further discussed five important conditions for advocacy. First, the members of the profession must communicate to clarify obligations and responsibilities. Second, open lines of communication among professionals about patient rights must be maintained. Third, it is essential for trust to be established and maintained between the nurse and the patient. Fourth, the nurse must be aware of all conditions and situations related to the health care decision. The fifth condition is that the nurse must remain educated about current legal and ethical trends.

The Nurse's Obligation to Self

According to Christensen,[14] ethical autonomy forms the basis for professional nursing practice. In this sense, autonomy denotes thinking for oneself, not unlimited freedom

of choice. There are both clinical practice and ethical elements inherent in professional nursing competence, and the nurse must incorporate both elements into practice.

Ethical dilemmas surround the critical care nurse on a daily basis. Exposure to frequent moral and ethical conflicts may affect the nurse in the form of burnout or resignation.[40] Dallery posited that there is a moral dilemma of mixed loyalties for the professional. Scientific and theoretical knowledge learned outside the practice setting are difficult to fully incorporate in a different social context, such as the critical care setting. "An ethics of responsibility, modeled on the caring process, is different from an ethics of discrete moral acts modeled on contractual obligations."[19] Nursing is based both on caring and on a contract with society to perform nursing. Thus a conflict in professional loyalties occurs.

Dallery[19] proposed a model of professional practice in which the professional orchestrates moral and ethical decisions. Professional loyalties are bound by time and are expressive and communicative compared to obligations that are absolute and rigid. The professional's primary responsibility is to care for the patient. This may require a great deal of soul searching, depending on the situation.

Jameton[36] described one's integrity as being compromised when professional and personal conflicts arise. This most frequently occurs when the nurse is highly dedicated, which leads to a conflict between professional care and self-care. The emotional strains of caring for the critically ill must balance with personal rewards for the nurse. "Nurses experience stress and anger as they attempt to reconcile their ideals about health care with its uncertainties, inadequacies, and abuses."[35] Personal values and principles may conflict with those of the profession or institution. This conflict with personal identity must be resolved. The duty to self in this situation is to express one's own moral convictions to others. Jameton purported, however, that integration of one's own personal identity with professional identity is possible.[36]

ETHICAL DECISION MAKING IN CRITICAL CARE

In general, ethical cases are not always clear-cut or black and white, but rather arise in settings and circumstances that involve innumerable side issues and distractions. The most common ethical dilemmas encountered in critical care are foregoing treatment and allocating the scarce resource of critical care. But how does one know that a true ethical dilemma exists?

What Is An Ethical Dilemma?

Before the application of any decision model, a decision must be made about the existence of a true ethical dilemma. Thompson and Thompson[58] delineated the following criteria for defining moral and ethical dilemmas in clinical practice:

1. Awareness of different options
2. An issue with different options
3. Two or more options with true or "good" aspects and the choice of one over the other compromises the option not chosen

Krekeler asserted that ethical situations arise when "the

STEPS IN ETHICAL DECISION MAKING

1. Identify the health problem.
2. Define the ethical issue.
3. Gather additional information.
4. Delineate the decision maker.
5. Examine ethical and moral principles.
6. Explore alternative options.
7. Implement decisions.
8. Evaluate and modify actions.

---

moral decision of one person conflicts with the moral decision of another. Both decisions may be good for each individual in question and undoubtedly are made according to their traditional values."[40] What complicates this process is when there is a third person involved, as is the case in most treatment care decisions in the critical care areas.

Steps in Ethical Decision Making

To facilitate the ethical decision process, a model or framework must be used so that all involved will consistently and clearly examine the multiple ethical issues that arise in critical care. Steps in ethical decision making are listed in the box above.

Step one. First, the major aspects of the medical and health problem must be identified. In other words, the scientific basis of the problem, potential sequelae, prognosis, and all data relevant to the health status must be examined.

Step two. The ethical problem must be clearly delineated from other types of problems. Systems problems, that is, those resulting from failures and inadequacies in the organization and operation of the health care facility and the health care system as a whole, are often misinterpreted as being ethical issues. Occasionally, a social problem that stems from conditions existing in the community, state, or country as a whole are also confused with ethical issues. Social problems can lead to a systemic problem, which can constrain responses to ethical problems.

Step three. Although categories of necessary additional information will vary, whatever is missing in the initial problem presentation should be obtained. If not already known, the health prognosis and potential sequelae should be clarified. Usual demographic data, such as age, ethnicity, religious preferences, and educational and economic status, may be considered in the decision process. The role of the family or extended family and other support systems needs to be examined. Any desires that the patient may have expressed either in writing or in conversation about treatment decisions are essential to obtain.

Step four. The patient is the primary decision maker and autonomously makes these decisions after receiving information about the alternatives and sequelae of treatments or lack of treatments. However, in many ethical dilemmas, the patient is not competent to make a decision, as occurs when he or she is comatose or otherwise physically or mentally unable to make a decision. It is in these situations that surrogates are designated or court appointed, because the urgency of the situation requires a quick decision. Although the decision process and ultimate decision are more important than who makes the decision, delineating the decision maker is an important step in the process.[58]

Others who are involved in the decision should also be identified at this time, such as family, nurse, physician, social worker, clergy, and any other members of disciplines having close contact with the patient. The role of the nurse should be examined. There may not be a need for a nurse decision; rather the nurse may provide additional information and support to the decision maker.

Step five. Personal values, beliefs, and moral convictions of all inolved in the decision process should be known. Whether actually achieved through a group meeting or through personal introspection, values clarification facilitates the decision process. Professional ethical codes of the nurse and physician will serve as a foundation for future decisions. At this time, legal constraints or previous legal decisions for circumstances at hand will need to be assessed and acknowledged.

General ethical principles need to be examined in relation to the case at hand. For instance, are veracity, informed consent, and autonomy promoted? Beneficence and nonmaleficence will be analyzed as they relate to the patient's condition and desires. Close examination of these principles will reveal any compromise of ethical or moral principles for either the patient or the health care provider and assist in decision making.

Step six. After the identification of alternative options, the outcome of each action must be predicted. This analysis helps one to select the option with the best "fit" for the specific situation or problem. Both short-range and long-range consequences of each action must be examined, and new or creative actions should be encouraged. Consideration should also be given to the "no action" option, which is also a choice.[58]

Step seven. When a decision has been reached, it is usually after much thought and consideration, and there is rarely complete agreement among all interested persons.[58] Krekeler described following the action until the actual results of the decision can be seen.[40] Fowler stated that the decision may need to be modified to meet legal or policy requirements.[30]

Step eight. Evaluation of an ethical decision serves to both assess the decision at hand and use it as a basis for future ethical decisions. If outcomes are not as predicted, it may be possible to modify the plan or to use an alternative that was not originally chosen.

STRATEGIES FOR PROMOTION OF ETHICAL DECISION MAKING

The complexity of health care and frequent ethical dilemmas encountered in clinical practice demand the establishment of mechanisms to address ethical issues found in hospitals and health care facilities. Four types of mechanisms will be discussed briefly in this chapter: institutional ethics committees, inservice and education, nursing ethics committees, and ethics rounds and conferences.

Institutional Ethics Committees (IECs)

Although not required by law, many health care facilities have developed IECs as a way to review ethical cases that are problematic for the practitioner. The three major functions of IECs are education, consultation, and recommendation to policy-making bodies. Kemp[37] identified three models of IECs. In the *Optional-Optional Model*, committees serve as consultants and make recommendations that are not binding. The *Optional-Mandatory Model* requires that health care providers consult with the committees when there is an ethical problem, but recommendations are again not binding. The *Mandatory-Mandatory Model* requires that ethical dilemmas be presented to the committee, and recommendations must be followed.

IECs are very often committees comprising executive medical staff. Membership may include staff physicians, administrators, legal counsel, nurses, social workers, clergy, and community public volunteers. To fulfill its requirement for consultation, the committee must include members that not only have expertise, but also are representative of various groups. Regardless of the type of committee model, consultation and support becomes available to the practitioners.

Inservice and Education

Basic education about ethical principles and decision making is an important first step in facilitating ethical decision making among nursing staff in the critical care area. It is important for nurses to examine their own values, beliefs, and moral convictions. The ANA *Code for Nurses* should be known and used by nurses in their daily clinical practice. Treatment choices for patients and ethical issues involving patients, nurses, and medical colleagues should be explored and discussed in the classroom setting where there are no time constraints or extraneous distractions to interrupt the decision process.

Nursing Ethics Committees

Nursing ethics committees provide a forum in which nurses can discuss ethical issues that are pertinent to nurses at the individual, unit, or department level.[5,28] Unlike the IEC, which involves treatment choices of patients, the nursing committee may or may not involve a patient situation. Depending on the specific goals of the committee, it can also serve as a resource to nursing staff, make recommendations to a policy-making body about a variety of professional issues, or actually formulate policies. It may also serve to educate the department on ethical and professional issues. Membership usually comprises representatives from all major clinical areas or divisions, educators, clinical nurse specialists, administrators, and other specialty staff. Some departments such as critical care may have their own unit or division committee.

Ethics Rounds and Conferences

Ethics rounds at the unit level on patients in the unit can be done by nurses on a weekly or otherwise established basis. Rounds educate the staff to problems and serve to be "preventive" when facilitated appropriately.[30] During the discussions, potential problems may be identified early, and actions taken to decrease or prevent a future problem. An individual patient ethics conference can be scheduled to include only the nursing staff or to include a multidisciplinary group to discuss unit issues. A patient ethics conference may either function as a liaison with the IEC or as an end in itself.

SUMMARY

The emergence of critical care as a specialty and the introduction of sophisticated technological innovations into critical care units have had a great impact on health care professional practices. Ethical dilemmas are encountered daily in the practice of critical care. The criticality of the situation and speed that is required to make decisions often prevent practitioners from gaining insight into the desires, values, and feelings of patients. The practitioner is often left with no clear ethical or legal guidelines, particularly in the fast-paced modern critical care unit. By assuming a solely technological approach, practitioners will violate the rights of patients and their professional codes of ethics.

By using an ethical decision-making process, the rights of the patient will be protected, and logical analysis of the case will lead to a decision that is made in the best interests of the patient. It is through moral reasoning and examining, weighing, justifying, and choosing ethical principles that patient rights and individuality will be upheld. The practice of nursing is built on a foundation of moral and ethical caring, and the critical care nurse is pivotal in identifying ethical patient situations and can participate in the decision-making process.

Ethical issues may be linked to *koans,* which are perplexing questions posed by Zen masters to students. The koan is designed to interrupt the thought process and reveal paradoxes of reality. It is not solved solely by the intellect, and it cannot be quickly derived. This concept is closely aligned with ethical decision-making in which alternative choices are sometimes painstakingly analyzed. As advocates for patients and families, the nurse is instrumental in ethical decisions and can facilitate the process in the critical care unit.

REFERENCES

1. American Nurses' Association: Code for nurses with interpretive statements, Kansas City, Mo, 1985.
2. American Nurses' Association: Ethics in nursing position statements and guidelines, Kansas City, Mo, 1988.
3. Annas GJ: The patient rights advocate: can nurses effectively fill the role? Supervisor Nurse 5:21, 1974.
4. Armstrong C: How will courts deal with costs in treatment decisions? Lecture presented at Rights, resource allocations and ethical integrity in critical care: an interdisciplinary approach, La Jolla, Calif, March 1988.
5. Aroskar M: Institutional ethics committees and nursing administration, Nurs Econ 2:130, 1984.
6. Aroskar M: Fidelity and veracity: questions of promise keeping, truth telling, and loyalty. In Fowler M and Levine-Ariff J, editors: Ethics at the bedside, Philadelphia, 1987, JB Lippincott Co.
7. Becker P: Advocacy in nursing: perils and possibilities, Holistic Nurs Prac 1:54, 1986.
8. Birkholz G: IABP: legal and ethical issues, Dimens Crit Care Nurs 4:285, 1985.
9. Bouressa G and O'Mara R: Ethical dilemmas in organ procurement

and donation, Crit Care Nurs 10:37, 1987.

10. Bresnahan J: Suffering and dying under intensive care: ethical disputes before the courts, Crit Care Nurs 10:11, 1987.

11. Callahan D: Terminating treatment: age as a standard. Hastings Cent Rep 17:21, 1987.

12. Caplan A: Ethical and policy issues in the procurement of cadaver organs for transplantation, New Engl J Med 311:981, 1984.

13. Caplan A: Equity in the selection of recipients for cardiac transplants, Circulation 75:10, 1987.

14. Christensen P: An ethical framework for nursing service administration, ANS 10:46, 1988.

15. Cooper M: Convenantal relationships: grounding for the nursing ethic, ANS 10:48, 1988.

16. Cranford R: The persistent vegetative state: the medical reality (getting the facts straight), Hastings Cent Rep 18:27, 1988.

17. Curtin L: The nurse as advocate: a philosophical foundation for nursing, ANS 1:1, 1979.

18. Curtin L: Ethics in nursing practice, Nurs Manage 19:7, 1988.

19. Dallery A: Professional loyalties, Holistic Nurs Prac 1:64, 1986.

20. Davis A and Aroskar M: Ethical dilemmas and nursing practice, Norwalk, Conn, 1983, Appleton-Century-Crofts.

21. Davison R and Davison L: Medical experimentation: ethics in high technology, Crit Care Nurse, 10:27, 1987.

22. Dracup K: Saying no and other ethical dilemmas, Heart Lung 15:1, 1986.

23. Engelhardt T: Shattuck lecture—allocating scarce medical resources and the availability of organ transplantation, New Engl J Med 311:66, 1984.

24. Engelhardt T and Rie M: Intensive care units, scarce resources, and conflicting principles of justice, JAMA 255:1159, 1986.

25. Evans R: Health care technology and the inevitability of resource allocation and rationing decisions. Part I. JAMA 249:2047, 1983.

26. Evans R: Health care technology and the inevitability of resource allocation and rationing decisions. Part II. JAMA 249:2208, 1983.

27. Flynn P: Questions of risk, duty, and paternalism: problems in beneficence. In Fowler M and Levine-Ariff J, editors: Ethics at the bedside, Philadelphia, 1987, JB Lippincott Co.

28. Fost N and Cranford R: Hospital ethics committees, JAMA 253:2687, 1985.

29. Fowler M: Introduction to ethics and ethical theory: a road map to the discipline. In Fowler M and Levine-Ariff J, editors: Ethics at the bedside, Philadelphia, 1987, JB Lippincott Co.

30. Fowler M: Piecing together the ethical puzzle: Operationalizing nursing's ethics in critical care. In Fowler M and Levine-Ariff J, editors: Ethics at the bedside, Philadelphia, 1987, JB Lippincott Co.

31. Fry S: Autonomy, advocacy, and accountability: ethics at the bedside. In Fowler M and Levine-Ariff J, editors: Ethics at the bedside, Philadelphia, 1987, JB Lippincott Co.

32. Fry S: New ANA guidelines on withdrawing or witholding food and fluid from patients, Nurs Outlook 36:122, 1988.

33. Guralnik D, editor: Webster's new world dictionary of the American language, New York, 1981, Simon & Schuster.

34. Huggins E and Scalzi C: Limitations and alternatives: ethical practice theory in nursing, ANS 10:43, 1988.

35. Jameton A: Nursing practice, the ethical issues, Englewood Cliffs, NJ, 1984, Prentice-Hall.

36. Jameton A: Duties to self: professional nursing in the critical care unit. In Fowler M and Levine-Ariff J, editors: Ethics at the bedside, Philadelphia, 1987, JB Lippicott Co.

37. Kemp V: The role of critical care nurses in the ethical decision-making process, Dimens Crit Care Nurs 4:354, 1985.

38. Knaus W: Rationing, justice, and the American physician, JAMA 255:1176, 1986.

39. Kohlberg L: The philosophy of moral development, San Francisco, 1981, Harper & Row Publishers, Inc.

40. Krekeler K: Critical care nursing and moral development, Crit Care Nurs 10:1, 1987.

41. Levine-Ariff J: Justice and the allocation of scarce nursing resources in critical care nursing. In Fowler M and Levine-Ariff J, editors: Ethics at the bedside, Philadelphia, 1987, JB Lippicott Co.

42. Luckenbill-Brett J and Stuhler-Schlag M: Mandatory reporting: legal and ethical issues, J Nurs Adm 17:32, 1987.

43. Marsden C: Ethical issues in a heart transplant program, Heart Lung 14:495, 1985.

44. Miller B: Autonomy and the refusal of lifesaving treatment, Hastings Cent Rep 11:22, 1981.

45. Murphy C: The changing role of nurses in making ethical decision, Law Medicine and Health Care 12:173, 1984.

46. Murray T: Gifts of the body and the needs of strangers, Hastings Cent Rep 17:30, 1987.

47. Nelson M: Advocacy in nursing, Nurs Outlook 36:136, 1988.

48. Nightingale F: Notes on nursing, Toronto, 1969, Dover Publications, Inc.

49. Nolan K: In death's shadow: the meanings of witholding resuscitation, Hastings Cent Rep 17:8, 1987.

50. O'Mara R: Dilemmas in cardiac surgery: artificial heart and left ventricular assist device, Crit Care Nurs 10:48, 1987.

51. O'Mara R: Ethical dilemmas with advance directives: living wills and do not resuscitate orders, Crit Care Nurs 10:17, 1987.

52. Omery A: Moral development: a differential evaluation of dominant values. In Chinn P, editor: Ethical issues in nursing, Denver, 1983, Aspen Publishers, Inc.

53. Packard J and Ferrara M: In search of the moral foundation of nursing, ANS 10:60, 1988.

54. Pinch W: Allocation of scarce resources: critical care nursing dilemma, Dimens Crit Care Nurs 4:164, 1985.

55. Robertson J: Supply and distribution of hearts for transplantation: legal, ethical and policy issues, Circulation 75:77, 1987.

56. Schmelzer M and Anema M: Should nurses ever lie to patients? Image J Nur Sch 20:110, 1988.

57. Shragg T and Albertson T: Moral, ethical, and legal dilemmas in the intensive care unit, Crit Care Med 12:62, 1984.

58. Thompson J and Thompson H: Bioethical decision-making for nurses, Norwalk, Conn, 1985, Appleton-Century-Crofts.

59. Veatch R: DRGs and the ethical reallocation of resources, Hastings Cent Rep 16:32, 1986.

60. Veatch R and Fry S: Case studies in nursing ethics, Philadelphia, 1987, JB Lippincott Co.

61. Winslow G: From loyalty to advocacy: a new metaphor for nursing, Hastings Cent Rep 14:32, 1984.

62. Wlody G and Smith S: Ethical dilemmas in critical care, Focus Crit Care 12:41, 1985.

63. Yarling R and McElmurry B: The moral foundation of nursing, ANS 8:63, 1986.

64. Young S: The nurse manager: clarifying ethical issues in professional role responsibility, Pediatr Nurs 13:430, 1987.

3

Legal Issues

CHAPTER OBJECTIVES

■ *Identify legal and professional obligations of critical care nurses*
■ *Describe the elements of several torts that might result from critical care nursing practice*
■ *Delineate types of liability*
■ *Relate critical care practices and risk management strategies*
■ *Characterize the state's role in critical care nursing practice*
■ *Recount special issues in critical care nursing practice*

CRITICAL CARE NURSING PRACTICE: LEGAL OBLIGATIONS OVERVIEW

The scope of critical care nursing practice has been defined by the American Association of Critical-Care Nurses (AACN), as follows[2]:

Critical care nursing practice is a dynamic process, the scope of which is defined in terms of the critically ill patient, the critical care nurse and the environment in which critical care nursing is delivered; all three components are essential elements for the practice of critical care nursing. The critically ill patient is characterized by the presence of real or potential life-threatening health problems and by the requirement for continuous observation and intervention to prevent complications and restore health. The concept of the critically ill patient includes the patient's family and/or significant others. The critical care nurse is a registered professional nurse committed to ensuring that all critically ill patients receive optimal care.

In *Nursing, A Social Policy Statement,* the American Nurses' Association (ANA) defines nursing as the diagnosis and treatment of human responses to actual or potential health problems. "Critical care nursing is that speciality within nursing which deals specifically with human responses to life-threatening problems."[2]

These definitions raise several pertinent legal and professional concerns:

1. The critical care nurse has legal obligations to the patient, the critical care setting, and the environment.
2. Both definitions speak to the fact that the nurse deals with life-threatening health problems. In this context, nursing mistakes are more likely than those made in situations that are not life-threatening to cause significant injuries, if not death, to a patient. Risk of suit is high.
3. The nurse is obligated to provided continuous observation and intervention.
4. The patient includes more than the individual for whom care is being provided; the family or significant other must also be cared for.
5. The nurse is licensed by the state and has legal obligations to the public to perform her or his duties safely.
6. The nurse's goal is to provide optimal care. This type of care is a professional obligation and is distinguishable from a reasonable level of care, which is the legal standard of care.
7. Critical care nursing is a specialty. Therefore the nurse's legal obligations are those of a specialist, one with special knowledge and skill. These obligations involve a higher standard of care.

These areas of concern are the focus of this chapter. Following a discussion of the types of liabilities and the law and legal processes that have an impact on critical care nursing, we will discuss the nurse's duty of reasonable care, obligations of state licensure, and special patient care issues.

Types of Liability and Responsibility

When a nurse takes a position in a critical care unit, a special relationship is created between patient and nurse and employer and nurse. Every state has a law that requires that a special course of study be taken, successfully completed, and an examination passed for one to practice nursing. A registered nursing position requires state registration and licensure as a registered nurse. The act of licensure creates a legal relationship between the nurse and the state.

These special relationships carry legal obligations. For example, the nurse owes a patient the duty of reasonable and prudent care, under the circumstances; the nurse owes an employer the duty of following policies and procedures, including any contractual duties that may exist between them; and the nurse owes the state and members of the

---

LAW AND ITS PROCESSES

LAW IS FOUND IN:
  Legislation
  Regulation
  Constitutions
  Judicial opinions

LAW IS ENFORCED THROUGH DIFFERENT PROCESSES:
  Civil
  Criminal
  Administrative

THERE ARE MANY TYPES OF LAW, SUCH AS:
  Torts
  Contracts
  Crimes
  Statutes and Rules

---

public the duty of providing safe, competent practice within the legally defined scope of nursing practice.

Membership in professional associations obliges the nurse to subscribe and adhere to standards defined by the associations. For example, the AACN states that "the critical care nurse adheres to the Code of Ethics of the American Nurses' Association."[3] This document contains statements of professional obligations.[4]

The critical care nurse's legal duties are enforced, and the nurse can be held legally accountable for violation of them, through a variety of laws and legal processes. The box above lists the sources of law and identifies several types of law and three legal processes. Nurses, hospitals, patients, and other health care providers have been involved in a wide range of legal disputes. Nurses have been involved in cases of negligence, malpractice, unprofessional conduct, workers' compensation, contract or other employment disputes, and a few cases of homicide, theft, patient abuse, and fraud.[5]

Nurses' professional duties may be enforced by the professional association to which a nurse belongs. For example, state nurses' associations are required to enforce ANA's Code for Nurses. This is an example of a type of private law—that of an association that determines its own rules for censuring its members.

The span of issues is broad. For example, in the last 15 years *health law* as a separate area of law practice has emerged, embracing over 60 topic areas.[6] Because of this, the chapter's focus has been narrowed to an exploration of unintentional tort liability, licensure law, and the laws surrounding consent, the refusal of treatment, and organ procurement. Nurses should always seek their own legal advice and counsel for any questions and concerns and not rely on the overview of material provided in this chapter.

Introduction to Civil and Tort Liability

The area of civil law is divided into many categories, two of which are torts and contracts. A *tort* is a type of civil wrong, meaning that the dispute resulted from an occurrence between private entities or individuals (referred to as parties to the dispute), and the wrong is the type that society does not consider criminal or a wrong against society as a whole. The *law of contracts* contains a set of rules governing the creation and enforcement of agreements between two or more parties (again, entities or individuals).

There are three types of torts. The box below catalogues the classifications of tort law and gives selected examples within each category. *Intentional torts* involve an intent and an act. The intent is not a malicious one; rather, it is the intent to achieve a particular outcome and consequence. Assault, battery, false imprisonment, trespassing, and infliction of emotional distress are all examples of intentional torts. In each of these torts, there is a specific act that is required. In *assault,* the act is any behavior that places the plaintiff (the one being wronged who later sues) in fear or apprehension of an offensive contact. The person being sued for wronging another in civil law is referred to as the defendant. *Battery* is the unlawful or offensive touching of another's physical being. *False imprisonment,* another intentional tort, involves isolating another against his or her will. There are two types of *trespassing*—one type involves a person's land; the other involves his or her personal property. These acts are defined as unauthorized entry onto land of another or unauthorized handling of another's personal property. In addition, the law protects a person's interest in peace of mind through the tort, *infliction of mental or emotional distress.* The act here, however, must be one of extreme misconduct or outrageous behavior.

Nurses can avoid allegations of intentional torts by:
1. Assuring patients, as far as possible, that the nursing care is part of an acceptable treatment plan
2. Asking patients for their consent before giving care (in addition, many hospital policies require that the nurse validate that the patient's physician has also received consent for medical treatment—this will be discussed more in a later section)
3. Determining if and when the patient needs self-protection or needs to be restrained to protect others from harm and

---

CLASSIFICATION OF TORTS

Intentional torts	Unintentional torts	Quasi-intentional torts
Assault	Negligence	Defamation
Battery	Malpractice	Slander
False imprison-ment	Abandon-ment	Libel
Trespassing		Invasion of privacy
Infliction of emotional distress		

taking steps to protect the patient or others by following established protocols, hospital policies, and state regulations governing the use of restraints

4. Handling the patient's personal effects in a safe, secure manner and following hospital policies about patient valuables

5. Avoiding extreme, outrageous behavior by delivering care according to generally accepted standards of care

Unintentional torts involve mistakes in nursing practice that lead to harm, including negligence, malpractice, and abandonment. *Negligence* is the failure to meet an ordinary standard of care, resulting in injury to the patient (here again, the allegedly injured person is referred to as the plaintiff). *Malpractice,* a type of negligence, is professional misconduct, illegal or immoral conduct, or a lack of reasonable skill, which leads to harm. A more complete outline of the elements of these two torts will follow. *Abandonment* is a type of negligence in which a duty to give care existed, was totally ignored, and resulted in harm to a patient. It is the absence of care and the failure to respond to a patient that can give rise to an allegation of abandonment.

Nurses can avoid allegations of unintentional torts by:

1. Identifying when a duty exists, knowing what the duty consists of, and providing nursing care that meets that expected duty

2. Documenting the care that was delivered and participating in other activities that decrease the chance of patient harm and a subsequent lawsuit (these are commonly known as risk management strategies, several of which will be discussed later)

Quasi-intentional torts protect interests one has in his or her reputation and privacy; defamation (including slander and libel) and invasion of privacy are both quasi-intentional torts. *Defamation* is actually made up of two torts, *slander* (oral defamation) and *libel* (written defamation). Defamation is not just saying or writing words that injure one's reputation or good name. The words must be communicated to another, and if the words are true this may provide a defense against a defamation lawsuit. *Invasion of privacy* is another type of tort that involves a violation of a person's right of privacy. Nurses can invade another's privacy by revealing confidential information without authorization or by failing to follow the patient's health care decisions. These issues are discussed under separate sections in this chapter.

Nurses can avoid allegations of quasi-intentional torts by:

1. Stating opinions of another's reputation only when objectively substantiated or privileged

2. Respecting another's privacy and autonomy and maintaining a confidential relationship with the patient

Introduction to Administrative and Licensure Law

A second type of law and legal process in which nurses have been involved is *administrative law.* This area of law governs the nurse's relationship to the government, either state or federal. Administrative law involves the rules of the government's activities in regulating health care delivery and practice. Generally, there are several sections of the government that are involved in regulatory activities.

A state has the power to regulate nursing because the state is responsible for the health, safety, and welfare of its citizens. Therefore establishing minimum standards of nursing practice, education, and competence is an acceptable state activity. The state legislatures create the laws governing nursing practice, and a unit of the state government within the executive branch of government is responsible for the enforcement of nursing laws. This unit is often called the state board of nursing. However, states do vary. This is another important reason that nurses must seek advice from counsel licensed to practice law within their own states.

For administrative law, the rules of investigation and procedure differ from civil law and criminal law. Each type of law has its own rules of procedure and evidence. Examples of disputes between the state and nurses will be provided below.

NEGLIGENCE AND MALPRACTICE

As defined earlier, negligence is an unintentional tort involving a failure (through either an act or a failure to act) to meet a standard of care, causing patient harm. Malpractice is negligence by a member of a profession in which the defendant is held accountable for a standard of care involving special knowledge and skill. These torts have several elements, all of which the plaintiff has the burden of proving.

Definition of Elements

Most legal scholars itemize four elements of negligence and malpractice, including:

1. Duty and standards of care
2. Breach of duty
3. Causation
4. Injury or damages

A *duty,* or legal obligation, must be one recognized by law, requiring the actor to conform to a certain standard of conduct, for the protection of others against unreasonable risks.[7] The critical care nurse's legal duty is to act in a reasonable and prudent manner, as any other critical care nurse would act under similar circumstances. The standard is that of a critical care nurse, one with special knowledge and skill in critical care. The standard is one that is owed at the time the incident occurred, not at the time of litigation. In most jurisdictions, the standard is a regional or even national standard, as opposed to a local, community standard.

Breach of duty involves a failure on the actor's part to conform to the standard required. *Causation,* the third element, involves proving that the actor's breach was reasonably close or causally connected to the resulting injury. This is also referred to as *legal cause,* or *proximate cause.*

The fourth element, *injury,* must involve an actual loss or damage to another or his or her interests. There are different types of damages that a plaintiff may claim, such as compensatory or punitive. Patient injury can range in value, depending on what happened to the patient. The plaintiff must produce evidence of the damages and their value. If the nurse breaches a standard of care, which leads to injury, the plaintiff must show what amount of money

LEGAL REVIEW

Confidentiality and human immunodeficiency virus and AIDS-related information

LEGISLATION EXAMPLE: New York Public Health Law Secs. 2780-2787 (McKinney's 1989)

State laws vary on the issue of confidentiality of HIV test results. Some states mandate that a positive HIV test result be reported to state health officials and the Centers for Disease Control; other states do not. Usually in states that mandate reporting test results, follow-up on all contacts is also mandated. In all states, however, a physician must report a patient who is diagnosed as having AIDS. Nurses in critical care, as in other areas of practice, employ universal precautions prescribed by the Centers for Disease Control guidelines.

Legislation discusses not only confidentiality, but also informed consent to an HIV test and disclosure of the results. Critical care policies should reflect the state's legislation, if any, in this area. Below are selected provisions of New York's legislation, presented here only as examples of one state's approach.

Informed consent to an HIV related test shall consist of a statement signed by the subject of the test who has capacity to consent or, when the subject lacks capacity to consent, by a person authorized pursuant to law to consent to health care for the subject which includes at least the following:

(a) an explanation of the test, including its purpose, the meaning of its results, and the benefits of early diagnosis and medical intervention; and

(b) an explanation of the procedures to be followed, including that the test is voluntary, that consent may be withdrawn at any time, and a statement advising the subject that anonymous testing is available; and

(c) an explanation of the confidentiality protections afforded confidential HIV related information under this article, including the circumstances under which and classes of persons to whom disclosure of such information may be required, authorized or permitted under this article or in accordance with other provisions of law or regulation.

■ ■ ■

Prior to the execution of a written informed consent, a person ordering the performance of an HIV related test shall provide to the subject of an HIV related test or if the subject lacks capacity to consent, to a person authorized pursuant to law to consent to health care for the subject, an explanation of the nature of AIDS and HIV related illness, information about discrimination problems that disclosure of the test result could cause and legal protections against such discrimination, and information about the behavior known to pose risks for transmission and contraction of HIV infection.

■ ■ ■

A person authorized pursuant to law to order the performance of an HIV related test shall provide to the person seeking such test an opportunity to remain anonymous and to provide written, informed consent through use of a coded system with no linking of individual identity to the test request or results. A health care provider who is not authorized by the commissioner to provide HIV related tests on an anonymous basis shall refer a person who requests an anonymous test to a test site which does provide anonymous testing.

■ ■ ■

At the time of communicating the test result to the subject of the test, a person ordering the performance of an HIV related test shall provide the subject of the test or, if the subject lacks capacity to consent, the person authorized pursuant to law to consent to health care for the subject with counseling or referrals for counseling:

(a) for coping with the emotional consequences of learning the result;

(b) regarding the discrimination problems that disclosure of the result could cause;

(c) for behavior change to prevent transmission or contraction of HIV infection;

(d) to inform such person of available medical treatments; and

(e) regarding the test subject's need to notify his or her contacts.

■ ■ ■

A physician may disclose confidential HIV related information under the following conditions:

(1) disclosure is made to a contact or to a public health officer for the purpose of making the disclosure to said contact; and

(2) the physician reasonably believes disclosure is medically appropriate and there is a significant risk of infection to the contact; and

(3) the physician has counseled the protected individual regarding the need to notify the contact, and the physician reasonably believes the protected individual will not inform the contact; and

(4) the physician has informed the protected individual of his or her intent to make such disclosure to a contact and has given the protected individual the opportunity to express a preference as to whether disclosure should be made by the physician directly or to a public health officer for the purpose of said disclosure. If the protected individual expresses a preference for disclosure by a public health officer or by the physician, the physician shall honor such preference.

■ ■ ■

When making such disclosure to the contact the physician or public health officer shall provide or make referrals for the provision of the appropriate medical advice and counseling for coping with the emotional consequences of learning the information and for changing behavior to prevent transmission or contraction of HIV infection. The physician or public health officer shall not disclose the identity of the protected individual or the identity of any other contact. A physician or public health officer making a notification pursuant to this subdivision shall make such disclosure in person, except where circumstances reasonably prevent doing so.

SAMPLE OF CRITICAL CARE NURSING ACTIONS INVOLVED IN NEGLIGENCE SUITS

- Failure to advise physician and/or supervisor of changes in patient's health status
- Failure to monitor patients
- Failure to adhere to protocols for monitoring oxygen levels
- Failure to adequately assess postoperative status
- Failure to respond to alarms
- Using malfunctioning equipment
- Refusing to provide supplemental oxygen when the ventilator could not be promptly reattached
- Allowing inappropriate use of the IV infusion equipment to extensively infuse fluids extravascularly
- Failure to monitor, recognize infiltration, and discontinue IV therapy
- Failure to recognize signs of intracranial bleeding
- Failure to investigate patient's complaint of pain and discover hematoma under blood pressure cuff

---

COMMON AREAS OF NURSING NEGLIGENCE

- Administration of treatments
- Medications
- Communication
- Supervision of patients
- Incorrect or inappropriate postoperative treatment, which can result in infections
- Foreign objects left in patient during surgery

---

will compensate for his or her injuries. The goal of the compensation is to provide the amount of money that will place the plaintiff back in the position he or she was in before the injury occurred.

Because critical care nurses deal with life-threatening patient care situations, patient injury could be severe, such as death. If this does occur, the nurse may be held accountable for the patient's death and also for the resulting loss to family members. All states have survival or wrongful death acts. Under these statutes, a lawsuit can be brought if the death was the result of a negligent act.

How often patients are injured by negligent nursing care and how frequently nurses are sued are two difficult questions to answer. In the studies reported in the nursing literature of general nursing negligence cases, critical care unit cases have been included. In Campazzi's study,[8] 1.3% of the cases were generated from critical care units. However, later studies found that 11% and 21% of the cases were generated from critical care units. The box above enumerates specific examples of critical care nurse actions that involved actual lawsuits. In these cases, the nurse's action was the center of the lawsuit, but in few instances was the nurse actually sued. Whether the nurse is actually sued depends on the situation and who else is responsible for the nurse's actions. This will be discussed further in another section.

Overall, nursing negligence cases discussed in the previously referenced studies have involved failures in relation to six general categories, which are found in the box at right. The first category includes the misuse of equipment or the failure to perform safety checks or proper maintenance checks. Nurses have made errors on medications, routes of administration, and dosages. Nurses have failed to communicate changes in patient status to physicians and have also failed to communicate to supervisors the physician's lack of response to the nurse's communication. The nurse's failure to prevent a patient's fall has also been the topic of nursing negligence. Changing dressings improperly (that is, not maintaining sterile technique) and incorrectly counting instruments and sponges in the operating room are areas of practice that have led to patient injury and lawsuits.

Types of Liability and Legal Doctrines

In tort and civil law, there are several rules of liability under which the nurse's actions may be examined, and responsibility defined. Types of liability include:
1. Personal
2. Vicarious: *respondeat superior*
3. Corporate
4. Other special doctrines, such as *res ipsa loquitur,* temporary or borrowed servant, and captain of the ship.

Personal liability means that each individual is responsible for his or her own actions. This includes the critical care nurse, the supervisor, the physician, the hospital, and the patient. Each has responsibilities that are uniquely his or her own. The opposite of personal liability is personal immunity. For some health care situations, Congress or state legislatures have determined that nurses do not have personal liability and are therefore immune from liability. Here again, it is wise to seek legal advice to review what specific rules apply to a particular situation.

Generally, however, mandated reported statutes include personal immunity provisions. For example, state child abuse statutes provide that a nurse who makes a good faith report will not be liable for making that report. Or, physicians and hospitals that are mandated to report communicable diseases to state or federal authorities are immune from liability for good faith reporting in a confidential manner. Also, nurses who render voluntary emergency care to a stranger are immune from liability for negligence under state good samaritan laws. Finally, federally employed nurses are immune from liability for negligence under the Federal Tort Claims Act.[10]

These personal immunities are not a guarantee of not being sued; rather, they are defenses for the nurse should the nurse be sued. The nurse-defendant must show how the immunity applies to her or his situation, and if so shown, the case against the nurse is dismissed.

Vicarious liability is sometimes referred to as employer liability. Under the doctrine of *respondeat superior,* an employer is responsible and liable for an employee's acts that are performed within the scope of the employee's employment. In critical care, the nurse is usually an employee of a hospital, but nurses may be independent contractors to the hospital through critical care nursing businesses. If the latter is the case, the nurse is not an employee of the hospital, so the hospital is not vicariously liable for the nurse's actions. Critical care nurses who are hospital employees are given work assignments and provided equipment and supplies to perform those assignments by the employer's agent, a supervisor. In fact, the hospital is responsible for the patient census and staffing in the critical care unit. Because of these responsibilities, the hospital-employer is responsible for the employee's performance within parameters that the employer determines. It would be unfair to hold the individual nurse solely responsible for patient care, which the nurse only partially controls.

Corporate liability is the liability that attaches to the corporate entity itself (in this case, the hospital) for its own decisions, such as patient census and staffing, budget, and hiring practices. These are corporate decisions for which the hospital is independently responsible.

There are other special doctrines, such as *res ipsa loquitur,* temporary or borrowed servant, and captain of the ship, which may apply to the critical care nurse and the critical care unit. The doctrine of *res ipsa loquitur* literally means "the thing speaks for itself." It is a doctrine that allows the plaintiff to introduce evidence of harm and imply negligence from the fact that the harm occurred. In this case, the type of injury incurred by the plaintiff is one that does not occur without someone's being negligent.

For example, negligence can be implied when muscle damage results from body positioning when applying restraints. Or negligence can be implied from a foreign object left in a patient's abdomen following surgery. The plaintiff must show that someone among the defendants was in exclusive control of the action that caused the injury. The burden of proof is shifted to the defendants to show how none of them was negligent.

The doctrines of *temporary or borrowed servant* and *captain of the ship* apply when the plaintiff argues that the physician is reponsible for the nurse's actions, even though the nurse is an employee of the hospital and not the physician. If it can be shown that the nurse acted under the

---

SAMPLE SOURCES OF CRITICAL CARE NURSING STANDARDS

Hospital policy and procedure manuals
Expert testimony
Education and experience
Professional association statements, such as:
AACN
  Standards for Nursing Care of the Critically Ill (1981)
  Position statements
    Certification in Cardiopulmonary Resuscitation for all Health Professionals (1981)
    Clarification of Resuscitation Status in Critical Care Settings (1985)
    Collaborative Practice Model: The Organization of Human Resources in Critical Care Units (1982)
    Definition of Critical Care Nursing (1984)
    Ethics in Critical Care Research (1984)
    Principles of Critical Care Nursing Practice (1981)
    Scope of Critical Care Nursing Practice (1980)
    Use of Technical Personnel in Critical Care Settings (1983)
ANA
  Standards for Nursing Practice
  Standards for Medical-Surgical Nursing Practice
  Code for Nurses with Interpretive Statements (1985)
  Nursing: A Social Policy Statement (1981)
  Position statements, such as:
    Guidelines on Withholding/Withdrawing Feedings
    HIV Testing in Health Care Workers

Literature, such as:
  Journals: Heart & Lung, Critical Care Nurse, Focus on Critical Care, Intensive Care Nursing, Intensive Critical Care, Critical Care Medicine, Anesthesia & Intensive Care
  Textbooks
Accreditation criteria, such as:
  Joint Commission on Accreditation of Health Care Organizations, particularly those for special care units, such as critical care units
State and federal laws, such as:
  Medicare laws
  Medicaid laws
  State Nurse Practice Act
  State and federal public health laws, such as:
    Occupational Safety and Health Act [OSHA]
State and federal regulations, such as:
  Conditions for Participation in Medicare
  State Board of Nursing Regulations
  State Hospital Regulations and Health Department Guidelines
  OSHA regulations enforcing CDC recommendations and other regulations enforcing the worker's right to a safe workplace.
Centers for Disease Control [CDC], Recommendations for Prevention of HIV Transmission in Health-Care Settings

STANDARDS FOR NURSING CARE OF THE CRITICALLY ILL

STRUCTURE

I. The critical care unit shall be designed to ensure a safe and supportive environment for critically ill patients and for the personnel who care for them.

II. The critical care unit shall be constructed, equipped, and operated in a manner that protects patients, visitors, and personnel from electrical hazards.

III. The critical care unit shall be constructed, equipped, and operated in a manner that protects patients, visitors, and personnel from fire hazards.

IV. The critical care unit shall have essential equipment and supplies immediately available at all times.

V. The critical care unit shall have a comprehensive infection control program.

VI. The critical care unit shall be managed in a manner that ensures the delivery of safe and effective care to the critically ill.

VII. The critical care unit shall have appropriately qualified staff to provide care on a 24-hour basis.

VIII. The critical care nurse shall be competent and have current knowledge in critical care nursing.

IX. The critical care nurse's performance appraisal shall be based on the roles and responsibilities identified in the job description.

X. The critical care unit shall have a well-defined, organized written program to evaluate care of the critically ill.

XI. Critical care nursing practice shall include both conducting and using clinical research.

XII. The critical care nurse shall ensure the delivery of safe nursing care to patients, being cognizant of the various "causes of action" for which she or he may be liable.

PROCESS

I. Data shall be collected continuously on all critically ill patients wherever they may be located.

II. The identification of patient problems or needs and their priority shall be based on collected data.

III. An appropriate plan of nursing care shall be formulated.

IV. The plan of nursing care shall be implemented according to the priority of identified problems or needs.

V. The results of nursing care shall be continuously evaluated.

OUTCOME

Value Statement: The critical care nurse shall be cognizant of the intended results of care provided to the critically ill.

For example: Critical care delivery is consistent with policies and procedures specific to the patient population.

Adapted from American Association of Critical-Care Nurses: Standards for nursing care of the critically ill, Newport Beach, Calif, 1989, The Association.

---

direction and control of the physician, it is possible that the physician may be accountable for the nurse's actions. These doctrines, however, are not applied very often.

Risk Management Activities

As previously mentioned, the nurse can avoid or decrease patient harm and the chance of being subsequently sued in a variety of ways. The best way is for the nurse to know the standard of care, deliver it, and document it, showing that the standard was met. Gaining knowledge of the standard of care occurs during basic nursing education. A nurse's education is an important source of evidence of the standard. However, the standard of care is not static—it evolves. Therefore critical care nurses must keep up with changes in health care delivery.

The box on p. 37 provides a comprehensive example of where critical care nursing standards can be found. The box entitled *Standards for Nursing Care of the Critically Ill* summarizes the critical care nursing standards of the AACN.

Any of these sources can be presented as evidence in negligence and malpractice litigation. The question for which these sources serve as measuring sticks of nursing action or inaction is "Did the nurse breach a standard of care?" Hospital policy and procedure manuals are also admissible as evidence of the standard of care.

Another important activity is the risk management (RM) program and system itself. Nurses should constantly be aware of potential harms to patients and take steps to avoid and correct deficiencies identified through the RM program. For example, most hospital RM programs require that reports or other documentation be completed for unusual incidents. Policy defines which incidents are to be reported. Nurses may wish to consider their own professional liability insurance as an RM strategy. Insurance is a mechanism whereby one can shift to another the economic burden of a lawsuit in which one is found negligent or to have committed malpractice. *Insurance* is a contract, an agreement between the insured (the nurse) and the insurer (the insurance company). Therefore the written agreement between these parties should be examined carefully. It spells out the premium, the coverage, the terms, and the requirements the nurse must fulfill if she or he is sued. For example, most policies state that the insurance company will pay the nurse's legal fees, expenses related to litigation, and the final award, but the nurse is under an obligation to notify the insurance company within a reasonable time of the lawsuit and to cooperate in the defense.

Peer review and quality assurance activities are also important processes that can decrease patient harm and the chance of a lawsuit. These activities involve self-review, self-evaluation, and the audit of others' actions and records. A significant way to improve documentation is to review records from 1 year earlier and ask, "Will I be able to adequately recount what I did for that patient from the charting?" This is particularly important, because patient charts are legal documents admissible as business records in court as evidence in negligence or malpractice lawsuits.

Other risk management techniques include strengthening communication skills and public relations. Those in the risk management field emphasize prompt information about an accident or injury being communicated directly to the patient involved. The rationale for this is that straightforward communication about what happened and what the hospital is doing in response to the injury will decrease the patient's likelihood of suing (maintains the patient's trust) and decrease the patient's injury and the hospital's exposure to financial loss.

NURSE PRACTICE ACTS

Every state has legislation that defines the legal scope of nursing practice and defines unprofessional conduct, conduct that may lead to investigation and disciplinary action by the state.

Generally, state law contains two definitions of nursing: one for the registered (or professional) nurse and one for the licensed practical (or vocational or technical) nurse. These definitions determine titles that may be used by nurses, the scope of nursing practice, and requirements for entering the nursing profession. In some states advanced registered nursing practice, prescriptive authority for some nurses, and third party reimbursement are also statutorily defined.

How critical care nursing practice fits within these legal definitions can be revealed by comparing the professional definitions and the job description of a nurse with the state law in the jurisdiction. In this way, nurses can avoid or defend themselves against allegations of practicing medicine without a license. The scope of medical practice is also statutorily defined, and in most states a physician is given broad discretion to delegate tasks to others. For critical care nurses, proper medical delegation may occur through written protocols or standing orders that exist for the critical care area.

These orders must be written, dated, and signed by the physician. They should be updated regularly, and the old orders should be kept with other older unit documents in archives. The nurse must be adequately prepared to perform each aspect of the protocol and is personally liable for performing each order in a reasonable and prudent manner under the circumstances. Protocols and standing orders should be established with formal recognition of the roles of hospital administration and nursing and medical staffs.

The state also defines unprofessional conduct and establishes mechanisms for enforcement of these rules. *Misconduct* generally includes fraud in obtaining a license or registration; negligence; incompetence; criminal acts; practicing while impaired (chemically, physically, or mentally); having been found guilty of misconduct in another jurisdiction; and violating the nursing practice act, including any

---

LEGAL REVIEW

Chemically impaired nurses

Of grave national concern to nurses and the public is the increase in the number of impaired nurses who are coming before boards of nursing for disciplinary action. In many states, chemically impaired nurses and other professionals have been provided an alternative to disciplinary action against their licenses as long as their impairment has not caused harm to a patient. Also, whether the reason is impairment or not, once the nurse is reported, the state is required to investigate the complaint, and this generally precludes the temporary surrender alternative.

The statutes that have created this option are known as voluntary or temporary surrender or diversion statutes. Under these statutes, a nurse makes an application to the state to temporarily surrender her or his license in exchange for agreeing to enter a rehabilitation or treatment program. Doing this allows the nurse to be "diverted"

from full investigation and disciplinary action into a program designed to support and oversee the nurse's return to competent, safe nursing practice. During this time, the license is surrendered to the state, and the nurse cannot practice.

When making the application to the state, the nurse also agrees to release treatment records and reports to the state, so the state can evaluate the nurse's progress. The nurse also agrees to be monitored by the state for a period of time, usually 2 years. Once the state deems the nurse to be making sufficient progress toward rehabilitation, it can reinstate the nurse's license. The reinstatement usually is contingent on reports of continued successful treatment and rehabilitation from the nurse's employer or other monitoring system that the state puts in place.

specific regulations, such as improper delegation of nursing responsibilities. A particular government unit is assigned to the investigation and the follow-up of complaints of nurses' misconduct. Complaints, reported both voluntarily and mandatorily, are initiated by patients, hospitals, other state agencies, or the criminal justice system. State investigators have broad powers and may conduct interviews and review and copy hospital charts and personnel files.

A nurse's license is an important property right that cannot be restricted without due process of the law. The amount of due process in administrative law differs from other legal processes. Due process basically involves notice to the nurse that a complaint has been made and investigated, and there is substantial (or in some states, a preponderance of) evidence in the state's view to support it. The notice is written and contains the exact charges against the nurse. Nurses in this situation should obtain legal advice; the state will not provide it. The nurse must be given an opportunity to be heard, often in more than one forum, and be given the right to present her or his own evidence of the situation.

Chemical impairment is a frequent cause of nurses' licenses being revoked. In some states, an impaired nurse may avoid disciplinary action by voluntarily surrendering her or his license in exchange for entering a rehabilitation program. This should be done with the advice of counsel (the nurse's own counsel). Generally, this option is available in the states that have it as long as no patient has been harmed because of the nurse's impaired practice.

SPECIAL PATIENT CARE ISSUES

There are many patient care issues that arise in critical care nursing. Critical care nurses manage some of the most complex, acute care in some of the most vulnerable situations for both nurses and patients alike. Questions often arise about consent, withholding or withdrawing of treatment, and organ procurement.

Consent, Informed Consent, and Refusing Treatment

Generally, patient consent is always an essential component of health care, including critical care. However, some exceptions do exist. For example, in life-threatening, emergency situations, patients give implied consent to treatment that will remove the threat to their lives. Consent as a legal doctrine recognizes the right of a patient to control his or her own body, privacy, and autonomy. As early as 1914, a court ruled that every adult of sound mind has a right to determine what shall be done with his or her own body (including consent and the right to refuse treatment), and a surgeon who performs an operation without consent commits an assault, for which he or she is liable in damages.[11]

Although consent can be either verbal or written, most hospital policies require that it be confirmed in writing that a patient agreed to treatment after being informed, that the patient agreed voluntarily, and that the patient was legally competent to agree to the treatment. These are the basic elements of consent and informed consent doctrines: voluntary, informed, and competent (having legal capacity). Consent is a process, not just the signing of a form.

Policies should set forth who should obtain the consent, how and when the consent should be obtained, and the documentation requirements. Obtaining the patient's consent is the responsibility of the patient's treating physician, who should explain the proposed procedure or treatment. However, if the treatment is going to be done by a specialist, that person, the one most knowledgeable about the risks and benefits of the procedure, should obtain the consent.

It is not advisable to delegate the physician's responsibility for obtaining the patient's consent to the hospital or its nursing staff.[12] Generally, though, critical care nurses may be given the task by their witnessing the signature of the patient and documenting that the consent form was completed. As in any witnessing role, one can be called on later to state her or his knowledge of the situation.

If the nurse has any doubts or questions about the patient's consent, those doubts should be discussed with the patient's physician and with the nursing supervisor. Hospitals are liable (under corporate liability doctrine) for injuries that result from their failure to rectify incompetent, unsafe practice of any member of its staff, employee or nonemployee. Once the nurse has told her or his supervisor, the hospital is alerted to a problem that it is obligated to investigate.

The right to consent and informed consent includes the right to refuse treatment. In most circumstances a competent adult's decision to refuse even life-sustaining treatment must be honored. There are a few situations in which the right to refuse treatment is not honored. These include, but are not limited to situations in which:

1. The treatment relates to a contagious illness that threatens the health of the public (for example, immunizations are required, even over religious objections, if the community danger is extreme)
2. The innocent third parties will suffer (for example, a mother's wish to refuse a blood transfusion was overruled to save the mother for her 9-month-old infant; these cases are often decided on a case-by-case basis, and legal counsel should always be sought)
3. The refusal violates ethical standards (for example, a Massachusetts court held that a hospital was not required to compromise its ethical principles by following a patient's decision but must cooperate in the transfer of the patient to a hospital that was willing to cooperate[13]; however, a New Jersey court ruled the opposite. A patient indicated that she did not want to be fed if she became incapacitated; the hospital opposed this. The court upheld the patient's right and refused to order her transfer.[14] Again, obtaining legal counsel in these instances is highly advisable)
4. Treatment must be instituted to prevent suicide and to preserve life (courts have clearly indicated, however, that terminally ill and/or comatose patients with no hope of recovery do not intend suicide when they refuse treatment)

When patients refuse treatment, complex ethical, legal, and practical problems arise. Hospitals should have specific policies to guide nurses in these areas. Ethics committees,

LEGAL REVIEW
The living will

The living will is a written document that states in advance a patient's wishes about the use of life-sustaining treatment when at a later time it becomes apparent that the patient is terminally ill. The document is signed by the maker of the document (the patient), witnessed by two adults, dated, and usually notarized. It is advisable that a patient review a living will periodically, making sure that it states current wishes about treatment, initialing it, and dating it. Some legal advisors recommend annual review. Legislation in some states provides that living wills are effective only for 5 years; therefore a living will should be reviewed at least every 5 years. A living will may be revoked at any time.

Physicians, nurses, and hospitals usually respect the document and adhere to it. State legislation provides civil and criminal immunity for good faith acts in carrying out a patient's living will. A copy of it can be inserted into the patient's chart to refer to when needed. The living will can be written to express individual needs and desires for a future time when the patient may not have capacity to speak. The treatments that are not wanted or those that are wanted can be specifically identified in the living will.

The living will can also have provisions for an appointment of a power of attorney to make medical care decisions, or a patient may have a separate document called the durable power of attorney. Both of these should become part of the patient's medical record.

The majority of states have legislation on living wills and on durable power of attorney for health care decisions. Critical care unit policies should reflect the laws of the jurisdiction where the unit exists.

A national resource for information on the living will is Concern for Dying, an educational council, located at 250 West 57th Street, New York, NY 10107. Two of their publications are "Questions and Answers about the Living Will" and "A Living Will." Below are provisions of the living will distributed by Concern for Dying.

My Living Will
To My Family, My Physician, My Lawyer and All Others Whom it May Concern

Death is as much a reality as birth, growth, maturity and old age—it is the one certainty of life. If the time comes when I can no longer take part in decisions for my own future, let this statement stand as an expression of my wishes and directions, while I am of sound mind. If at such a time the situation should arise in which there is no reasonable expectation of my recovery from extreme physical or mental disability, I direct that I be allowed to die and not be kept alive by medications, artificial means or "heroic measures". I do however, ask that medication be mercifully administered to me to alleviate suffering even though this may shorten my remaining life.

This statement is made after careful consideration and is in accordance with my strong convictions and beliefs. I want the wishes and directions here expressed carried out to the extent permitted by law. Insofar as they are not legally enforceable, I hope that those to whom this Will is addressed will regard themselves as morally bound by these provisions.

Measures of artificial life-support in the face of impending death that I specifically refuse are [patients can insert their own specific wishes, such as]:
(a) electrical or mechanical resuscitation of my heart when it has stopped beating.
(b) mechanical respiration when I am no longer able to sustain my own breathing.

If any of my tissues are sound and would be of value as transplants to other people, I freely give my permission for such donation.

---

case conferences, and careful medical and legal evaluation can provide direction on how to proceed; these are discussed in Chapter 2.

Tools for indicating wishes. Patients themselves can provide clear direction by preparing in advance written documents that specify their wishes. Tools for indicating wishes include the living will and durable power of attorney. To be effective in a jurisdiction, both of these tools must be statutorily or judicially recognized. The *living will* specifies that if certain circumstances occur, such as terminal illness, the patient will decline specific treatments, such as cardiopulmonary resuscitation. The living will does not cover all treatment. For example, in some states nutritional support may not be declined through a living will. The *durable power of attorney* is a tool through which a patient designates a spokesperson, someone who will speak for the patient if he or she becomes unable to speak on his or her

own. Both the living will and the durable power of attorney have statutory requirements, such as number of witnesses and the time for which the document is effective.

Critical care nurses whose patients have these or other tools should follow the policies that the hospital has about them. For example, special sections are set aside for these tools in the patient's medical record. Risk management staff or specialists, the administration, and legal counsel should review them and answer any questions nurses have about implementing them. Most statutes, for example, have immunity provisions, which protect nurses from liability for following the patient's wishes in good faith.

Working with substituted decision makers. A person identified by a patient as holding his or her durable power of attorney is authorized to speak for that patient. In some situations, a patient may have a legal guardian. This person is appointed by the court following a formal determination

---

PRINCIPLES FOR DECISION MAKING REGARDING THE USE OF LIFE-SUSTAINING TECHNOLOGIES FOR ELDERLY PERSONS

- An adult patient who is capable of making decisions has the right to decline any form of medical treatment or intervention. However, an individual does not necessarily have a right to unlimited medical treatment or intervention.
- Decisions regarding the use of life-sustaining treatments must be made on an individual basis and should never be based on chronological age alone. Chronological age per se is a poor criterion on which to base individual medical decision; however, age may be a legitimate modifier regarding appropriate utilization of life-sustaining medical technologies.
- Diagnosis alone is a poor criterion for decisions about the use of life-sustaining technologies. Because of the great variability among patients with the same diagnosis, patient assessment must also include measure of functional impairment and severity of illness.
- Cognitive function is an important marker of the quality of life.
- The courts are not and should not be the usual route or determinant for making decisions about the use of life-sustaining technologies or for resolving the dilemmas these may create.
- There is little need or room for federal legislation concerning the initiation, withholding, or withdrawal of specific life-sustaining technologies.
- There is a major need for a clear, workable definition of the appropriate role of surrogates in health care decision making, including the nature of their responsibilities and their suitability to make decisions.
- There is a need to recognize that a decision making process exists, or should exist, for making decisions about the use of life-sustaining technologies. The process described by the President's Commission for the Study of Ethical Problems in Medicine and Biomedical and Behavioral Research could serve as a model.
- A physician or other health care professional who does not want to follow the wishes of a patient who is capable of making decisions regarding his or her treatment should withdraw from that case.
- Socioeconomic status should not be a barrier to access to health care, including life-sustaining technologies.
- There is an important need for education of the public and health care providers regarding the nature and appropriate use of life-sustaining technologies.
- There is a specific need for improved clinical information that would predict the probability of a critically or seriously ill patient's survival, functional status, and subsequent quality of life.
- There is a wide range of medical and legal disagreement and varying levels of emotional strain and moral conflict about the appropriate use of life-sustaining technologies. The great heterogeneity of the American population makes consensus difficult and increases the likelihood of formal institutional decision-making procedures.

Developed by Project Advisory Panel, US Congress, Office of Technology Assessment: Life-sustaining technologies and the elderly 23, OTA-BA-306, Washington, DC, 1987, US Government Printing Office.

---

by the court that the patient is legally incompetent. A few states have family consent laws that allow relatives of adults who do not have decision making capabilities to make legally binding decisions on behalf of those patients without a formal judicial proceeding.[15] New York has yet another option—specific legislation has been enacted entitled *Orders Not to Resuscitate*.[16] Under this law, if two physicians decide a patient does not have the capability to consent, a surrogate decision maker can be selected from a priority list established by the law. This can be done without a formal judicial determination of the patient's legal competency.

In fact, the only way an adult loses legal competency is through a formal judicial proceeding. And even after a formal proceeding determines that a patient should be involuntarily committed, the patient still has important rights in treatment decisions, such as the right to refuse antipsychotic medications.

The first step in working with substitute decision makers is to be assured that they have the authority to speak for the patient. This authority should be documented in the patient's chart. Clearly identifying who speaks for the patient is important for the patient's care and for respect of the patient's privacy. If the patient's surrogate has authority to speak on the patient's behalf, then nurses avoid allegations of invasion of privacy and breach of confidentiality, because the surrogate is an authorized person, entitled to knowledge of private facts and information about the patient.

Withholding and Withdrawing Treatment

As indicated earlier, an adult has the right to refuse treatment, even treatment that sustains life. This right means that the critical care nurse may participate in withholding or withdrawing treatments. Initially, the distinction between withholding and withdrawing treatments was considered important, but that is no longer the case. These health care decisions become most complex when patients lose capacity to personally make their own decisions.

Two important and helpful reports for this area of concern were issued in 1987 by the Office of Technology Assessment (OTA), U.S. Congress[17] and by The Hastings Center.[18] Among the topics discussed were types of treatment and decision-making processes. The box on p. 42 contains a set of principles for decision making about the use of life-sustaining technologies developed by the OTA's Project Advisory Panel.

Orders not to resuscitate and other orders. Hospital policies that discuss orders to withhold or withdraw treatment should exist in all critical care units. For example, orders not to resuscitate, commonly referred to by nurses as DNR (do not resuscitate) orders, should be governed by written policies, including, but not limited to, the following:

1. DNR orders should be entered in the patient's record with full documentation by the responsible physician about the patient's prognosis, the patient's agreement (if he or she is capable), or the family's concurrence (for incapacitated patients).
2. DNR orders should have the concurrence of another physician, designated in the policy.
3. Policies should specify that orders are reviewed periodically (some policies require daily review).
4. Patients with capacity must give their informed consent.
5. For patients without capacity, that incapacity must be thoroughly documented, along with the diagnosis and prognosis, and family agreement.
6. Judicial intervention before writing a DNR order is usually indicated when the patient's family does not agree,

---

LEGAL REVIEW

Withholding treatment decisions in the critical care unit

CASE EXAMPLE: *Morgan v. Olds,* 417 N.W.2d 232 (Iowa App 1987).

Dwaine Morgan was admitted to Iowa Methodist Medical Center on May 22, 1981, following an episode of cardiac arrest. CPR was successful, and Mr. Morgan regained conscious functioning. However, he suffered two more cardiac arrests. Resuscitation was again successful; however, he suffered brain damage resulting from a lack of oxygen and lapsed into a coma from which he never awoke. It became apparent to his physicians that the prognosis was bleak. Neurological testing showed severe damage to the cerebral cortex. However, he was not brain dead, because he retained brainstem function. The brain damage was irreversible, and he was considered vegetative.

Because of the poor prognosis, the physicians decided to recommend to Mrs. Morgan that further life-sustaining treatment be withheld in the event such treatment became necessary. A conference was held June 2 among three doctors, a social worker, Mrs. Morgan, and another relative. During the conference, the doctors suggested that Mr. Morgan be weaned from the ventilator to see whether he would be able to breathe on his own, but after this was accomplished, he should not be placed back on the ventilator or otherwise resuscitated if his condition deteriorated. On June 7, Morgan was successfully weaned from the ventilator. Later in the day, he began to have difficulty breathing, and his condition deteriorated. In conformance with the plan, no additional life-sustaining procedures were provided, and he died.

At trial Mrs. Morgan testified that she did not consent to this plan, because she had not received information justifying the decision. The doctors testified that Mrs. Morgan did consent. Mrs. Morgan testified that she was aware at the time of the discussion that the brain damage was probably irreversible but that the medical information she had received did not convince her the decision was appropriate or necessary. She had been informed of the results of only one of two planned EEGs that, while grim, indicated to her that there was still hope. She had been told that her husband could probably survive a long time in a chronic vegetative state. Even though this would probably be the highest level of recovery, she felt it was not a good reason to allow her husband to die. She felt this would have been his preference.

A letter Mrs. Morgan prepared after the conference (mentioned above) and directed to the physician stated in part: "You have the whole picture, plus the experience and I will stand by the decision. Need more details for me, for later." The court stated that it did not appear from the evidence that Mrs. Morgan withdrew her consent or objected to the decision.

One of the questions raised in this case was whether the attending doctors have an independent duty to the patient's family to employ reasonable care in consulting with them and obtaining their consent before making any decision about the treatment of a patient who does not have the capacity to consent. Although this Iowa court held that no such duty existed, the court stated that the doctor, as part of his or her duty to a patient without capacity, must consult with the patient's surrogate decision maker before implementing a course of treatment. When a doctor implements a course of treatment without obtaining the patient's consent, he or she breaches a duty and is liable to the patient for any resultant damages. Similarly, when a doctor fails to obtain the consent of the patient's surrogate decision maker, a duty to the patient is breached and the physician will be liable for any resultant damages.

or there is uncertainty or disagreement about the patient's prognosis or mental status.

7. Policies should specify who is to be contacted and notified within the hospital administration.

Other orders to withhold or withdraw treatment may involve mechanical ventilation, dialysis, nutritional support, hydration, and medications, such as antibiotics. The legal and ethical implications of these orders for each patient must be carefully considered. Hospitals should have written policies on all orders to withhold or withdraw treatment. Policies must cover how decisions will be made; who will decide; and what the roles of patient, family, health care providers, and the institution will be. Policies must be developed that take into consideration state laws and judicial opinions, such as those governing neglect or abuse of patients.

Organ Procurement

Critical care nurses are often involved in organ procurement for donation and transplantation. State and federal laws regulate this area. For example, before an organ can be procured, a patient must first be declared dead. State laws and regulations define death. Traditionally, death was defined as cessation of circulation and respiration; today, laws define death to include irreversible cessation of all functions of the entire brain, including the brain stem. Laws state that a determination of death must be made in accordance with accepted medical standards and is deemed to have occurred when the determination of death is completed. In the critical care unit, a physician determines that death has occurred for all legal purposes, including organ procurement.

The federal law on organ transplants establishes a national network of procurement centers, encourages and funds coordination of organ donation, and prohibits the sale of organs. It is unlawful for any person to knowingly acquire, receive, or otherwise transfer any human organ for valuable consideration for use in human transplantation if the transfer affects interstate commerce. Any person violating this law shall be fined not more than $50,000 or imprisoned not more than 5 years, or both.[19]

The state law governing organ procurement is referred to as the Uniform Anatomical Gift Act.[20] Each state has adopted a variation of this uniform statute. Generally, the law provides that any individual of sound mind and over 18 years of age may donate any part or all of his or her body. In most states, the individual's decision in this regard cannot be overruled after death by a family member. However, in some states family members can do this.[21] State law also specifies who else may donate, who may receive the anatomical gift, and how the gift is made; state law also includes restrictions. For example, the physician who determines time of death may not participate in the removal or transplantation of organs.

To increase the availability of organs, state and federal laws and regulations have been passed that require hospitals to ask patients or their family members about organ donation. From the federal level, under Medicare regulations, hospitals participating in Medicare or Medicaid must establish written protocols for the identification of potential donors. From the state level, through amendments to the anatomical gift act, hospital administrators must establish a policy to ask patient's or their family members to make an organ donation. These policies should specify clearly the nurse's involvement in organ procurement, how it is to be carried out, and what documentation requirements exist. For example, in New York, Section 4351 of the Public Health Law requires that a request for consent for an anatomical gift must be made to the authorized family members of patients who die in hospitals if those patients are medically suitable donors of at least one organ, tissue, or other body part, unless (1) there is actual notice of contrary intentions or opposition by the decedent [one who has died] or an authorized family member or (2) reason to believe that an anatomical gift is contrary to the decedent's religious or moral beliefs.

SUPPORTING STANDARDS OF STANDARD XII

The critical care nurse shall ensure the delivery of safe nursing care to patients, being cognizant of the various "causes of action" for which the nurse may be liable.

1. Patients shall be fully advised in advance of all nursing and/or medical procedures to which they are subjected, signing a written informed consent when required. (Causes of action: assault, battery.)
2. Patients shall be allowed freedom of movement within their hospital rooms and are allowed to discharge themselves from the hospital. (Causes of action: false imprisonment.)
3. Patients shall receive nursing care in accordance with good nursing practice and those policies specifically established by the hospital. (Causes of action: negligence.)
4. Patients shall be assured that any medical information will be shared only with health professionals treating the patient, and any other communication is restricted or occurs only with the consent of the patient. (Causes of action: defamation.)
5. The patient's family members shall not be subjected to incorrect information concerning the patient or careless treatment of the patient. (Causes of action: infliction of mental distress.)
6. Patients shall be treated in a dignified manner; only those professionals directly involved in their care have access to their medical information, and this information will not be released or disclosed to others without the approval of the patients. (Causes of action: invasion of privacy.)

Adapted from the American Association of Critical-Care Nurses: Standards for nursing care of the critically ill, Newport Beach, Calif, 1989, The Association.

SUMMARY

This chapter began with definitions of critical care nursing, drawing out of them specific legal and professional concerns. After an overview of law, legal processes, civil and administrative law, attention turned to negligence and malpractice, nursing practice acts, and specific practice issues.

Critical care nurses have been urged by their professional association to ensure the delivery of safe nursing care to patients. To that end, their standards of care include being cognizant of "causes of action" for which the nurse may be liable. The box on p. 44 summarizes this standard and serves as a reminder and a review of the important legal responsibilities of critical care nurses.

REFERENCES

1. American Association of Critical-Care Nurses, Standards for nursing care of the critically ill 5 (1989).
2. American Association of Critical-Care Nurses: Position statement: definition of critical care nursing (Feb 1984).
3. American Association of Critical-Care Nurses: Position statement: principles of critical care nursing practice Item 7. [1981].
4. American Nurses' Association: Code for nurses with interpretive statements (1985).
5. For a comprehensive handling of nursing legal issues see Northrop and Kelly, Legal issues in nursing (CV Mosby 1987).
6. Tom Christoffel, Health and the Law 8 (Macmillan 1982).
7. William Prosser, Law of torts 143 (4th ed, West 1971).
8. Betty Campazzi, Nurses, nursing and malpractice litigation: 1967-77, 5 Nurs Admin Q 1 (No 1 1981).
9. Cynthia Northrop, Status of recent nursing litigation, 2 Nurs Econ 423 (Nov-Dec 1984); Cynthia Northrop, Nursing actions in litigation, in Special Publication of qual rev bull: risk management and quality assurance: issues and interactions 24 (Sept 1986).
10. 28 United States Code Sections 2671-2680 (1986).
11. *Schloendorff v Society of New York Hospital,* 105 N.E. 92 (1914).
12. Mcdonald, Meyer, Essig, Health care law Section 18.03[2][2] (1987).
13. *Brophy v New England Sinai Hospital,* 497 N.E.2d 626 (Mass 1986).
14. *In re Requena,* 517 A.2d 869 (NJ App Div 1986).
15. Northrop, Nursing practice and the legal presumption of competency, 36 Nurs Outlook 112 (No 2 Mar-Apr 1988).
16. New York public health law §2960-2978 (McKinney Supp 1988).
17. US Congress, Office of Technology Assessment, Life-sustaining technologies and the elderly, OTA-BA-306 (Washington, DC, US Government Printing Office, July 1987).
18. The Hastings Center, Guidelines on the termination of life-sustaining treatment and the care of the dying (1987). The Hastings Center, 255 Elm Road, Briarcliff Manor, NY 10510.
19. 42 United States Code Section 274e (1986).
20. 8A Uniform Law Acts [ULA] (1983).
21. New York, for example, says that if the donee (one receiving the donation) has actual notice that the gift is opposed by a member of the family the donee shall not accept the gift. NY Pub Health Law Section 4301(3) (McKinney's 1987).

CHAPTER

4

Cultural Issues

CHAPTER OBJECTIVES

- *Define the term* stereotyping *and explain how this practice can interfere with the accurate perception of the critical care patient.*
- *List five questions to ask oneself to become aware of one's own cultural values.*
- *List two ways in which patients' feelings of powerlessness can interfere with the delivery of effective critical care.*
- *Explain how the doctrine of fatalism can affect the attitude of the critically ill patient.*
- *List three ethnic groups to whom visits from the extended family are very important in the healing process.*
- *Explain 10 possible reasons for a patient to cry out in pain and propose appropriate interventions.*
- *Explain 15 possible reasons a patient might strive to conceal his or her pain and propose appropriate interventions.*
- *Propose seven techniques for improving communication despite the presence of language barriers.*

The impact of cultural and ethnic diversity on both American society and the nursing profession has intensified as the number of immigrants and refugees has steadily increased throughout recent decades.

While enriching the lives of us all, diversity has generated numerous challenges for health care professionals who are attempting to deliver effective, compassionate care to patients whose values, beliefs, and language can be very different from their own. Although much remains to be done, in recent years there has developed a substantial body of theoretical and applied literature designed to help overcome the challenges of what has become known as "transcultural nursing." A select bibliography of these materials is found at the end of this chapter.

This chapter attempts to cover the most commonly encountered challenges in this new and growing field. After discussing some of the general principles behind successful cross-cultural communication (for example, the importance

of overcoming ethnocentrism and the danger of making unwarranted generalities), we will survey the perspective and values of the patient. Emphasis is placed on patients' attitudes toward the health care professional, family roles, and responses to pain and grief and finally, techniques for overcoming accent and language barriers.

THE CHALLENGE OF DIVERSITY

Culture consists of socially transmitted beliefs about the proper ways of behaving, the nature of the world, and the structure and purpose of the universe. On a more practical level, culture supplies a design for living that delineates how to interpret and react to the world.

Before discussing the challenges presented to the critical care nurse by cultural diversity, an even more fundamental difficulty must be addressed—the resistance that many individuals feel to admitting that cultural diversity does indeed exist. It may seem like an easy matter to see diversity, but some who come into regular contact with people from other cultures are reluctant to recognize that cultural differences are interfering with communication and mutual understanding. There is a tendency to feel that if language differences could be eliminated, so would communication difficulties.

There are many reasons why people deny the impact that cultural diversity can have on effective human and professional relationships. Perhaps the most common cause is the fear that to admit that people's values, etiquette, and even world views might be different is to appear guilty of stereotyping the population in question. Quite the contrary is true. To deny a person his or her cultural distinctiveness is to deny an important part of the individual's being and to limit dramatically one's accurate perception of that person.

Another reason that people tend to deny the importance of cultural diversity is that to do so necessitates confronting and dealing with a complex set of behavioral variables that otherwise could be ignored. The information that follows focuses on those culturally generated behavioral variables that most often arise in critical care settings. Cultural assessment guidelines are described for use in planning care. Particular emphasis is placed on the importance of understanding one's own culture, the perspectives of the immigrant patient and family, cultural variations in the pain response, and techniques for minimizing the difficulties created by language barriers.

THE NURSE'S PERSPECTIVE

Culture is a phenomenon that is common to all human beings. The critical care nurse has personal beliefs, attitudes, perspectives, and behaviors that depend on ancestral and geographical background. For example, the nurse of Italian ancestry who was brought up in New York but currently lives in southern California is a representative of the cultural styles of Italy, New York, and California. In addition to these layers of culture, the hospital in which the nurse works also has a culture of its own that can be quite distinct from other facilities. The hospital culture consists of goals, priorities, heroes, traditional ways of doing things, and even terminology that becomes a part of each health professional's cultural "baggage."

Culture, in short, is not just something that belongs to the ethnic or immigrant patient and family, but it affects, often in very subtle ways, the manner in which each nurse responds to colleagues, patients, and families. Within these culturally conditioned responses lie a great many of the pitfalls to cross-cultural communication. The primary reasons for these pitfalls are (1) the tendency to be ethnocentric and (2) the temptation to stereotype others as a means of eliminating ambiguity from the environment.[12]

Ethnocentrism

Ethnocentrism is the view that one's own culture does things in the best way possible and that cultures that appear different are merely lesser versions of one's own. The dangerous corollary of this belief—that all cultures are striving to be more like his or her own—leads to the assumption that the behavior of culturally diverse patients can be accurately interpreted in the light of traditional American values and priorities. In short, it is easy to forget that the patient's behavior, developed in the context of a certain culture, is based on a different perspective of the world, and behaviors might have very different meanings from those ordinarily expected.

One simple example can clarify how this type of misunderstanding can arise. Although it is always dangerous to generalize about the behavior of any group, it is nonetheless not unusual for critical care nurses to encounter Hispanic males who do not initially express much grief at the loss of a wife. According to mainstream American notions of appropriate grief responses, this lack of response would indicate that the husband cared little for his wife and was feeling little grief. This interpretation would probably be inaccurate; the ethnocentric view that all cultures teach the same responses to grief causes the nurse to project personal values onto the Hispanic man and therefore arrive at the wrong conclusion.

The correct conclusion can be reached only when the Hispanic man's lack of response is interpreted in the context of Hispanic cultural mores. In Hispanic culture, although grieving is generally done quite openly, it is not uncommon to find the male head of the household exhibiting little emo-

---

PROMOTING CULTURAL SELF-AWARENESS

Before arriving at any conclusions regarding the behavior of someone from a different culture, become aware of your own culturally conditioned perspective by asking yourself the following:
- If I observed my parents behaving in this way, what would the behavior have meant for them?
- How was I raised to behave in a similar situation?
- How would I behave now if I were in the patient's position?
- If I were to behave just as the patient has, what would my motivation be?
- What is my idea of "proper" behavior in a situation such as this?

---

tion on the death of a loved one, because he feels his duty as head of the household keenly and postpones his expression of grief until the rest of the family has recovered enough to cope with the duties of everyday life.[9] The cultural value is that someone (the male) must stay in charge and in control until calm has been restored.

Once the Hispanic culture is examined and the behavior evaluated in the light of this newfound knowledge, it becomes clear that the initial conclusion that the husband cared little for his wife is probably quite incorrect. Instead, the Hispanic husband was probably feeling a great deal of love, not only for the deceased wife, but for his entire family to whom he owed a most difficult duty. This case illustrates clearly the danger of projecting one's own cultural values onto another.

It is not an easy task to avoid this trap. Indeed, culture is so much a part of us that it is almost impossible to be aware of it—it is like the air we breathe; we experience it but are not conscious of its existence. The key to avoiding the pitfalls of ethnocentrism is to become as aware as possible of how one's own culture stands on the situation being considered. The box above contains a list of questions designed to help facilitate this process of cultural self-awareness and is to be used anytime a situation arises in which the nurse suspects that cultural differences may be involved. Becoming aware of how one's own culture feels about a given behavior enables the nurse to separate her own views from those of the patient. Thus the automatic process of projection and ethnocentrism is short-circuited.

Working Generalities Versus Stereotypes

The second primary pitfall to effective cross-cultural communication involves the human tendency to place people and events into neat, unambiguous categories. Stereotyping involves the assumption that all members of a given group will behave in the same way and for the same reasons. Generally, these stereotypes are created out of the values and fears of one's own culture.

For practical purposes, it is important to distinguish between working generalities and stereotypes. A *working generality* is a guideline—a starting point—formed from intelligently considered experiences and study. These generalities help sort out the universe and help predict, with some reasonable accuracy, what to expect from others. Without them, it would be impossible for human beings to carry out even the simplest interaction.

The main feature of a working generality is that it is abandoned immediately when one suspects that the assumptions on which the generality was based are incorrect. For example, nothing is intrinsically wrong in assuming that newly arrived Vietnamese families prefer a more formal approach from a health professional; this guideline helps us know what tone to strike when approaching people with whom we are not familiar.[13] If it is discovered, however, once the family is met, that the individuals are casual and spontaneous and prefer to be addressed by first names, the culturally aware nurse will quickly abandon the initial guideline and relate to that particular family less formally.

A *stereotype* differs from a working generality in that it is rarely abandoned in the face of contradictory evidence. One reason stereotypes are adhered to so tenaciously is they make the believer feel more secure by providing a systematic, static way of sorting the world and its inhabitants. Stereotypes also differ from working, flexible generalities in that they tend to limit one's definition of the individual toward whom they are directed. It does not matter whether the stereotypical statement is negative or positive—it still draws limits on who and what the observer believes that person can be. There is, for example, nothing negative in saying that Asians prefer a holistic approach to medicine, Hispanics tend to value the present moment over the future, and Moslems believe in the will of Allah when it comes to matters of illness and death. The problem arises when such statements are used to limit a definition of the person and to distort an accurate perception of who and what that individual really is. The result of an inflexible stereotype is that it causes one to see what is expected, that is, the stereotype, not the real individual.

Just like ethnocentrism, which distorts the accurate perception of the individual because of the cultural screen it erects, stereotypical thinking distorts reality by causing us to see what we are predisposed to see, not what is actually there. Nurses who can avoid the temptation to categorize people and behaviors into inflexible boxes will function most effectively in a multicultural hospital setting.

THE PATIENT'S PERSPECTIVE

Some of the greatest challenges ethnic and cultural diversity presents to the critical care nurse arise out of differing attitudes toward health care and toward the health care professional. These variations in attitude include differing views on the position and responsibility of the health care professional and differing beliefs about the patient's ability to control health and destiny.

The Nurse as Authority Figure

It is impossible to generalize about patient attitudes toward health care professionals. However, two perspectives

vary so dramatically from those found among mainstream, native-born Americans that they must be mentioned. They are the patient's perception of the health professional as an authority figure and as the individual who is ultimately responsible for the success or failure of treatment.

One manifestation of this attitude is the tendency for some patients—and their families—to resist, when given the opportunity, making choices about their treatment. During recent years in the United States, there has been a growing trend toward patient involvement and patient responsibility in the treatment process.[1] Indeed, the provision of choice, whenever possible, has become one of the basic tenets of sound, effective nursing care.

In many nations of the world, the movement toward patient involvement and decision making has yet to manifest itself. The patient, instead, looks to the health professional to make decisions and accept full responsibility for these decisions. In short, it cannot be assumed that the patient and family are ignorant, lazy, or unintelligent when its members do not wish to participate in the decision-making process. This behavior quite simply reflects a different health care hierarchy.

Powerlessness and Fatalism

Related to the desire to give the responsiblity for treatment to health professionals is a psychological phenomenon known as powerlessness. *Powerlessness* is an acquired belief that the individual has little or no control over his or her life. Although this belief is usually not based on reality, its emotional roots lie in historical situations that have left individuals and entire populations with a sense of being out of control.

Decades of discrimination, for example, can leave a people with the belief that it cannot succeed no matter what efforts are forthcoming. In addition, living for generations at the poverty level can result in the overwhelming and paralyzing belief that no effort will allow the individual to break out of this pattern.[5] Short-term historical events can have an equally devastating impact on individual and group feelings of control. Southeast Asian immigrants, for example, who have spent as long as 5 years in refugee camps where every effort at planning for the future was thwarted, experience the same feelings of powerlessness that have taken decades to develop in other peoples.

The ramifications of powerlessness for effective critical care nursing can be dramatic. Foremost is the fact that feelings of powerlessness interfere with a patient's willingness to participate in ongoing treatment. When a patient or family member believes that he or she has no control over the future, lengthy and sometimes uncomfortable treatment seems pointless and fruitless.

The problems created by this perspective for patient compliance and morale are obvious; the solutions can be more obscure. Ordinarily, the best way to restore power to the "powerless" patient is to supply him or her with decision-making power and with information. Although these techniques sometimes apply, there is often a disinterest in choice and information among these population groups. Supplying the patient and family with the opportunity to exhibit personal power in a way that is meaningful to them is one of the most effective ways of overcoming this difficulty and, in turn, improving compliance. The nurse must be careful to first assess what the "perceived needs" of the patient and family member really are.

To accurately ascertain the ways in which the patient or family would most like to exhibit power, the nurse must first learn as much as possible about the culture in question. The importance, for example, of allowing the extended family to gather around the patient cannot be overemphasized. Likewise, appointing one individual as the hospital spokesperson so that the family always knows whom to approach for information can have a dramatic effect on how powerful, and therefore cooperative, the family feels. A hospital ombudsman or patient representative could serve this function. The patient and family must be allowed to exhibit power in a way that is meaningful to them, in the context of their culture, not in a way that would be important to persons born and raised in mainstream American culture.

Fatalism—that is, the view that the course of life is dictated by a higher power—is a positive version of powerlessness. The difference between the two is that feelings of powerlessness arise out of discrimination, poverty, and historical adversity and fatalism is generated out of faith in a higher power and in the preordained perfection of the universe. Although the impact of fatalism on health care can sometimes be adverse (for example, resistance to invoking heroic measures during critical illness), the effect is a positive one, because it leaves the patient and family in a more peaceful, accepting state of mind.

The impact of fatalism is seen most dramatically in those who are critically ill. The notion of calling on the individual's "will to live" is an important feature of American health care attitudes. The fatalistic attitudes found among Hispanic and Middle Eastern immigrants, on the other hand, hold that the will of God dictates the fate of the critically ill.[6] The Arabic phrase *in shallah* (if God wills it) sums up this perspective and illustrates the importance of critical care nurses' recognizing and honoring this distinction.

To speak, for example, to the Hispanic patient of his or her "will to live" will, in all probability, be fruitless and misunderstood. To speak, on the other hand, of the importance of relying on and having faith in God's will may prove both comforting and productive. However, this reliance on God's will among the terminally ill can create problems for the nursing staff. Because in many cultures it is considered God's will whether a person lives or dies, many family members will not want the patient told that he or she is terminal because this, in their eyes, would be second-guessing God and therefore defying His will.[6] There is little that the critical care nurse can or should do about this preference. However, awareness is necessary so that misunderstandings that could result in family alienation can be avoided.

THE FAMILY'S PERSPECTIVE

The ability to communicate effectively with the family of the critical care patient is a most important psychosocial element for the critical care nurse. To succeed at this task, the nurse must understand the structure of the family, who its leaders are, and who its members are.

In contrast to traditional Anglo-American families that consist of comparatively few important members, immigrant families are generally *extended units* in which aunts, uncles, cousins, and grandparents are closely bound and have a central importance in each other's eyes. Many families extend even beyond blood relatives to include *fictive kin*—individuals who are loved and regarded as family members but who are not related by biology or marriage—especially within Black culture, as well as within the *compadres* and *comadres* (godparents) tradition of the Hispanic culture.

The implication for critical care of the extended and fictive family lies primarily in the importance of respecting the wishes of the patient concerning visiting rights. Hospital rules must also be respected, but the nurse should make no rash judgments about who really matters to the patient, who is capable of rendering valuable support, and who is not. In addition, the nurse must not believe that she or he has been lied to if a patient refers to a nonblood "relative" as "brother," "sister," "aunt," or "uncle." These designations are merely affectionate and are not meant to manipulate the nurse into allowing a nonfamily member to visit the patient.

With respect to visitation, the importance of family support to the critically ill immigrant patient cannot be overemphasized. In Gypsy culture, to cite an extreme, the presence of the family is believed to bring healing energy to the patient. Among those from the Middle East, the family brings very tangible hope to the critically ill.[6] In short, the family functions not just as a support system but as a central component in the healing process.[4]

Because of the central role played by the extended family in the care of the immigrant patient, the nurse must know how to address the family to ensure mutual respect and cooperation.[4] Above all else, the nurse must use last names, proceed slowly, and generally respect the more formal social rules of immigrant culture. The nurse must also be able to establish who the spokesperson and decision maker is for the family. Only in this way will the professional be able to establish rapport and ensure good communication.

Within Middle Eastern families, for example, the spokesperson is likely to be the father or eldest brother, although the eldest female is likely to hold a great deal of power within the home. This distinction between public power and private control is an important one and must be honored by the health worker. In Hispanic culture, the public head of the household is very likely the father, but within the home, it is the woman who controls many of the decisions. A similar situation occurs within the Italian household.[11] Despite this covert power of the woman, the nurse must respect the male in public and address him with respect and formality.

The issue of whom to address becomes even more complicated when considering the existence of tribal systems within certain immigrant cultures. The Samoans, Laotians, and Gypsies, for example, each practice a form of tribal culture that has as one of its components a tribal leader who functions as the spokesperson and decision maker for the community. By showing respect for the family and the tribal structure of the group, the nurse can dramatically improve patient and family cooperation.

THE PAIN RESPONSE

One of the most bewildering aspects of cultural diversity is the cultural variations that critical care nurses observe in the response to pain. However, a careful distinction must be drawn between the pain threshold and the pain response. The *pain threshold* is that point at which a given sensation is physically perceived as painful. Pain thresholds vary from individual to individual but do not vary along ethnic or cultural lines.

The *pain response* does vary along cultural lines, because it reflects the patient's attitude toward the pain and a learned behavior in response to the pain. Pain response is a behavior that reflects the values and priorities of the culture in which the patient was reared. The response is learned both through observation of how parents responded to pain and through the experience of how parents reacted to children in pain.

Responses to pain can be divided into two broad categories—emotive and stoic. As a working generality, immigrants from the Latin countries, southern Europe, and the Middle East tend to be emotive. Those from northern Europe and Asia and the Native American (American Indian) tend to be more stoic in responding to discomfort. There are, of course, numerous exceptions to these guidelines. Factors such as gender, degree of assimilation into mainstream American culture, socioeconomic status, age, and individual personality create considerable diversity within any one cultural group. Nevertheless, these guidelines can be a good starting point in evaluating the behavior of a given patient.

Before examining some of the reasons for an emotive or stoic response to pain and some possible interventions, it must be noted that there is no intrinsic right or wrong in either of these responses—the patient is behaving in a fashion that, because of cultural background, works under the circumstances. The danger of the nurse's projecting personal cultural beliefs onto the patient again comes into play. It is not uncommon for the Anglo-American nurse who has been taught to restrain the expression of pain and "act like a big girl or boy" to assume that those who express pain are being childlike or self-indulgent.[3] This conclusion merely reflects the nurse's culture and has little to do with the motivation or motives of the patient. The behavior must be evaluated in the context of the patient's culture—not by comparison to American values and norms.

The box at right lists some of the possible reasons that a patient might emote when in pain and the appropriate nursing interventions for emotive patients. The item "grief over loss of role" deserves special attention, because it addresses one of the most important values of many immigrant cultures: the desire to properly fulfill one's role as a man or a woman. It is not unusual to see a male patient whose critical illness has deprived him of potency or of the ability to support his family display a great deal of apparent pain even in the absence of actual physical discomfort, in which case, he is probably grieving over loss of manhood and not, as it may appear on the surface, crying out in physical pain. The obvious intervention, as indicated in the second part of the box, is to reassure the patient about the severity of his affliction. If the perceived loss has indeed taken place, suggestions about alternative ways of performing the desired role might be provided.

THE EMOTIVE PATIENT

REASONS FOR EMOTING

Fear of the situation
Desire for help and fear of not receiving it
Loneliness and need for attention
Grief over loss of role, dignity, life
Anger
Desire to pay a price
Exorcism of pain through the act of crying out
Appropriateness of emotive behavior
Self-absorption
Great pain

APPROPRIATE INTERVENTIONS

Ask what is needed
Listen carefully to the reply
Provide information about medications, procedures, pain
Provide attention promptly
Be prompt with medications and treatments
Provide distractions
Provide the chance to give to others
Reassure patient about role fulfillment
Speak softly
Touch (if culturally appropriate)
Use relaxation techniques
Contact consultant, spiritual leader, family member
Provide appropriate pain medications

The intervention listed in the box as "Provide attention promptly" cannot be overemphasized. When the patient is feeling frightened and lonely and is needing attention and is afraid of not getting it, nothing can be more distressing than having to wait for the desired help. The more the patient has to wait, the more his or her fear that the help will not be forthcoming increases. The realities of a busy unit are not to be denied, but so too are the realities of punctuality when it comes to relieving patient anxiety.

The box on p. 51 addresses the stoic patient—the individual who will not push the button to ask for help and will not admit to any discomfort when asked. On the surface, this sort of patient may seem the ideal, but in reality, the concealment of pain can create many problems for the critical care nurse. For one thing, if the nurse does not know that the patient is in pain, the proper medications will not be administered and, in turn, the proper rest and its healing effects will not be experienced by the patient. Providing explanations to the patient who is afraid to take pain medications can be very helpful in improving communication. Many immigrant patients are fearful that medications will become addictive and that too much will be given. Particularly, an Asian who has a small body stature may fear that the effects of the drug will put the patient out of control, or he or she may believe that pain is an essential part of the healing process.

THE STOIC PATIENT

REASONS FOR STOICISM

To facilitate denial
To perform as the "perfect patient"
To gain self-worth and power
To avoid loss of control
Fear of addiction
Fear of overdose and side effects
Fear of intravenous treatment
To avoid calling attention to oneself
To avoid worrying family
To pay a price for past sins and future joys
Low self-esteem
Desire to experience the process
Desire for meditation
Acceptance of condition
No pain

APPROPRIATE INTERVENTIONS

Careful observation

Check the patient frequently for symptoms of pain
Observe for objective symptoms of distress

Elicitation of patient cooperation

Explain that pain retards healing
Explain that medication is more effeceive if given at onset of pain
Explain that medications are safe
Describe what to expect from pain medication
Give praise when appropriate

Intervention in these cases obviously involves providing correct information about these concerns. It is particularly helpful for nurses to ask the patient to help them do their job by revealing the amount of pain, explaining that only in this way can the nurse, as the person responsible for the patient's well-being, do a good job. This approach, particularly in view of the Asian emphasis on avoiding failure or embarrassment for all concerned, can have remarkable results.

Observing objective symptoms and noting recent procedures that might cause extreme pain are two of the best ways to assess the amount of pain being experienced. Clenched fists, raised blood pressure, flush, pallor, lack of movement, grimace, rapid pulse, and perspiration are a few of the ways in which the presence of pain can be determined. Even the patient (particularly if he or she is Asian) who smiles perpetually should be suspected as one who is trying to maintain dignity and stoicism at all costs.

CULTURAL VARIATIONS IN THE GRIEF RESPONSE

Just as it is necessary for the critical care nurse to understand cultural variations in the response to physical pain,

it is equally important to be aware of culturally specific ways of expressing grief and emotional loss, especially if the nurse is to avoid the danger of misinterpreting the meaning of a family's reaction, or lack of reaction, to a loved one's critical condition or death. As in the case of the Hispanic husband mentioned previously, if an individual does not react as expected, it is very easy to label the behavior as callousness, denial, or overreaction. In short, the norms for proper grief behavior in one culture may appear strange or even repugnant in the context of another culture. Table 4-1 delineates death-related behaviors associated with six cultural groups.

East Indian culture, for example, allows and indeed calls for a public display of grief. The "stiff upper lip" and brave face that is often called for in British and Anglo-American culture is considered by East Indians as neither appropriate nor necessary.[7]

Although it is impossible to generalize about grief behavior, a good "working generality" with respect to the Jewish family is that in its culture, too, open grieving is encouraged. This grieving is generally confined to a prescribed period of time, which begins with the first 7 days of intense mourning and terminates after 1 year when the official season of mourning has ended.[15] During the initial period of mourning, Jewish culture dictates that those who are present to comfort the bereaved would do well to simply listen rather than attempt to mouth empty words of consolation. For this reason, it is important that the family be allowed to congregate at the time of death to provide this necessary support.[14]

Because of the great diversity of Asian cultures within the United States today, it is very difficult to predict the grieving pattern of any given Asian family. The Japanese, for example, are likely to be stoic when grieving, whereas certain Chinese will feel comfortable venting their feelings even when in public.[14,16] The critical care nurse needs to bear in mind that the stoicism that is often seen among Asian patients when in physical pain is likely to be missing when that pain is emotional.

Dr. Lois Davitz and colleagues[3] raised an interesting question during their research into nurses' responses to patient pain. She pointed out that Anglo-American nurses tend to be less tolerant of patients who emote when in physical and psychological pain than they are of those who are more stoic.[3] This attitude can raise serious problems for the nurse who comes in contact with large numbers of Hispanic families whose culture dictates a very open expression of grief.[16] It must be remembered that each individual learns to react to emotional pain in a way that provides the most effective relief and elicits the most desired support. Hispanic, Black, and emotive Asian families must be allowed the time and the physical room in which to express their pain. For the nurse to assume that these people are weak, overindulgent, or childlike is to miss one of the most important concepts of transcultural nursing.

THE LANGUAGE BARRIER

Although language differences form the most obvious barrier to effective cross-cultural communication, they are,

Table 4-1 Death-related behaviors in six cultural groups

Culture	Religious attitudes	Grief expressions	Death rituals	Resources for support
Japanese/Chinese	Very protective of people's feelings Believe in afterlife Decedents return to Nirvana	Not publicly expressive	Chanting ceremony at bedside after death Accepting clothes of deceased may not be appropriate Japanese prepare gift food packs for mourners	Families
Indo-Chinese	After death, soul lives in land of Tian	May weep/wail aloud	Mourning attire consists of white outfit worn by women mourners and black armband worn by men	Families
Black Americans	Commonly recognized Western concept of heaven/hell Deceased do not watch over earthlings	Very expressive	Funeral rite is an informal gathering, including prayers, scripture reading, songs, crying/screaming	Minister, family, friends Strong family kinship
Mexican-Americans	Illness/death are God's will	Very expressive	Dependent on religious beliefs	Families
Native Americans	No life after death—return to ancestors Navajos are fearful of death; will burn decedent's possessions Belief in spirits and need to be in harmony with nature	May or may not be publicly expressive	May take form of beasts chanting, monotonous singing over the dead to frighten away evil spirits	Families, shaman, tribal group
Arabs	Anticipatory grief work not acceptable Children are integral part of family activities	Express grief openly Much touching of decedent's body	Remain with body until transported to funeral home Do life review at decedent's bedside	Family

Modified from York C and Stichler J: Dimens Crit Care Nurs 4(2):122, 1985.

paradoxically, among the easiest to overcome, because actual verbiage is only one relatively small element in the communication process. Researchers have indicated that nonverbal communication accounts for 70% to 90% of the communication. Gestures, facial expression, bodily stance and space, eye contact, touch, and tone of voice can go far to sooth the foreign-speaking patient's fears and to establish rapport.[10]

An awareness of the meaning of nonverbal communication can also help the critical care nurse overcome one of the most serious barriers to patient compliance and family cooperation—the tendency for newly arrived immigrants to pretend to understand an instruction when in fact they do not.[8] Although this behavior can be very frustrating to the attending nurse, understanding the reasons behind the behavior and some techniques for dealing with it can diffuse this frustration.

Immigrants will pretend to understand for a number of reasons. First, they do not wish to appear inadequate by admitting that their English comprehension is incomplete. Second, they do not wish to have the nurse repeat the material because it is likely that they will still not understand

and will therefore feel even more inadequate. Finally, they will pretend comprehension because to not do so would be insulting to the nurse, who, it might be said, failed to explain the material adequately.

Once the motivation of the foreign-born patient is understood, it becomes much easier both to be compassionate and to devise effective interventions. Before interventions can be devised, it is necessary to assess whether or not the learner does understand what you are saying. To simply ask "Do you understand?" is not a very effective means of assessment, for the immigrant will possibly say "yes" to please the nurse and avoid embarrassment for all concerned.

Nonverbal communication is one of the most valuable tools available in dealing with this problem. By observing body language closely, the nurse can readily perceive that the patient or relative does not understand. Signs such as a blank expression, constant nodding of the head and smiling, and a quizzical expression can indicate that true understanding is not taking place. Contrary to popular belief, the avoidance of eye contact (particularly if the family is Asian) does not always mean that the listener is not comprehending. Such behavior is often merely a way of showing respect

<table>
<tr><td>

CROSSING LANGUAGE BARRIERS

Face the patient or relative
Observe and use nonverbal cues
Speak simply
Avoid slang
Speak slowly
Speak in short units
Learn a few words of the language (e.g., "I'm here to help you"; "Do not be afraid"; "You will be all right.")

</td></tr>
</table>

and deference to the speaker. Another means of assessing the degree of understanding is by the number of questions asked. Paradoxically, if few questions are asked, it can often indicate a lack of understanding, not the opposite. In this case, the patient has not understood enough material to formulate a worthwhile question.

If it appears that the patient or relative has indeed not understood the information, the box above contains a number of suggestions for facilitating mutual understanding. The final item ("Learn a few words of the language") is a particularly valuable suggestion. By learning just a few words of the languages most often encountered, the nurse is able to improve rapport with the foreign speaker, make the patient feel emotionally and physically more comfortable, and, perhaps most important, communicate a respect for the patient's own culture.

It is not always necessary to use an interpreter to communicate effectively. On the occasions, however, when an interpreter is necessary, a few guidelines are indicated. If possible, do not use family members as interpreters, because relatives frequently will keep information from each other in an attempt to spare feelings or avoid conflict.[2] Further, be certain that the interpreter speaks the correct dialect. This may seem obvious, but numerous errors in this regard are being reported. It is not unknown, for example, for hospitals to have called in an Arabic interpreter when dealing with an Iranian Farsi-speaking family. Finally, if at all possible, arrange for the interpreter and patient to be of the same class, because differences in class can result in severe discomfort and reticence for both parties.[13]

SUMMARY

The key to overcoming cultural barriers to effective critical care nursing lies in the nurse's willingness to examine with an open mind the perspective of the immigrant patient and family. The ability to understand another's way of looking at the world arises, not only out of experience and repeated interaction, but also from careful study of the literature in the field. At the end of this chapter is a bibliography of the most clinically applicable material in the field of cross-cultural nursing. The selective reading of these materials will prepare the critical care nurse for the inevitable challenges and joys of bridging cultural gaps with compassion and understanding.

REFERENCES

1. Balsmeyer B: Locus of control and the use of strategies to promote self-care, J Commun Health Nurs, 1(3):171, 1984.
2. Castro F and Wagner N: The Chicano community and its aged. In Reinhardt A and Quinn M, editors: Current practice in gerontological nursing, St Louis, 1979, The CV Mosby Co.
3. Davitz L, Davitz L, and Higuchi Y: Cross-cultural inferences of physical pain and psychological distress-2, Nurs Times 73:556, 1977.
4. Hartog J and Hartog E: Cultural aspects of health and illness behaviors in the hospital, West J Med 139(6):901, 1983.
5. Lattimore V: The positive contributions of Black cultural values to pastoral counseling, J Pastoral Care 36(2):105, 1982.
6. Lipson J and Afaf I: Issues in health care of Middle-Eastern patients, West J Med 139(6):854, 1983.
7. Mayor V: The family, bereavement and dietary beliefs, Nurs Times 80:40, 1984.
8. Muecke M: In search of healers—South East Asian refugees in the American health care system, West J Med 139(6):835, 1983.
9. Murilla N: The Mexican-American family. In Martinez A, editor: Hispanic culture and health care, St Louis, 1978, The CV Mosby Co.
10. Orque M, Bloch B, and Monrroy L, editors: Ethnic nursing care: a multi-cultural approach, St Louis, 1983, The CV Mosby Co.
11. Quadagno J: The Italian-American family. In Mindel C and Habenstein R, editors: Ethnic families in America, ed 2, New York, 1981, Elsevier Science Publishing Co, Inc.
12. Ruiz M: Open-closed mindedness, intolerance of ambiguity and nursing faculty attitudes toward culturally different patients, Nurs Res 30(3):177, 1981.
13. Santopietro M: How to get through to a refugee patient, RN 44:43, 1981.
14. Speck P: Loss and grief in medicine, London, 1978, Bailliere Tindall.
15. Walker C: Attitudes to death and bereavement among cultural minority groups, Nurs Times 78(50):2106, 1982.
16. York C and Stichler J: Cultural grief expressions following infant death, Dimens Crit Care Nurs 4(2):120, 1985.

ADDITIONAL READING
General Works

Baxter C: Culture shock, Nurs Times 84:36, 1988.
Bullough V and Bullough B: Health care for the other Americans, New York, 1982, Appleton-Century-Crofts.
Chrisman N and Maretzki T, editors: Clinically applied anthropology, Boston, 1982, D Reidel Publishing Co.
Fong C: Ethnicity and nursing practice, Top Clin Nurs 7:1, 1985.
Harwood A: Ethnicity and medical care, Cambridge, Mass, 1981, Harvard University Press.
Henderson G and Primeaux M: Transcultural health care, Menlo Park, Cal, 1981, Addison-Wesley Publishing Co.
Johnson T and others: Providing culturally sensitive care: intervention by a consultation-liaison team, Hosp Community Psychiatry 39(2):200, 1988.
Leininger M: Transcultural nursing: concepts, theories, and practices, New York, 1978, John Wiley & Sons, Inc.
Madjar I: Pain and the surgical patient: a cross-cultural perspective, Aust J Adv Nurs 2:29, 1985.
Mindel C and Habenstein, R, editors: Ethnic families in America, ed 2, New York, 1982, Elsevier Science Publishing Co, Inc.
Qureshi B: Pediatric problems in multi-ethnic groups, Matern Child Health 1:15, 1987.
Sward K: Cultural diversity in health care: an introduction, J NY State Nurses Assoc 17:5, 1986.
Vavasseur J: Psychosocial aspects of chronic disease: cultural and ethnic implications. Birth Defects 23:144, 1987.

Hispanic Culture

Chesney A: Mexican-American folk medicine: implications for the family physician, J Fam Pract 11(4):567, 1980.

Gomez G and Gomez E: Folk healing among Hispanic Americans, Public Health Nurse 2:245, 1985.

Herrera J: The effectiveness of a cultrual milieu on hospitalized Hispanic patients, Int J Psychosom 34:6, 1987.

Martinez R, editor: Hispanic culture and health care, St Louis, 1978, The CV Mosby Co.

Reinert B: The health care beliefs and values of Mexican-Americans, Home Health Care Update 4:23, 1986.

Ross C, Mirowsky J, and Cockerham W: Social class, Mexican culture, and fatalism: their effects on psychological distress, Am J Community Psychol 11(4):383, 1983.

Rubel A, O'Neill C, and Collado-Ardon R: Susto, a folk illness, Berkeley, Cal, 1984, University of California Press.

Trotter R and Chavira J: Curanderismo: Mexican-American folk healing, Athens, Ga, 1981, University of Georgia Press.

Asian Culture

Anderson J: Health and illness in Filipino immigrants, West J Med 139(6):811, 1983.

Eyton J and Neuwirth G: Cross-cultural validity: ethnocentrism in health studies with special reference to the Vietnamese, Soc Sci Med 18:447, 1984.

Louie K: Providing health care to Chinese clients, Top Clin Nurs 7:18, 1985.

Ludman E and Newman J: Yin and yang in the health-related food practices of three Chinese groups, J Nutr Educ 16:3, 1984.

Muecke M: Caring for Southeast Asian refugee patients in the USA, Am J Pub Health 73(4):431, 1983.

Muecke M: In search of healers—Southeast Asian refugees in the American health care system, West J Med 139(6):835, 1983.

Nguyen M: Culture shock—a review of Vietnamese culture and its concepts of health and disease, West J Med 139(6):835, 1983.

Rosenberg J: Health care for Cambodian children: integrating treatment plans, Pediatr Nurs 12(2):118, 1986.

Sue D and Sue S: Cultural factors in the clinical assessment of Asian Americans, J Consult Clin Psychol 55(4):479, 1987.

Tung T: Indochinese patients: cultural aspects of the medical and psychiatric care of Indochinese refugees, Washington, DC, 1980, Action for South East Asians, Inc.

Yeatman G and Dang V: Cao gio (coin rubbing): Vietnamese attitudes toward health care, JAMA 244(24):2748, 1980.

Black Culture

Bailey E: Sociocultural factors and health care–seeking behavior among Black Americans, J Natl Med Assoc 79:389, 1987.

Capers F: Nursing and the Afro-American diet, Top Clin Nurs 7:11, 1985.

Dressler W: The social and cultural context of coping: action, gender and symptoms in a southern Black community, Soc Sci Med 21:499, 1985.

Mahon R: Psychological factors in providing health care to Blacks. In Jospe M, Nieberding J, and Cohen G, editors: Psychological factors in health care, Toronto, 1980, Lexington Books.

Mays V: Identity developing of Black Americans: the role of history and the importance of ethnicity, Am J Psychother 40(4):582, 1986.

Snow L: Traditional health beliefs and practices among lower class Black Americans, West J Med 136(6):820, 1983.

Williams R: The testbook of Black-related diseases, New York, 1975, McGraw Hill Book Co.

The Pain Response

Flannery R, Sos J, and McGovern P: Ethnicity as a factor in the expression of pain, Psychosomatics 22:39, 1981.

Zola I: Culture and symptoms— an analysis of patients' presenting complaints, Am Sociol Rev 31(5):615, 1966.

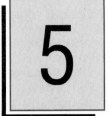

Health Promotion and Patient Education

CHAPTER OBJECTIVES

- *Describe the role of the critical care nurse in health pro- motion activities.*
- *List three factors that influence an individual's health- maintenance practices.*
- *Adapt and apply teaching-learning theory to the critical care setting.*
- *Describe the stages of adaptation to illness and the im- plications of each for the patient teaching plan.*
- *Perform a learning needs assessment.*
- *Construct a teaching plan for a patient in the critical care unit.*
- *Discuss four methods of instruction and the appropriate- ness of each to the critical care setting.*

Persons entering the health care system bring with them unique medical, social, and educational histories that affect their interactions with health care providers. These past experiences also form the basis of the philosophies and perceptions of health, illness, and wellness and, therefore, of behaviors related to health maintenance and management. When a patient is admitted to the hospital with an acute or critical problem, it is often the result of a failure to manage and maintain his or her own health. In adition, the illness often creates new requirements in the areas of health man- agement and self-care that must be practiced by the patient during recovery and sometimes for a lifetime. The nurse in the critical and acute care units has many opportunities to incorporate health promotion activities into daily practice. This chapter is intended to assist the nurse in identifying health perception and health management issues that affect the plan of care and the patient's response in the critical care unit. It presents theory related to health promotion and criteria through which a patient's health maintenance skills can be assessed. Compliance and noncompliance with the

health care plan are discussed. Finally, the role of patient education in the critical care unit is covered.

HEALTH MAINTENANCE AS A NURSING RESPONSIBILITY

Nursing has played a major role in health promotion since the mid-nineteenth centruy.[35] In 1980 the American Nurses' Association published its *Social Policy Statement* for nurs- ing, which outlined the social context of nursing and the nature and scope of nursing practice. This document high- lights the importance of health promotion and maintenance as a responsibility of the nursing profession. Health pro- motion refers to activities directed toward developing the client resources that maintain or enhance well-being. In the past several years there has been a shift of focus from a disease-oriented system of care to one that values wellness and optimal health, including the prevention or control of disease, with a focus on gaining, attaining, and maintaining health. At the same time both health professionals and the public have recognized an increasing responsibility on the part of the individual and family for health maintenance. Nevertheless, the Surgeon General in 1980 stated that half the mortality in the United States is caused by unhealthy lifestyles.[43] Nurses continue to make major contributions to the evolution of the health-oriented system of care and are uniquely qualified to assist patients in planning for short- term and long-term health management and maintenance needs, while at the same time treating the condition for which the patient was admitted.[1]

HEALTH PROMOTION IN THE CRITICAL CARE SETTING

Nurses in the critical care areas usually focus on the life- threatening physiological problems of their patients. Con- straints of time and the necessity to prioritize care have limited health promotion activities of the critical care nurse.

However, in the current climate of health care, with hospitalized patients more acutely ill and generally in the hospital for a shorter time, the role of health promotion in the hospitals and in the critical care areas must be examined. Priorities set by the critical care nurse must place maintenance of immediate physical and psychological safety above long-term health promotion needs. However, the relationship that often develops between patient and nurse in the critical care unit provides an excellent environment for discussion of health promotion needs when the patient's situation allows.

Hospitalization may be the patient's first encounter with health care professionals and health promotion information. The nurses with whom the patient interacts have the potential to influence perceptions about future health care practices.[18] Critical care nurses must recognize that their attitudes directly affect patients' decisions about future health behaviors. If health teaching, role modeling, effective communication, and skilled nursing care are combined in the experience of the critically ill patient, the patient may begin to identify his or her continuing role in health maintenance as recovery continues and discharge nears. Families, too, can benefit from health promotion activities during the hospitalization, and valuable information concerning the family environment to which the patient will return can be gained during health promotion assessment and teaching.[27] Creative nursing strategies that combine the holistic, long-term goals of health promotion with the critical short-term goals and behaviors in the critical care setting can add an important and satisfying aspect to the care of the acutely ill.

Factors Influencing Health Practices

Assessment of factors influencing an individual's health practices provides information regarding the patient's overall health status and the effectiveness of the methods used to maintain health. This information provides insight into the patient's perceived health status, the importance he or she places on health, and the level of his or her commitment to health maintenance. Careful assessment in this area also identifies actual or potential health problems or risks that are unrelated to the reason for admission but may adversely affect recovery or future self-care. For this reason, the nursing assessment in the critical care unit should include information related to these primarily nonacute health patterns. The patient's health perceptions provide some guidance in the planning of care in the critical care unit and in later stages of recovery. The care plan and teaching plan in the critical care unit should take into consideration individual differences in these beliefs.

The box at right gives general information about health perception and management that should be obtained during the nursing history gathered for the assessment.[23] This assessment should be carried out as soon after admission as the patient's condition allows.

Health Belief Model. All human behavior is motivated by one or more factors. The Health Belief Model is one framework to explain predictable sources of motivation for specific health behaviors.

The Health Belief Model was developed in its original form in the 1950s. It was designed to predict those

---

> ### NURSING HISTORY OF HEALTH PERCEPTION AND MANAGEMENT
>
> How has the patient's general health been?
>
> Has the patient had any other illnesses in the past year, including colds and minor illnesses?
>
> What are the most important things the patient does to keep healthy? Do these things make a difference? Include folk remedies if appropriate.
>
> Does the patient use cigarettes, alcohol, or drugs? Are appropriate self-screening examinations performed (e.g., regular breast self-examinations for women)?
>
> In the past, has the patient found it easy to follow the advice of health professionals?
>
> Are there financial, social, cultural, or geographical barriers to access to proper health care?
>
> What caused this illness? What actions were taken when the symptoms were noticed? What were the results of those actions?
>
> What things are most important to the patient while in the hospital? How can the staff be most helpful?

---

individuals who would or would not use the growing resources in disease prevention. In the 1970s, Becker revised the model to the form that is used today. It identifies the individual perceptions, modifying factors, and variables that affect the likelihood of taking preventive action.

Individual perceptions. Individual perceptions refers to the degree to which individuals perceive that they are susceptible to a particular disease and how serious it is believed to be. Research has shown that the more individuals perceive they are susceptible, the greater the likelihood of their engaging in preventive behaviors.[36] This concept also extends to continued or renewed susceptibility to an illness experienced in the past. While less strongly supported as a motivator of preventive behavior, the degree to which the disease is perceived as serious can affect the health care seeking actions.[36]

Studies have shown that the greater the perceived threat of an illness, the more likely are preventive behaviors.[36] However, a very high level of perceived severity can produce overwhelming threats and subsequent avoidance of preventive behavior because of the immobilizing effects of severe anxiety.[2]

Modifying factors. Modifying factors are those demographic, sociopsychological, and structural variables that may affect an individual's likelihood of practicing behaviors. These factors may include gender, socioeconomic status, race, ethnicity, or level of education. Pressure to conform to social norms appears to play a role in promoting use of preventive measures, as does the expectation of significant others. Structural variables such as knowledge about the disease and prior contact with it are motivating factors.

Also considered modifying factors are various cues to

action that may trigger preventive action. These may be internal clues such as uncomfortable symptoms or unpleasant memories of a family member's illness. External cues include reminder cards from health professionals or exposure to media campaigns, news articles, or advice from others.

Likelihood of action. The likelihood of practicing the recommended preventive health action also depends on the perceived benefits and barriers. The belief that the action taken will be effective in preventing illness is an important determining factor of the preventive behavior. In addition, barriers such as cost, inconvenience, fear of pain, or significant changes in lifestyle are negative motivators for health promotion.

NONCOMPLIANCE

Compliance is defined as "the extent to which a person's behavior coincides with medical or health advice."[22] This concept and that of noncompliance are generally discussed in reference to the chronically ill patient whose care and treatment regimen continues past hospitalization and requires commitment and energy by the patient and family. The use of the nursing diagnosis of Noncompliance, however, refers to the individual who wants to comply, but the presence of certain factors prevents him or her from doing so.[10] Using this definition, noncompliance issues concerning the hospitalized patient and the short-term problems of compliance with the medical and nursing treatments in the critical care unit can be considered. Thus the nurse can concentrate on identifying, reducing, or eliminating the factors that affect the patient's ability to comply with treatment.

Factors Influencing Compliance

Alteration in cognition. Patients may be noncompliant because they do not know the reason for or the importance of the recommended behaviors. This group of patients includes those who, for whatever reason, do not want information that would lead to compliance. In addition, patients may have false or inaccurate information on which they are basing their behaviors. Some hold to folk beliefs that interfere with their motivation to follow the prescribed medical treatments. Any disturbance in thought processes such as memory loss, inability to concentrate, and inability to solve problems or to follow directions can affect compliance. This very often occurs in the critical care areas because of side effects of pain medications, sleep deprivation, sensory overload, anxiety, or neurological deficits. Nurses must also consider the patient's ability to read, write, and understand the language and any real or potential visual or hearing deficits.

Alteration in perception. Beliefs, feelings, and values may affect compliance. The Health Belief Model, one theory explaining motivation for compliance, has been discussed on p. 56 of this chapter. Psychological and emotional responses to illness are often seen in the critical care areas and can adversely affect the patient's ability to comply. For example, the defense mechanism of denial, although serving a useful purpose in protecting the patient from unmanageable levels of anxiety, allows him or her to discount the

illness, its severity, or the need for cooperation with health care personnel or for making lifestyle changes. Depression, anger, or fear can also establish barriers to compliant behavior, as can a conflict in values. In this case, the patient agrees with the desirability of a behavior, but the necessary time, money, or energy resources are not available, or the goals are low priority. Finally, some patients agree with the need to comply but feel unable to make the required changes. This is often seen as a return to habitual behaviors despite the attempt to change. In the case of the dependent individual, including children and many of the disabled and elderly, the health beliefs and attitudes of the responsible party determine the extent to which the treatment regimen is followed.[4]

Inadequacies in the social system. Factors related to the patient's environment, including significant others, job, community, religious beliefs, and material resources, may affect the ability to comply with treatment. The support of significant others may be the important determinant in the patient's compliance, especially in long-term compliance.[22] Inadequate financial resources may be a barrier to compliance (for example, an individual on a fixed income who has been prescribed a very expensive medication). Adequate financial resources, however, do not ensure compliance. Geographical and transportation difficulties may also affect the ability to comply in some cases.

Deficits in the health care system. Health care system deficits that may affect compliance include a treatment regimen that is perceived by the patient as too complex or unmanageable, the failure of the system to provide specific and complete instructions, and a patient–health provider relationship that is not supportive and mutually respectful. It is therefore necessary to examine the system and the caregivers as possible factors in patient compliance.

Discontinuation of Treatment

A discussion of noncompliance in the critical care setting must include cases in which patients choose to discontinue treatment. This is occasionally seen in the critical care unit when a chronically ill patient with cancer, renal failure, or some other chronic or terminal illness is admitted with an exacerbation of the disease or for some unrelated condition. Although a thoughtful decision to terminate treatment by a person with advanced disease is not universally viewed as noncompliance,[32] it does represent a rejection of medical advice and can be frustrating to the nurse whose goals are the restoration of optimal health and functional status. Patients, families, and health professionals face difficult decisions when the patient in the critical care unit has an advanced, incurable disease.

PATIENT EDUCATION

The education of the patient and family is now universally accepted as an important nursing function in all settings of practice. Nowhere is this more important than in the critical care unit, which is often foreign and very threatening to the patient, who depends on the nurses to provide the information necessary to survive in this environment. In addition, nursing has a legal and ethical responsibility to meet stan-

RESEARCH ABSTRACT
Patient perception of cardiovascular surgical patient education

Grady KL, Cisar NS, and Ryan SD: Heart Lung 17(4):349, 1988.

PURPOSE

The purpose of this study was to determine from patients undergoing coronary artery bypass (CAB) their perceptions of the importance and the adequacy of preparation about preoperative and postoperative information.

FRAMEWORK

Knowles's teaching-learning theory formed the basis for the study. The theory asserts that adults need to be independent, self-directed, and interested in learning from an experience. They learn best when education is based on practical life problems, and they want to apply their new knowledge and skills immediately.

METHODS

English-speaking patients who had not had a prior CAB or whose spouse had not had CAB were selected on a nonrandom volunteer basis from individuals undergoing nonemergent CAB surgery. Instruments were formulated to collect data about the patient's knowledge preoperative and postdischarge of what to expect before the surgery and after discharge from the hospital. The questionnaires consisted of closed-ended questions and a four-point Likert-type scale to evaluate patient perceptions of the importance of information and the level of preparedness. The predischarge questionnaire consisted of questions that focused on an explanation of preoperative preparation, the surgical procedure, equipment, treatments and procedures, the critical care unit environment, and an overview of the postoperative period. The postdischarge questionnaire contained questions about general categories of self-care instructions, exercise programs, activity limitations, and knowledge of cardiac risk factors. Validity and reliability were established on both instruments. The patient completed the predischarge questionnaire between the fifth and tenth postoperative day in the hospital. A demographic form was also completed. One to 4 weeks after discharge, the patient completed the postoperative questionnaire during a return visit to the clinic.

RESULTS

One-hundred patients, ranging from 30 to 70 years of age, completed the predischarge questionnaire, and 54 of them completed the postdischarge questionnaire. Data analyses were performed using item frequencies, rank orders, t-tests, analysis of variance, and Pearson product correlations. The data from the preoperative and postoperative questionnaire were ranked by using means for importance and for preparedness for information received. On the predischarge questionnaire, three items were above the median for both importance and preparedness: (1) explanation of the type of surgery, (2) intensive care environment, and (3) coughing and deep breathing exercises. On the postdischarge questionnaire, only exercise at home was ranked in the top third of all items for both importance and preparedness. Patients also indicated that side effects of medication, whom to contact with medication questions, and diet planning were all important but that they were not adequately prepared about these areas. Limitations regarding sexual activity and potential emotional changes were ranked in the lower third for both importance and preparedness.

IMPLICATIONS

Nurses need to identify what information patients perceive as important so that educational programs can be appropriately formulated. Patient education should be structured, as well as individualized, in a setting in which length of hospital stay is shortened. Hospital teaching methods must be examined so that patient learning is individualized and is available at a time when the patient is ready to learn. Side effects of medication, diet planning, and whom to call with medication questions were important areas about which patients in this study desired more information and that they considered important. Future research areas include longitudinal studies to assess patients' learning needs as they rehabilitate and studies that examine differentiation of learning needs with variables such as age, gender, and previous CAB surgeries.

dards of care related to patient education. These standards include identifying the patient's and family's learning needs, assessing their readiness to learn, teaching the appropriate content, documenting the teaching plan as part of the nursing care plan, and evaluating and documenting the results of the patient teaching.[39] In 1982 the American Association of Critical Care Nurses highlighted the importance of patient education in critical care by stating in their "Standards of Care": "The critical care nurse shall identify areas of education of the patient and significant others."[44] Subsequently authors have explored the questions of whether critically ill patients can be taught[25] and how best to approach patient and family education in the critical care areas.[8,26,27,37,41]

The basis for all educational activities for patients and

families is the belief that they have the right to information regarding diagnosis, treatment, and prognosis in terms that are understandable to them.[38] Part of this belief is that rational individuals can, on some level, understand all but the most technical aspects of their care.[41] It also involves the knowledge that each patient is unique, learns in a unique way, and has motivation and skill in applying new knowledge that differs from that of other patients. These individual differences are the reasons for varied responses to the same teaching strategies.

Traditional views of teaching and learning involve the idea of providing information (teaching) that causes a lasting change in behavior (learning).[9] Effectiveness of the educational interaction is measured by the specific objectives that are met. If the nurse in the critical care setting limits measurement of teaching effectiveness to long-term behavior changes, many critical educational activities necessary for the well-being of the patient will be judged failures. It may be more appropriate to expand the view of successful educational outcomes to not only long-term behavior change but also to less concrete but equally valuable outcomes such as decreased anxiety or greater participation in self-care. This approach recognizes that there are real and valuable aspects of learning that cannot be easily measured by objective criteria. It does not negate the fact that in many situations written measurable objectives are necessary and useful, but it does mean that they should not be the sole measures of educational success.[6] A good example of this is the interaction that occurs when a patient is taught about the cardiac monitor on admission to the critical care unit. In teaching the reason for and function of this equipment, the nurse not only increases the patient's knowledge about cardiac monitoring but may also decrease his or her anxiety about the critical care setting, thereby promoting rest and healing.

Along with a belief in the patient's right to know, the patient's right not to know must also be recognized in some cases. It must be respected in those cases in which patients prefer not to learn about their illnesses. Simple basic information about monitors and unit policy, for example, usually suffices in these cases. Indeed, more information than can be processed and integrated can greatly increase anxiety and may result in slower recovery.[9,41] Individuals have the right to accept, adopt, or reject the information provided in educational encounters, however frustrating this may be to the nurse.[9]

Teaching-Learning Process

The teaching-learning process used in the health care setting can be defined as a set of activities organized and structured to maximize the results for the patient and to minimize the amount of time and effort on the part of the health care practitioner.[5] It can be divided into the five steps summarized in the box at right. These steps can be closely related to the nursing process. Table 5-1 shows the application of the nursing process to the teaching-learning process in the care of the critically ill patient.

Stressors

Physiological stressors. Many physiological stressors for the critically ill patient are obvious. First and foremost is the illness for which the patient was admitted. This is often

---

THE TEACHING-LEARNING PROCESS

1. Assessment of the need to learn
2. Assessment of readiness to learn
3. Setting of objectives
4. Teaching-learning activities
5. Evaluation and reteaching if necessary

Table 5-1   Application of the nursing process to the teaching-learning process

Nursing process	Teaching-learning process
Assessment	Physiological
	Psychological
	Environmental
	Sociocultural
	Assessment of physiological and psychological stress response
	Physiological
	Heart rate
	Blood pressure
	Peristalsis
	Mental acuity
	Blood glucose
	Dilated pupils
	Psychological
	Anxiety
	Depression
	Panic
	Withdrawal
	Denial
	Hostility
	Regression
	Frustration
	Assessment of readiness to learn
Nursing diagnosis and plan	Identification of specific knowledge deficit
	Identification of causes and associated factors
	Identification of expected outcomes and behavioral objectives
	Development of teaching plan
Nursing intervention	Teaching-learning activities and experience
Evaluation	Evaluation and documentation of effectiveness of teaching-learning process
	Measurement of knowledge gain
	Measurement of behavior changes

a life-threatening situation, and the patient will respond to the stress with all of his or her energy in an attempt to cope with the crisis. In addition, there are usually other physiological changes in critically ill patients that act as further stressors; they may include pain, hypoxia, cardiac dysrhythmias, hypotension, fluid and electrolyte imbalances, infection, fever, or neurological deficits. The presence of these stressors may completely consume the patient's available energy and leave none for any type of orientation to stimuli.

Psychological stressors. Serious illness affects a patient not only physically, but also psychologically. Intense emotions can alter a person's normal way of coping and ability to learn and retain information. Psychological stressors often present in the critically ill include helplessness, powerlessness, loneliness, changes in role in the family and at work, changes in body image, fear of future lifestyle changes, and fear of death. These and other psychological stressors can result not only in physiological changes but can trigger behavior consistent with anxiety, denial, and depression. These behaviors are examined in "Psychological Assessment."

Environmental stressors. The physical surroundings in a critical care unit contribute to the stress of the experience for a patient. Factors such as sleep deprivation, observation of other patients, loss of privacy, bright lights, unfamiliar noises, unpleasant odors, and loss of contact with loved ones are some of the factors that contribute to stress. Management and control of these factors have become important nursing functions.

Sociocultural stressors. Variables such as age, sex, ethnic origin, economic status, religious beliefs, level of education, and occupation may add to the stress of illness and alter learning ability. The nurse-patient interaction should be structured to recognize the effects of these variables on the process and outcome of the teaching-learning experience.

Assessment. The assessment step in patient teaching involves gathering a data base to assist the nurse in meeting the patient's and family's learning needs.[5] It is a vital part of any successful teaching plan. Among the components of this assessment in the critical care unit are identification of the various stressors present, assessment of biopsychosocial issues and adaptation to illness, and an examination of motivation and readiness to learn. In reality, these issues are often related to one another and cannot be assessed as separate entities. For ease of illustration, however, they are discussed separately.

Biopsychosocial assessment. Following identification of actual and potential stressors, an assessment of their effect on the patient's biopsychosocial integrity should be undertaken.

PHYSICAL ASSESSMENT. A physical assessment will yield information about physiological reactions to stress. The following factors should be considered: Is the patient in pain or some other type of distress? What is his or her level of consciousness and orientation? Has he or she been sedated? Is the patient hypoxic or hypercapnic? Are the heart rate, blood pressure, cardiac output, and perfusion adequate? Can the patient see and hear? These questions add to the data base for formulation of an effective teaching plan.

PSYCHOLOGICAL ASSESSMENT. The psychological assessment is also important in determining the patient's ability to respond to the teaching-learning experience. A very important factor is the patient's stage in adaptation to illness during the time teaching is undertaken. The general characteristics of the *stages of adaptation to illness* are outlined in Table 5-2 with corresponding applications for the teaching-learning process. Salient points are reviewed here. It should be noted that each individual moves at his or her own pace through the stages, and it is not uncommon to skip or move back and forth through the stages.

Disbelief and denial. The first response to acute illness

Table 5-2 Teaching-learning process in adaptation to illness

Stage of adaptation	Characteristic patient response	Implications for teaching-learning process
Disbelief	Denial	Orient teaching to present. Teach during other nursing activities. Reassure patient about safety. Explain all procedures and activities clearly and concisely.
Developing awareness	Anger	Continue to orient teaching to present. Avoid long lists of facts. Continue to foster development of trust and rapport through good physical care.
Reorganization	Acceptance of sick role	Orient teaching to meet patient needs. Teach whatever patient wants to learn. Provide necessary self-care information. Reinforce with written material.
Resolution	Identification with others with same problem; recognition of loss	Use group instruction. Use patient support groups and visits by recovered patients with same problem.
Identify change	Definition of self as one who has undergone change and is now different	Answer patient's questions as they arise. Recognize that as basic needs are met more mature needs will arise.

is generally disbelief and denial. The shock and threat of the condition or illness are so great that the patient denies the condition's existence and severity in an attempt to ease the emotional impact or to conserve energy by avoiding the work of worrying. During this phase patients may say, "I can't believe this is really happening," or "I'm not that sick—I'll be fine in a day or two." Although this response has some psychological benefit for the patient, it acts as a barrier to learning. Patients who do not believe they are ill or do not believe their condition will affect their lives will have little motivation to learn. During this stage it is acceptable for the nurse to allow denial if it does not put the patient in danger. Teaching should be focused on the present, and comments referring to the future should be avoided.

Developing awareness. After a few days, the denial mechanism usually breaks down, and the patient moves into the stage of developing awareness. This can occur while the patient is still in the critical care unit. Often, in fact, this setting accelerates the process because the stark reality of seeing other sick people, being treated like them, and often being in pain or having multiple medical treatments strips the patient of the power to continue to deny. The patient must accept that he or she is ill. This stage generally coincides with the assumption of the sick role.

At this time, a patient may respond with anger or guilt. If these emotions are turned inward, he or she may experience depression. If emotions are expressed outwardly, behavior may be hostile toward persons and things in the environment, including the nurse. Depending on the particular response, patients may ask, "Why didn't I do things differently—then I wouldn't be sick now," or "They don't know what they're doing around here." It is important at this time to listen to the expressions of anger but not to argue with the patient. Remember that the patient is reacting to factors other than the nurse. Teaching during this time should continue to be oriented to the present but may relate more to the disease process, which is now recognized by the patient. He or she is still too anxious to learn and assimilate lists of facts but may be interested in the meaning of symptoms and treatments as they relate to his or her experience at the moment.

Reorganization. The third stage of adaptation to illness is reorganization. At this time the patient has begun to work through the anger and guilt and to reorganize his or her self-concept and relationships with others consistent with the acceptance of the sick role. During this time the nurse should teach whatever the patient wants to learn, thus helping the patient to achieve the reorganization necessary to move on to adaptation. Some patients, especially those in the critical care unit for several weeks, may experience this stage during the stay in the unit.

Resolution and identity change. The final stages of adaptation are resolution and identity change. They occur late in recovery, even as late as the sixth week in the case of a patient with a myocardial infarction.[34] During these times the patient is more receptive to teaching based on objectives and to learning about long-term needs. Group instruction that includes the spouse and significant others can be an effective method at this time. These stages will rarely be reached during the critical care stay but may be identified by nurses working in step-down or telemetry units.

The nurse should consider that the family go through the stages of adaptation to their loved one's illness as well. Family members may or may not progress at the same rates as the patient, so teaching strategies may need modification to ensure meeting the individual needs of both the patient and the significant others.

Assessment of motivation and readiness to learn. Evaluation of motivation and readiness to learn are important parts of the teaching-learning assessment. They are more difficult to measure and assess than the other variables discussed. One well-known and important theory describing human behavior motivation is Maslow's hierarchy of needs, which provides background for the discussion of motivation to learn.

Maslow described a number of needs that were postulated as motivating all behavior. According to this theory, human beings have a number of needs that are interrelated and hierarchical. In other words, the lower-level needs must be met before higher-level needs can emerge and be satisfied. The following needs were identified as basic to human motivation: physiological needs, safety and security, love and belongingness, self-esteem, and self-actualization.[31] The physiological needs are the most basic and powerful, and if they are not at least minimally met, higher-level needs will not become apparent. As soon as the physiological needs are satisfied, the group of needs for safety emerges, including both physical and psychological security. Following satisfaction of safety needs, the need for love and belongingness emerge, followed in turn by the need for self-esteem and self-actualization.

The need to know and understand are among the highest-level needs.[31] During a time of critical illness, a patient's energy is often consumed by the lower-level physiological and safety needs, and it would be impossible for the patient to attend to learning interactions. Attempting to teach a patient who fears for his or her life and safety is of little use unless the patient is being taught that he or she is safe and in no immediate danger of dying. Once the lower-level needs are met and the patient feels out of danger, he or she will have more resources to devote to learning and meeting higher-level needs.

The basic physiological needs to be assessed include the need for oxygen, liquid, food, shelter, and sleep. Table 5-3 identifies assessment areas for the lower-level physiological and safety needs and some indicators of unmet needs in these areas. If the assessment discloses significant needs in these areas, the nurse should address those needs before attempting any teaching. Once met, these needs cease to be the primary motivators of behavior, and the patient can attend to his or her learning and other higher-level needs.

Factors that motivate behavior change related to preventive health practices also influence a patient's motivation to learn about health and health practices in the hospital setting. The assessment of readiness and motivation to learn, then, should include information about individual perceptions, modifying factors, and perceived benefits and barriers.

Assessment of external barriers. Patient barriers to learning related to physiological, emotional, and motivational factors have been identified. To structure a successful teaching-learning experience in a critical care area, the nurse must also carefully assess the environmental and iatrogenic

Table 5-3 Assessment of satisfaction of basic needs

Need	Indicators of unmet needs
Physiological	Tachycardia
Oxygen	Dyspnea
	Pallor/cyanosis
	Confusion or apprehension
Fluids	Poor skin turgor
	Dryness of mouth, skin, lips
	Constipation
	Concentrated urine with increased specific gravity
	Confusion, irritability, sluggishness (if electrolyte imbalance exists)
Food	Unplanned weight loss
	Signs of malnutrition (pallid skin, dull hair, lack of energy)
	Poor appetite or food intake
Shelter and temperature maintenance	Body temperature
	Discomfort caused by feeling too warm or cold
Sleep	Low energy
	Sleepiness
	Slow reactions
	Decreased mental acuity
	Insomnia or inability to sleep caused by therapeutic interventions
Safety	Frequent and repetitious questions
Psychological	Frequent or seemingly unreasonable requests
	Unusually passive compliance or refusal to comply without extensive explanations
	Demands for a ritualized schedule or rigid routine
	Physiological signs of fear or anxiety
Physical	Questions such as "will it hurt?"
	May be no indicators until injury, such as joint contractures, bedsores, fever from nosocomial infections, is present

barriers that affect the interaction. Bright lights, unpleasant odors, unfamiliar noises, and untidy surroundings can distract patients and add to cognitive impairment. Control of these factors can facilitate the learning process. Factors that cannot be controlled should be explained to the patient to alleviate anxiety and facilitate a trusting relationship between patient and nurse.

Finally, the nurse should examine possible barriers to learning that he or she brings to the interaction. Nurses have been found to set up barriers both consciously and unconsciously to the patient's learning and understanding.[34] The use of medical terms that are not understood by the patient and the use of language inappropriate to the patient's educational level are examples of ways in which nurses may adversely affect the teaching-learning process.[15] There may also be a failure to set aside time just for teaching, resulting in hurried and fragmented sessions. Nonverbal cues on the part of the nurse, such as glancing at the clock or breaking eye contact, may interrupt patient interactions. The manner in which the teaching sessions are planned and executed can have as important an effect on patient learning as the material presented.

The Teaching-Learning Experience

Once the process of the initial educational assessment is completed, the nurse will have an adequate data base from which to determine a teaching plan and decide on appropriate teaching methods. Patient teaching and nursing care are, in many ways, inseparable. Patients are educated in many informal interactions with the nurse, and knowledge gained greatly fosters patient understanding and well-being. Educational opportunities can be present during various nursing care activities such as bathing and administration of medication. Each encounter with the patient and family should be viewed as a teaching opportunity. There are times, however, during the acute care experience when more formal or structured educational experiences are in order. For this reason, a discussion of objectives, methods, evaluation of the teaching-learning experience, and some suggested content for education in the critical care setting follow.

Objectives. Objectives state the desired behaviors expected from the learning process.[38] They are based on the patient's learning needs and serve as a guide for the teaching-learning process. Objectives are written in behavioral terms that are measurable and are stated in terms of what the patient is to learn, rather than what the nurse is to teach. Terms such as to know, understand, be familiar with, realize, and appreciate are open to many interpretations and are difficult to measure. Rather, active verbs such as to *identify, state, list, describe,* or *demonstrate* should be used, because they are readily understood by all and easily lend themselves to evaluation.

Both long-term and short-term objectives are appropriate, in many cases it takes days, weeks, or even months of repetition and practice for a new skill to be mastered. A nurse in the critical care setting should not hesitate to identify goals that are long-term. Often it is appropriate to begin the teaching early and continue to evaluate it later in the hospitalization. Generalized objectives have been developed for teaching programs used for large numbers of patients, such as cardiac teaching plans for patients recovering from myocardial infarctions. Standardized plans can be useful resource materials in developing a teaching plan but must not take the place of individualized, specific objectives designed for each patient.

Teaching methods. The three basic methods of teaching are lecture, discussion, and demonstration.[9] The choice of method depends on the material to be taught.

Lecture. Lecture is the presentation of information in a highly structured format to a group. In this method the teacher provides a great deal of material but may not provide ample opportunities for teacher-learner interaction. Although this method can be used for patient teaching in outpatient settings, it is not a good choice for hospitalized patients and is inappropriate for acutely ill individuals.

Discussion. Discussion is less structured than lecturing and allows an exchange and feedback between the teacher and learner. The teacher can adapt the material to meet the needs of the individual or group. The discussion approach is probably most useful when learning should result in behavior change or in development of an attitude.[9] Discussion groups can be effective with hospitalized patients when a group with similar problems and at similar stages of adaptation can be gathered. Individual discussion with patients and families is appropriate and valuable during the acute phase of illness because it allows them to express their feelings and interpretations. This approach is the ideal way to teach about sensitive issues such as resuming sexual activity after myocardial infarction.[9]

Demonstration. Demonstration involves acting out a procedure while giving appropriate explanations to provide the learner with a clear idea of how to perform a task. The patient can then practice the skill and be given feedback about his performance. This method is often used in the acute care setting such as when coughing and deep breathing or taking one's own pulse is taught.

Other methods of instruction. In addition to the three basic methods just presented, several other approaches to delivering or augmenting information in a patient teaching program are available. They include commercially prepared or custom-designed printed materials, bedside videotape programs, and computer-assisted patient education programs. Computer programs, relatively new to health education, have been used in community-based education programs, in hospital waiting rooms or designated teaching rooms, and, in some cases, at the bedside with microcomputers on transportable carts.[3] These programs allow the learner to set the program pace and are generally presented in an attractive, colorful format.[12]

Written materials can be very useful tools in patient and family education. They allow repetition and reinforcement of content and provide basic information in printed form for reference at a later time. To be useful, however, the content must be accurate and current, and the patient and family must be able to read and understand it.

It is estimated that the median literacy level of the United States' population is at the tenth grade level, with about 20% of the population having reading skills at the fifth grade level or lower.[38] Other research indicates that approximately 50% of health care clients have serious difficulty reading instructional materials written at the fifth grade level.[13] The vast majority of patient education materials are written at or above the eighth grade level.[42] To ensure that the reading level of the educational material and the learner are well matched, the patients should be questioned about the last grade level completed in school. Because this level may not equal the grade level in reading ability, written material two to four grade levels below that should be selected.[7] The box below shows examples of an instruction written at various reading levels.

In recent years the use of educational videotapes at the bedside or in group settings has gained increasing popularity. A recent review of the literature on the use of videotapes verifies that the medium can be used to address the basic and repetitive aspects of patient education and that it is effective for short-term knowledge gain.[33] The use of videotapes, however, should not be considered a substitute for individualized patient teaching, and it is most effective when it is promoted by staff as reinforcing other educational activities.[14,33] Staff should preview the tapes before showing them to patients to ensure the accuracy and appropriateness of the content and to assess the best way to introduce and reinforce the material.

Teaching the critically ill patient may require modification of traditional teaching methods and strategies. In critical care units, patient goals are generally short-term and ob-

---

SAMPLES OF DIFFERENT READING LEVELS

COLLEGE READING LEVEL

With the onset of nausea, diarrhea, or other gastrointestinal disturbances, consult your physician immediately.

TWELFTH GRADE READING LEVEL

If you experience nausea, diarrhea, or other stomach or bowel problems, call your physician immediately.

EIGHTH GRADE READING LEVEL

If you start having nausea, loose bowel movements, or other stomach or bowel problems, call your doctor immediately.

FOURTH GRADE READING LEVEL

If you start having an upset stomach, loose bowel movements, or other problems, call your doctor right away.

From Boyd MD: Nurs Management 18(7):57, 1987.

jectives are concrete. Teaching should be kept brief and concise and should be in terms the patient can understand. The many stressors of illness and critical care and the effects of sedation and other drugs may cause the patient to require frequent repetitions and reinforcement of information. This is to be expected with the critically ill person and is not considered failure of the teaching experience. Each educational interaction between patient and nurse is of value, despite the fact it often will not result in long-term behavior change. Nurses should remember that family members are also stressed and may forget pertinent information that has been provided about visiting hours, unit policies, and how to contact a staff member for information about the patient. It is helpful to provide them with written information to supplement and reinforce verbal instructions.[8,19]

Evaluation. Traditionally, the teaching-learning process has been evaluated by measurable behavior changes, in other words, how well the predetermined objectives were met. This evaluation is appropriate for some teaching in critical care, but often the traditional criteria do not apply. If the teaching meets a momentary need, the effect may not be measurable or quantifiable but is no less valuable and successful. Evaluating only the "product of teaching" does not do justice to the entire range of educational experiences provided by the critical care nurse. The effectiveness of teaching can also be measured by observation of subtle changes in patients such as signs of relaxation when the information provided decreases anxiety.

Teaching Content in the Critical Area

Determination of the content presented in the critical care unit will depend on the patient's clinical and emotional status and will vary with each patient. The nurse prioritizes learning needs based on the assessment as soon as possible. However, at times an acute event precludes full assessment at the time of admission. In this case, behavior crucial to the patient's treatment and his or her participation in care can be taught as soon as they are appropriate. The teaching should be guided by the patient and family—that is, teach what they want to know when they want to know it. If the patient's questions and concerns are left unanswered during this time of high anxiety, the unmet needs will serve as a block to further communication and prevent the patient from focusing his or her energy appropriately.

Although the specific content taught will vary, depending on the condition for which the patient was admitted, there are certain areas that should be covered with any patient who is conscious. Environmental factors in a critical care unit can be frightening to patients and should be explained as soon as possible. Cardiac monitors, oxygen equipment, indwelling lines and catheters, frequent laboratory tests, and checking vital signs may cause the patient undue anxiety unless their purpose or function is understood. The reason for procedures, as well as their associated sensations or discomfort, should be briefly explained. This information may not be retained and may require several repetitions, but it will assist in decreasing anxiety and providing a sense of control for the moment.

Most of the time it is appropriate to give information about the illness or diagnosis in the critical phase of care. The nurse must often interpret and explain information pro-

vided by physicians. Despite the denial often present, some patients want to know about their illness, prognosis, complications, and reason for admission to the critical care unit. A patient may ask if he or she is going to die. This is a traumatic question for both the patient and the nurse. Nurses may reluctantly talk about death with colleagues or a family but are often very uncomfortable in discussing it with patients. It is important for the nurse to remember that the entire experience of the critical care unit, although routine for the staff, is frightening for the patient who may be confronting mortality for the first time. Questions should be answered as honestly, compassionately, and sensitively as possible and should be followed by supportive care as necessary.

Two specific instances in which patient teaching in the critical care area is especially important are in preparing the patient for surgery with preoperative teaching and preparing patients for other stressful medical procedures, which are performed often in critical care units. The effect of preoperative teaching on selected measures of patient recovery has been of interest to nurses for many years.[28,29] More recently, nurses have studied the effect of preoperative teaching on a wider variety of variables, including psychological well-being, satisfaction with care, patient understanding of informed consent, and cost relevant benefits.[11,40]

Critical care nurses are in a position to positively influence many aspects of recovery and patient outcome through implementation of a carefully planned preoperative teaching program when the patient's condition and situation allows. Patient benefits from preoperative teaching include quicker return of functional capacity, prevention of postoperative complications, increased self-esteem, decreased anxiety, decreased hospitalization costs, and a decrease in immediate and residual pain.[20] Whenever possible, families should be included in the teaching session to decrease their anxiety and to foster a feeling of support for the family unit.[20]

Although specific content for preoperative teaching sessions depends on the patient's physical and psychological condition, the specific operative procedure, and the time available for teaching, these general topics should be considered when planning the teaching session: preoperative medications and treatments such as enemas, skin preparation, urinary catheters, and intravenous catheters; the experience of anesthesia; postoperative treatments, including coughing, deep breathing, use of incentive spirometer, pain medications, tubes, drains, and dressings; and information about arrangements for care of the family during surgery and their sources of information about the patient's progress and condition. Whenever possible, the session should be private and unhurried to allow ample time for questions and emotional support of the patient and family.

Patients in critical care units experience many stressful medical procedures during the course of their care, including radiological procedures, placement of vascular access or monitoring devices, intubation, suctioning, spinal taps, and many others. Educational and psychological preparation for these procedures can decrease anxiety and increase patient cooperation with care. Two types of information can be offered to patients in preparation for these procedures. *Procedural* information refers to what will be done, when and where it will happen, and who will provide the service.

Sensory information refers to what the patient should expect to feel during and after the procedure.[46] When time permits, allowing the patient to ask questions, see equipment that will be used, and practice movements or body positions that will be required can be very helpful in reducing anxiety. In addition, teaching the patient basic relaxation techniques such as deep breathing or guided imagery can be effective in helping patients relax during a stressful or uncomfortable procedure.[21,46] When these procedures must occur on an emergent basis without time for patient preparation, the nurse should explain what happened and why as soon as the patient has stabilized and is able to understand the information.

Transfer from the Critical Care Unit

Transfer from the critical care unit can be an anxiety-producing time for the patients. During the stay in the unit, constant interaction with the nurse, monitoring devices, and controlled environment has offered security to the patient. Transfer from that environment can destroy the sense of security and create acute anxiety.[41] To avoid this anxiety, nurses should prepare patients for imminent or eventual transfer, that is, teach toward transfer. To do this, the nurse should point out early in the stay that the patient will be there only temporarily until his or her condition is improved and stable, and these improvements should be made known to the patient on an ongoing basis. As the time for transfer approaches, careful explanations can reassure patients and families that close observation and monitoring are no longer necessary. When possible, tubes, machines, and equipment used in the critical care unit, which the patient may see as important to his or her survival, should be removed gradually rather than discontinued all at once. This will alleviate feelings of dependence on equipment.

At the time of transfer, patients can be told how care will change and what changes in activity, self-care, and visiting hours to expect. The critical care unit nurse should accompany the patient to the new floor and introduce the new staff members to the patient. The patient can be told that a complete report on his or her condition will be given and that nursing care needs at this stage of recovery will be met in the new setting. Family members should be contacted and informed of the transfer. The care plan and teaching plan developed in the critical care area should accompany the patient to the floor and the new nurses informed about current short-term and long-term goals and the patient's progress. Although careful preparation and planning for transfer are always desirable, a patient may be transferred unexpectedly to make room for a more critically ill admission. When this situation occurs, the patient to be moved from the unit must be notified and prepared for the possibility of a quick transfer. Tangible evidence of improvement such as improvement in vital signs, fewer medications, or fewer tubes can be helpful in pointing out advances in condition before unplanned transfers.

SAMPLE TEACHING PLANS AND CARE PLANS

Examples of teaching plans appropriate for the acutely ill patient begin below, including suggested content and time frames for teaching. In addition, care plans are provided for the following nursing diagnoses: Altered Health Maintenance, Noncompliance, and Knowledge Deficit—to assist the nurse in using the theoretical concepts presented.

Teaching Plan for the Patient Taking Warfarin (Coumadin)

Education of the patient taking an anticoagulant medication is important to reassure the patient, secure compliance, and minimize risks.

During the critical care unit stay, limit teaching to simple statements such as "This is Coumadin. It is a blood thinner."

During the hospitalization the following points should be covered:

■ Basic physiology of coagulation
■ Action of warfarin
■ Importance of taking the medication exactly as prescribed and at the same time each day
■ Importance of regular laboratory work
■ Use of dosage calendar to verify dosage and schedule
■ Use of Medic-Alert or some other system of identification
■ Recognition of following signs and symptoms of bleeding to be reported:
  Prolonged bleeding from cuts
  Nosebleeds
  Bleeding gums
  Hemoptysis or hematemesis
  Spontaneous bruising
  Red or black stools
  Red or dark brown urine
  Prolonged headache, severe abdominal pain, or backache
■ Use of electric razor only
■ Application of 5 to 10 minutes of pressure to cuts
■ Notification of all health care providers, including dentists, of anticoagulation medication
■ Avoidance of aspirin and aspirin-containing products
■ Impact of diet on warfarin therapy:
  Maintenance of steady diet is important.
  Vitamin K affects anticoagulation.
  Foods high in vitamin K (fish, green leafy vegetables) must be eaten.
  Fasting or prolonged diarrhea should be reported.
  Alcoholic beverages may alter clotting time; drink only with physician's approval.
■ Possibility of drug interactions (suggest having all prescriptions filled at the same pharmacy)
  Provide wallet identification card and printed material to reinforce learning.

Teaching Plan for the Patient Undergoing Coronary Artery Bypass Surgery

PREOPERATIVE PHASE

During the preoperative educational interactions, the nurse should assess the patient's and family's levels of anxiety and their effect on the ability or desire to learn. The preoperative education should be individualized to prepare the patient appropriately for the surgery, to educate him or her about postoperative care, and to minimize anxiety. Before the teaching-learning experience, the nurse:

- Assesses the patient's level of anxiety and desire to learn about the upcoming surgery.
- Individualizes the preoperative teaching plan, based on assessment findings.

The following content may be included in the preoperative teaching session:

- Review of the coronary artery bypass graft (CABG) procedure
- Time leaving room for surgery, length of surgery
- Location of family waiting area
- Surgical preparation and shave
- Nothing by mouth after midnight
- What to expect when awakening from anesthesia
- Sights and sounds of the recovery room and/or critical care unit
- Tubes and drains: chest tubes, hemodynamic monitoring lines, Foley catheter, intravenous lines, pacemaker wires (if appropriate), endotracheal tube
- Inability to speak with endotracheal tube in place
- Discomfort to expect from incisions, availability of pain medication
- Coughing and deep breathing practice
- Use of incentive spirometer
- When family can visit, how long, how often
- Usual length of critical care unit stay

In addition to this content, the nurse:

- Reassures patient that many staff members and much activity around bedside is normal and does not indicate complications.
- Elicits and answers any specific questions patient and family have at that time.
- Determines specific needs and desires for day of surgery (e.g., patient needs hearing aid or glasses as soon as possible).
- Meets with the family alone to offer support and address concerns they may not wish to voice to the patient.

CRITICAL CARE UNIT PHASE

During the critical care unit phase, education is designed to meet immediate needs and reduce anxiety. The following are examples of content appropriate for this time:

- Basic explanation of bedside equipment
- Review of tubes and drains
- Turning, coughing, deep breathing
- Use of incentive spirometer
- Use of oxygen equipment
- Orientation to time, place, situation

- Explanation of procedures
- Basic purpose of medications
- Explanation of normal progression in early postoperative period
- Basic range-of-motion exercises (e.g., ankle circles, point and flex)

During this phase, the nurse also:

- Reassures patient and family of normal progression.
- Repeats and reinforces information as necessary.
- Answers questions as they arise.
- Begins early to prepare patient for transfer to prevent transfer anxiety.
- Determines family learning needs and addresses them together with patient or in separate teaching sessions as appropriate.

STEP-DOWN UNIT PHASE

After transfer from the critical care unit, the patient's and family's educational needs increase. Short daily educational sessions should be planned to cover the following content:

- Basic pathophysiology of coronary artery disease
- Review of surgical procedure
- Risk factors for coronary artery disease
- Upper-extremity range of motion exercises
- Dietary recommendations (salt- and fat/cholesterol-modified diet)
- Taking of own pulse
- Recognition and treatment of angina (use of nitroglycerin)

During this phase, the nurse also:

- Uses audiovisual materials in teaching sessions or as reinforcement of content.
- Provides printed take-home materials outlining important content.
- Answers questions as they arise.

DISCHARGE TEACHING

Before discharge, the following content should be covered with the patient and family:

- Activity guidelines
- Lifting restrictions
- Incisional care
- Possibility of patient being extremely fatigued or depressed after discharge
- Guidelines for return to work, driving, sexual activity
- Medication safety and administration

Before discharge, the nurse also:

- Reassures patient that ups and downs are normal.
- If necessary, reassures patient and family that likelihood of cardiac emergencies at home is small.
- Provides printed material for further study by patient and family.
- Answers questions as they arise.
- Provides phone number for patient or family to call when further questions arise.

Altered Health Maintenance

Definition: Inability to identify, manage, or seek out help to maintain health.

Altered Health Maintenance related to lack of resources (financial, interpersonal support systems, health care access)

DEFINING CHARACTERISTICS

■ Lack of participation in primary and/or secondary preventive activities such as obtaining appropriate screenings, proper nutrition, routine medical and dental care
■ Finances inadequate to support medical care
■ Health maintenance behaviors of low priority to family or significant others
■ Access to health care limited because of geographical, transportation, or social barriers
■ Frequent or chronic health problems such as chronic cough, loss of teeth at an early age, frequent infections, chronic fatigue, or anemia
■ Physical signs such as poor hygiene or lesions associated with lack of oral care

OUTCOME CRITERIA

■ Patient gains access to necessary health care.
■ Patient can state self-care and health maintenance behaviors appropriate to his or her age and developmental level.

NURSING INTERVENTIONS *AND RATIONALE*

1. Continue to monitor the assessment parameters listed under "Defining Characteristics."
2. Assist patient and family in identifying social, financial, and environmental factors that limit ability to practice appropriate health maintenance measures.
3. Assist patient and family in identifying appropriate self-care and health maintenance behaviors (e.g., dental hygiene every 6 to 12 months, monthly breast self-examination for women, or complete physical examinations every 2 years for adults aged 60 years or older).
4. Include family and/or other support systems in the planning for immediate and long-term health needs.
5. Provide early referral to social services if indicated *so that appropriate resources and assistance can be obtained.*

Altered Health Maintenance related to lack of perceived threat to health

DEFINING CHARACTERISTICS

■ Lack of participation in primary and/or secondary preventive activities such as obtaining appropriate screenings, proper nutrition, routine medical and dental care
■ Denial of susceptibility to a particular disease or problem
■ Denial of the seriousness of a health problem or its consequences
■ Absence of cues for action such as uncomfortable symptoms
■ Failure to assume appropriate sick role behaviors

OUTCOME CRITERIA

■ Patient is able to state the health consequences of specific behaviors (e.g., smoking is directly related to the onset of heart and lung disease).
■ Patient assumes appropriate sick role behaviors.
■ Patient states plans for appropriate primary and secondary preventive activities after discharge.

NURSING INTERVENTIONS *AND RATIONALE*

1. Continue to monitor the assessment parameters listed under "Defining Characteristics."
2. Assist patient to see the connection between specific behaviors and the short-term onset of symptoms or long-term progression of disease.
3. Assist patient to set short-term and long-term health management goals related to self-care and lifestyle.
4. Assist patient to prioritize goals and to make plans to pursue them in a manageable and realistic fashion.
5. Initiate health education *to give the patient skills necessary to meet the immediate goals.* (See care plans for Knowledge Deficit.)
6. Initiate referrals for long-term follow-up after discharge (e.g., health educators, counselors, home health personnel, primary care practitioners, or rehabilitation programs).

Noncompliance

Definition: Personal behavior that deviates from health-related advice given by health care professionals.

Noncompliance _____ (Specify) related to knowledge deficit

DEFINING CHARACTERISTICS

- Lack of participation in necessary therapeutic measures
- Lack of prior experience with the recommended treatment or action
- Verbalization of inadequate knowledge or skills
- Questioning the need for the treatment or action

OUTCOME CRITERIA

- Patient verbalizes adequate knowledge or demonstrates adequate skills necessary for participation in treatment.
- Patient demonstrates compliance with treatment.

NURSING INTERVENTIONS *AND RATIONALE*

1. Continue to monitor the assessment parameters listed under "Defining Characteristics."
2. Determine specific knowledge or skills necessary *for adherence to therapeutic plan.*

For other interventions, see care plan for Knowledge Deficit, p. 69.

Noncompliance _____ (Specify) related to lack of resources (see Altered Health Maintenance)

DEFINING CHARACTERISTICS

- Lack of participation in necessary therapeutic measures
- Interpersonal or financial resources inadequate to support patient's appropriate participation in treatment
- Expression of concern about the cost of hospitalization and treatments
- Reinforcement of patient's behaviors and lack of proper participation in therapy by family/significant others

OUTCOME CRITERIA

- Patient demonstrates compliance with treatment.
- Family/significant others appropriately support and encourage patient in health-related and treatment-related behaviors.

NURSING INTERVENTIONS *AND RATIONALE*

1. Continue to monitor the assessment parameters listed under "Defining Characteristics."
2. Educate family and significant others about the prescribed treatments, their importance, and patient's need to participate *so that support and assistance can be given to the patient.*
3. Assist family/significant others to identify specific ways in which they can assist patient *so that he or she can comply with plan.*

For other interventions, see care plan for Altered Health Maintenance related to lack of resources, p. 67.

Knowledge Deficit

Definition: The state in which the individual experiences a decrease in cognitive knowledge or psychomotor skills that alters or may alter health maintenance.

Knowledge Deficit _____ (Specify) related to lack of previous exposure to information

DEFINING CHARACTERISTICS

- Verbalized statement of inadequate knowledge or skills
- New diagnosis or health problem requiring self-management or care
- Lack of prior formal or informal education about the specific health problem
- Demonstration of inappropriate behaviors related to management of health problem

OUTCOME CRITERIA

- Patient verbalizes adequate knowledge about or performs skills related to disease process, its causes, factors related to onset of symptoms, and self-management of disease or health problem.
- Patient actively participates in health behaviors required for performance of a procedure or in those behaviors enhancing recovery from illness and preventing recurrence or complications.

NURSING INTERVENTIONS *AND RATIONALE*

1. Continue to monitor the assessment parameters listed under "Defining Characteristics."
2. Determine existing level of knowledge or skill.
3. Assess factors affecting the knowledge deficit:
   Learning needs, including patient's priorities and the necessary knowledge and skills for safety
   Learning ability of client, including language skills, level of education, ability to read, preferred learning style
   Physical ability to perform prescribed skills or procedures; consider effect of limitations imposed by treatment such as bedrest, restriction of movement by intravenous or other equipment, or effect of sedatives or analgesics
   Psychological effect of stage of adaptation to disease
   Activity tolerance and ability to concentrate
   Motivation to learn new skills or gain new knowledge
4. Reduce or limit barriers to learning:
   Provide consistent nurse-patient contact *to encourage development of trusting and therapeutic relationship.*
   Structure environment *to enhance learning;* control unnecessary noise, interruptions.
   Individualize teaching plan *to fit patient's current physical and psychological status.*
   Delay teaching until patient is ready to learn.
   Conduct teaching sessions during period of day when patient is most alert and receptive.
   Meet patient's immediate learning needs as they arise, e.g., give brief explanation of procedures when they are performed.
5. Promote active participation in the teaching plan by the patient and family:
   Solicit input during development of plan.
   Develop mutually acceptable goals and outcomes.
   Solicit expression of feelings and emotions related to new responsibilities.
   Encourage questions.
6. Conduct teaching sessions, using the most appropriate teaching methods:
   Discussion
   Lecture
   Demonstration/return demonstration
   Use of audiovisual or printed educational materials
7. Repeat key principles and provide them in printed form *for reference at a later time.*
8. Give frequent feedback to patient when practicing new skills.
9. Use several teaching sessions when appropriate. *New information and skills should be reinforced several times after initial learning.*
10. Initiate referrals for follow-up *if necessary:*
    Health educators
    Home health care
    Rehabilitation programs
    Social services
11. Evaluate effectiveness of teaching plan, based on patient's ability to meet preset goals and objectives:
    Determine need for further teaching.

Knowledge Deficit _____(Specify) related to cognitive/perceptual learning limitations (e.g., sensory overload, sleep deprivation, medications, anxiety, sensory deficits, language barrier)

DEFINING CHARACTERISTICS

- Verbalized statement of inadequate knowledge of skills
- Verbalization of inadequate recall of information
- Verbalization of inadequate understanding of information
- Evidence of inaccurate follow-through of instructions
- Inadequate demonstration of a skill
- Lack of compliance with prescribed behavior

OUTCOME CRITERIA

- Patient participates actively in necessary and prescribed health behaviors.
- Patient verbalizes adequate knowledge or demonstrates adequate skills.

NURSING INTERVENTIONS *AND RATIONALE*

1. Continue to monitor the assessment parameters listed under "Defining Characteristics."
2. Determine specific cause of patient's cognitive or perceptual limitation. (See also table of contents for Impaired Verbal Communication, Anxiety, Sleep Pattern Disturbances, Sensory-Perceptual Alterations.)
3. Provide uninterrupted rest period before teaching session *to decrease fatique and encourage optimal state for learning and retention.*
4. Manipulate environment as much as possible *to provide quiet and uninterrupted learning sessions:*
   Ensure lights are bright enough to see teaching aids but not too bright.
   Close door if necessary *to provide quiet environment.*
   Schedule care and medications *to allow uninterrupted teaching periods.*
   Move patient to quiet, private room for teaching *if possible.*

5. Adapt teaching sessions and materials to patient's and family's levels of education and ability to understand:
   Provide printed material appropriate to reading level.
   Use terminology understood by the patient.
   Provide printed materials in patient's primary language *if possible.*
   Use interpreters during teaching sessions *when necessary.*
6. Teach only present-tense focus during periods of sensory overload.
7. Determine potential effects of medications on ability to retain or recall information. Avoid teaching critical content while patient is taking sedatives, analgesics, or other medications affecting memory.
8. Reinforce new skills and information in several teaching sessions. Use several senses when possible in teaching session (e.g., see a film, hear a discussion, read printed information, and demonstrate skills related to self-injection of insulin).
9. Reduce patient's anxiety:
   Listen attentively and encourage verbalization of feelings.
   Answer questions as they arise in a clear and succinct manner.
   Elicit patient's concerns and address those issues first.
   Give only correct and relevant information.
   Continually assess response to teaching session and discontinue if anxiety increases or physical condition becomes unstable.
   Provide nonthreatening information before more anxiety-producing information is presented.
   Plan for several teaching sessions so information can be divided into small manageable packages.

SUMMARY

This chapter has outlined and discussed theory and assessment of health perception and health management issues important in the care of the critically ill patient, as well as the role of health promotion in the acute care setting. Factors influencing patient compliance have been identified, and strategies for optimizing patient compliance have been suggested. Finally, the role of patient education in the critical care area has been reviewed. A detailed educational assessment has been outlined, and suggestions for content and teaching methods appropriate to the critical care area have been offered. Sample teaching plans and care plans have been provided.

REFERENCES

1. American Nurses' Association: A Social Policy Statement, Kansas City, Mo, 1980, The Association.
2. Becker MH and others: Some influences on program participation in a genetic screening program, Community Health 1:3, 1975.
3. Bell JA: The role of microcomputers in patient education, Comput Nurs 4(6):255, 1986.
4. Bertakis KD: An application of the health belief model to patient education and compliance: acute otitis media, Fam Med 18(6):347, 1986.
5. Billie DA: The teaching-learning process. In Billie DA: Practical approaches of patient teaching, Boston, 1981, Little, Brown & Co., Inc.
6. Billie DA: Process oriented patient education. Dimens Crit Care Nurs 2:2, 1983.
7. Boyd MD: A guide to writing effective patient education materials, Nurs Management 18(7):56, 1987.
8. Burke LE: Learning and retention in the acute care setting, Crit Care Q 4:3, 1981.
9. Burke LE and Scalzi CC: Education of the patient and family. In Underhill S and others: Cardiac Nursing, Philadelphia, 1982, JB Lippincott Co.
10. Carpenito L: Nursing diagnosis: application to clinical practice, Philadelphia, 1988, JB Lippincott Co.
11. Devine EC and Cook TD: Clinical and cost-saving effects of psycho-educational interventions with surgical patients: a meta-analysis, Res Nurs Health 9:89, 1986.
12. Dobberstein K: Computer-assisted patient education, Am J Nurs 87(5):697, 1987.
13. Doak L and Doak C: Patient comprehension profiles: recent findings and strategies, Patient Coun Health Educ 3:101, 1980.
14. Durand RP and Counts CS: Developing audio-visual programs for patient education, Am Neph Nurs Assoc 13(3):158, 1986.
15. Eaton S, Davis G, and Brenner P: Discussion stoppers in teaching, Nurs Outlook 25(9):578, 1977.
16. Edelman C and Milio N: Health defined: promotion and specific protection. In Eidelman C and Mandle CL: Health promotion throughout the lifespan, St Louis, 1986, The CV Mosby Co.
17. Elsberry NL and Sorensen ME: Using analogies in patient teaching, Am J Nurs 86(10):1171, 1986.
18. Flynn JB and Griffin PA: Health promotion in acute care settings, Nurs Clin North Am 19(2):239, 1984.
19. Foster DS: Written reinforcement for teaching, MCN 11(5):347, 1986.
20. Fox V: Patient teaching—understanding the needs of the adult learner, AORN 44(2):234, 1986.
21. Frenn M, Fehring R, and Kartes S: Reducing the stress of cardiac catheterization by teaching relaxation, Dimens Crit Care Nurs 5(2):108, 1986.
22. Gerber KE: Compliance in the chronically ill: an introduction to the problem. In Gerber KE and Nehemkis A: Compliance—the dilemma of the chronically ill, New York, 1986, Springer-Verlag New York, Inc.
23. Gordon M: Nursing diagnosis: process and application, New York, 1982, McGraw-Hill Book Co.
24. Gruber-Wood R and Mandel C: Health promotion and the individual. In Edelman C and Mandle CL: Health promotion throughout the lifespan, St Louis, 1986, The CV Mosby Co.
25. Guzzetta CE: Can critically ill patients be taught? In Billie DA: Practical approaches to patient teaching, Boston, 1981, Little, Brown & Co, Inc.
26. Informational needs of families of intensive care unit patients, Quality Rev Bull 12:1, 1986.
27. Keeling AW: Health promotion in coronary care and step down units: focus on the family—linking research to practice, Heart Lung 17(1):28, 1988.
28. Lindeman CA: Influencing recovery through preoperative teaching, Heart Lung 2(4):515, 1973.
29. Lindeman CA and Van Aernam B: Nursing intervention with the presurgical patient—the effects of structured and unstructured preoperative teaching, Nurs Res 20(4):319, 1971.
30. Murdaugh C: Barriers to patient education in the coronary care unit, Cardiovasc Nurs 18(6):31, 1982.
31. Narrow B: Patient teaching in nursing practice, Salt Lake City, 1978, John Wiley & Sons, Inc.
32. Nehemkis AM and Gerber KE: Compliance and the quality of life. In Gerber KE and Nehemkis AM: Compliance—the dilemma of the chronically ill, New York, 1986, Springer-Verlag New York, Inc.
33. Neilsen E and Sheppard MA: Television as a patient education tool: a review of its effectiveness, Patient Educ Coun 11:3, 1988.
34. Nite G and Willis F: The coronary patient: hospital care and rehabilitation, New York, 1964, Macmillan, Inc.
35. Novak J: The social mandate and historical basis for nursing's role in health promotion, J Prof Nurs 4(2):80, 1988.
36. Pender NJ: Health promotion in nursing practice, Norwalk, Conn, 1982, Appleton-Century-Crofts.
37. Provine R: The challenge of patient education in critical care, Crit Care Nurs 6(2):22, 1986.
38. Redman BK: The process of patient teaching in nursing, St Louis, 1984, The CV Mosby Co.
39. Smith E: Patient teaching—it's the law, Nursing 87 17(7):67, 1987.
40. Solomon S and Schwegman-Melton K: Structured teaching and patient understanding of informed consent, Crit Care Nurs 7(3):74, 1987.
41. Storlie F: Patient teaching in critical care, New York, 1975, Appleton-Century-Crofts.
42. Streiff LD: Can clients understand our instructions? Image: J Nurs Schol 18(2):48, 1986.
43. Surgeon General: Healthy people: the Surgeon General's report on health promotion and disease prevention, Washington, DC, 1980, Department of Public Health and Human Service.
44. Theirer J and others: Standards for nursing care of the critically ill, Englewood Cliffs, NJ, 1981, Reston Publishing Co.
45. Thompson J and others: Clinical nursing, ed 2, St Louis, 1989, The CV Mosby Co.
46. Williams CL and Kendall PC: Psychological aspects of education for stressful medical procedures, Health Educ Q 12(3):135, 1985.

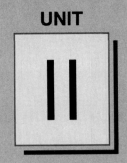
SLEEP ALTERATIONS

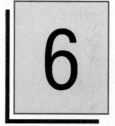

Sleep Physiology and Assessment

CHAPTER OBJECTIVES

- *State the stages of sleep.*
- *Explain three physiological effects that occur during rapid eye movement (REM) sleep.*
- *State two major physiological effects of slow wave sleep.*
- *Describe desynchronized sleep and its primary effects.*
- *Describe the changes in sleep resulting from the aging process.*
- *State the two major methods that accurately measure sleep.*

William Shakespeare early recognized the therapeutic value of sleep: "O sleep, o gentle sleep, nature's soft nurse!" Patients admitted to critical care units, because their critical illnesses require frequent treatments and 24-hour intensive monitoring, will probably suffer an alteration in sleep pattern. Henderson[9] described the inability to rest and sleep as "one of the causes, as well as one of the accompaniments of disease." Bahr[2] stated, "The phenomenon of sleep has the potential for relieving an individual of stress and responsibility when a break is needed to recharge the person's spirit, mind and body; or, it can remain maddeningly aloof when it is needed most." A lack of sleep can have disastrous results for the critically ill patient. The critical care nurse can promote recovery and healing through facilitating sleep for patients. To do this, the nurse must understand the physiology of normal sleep and recognize events that can potentially disrupt sleep in the critical care environment. The purpose of this chapter is to familiarize the reader with the phenomenon of sleep and the types of sleep pattern disturbances that may occur in critical care and to describe the assessment of sleep pattern disturbances in critically ill patients.

PHYSIOLOGY OF SLEEP

Sleep has been defined as "a state of unconsciousness from which a person can be aroused by appropriate sensory or other stimuli."[6] Adults normally spend approximately one third of their lives asleep. Research involving the simultaneous monitoring of the electroencephalogram (EEG), electrooculogram (EOG), and electromyogram (EMG) has shown that there are two distinct stages of sleep: *REM (rapid eye movement)* and *NREM (non–rapid eye movement)*.[5]

NREM Sleep

NREM sleep is divided into four stages (NREM 1 through 4), which are associated with progressive relaxation. NREM stage 1 is a transitional state, with the EEG being similar to that seen in the awake stage. See Fig. 6-1 for a comparison of EEG patterns of subjects that were either awake or asleep. Stage 1 is the lightest level of sleep, lasting only 1 to 2 minutes (Fig. 6-2). This stage is characterized by aimless thoughts, a feeling of drifting, and frequently, myoclonic jerks of the face, hands, and feet. The individual is easily awakened during this stage.[3]

NREM stage 2 differs from stage 1 in that the background wave frequency on the EEG is slower with *sleep spindles* (characteristic waveforms) superimposed and high voltage spikes known as K-complexes (Fig. 6-3). This stage lasts from 5 to 15 minutes, during which time the individual becomes more relaxed but is still easily awakened. Stages 1 and 2 in the average young adult constitute 50% to 60% of the total sleep time.[2]

Stages 3 and 4 are characterized by large, slow-frequency delta waves on the EEG and are primarily differentiated by the relative percentage of these waves (Figs. 6-4 and 6-5).[17] Random stimuli do not arouse the individual from these deepest levels of sleep. The length of time spent in stages 3 and 4 varies from 15 to 30 minutes and constitutes approximately 20% of the total sleep time. During NREM sleep, the EOG gradually slows and eye movements cease. The EMG also declines, indicating profound muscle relaxation; however, it does not reach the low levels that it does in REM sleep.[18] The parasympathetic nervous system predominates during NREM sleep. The cardiac and respiratory rates, the metabolic rate, and the blood pressure decrease to basal levels. Thus the supply/demand ratio of coronary blood flow is likely to improve.[9]

In addition, during slow wave sleep, growth hormone (GH) is secreted by the anterior pituitary and functions to promote protein synthesis while sparing catabolic breakdown. Elevated GH and other anabolic hormones, such as

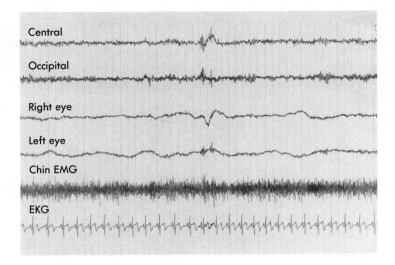

Fig. 6-1 Awake.

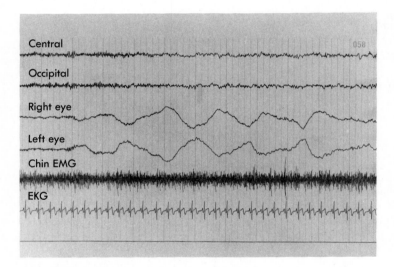

Fig. 6-2 NREM stage 1 sleep.

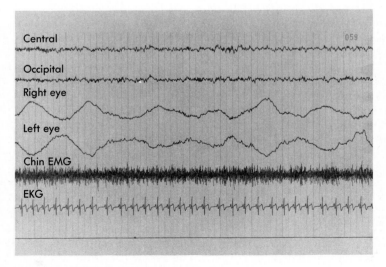

Fig. 6-3 NREM stage 2 sleep.

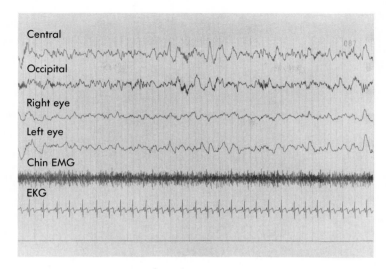

Fig. 6-4 Delta sleep NREM stage 3.

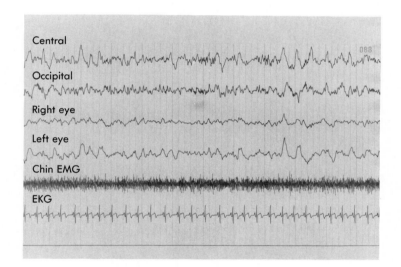

Fig. 6-5 Delta sleep NREM stage 4.

prolactin and testosterone, imply that anabolism is taking place during NREM stage 4, particularly in tissues with a high protein content. Thus activities associated with NREM stage 4 include protein synthesis and tissue repair, such as the repair of epithelial and specialized cells of the brain.[7] NREM dreams are often realistic and thoughtlike, rarely in color, and often similar to a recent activity. These dreams are generally more difficult to remember than REM dreams.[22] NREM sleep, then, is a time of energy conservation.

REM Sleep

REM, or *paradoxical*, sleep constitutes 20% to 25% of the total sleep time in the young adult.[18] This type of sleep is paradoxical in that some areas of the brain are quite active during REM sleep, while other areas are suppressed. During REM sleep, there are bursts of eye movements seen on the EOG that are often associated with periods of dreaming. The EMG becomes essentially flat, indicating immobility

and functional paralysis of the skeletal muscles. The cerebral cortical activity increases during REM so that the EEG resembles one taken during the waking state.[5] (See Fig. 6-6.) During REM sleep, the individual is more difficult to awaken than in any other stage of sleep.[18] In this regard, REM sleep can be thought of as a "dissociative state."

The sympathetic nervous system predominates during REM sleep. Oxygen consumption increases, and cardiac output, blood pressure, heart rate, and respiratory rate may become erratic.[17] An increase in premature ventricular contractions (PVCs) and tachydysrhythmias associated with respiratory pauses may occur during REM sleep.[22] Serum cholesterol and antidiuretic hormone levels increase, and perfusion to the gray matter in the brain doubles.[3] The dreams of REM sleep tend to be colorful, vivid, and implausible, often containing an element of paralysis.[16] REM sleep filters information stored from the day's activities, sifting the important from the trivial, helping to psychologically integrate activities such as problem solving.[18] REM

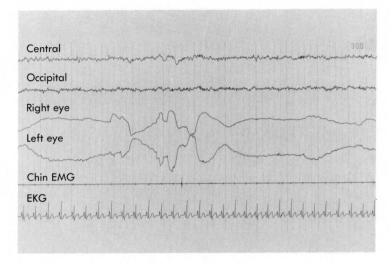

Fig. 6-6 REM sleep.

sleep seems to facilitate emotional adaptation to the physical and psychological environment and is needed in large quantities after periods of stress or learning.[19] The adequacy of sleep is judged by the relative periods of time spent in each of the stages of sleep.[8]

REM sleep, like the other stages of sleep, is essential to physiological and psychological well-being. REM sleep is of great importance to nurses because as the patient is entering this stage of sleep, the nurse may notice a change in vital signs and become concerned that the patient's condition is worsening. If the nurse increases the monitoring of the patient, adjusts drips, and measures vital signs in response to this perceived change in condition, she or he may awaken the patient. Thus the patient may not get the REM sleep he or she needs. Further research must address the ways in which the nurse can assess sleep and all of its stages without unnecessarily disrupting the patient from the much needed REM sleep. An accurate knowledge of sleep will assist nurses in monitoring patients safely.

Cyclical Aspects

At the onset of sleep, the individual normally progresses through repetitive cycles beginning with NREM stages 1 through 4 and then back again to stage 2. From stage 2, the individual enters REM. Stage 2 is then reentered, and the cycle repeats (see Fig. 6-7). These cycles occur at approximately 90-minute intervals, so that four to five cycles are normally completed in the sleep period. Early in the sleep period, NREM predominates. During the end of the sleep period, REM periods tend to be of longer duration than those of NREM sleep.[5]

The rhythmic nature of sleep is not unique. The body experiences rhythms in temperature, blood pressure, heart rate, respiratory rate, and hormone secretion. This cyclical 24-hour rhythm has been termed the circadian rhythm. Sleep normally occupies the low phase of the circadian rhythm, while wakefulness and activity normally occupy the higher phase.[19]

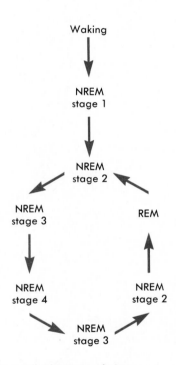

Fig. 6-7 The cyclical nature of sleep.

The cyclical nature of sleep and wakefulness is thought to be regulated by neurotransmitters. Excitation of an area in the pons called the locus ceruleus stimulates neurons to secrete norepinephrine, a major neurotransmitter of the sympathetic nervous system. Norepinephrine along with dopamine and epinephrine are believed to play a role in the waking process. Excitation of the raphe nuclei in the pons and the medulla leads to natural sleep. These cells secrete serotonin, a neurotransmitter that is therefore thought to be associated with the inducement of sleep.[6]

In addition to their role in the sleep-wake cycle, the catecholamine neurotransmitters are postulated to play a role in the cycles of REM and NREM sleep. Norepinephrine and dopamine secreted by the locus ceruleus and dorsal raphe nuclei of the brainstem fire more slowly during REM sleep ("REM off" cells). In contrast, the major neurotransmitter of the parasympathetic nervous system, acetylcholine (ACh) is secreted more rapidly from the gigantocellular tegmental field (FTG) in the reticular formation during the initiation of REM ("REM on" cells). A negative feedback mechanism is theorized to be responsible for REM-NREM cycling in sleep. Thus both of the major neurotransmitters of the autonomic nervous system are hypothesized to play important roles in the cyclical regulation of sleep, including both the sleep-wake cycle and REM-NREM cycles.[13]

It is interesting to note that the neurotransmitters dopamine and serotonin are major determinants of mood and affect. The changes in mood and affect in persons with sleep deprivation and desynchronization may partially be explained by the functioning of these transmitters. It is also interesting to note in light of the major role of neurotransmitters in sleep that sleep disorders are frequently seen in psychiatric illness; that is, early morning awakenings are classically found with major depressive disorders that are thought to be biochemically induced.

The sleep-wake cycle follows the circadian rhythm in a 24-hour cycle synchronized with other biological rhythms.[17] Nighttime sleep is the normal pattern for most adults. Serotonin, for example, is usually released around 8 PM to prepare the body for sleep. Conversely, adrenocorticotropic hormone (ACTH), corticotropin-releasing hormone (CRH), and cortisol all normally peak in the early morning hours to prepare the individual for the day's stresses. If a person is deprived of sleep, especially the deeper stages, these hormones will still be released, but at times that may or may not coordinate approximately with the stresses he or she is about to face. Thus an abnormal sleep pattern will compromise the patient's ability to cope with the stress of critical illness, thereby possibly complicating his or her recovery.[17] When sleep occurs during the low phase of the circadian rhythm, circadian synchronization is present. Sleep that occurs during normal waking hours is out of phase or desynchronized (see Fig. 6-8). Desynchronized sleep is rated as poor-quality sleep and causes a decreased arousal threshold; therefore frequent awakenings are more likely. Irritability, restlessness, depression, anxiety, and decreased accuracy in task performance are characteristic effects of desyncrhonized sleep.[20] Resynchronization with the circadian rhythm must occur whenever sleep has become desynchronized for the individual to establish a normal sleep-activity pattern. Although variable among individuals, the resynchronization process is thought to require a minimum of 3 days with a consistent sleep-wake schedule. During resynchronization, the individual often feels fatigued and unable to perform all of his or her activities of daily living.[20]

SLEEP CHANGES WITH AGE

Of the factors that influence the quality of sleep, age is one of the most prominent. The sleep of a normal infant is divided into two types. The first is characterized by no eye or body movements and regular respirations. The second type is associated with eye and body movements and a predominant suck reflex. The first type of sleep develops into NREM sleep and the latter into REM sleep. The infant, unlike the adult, goes from wakefulness directly into REM sleep. By approximately 3 months of age, the full-term infant develops the normal adult pattern of falling from wakefulness into NREM sleep.[5] Infants spend a relatively large proportion of their sleep time in REM sleep. For the full-term newborn this percentage is approximately 40% to 50% of total sleep time.[15]

As the biological systems change during the normal aging process, stress is placed on the human system, and the delicate mechanism of sleep is altered.[12] Hayter[8], in a study of 212 healthy, noninstitutionalized older adults aged 65 to 93, found extreme variability in the sleep behaviors of different subjects within age-groups. Sleep behaviors between men and women had few differences, though women did report more difficulty getting to sleep and more frequent use of sleep aids than did men. The number of daytime naps and nighttime awakenings and variability in sleep behaviors increased with age. By age 75, the number of naps and length of naptime increased, resulting in a gradual increase in the total sleep time. Therefore both the time needed to fall asleep and the amount of time spent in bed increased with age.

The number of awakenings increases significantly, from one or two to as many as six per night; thus the elderly experience an increase in the total duration of NREM stage 1 sleep and an increase in the number of shifts into stage

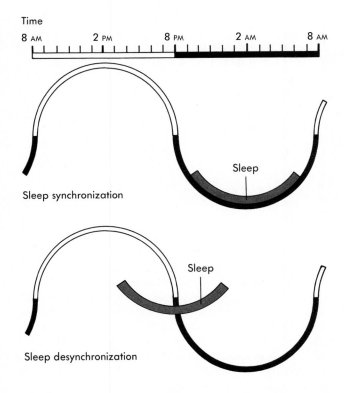

Fig. 6-8 Sleep synchronization and desynchronization with circadian rhythm.

1. The duration of stage 2 sleep changes very little; however, awakenings from stage 2 sleep become more frequent. NREM stage 3 tends to be normal. The duration of NREM stage 4, however, declines rapidly so that by age 50 it is reduced by 50%. Little or no stage 4 sleep may be found in 25% of the population in the sixth decade of life.[21] Stage 4 sleep is virtually absent in old age, and the proportion of REM begins to decline in relation to total sleep time.[14] The circadian rhythm in the elderly appears to shift to the earlier part of the night so that distribution of REM sleep throughout the night is unusually uniform.[2] These changes, along with more fragmentation and frequent long periods of wakefulness at night, cause the elderly to perceive an impairment in their quality of sleep.

Advanced age involves losses: of functional capabilities, friends, spouse, and material belongings.[18] Because these losses can lead to depression, a state that is relatively common in the older population, the relationship between depression and sleep disturbance is important for the nurse to consider when working with the elderly. These losses, by disrupting the psychological state of the elderly patient, may also compound existing sleep difficulties.

SLEEP CHANGES WITH CHRONIC ILLNESS

Chronic illnesses, common in the elderly, tend to increase the frequency and severity of sleep disorders. Illnesses that commonly affect sleep are arthritis, angina pectoris, chronic obstructive pulmonary disease (COPD), congestive heart failure, diabetes mellitus, peptic ulcers, alcoholism, parkinsonism, thyroid disorders, altered sensory perceptions, and depression. Both situational stress and long-term anxiety are causes of disrupted and restless sleep.[18]

ASSESSMENT OF SLEEP PATTERN DISTURBANCE

Assessment of the patient on admission to the critical care unit should include a description of the normal sleep pattern, including awakenings, naps, normal bedtime and waking time, and customary habits that enhance sleep (for example, number of pillows, extra blankets, bedtime rituals, and medications); any recent changes in the patient's normal pattern resulting from the acute illness; recent and past history of sleep disturbances; the severity, duration, and frequency of the problem; and history of chronic illnesses and physical conditions that may disturb sleep, such as COPD, bronchial asthma, bronchitis, arthritis, nocturnal angina, hyperthyroidism, hypertension, duodenal ulcer, or reflux esophagitis and nocturia. The patient's response to the critical care environment should be assessed, along with the noise level in the patient's immediate environment. The critical care nurse should elicit history of snoring because of its relationship to sleep apnea and sleep disturbances. One effective way to assess the quality of the patient's sleep is for the nurse to ask how his or her sleep in the hospital compares to sleep at home. Because of the extreme variations in sleep behaviors, individual differences must be recognized, and

a flexible, individualized plan of care formulated to promote rest and sleep. Sleep, like pain, is a multidimensional process with considerable individual variations making the assessment of sleep a difficult process. For this reason, both qualitative and physiological indices are needed to measure sleep.[4] The scientific standard for the measurement of sleep is the polysomnogram (PSG). While the PSG is considered a medical diagnostic and research tool, the nurse can employ it to validate the results of observational and perceptual tools used to measure sleep. In normal healthy individuals, a high correlation exists between the person's subjective assessment of sleep recorded on a sleep log or questionnaire and PSG data.[1] However, in hospitalized persons this correlation does not always exist.[11]

Another problem in the measurement of sleep is that nurses' observations of patients' sleep have demonstrated both overestimation and underestimation of sleep when compared to PSG recordings. When a tool with specific sleep criteria was used, however, the amount of time a patient actually spent awake during the night (a measure of sleep efficiency) was valid when compared to PSG data.[4]

Sleep efficiency is an important sleep variable—it is defined as the proportion of actual sleep time in the total sleep period. Usual adult sleep efficiency is 95% of actual sleep time, whereas in multisystem trauma patients in the critical care area, it may be as low as 65%.[4]

For patients most at risk for a sleep pattern disturbance (for example, patients with invasive monitoring, those requiring hourly or more frequent assessments and interventions, patients whose illness will require an extended stay in critical care, or patients exhibiting initial signs of sleep deprivation), the nurse's keeping a sleep chart for 48 to 72 hours may assist in assessing actual quantity of sleep in addition to assessing necessary and unnecessary wakenings. The sleep chart should include the date and time, whether the patient was awake or asleep, and any procedures for which it was necessary to awaken the patient. A 24-hour flow sheet such as is common in critical care units could have an area for documentation of sleep. Just as nurses document other data relevant to the patient's recovery, sleep periods of more than 90 minutes in duration and total sleep time should be recorded and evaluated. An example of such a documentation system is provided in Chapter 8 (see Fig. 8-2).

SUMMARY

Sleep patterns usually change in the critically ill patient. An understanding of these changes and an awareness of potential problems for the critically ill patient in the critical care environment will contribute to the health and well-being of patients. The critical care nurse is in a position to monitor, coordinate, and control the patient's 24-hour environment. Carefully planned and individualized interventions will maximize the quality and quantity of restorative sleep, thus enhancing recovery for the critically ill. Refer to Chapter 8 for nursing interventions for the nursing diagnosis Sleep Pattern Disturbance.

REFERENCES

1. Baekeland F and Hoy P: Reported vs. recorded sleep characteristics, Arch Gen Psychiatry 24:548, 1971.
2. Bahr R: Sleep-wake patterns in the aged, J Gerontol Nurs 9(10):534, 1983.
3. Fabijan N and Gosselin M: How to recognize sleep deprivation in your ICU patient and what to do about it, Can Nurse 4:20, 1982.
4. Fontaine D: Measurement of nocturnal sleep patterns in multisystem trauma patients, unpublished doctoral dissertation, Washington, DC, 1987, The Catholic University of America.
5. Freemon F: Sleep research, Springfield, 1972, Charles C Thomas, Publisher.
6. Guyton AC: Medical physiology, ed 6, Philadelphia, 1981, WB Saunders Co.
7. Hartmann E: The sleeping pill, London, 1978, Yale University Press.
8. Hayter J: Sleep behaviors of older persons, Nurs Res 32(4):242, 1983.
9. Hemenway J: Sleep and the cardiac patient, Heart Lung 9(3):453, 1980.
10. Henderson V: Basic principles of nursing care, New York, 1969, Macmillan Publishing Co.
11. Kavey NB and Altshuler KZ: Sleep in herniorrhaphy patients, Am J Surg 138:682, 1979.
12. Lerner R: Sleep loss in the aged: implications for nursing practice, J Gerontol Nurs 8(6):323, 1982.
13. Mendelson W: Human sleep, New York, 1987, Plenum Publishing Co.
14. Pacini C and Fitzpatrick J: Sleep patterns of hospitalized and non-hospitalized aged individuals, J Gerontol Nurs 8(6):327, 1982.
15. Roffwarg HP, Muzio JN, and Dement WC: Ontogenetic development of the human sleep-dream cycle, Science, 152:604, 1966.
16. Salamy JG: Sleep: some concepts and constructs. In Williams RL and Karacan I, editors: Pharmacology of Sleep, New York, 1976, John Wiley & Sons.
17. Sanford S: Sleep and the cardiac patient, Cardiovasc Nur 19(5):19, 1983.
18. Schirmer M: When sleep won't come, J Gerontol Nurs 9(1):16, 1983.
19. Sebilia A: Sleep deprivation and biological rhythms in the critical care unit, Crit Care Nurse 3:19, 1981.
20. Taub J: Acute shifts in the sleep-wakefulness: effects on performance and moods, Psychosom Med 36(2):164, 1974.
21. Wotring K: Using research in practice, Focus 9(5):34, 1982.

CHAPTER

7

Sleep Disorders

CHAPTER OBJECTIVES

- *State the four major categories for classifying sleep disorders.*
- *Define obstructive sleep apnea syndrome.*
- *State the major complications of obstructive sleep apnea and the implications for critical care nursing practice.*
- *Describe the treatment of sleep apnea syndrome and state the implications for critical care nursing practice.*
- *Define central sleep apnea.*
- *Describe how the medical treatment for central sleep apnea differs from that of obstructive sleep apnea.*

CLASSIFICATION OF SLEEP DISORDERS

Sleep disorders have been classified by the Association of Sleep Disorders Centers.[1] In this classification, sleep disorders are divided into four major groups (see the box on p. 81). The first is "disorders of initiating and maintaining sleep" (DIMS). The second major category is "disorders of excessive somnolence" (DOES). The third and fourth categories are "disorders of sleep-wake schedule" and "dysfunctions associated with sleep, sleep stages, or partial arousals." This chapter will focus exclusively on sleep apnea syndrome and its management.

SLEEP APNEA SYNDROME

Sleep apnea syndrome (SAS) can be periodic cessation of breathing that results from upper airway obstruction (obstructive apnea), a lack of respiratory muscle activity (central apnea), or a combination of both (mixed apnea). Guilleminault and others[3] has suggested that in all populations except the elderly more than 30 episodes of apnea per 7 hours of sleep or an *apnea index* (the number of apneas per hour) of 5 or greater is diagnostic of SAS. Because there is a relationship between advanced age and sleep apnea episodes, further research must be done to determine diagnostic criteria for every age group. SAS results in daytime

somnolence, systemic or pulmonary hypertension, arterial blood gas abnormalities, life-threatening dysrhythmias, chronic respiratory failure, sexual dysfunction, and mental insufficiency. Hence, it is clearly a life-threatening disorder that requires proper diagnosis and treatment.[4]

Obstructive Sleep Apnea

Definition. Obstructive sleep apnea is the most common form of sleep apnea. Obstructive apnea is characterized by cessation of air flow resulting from upper airway obstruction although respiratory effort is exerted. Manifestations can range from a few mild symptoms to very severe symptoms that often constitute Pickwickian syndrome. The syndrome most commonly affects men over age 50 and postmenopausal women, with predominant symptoms of snoring and daytime somnolence. Other symptoms include systemic and pulmonary hypertension, arterial blood gas abnormalities, life-threatening cardiac dysrhythmias, chronic respiratory failure, sexual dysfunction, and mental insufficiency. An understanding of SAS is helpful to the critical care nurse, because the physiological effects of the syndrome can be life threatening.

Etiological factors. The cause of obstructive sleep apnea is not entirely understood; however, upper airway structure, hormonal balance, and neural control are implicated. Computerized tomographies of awake subjects have shown that patients with SAS have narrower airways than do normal subjects. The narrower the airway, the more easily it becomes obstructed.

Upper airway patency is also affected by upper airway function, which is under the control of the respiratory motor neurons. During sleep, this control varies and causes decreased neural activity, thereby narrowing the airway. This effect is especially prevalent during REM sleep when the motor neurons are hypotonic. Unstable control of the respiratory nerves of the diaphragm, intercostal, and upper airway muscles can cause sleep apneas. In addition, sex hormone balance contributes to airway status. Increased levels of testosterone may trigger sleep apnea.[6] Hypothyroidism can alter respiratory controls and therefore contribute to sleep apnea. Other contributing disorders are exog-

---

CLASSIFICATION OF SLEEP DISORDERS

I. DIMS (disorders of initiating and maintaining sleep)
   A. Psychophysiological DIMS
   B. DIMS with affective disorders
   C. DIMS with tolerance to or withdrawal from central nervous system (CNS) depressants
   D. DIMS with sustained use of CNS stimulants
   E. DIMS with chronic alcoholism
   F. Sleep apnea DIMS syndrome
   G. Alveolar hypoventilation DIMS syndrome
   H. Sleep-related (nocturnal) myoclonus DIMS syndrome
   I. "Restless legs" DIMS syndrome
   J. Etc.

II. DOES (disorders of excessive somnolence)
   A. Psychophysiological DOES
   B. DOES with affective disorders
   C. DOES with sustained use of CNS depressants
   D. Sleep apnea DOES syndrome
   E. Alveolar hypoventilation DOES syndrome
   F. Sleep-related (nocturnal) myoclonus DOES syndrome
   G. "Restless legs" DOES syndrome
   H. Narcolepsy
   I. Idiopathic CNS hypersomnolence
   J. Etc.

III. Disorders of the sleep-wake pattern
   A. Rapid time-zone change ("jet lag") syndrome
   B. "Work shift" change in conventional sleep-wake schedule
   C. Frequently changing sleep-wake schedule
   D. Non-24-hour sleep-wake schedule
   E. Irregular sleep-wake pattern
   F. Etc.

IV. Dysfunctions associated with sleep, sleep stages, or partial arousals (parasomnias)
   A. Sleepwalking (somnambulism)
   B. Sleep-related enuresis
   C. Dream anxiety attacks (nightmares)
   D. Sleep-related epileptic seizures
   E. Familial sleep paralysis
   F. Sleep-related painful erections
   G. Sleep-related cluster headaches
   H. Sleep-related asthma
   I. Sleep-related cardiovascular symptoms
   J. Sleep-related hemolysis
   K. Etc.

From Williams and others: Heart Lung II(3):263, 1982.

---

enous obesity, kyphoscoliosis, and autonomic dysfunction.

Pathophysiology. Although the pathophysiology of SAS is unclear, hypotheses suggest that the various types of sleep apnea are all actually part of a disease continuum.[2] Failure of the central respiratory rhythm control center to generate a stable rhythm is thought to be the basic defect responsible for sleep apnea syndrome. Cyclical oscillations occur with greater frequency at night and are further exacerbated by mouth breathing.[2]

The patient with sleep apnea develops cycles of hypoxemia, hypercapnea, and acidosis with each episode of apnea until he or she is aroused and resumes breathing. Alveolar hypoventilation accompanies each episode of apnea and results in hypercapnea. Between episodes, alveolar ventilation improves so that overall there is not retention of CO_2. Morning headaches may result from lingering hypercapnea.

All types of sleep apnea are accompanied by arterial desaturation and hypoxemia, which may cause pulmonary vasoconstriction and an increased systemic vascular resistance. However, desaturation and hypoxemia are most severe in the obstructive type. With obstruction, inspiratory subatmospheric intrathoracic pressures are abnormally elevated. This leads to a tendency for airways to collapse, resulting in both hemodynamic and electrocardiographic changes.

The extremely elevated pressures that occur in individuals with obstructive sleep apnea who have apneic spells in both REM and NREM stages cause systemic and pulmonary hypertension. Systemic pressures of 200/120 mm Hg (awake control: 130/80 mm Hg) and pulmonary artery pressures of 80/54 mm Hg (awake control: 30/20 mm Hg) have been reported.[6] Cardiac dysrhythmias associated with obstructive apnea include bradycardias, sinus arrest, and occasionally, second-degree heart blocks. Following resumption of air flow, tachycardias commonly occur. Thus bradycardia-tachycardia syndrome is associated with obstructive sleep apnea. Hemodynamic monitoring can help the nurse identify this syndrome and assist in its diagnosis and treatment.

Assessment and diagnosis. The classic features of sleep apnea syndrome are daytime sleepiness and nocturnal snoring. Often the patient's partner originally reports the disrupted sleep, because of episodes of apnea and loud, abrupt sounds as breathing resumes. Patients become excessively sleepy during the day because of sleep fragmentation. Daytime napping and dozing at inappropriate times may be reported. Morning headaches are a complaint of many patients with SAS. The headache is frontal and diffuse, disappearing in several hours. Patients with SAS have increased motor activity during sleep. One significant difference between SAS and narcolepsy is that with the former, patients are able to keep themselves awake, whereas patients with narcolepsy cannot. Memory loss, poor judgment, decreased attention span, irritability, personality changes, exercise intolerance, and impotence often lead to employment difficulties and marital problems for sleep apnea patients.[6] Examination of the throat typically reveals enlarged tonsils, uvula, or tongue or excessive pharyngeal tissue.

Diagnosis of SAS is made by polysomnogram, a sleep study. The polysomnogram is used to determine the number and length of apnea episodes and sleep stages, number of arousals, air flow, respiratory effort, oxygen desaturation, and vital signs. This monitoring is done using the electroencephalogram, electrooculogram, electromyogram, and electrocardiogram. Respiratory air flow and effort is measured with nasal and oral thermistors and thoracic and abdominal strain gauges respectively. Gas exchange is monitored with an ear oximeter or a transcutaneous CO_2 electrode.

After SAS is diagnosed, the patient's hematocrit levels will be checked for signs of hypoxia-induced polycythemia. Arterial blood gases will be checked to assess for daytime hypoxia or hypercapnea. Thyroid function and the pharynx will be evaluated for causes of sleep apnea that can possibly be surgically corrected.

Medical treatment. Medical treatment includes surgical, medical, and mechanical approaches. The treatment is multiple and varied, depending on the type and extent of the patient's illness. Alcohol should be avoided, and weight loss should be encouraged. Medroxyprogesterone acetate (Provera), a central respiratory stimulant, has been shown to improve waking CO_2 retention. Protriptyline HCl (Vivactil), a nonsedating tricyclic antidepressant that supresses REM sleep, has been shown to decrease the number of apnea episodes and reduce daytime hypersomnolence. Acetozolamide is a respiratory stimulant that works by producing metabolic acidosis. Theophylline also has a stimulating effect and may be useful in some cases of SAS. Oxygen may be used to relieve hypoxemia and relieve nocturnal desaturations. In general, however, drug therapy has been disappointing in the treatment of SAS.[6]

Other therapies available include various appliances, such as nasal trumpets, tongue-retaining devices, nasal CPAP (continuous positive airway pressure), tracheostomy, and uvulopalatopharyngoplasty (UPPP). Nasal CPAP has been the most exciting development in recent years in the treatment of sleep apnea. Positive pressure is delivered via a mask placed over the nose that splints the airways open, improves oxygenation, and stimulates afferent impulses from the upper airways, resulting in reflex dilation of the upper airways and stimulation of ventilation. Obstructive sleep apnea is improved by nasal CPAP, which in turn improves the architecture of sleep and decreases daytime hypersomnolence.

Uvulopalatopharyngoplasty (UPPP) is a surgical approach to the treatment of obstructive sleep apnea. Essentially, a large tonsillectomy is performed, and redundant tissue is removed. Most patients following this procedure no longer snore; however, only 50% have their sleep apnea improved.[5] Because of the extensive resection of the posterior pharynx, regurgitation may be a problem for up to 33% of patients. Patient selection is important to the success of UPPP. By means of cephalometry or pharyngoscopy, the site of upper airway obstruction is identified.

Tracheostomy was the standard operation for obstructive sleep apnea but now is rarely used since the development of nasal CPAP. It is presently indicated for severe apnea with severe life-threatening dysrhythmias, cor pulmonale, hypersomnolence, and failure of conservative treatment. The complications of tracheostomy are significant, including infection, bleeding, bronchitis, and granulation tissue, as well as the psychosocial complications of an altered body image.

Nursing Diagnosis and Management
Status post uvulopalatopharyngoplasty (UPPP)

- Potential for Aspiration risk factors: impaired swallowing, altered gag reflex, gastrointestinal tube, p. 489

- Pain related to transmission and perception of noxious stimuli secondary to UPPP, p. 594

- Sleep Pattern Disturbance related to fragmented sleep, p. 88

- Anxiety related to threat to biological, psychological, and/or social integrity secondary to uncertain outcome of UPPP, p. 852

- Knowledge Deficit: Reportable Symptoms related to lack of previous exposure to information, p. 69

Nursing management Nursing care for patients diagnosed with SAS includes educating the patient, monitoring the effects of drug therapy, providing preoperative teaching, and monitoring for and preventing postoperative complications of UPPP or tracheostomy. Medroxyprogesterone acetate stimulates alveolar hypoventilation but in the dosages required for sleep apnea may be too expensive for some patients, and it may have feminizing effects in men. For these reasons, patient compliance with therapy may be jeopardized. Protryptyline reduces daytime hypersomnolence and nocturnal apneas. In addition to these effects, however, it has the anticholinergic effects of urinary retention and tolerance with prolonged use. Oxygen, as with other drugs, needs careful monitoring to verify its effectiveness and proper dosage.

Nasal CPAP is most effective when patients are properly fitted with the nasal mask and have adequate instruction in the application of the mask and blower. Allowing patients to develop comfort with the equipment facilitates the success of the therapy.

UPPP reduces the number of apneas. Complications of UPPP include bleeding, infection, swallowing difficulty, impaired speech, nasal reflux, dry mouth, increased gag reflex, and recurrence of snoring.[4] Patients need close postoperative observation of their airways because of airway edema (refer to Chapter 22, Ineffective Airway Clearance). Postoperative pain is common but manageable with analgesics. Precautions to avoid respiratory depression in this group of patients is imperative. Patients should be observed for regurgitation phenomena and signs of infection.

In the event that a tracheostomy is indicated, patients need to be evaluated for their ability to care for the tracheostomy at home. Careful preoperative instruction should include airway management techniques, such as suctioning and routine tracheostomy changes; information about communication techniques with the trach; explanation of comfort measures, such as pain relief; and close nursing observation. Emphasis should be placed on the relief of the apnea symptoms accomplished by the tracheostomy. Patients with UPPP may temporarily require a tracheostomy for airway management after the UPPP procedure. The critical care nurse must support the patient and family during the critical phase after the operation and be especially sensitive to long-term adjustments to changes in body image. In this case, the nurse can assist the patient to deal with possible disenchantment in the recovery phase.

Central Sleep Apnea

Definition, etiology, pathophysiology, assessment, and diagnosis. Central sleep apnea is the least common form of SAS. It is characterized by decreased respiratory output, resulting in absence of thoracic and abdominal movements. Patients complain of disrupted sleep and waking with a choking feeling. Snoring is absent. Patients tend to be older and have less-pronounced oxygen desaturation and hemodynamic effects.[4] Central apnea is associated with encephalitis, brainstem neoplasm or infarction, spinal cord injury, and bulbar poliomyelitis.

In the mixed type of SAS, there is no initial respiratory effort, but a progressive return of respiratory effort follows, thereby creating an air flow.[6] Mixed apneas are more common than central sleep apnea but less common than the obstructive type. Diagnosis is again made by polysomnography.

Medical treatment. Patients whose central sleep apnea is caused by a neurological deficit combined with chronic respiratory failure may require ventilatory support at night. This can be accomplished by a rocking bed, chest cuirass, iron lung, or portable ventilator. Phrenic nerve stimulation works for some patients. Medications used for central sleep apnea include acetazolamide (Diamox). The metabolic acidosis produced by medication stimulates the diaphragm.

Nursing management. The nursing management of the patient with a pure type of central sleep apnea involves careful nighttime observation and assessement of breathing pattern. Anxiety about or fear of sleep because of apneic episodes is common and should be confronted. Patient reassurance of continuous nursing observation and monitoring is helpful.

For the patient with a chest cuirass or iron lung, observation for upper airway collapse as a result of this treatment is essential. Supplemental oxygen may help some patients.[6]

REFERENCES

1. Association of Sleep Disorders Centers, prepared by the Sleep Disorders Classification Committee, Roffwarg HP, chairman: Diagnostic classification of sleep and arousal disorders, Sleep 2:1, 1979.
2. Bjurstrom R, Schoene R, and Pierson D: The control of ventilatory drives: physiology and clinical applications, Respir Care 31(11):1128, 1986.
3. Guilleminault C, van den Hoed J, and Milter M: Clinical overview of sleep apnea syndrome. In Guilleminault C and Dement WC, editors: Sleep apnea syndromes, New York, 1978, Alan R Liss Inc.
4. Mishoe S: The diagnosis and treatment of sleep apnea syndrome, Respir Care 32(3):183, 1987.
5. Sanders M and others: The acute effects of uvulopalatopharyngoplasty on breathing during sleep in sleep apnea patients, Sleep 11(1):75, 1988.
6. Weaver T and Millman R: Broken sleep. Am J Nurs 86(2):146, 1986.
7. Williams RL and Jackson D: Problems with sleep, Heart Lung 11(3):262, 1982.

Sleep Care Plans

THEORETICAL BASIS AND MANAGEMENT

CHAPTER OBJECTIVES

- *Define dysfunctional sleep.*
- *Define circadian desynchronization.*
- *Name three commonly prescribed critical care medications that decrease REM sleep.*
- *Describe common symptoms of sleep deprivation.*
- *Identify four interventions for sleep pattern disturbance related to fragmented sleep.*
- *Name two interventions for sleep pattern disturbance related to circadian desynchronization.*

THEORETICAL CONCEPTS ON SLEEP PATTERN DISTURBANCE
Dysfunctional Sleep

In the acutely ill patient, the amount, quality, and consistency of sleep may all decrease. Total sleep deprivation rarely occurs outside the experimental setting; however, in the critical care unit sleep is often interrupted or fragmented, which alters the normal stages and cycles and produces dysfunctional sleep. With frequent interruptions in sleep, the patient spends a larger proportion of time in the transitional stages (that is, NREM stages 1 and 2) and less time in the deeper stages of sleep (NREM stages 3 and 4 and REM). Thus patients may suffer a decrease in total sleep time (TST) if they do not receive their usual amount of sleep, and they may also experience selective deprivation of the deeper stages of sleep.[11]

Circadian Desynchronization

Circadian disruption or desynchronization is another form of sleep pattern disturbance that may affect critically ill patients. The loss of rhythmicity may result from external stressors, which then alters the timing relationships of neural, hormonal, and cellular systems. Animals and humans respond to stressors such as surgery, immobilization, and pain with increased levels and altered timing of adrenal

hormones and other hormones.[4] Farr[4] reported that circadian levels; the timing of temperature, blood pressure, and heart rate; and urinary excretion of catecholamines, sodium, and potassium were altered following surgery in hospitalized patients. Nurses should closely observe patients for signs and symptoms of such alterations and anticipate problems such as poor responses to physiological challenges, disruption of sleep, gastrointestinal disturbances, decreased vigilance and attention span, and malaise. Nursing interventions that maintain normal rhythmicity of the day-night cycle, such as opening window blinds, placing clocks and calendars within the patient's view, and allowing the patient to retire and rise at familiar times should be encouraged. Attention should be given to minimizing disruption during rest periods.[4]

PHARMACOLOGY AND SLEEP

Patients hospitalized in critical care units often receive pharmacological therapy, which may affect their quality of sleep and compound sleep disturbances. The critical care nurse should be aware of the effects that commonly used drugs have on sleep. In fact, hypnotic drugs have been found to promote the lighter stages of sleep (that is, NREM stage 2) and may, paradoxically, be the cause of night terrors, hallucinations, and agitation in the elderly.[8] This is an area that has great potential for nursing research.

Barbiturates and sedative-hypnotic and analgesic medications may compound sleep disorders by further decreasing NREM stages 3 and 4 and REM sleep. Amobarbital, secobarbital, and pentobarbital reduce REM and increase NREM stage 2 sleep. Phenobarbital facilitates stage 4 NREM but decreases REM in doses greater than 200 mg. *REM rebound* (discussed later in this chapter) has been documented after the patient is withdrawn from phenobarbital therapy.[11]

Diazepam increases NREM stage 1 and reduces both NREM stages 3 and 4 and REM. REM suppression depends on the dose, with the larger doses leading to greater suppression. Flurazepam hydrochloride may be an effective hypnotic if administered in dosages equaling less than 60 mg/

day. However, the long half-life of flurazepam may lead to morning drowsiness and may increase sleep apneic episodes in susceptible persons. Chloral hydrate has been shown to be an effective sedative that does not simultaneously disrupt sleep. Chlordiazepoxide and methaqualone also minimally disrupt sleep. Triazolam is effective for short-term use in increasing the total sleep time and decreasing the number of nocturnal awakenings, although it decreases REM sleep during the first 6 hours of sleep. These REM changes have been predominantly noted in young adults. An early morning "hangover" may occur with triazolam, and rebound insomnia may occur in the first 2 nights following discontinuation of the drug.[1] Morphine increases spontaneous arousals during sleep and shortens the sleep time by reducing both REM and NREM stages 3 and 4, resulting in overall lighter sleep.[14]

The prolonged half-life of medications, coupled with altered metabolism or decreased excretion of the drug resulting from renal or liver disease that may occur in the elderly, can cause the effects of sedatives to continue into the daytime, leading to confusion and sluggishness. Sedative and analgesic medications should not be withheld, but rather, drugs that minimally disrupt sleep should be used to complement comfort measures with dosages reduced gradually as the medication is no longer necessary. It is the responsibility of the critical care nurse to assess the need for sedative and analgesic medication, to administer them in the most effective manner to promote sleep, and to monitor their effectiveness (see Table 8-1).

SLEEP DEPRIVATION

Much of what is known about the function of sleep has been learned from observations made when people are deprived of sleep in the laboratory setting. Both physiological and psychological symptoms of sleep deprivation have been reported.[1] (See the box on p. 86.) These symptoms may be, but are not always, associated with the length of sleep deprivation. The symptoms vary among individuals with such factors as age, premorbid personality, motivation, and environmental factors.[5]

Table 8-1 Common drugs that affect sleep

Drug	Effect on sleep	Comments
BARBITURATES		
Amobarbital	Increase NREM 2	Not considered drugs of choice because of toxicity
Pentobarbital	Suppress REM	and long-lasting effects.
Secobarbital		Often patients experience rebound insomnia, restless sleep, and frequent dreaming and nightmares when drugs are discontinued.
Phenobarbital	Facilitates NREM 4	REM rebound (increased REM in subsequent
	Decreases REM in doses greater than 200 mg.	sleep) after withdrawal of phenobarbital.
BENZODIAZEPINES		
Diazepam	Increases NREM 1	NREM suppression is not dose related.
	Decreases NREM 3 and 4	REM suppression is dose related.
	Decreases REM	May increase sleep apneic episodes.
Flurazepam	Increases total sleep time	Conflicting reports about effects on sleep.
	Decreases NREM 2, 3, and 4	Long half-life may produce daytime drowsiness.
	Decreases REM	
Midazolam hydrochloride	No reports available as yet	
Triazolam	Decreases sleep latency (time it takes to get to sleep)	Drug has a short half-life.
	Decreases awakenings	Should not be used for a prolonged time because of decreased effectiveness.
	Increases total sleep time	
MISCELLANEOUS		
Chloral hydrate	Thought to be an effective sedative that does not disrupt sleep	Drug has a short half-life, and some reports of nightmares.
		Increased daytime drowsiness.
Chlordiazepoxide	Minimally disrupt sleep	
Methaqualone		
Morphine sulfate	Decreases NREM 3 and 4	Results in increased spontaneous arousals and
	Decreases REM	overall lighter sleep.

EFFECTS OF SELECTIVE
SLEEP DEPRIVATION

SYMPTOMS OF NREM SLEEP DEPRIVATION

Fatigue
Anxiety
Increased illness

SYMPTOMS OF REM SLEEP DEPRIVATION

Restlessness
Disorientation
Combativeness
Delusions
Hallucinations

Selective *REM deprivation* leads to irritability, apathy, decreased alertness, and increased sensitivity to pain. Continued loss of REM sleep may lead to perceptual distortion and significant disturbance in mental-emotional function, often within 72 hours of REM deprivation. Manifestations of sleep deprivation range from disorientation and restlessness to frank auditory and visual hallucinations, with personality changes including withdrawal and paranoia.[5]

Selective *NREM deprivation* is less well studied, but it appears that fatigue is the primary result of NREM deprivation.[14] Because of the renewal, repair, and conservation functions of NREM sleep, deprivation impairs the immune system and depresses the body's defenses, rendering the individual vulnerable to disease.[12]

The critical care environment affects both the quantity and quality of sleep the critically ill patient receives. The patient admitted to a critical care unit is bombarded with combined sensory overload and deprivation and unfamiliar sights, sounds, people, and perceptions. Such environmental conditions have been shown to be of primary importance in sleep deprivation in the critical care unit. Dlin, Rosen, and Dickstein[2] showed the chief deterrents to sleep in the critical care unit in order of importance were activity and noise, pain and physical condition, nursing procedures, lights, vapor tents, and hypothermia. Woods and Falk[13] found that 10% to 17% of noises in the critical care unit were of a level capable of arousing patients from sleep (greater than 70 decibels).

Using EEGs, Hilton[7] documented quantity and quality of sleep of nine patients in a respiratory critical care unit. Total sleep time ranged from 6 minutes to 13.3 hours. Only 50% to 60% of the sleep occurred at night, and no patients had complete sleep cycles. NREM stage 1 sleep predominated, to the deprivation of all other stages. Significant deprivation of restorative sleep (NREM stages 3 and 4) was demonstrated by only 4.7% to 10.5% of sleep time being spent in these stages (normally 30% to 35%). Sleep-disturbing events validated by EEG were mainly staff and environmental noise, which occurred on the average of every 20 minutes. Quality and quantity of sleep were reported as poor in all subjects. Nightmares, hallucinations, restlessness, or other

behavioral changes were observed in 60% of the patients in the sample.

Psychological stresses and fear associated with the critical care environment and the critical illness make it difficult for patients to relax and fall asleep. Fear and stress precipitate sympathetic nervous system stimulation, which decreases the arousal threshold and results in frequent awakenings and sleep stage transitions.[11]

The relationship between sleep deprivation and delirium in the critical care unit has been shown to be significant.[6] In a study of 62 patients in critical care units and surgical critical care units who ranged in age from 16 to 70 years, Helton, Gordon, and Nunnery[6] correlated mental status alterations (disorientation, combativeness, hallucinations, paranoia, and delusions) and sleep deprivation. A 33% increase in mental status alterations was found in severely sleep-deprived patients, defined as those who received less than 50% of their normal sleep time.

Mortality is higher in critical care patients who exhibit symptoms of psychosis or delirium.[9] Perhaps persons experiencing hallucinations and paranoia (the most severe consequences of sleep deprivation and critical care unit psychosis) are in fact dreaming in the awake state. This hypothesis remains to be verified by research; however, caution needs to be taken in diagnosing a previously nonconfused elderly patient as having organic mental disorder (OMD) until the possibility of sleep deprivation has been ruled out.

"There is substantial evidence to support the fact that 4 days of sleep deprivation results in a decreased production of ATP, the critical energy substance. Sleep returns this balance to normal."[3] An understanding of the stages of sleep and the effects of sleep deprivation assists the nurse in evaluating the quantity and quality of sleep her or his patients receive (see Fig. 8-1).

RECOVERY SLEEP

When an individual has sleep deprivation, the changes in physiological and psychological performance can be reversed through recovery sleep. Rosa, Bonnet, and Warm[10] found that recall returned to baseline with 4 to 8 hours of recovery sleep after 40 to 64 hours of total sleep deprivation (see Fig. 8-2).

Deprivation of REM and NREM stage 4 results in rebounds in an attempt to compensate for "debts." The phenomenon of *REM rebound* occurs following selective REM deprivation. In an attempt to make up for lost REM and NREM stage 4 sleep, REM and NREM stage 4 periods quantitatively increase in the sleep periods following the deprivation. NREM stage 4 sleep is preferentially restored first, presumably because of its anabolic function. Because REM sleep is replenished last, it is more likely that REM debts will occur. REM rebound can exacerbate angina, dysrhythmias, duodenal ulcer pain, or sleep apneic episodes.[11] When a patient is exhibiting any of these symptoms and has had a period of sleep deprivation, REM rebound should be considered when determining the cause. Although the symptoms of angina, dysrhythmias, duodenal ulcer pain, and sleep apnea are treated as usual, further REM deprivation should be avoided.

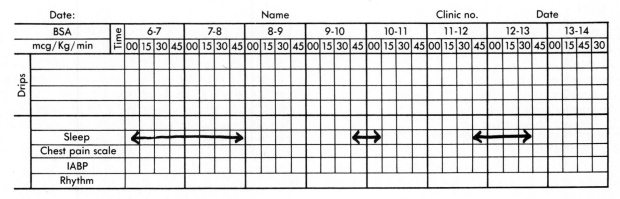

Date:		Time	6-7				7-8				8-9				9-10				10-11				11-12				12-13				13-14			
BSA																																			
mcg/Kg/min			00	15	30	45	00	15	30	45	00	15	30	45	00	15	30	45	00	15	30	45	00	15	30	45	00	15	30	45	00	15	45	30
Drips																																			
	Sleep																																	
	Chest pain scale																																	
	IABP																																	
	Rhythm																																	

Fig. 8-1   Sample critical care flow sheet.

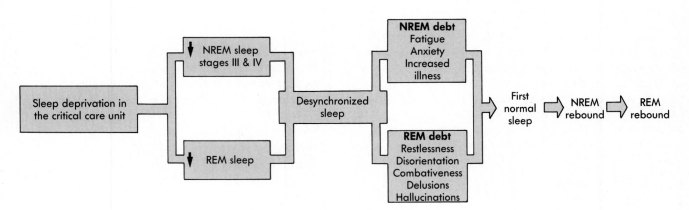

Fig. 8-2   The effects of sleep deprivation on sleep cycling, debt, and rebound.
(Modified from Slota M: Focus Crit Care 15(3):41, 1988).

Sleep Pattern Disturbance related to fragmented sleep

DEFINING CHARACTERISTICS

- Decreased sleep during one block of sleep time
- Daytime sleepiness
- Sleep deprivation
  Less than one half normal total sleep time
  Decreased slow wave or REM sleep
- Anxiety
- Fatigue
- Restlessness
- Disorientation and hallucinations
- Combativeness
- Frequent wakenings
- Decreased arousal threshold

OUTCOME CRITERIA

- Patient's total sleep time approximates patient's normal.
- Patient is able to complete sleep cycles of 90 minutes without interruption.
- Patient has no delusions, hallucinations, illusions.
- Patient has reality-based thought content.
- Patient is oriented to four spheres.

NURSING INTERVENTIONS *AND RATIONALE*

1. Continue to monitor the assessment parameters listed under "Defining Characteristics."
2. Assess normal sleep pattern on admission and any history of sleep disturbance or chronic illness that may affect sleep or sedative/hypnotic use. Promote normal sleep activity while patient is in critical care unit. Assess sleep effectiveness by asking patient how his or her sleep in the hospital compares to sleep at home. (Refer to Chapter 28, *Sensory-Perceptual Alterations*, for the management of acutely psychotic/suspicious patient.)
3. Minimize awakenings *to allow for at least 90 minute sleep cycles.* Continually assess the need to awaken the patient, particularly at night. Distinguish between essential and nonessential nursing tasks. Organize nursing care to allow for maximum amount of uninterrupted sleep while ensuring close monitoring of the patient's condition. Whenever possible, monitor physiological parameters without waking the patient. Coordinate awakenings with other departments such as respiratory therapy, laboratory, and x-ray *to minimize sleep interruptions.*
4. Minimize noise, particularly that of the staff and noisy equipment. Reduce the level of environmental stimuli. Refer to interventions to minimize sensory overload, p. 601.
5. Plan nap times to assist in equilibrating the normal total sleep time. Discourage or prevent catnaps (sleep lasting longer than 90 minutes at a time) as *these physically refresh the individual and thereby decrease the stimulus for longer sleep cycles in which REM sleep is obtained.* Early morning naps, however, may be beneficial in promoting REM sleep *as a greater proportion of early morning sleep is allocated to REM activity.*
6. Promote comfort, relaxation, and a sense of well-being. Treat pain. Eliminate stressful situations before bedtime. Use of relaxation techniques, imagery, backrubs, or warm blankets may be helpful. Other interventions may include increased privacy or a private room. Individual patients may prefer quiet or may prefer the background noise of the television *to best promote sleep.*
7. Be aware of the effects of commonly used medications on sleep. *Many sedative and hypnotic medications decrease REM sleep.* Sedative and analgesic medications should not be withheld, but rather, drugs that minimally disrupt sleep should be used to complement comfort measures, with dosages reduced gradually as the medication is no longer necessary. Do not abruptly withdraw REM-suppressing medications, because *this can result in "REM rebound."*
8. Foods containing tryptophan, e.g., milk or turkey, may be appropriate because *these promote sleep.*
9. Be aware that the best treatment for sleep deprivation is prevention.
10. Facilitate staff awareness that sleep is essential and health promoting. Assess for the critical care unit sleep-reducing stimuli and work to minimize them.
11. Document amount of uninterrupted sleep per shift, especially sleep episodes lasting longer than 2 hours. This can be effectively documented as part of the 24-hour flow sheet and reported routinely, shift to shift. *Sleep pattern disturbance is diagnosed, treated, and resolved more efficiently when formally documented in this manner.*

Sleep Pattern Disturbance related to circadian desynchronization

DEFINING CHARACTERISTICS

- Sleep is out of synchronization with biological rhythms, resulting in sleeping during the day and awakening at night
- Anxiety and restlessness
- Decreased arousal threshold

OUTCOME CRITERIA

- Majority of patient's sleep time will fall during low cycle of the circadian rhythm (normally at night).

NURSING INTERVENTIONS *AND RATIONALE*

1. Continue to monitor the assessment parameters listed under "Defining Characteristics."
2. Assist patient to maintain normal day-night cycles by decreasing lighting, noise, and sensory stimulation at night and critically evaluating the need to awaken the patient at night.
3. Activity during the daytime should be increased to stimulate wakefulness. Increased physical activity until 2 hours before bedtime is useful in *promoting naturally induced sleep.* Limiting caffeine intake after early afternoon will promote sleep in the evening.
4. Do not schedule routine procedures at night.
5. Be aware that cardiac dysrhythmias can be precipitated by the decreased arousal threshold secondary to desynchronization.
6. If desynchronization occurs, plan for resynchronization by maintaining constancy in day-night pattern for at least 3 days (may require 5 to 12 days to reacclimatize). Plan for activities during the day *to stimulate wakefulness* and use comfort measures (comfortable body position, warm blankets, backrub, etc.) *to promote sleep* at night. Resynchronization is characteristically associated with chronic fatigue, malaise, and a decreased ability to perform life tasks.[11]

REFERENCES

1. Brewer MJ: To sleep or not to sleep: the consequences of sleep deprivation, Crit Care Nurse 5(6):35, 1985.
2. Dlin B, Rosen H, and Dickstein K: The problems of sleep and rest in the intensive care unit, Psychosomatics 12:155, 1971.
3. Fabijan M and Gosselin M: How to recognize sleep deprivation in your ICU patient and what to do about it, Can Nurse 4:20, 1982.
4. Farr LA, Campbell-Grossman C, and Mack JM: Circadian disruption and surgical recovery, Nurs Res 37(3):170, 1988.
5. Freemon F: Sleep research, Springfield, Ill, 1972, Charles C Thomas, Publisher.
6. Helton M, Gordon S, and Nunnery S: The correlation between sleep deprivation and ICU syndrome, Heart Lung 9(3):464, 1980.
7. Hilton B: Quantity and quality of patient's sleep and sleep disturbing factors in a respiratory intensive care unit, Adv Nurs 1:453, 1976.
8. Lerner R: Sleep loss in the aged: implications for nursing practice, J Gerontol Nurs 8(6):323, 1982.
9. Noble M: Communication in the ICU: therapeutic or disturbing, Nurs Outlook 27:195, 1979.
10. Rosa R, Bonnet M, and Warm J: Recovery of performance during sleep following sleep deprivation, Psychophysiology 20:152, 1983.
11. Sanford S: Sleep and the cardiac patient, Cardiovasc Nurs 19(5):19, 1983.
12. Schirmer M: When sleep won't come, J Gerontol Nurs 9(1):16, 1983.
13. Woods N and Falk S: Noise stimuli in the acute care area, Nurs Res 23:144, 1974.
14. Wotring K: Using research in practice, Focus Crit Care 9(5):34, 1982.

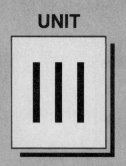

UNIT

III

NUTRITIONAL ALTERATIONS

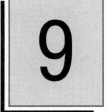

CHAPTER

9

Nutritional Assessment and Support

CHAPTER OBJECTIVES

- Describe the adverse effects of nutritional impairments on critically ill patients.
- Assess the nutritional status of critically ill patients.
- Participate with other health care team members in designing an effective nutrition support program for a patient in the critical care unit.
- Develop a nursing care plan for the patient receiving nutrition support.
- Identify complications of nutrition support and nursing measures for prevention and treatment of these complications.
- Evaluate the patient's response to nutrition support.

Extreme underfeeding or starvation of a healthy adult results in an initial decline in metabolic rate, which serves to protect the body from excessive tissue catabolism. Early in starvation, serum glucose levels drop by 10% to 15%. This drop causes a decrease in insulin release and an increase in glucagon, which in turn results in an increase in the following processes: glycogenolysis (glycogen breakdown), lipolysis (fat breakdown), and gluconeogenesis (catabolism of amino acids to produce glucose). There are limitations in the ability of body carbohydrate and fat stores to provide metabolic fuel for the body. Glycogen stores are essentially used up within a few hours of fasting. Although fat reserves are almost unlimited in many adults, not all body tissues can utilize fat. Initially, tissues such as the brain, peripheral nervous system, leukocytes, and erythrocytes depend solely on glucose. Although some of these tissues are eventually able to adapt so that they rely primarily on ketone bodies derived from fats, some (such as the erythrocytes) continue to utilize glucose, which can only be supplied by protein.

When stress (for example, major surgery, trauma, burns, or infection) accompanies starvation, sympathetic stimulation triggers the release of the catecholamines norepinephrine and epinephrine. These catecholamines increase the metabolic rate and thus the amount of catabolism required to provide sufficient fuel for the body. This can rapidly exacerbate the deterioration that accompanies starvation.

Prolonged starvation can be detrimental. Skeletal muscle catabolism weakens and debilitates the patient. Wasting of the diaphragm and intercostal muscles, for instance, impairs the ability to breathe deeply and cough and may contribute to development of atelectasis and pneumonia. Even more serious is the loss of visceral proteins such as serum proteins, immunoglobulins, and leukocytes. These proteins have critical roles, including the transport of some nutrients to the cells, maintenance of immunocompetence, and maintenance of plasma oncotic pressure.

Surveys of hospitalized patients have revealed that 12% to 48% of them show signs of malnutrition or starvation at admission.[15,37,38] Critically ill patients are especially vulnerable, with more than 40% of these patients being malnourished at the time of admission.[10] An even more ominous finding is that the nutritional status of more than two thirds of medical patients hospitalized for 2 weeks or longer deteriorates during hospitalization.[38] Patients who are hospitalized for longer than 2 weeks tend to be the sickest patients, and some of the nutritional deterioration may be ascribed to the severity of their illnesses. Other possible contributing factors include lack of communication among the nurses, physicians, and dietitians responsible for the care of these patients; frequent diagnostic testing, which causes patients to miss meals or to be too exhausted for meals; medications and other therapies that cause anorexia, nausea, or vomiting and thus interfere with food intake; or inadequate use of tube feedings or total parenteral nutrition to maintain the nutritional status of these patients.

When protein and calorie intake are inadequate for more than a few hours, existing body proteins will be broken down to meet the body's needs. Even when the individual has large fat reserves, catabolism of body proteins will occur. Unlike fat, proteins can provide the amino acids that are needed for tissue synthesis and repair and can also provide a significant source of glucose. The well-nourished individual tolerates a few days of starvation when not exposed to stress, but a patient with trauma, surgery, burns,

91

or infection, along with inadequate nutritional intake will have accelerated catabolism. An already undernourished patient exposed to stress (for example, a cancer patient with anorexia and weight loss who undergoes surgery) will be especially vulnerable.

Malnutrition is an ominous finding among the very ill. Undernourished patients are three times as likely as well-nourished patients to have major surgical complications.[37] Wound dehiscence, decubitus ulcers, sepsis, and pulmonary infections are more common among the undernourished. Hospital stays of medical patients with evidence of malnutrition are approximately two thirds longer than those of well-nourished patients, and mortality is three times greater.[38]

Nutrition assessment is the process of obtaining and interpreting patient data about nutritional status. It provides a basis for identifying patients who are malnourished or at risk of becoming malnourished, determining the nutritional needs of individual patients, and selecting the most appropriate methods of nutritional support for patients with or at risk of developing nutritional deficits. Nutrition support (the provision of specially formulated or delivered enteral or intravenous nutrients to prevent or treat malnutrition)[1] provides a method of coping with the nutritional problems of very ill patients both in the hospital and at home.

ASSESSING NUTRITIONAL STATUS

Nutrition assessment is a multistep process involving the collection and evaluation of pertinent information from the patient's diet and medical history, physical examination, and laboratory values. The assessment can be performed by a designated member of the health care team, such as the dietitian or the nurse, or it can be a team effort.

History

Information about dietary intake and significant variations in weight are vital parts of the history. A change of 10% or more in body weight during the past year or 5% to 6% during the last 3 months is usually considered significant. Dietary intake can be evaluated in several ways, including a diet record, a 24-hour recall, and a diet history. The diet record, a listing of the type and amount of all foods and beverages consumed for some period of time (usually 3 days), is useful for evaluating the patient's intake in the critical care setting if there is a question of the adequacy of intake. However, it tends to reveal little about the patient's habitual intake before the illness or injury. The 24-hour recall of all food and beverage intake is easily and quickly performed, but it, too, may not reflect the patient's usual intake and thus has limited usefulness. The diet history consists of a detailed interview about the patient's usual

Table 9-1 Nutrition history information

Area of concern	Significant findings	Nutrients of special concern
Inadequate intake of nutrients	Avoidance of specific food groups because of poverty or poor dentition	Protein, iron
	Alcohol abuse	Protein; vitamin B$_1$, niacin, folate
	Anorexia, nausea, vomiting	Most nutrients, particularly protein, electrolytes
	Confusion, coma	All nutrients
Inadequate absorption of nutrients	Previous GI surgeries:	
	Gastrectomy	Vitamin B$_{12}$, minerals, calories (if the patient experiences dumping syndrome)
	Ileal resection	Vitamins B$_{12}$, A, E; minerals; calories (in extensive small bowel resection)
	Certain medications:	
	Antacids, cimetidine (reduce upper duodenal acidity)	Minerals
	Cholestyramine (binds fat soluble nutrients)	Vitamins A, D, E, K
	Corticosteroids	Protein
	Anticonvulsants	Calcium
Increased nutrient losses	Chronic or acute blood loss	Iron
	Severe diarrhea	Fluid, electrolytes
	Fistula, draining abscesses, wounds	Protein, zinc
	Nephrotic syndrome	Protein, zinc
	Peritoneal dialysis or hemodialysis	Protein, zinc, water soluble vitamins
Increased nutrient requirements	Fever	Calories
	Surgery, trauma, burns, infection	Calories, protein, zinc, vitamin C
	Neoplasms (some types)	Calories, protein
	Physiological demands (pregnancy, lactation, growth)	Calories, protein, iron

*Each 1° C (1.8° F) elevation in temperature increases caloric needs approximately 13%.

intake, along with social, familial, cultural, economic, educational, and health-related factors that may affect intake. Although the diet history is time consuming to perform and may be too stressful for the acutely ill patient, it provides a wealth of information about food habits over a prolonged period and provides a basis for planning specific patient teaching, if changes in eating habits are desirable. Other information to include in a nutrition history is listed in Table 9-1.

Physical Assessment

Anthropometric measurements. Obtaining anthropometric or body measurements, of which height and weight are the most important, is the first step in physical evaluation. If at all possible, height and weight should be measured, rather than obtained through patient or family report. Skinfold measurements, another anthropometrical parameter, provide an estimate of body fat, which is helpful in diagnosing obesity and malnutrition. The triceps skinfold is the most commonly used (see Fig. 9-1). The triceps skinfold (TSF) is measured at the midpoint of the upper arm, which is located by taking half the distance between the olecranon and acromion. The TSF is obtained by grasping the skin and subcutaneous tissue at the back of the arm about 1 cm from the midpoint. Special calipers are then applied to the skinfold at the midpoint, and the skinfold reading is taken to the nearest millimeter. Skinfold measurements are best

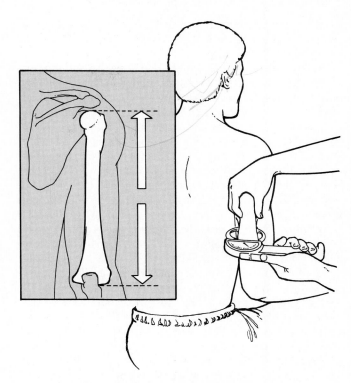

Fig. 9-1 Measuring the triceps skinfold.

Table 9-2 Signs and symptoms of nutritional alterations

Finding	Possible deficiency	Possible excess of
HEAD AND NECK		
Hair loss	Protein, zinc, biotin	Vitamin A
Dull, dry, brittle hair; loss of hair pigment	Protein	
Conjunctival and corneal dryness	Vitamin A	
Blue sclerae	Iron	
Pale conjunctiva	Iron	
Gingivitis	Vitamin C	
Cheilosis or angular stomatitis (lesions at corners of mouth)	Vitamin B_2	
Glossitis	Niacin, folate, vitamin B_{12}, other B vitamins	
Hypogeusia (poor sense of taste), dysgeusia (bad taste)	Zinc	
SKIN AND NAILS		
Dry, scaly	Vitamin A, zinc, essential fatty acids	Vitamin A
Follicular hyperkeratosis (resembles gooseflesh)	Vitamin A	
Eczematous lesions	Zinc	
Petechiae, ecchymoses	Vitamin C or K	
Poor wound healing	Protein, zinc, vitamin C	
Koilonychia (spoon-shaped nails)	Iron	
ABDOMEN		
Hepatomegaly	Protein	Vitamin A
MUSCULOSKELETAL AND EXTREMITIES		
Muscle wasting	Calories	
Edema	Protein, vitamin B_1	
Paresthesias	Vitamins B_1, B_6, B_{12}, biotin	

performed by specially trained nurses and dietitians, because the measurements tend to vary greatly when performed by inexperienced personnel.

Anthropometric measurements are sometimes compared with tables of standard values for large numbers of healthy people. Generally, measurements are considered abnormal if less than the 10th percentile or greater than the 90th. A guideline often used for evaluating body weight states that ideal weight for men is 106 pounds plus 6 pounds for every inch in height over 5 feet, and ideal weight for women is 100 pounds plus 5 pounds for every inch over 5 feet. Thus a man 6 feet 2 inches tall would be expected to weigh 190 pounds (86.4 kilograms). However, standard tables are not always reliable. For instance, an obese woman who has lost 33 pounds (15 kilograms) over the previous 4 months may be within the normal range for weight while suffering from malnutrition. Furthermore, standard tables fail to take into account variations in weight with body build. The best use of anthropometric measurements is for comparison of changes in an individual over a period of time. Good judgment must be used in interpreting anthropometric data. As an example, edema may mask significant weight loss and may also falsely elevate skinfold readings.

Physical examination. A thorough physical examination is an essential part of nutrition assessment. Table 9-2 lists some of the more common findings that may indicate an altered nutritional state. It is especially important for the nurse to check for signs of muscle wasting, loss of subcutaneous fat, skin or hair changes, and impairment of wound healing.

Laboratory Data

A wide range of diagnostic tests can provide information about nutritional status. Those most often used in the clinical setting are described in Table 9-3. As the table emphasizes, there are no perfect diagnostic tests for evaluation of nutrition, and care must be taken in interpreting the results of the tests.

Evaluating Nutritional Assessment Findings and Determining Nutritional Needs

It is rare for a patient to exhibit a lack of only one nutrient. Usually nutritional deficiencies are combined, with the patient lacking adequate amounts of protein and calories and possibly vitamins and minerals. A common form of combined nutritional deficit among hospitalized patients is protein-calorie malnutrition. Protein deficits, sometimes referred to as *kwashiorkor,* are evidenced by low levels of the serum proteins albumin, transferrin, and prealbumin; low total lymphocyte count; impaired immunity; loss of hair or hair pigment; edema; and an enlarged, fatty liver. Calorie deficits, termed *marasmus,* are recognizable by weight loss, a decrease in skinfold measurements, loss of subcutaneous fat, muscle wasting, and low levels of creatinine excretion. Since protein-calorie malnutrition weakens musculature, increases vulnerability to infection, and can prolong hospital stays, the health care team should diagnose this serious disorder as quickly as possible so that appropriate nutritional intervention can be implemented.

Nutrition assessment provides a basis for estimating nutritional needs. Table 9-4 demonstrates methods that are frequently used in estimating the calorie and protein needs of patients.

ADMINISTERING NUTRITION SUPPORT
Enteral Nutrition Support

The enteral route is the preferred method of feeding whenever possible, because this route is generally safer, more physiological, and much less expensive than parenteral feeding. There are a variety of enteral feeding products, some of which are designed to meet the specialized needs of very sick patients. Some products can be consumed orally, but many of the specialized ones are so unpalatable that they are solely reserved for tube feeding. Table 9-5 provides more information about the major categories of products.

Oral supplementation. For patients who can eat and have normal digestion and absorption, but simply cannot consume enough regular foods to meet caloric and protein needs, oral supplementation may be necessary. Patients with mild to moderate anorexia, burns, or trauma sometimes fall into this category. To improve intake and tolerance of supplements, the critical care nurse should:

1. Collaborate with the dietitian to choose appropriate products and allow the patient to participate in the selection process if possible. Milk shakes made with ice cream and half-and-half; powdered milk added to cereal and fluid milk; and instant breakfast are often more palatable and economical than commercial supplements. However, intolerance of lactose (milk sugar) is common among adults, especially blacks, Orientals, American Indians, and Eskimos. Furthermore, many disease processes (for example, Crohn's disease, radiation enteritis, and severe gastroenteritis) are associated with lactose intolerance. Individuals with this problem experience abdominal cramping, bloating, and diarrhea after lactose ingestion and may require commercial lactose-free supplements.

2. Serve commercial supplements well chilled or on ice, because this improves flavor.

3. Advise patients to sip formulas slowly, consuming no more than 240 ml over 30 to 45 minutes. These products contain easily digested carbohydrates. If formulas are consumed too quickly, rapid hydrolysis of the carbohydrate in the duodenum can contribute to dumping syndrome, characterized by abdominal cramping, weakness, tachycardia, and diarrhea.

4. Record all supplement intake separately on the intake and output sheet so that it can be differentiated from intake of water and other liquids.

Enteral tube feedings. Tube feedings are used for patients who have at least some digestive and absorptive capability but are unwilling or unable to consume enough by mouth. Patients with profound anorexia and those experiencing severe stress (for instance, major burns or trauma) that greatly increases their nutritional needs often benefit from tube feedings. Individuals who require elemental formulas or the specialized formulas for altered metabolic conditions (see Table 9-5) usually require tube feeding because the unpleasant flavors of the free amino acids, peptides, or

Table 9-3 Diagnostic tests used in nutrition assessment

Area of concern	Possible deficiency	Comments
SERUM PROTEINS		
*Decrease of serum albumin, transferrin (iron transport protein), or thyroxine-binding prealbumin	Protein	These proteins are produced in the liver, depressed in hepatic failure, and are falsely low in fluid volume excess and elevated in volume deficit. Albumin has long half-life (14-20 days) and is slow to change in malnutrition and repletion; transferrin has a half-life of 7-8 days, but levels increase in iron deficiency, and prevalence of iron deficiency limits usefulness in diagnosing protein deficits; prealbumin half-life is 2-3 days, levels fall in trauma and infection
HEMATOLOGICAL VALUES		
Anemia (decreased Hct, Hgb)		Hct and Hgb are falsely low in fluid volume excess and falsely high in fluid volume deficit
Normocytic (normal MCV, MCHC)	Protein	
Microcytic (decreased MCV, MCH, MCHC)	Iron, copper	
Macrocytic (increased MCV)	Folate, vitamin B_{12}	
Total lymphocyte count (TLC) = WBC × % lymphocytes		
TLC <1200 mm³	Protein	Decreased in severe debilitating disease
URINARY CREATININE		
Creatinine excretion <17 mg/kg/day (women), <23 mg/kg/day (men)	Protein (reflects lean body mass)	Difficult to collect accurate 24-hr urine; wide variation in creatinine excretion from day to day; levels decline with age as percentage of lean body mass declines
NITROGEN BALANCE†		
Negative values	Protein, calories (during calorie deficit, protein is metabolized to provide calories)	Negative values occur when more nitrogen is excreted than is consumed (reflects inadequate intake or increased needs); positive values occur when more is consumed than lost (e.g., during nutrition repletion, growth, or pregnancy); normal healthy adults excrete exactly what they consume. Limitations: difficult to collect accurate 24-hr urine; retention of nitrogen does not necessarily mean that it is being used for tissue synthesis

*Evaluation of at least one of these is a part of almost every nutritional assessment.
†Protein is 16% nitrogen. Thus nitrogen balance = [24-hr protein intake (g) × 0.16] − [24-hr urine nitrogen (g) + 4g]. The 4 g is an estimate of fecal, skin, and other minor losses.

Table 9-4 Estimating nutritional requirements

ESTIMATING CALORIC NEEDS

1. Calculate basal energy expenditure (BEE). This is the energy needed for basic life processes such as respiration, cardiac function, and maintenance of body temperature.

   Women: BEE = 655 + (9.6 × W) + (1.7 × H) − (4.7 × A)

   Men: BEE = 66 + (13.7 × W) + (5 × H) − (6.8 × A)

   W = Current weight in kg; H = Height in cm; A = Age in yr

2. Multiply BEE by an appropriate activity factor.

Level of activity	Multiply BEE by
Bed rest	1.2
Light (e.g., sedentary office work)	1.3
Moderate (e.g., nursing)	1.4
Strenuous (e.g., manual labor)	1.5 or more

3. Multiply by an appropriate stress factor to meet the needs of the ill or injured patient.

Type of stress	Multiply the value obtained in step 2 by
Fever	1 + 0.13/°C elevation above normal (or 0.07/°F)
Pneumonia	1.2
Major injury	1.3
Severe sepsis	1.5-1.6
Major burns	1.8-2

ESTIMATING PROTEIN NEEDS

Protein needs vary with degree of malnutrition and stress.

Condition	Multiply desirable body weight (kg) by
Healthy individual or well-nourished elective surgery patient	0.8-1 g protein
Malnourished or catabolic state (e.g., sepsis, major injury, burns)	1.2-2+ g protein

Example of calculation of needs

A 38-year-old male patient with pelvic, rib, and long-bone fractures; pneumothorax, and a ruptured spleen following a motor vehicle accident. Height 180 cm (5'11"), current weight 81.8 kg (180 lb), desirable weight 72.7 kg (160 lb).

Energy needs

1. BEE = 66 + (13.7 × 81.8) + (5 × 180) − (6.8 × 38) = 1829 calories/day
2. Energy needs for bed rest = 1829 calories × 1.2 = 2195 calories/day
3. Energy needs for injury = 2195 calories × 1.3 = 2853 calories/day

Protein needs = 72.7 kg × 1.5 g = 109 g/day

Table 9-5 Enteral formulas

Formula type	Examples of formulas	Oral or tube feeding	Nutritional problem	Clinical examples
Complete diet with intact protein and LCT,*† (some contain blended foods)	Ensure and Osmolite (Ross), Sustacal and Isocal (Mead Johnson Nutritional), Meritene and Compleat (Sandoz), Entrition (Biosearch). For fluid restriction: Magnacal (Sherwood Medical), Isocal HCN (Mead Johnson Nutritional), TwoCal HN (Ross)	Some are suited to both (e.g., Ensure), some primarily to oral (Sustacal, Meritene), and some primarily to tube feeding (Compleat, Osmolite, Isocal)	Inability to ingest food Inability to ingest enough food to meet needs	Oral or esophageal cancer Coma Anorexia resulting from chronic illness Burns or trauma
Elemental diets‡	Criticare HN (Mead Johnson Nutritional), Vital High Nitrogen (Ross), Reabilan (O'Brien), Vivonex and Vivonex T.E.N. (Norwich Eaton), Travasorb HN (Clintec Nutrition)	Tube feeding	Impaired digestion and/or absorption Hypoalbuminemia	Pancreatitis Inflammatory bowel disease Radiation enteritis Short bowel syndrome Malnutrition

SPECIALIZED DIETS FOR METABOLIC ALTERATIONS

Formula type	Examples of formulas	Oral or tube feeding	Nutritional problem	Clinical examples
Diets high in essential amino acids, low in nonessential amino acids	Amin-Aid (Kendall McGaw), Travasorb Renal (Clintec Nutrition)	Both (especially tube)	Renal failure	Undialyzed end stage renal disease
Diets high in branched chain amino acids, low in aromatic amino acids	Hepatic-Aid II (Kendal McGaw), Travasorb Hepatic (Clintec Nutrition)	Both (especially tube)	Hepatic failure	Impending hepatic coma
Diets high in branched chain amino acids§	Stresstein (Sandoz), TraumaCal (Mead Johnson Nutritional), Traum-Aid HBC (Kendall McGaw)	Both (especially tube)	Stress	Trauma and injury Sepsis

*LCT = Long-chain triglycerides or fat, used in formulas for patients with no digestive or absorptive abnormality.

†Some of these formulas contain lactose. If the patient has a lactose intolerance, the dietitian can recommend an appropriate lactose-free formula.

‡Contain "predigested" nutrients: protein in the form of amino acids and/or peptides or protein hydrolysates, fat as medium chain triglycerides (which require less emulsification by bile salts and enzymatic digestion than LCT) or minimal fat, and easily digested carbohydrates (no lactose).

§Branched-chain amino acids (leucine, isoleucine, and valine) contain a branch in their carbon chain structure. They are required for protein synthesis, but they are especially important because they serve as a valuable energy source following injury.

protein hydrolysates used in these formulas are very difficult to mask.

Location and type of feeding tube. Whether temporary tubes (nasogastric or nasoduodenal/nasojejunal) or more permanent ones (gastrostomy or jejunostomy) are used depends largely on the length of time that feedings are anticipated to be needed. Usually 3 months or longer constitutes long-term feedings. However, the patient who is extremely agitated or confused or for some other reason does not tolerate nasal intubation may require a permanent tube earlier. In addition, the advent of the percutaneous gastrostomy tube, which can be inserted with local anesthesia, has made gastrostomy increasingly popular, even in patients who do not require long-term feeding.

The site for intubation is also determined by patient need. Nasoduodenal, nasojejunal, or jejunostomy tubes are most often used when there is danger of pulmonary aspiration, because the pyloric sphincter provides a barrier which appears to lessen the risk of regurgitation and aspiration.[25] Jejunostomy tubes have the added advantage of being able to bypass an upper gastrointestinal (GI) obstruction.

Nursing responsibilities. The nurse's role in delivery of tube feedings usually includes insertion of the tube, if a temporary tube is used; maintenance of the tube; administration of the feedings; prevention of complications associated with this form of therapy; and participation in assessment of the patient's response to tube feedings. Assessment of response will be discussed later in this chapter.

Critical care nurses are usually familiar with tube insertion, and therefore this topic will not be discussed in depth here. However, transpyloric passage of tubes deserves special mention. Tubes with mercury, stainless steel, or tung-

---

RESEARCH ABSTRACT
Clogging of feeding tubes

Marcuard SP and Perkins AM: J Parenter Enter Nutr 12(4): 403, 1988.

PURPOSE

The purpose of this study was to determine the in vitro clotting ability of frequently used formulas and to occlude feeding tubes in vitro by acid precipitation of formula.

FRAMEWORK

Feeding tube obstruction can occur with long- and short-term therapy. Early obstruction is usually caused by pump malfunction, high formula viscosity, or a failure to irrigate the tube when using intermittent administration. Tube replacement is frequently necessary in this situation, which results in added cost, radiation exposure, and possible trauma to the patient. A better understanding of the possible causes of tube occlusion may help in preventing the problem, thereby preventing trauma to the patient.

METHODS

The following 10 products were tested: Ensure Plus, Ensure, Enrich, Osmolite, Pulmocare, Citrotein, Resource, Vivonex TEN, Vital High Nitrogen, and Hepatic Acid II. Protein (ProMod) was added to Citrotein and Ensure Plus in concentrations of 10 and 20 g/l. All samples were mixed by turning the test tube twice, and a clotting score was assigned to each mixture by five volunteers who did not know the content of the test tubes. Ten feeding tubes (Dobhoff, size 8 Fr) were filled with Ensure Plus, and the tips were placed in a 0.1 N HCl solution. One half of the contents of each tube was then aspirated, and the tubes were again filled with formula and left 1 hour. This procedure was repeated six times per tube, and if the tube was still patent, it was left standing overnight and the procedure was again repeated six times the next day until the feeding tube occluded.

RESULTS

Clotting was observed in all intact protein formulas with the exception of Citrotein. The strongest clotting was observed for Pulmocare (mean score = 3.7), followed by Ensure Plus and Osmolite. Diluting the formulas to half strength reduced the clotting score by 23% for Ensure Plus, 22% for Osmolite, and 14% for Pulmocare. Adding protein failed to increase the clotting score. The average pH when the formula began to clot was 4.5. Of the 10 tested feeding tubes, 6 were occluded after the first 24 hours; 2 tubes clogged after 2 days; and the remaining 2 tubes were obstructed after 3 days.

IMPLICATIONS

Clotting of some liquid formula diets may possibly cause gastric feeding tube occlusion. The following measures may help in preventing this problem: flushing the tube before and after aspirating for gastric residuals to eliminate acid precipitation of formula in the feeding tube, advancing the nasogastric feeding tube into the duodenum, and avoiding mixing these products with liquid medications having a pH value of 5.0 or less. In addition, it is important to crush tablets into a fine powder before mixing with water, because the tablet particles may easily block the ports at the end of the tube.

sten weights on the proximal end are often used when transpyloric tube placement is desired, in the belief that the weight will encourage transpyloric passage of the tube or that the weight will help the tube maintain its position once it passes into the bowel. Two groups of investigators, however, have independently noted that unweighted tubes are just as likely as weighted ones to migrate through the pylorus.[19,29] Furthermore, weighted tubes appear to offer no advantage over unweighted ones in regard to remaining in place.[29,34] Because the weights increase manufacturing costs and sometimes cause discomfort while being inserted through the nares, unweighted tubes may be preferable. One technique that has been shown to promote transpyloric passage of tubes is the administration of metoclopramide hydrochloride before tube insertion. Administering the drug after the tube's proximal tip is already in the stomach is much less effective.[18,40]

Maintenance of the tube includes regular irrigation of the tube to maintain patency, skin care around the insertion site, and mouth care. The newer small-bore (usually 8 French) "nonreactive" tubes made of polyurethane, silicone rubber, and similar materials are much more comfortable for the patient than the older polyethylene or polyvinylchloride tubes (usually 12 to 16 French), and patient complaints of discomfort[11] and nasal and skin erosion have decreased with the use of the nonreactive tubes. Unfortunately, these small tubes tend to clog readily. Regular irrigation helps to prevent tube occlusion. Generally, 30 to 60 ml of irrigant every 3 to 4 hours or after each feeding is appropriate. The volume of irrigant may have to be reduced during fluid restriction. The irrigant is usually water, but other fluids such as cranberry juice or cola beverages are sometimes used in an effort to reduce the incidence of tube occlusion. However, cranberry juice is inferior to, and cola beverages appear no better than, water for irrigating tubes.[24] Furthermore, once a tube has occluded, cranberry juice and cola are of little use in clearing the occlusion. In vitro studies[21,27] have shown that pancreatic enzymes, and sometimes papain (an enzyme from fresh papaya, commonly used in meat tenderizers), can be effective in clearing occlusions, but no reports exist about the safety and efficacy of enzymes in clearing occlusions in the clinical setting. Polyurethane tubes clog less readily than silicone rubber, an important consideration for the nurse in selecting a feeding tube.[24]

The skin around the tube should be cleaned at least daily, and the tape around the tube replaced whenever loosened or soiled. Secure taping helps to prevent movement of the tube, which may irritate the nares or skin or result in accidental dislodgement of the tube. Dressings are used initially around gastrostomy insertion sites. The dressing should be changed daily and the skin cleansed with half-strength hyrogen peroxide. If leakage of gastric fluid occurs around a gastrostomy tube, the skin can be protected with karaya.

To prevent dryness of the mouth (a common complaint during tube feeding), the patient should be encouraged to breathe through the nose as much as possible, drink and eat as much as desired (if compatible with the patient's nutrition orders), suck sugarfree candies or chew sugarfree gum (if allowed), and perform regular mouth care. If the patient is unconscious or otherwise unable to perform mouth care, the nurse should do it or should enlist the family in performing it. Patients often report that they can "taste" the tube feedings, and frequent mouth care will clear the palate of unpleasant flavors from the formula, as well as cleaning the teeth, tongue, and oral mucous membranes.

Careful attention to administration of tube feedings can prevent many complications. Very clean techniques in the handling and administration of the formula can help prevent bacterial contamination and a resultant infection. Routinely monitoring the patient's gastric residuals (especially if feedings are delivered into the stomch) can prevent gastric distention, which could cause patient discomfort, vomiting, and pulmonary aspiration. The schedule for delivery of feedings is also important. Tube feedings may be administered intermittently or continuously. Intermittent feedings are best suited to those patients who are disoriented and attempt to remove the feeding tube when they are alone. Bolus feedings, which are intermittent feedings delivered rapidly into the stomach or small bowel, are likely to cause distention, vomiting, and dumping syndrome with diarrhea. Instead of using bolus feedings, nurses should gradually drip intermittent feedings, with each feeding lasting 20 to 30 minutes or longer, to promote optimal assimilation. Regardless of how slowly intermittent feedings are given, however, continuous feedings are usually better absorbed by patients who have compromised digestion or absorption. Even patients who might be expected to have normal GI function, such as those with burns or trauma, have been shown to absorb the feedings better, tolerate larger volumes of formula, and experience less diarrhea with continuous feedings than with intermittent ones.[13] Therefore, continuous feedings are usually preferable for very sick patients.

Prevention and correction of complications. Some of the more common and serious complications of tube feeding are pulmonary aspiration, diarrhea, constipation, tube occlusion, and delayed gastric emptying. Delayed gastric emptying limits the amount of feeding that the patient can tolerate and thus interferes with adequate nutrition support. Nursing management of these problems is detailed in Table 9-6.

Total Parenteral Nutrition

Total parenteral nutrition (TPN) refers to the delivery of all nutrients by the intravenous route. TPN is generally not worthwhile when enteral intake is expected to be adequate within 5 to 7 days. Likely candidates for TPN include patients who are unable to ingest or absorb nutrients via the GI tract, as in short bowel syndrome, severe disease of the small bowel (for instance, inflammatory bowel disease, collagen-vascular diseases, intestinal pseudo-obstruction, or radiation enteritis), or intractable vomiting. TPN may be warranted in patients receiving high-dose chemotherapy, radiation, and bone marrow transplantation, where nutritional intake is apt to be poor for several weeks resulting from a combination of stomatitis, nausea, vomiting, diarrhea, and anorexia. It may also be useful in patients who can benefit from a period of bowel rest, including those with moderate to severe pancreatitis or with enterocutaneous fistulae. In

Table 9-6 Nursing management of enteral tube feeding complications

Complication	Contributing factor(s)	Prevention/correction
Pulmonary aspiration	Feeding tube positioned in esophagus or respiratory tract	Check tube placement before intermittent feeding and every 4-6 hr during continuous feedings; be aware that an in-rush of air can sometimes be auscultated over the right upper quadrant even when the distal tip of the tube is in the esophagus or respiratory tract[20,26,35]; if there is a question about the tube position, check the pH of fluid aspirated from the tube (usually gastric juice pH is 1.0-3.5) or obtain an x-ray[23]
	Regurgitation of formula (most common in patients with inadequate gag reflex, artificial airways, or altered state of consciousness and also in those with delayed gastric emptying[11,25])	Add food coloring (usually blue, to avoid mistaking it for any body secretion) to all formula to facilitate diagnosis of aspiration
		Elevate head to 30 degrees during feedings; if it is impossible to raise the head, position patient in lateral or prone position to improve drainage of vomitus from the mouth (the right lateral position is especially advantageous because it facilitates gastric emptying); if head must be in a dependent position (e.g., for postural drainage), discontinue feedings 30-60 min earlier and restart them only when the head can be raised
		Keep cuff of endotracheal or tracheostomy tube inflated during feedings, if possible[34]
		Measure gastric residual before each intermittent feeding and at least every 4-6 hr during continuous feedings; guidelines vary, but often a volume greater than 150 ml or more than 110%-120% of the hourly rate is considered excessive;[25] it is difficult to aspirate GI contents via small-bore nonreactive tubes without collapsing the tube, but use of large syringes (35-60 ml) is least likely to cause tube collapse. If a patient is at risk for pulmonary aspiration and it proves impossible to measure gastric residuals with an 8 French tube, substitute a 10 or 12 French one[24]
Diarrhea	Medications with GI side effects (antibiotics, which can alter gut flora, are common culprits,[17] but others include digitalis, laxatives,[33] magnesium-containing antacids, and quinidine)	Evaluate the patient's medications to determine their potential for causing diarrhea, consulting the pharmacist if necessary; if the possibility of pseudomembranous colitis is ruled out, consult with the physician about adding pectin (a soluble fiber that may result in formation of firmer stools) to the formula or the use of antidiarrheal medications
	Hypertonic formula or medications (e.g., oral suspensions of antibiotics, potassium, or other electrolytes),[28] which cause fluid to be drawn into the gut to dilute the hypertonic load	Consult the physician about using continuous feedings (if feedings are currently intermittent) or diluting or slowing tube feedings temporarily; dilute enteral medications well

Table 9-6   Nursing management of enteral tube feeding complications—*cont'd*

Complication	Contributing factor(s)	Prevention/correction
Diarrhea—cont'd	Malnutrition (hypoalbuminemia impairs absorption by decreasing plasma oncotic pressure; malnutrition also results in loss of intestinal microvilli, reducing brush border enzymes needed for digestion, as well as the absorptive area[4])	Consult with the physician about using an elemental formula, which may be more readily absorbed by the malnourished patient,[3] and utilizing continuous feedings[39,41]
	Cold formula[14]	Allow formula for intermittent feeding to come to room temperature before use (usually formula warms sufficiently during continuous infusions so that there is no need for prewarming.)
	Bacterial contamination[6]	Use scrupulously clean technique in administering tube feedings; keep opened containers of formula refrigerated and discard them within 24 hr; discard enteral feeding containers and administration sets every 24 hr[2]; hang formula no more than 4-8 hr unless it comes prepackaged in sterile administration sets; be especially careful with feedings given to patients being fed transpylorically or those receiving cimetidine or antacids, because these patients lack the normal antibacterial barrier of the stomach's hydrochloric acid[9]
	Fecal impaction with seepage of liquid stool around the impaction	Perform a digital rectal examination to rule out impaction; see guidelines for prevention of constipation (below)
Constipation	Low residue formula, creating little fecal bulk	Consult with the physician regarding the use of fiber-containing formula (e.g., Enrich [Ross], Compleat [Sandoz]), although this is not possible if the patient requires an elemental diet; consult with the physician about adding bran or bulk-type laxatives to the patient's regimen
	Inadequate fluid intake	Check patient's fluid intake to see that it totals 50 ml/kg/day, unless there is need for fluid restriction
Tube occlusion	Giving medications via tube (medications may physically plug the tube or may coagulate the formula, causing it to clog the tube)[7,22]	If medications must be given by tube, avoid use of crushed tablets; consult with the pharmacist to see whether medications can be dispensed as elixirs or suspensions; irrigate tube with water before and after administering any medication; never add any medication to the tube feeding formula unless the two are known to be compatible
	Sedimentation of formula	Irrigate tube every 4-8 hr during continuous feedings and after every intermittent feeding
Gastric retention	Delayed gastric emptying resulting from neural impairment or serious illness (e.g., diabetic gastroparesis, trauma)	Measure gastric residual at least every 4-6 hr or before every feeding; consult with physician regarding use of transpyloric feedings, temporary reduction of formula volume, or metoclopramide hydrochloride to stimulate gastric emptying; encourage patient to lie in right lateral position frequently, unless contraindicated

Table 9-7 Nursing management of TPN complications

Complication	Signs/symptoms	Prevention/correction
Catheter-related sepsis	Fever, chills, glucose intolerance, positive blood culture	Maintain an intact dressing, change if contaminated by vomitus, sputum, etc.; use aseptic technique when handling catheter, IV tubing, and TPN solutions; hang a bottle of TPN no longer than 24 hr, lipid emulsion no longer than 12-24 hr; use an in-line 0.22 μm filter with TPN to remove microorganisms; avoid drawing blood, infusing blood or blood products, piggybacking other IV solutions or medications into TPN IV tubing, or attaching manometers or tranducers via the TPN infusion line, if at all possible If catheter-related sepsis is suspected, remove catheter or assist in changing the catheter over a guidewire and administer antibiotics as ordered
Air embolism	Dyspnea, cyanosis, apnea, tachycardia, hypotension, "mill-wheel" heart murmur; mortality estimated at 50% (depends on quantity of air entering)	Use Luer-Lok syringe or secure all connections well; use an in-line 0.22 μm air-eliminating filter; have patient perform Val-salva maneuver during tubing changes; if the patient is on a ventilator, change tubing quickly at end expiration; maintain occlusive dressing over catheter site for at least 24 hr after discontinuing catheter to prevent air entry through catheter tract If air embolism is suspected, place patient in left lateral decubitus and Trendelenburg position (to trap air in the apex of the right ventricle, away from the outflow tract) and administer oxygen and CPR as needed; immediately notify physician, who may attempt to aspirate air from the heart
Pneumothorax	Chest pain, dyspnea, hypoxemia, hypotension, radiographical evidence, needle aspiration of air from pleural space	Throughly explain catheter insertion procedure to patient, because when a patient moves or breathes erratically he or she is more likely to sustain pleural damage; perform x-ray examination following insertion or insertion attempt If pneumothorax is suspected, assist with needle aspiration or chest tube insertion, if necessary; chest tubes are usually used for pneumothorax >25%
Central venous thrombosis	Edema of neck, shoulder, and arm on same side as catheter; development of collateral circulation on chest; pain in insertion site; drainage of TPN from the insertion site; positive findings on venogram	Follow measures to prevent sepsis; repeated or traumatic catheterizations are most likely to result in thrombosis If thrombosis is suspected, remove catheter and administer anticoagulants and antibiotics as ordered
Catheter occlusion or semiocclusion	No flow or a sluggish flow through the catheter	If infusion is stopped temporarily, flush catheter with heparinized saline. If catheter appears to be occluded, attempt to aspirate the clot; if this is ineffective, physician may order thrombolytic agent such as streptokinase or urokinase instilled in the catheter
Hypoglycemia	Diaphoresis, shakiness, confusion, loss of consciousness	Infuse TPN within 10% of ordered rate; observe patient carefully for signs of hypoglycemia following discontinuance of TPN* If hypoglycemia is suspected, administer oral carbohydrate; if the patient is unconscious or oral intake is contraindicated, the physician may order a bolus of IV dextrose
Hyperglycemia	Thirst, headache, lethargy, increased urinary output	Administer TPN within 10% of ordered rate; monitor blood glucose at least daily until stable; the patient may require insulin added to the TPN if hyperglycemia is persistent; sudden appearance of hyperglycemia in a patient who was previously tolerating the same glucose load may indicate onset of sepsis

*The nurse should observe the patient especially closely for the first 1-2 hr after abrupt discontinuance of TPN (without tapering of the rate), because hypoglycemia is most probable at this time.[36]

Table 9-8 Evaluating response to nutrition support

Parameter	Frequency of measurement*	Purpose/comments
ANTHROPOMETRIC MEASUREMENTS		
Weight	Daily	Indicator of efficacy or of overfeeding; underweight patient should have steady gain, and normal weight or overweight patient should maintain current weight Detection of overhydration: a consistent gain of >0.11-0.22 kg (0.25-0.5 lb)/day usually indicates fluid retention
Skinfolds	Weekly, if trained personnel available	Indicator of efficacy
PHYSICAL ASSESSMENT		
State of hydration	Daily	Detection of overhydration: check for edema of dependent body parts, shortness of breath, rales in lungs, fluid intake consistently >output Detection of dehyration: look for poor skin turgor, dry mucous membranes, complaints of thirst, output > intake (measure stool volumes if liquid), >10% difference between blood pressure when lying and standing
Bowel motility	Daily	Detect hypermotility or hypomotility: auscultate bowel sounds to be sure that peristalsis is present in patients receiving enteral feedings and to help determine when feedings can start in those not being enterally fed; evaluate stool consistency: hard, dry stools, decreased stool frequency, or <3 stools/wk may indicate constipation in the tube-fed patient, although infrequent stools are expected in the patient who is receiving nothing by mouth; loose or liquid stools, increased frequency or >3 stools/day may indicate diarrhea
Gastric emptying (tube-fed patients)	Every 4-6 hr or as indicated	Detect gastric retention: measure gastric residual as described in the discussion of tube feeding complications. Measure distance between the two anterior iliac crests; an increase of 8-10 cm is excessive and may necessitate temporarily stopping feedings[25]
HEMATOLOGICAL AND BIOCHEMICAL MEASUREMENT		
Serum albumin, transferrin, or prealbumin	Weekly	Indicator of efficacy: levels should be maintained or improved if protein nutriture is adequate
Serum glucose and electrolytes	Daily until stable, then 2-3/wk	Indicates whether intake is adequate or excessive
Blood urea nitrogen (BUN)	1-2/wk	Increased: inadequate fluid intake, renal impairment, or excessive protein intake
Serum calcium, phosphorous, magnesium	1-2/wk	Measure of adequacy of intake
Serum triglycerides (patients receiving IV lipid emulsions)	After each increase in lipid dosage; then 2-3/wk when stable	Elevated levels: inadequate lipid clearance and possibly a need for reduction in lipid dosage
REE (resting energy expenditure—measured by indirect calorimetry, not available in all institutions)	At beginning of nutrition support and as indicated	Permits very accurate determination of energy expenditure, allowing the nutrition support regimen to be planned to avoid overfeeding or underfeeding

*These are suggested frequencies only; individual patients may need more or less frequent assessment.
Adapted from Moore MC: Pocket guide to nutrition and diet therapy, St Louis, 1988, The CV Mosby.

both cases, enteral intake (which stimulates secretion of digestive enzymes) is likely to exacerbate the condition, whereas bowel rest may promote healing. In addition, some postoperative, trauma, or burn patients may need temporary TPN.[1]

Routes for TPN. TPN may be delivered through either central or peripheral veins. Because it requires an indwelling catheter, central vein TPN carries an increased risk of sepsis, as well as potential insertion-related complications such as pneumothorax and hemothorax. Air embolism is also more likely with central vein TPN. However, central venous catheters provide very secure IV access and allow delivery of more hyperosmolar solutions than peripheral TPN. TPN solutions containing 25% to 35% dextrose are commonly used via central veins, and this provides an inexpensive source of calories. It is increasingly common for patients requiring multiple IV therapies and frequent blood sampling to have multilumen central venous catheters and for TPN to be infused via these catheters. Infection rates in patients receiving TPN via multilumen catheters have been reported to be as much as three times higher than those in patients with single lumen catheters.[30,32] Scrupulous aseptic technique is essential in maintaining multilumen catheters; the manipulation involved in frequent changes of intravenous (IV) fluid and blood drawing through these catheters increases the risk of catheter contamination. Also, patients requiring these catheters are likely to be very ill and immunocompromised.

Peripheral TPN is rarely associated with serious infectious or mechanical complications, but it does necessitate good peripheral venous access. Therefore, it may not be appropriate for long-term nutrition support or for patients receiving multiple IV therapies. Furthermore, peripheral veins tolerate very hyperosmolar solutions poorly, and thus peripheral solutions are limited to about 10% dextrose. Daily use of IV lipid emulsions, which are isotonic, is necessary to provide adequate calories during peripheral TPN, unless the patient is consuming substantial amounts by mouth and the TPN is being used only as a supplement.

Nursing responsibilities. Nursing care of the patient receiving TPN includes catheter care, administration of solutions, prevention or correction of complications, and evaluation of patient responses to IV feedings. Evaluation of patient response will be discussed later in this chapter.

The indwelling central venous catheter provides an excellent nidus for infection. The nurse has a major role in preventing this complication of TPN therapy. Catheter care includes maintaining an intact dressing at the catheter insertion site and manipulating the catheter and administration tubing with aseptic technique. Dressings for TPN catheters may consist either of gauze and tape or transparent film. Usually gauze dressings are changed three times weekly, and transparent dressings are changed every 5 to 7 days. Both types are also changed whenever they become wet, soiled, or nonadherent. These types of dressings are associated with comparable rates of catheter-related sepsis,[16,31,42] but the transparent dressings usually decrease nursing time spent on dressing changes and may reduce irritation of sensitive skin.[16,42] After removal of the old dressing, the skin at the insertion site is commonly cleansed with povidone iodine, which is used because it has both antibacterial and antifungal activity. Chlorhexidine hydrochloride can be substituted for povidone iodine for patients allergic to iodine.

TPN solutions usually consist of amino acids, dextrose, electrolytes, vitamins, minerals, and trace elements. Although dextrose-amino acid solutions are commonly thought of as good growth media for microorganisms, they actually suppress the growth of most organisms usually associated with catheter-related sepsis, except yeasts.[8] However, because the many manipulations required to prepare solutions increase the possibility of contamination, TPN solutions are best used with caution. They should be prepared under laminar flow conditions in the pharmacy, with avoidance of additions on the nursing unit. Solution containers should be inspected for cracks or leaks before hanging, and solutions should be discarded within 24 hours of hanging. A 0.22 μm-line filter, which eliminates all microorganisms but not endotoxins, may be used in administration of solutions. Use of the filter, however, should not be substituted for scrupulous aseptic technique, because there is no conclusive evidence that filters decrease sepsis rates.[12]

In contrast to dextrose–amino acid solutions, IV lipid emulsions support the proliferation of many microorganisms.[5] Furthermore, lipid emulsions cannot be filtered, because some particles in the emulsions are larger than 0.22 μm. Lipid emulsions should be handled with strict asepsis, and they should be discarded within 12 to 24 hours of hanging. There is a trend toward mixing lipid emulsions with dextrose–amino acid TPN solutions. Although this saves nursing time, the nurse must be extremely careful in administering these solutions. TPN solutions containing lipids cannot be filtered, and they support the growth of most bacteria and *Candida albicans* better than dextrose–amino acid TPN solutions.[8]

Prevention or correction of complications. Some of the more common and serious complications of TPN include catheter-related sepsis, air embolism, pneumothorax, central venous thrombosis, catheter occlusion, and metabolic imbalances such as hypoglycemia and hyperglycemia. These complications, along with nursing approaches to their management, are described in Table 9-7.

EVALUATING RESPONSE TO NUTRITION SUPPORT

Assessment of response to nutrition support is an ongoing process that involves anthropometric measurements, physical assessment, and biochemical evaluation. Table 9-8 summarizes some of the parameters that are used most frequently. Daily weighings and the maintenance of accurate intake and output records are especially crucial for evaluating nutritional progress and state of hydration in the patient receiving nutrition support. In addition, the nurse, as the health care team member having the most constant contact with the patient, is uniquely qualified to evaluate bowel function, determining whether the patient has enough diarrhea to preclude advancement of enteral feedings or whether the patient is at risk of pulmonary aspiration because of slow gastric emptying. Also, the nurse should alert other team members to changes in laboratory parameters.

REFERENCES

1. American Society for Parenteral and Enteral Nutrition: Guidelines for use of total parenteral nutrition in the hospitalized adult patient, J Parent Ent Nutr 10:441, 1986.
2. American Society for Parenteral and Enteral Nutrition: Standards for nutrition support: hospitalized patients, Nutr Clin Prac 3:28, 1988.
3. Brinson R, Curtis WD, and Singh M: Diarrhea in the intensive care unit: the role of hypoalbuminemia and the response to a peptide-based, chemically defined diet, J Am Coll Nutr 6:517, 1987.
4. Coale M and Robson J: Dietary management of intractable diarrhea in malnourished patients, J Am Diet Assoc 76:444, 1980.
5. Crocker KS and others: Microbial growth comparisons of five commercial parenteral lipid emulsions, J Parent Ent Nutr 8:391, 1984.
6. Crocker KS and others: Microbial growth in clinically used enteral delivery systems, Am J Infect Control 14:250, 1986.
7. Cutie AJ, Altman E, and Lenkel L: Compatibility of enteral products with commonly employed drug additives, J Parent Ent Nutr 7:186, 1983.
8. D'Angio R and others: The growth of microorganisms in total parenteral nutrition admixtures, J Parent Ent Nutr 11:394, 1987.
9. Donowitz LG and others: Alteration of normal gastric flora in critical care patients receiving antacid and cimetidine therapy, Infect Control 7:23, 1986.
10. Driver AG and LeBrun M: Iatrogenic malnutrition in patients receiving ventilatory support, JAMA 244:2195, 1980.
11. Flynn KT, Norton LC, and Fisher RL: Enteral tube feeding: indications, practices and outcomes, Image J Nurs Sch 19:16, 1987.
12. Goldman DA and Maki DG: Infection control in total parenteral nutrition, JAMA 223:1360, 1973.
13. Hiebert JM and others: Comparison of continuous vs intermittent tube feedings in adult burn patients, J Parent Ent Nutr 5:73, 1981.
14. Kagawa-Busby KS and others: Effects of diet temperature on tolerance of enteral feedings, Nurs Res 29:276, 1980.
15. Kamath SK and others: Hospital malnutrition: a 33-hospital screening study, J Am Diet Assoc 86:203, 1986.
16. Kellam B, Fraze DE, and Kanarek KS: Central line dressing material and neonatal skin integrity, Nutr Clin Prac 3:65, 1988.
17. Keohane P and others: Relation between osmolality of diet and gastrointestinal side effects in enteral nutrition, Br Med J 288:678, 1984.
18. Kittinger JW, Sandler RS, and Heizer WD: Efficacy of metoclopramide as an adjunct to duodenal placement of small-bore feeding tubes: a randomized, placebo-controlled, double-blind study, J Parent Ent Nutr 11:33, 1987.
19. Levenson R and others: Do weighted nasoenteric feeding tubes facilitate duodenal intubations? J Parent Ent Nutr 12:135, 1988.
20. Lipman TO, Kessler T, and Arabian A: Nasopulmonary intubation with feeding tubes: case reports and review of the literature, J Parent Ent Nutr 9:618, 1985.
21. Marcuard SP: Dissolution of clotted enteral feeding, J Parent Ent Nutr 11:16S, 1987.
22. Marcuard SP and Perkins AM: Clogging of feeding tubes, J Parent Ent Nutr 12:403, 1988.
23. Metheny, N: Measures to test placement of nasogastric and nasointestinal feeding tubes: A review. Nurs Res 37:324-329, 1988.
24. Metheny N, Eisenberg P, and McSweeney M: Effect of feeding tube properties and three irrigants on clogging rates, Nurs Res 37:165, 1988.
25. Metheny NA, Eisenberg P, and Spies M: Aspiration pneumonia in patients fed through nasoenteral tubes, Heart Lung 15:256, 1986.
26. Metheny NA, Spies MA, and Eisenberg P: Measures to test placement of nasoenteral feeding tubes, West J Nurs Res 10:367, 1988.
27. Nicholson LJ: Declogging small-bore feeding tubes, J Parent Ent Nutr 11:594, 1987.
28. Niemiec PW and others: Gastrointestinal disorders caused by medication and electrolyte solution osmolality during enteral nutrition, J Parent Ent Nutr 7:387, 1983.
29. Payne-James JJ and others: Enteral tube design and its effect on spontaneous transpyloric passage and duration of tube usage, J Parent Ent Nutr 12:21S, 1988.
30. Pemberton LB and others: Sepsis from triple- vs single-lumen catheters during total parenteral nutrition in surgical or critically ill patients, Arch Surg 121:591, 1986.
31. Powell C and others: Op-Site dressing study: a prospective randomized study evaluating povidone iodine ointment and extension set changes with 7-day Op-Site dressings applied to total parenteral nutrition subclavian sites, J Parent Ent Nutr 9:443, 1985.
32. Powell C, Fabri PJ, and Kudsk KA: Risk of infection accompanying the use of single-lumen vs double-lumen subclavian catheters: a prospective randomized study, J Parent Ent Nutr 12:127, 1988.
33. Taylor TT: A comparison of two methods of nasogastric tube feedings, J Neurosurg Nurs 14:49, 1982.
34. Treloar DM and Stechmiller J: Pulmonary aspiration in tube-fed patients with artifical airways, Heart Lung 13:667, 1984.
35. Valentine RJ and Turner WW: Pleural complications of nasoenteric feeding tubes, J Parent Ent Nutr 9:605, 1985.
36. Wagman LD and others: The effect of acute discontinuation of total parenteral nutrition, Ann Surg 204:524, 1986.
37. Warnold I and Lundhold K: Clinical significance of preoperative nutritional status in 215 noncancer patients, Ann Surg 199:299, 1984.
38. Weinsier RL and others: Hospital malnutrition: a prospective evaluation of general medical patients during the course of hospitalization, Am J Clin Nutr 32:418, 1979.
39. Weizman Z, Schmueli A, and Deckelbaum RJ: Continuous nasogastric drip elemental feeding: alternative for prolonged parenteral nutrition in severe prolonged diarrhea, Am J Dis Child 137:253, 1983.
40. Whatley K and others: When does metoclopramide facilitate transpyloric intubation? J Parent Ent Nutr 8:679, 1984.
41. Wrobel J and Bodin T: Are serum albumin levels detrimental to enteral formulation tolerance? J Parent Ent Nutr 12:21S, 1988.
42. Young GP and others: Catheter sepsis during parenteral nutrition: the safety of long-term OpSite dressings, J Parent Ent Nutr 12:365, 1988.

CHAPTER

10

Nutritional Management by Systems

CHAPTER OBJECTIVES

- *Recognize nutritional alterations commonly associated with cardiovascular, pulmonary, neurological, fluid and renal, gastrointestinal, and endocrine systems.*
- *Assess the nutritional status of a patient with cardiovascular, pulmonary, neurological, fluid and renal, gastrointestinal, and/or endocrine system dysfunction(s).*
- *Develop and follow a nursing care plan for a patient with cardiovascular, pulmonary, neurological, fluid and renal, gastrointestinal, and/or endocrine system dysfunction(s).*
- *Develop a nutritional teaching plan for a critically ill patient.*
- *Evaluate the success of and make the necessary changes in the nursing care plan/nutritional teaching plan for a critically ill patient.*

Chapter 9 dealt with generalized nutrition assessment and nutrition support for a wide variety of sick or injured patients. This chapter focuses on specific aspects of nutrition assessment, intervention, and teaching for patients with selected cardiovascular, pulmonary, neurological, renal, gastrointestinal, endocrine, and immune alterations.

NUTRITION AND CARDIOVASCULAR ALTERATIONS

Diet and cardiovascular disease may interact in a variety of ways. In one situation, excessive nutrient intake, manifested by overweight or obesity and a diet rich in cholesterol and saturated fat, is a risk factor for development of arteriosclerotic heart disease. Conversely, the consequences of chronic myocardial insufficiency can include malnutrition.

Nutrition Assessment in Cardiovascular Alterations

A nutrition assessment provides the nurse and other members of the health care team the information necessary to plan the patient's nutrition care and teaching. Key points of the nutrition assessment of the cardiovascular patient are summarized in Table 10-1. The major nutritional concerns

relate to appropriateness of body weight, serum lipid levels, and blood pressure.

Nutrition Intervention in Cardiovascular Alterations

Myocardial infarction. The following guidelines will assist the nurse in providing appropriate nutritional care for the patient in the immediate post–myocardial infarction (MI) period:

1. Limit meal size for the patient with severe myocardial compromise or postprandial angina. While typical size meals are less stressful than a bed bath or shower for the patient with an uncomplicated condition, these meals increase cardiac index, stroke volume, heart rate, myocardial oxygen consumption, and whole body oxygen consumption; thus they increase cardiac work. Five to six small meals daily are less likely than three larger meals to increase myocardial work, promote ischemia, and cause angina.[2]

2. Monitor the effect of caffeine on the patient, if caffeine is included in the diet. Because caffeine is a stimulant, it might be expected to increase heart rate and myocardial oxygen demand. In the United States and in most industrial nations, coffee is the richest source of caffeine in the diet, with about 150 mg of caffeine per 180 ml (6 fluid ounces) of coffee. In comparison, the caffeine content of the same volume of tea or cola is approximately 50 mg or 20 mg, respectively. Schneider[13] found that one cup of caffeine-containing coffee had no effect on heart rate, blood pressure, myocardial oxygen consumption, and cardiac rhythm in patients convalescing from acute MI. Similarly, a double-blind study in which patients recovering from MI received 300 mg caffeine or a placebo revealed no increase in ventricular dysrhythmias after caffeine intake.[7] However, the acute MI patient should be carefully monitored during and after coffee consumption to rule out any adverse effects.

3. Avoid serving foods at temperature extremes. Very hot or very cold foods could potentially trigger vagal or other neural input and cause cardiac dysrhythmias.

Hypertension. The primary nutritional intervention for hypertensive patients is to limit sodium intake, usually to no more than 2 g/day. To achieve this level of intake, the patient usually must be helped to avoid the foods listed in

Table 10-1 Nutrition assessment of the cardiovascular patient

Area of concern	Significant findings		
	History	Physical assessment	Laboratory data
Overweight/obesity	Excessive kcal intake (consult dietitian regarding nutrition history) Sedentary lifestyle	Weight >120% of desirable Triceps skinfold >90th percentile*	
Protein-calorie malnutrition (cardiac cachexia)	Chronic cardiopulmonary disease causing: Decreased food intake related to angina, respiratory embarrassment, or fatigue during eating Malabsorption of nutrients (hypoxia of the gut impairs absorption,[4] in chronic congestive heart failure or cardiomyopathy, the amount of malabsorption may be significant) Medications that impair appetite, e.g., digitalis, quinidine	Weight <85% of desirable Triceps skinfold <10th percentile† Muscle wasting Loss of subcutaneous fat	Serum albumin <3.5 g/dl (or low serum transferrin or prealbumin) Negative nitrogen balance Creatinine excretion <17 mg/kg/day (women) or 23 mg/kg/day (men)
Elevated serum lipid levels	Frequent or daily use of foods high in cholesterol and saturated fat, including red meat, cold cuts, bacon or sausage, butter, cream or nondairy creamer, foods containing shortening or lard or fried in those products, eggs, organ meats, cheese, ice cream Sedentary lifestyle Family history of hyperlipidemia Overweight or obesity	Xanthomas, or yellowish plaques deposited in the skin (uncommon)	Serum cholesterol >200 mg/dl (age 20-29), >220 (age 30-39), >240 (>40 yr)[8] Low-density lipoprotein cholesterol >130 mg/dl[9]
Elevated blood pressure	Daily use of high-sodium foods and salt at the table Consumption of >2 ounces of alcohol/day		

Adapted from Moore MC: Pocket guide to nutrition and diet therapy, St. Louis, 1988, The CV Mosby Co.
Chapter 9 provides additional information regarding nutrition assessment techniques and interpretation of findings.
*20 mm for men and 34 mm for women.
†6 mm for men and 14 for women.

the box on p. 108. The primary sodium source in the American diet is salt (sodium chloride) added during food processing and food preparation or at the table. One teaspoon of salt provides about 2.3 g of sodium. Most salt substitutes contain potassium chloride and may be used with the physician's approval by the patient who has no renal impairment. "Lite salt" is about half sodium chloride and half potassium chloride. It too may be used if the physician agrees, but it must be used very sparingly to achieve a sodium intake of 2 g or less daily.

Caffeine causes an acute increase in blood pressure but apparently has no sustained effect, and the incidence of hypertension is no higher among caffeine users than nonusers. Therefore restriction of the caffeine intake of hyper-

tensive patients does not appear to be necessary.[10]

Congestive heart failure. Nutrition intervention in congestive heart failure is designed to reduce fluid retained within the body and thus reduce the preload.[11] Since fluid accompanies sodium, limitation of sodium is necessary in order to reduce fluid retention. Specific interventions include (1) limiting sodium intake, usually to 2 g/day or less (see the box on p. 108), and (2) limiting fluid intake as appropriate. The amount ordered is usually 1.5 to 2 L/day, to include both fluids in the diet and those given with medications and for other purposes. The nurse should remember that some foods that are normally served as solids are actually liquids at body temperature. These include gelatins (100% water), custard (75% water), sherbet and fruit ices

---

FOODS TO AVOID ON A SODIUM-RESTRICTED DIET

Salt

Smoked, processed, or cured meats and fish (e.g., ham, bacon, sausage, cold cuts, corned beef, frankfurters, salt pork, pickled fish, anchovies, and sardines)

Salted foods such as pretzels, chips, nuts, and popcorn

Soups, bouillon, meat extracts, and gravies unless prepared without salt

Canned meats and vegetables unless prepared without salt

Prepared mixes for baked goods, entrees, and side dishes; frozen entrees; frozen vegetable dishes with sauce

Condiments (catsup; prepared mustard; steak, soy, Worcestershire, or similar sauces), relishes, olives, pickles

Butter, margarine, cheese, and peanut butter unless prepared without salt

Buttermilk

Celery, onion, or garlic salt; barbecue seasonings; chili powder

Mineral water

STRATEGIES FOR INCREASING ORAL INTAKE

Schedule five or six small meals and snacks daily, rather than three main meals. Smaller feedings are more likely to be acceptable to patients with anorexia.

Schedule painful or tiring treatments and activities so that they do not interfere with meals and the patient has time to rest before and after eating.

Encourage the patient to consume calorie-dense foods and supplements.

Fat is the most concentrated source of calories, and it should be used liberally. Examples of ways to increase fat intake*:

Serve breads hot, because more butter or margarine is used when it melts into the bread.

Add sour cream, cream cheese, butter, or sauces to cooked vegetables.

Serve meats with gravy.

Provide half-and-half or cream rather than milk for use with cereal and in hot beverages.

Encourage snacking on nuts, ice cream, frozen yogurt (not low fat), pudding, granola, cheese, or peanut butter.

Some patients with moderate to severe dyspnea may find it easier to sip liquids rather than to eat. Shakes, instant breakfast, and commercial supplements can be used for these patients.

Avoid the use of bulky foods that fill the patient up without providing many calories. This includes salads, raw vegetables, and most beverages. If the patient wants these, encourage consumption at the end of the meal and increase the caloric content as much as possible. For example, add dressing, cheese, chopped egg, or legumes to salads. Add sugar and cream to beverages; for sweet beverages such as fruit juice and for the patient who prefers unsweetened coffee or tea, add glucose polymers (a carbohydrate caloric supplement that has the advantage of not being sweet; 15 ml [1 tablespoon] or more per 240 ml [1 cup] of beverage is usually well accepted.

---

*The patient with arteriosclerotic heart disease or hyperlipidemia will need to utilize polyunsaturated fats primarily (e.g., tub margarine rather than butter, foods fried or sauteed in polyunsaturated oils) and omit items such as cream, gravies containing meat drippings, ice cream, and high-fat cheeses.

(50% water), and ice cream (33% water).

Cardiac cachexia. The severely malnourished cardiac patient often suffers from congestive heart failure. Therefore sodium and fluid restriction, as previously described, are appropriate. It is important to concentrate nutrients into as small a volume as possible and to serve small amounts frequently, rather than three large daily meals that may overwhelm the patient (see box at right).

Because the patient is likely to tire quickly and to suffer from anorexia, tube feeding or total parenteral nutrition (TPN) may be necessary. When tube feeding is needed, formulas with 2 or more calories/ml are preferable. (Most commonly used formulas provide 1 calorie/ml.) Formulas appropriate for the fluid-restricted patient include Magnacal (Biosearch), Isocal HCN (Mead Johnson), TwoCal HN (Ross), and Nutrisource (Sandoz). During TPN, 20% lipid emulsions with 2 calories/ml provide a concentrated energy source. (The 10% emulsions, in contrast, contain only 1.1 calorie/ml.)

The nurse must monitor the fluid status of these patients carefully when they are receiving nutrition support. Body weight must be recorded daily; a consistent gain of more than 0.11 to 0.22 kg (¼ to ½ pounds) a day usually indicates fluid retention rather than gain of fat and muscle mass. The nurse must also check the patient frequently for increasing pulmonary and peripheral edema.

Nutrition Teaching in Cardiovascular Alterations

Myocardial infarction. The patient recovering from MI must recognize the need for permanent changes in diet and lifestyle to reduce the risk of additional MIs. These changes include:

1. Weight reduction, if the patient is overweight. Gradual loss of 0.45 to 0.9 kg (1-2 pounds) per week should be the goal. This can be achieved through moderate exercise and reduction of dietary intake, in particular, reducing intake of fried and fatty foods, because fat is the most concentrated source of calories. In addition, although there is no concrete evidence that a high-fiber diet is effective in promoting

SUGGESTIONS FOR REDUCING CALORIC INTAKE

Increase intake of bulky, high-fiber foods such as raw vegetables and fruits, legumes, and whole grains.

Serve meats, fish, and poultry broiled or baked with little or no added fat. "Protein" foods often contain a surprisingly high percentage of fat. Keep serving sizes moderate—usually no larger than a deck of cards.

Reduce intake of fatty foods—butter, margarine, salad dressing, mayonnaise, sour cream, sauces, gravy, bacon, sausage, cold cuts, fried foods, and snack foods, such as chips. Be aware that there are hidden sources of fat, such as chocolate, doughnuts, pie crust, croissants, and other pastries.

Drink a large glass of water or other low-carlorie or no-calorie beverage a few minutes before eating to help reduce appetite.

Avoid eating while performing any other activity, such as watching television. Eat in a designated place, such as the dining room, and eat slowly, laying down the utensils after each bite and chewing each mouthful thoroughly.

Keep low-calorie snacks available at all times. Some suggestions are fresh fruit, low-fat cottage cheese, nonfat yogurt, popcorn (served unbuttered and preferably popped without added oil), and low-calorie fruit ices.

weight loss,[14] the patient should be encouraged to choose high-fiber foods. Foods high in fiber or "bulk" are usually low in caloric density. They also take longer to consume than more refined foods, allowing the patient to attain satiety before he or she has consumed large numbers of calories. Studies of the use of fiber supplements to produce weight loss have yielded inconclusive results; therefore fiber supplements should not be relied on.[14]

The box above provides specific suggestions that can be used in patient teaching to produce gradual weight loss while relying on a diet of normal foods. "Crash" diets or fad diets that promise rapid loss generally cause more loss of muscle and water than body fat. Moreover, their use does not require the development of modified eating habits, and the weight lost is usually regained.[12]

2. Reduction of cholesterol and saturated fat intake. The American Heart Association recommends that healthy adults consume no more than 30% of calories as fat (with less than 10% as saturated fat, since this contributes to elevation of blood cholesterol) and no more than 300 mg cholesterol per day.[1] Adults with a history of heart disease may need to restrict intake even further. To achieve this level of intake, the patient can follow the guidelines for reduction of cholesterol and saturated fat intake in the box on p. 118. Oat bran, barley, and most fruits and vegetables contain "soluble fiber," which lowers cholesterol, probably by inhibiting absorption of bile salts (which are manufactured from cho-

lesterol and are normally recycled within the body) or dietary cholesterol. Sources of soluble fiber should be especially encouraged. It is important to emphasize to the patient that this diet does not have to be unpleasant. Fruits and vegetables, whole-grain and enriched bread and pasta products, legumes, lean meats, poultry, and fish can be used to create attractive and tasty meals. There is little reason for the patient to feel deprived.

3. Increase fish consumption. The patient may ask about the use of fish oils to reduce the risk of MI. There is evidence that consumption of fish once or twice a week may reduce the incidence of MI, possibly by altering platelet membrane lipids and thus decreasing platelet aggregation.[5,6] While consumption of fish as a part of a balanced diet may be advantageous and at least is unlikely to be harmful, regular use of fish oil supplements should be carried out only under a physician's supervision. Excessive use of supplements might result in prolonged bleeding and increased risk of cerebrovascular accident. The patient should be cautioned not to self-medicate with cod liver oil, since the high levels of vitamins A and D in this oil may be toxic.

Hypertension. The patient must understand the rationale for the necessary dietary changes, as well as the risks associated with noncompliance. Recommended dietary changes include:

1. Reduce weight, if overweight or obese. Even if the patient does not achieve the ideal weight, each kilogram lost by the obese patient may lower both systolic and diastolic pressures by as much as 1 mm Hg.[3]

2. Restrict sodium intake. The measures in the box on p. 108 can be used to help the patient understand the dietary changes necessary. Although the patient with no renal impairment may use a salt substitute with the physician's approval, many patients do not care for the taste of the substitutes. The patient and/or the person normally responsible for the patient's food preparation can be encouraged to experiment with the use of low-sodium herbs and seasonings to replace salt. Examples of suggested seasonings are horseradish, dry mustard, pepper, bay, and garlic for beef; curry, sage, coriander, and ginger for poultry; and lemon juice, mace, nutmeg, dill, rosemary, and savory for vegetables. The patient may be encouraged to know that the taste for sodium declines after about 3 months if the low-sodium regimen is followed conscientiously.[3]

Almost all fresh fruits and vegetables are low in sodium and can be used to provide interest in the diet. These foods are also a good source of potassium, and some evidence suggests that a high potassium intake helps to maintain a normal blood pressure, although this has not been proved.[3]

3. Consume no more than 2 ounces of alcohol daily. One ounce of alcohol is the equivalent of 2 ounces of 100-proof whiskey, 8 ounces of wine, or 24 ounces of beer. Alcohol has a direct pressor effect.[10]

Congestive heart failure. Recommended dietary changes include:

1. Restrict sodium intake. This teaching is the same as that for the hypertensive patient.

2. Restrict fluid intake, if appropriate. The patient and family will need help in learning to measure and record fluid intake, including those foods such as ice cream, custard, and sherbet that are commonly consumed as solids.

3. Consume a balanced, nutritious diet if cachectic or undernourished. Patient teaching should include the suggestions presented in the box on increasing oral intake.

NUTRITION AND PULMONARY ALTERATIONS

Malnutrition has extremely adverse effects on respiratory function, decreasing both surfactant production and vital capacity.[19] Moreover, individuals who lose weight lose proportionately more mass from the diaphragm than total body mass, and this further impairs ventilation.[16] Early detection and treatment of nutritional deficits seems to be especially important in patients with pulmonary alterations. Patients with acute respiratory disorders find it difficult to consume adequate oral nutrients and can rapidly become malnourished. Patients with chronic disorders and long-term weight loss have proved challenging to rehabilitate nutritionally. Goldstein and others[16] have shown that patients who do tolerate nutritional repletion demonstrate significant improvements in forced expiratory volume at 1 minute (FEV_1) and forced vital capacity (FVC), as well as increased sensitivity to $Paco_2$ levels. Patients with undernutrition and end-stage chronic obstructive pulmonary disease (COPD), however, are unable to tolerate the increase in metabolic demand that occurs during refeeding. Also, they are at significant risk for development of cor pulmonale and often fail to tolerate the fluid required for delivery of enteral or parenteral nutrition support. Prevention of severe nutritional deficits, rather than correction of deficits once they have occurred, is the key to nutritional management of these patients.

Nutrition Assessment in Pulmonary Alterations

Nutrition assessment is summarized in Table 10-2. The patient with respiratory compromise is especially vulnerable to the effects of fluid volume and carbohydrate excess and must be assessed continually for these complications.

Table 10-2   Nutrition assessment of the pulmonary patient

Area of concern	Significant findings		
	History	**Physical assessment**	**Laboratory data**

Protein-calorie malnutrition	Chronic lung disease: Poor intake of protein and calories because of:
	   Breathing difficulty from pressure of a full stomach on the diaphragm
	   Unpleasant taste in the mouth from chronic sputum production
	   Gastric irritation from bronchodilator therapy
	   Increased energy expenditure from increased work of breathing[16]
		Muscle wasting
		 Loss of subcutaneous fat
		 Recent weight loss, or weight <90% of desirable
		 Triceps skinfold <10th percentile*
			Serum albumin <3.5 g/dl, or low transferrin or prealbumin
			 Total lymphocyte count <1200/mm³
			 Creatinine excretion <17 mg/kg (women) or 23 mg/kg (men)

	Acute respiratory alterations:
	   Inadequate intake of protein and calories because of:
	   Upper airway intubation
	   Altered state of consciousness
		Same as for chronic disease	Same as for chronic disease

Chapter 9 provides further information about nutrition assessment techniques and interpretation of findings.
*6 mm for men and 14 mm for women.
†20 mm for men and 34 mm for women.
‡RQ, or CO_2 produced ÷ O_2 consumed, is measured by indirect calorimetry, which is not available in all institutions. However, pulmonary function tests can provide some indication of RQ, as the "laboratory data" column demonstrates. Carbon dioxide production (and RQ) rises in the patient who is depending primarily on carbohydrate for fuel (e.g., the patient receiving TPN in whom dextrose is supplying almost all calories, rather than receiving a balance between dextrose and lipid calories) and especially the patient who is being overfed so that adipose tissue is being accumulated.
§The defect is not usually sufficient to alter Pao_2 or $Paco_2$ except in patients with the most severe lung disease.[17]

Table 10-2 Nutrition assessment of the pulmonary patient—cont'd

Area of concern	Significant findings		
	History	Physical assessment	Laboratory data
Protein-calorie malnutrition—cont'd	Dyspnea Increased protein and calorie requirements due to increased work of breathing or acute pulmonary infections Catabolism resulting from corticosteroid use		
Overweight/obesity (in patients with chronic lung disease)	Decreased caloric needs resulting from decreasing metabolic rate with aging (metabolic rate declines 2%/decade after age 30) or decreased activity to compensate for impaired respiratory function	Weight >120% of desirable Triceps skinfold >90th percentile†	
Elevated respiratory quotient (RQ)‡	Use of glucose or other carbohydrate to provide 70% or more of nonprotein calories Consumption of excess calories	Tachypnea, shortness of breath	RQ ≥1 Elevated $\dot{V}O_2$ and $\dot{V}CO_2$ Elevated $PaCO_2$ (not always present)
Fluid volume excess	Administration of more than 35-50 ml fluid/kg/day Increased antidiuretic hormone (ADH) release resulting from stress and ventilator dependency	Dependent edema Pulmonary rales Bounding pulse Shortness of breath	Serum sodium <135 mEq/L BUN, hematocrit, and serum albumin decreased from previous values
Excess lipid intake	Administration of IV lipids		Serum triglycerides >150 mg/dl Low $\dot{V}A/\dot{Q}$§

Nutrition Intervention in Pulmonary Alterations

Prevent or correct undernutrition and underweight. The nurse and dietitian can work together to encourage oral intake in the undernourished or potentially undernourished patient who is capable of eating. Small, frequent feedings are especially important, since a very full stomach can interfere with diaphragmatic movement. Mouth care needs to be provided before meals and snacks to clear the palate of the flavors of sputum and medications. Administering bronchodilators with food can help to reduce gastric irritation. Consult the box on p. 108 for additional suggestions.

Because of anorexia, dyspnea, and debilitation, however, many patients will require tube feeding or TPN. Some, but not all, investigators[15,18,22] have found pulmonary aspiration to be increased in patients with artificial airways who are receiving tube feedings, and it is especially important for the nurse to be alert to the risk of pulmonary aspiration. To reduce the risk of this complication, the nurse should keep the patient's head elevated at least 30 degrees during feed-

ings, unless contraindicated; discontinue feedings 30 to 60 minutes before any procedures that require lowering the head; keep the cuff of the artificial airway inflated during feeding, if possible; measure the patient's gastric residuals at frequent intervals and discontinue feedings if residuals exceed the guidelines established for the patient (if no guidelines are set, 150 ml is often considered excessive for intermittently fed and 10% to 20% more than the hourly flow rate is considered excessive for continuously fed patients); and monitor the patient for increasing abdominal distension.[18,21,22]

Avoid excess carbohydrate administration. The production of carbon dioxide increases when carbohydrate is relied on as the primary energy source, and this raises the respiratory quotient (see the section on assessment). This is unlikely to be significant in the patient who is eating foods. Instead, it is an iatrogenic complication of TPN in which glucose is often the predominant calorie source, or occasionally of tube feeding in a patient with a very high car-

Table 10-3 Sample TPN prescription for a patient with acute respiratory failure

PATIENT INFORMATION

Estimated nonprotein calorie need = 2600 calories/day
Estimated protein need = 100 g/day

NUTRIENT SOLUTIONS

Glucose–amino acid TPN solution, each liter containing:

	Nonprotein calories/L	Protein (g/L)
70% glucose, 300 ml	714	0
8.5% amino acids, 700 ml	0	60
Vitamins, minerals, and electrolytes to meet patient requirements	0	0
20% lipid emulsion	2000	0

NUTRITION ORDERS

Infuse 1.8 L glucose–amino acid solution (1285 calories and 107 g amino acids) and 650 ml lipid emulsion (1300 calories) daily. Glucose and lipid will each provide approximately 50% of the nonprotein calories.

---

bohydrate formula.[20] Excessive carbohydrate intake can raise $PaCO_2$ sufficiently to make it difficult to wean a patient from the ventilator. Patients not dependent on a ventilator may experience tachypnea or shortness of breath on a high carbohydrate regimen.

The nurse who notes an increasing $PaCO_2$ in a patient receiving carbohydrate-based TPN should discuss with the physician the possibility of providing daily lipid infusions for the patient. A regimen with approximately equal amounts of the nonprotein calories from lipid and carbohydrate is probably optimal for the patient with respiratory compromise. Table 10-3 illustrates a sample TPN prescription for a patient with acute respiratory failure.

Avoid excessive serum lipid levels. Excessive lipid intake can impair capillary gas exchange in the lungs, although this is not usually sufficient to produce an increase in $PaCO_2$ or decrease in PaO_2.[17] However, the patient with severe respiratory alteration may be further compromised by lipid overdose. If lipid intake is maintained at no more than 2 g/kg/day, lipid excess is rarely a problem. (Lipids are available as 20 g lipid per 100 ml of 20% lipid emulsion and 10 g/100 ml of 10% emulsion.) Serum triglycerides should be maintained less than 150 mg/dl. Higher levels may indicate inadequate clearance and a need to decrease the lipid dosage.

Prevent fluid volume excess. Pulmonary edema and right heart failure, which may result from fluid volume excess, further worsen the status of the patient with respiratory compromise. Strict intake records must be maintained to allow for accurate totals of fluid intake. Usually the patient requires no more than 35 to 50 ml/kg/day of fluid.

For the patient receiving nutrition support, fluid intake can be reduced by using 20% lipid emulsions as a source of calories, using tube feeding formulas providing at least 2 calories/ml (the dietitian can suggest appropriate choices), and choosing oral supplements that are low in fluid. Some examples are cottonseed oil (Lipomul, Upjohn), an oral lipid supplement providing 6 calories/ml, and powdered glucose polymers, which increase caloric intake without increasing volume. The nurse plays a valuable role in continually reassessing the patient's state of hydration and alerting other team members to changes that may dictate an increase or decrease in fluid intake.

Nutrition Teaching in Pulmonary Alterations

Teaching focuses on achieving or maintaining the desirable body weight and avoiding nutritional deficits.

Undernourished patients and patients at risk of undernutrition. Undernourished patients should be encouraged to follow the previously outlined suggestions concerning nutrition intervention. Specifically, they should continue to eat frequent small meals and choose calorie-dense foods. They may need help in determining which foods are good calorie sources and in learning to increase calories by adding fat or by using nutritional supplements.

Overweight or obese patients. Some patients with chronic lung disease become overweight or obese, rather than underweight, primarily because they restrict their activity because of their disease. The nurse can help them to reduce their weight, which often improves their activity tolerance, with the suggestions in the box on p. 109. In addition, with the physician's agreement, the nurse may recommend a graduated exercise program designed to assist the patient in increasing the metabolic rate and the number of calories used.

NUTRITION AND NEUROLOGICAL ALTERATIONS

Because neurological disorders tend to be long-term problems, they necessitate good nutritional care to prevent nutritional deficits and promote well-being.

Nutrition Assessment in Neurological Alterations

Nutrition-related assessment findings vary widely in the patient with neurological alterations, depending on the type of disorder present. Some common findings are shown in Table 10-4.

Nutrition Intervention in Neurological Alterations

Prevention or correction of nutritional deficits

Oral feedings. Patients with dysphagia or weakness often experience the greatest difficulty in swallowing foods that are dry or thin liquids such as water that are difficult to control. For these patients, the nurse and dietitian can work together to plan suitable meals and evaluate patient acceptance and tolerance. Some suggestions that may help the patient with dysphagia or weakness of the swallowing musculature include the following.

1. Serve soft, moist foods. Tender chopped meats and poultry; casseroles; gravies and sauces over meats and veg-

Area of concern	Significant findings		
	History	**Physical assessment**	**Laboratory data**

DISORDERS OF PROTEIN AND CALORIE NUTRITURE

Area of concern	History	Physical assessment	Laboratory data

Protein-calorie malnutrition	Decreased intake because of:
	  Coma or confusion
	  Feeding/swallowing difficulties such as dribbling of food and beverages from mouth, dysphagia, weakness of muscles involved in chewing and swallowing
	  Ileus resulting from spinal cord injury or use of pentobarbital
	  Anorexia resulting from depression
	Increased needs because of:
	  Hypermetabolism and catabolism following head injury
	  Increased needs for protein and calories to heal trauma and surgical wounds
	  Loss of protein from decubitus ulcers
		Muscle wasting
		Loss of subcutaneous fat
		Weight <90% of desirable
		Triceps skinfold <10th percentile*
		Change in hair texture, loss of hair
			Serum albumin <3.5 g/dl (or low transferrin or prealbumin values)
			Negative nitrogen balance
			Total lymphocyte count <1200/mm³
			Creatinine excretion <17 mg/kg/day (women) or <23 mg/kg/day (men)

Overweight/obesity	Decreased caloric needs resulting from inactivity Reliance on soft or pureed foods, which are often more dense in calories than higher fiber foods Increased food intake resulting from depression/boredom	Weight >120% of desirable Triceps skinfold >90th percentile†	

VITAMIN AND MINERAL DEFICIENCIES

Area of concern	History	Physical assessment	Laboratory data
Iron (Fe)	Poor intake of meats resulting from chewing difficulties (e.g., myasthenia gravis) Loss of blood in trauma	Pallor, blue sclerae Koilonychia	Microcytic anemia (low hct, hgb, MCV, MCH, MCHC) Serum Fe <50 µg/ml
Zinc (Zn)	Poor intake of meat resulting from chewing problems Increased needs for healing decubitus ulcers, trauma, or surgical wounds	Hypogeusia, dysgeusia Diarrhea Seborrheic dermatitis Alopecia	Serum Zn <60 µg/ml

FLUID ALTERATIONS

Area of concern	History	Physical assessment	Laboratory data
Fluid volume deficit	Poor intake resulting from difficulty swallowing (e.g., in cerebral vascular accident), inability to express thirst, fluid restriction in an effort to reduce intracranial edema	Poor skin turgor Decreased urinary output Dry, sticky mucous membranes	Serum sodium >145 mEq/L Serum osmolality >300 mOsm/kg Increased BUN and hct Urine specific gravity >1.030

Adapted from Moore MC: Pocket guide to nutrition and diet therapy, St Louis, 1988, The CV Mosby Co.
Chapter 9 provides additional information regarding nutrition support techniques and interpretation of findings.
hct, hematocrit; hgb, hemoglobin; MCV, mean cell volume; MCH, mean cell hemoglobin; MCHC, mean cell hemoglobin concentration; BUN, blood urea nitrogen.
*6 mm (men) or 14 mm (women).
†20 mm (men) or 34 mm (women).

etables; applesauce; cooked or canned fruits; ripe banana; cottage cheese; yogurt; poached, soft-cooked, or scrambled egg; mashed potatoes; cooked cereals; pudding; and custard are examples.

2. Thicken beverages with infant cereal, yogurt, or ice cream if the patient has difficulty swallowing fluids or chokes on water and other thin liquids. Alternatively, fluid can be provided by gelatin, sherbet, sorbet, fruit ices, popsicles, and ice cream. Fruit nectars may be better tolerated than juices.

3. Do not rush the patient who is eating, because this may increase the risk of pulmonary aspiration. Providing small amounts of food at frequent intervals, rather than larger amounts only at mealtimes, may help the patient feel less need to hurry. Keep suction equipment available in case aspiration does occur.

4. Place the patient in Fowler's position before feedings, if possible, to allow gravity to encourage effective swallowing.

5. Serve the main meal early in the day to the patient with myasthenia gravis, because muscle strength is greatest at that time.

Tube feedings or TPN. Patients who are unconscious or unable to eat because of severe dysphagia, weakness, ileus, or other reasons will need tube feedings or TPN. Prompt initiation of nutrition support must be a priority in the patient with neurological impairments. Needs for protein and calories are increased by infection and fever, as may occur in the patient with encephalitis and meningitis. Needs for protein, calories, zinc, and vitamin C are increased during wound healing, as in the trauma patient and the patient with decubitus ulcers.

Tube feeding can be successful in many patients with neurological impairment. Because these patients have an increased risk of certain complications, particularly pulmonary aspiration, they require especially careful nursing care, however. Patients of most concern are (1) those with an impaired gag reflex, such as some patients with cerebral vascular accident, (2) those with delayed gastric emptying, such as patients in the early period after spinal cord injury and patients with head injury treated with barbiturate coma, and (3) patients likely to experience seizures. To prevent aspiration, feedings must not be initiated until bowel sounds are present and should be discontinued if bowel sounds cease. Furthermore, gastric residuals must be measured at least every 4 hours in neurologically impaired patients.[28] If residuals are difficult to aspirate from the stomach via the small-bore (8 Fr diameter) feeding tubes often used now for tube feedings, it may be necessary to insert a 10 or 12 Fr tube instead.[30] Tubes of 16 Fr or larger diameter are associated with a very high incidence of pulmonary aspiration in patients with neurological disorders and therefore are not recommended.[36] Abdominal distension, evaluated by measuring between the anterior iliac crests, should also be assessed regularly. If the measurement increases by 8 to 10 cm, feedings may need to be halted temporarily.[29] To help prevent pulmonary aspiration, the patient's head should be kept elevated at 30 degrees, if possible; when elevation of the head is not possible, administering feedings with the patient in the prone or lateral positions will allow free drainage of emesis from the mouth and decrease the risk of aspiration. In patients in whom pulmonary aspiration is likely, the nurse may want to discuss with the physician the possibility of delivering feedings below the pylorus, rather than intragastrically. Evidence suggests that feedings delivered below the pylorus are less likely to result in pulmonary aspiration than intragastric feedings.[27]

Continuous tube feedings decrease absorption of oral phenytoin as much as 70%. While it might be possible to increase the phenytoin dose to compensate for the impaired absorption, this poses a danger of drug toxicity if the tube feeding is abruptly halted.[35] Current recommendations are that tube feedings not be given for 2 hours before and 2 hours after a single daily dose of phenytoin and that blood levels of phenytoin be monitored carefully in patients receiving continuous feedings.[23,35]

Hyperglycemia is a common complication in patients receiving corticosteroids. Patients treated with these drugs should have blood glucose levels monitored regularly and may require insulin to prevent substantial loss of glucose in the urine, as well as osmotic diuresis, loss of excessive amounts of potassium, and other fluid and electrolyte disturbances.

Tube feedings may not be possible in some patients with neurological alterations. Certain patients with head injury may not tolerate tube feedings for a prolonged period of time because of vomiting and poor gastrointestinal motility. Intolerance of enteral feedings seems to be related to the severity of the injury and to increased intracranial pressure.[31] Another group of patients who are not good candidates for enteral feedings are those with frequent or uncontrolled seizures.

TPN is needed by most patients who fail to tolerate tube feedings or those who cannot be enterally fed for at least 5 to 7 days. Prompt use of TPN is especially important for patients with head injuries, because head injury causes marked catabolism,[33] even in patients who receive barbiturates, which should decrease metabolic demands.[24,28] Head-injured patients rapidly exhaust glycogen stores and begin to utilize body proteins to meet energy needs, a process that can quickly cause protein-calorie malnutrition. The catabolic response to head injury is partly a result of the corticosteroids often used in treatment.[26] However, the hypermetabolism and hypercatabolism is also caused by dramatic hormonal responses to this type of injury.[33] Levels of cortisol, epinephrine, and norepinephrine increase, with levels of norepinephrine elevating as much as seven times normal. These hormones increase the metabolic rate and caloric demands, causing mobilization of body fat and proteins to meet the increased energy needs. Furthermore, head-injured patients undergo an inflammatory response and may be febrile, creating increased needs for protein and calories. Improved survival has been observed in head-injured patients who received TPN early in the hospital course, rather than being deprived of adequate nutrition or provided with only enteral feedings for several days or weeks after injury.[32,34]

As mentioned previously, patients receiving corticosteroids are especially prone to hyperglycemia, and they must be monitored carefully for development of this complication while receiving TPN. Administering insulin, usually as an additive in the TPN, or decreasing the glucose intake and substituting increased amounts of calories from intravenous lipid emulsions will help to control blood glucose.

Prevention of overweight and obesity. Many stable patients with neurological disorders are less active than their healthy counterparts and require fewer calories. Thus they may become overweight or obese if given normal amounts of calories for their age and sex. An example is the patient with spinal cord injury. For the first few weeks after injury, caloric needs can be calculated as for any traumatized patient (see Table 9-4). However, within 1 or 2 months, substantial amounts of muscle atrophy and loss of body mass begin to occur as a result of denervation and disuse.[37] Consequently, body weight and caloric needs decline. Ideal body weights for paraplegics and quadriplegics are 4.5 kg and 9 kg, respectively, less than those for healthy adults of the same height. Stable, rehabilitating paraplegics need approximately 27.9 calories/kg/day, and quadriplegics need 22.7 calories/kg/day.[25] Patients with dysphagia or extreme weakness may rely on very soft, easy to chew foods that are usually more dense in calories than bulky, high-fiber foods. Thus they also may gain unneeded weight that will hamper their care and impede mobility. Decreased use of high-fat foods, such as shakes, ice cream, butter, margarine, and pastries, will help to reduce calorie intake. Unsweetened canned or fresh fruits, fruit ices, low-calorie margarine, and vegetables cooked without added fat are good choices for the very sedentary patient. Drinking water, tea, coffee, or another no-calorie beverage a few minutes before mealtime will help the patient to feel less hungry and eat less.

Nutrition Teaching in Neurological Alterations

The primary nutrition teaching needs of the patient and family are coping with dysphagia and preventing unwanted weight gain. The nurse can share with them the suggestions for dealing with dysphagia that are described in the section concerning nutrition interventions in neurological alterations (pp. 112 and 114). Dysphagia is frustrating and frightening for the patient and requires much understanding and patience by the family. Support and empathy on the part of the nurse can make their coping process easier. For the patient who is at risk of overweight or obesity, see the box on p. 109 outlining suggestions for reducing caloric intake provides a basis for teaching.

NUTRITION AND RENAL/FLUIDS ALTERATIONS

Providing adequate nutritional care for the patient with renal disease can be extremely challenging. While renal disturbances and their treatments can markedly increase needs for nutrients, necessary restrictions in intake of fluid, protein, phosphorus, and potassium make delivery of adequate calories, vitamins, and minerals difficult. Thorough nutrition assessment provides the basis for successful nutritional care in patients with renal disease.

Nutrition Assessment in Renal/Fluids Alterations

Assessment is summarized in Table 10-5.

Nutrition Intervention in Renal/Fluids Alterations

The goal of nutritional interventions is to administer adequate nutrients, including calories, protein, vitamins, and minerals, while avoiding excesses of fluid, protein, electrolytes, and other nutrients with potential toxicity.

Protein. Evidence suggests that a low-protein diet retards the progression of renal damage. It is postulated that a high-protein intake increases glomerular flow and pressures, as the kidney attempts to excrete the urea and other nitrogenous products derived from the protein. The increase in glomerular pressures may hasten the death of the glomeruli.[38] Consequently, decreased protein intake (0.6 g/kg/day compared with the 0.8 g/kg/day recommended for the healthy person and the 1.7 g/kg/day actually consumed by the average American) is recommended for the undialyzed patient with renal failure.[46] Although uremia necessitates control of protein intake, the patient with renal failure often has many problems that actually increase protein/amino acid needs: losses in dialysis, wounds, and fistulae; use of corticosteroid drugs that exert a catabolic effect; increased endogenous secretion of catecholamines, corticosteroids, glucagon, and parathyroid hormone, all of which can cause or aggravate catabolism; and catabolic conditions such as trauma, surgery, and sepsis associated or coincident with the renal disturbances.[39,48] Therefore, protein needs may actually be increased. During hemodialysis and arteriovenous hemofiltration, amino acids are freely filtered and lost, but proteins such as albumin and immunoglobulins are not. Both proteins and amino acids are removed during peritoneal dialysis, creating a greater nutritional requirement for protein.[49] Protein needs are estimated at 1 to 1.2 or more g/kg/day for patients receiving hemodialysis or hemofiltration, and 1.2 to 1.4 or more g/kg/day for those receiving peritoneal dialysis.[44] Although these amounts are greater than the recommended daily level for healthy adults, they are probably lower than the amount found in the diet before the patient's illness, and thus most patients will perceive them as restrictions.

Controversy exists regarding the type of amino acids to be provided to the patient in renal failure. Some authorities advocate using primarily essential amino acids, those which the body cannot make, with the idea that the patient will form adequate amounts of nonessential amino acids via the process of transamination (transfer of amine groups from one carbon backbone to another). Foods containing protein of high biological value, such as eggs, milk, beef, poultry, and fish, are richer in essential amino acids than foods with lower biological value protein, such as grains, legumes, and vegetables. Therefore foods containing lower biological value protein would need to be especially restricted. Specialized essential amino acid products have been developed for nutrition support. These include Amin-Aid (Kendall McGaw) and Travasorb Renal (Travenol) for enteral feedings and Aminosyn RF (Abbott), RenAmin (Travenol), and Nephramine (Kendall McGaw) for use in preparation in TPN. Reliance on these solutions may delay the need for dialysis. However, it is not clear that outcome is improved in patients receiving essential amino acid preparations, and many physicians now recommend the use of more balanced preparations, containing both essential and nonessential

Table 10-5 Nutrition assessment of the renal patient

Area of concern	History	Physical assessment	Laboratory data
Protein-calorie mal-nutrition	Poor dietary intake because of: Dietary restrictions on protein-containing foods Anorexia caused by zinc deficiency (lost in dialysis or decreased in diet because of restrictions on meats, whole grains, legumes) Increased protein and amino acid losses from: Dialysis (hemodialysis losses ≈ 14 g/session; CAPD losses ≈ 9-12 g/day) Tissue catabolism resulting from corticosteroid use Proteinuria (e.g., nephrotic syndrome) Increased needs for protein and calories during peritonitis and other infections	Muscle wasting Loss of subcutaneous tissue Weight <90% of desirable Triceps skinfold <10th percentile* (Loss of weight and subcutaneous fat may be masked by edema) Loss of hair, change of texture	Serum albumin <3.5 g/dl or low transferrin or prealbumin levels Total lymphocyte count <1200/mm³ Negative nitrogen balance
Altered lipid metabolism	Nephrotic syndrome, with elevated cholesterol levels Excess carbohydrate (CHO) consumption from: Emphasis on CHO in the diet to replace some of the calories normally provided by protein Use of glucose as an osmotic agent in dialysis		Serum cholesterol >250 mg/dl Serum triglycerides >180 mg/dl
Potential fluid volume excess	Oliguria or anuria Patient knowledge deficit about or noncompliance with fluid restriction	Edema Hypertension Acute weight gain (≥1%-2% of body weight)	Hematocrit decreased from previous levels

Adapted from Moore, MC: Pocket guide to nutrition and diet therapy, St. Louis, 1988, The CV Mosby Co.
Chapter 9 provides additional information regarding nutrition assessment techniques and interpretation of findings.
CAPD, continuous ambulatory peritoneal dialysis; MCV, mean cell volume; MCH, mean cell hemoglobin; MCHC, mean cell hemoglobin concentration.
*6 mm for men and 14 mm for women.

amino acids, in settings in which dialysis is available.[39,40] For the stressed, catabolic renal patient, provision of adequate amounts of all types of amino acids required for anabolism appears to be more important than delaying initiation of dialysis.

Some nephrologists advocate the use of ketoanalogues (carbon structures related to the amino acids, but lacking the amine group) rather than or in addition to essential amino acids. Patients can form amino acids from the ketoanalogues and circulating nitrogenous compounds. Use of ketoanalogues requires reduction of protein intake to at least 0.4 g/kg/day.[45,47] Because these compounds are relatively unpalatable, they may need to be given by tube.

Fluid. Patients are usually limited to a fluid intake resulting in a gain of no more than 0.45 kg (1 pound) per day on the days between dialysis. This generally means a daily intake of 500 ml plus the volume lost in urine, diarrhea, and vomitus. With the use of continuous peritoneal dialysis, hemofiltration, or arteriovenous hemodialysis, the fluid intake can be liberalized. A liberal fluid allowance permits more adequate nutrient delivery, whether by oral, tube, or parenteral feedings. Enteral formulas providing 2 calories/ml or more, such as Nutrisource (Sandoz), TwoCal HN (Ross), Isocal HCN (Mead Johnson), and Magnacal (Biosearch), are useful in providing a concentrated source of calories for tube-fed patients who require fluid restriction. Intravenous lipids, particularly 20% emulsions, can be used to supply concentrated calories for the TPN patient.

Table 10-5 Nutrition assessment of the renal patient—cont'd

Area of concern	History	Physical assessment	Laboratory data
DISORDERS OF MINERALS/ELECTROLYTES			
Phosphorus (P) excess	Oliguria or anuria	Tetany	Serum P > 4.5 mg/dl Calcium × P product (Ca in mg/dl × P in mg/dl) >70
Zinc (Zn) deficit	Poor intake because of restriction of protein-containing foods Loss in dialysis	Hypogeusia, dysgeusia Alopecia Seborrheic dermatitis Diarrhea	Serum Zn < 60 μg/ml
Iron (Fe) deficit	Decreased intake because of restriction of protein-containing foods Loss of blood in dialysis tubing	Fatigue Pallor, blue sclerae Koilonychia	Hematocrit < 37% (women) or 42% (men), hemoglobin < 12 g/dl (women) or 14 g/dl (men), low MCV, MCH, MCHC
Sodium excess	Oliguria or anuria	Edema Hypertension	
Potassium (K⁺) excess	Oliguria or anuria	Weakness, flaccid muscles	Serum K^+ > 5 mEq/L Elevated T wave and depressed ST segment on ECG
Aluminum (Al) excess	Use of aluminum-containing phosphate binders Al contamination of TPN constituents, especially Ca and vitamins[43]	Ataxia, seizures Dementia Renal osteodystrophy with bone pain and deformities	Plasma Al > 100 μg/L
DISORDERS OF VITAMIN NUTRITURE			
A excess	Oliguria or anuria Daily administration of tube feedings, TPN, or oral supplement with vitamin A	Anorexia Alopecia, dry skin Hepatomegaly Fatigue, irritability	Serum retinol > 80 μg/dl
C deficit	Loss in dialysis Decreased intake due to restriction of K^+-containing fruits and vegetables	Gingivitis Petechiae, ecchymoses	Serum ascorbate < 0.4 mg/dl
B₆ deficit	Failure of the diseased kidney to activate vitamin B_6 Loss in dialysis	Dermatitis Ataxia Irritability, seizures	Plasma pyridoxal phosphate < 34 nmol (normal values not well established)
Folic acid	Loss in dialysis Decreased intake resulting from restriction of meats, fruits, and vegetables	Glossitis (inflamed tongue) Pallor	Hematocrit < 37% (women) or 42% (men), elevated MCV Serum folate < 6 ng/ml

Calories. It is essential that the renal patient receive adequate amounts of calories to prevent catabolism of body tissues to meet energy needs. Catabolism not only reduces the mass of muscle and other functional body tissues but also releases nitrogen that must be excreted by the kidney. Adults with renal failure need about 35 to 45 calories/kg/day, compared with the 25 to 30 calories/kg needed by healthy adults, in order to prevent catabolism and ensure that all protein consumed is used for anabolism rather than to meet energy needs. After renal transplantation, when the patient usually receives large doses of corticosteroids, it is especially important to ensure that adequate caloric intake continue to prevent undue catabolism.[48]

High-carbohydrate foods such as hard candies, sugar, honey, jelly, jellybeans, and gumdrops are often used as a means of supplying calories to the patient with renal failure, because these foods are low in sodium and potassium, which are retained in renal failure. However, hypertriglyceridemia is found in a substantial number of patients with renal disorders. This condition is worsened by excessive intake of simple refined sugars such as sucrose (table sugar) or glucose. To help control hypertriglyceridemia, only about 35% of the patient's calories should come from carbohydrates, with the emphasis placed on complex carbohydrates (starches and fibers). Breads, pastas, and cereals can provide most of these complex carbohydrates, with some also being

GUIDELINES FOR REDUCING CHOLESTEROL AND SATURATED FAT INTAKE

Substitute skim milk and dairy products made with skim milk for full-fat milk or dairy products. If this is too difficult at first, use 2% or "part skim" products initially and then gradually change to skim.

Choose lean cuts of meat and trim all visible fat; choose ground beef that is at least 85% lean. Avoid fatty meats such as frankfurters, most cold cuts, bacon, and sausage, as well as organ meats—liver, kidney, sweetbreads—which are especially high in cholesterol.

Remove skin and fat from poultry.

Limit serving sizes of meat, poultry, or fish to a piece about the size of a deck of cards.

Limit egg yolk consumption, including eggs used in preparing recipes, to 2 to 3 per week. Egg white is devoid of cholesterol and fat and may be used as desired. Two egg whites can be substituted for one whole egg in recipes.

Cool soups and stews before eating and remove the fat layer on the top.

Substitute soft (tub) margarines for hard margarines or butter. (The softer a spread, the more likely it is to contain polyunsaturated oils that help to decrease serum cholesterol.)

Substitute polyunsaturated oils—corn, soy, sunflower, safflower, and cottonseed—for lard, shortening, coconut oil, palm oil, or "vegetable oil" (that is usually coconut or palm) in cooking.

Avoid doughnuts, croissants, pie crust, muffins, or other pastries prepared with or fried in butter, shortening, or lard.

Avoid cashews and macadamia nuts, which are high in saturated fat. Use walnuts and pecans instead, since these are rich in polyunsaturates.

Substitute hard candies for chocolate, cream-filled, or coconut varieties. (Cocoa butter and coconut contain saturated fat.)

Increase use of legumes, whole grains, fruits, and vegetables, which are good sources of fiber. Try to include one or more "meatless" meals per week, with a main dish of legumes and grains.

---

supplied by vegetables. (In general, bread and pasta made from white flour are preferred, because the bran portion of grains is high in phosphorus. Low-protein breads, pasta, and cereals are available for cases in which regular products would provide excessive amounts of protein.) When glucose is used as the osmotic agent in peritoneal dialysis and arteriovenous hemodialysis, approximately 70% of the glucose in the dialysate may be absorbed, and this must be considered part of the patient's carbohydrate intake.[39,44] For the tube-fed patient, enteral formulas that contain some fiber, such as Compleat (Sandoz) and Enrich (Ross), may help to control hypertriglyceridemia.

To help control hypertriglyceridemia and to provide concentrated calories in minimal fluid, fat should supply about half or more of the patient's calories. Because hypercholesterolemia is frequently found in patients with renal failure, polyunsaturated fats and oils—corn, soy, cottonseed, safflower, and sunflower—are preferred over saturated fats, which tend to raise cholesterol levels. The necessary restriction of meat, milk, and other protein foods in the diet will help to lower cholesterol and saturated fat intake. The box at left provides further information. For patients who need a caloric supplement, Lipomul (Upjohn) is a palatable oral lipid supplement providing 6 calories/ml with minimal sodium and potassium. Intravenous lipids and the long-chain fats found in most enteral formulas, except those prepared from blended foods, are primarily polyunsaturated. Some formulas are rich in medium-chain triglycerides, or fats. Although these triglycerides are saturated, they do not contribute to hypercholesterolemia and thus may be used for the renal patient.

Other nutrients. Table 10-6 is a summary of the recommended nutrient intake for patients with renal disorders, where recommendations are different from those for healthy adults. The recommendations for healthy adults are included to provide a basis for comparison. Certain nutrients are restricted because they are excreted by the kidney. Phosphorus is one example; its restriction appears to delay progression of renal damage.[46] Phosphorus is found primarily in meat, milk, nuts, and whole grains, so that limitation of protein intake will also help to lower phosphorus levels. The patient has no specific requirement for the fat-soluble vitamins A, E, and K because they are not removed in appreciable amounts by dialysis, and restriction prevents development of toxicity. Elevated levels of vitamin A are a common finding in dialyzed patients.[41,42] On the other hand, needs for several water-soluble vitamins and trace minerals are increased in the dialysis patient because they are small enough to pass freely through the dialysis filter. If the patient is not receiving supplements of the water-soluble vitamins listed in Table 10-6, or, if levels of trace elements are not being monitored, the nurses should consult with the physician about the need for such measures. Similarly, if the patient is receiving vitamin A–containing TPN or tube feeding daily, the nurse can discuss with the physician, pharmacist, and dietitian the desirability of devising nutrient solutions providing only the water-soluble vitamins.

Nutrition Teaching in Renal and Fluid Alterations

Although the primary nutrition teaching for such a complex dietary regimen will normally be performed by the dietitian, the nurse can reinforce and supplement the dietary instruction. The patient and family may have special difficulty understanding the rationale for the dietary modifications. For example, laypersons often perceive protein as the most important nutrient, and patients may feel that a protein restriction will result in an inadequate diet. The nurse can reassure them that their diets are planned to provide all the necessary nutrients and explain that they should not

Table 10-6 Daily nutritional recommendations for patients with renal failure

Nutrient	Recommended dietary allowance (RDA) for healthy persons	Daily amount in renal failure
Protein or amino acids (g/kg)	0.8	0.6 (undialyzed)* 1-1.2+ (hemodialysis)* 1.2-1.4+ (peritoneal dialysis)*
Calories/kg	25-30	35-45
Electrolytes and minerals†		
Sodium	Unspecified	87-109 mEq (2-2.5 g)‡
Potassium	Unspecified	70-80 mEq (2.7-3.1 g)
Calcium (mg)	800	1000-1500
Phosphorus (mg)	800	700-800
Magnesium (mg)	300-350	200-300
Trace minerals		
Iron (mg)	10-18	18 mg +, as needed to prevent deficiency
Zinc (mg)	15	15 mg +, as needed to prevent deficiency
Vitamins		
C (mg)	60	70-100
B_6 (mg)	2-2.2	5-10
Folic acid (mg)	0.4	1

Adapted from Feinstein EI: Nutr Clin Prac 3:9, 1988; Kopple JD and Blumenkrantz MJ: Kidney Int (suppl) 16:S295, 1983; and Maschio G and others: Kidney Int 22:371, 1982.
*Based on estimated dry weight.
†Dosages given are representative ranges; serum levels and physical findings help to determine actual individual intake. For instance, the presence of edema and hypertension usually necessitates a reduced sodium allowance. These are enteral recommendations, and parenteral levels may be lower.
‡Levels for continuous ambulatory peritoneal dialysis (CAPD) may be higher.

compare their protein allowances with the amount of protein consumed by the average American, which is actually quite excessive. In addition, an understanding of the need for a generous caloric intake may make the patient more cooperative in consuming meals and supplements or in cooperating when it is apparent that tube feeding or TPN is necessary.

The nurse can help the patient and family learn to recognize sources of high and low biological value protein and to select moderate amounts of the high biological value, to measure all fluid intake and maintain daily records of all fluid intake, and to control sodium (see the box on p. 108) and potassium intake as necessary. Rich sources of potassium include meats, vegetables, and fruits. Potassium content can be reduced by cutting foods into small pieces, soaking them in water, and then draining off the water before cooking the foods or eating them raw. Canned fruits and vegetables (unsalted if the patient requires a sodium restriction) drained of all liquid are lower in potassium than fresh ones.

NUTRITION IN GASTROINTESTINAL ALTERATIONS

Because the gastrointestinal (GI) tract is so inherently related to nutrition, it is not surprising that catastrophic occurrences in the GI tract—hemorrhage, perforation, infarct, or related organ failure—have acute and severe adverse effects on nutritional status.

Nutrition Assessment in Gastrointestinal Alterations

Assessment is summarized in Table 10-7. A fuller explanation of the techniques and terms used in nutritional evaluation may be found in Chapter 9. The area and amount of the GI tract affected determine, to a large extent, the likelihood and degree of nutritional deficits. The ileum is among the most nutritionally important areas. Fat and bile salt absorption occurs in this area, as does absorption of fat-soluble vitamins and vitamin B_{12}. Patients with ileal disease or resection are likely to become malnourished as a result of significant loss of calories, as well as vitamins and minerals, in the feces. The ileocecal valve is especially critical in maintaining adequate nutrition. Not only does it slow entry of GI contents into the large bowel, allowing more time for absorption to take place in the small bowel, but it also helps prevent migration of the microorganisms from the large bowel into the small bowel. Proliferating microorganisms in the small bowel deconjugate the bile salts, impairing fat absorption. Deconjugated bile salts also irritate the intestinal mucosa and raise the osmolality within the bowel, promoting diarrhea.[54]

Nutrition Intervention in Gastrointestinal Alterations

The GI tract is the preferred route for delivery of nutrients in GI disease, as it is in all other disease states. However, following damage or resection, enteral nutrition support may be inadequate or impossible, at least temporarily. The most

Table 10-7 Nutrition assessment of the patient with a gastrointestinal disorder

Area of concern	History	Physical assessment	Laboratory data
Protein-calorie malnutrition	Decreased oral intake caused by: Fear of symptoms—pain, cramping, diarrhea—associated with eating (e.g., peptic ulcer, dumping syndrome) Alcohol abuse Nausea, vomiting, anorexia Increased losses because of: Maldigestion or malabsorption (e.g., inadequate bile salt production, increased loss of bile salts in short bowel syndrome, diarrhea, inadequate absorptive area in short bowel syndrome) GI bleeding Fistula drainage Increased requirements caused by: Needs for healing (e.g., surgical wounds, fistulae)	Muscle wasting Loss of subcutaneous fat Weight <90% of desirable or recent weight loss Triceps skinfold <10th percentile* Hair loss or change in texture	Serum albumin <3.5 g/dl or low transferrin Total lymphocyte count <1200/mm³ Creatinine excretion <17 mg/kg/day (women) or 23 mg/kg/day (men) Negative nitrogen balance Fecal fat >5 g/day or >5% of intake
Potential fluid volume deficit	Losses caused by severe vomiting or diarrhea (e.g., GI obstruction, short bowel syndrome)	Poor skin turgor Dry, sticky mucous membranes Complaint of thirst Loss of ≥0.23 kg (0.5 pounds) in 24 hr	Hct >52% (men) or 47% (women) BUN >20 mg/dl Serum sodium >145 mEq/L Serum osmolality >300 mOsm/kg Urine specific gravity >1.030

DISORDERS OF MINERAL/ELECTROLYTE NUTRITURE

Calcium (Ca)	Increased loss because of steatorrhea (Ca forms soaps with fat in the stool and thus becomes unabsorbable)	Tingling of fingers Muscular tetany and cramps Carpopedal spasm Convulsions	Serum Ca <8.5 mg/dl (Severe deficits only)
Magnesium (Mg)	Inadequate intake because of poor diet in alcoholism Increased losses because of: Diarrhea or steatorrhea Loss of small bowel fluid (e.g., in short bowel syndrome, fistulae)	Tremor Hyperactive deep reflexes Convulsions	Serum Mg <1.5 mEq/L

Adapted from Moore MC: Pocket guide to nutrition and diet therapy, St. Louis, 1988, The CV Mosby Co.
hct, hematocrit; BUN, blood urea nitrogen; hgb, hemoglobin; MCV, mean cell volume; MCH, mean cell hemoglobin; MCHC, mean cell hemoglobin concentration; Ca, calcium.
See Chapter 9 for explanation of nutrition assessment techniques and their interpretation.
*6 mm for men and 14 mm for women.

Table 10-7 Nutrition assessment of the patient with a gastrointestinal disorder—cont'd

Area of concern	History	Physical assessment	Laboratory data
DISORDERS OF MINERAL/ELECTROLYTE NUTRITURE—cont'd			
Iron (Fe)	Blood loss Impaired absorption because of decreased upper GI acidity with gastrectomy or use of antacids and cimetidine Inadequate intake (e.g., restriction of protein foods in hepatic failure)	Pallor, blue sclerae Fatigue Koilonychia	Hct <42% (men) or 37% (women), hgb <14 g/dl (men) or 12 g/dl (women), low MCV, MCH, MCHC Serum Fe <60 μg/dl

Zinc (Zn)	Increased losses caused by:
	  Diarrhea, steatorrhea
	  Loss of small bowel fluid
	  Diuretic use (in hepatic failure)
	  Increased urinary losses in alcoholism
	Inadequate intake caused by:
	  Protein restriction in hepatic failure
	  Poor diet in alcoholism
		Anorexia
		Hypogeusia, dysgeusia
		Seborrheic dermatitis
			Serum Zn <60 μg/ml

Potassium (K⁺)	Increased loss caused by:
	  Diarrhea
	  Diuretic use
	  Hyperaldosteronism (in hepatic failure)
	  GI suction
		Muscle weakness, ileus
		Diminished reflexes
			Serum K^+ <3.5 mEq/L

DISORDERS OF VITAMIN NUTRITURE			
A	Increased loss in steatorrhea (vitamin A dissolves in fatty stools) Impaired release of vitamin A from storage in the liver because of inadequate production of retinol-binding protein, the transport protein, in malnutrition or liver failure)	Drying of skin and cornea Poor wound healing Follicular hyperkeratosis (resembles gooseflesh)	Serum retinol <20 μg/dl
K	Impaired absorption in steatorrhea Decreased production because of destruction of intestinal bacteria by antibiotic usage	Petechiae, ecchymoses Prolonged bleeding	Prothrombin time >12.5 sec (not accurate in liver failure)

INDICATIONS FOR SPECIALIZED NUTRITION SUPPORT IN GI ALTERATIONS

PARENTERAL NUTRITION

Complete obstruction of the small or large bowel
Ileus or severe hypomotility of the intestine
Short bowel syndrome (>50% small bowel resection)
High output (>500 ml/day) enterocutaneous fistulae, where bowel rest may reduce GI secretions and promote healing
Severe diarrhea unresponsive to pharmacological therapy

ENTERAL NUTRITION

Short bowel syndrome (50% to 90% small bowel resection), in conjunction with TPN
Low output enterocutaneous fistulae, especially if feedings can be given distal to the fistulae
Anorexia caused by hepatic failure and the unpalatable diet required for its treatment
Stupor or coma

---

common indications for parenteral and enteral feedings in GI patients are listed in the box above. Nursing care of patients receiving enteral feedings and TPN has already been described. Since bowel resection and hepatic failure are two of the most nutritionally challenging GI alterations, most of this discussion will be devoted to them.

Short bowel syndrome

Administration of fluids and electrolytes. Extensive bowel resection is associated with marked gastric hypersecretion. The increase in gastric juices, coupled with the sudden loss of absorptive area, results in the loss of several liters of fluid daily, along with potassium, magnesium, and zinc. The nurse's role in management of these patients includes (1) strict intake and output records, including volume or weight of stools if they are frequent or loose, (2) ongoing assessment of the patient's state of hydration, and (3) administration of fluids and electrolytes and evaluation of the patient's response, including daily weight measurements to evaluate the adequacy of fluid replacement.

Administration of nutrition support. The major nutritional problems associated with bowel resection are loss of absorptive area, with increased fecal losses of fluids, electrolytes, fat, protein, and other nutrients; increased loss of bile salts, especially if the terminal ileum was resected, with further malabsorption of fat; and micronutrient deficiencies resulting from trapping of minerals and fat-soluble vitamins within the excreted fat. Following bowel resection, the remaining intestine undergoes marked hyperplasia, with increasing length of the remaining villi, which increases the available absorptive area. The result is improved absorption of water, electrolytes, and glucose.[52] Some patients with 70% to 80% resection of the small bowel can eventually be

maintained on enteral feedings only, especially if the terminal ileum and ileocecal valve are retained, but patients with resection of more than 90% of the small bowel usually require permanent TPN.[50,54] The small bowel is estimated to be approximately 350 to 650 cm in length, depending on whether measurements are made during surgery, when the GI tract retains much of the muscle tonus, or on postmortem examination, when minimal tone is present.[54] It is difficult to estimate the amount remaining at the time of intestinal resection, and thus many patients undergo contrast radiographs when stable to determine the length of the remaining bowel. The adaptive response may take up to a year to become complete, and it does not occur without the presence of nutrients within the gut.[52] Therefore every attempt is made to introduce some enteral feedings early in the course of recovery.

Patients are supported with TPN until fecal output declines, usually to less than 1 L/day. At that point, very small amounts of enteral feedings are begun. Feedings may consist of an elemental, or predigested, diet given by tube. Fat is the most difficult nutrient to absorb, and the formula will ordinarily be very low in fat or will be high in medium-chain triglycerides (MCTs), which are more readily absorbed than the long-chain triglycerides predominating in most foods. Tube feedings should be given on a continuous basis, to promote optimal absorption. Intragastric rather than transpyloric feedings are preferable to utilize every available centimeter of intestinal surface area. Alternatively, a low-fat, high-starch diet may be given by mouth. Foods such as white rice; enriched white bread and toast; plain pasta; and peeled boiled or baked potato, without added milk, cheese, butter, margarine, or other fat are examples of those allowed initially. Low-fat meats such as chicken without skin are gradually added, and then small amounts of fruits and vegetables are introduced.[51] Lactose, or milk sugar, is often tolerated poorly by patients with bowel resection, but low-fat cottage cheese or yogurt, which are relatively low in lactose, may be tolerated. MCTs can be served in juice or used in food preparation to increase caloric intake. Patients receiving oral feedings often require much encouragement to eat, because they may associate eating with worsening of diarrhea. As more and more enteral intake is tolerated, TPN is gradually tapered. Careful records must be kept of all enteral and parenteral intake to determine when TPN can be decreased or discontinued.

Administration of medications. The nurse may need to discuss with the physician the possibility of using medications to control severe, watery diarrhea. In some patients with short bowel syndrome, in whom diarrhea is prolonged or especially severe and causes anal excoriation or copious ostomy output, antidiarrheal agents such as diphenoxylate with atropine or codeine may be beneficial. Anticholinergic drugs such as glycopyrrolate can also be used to counteract the gastric hypersecretion.

Hepatic failure.
Hepatic failure is associated with a wide spectrum of metabolic alterations. Because the diseased liver has impaired ability to deactivate hormones, there are elevated levels of circulating glucagon, epinephrine, and

cortisol. These hormones promote catabolism of body tissues. Glycogen stores are rapidly exhausted. Although release of lipids from their storage depots is accelerated, the liver has decreased ability to metabolize them for energy. Furthermore, as many as half of the patients with hepatic failure may have malabsorption of fat because of inadequate production of bile salts by the liver. Therefore body proteins are increasingly utilized for energy sources, producing rapid tissue wasting. The branched chain amino acids (BCAA), leucine, isoleucine, and valine, are especially well utilized for energy, and their levels in the blood decline. Conversely, levels of the aromatic amino acids (AAA), phenylalanine, tyrosine, and tryptophan, rise as a result of tissue catabolism and impaired ability of the liver to clear them from the blood. While hyperammonemia is a feature of hepatic failure, it probably is not the causative agent in encephalopathy; instead, AAAs appear to be the culprits. After transport across the blood-brain barrier, they can be converted to "false neurotransmitters," which compete with the normal neurotransmitters for binding sites. The net result is to impede normal neurotransmission and produce hepatic encephalopathy.[56]

Monitoring of fluid and electrolyte status. Ascites and edema occur because of decreased colloid osmotic pressure in the plasma as the diseased liver produces less albumin and other plasma proteins, increased portal pressure caused by obstruction, and renal sodium retention from secondary hyperaldosteronism. To control the fluid retention, restriction of sodium (usually 500 to 1500 mg, or 20 to 65 mEq, daily) and fluid (1500 ml or less) is generally necessary, in conjunction with administration of diuretics. Patients must be weighed daily to evaluate the success of treatment. In addition, laboratory and physical status must be closely observed for potassium deficits caused by diuretic therapy and hyperaldosteronism.

Provision of a nutritious diet and evaluation of response to dietary protein. Nutrition intervention in hepatic failure is based on the metabolic alterations. Initially, protein allowances are increased to 1 to 1.5 g/kg/day, in an effort to suppress catabolism and promote liver regeneration. However, if encephalopathy occurs or appears to be impending, protein intake is reduced to 0.5 g/kg/day or less. A high-calorie diet (45 to 50 calories/kg/day compared with about 25 to 30 calories for the healthy adult) is provided to help prevent catabolism and to prevent the use of dietary protein for energy needs. Moderate amounts of fat are given, unless the patient has steatorrhea, in which case it is necessary to rely heavily on carbohydrates and MCTs to meet caloric needs. Soft foods are preferred, because the patient may have esophageal varices that might be irritated by high-fiber foods. Since alcoholism is so often the cause of hepatic failure and the diets of alcoholics have been shown to be low in zinc, vitamin B complex, folate, and magnesium, supplements of these nutrients are usually provided daily.[56] Anorexia, malaise, and confusion may interfere with oral intake, and the nurse may need to provide much encouragement to the patient to ensure intake of an adequate diet. Small, frequent feedings are usually better accepted by the anorexic patient than three large daily meals. The nurse must assess the patient's neurological status daily to evaluate tolerance of dietary protein. Increasing lethargy, confusion, or asterixis may signal a need for decreased protein intake. Anorexia, coupled with the unpalatable nature of the very low-sodium, low-protein diet required in impending coma, may result in a need for tube feedings.

Although experimental results are conflicting,[53,58,59] some authorities feel that administration of increased amounts of BCAA in encephalopathy may improve electroencephalograms, arousal, and survival, as well as nutritional status. BCAA-enriched enteral formulas (Hepatic-Aid II [Kendall McGaw] and Travasorb Hepatic [Travenol]) and parenteral amino acid solutions (Hepatamine [Kendall McGaw]) are available. Diarrhea from concurrent administration of lactulose should not be confused with intolerance of the enteral formulations. Thus far evidence is lacking that BCAA-enriched formulas are beneficial in hepatic failure without encephalopathy.

Nutrition Teaching in Gastrointestinal Alterations

Teaching usually focuses on three areas: the rationale for dietary modifications and nutrition support, components of a nutritious and balanced diet, and the need to take vitamin/mineral supplements as ordered. Both the patient with hepatic failure and the one with short bowel syndrome require high-calorie, high-protein diets during convalescence. In addition, the patient with short bowel syndrome should adhere to a low-fiber diet with generous amounts of fluids. Although fat is an excellent source of calories, fat malabsorption is a problem for both groups of patients. Even with intestinal adaptation and hyperplasia, fat absorption may never normalize in the patient with short bowel syndrome, and the patient may experience less diarrhea and discomfort if a low-fat diet is followed permanently.[51] Fried foods, visible fat in meats, butter, margarine, salad dressings, and ice cream are obvious sources of fat. Patients may need help in recognizing "hidden" sources of fat, such as nuts, pastries, marbling in meats, and egg yolks. Energy needs can be met by cereals and breads, starchy vegetables, and dairy products made from skim milk. Glucose oligosaccharides (for example, Polycose [Ross] and Moducal [Mead Johnson]), which can be added to beverages, cereals, or soups without increasing the sweetness, and MCT oil are two caloric supplements that can also be used. Patients with steatorrhea usually need daily oral water-miscible supplements of the fat-soluble vitamins to prevent deficiencies. Supplements of calcium, zinc, and magnesium may also be needed. The nurse needs to be sure that the patient understands the dosage and is capable of administering these supplements.

In addition, patients who will be discharged on tube feedings or TPN (usually those with short bowel syndrome) must be taught the mechanics of administering their feedings and maintaining their feeding tube or catheter, as well as methods of preventing and coping with problems and complications. The need for long-term nutrition support may have severe emotional and financial impacts. Emotional support

Table 10-8 Nutrition assessment of the patient with an endocrine disorder

Area of concern	History	Physical findings	Laboratory data
Underweight or protein-calorie malnutrition	Increased losses of calories in urine or feces caused by: Impaired glucose metabolism and glucosuria in type I diabetes mellitus Steatorrhea in pancreatitis Decreased intake because of: Discomfort with eating (in pancreatitis) Alcoholism (often a cause of pancreatitis)	Weight less than 90% of desirable Recent weight loss Wasting of muscle and subcutaneous tissue Triceps skinfold <10th percentile*	Urine glucose >0.5% Fecal fat >5 g/24 hr or <95% of intake Serum albumin <3.5 g/dl, or low transferrin or prealbumin levels Total lymphocyte count <1200/mm³ Creatinine excretion <17 mg/kg/day (women) or 23 mg/kg/day (men)
Overweight	NIDDM Sedentary lifestyle	Weight >120% of desirable Triceps skinfold >90th percentile†	
Potential fluid volume deficit	Diuresis (from diabetes insipidus or osmotic diuresis of HHNK or ketoacidosis)	Poor skin turgor Dry, sticky mucous membranes Thirst Loss of >0.23 kg (0.5 pounds) in 24 hr Increased urine output	Serum glucose >250 mg/dl Urine glucose >0.5% Serum sodium >145 mEq/L Increasing hct BUN >20 mg/dl
Potential fluid volume excess	Fluid retention caused by SIADH	Edema (peripheral and/or pulmonary) Gain of >0.23 kg (0.5 pounds) in 24 hr	Serum sodium <135 mEq/L Decreasing hct
Potential zinc deficiency	Impaired absorption in steatorrhea Increased urinary losses in diuresis, diabetes mellitus, and alcoholism Poor intake in alcoholism	Hypogeusia, dysgeusia Alopecia Seborrheic dermatitis Impaired wound healing	Serum zinc <60 μg/ml

Adapted from Moore MC: Pocket guide to nutrition and diet therapy, St. Louis, 1988, The CV Mosby Co.
See Chapter 9 for further information on laboratory and physical findings and their interpretation in nutrition assessment.
Hct, hematocrit; BUN, blood urea nitrogen; SIADH, syndrome of inappropriate secretion of antidiuretic hormone.
*6 mm for men and 14 mm for women.
†20 mm for men and 34 mm for women.

and counseling are among the nurse's most important roles in assisting these patients. In an effort to encourage resumption of normal activity patterns, many patients are begun on cyclical feedings, usually administered nocturnally, as discharge is anticipated. In stable patients, cyclical feedings appear to be nutritionally adequate.[57] The patient may feel deprived of sensory pleasures and interaction with family and friends at mealtimes and events where food is served. If at all possible, the patient should be encouraged to join family and friends at mealtimes or social events and to eat, even if only small amounts.[55] The costs of long-term home nutrition support are high, although not nearly as high as continued hospitalization, and the social worker or financial counselor should be involved early in the patient's hospitalization in exploring routes of payment, as plans are made for discharge.

NUTRITION AND ENDOCRINE ALTERATIONS

Because of the far-reaching effects on all body systems, endocrine alterations have an impact on nutritional status in a variety of ways.

Nutrition Assessment in Endocrine Alterations

The nutrition assessment process is summarized in Table 10-8. Because of the prevalence of non–insulin-dependent diabetes mellitus (NIDDM) patients among the hospitalized population, the nutritional problems most commonly noted in patients with endocrine alterations are overweight and obesity.

Nutrition Intervention in Endocrine Alterations

Underweight and malnourished patients. The most severely undernourished patients are usually those with pancreatitis, because of loss of pancreatic exocrine function. Pancreatic insufficiency, with inadequate release of trypsin, chymotrypsin, and pancreatic lipase and amylase, results in impaired digestion and subsequent loss of nutrients in the stool. Fat malabsorption is the most marked effect of pancreatic insufficiency. Fat lost in the stools is accompanied by calcium, zinc, and other minerals, along with the fat-soluble vitamins. Nutritional care in malabsorptive disorders is discussed more thoroughly in the section concerning nutrition in gastrointestinal alterations.

Patients with insulin-dependent diabetes mellitus (IDDM) or endocrine dysfunction caused by pancreatitis often have weight loss and malnutrition as a result of tissue catabolism, because they cannot utilize dietary carbohydrate to meet energy needs. Although patients with NIDDM are more likely to be overweight than underweight, they too may become malnourished as a result of chronic or acute infections, trauma, major surgery, or other illnesses. Delivery of nutrition support in these patients, especially control of blood glucose, can be challenging. Blood glucose should be monitored regularly, usually several times a day until the patient is stable. Regular insulin added to the solution is the most common method of managing hyperglycemia in the patient receiving TPN. The dosage required is almost always larger than the patient's usual subcutaneous dose, because some of the insulin adheres to glass bottles and plastic bags

or administration sets. Continuous subcutaneous infusion of insulin may also be used. Hyperglycemia is also a common problem in tube-fed patients, particularly when feedings are given continuously. Twice-daily doses of intermediate-acting insulin or more frequent doses of regular insulin may be inadequate to control hyperglycemia in continuously fed patients. One solution is to administer feedings intermittently, on a "meal-type" schedule, and to administer oral hypoglycemics, regular insulin, or intermediate-acting insulin based on this schedule.[66] However, some diabetic patients require continuous feedings. For example, patients with severe gastroparesis may need transpyloric feedings because poor gastric emptying makes intragastric feedings impossible or inadequate. Transpyloric feedings must almost always be given continuously, since dumping syndrome and poor absorption often occur if feedings are given rapidly into the small bowel. For the continuously tube-fed diabetic patient, control of blood glucose may be improved either with continuous insulin infusion or by use of a formula containing fiber, if possible. Examples are Compleat (Sandoz) and Enrich (Ross). Fiber slows the absorption of the carbohydrate in the formula, producing a more delayed and sustained glycemic response.

Overweight patients. Aggressive attempts at weight loss are rarely warranted among very ill patients, although weight loss in overweight patients with NIDDM improves glucose tolerance. Instead of suggesting a low-calorie diet, nurses should encourage patients to select foods providing fiber and starches (for example, dried beans and peas, whole-grain breads and cereals, pasta, fresh fruits and vegetables) rather than more refined carbohydrates (for example, white bread, fruit juice, and "instant" mashed potatoes). Diets rich in complex carbohydrates have been shown to lower insulin requirements, increase the sensitivity of the peripheral tissues to insulin, and decrease serum cholesterol levels.[61] Although results of studies of the use of high-fiber diets in an effort to promote weight loss are inconclusive,[68] it appears that reliance on bulky, high-fiber foods may help to reduce caloric intake.[60,65] Weight loss may occur because fiber delays gastric emptying and increases satiety, so the patient is satisfied with less food. Also, absorption of nutrients such as starch and fats from a high-fiber diet may be less complete than absorption from a low-fiber diet.[65,70]

Nutrition support should not be neglected simply because a patient is obese, because protein-calorie malnutrition develops even among such patients. When a patient is not expected to be able to eat for at least 5 to 7 days, or inadequate intake persists for that period of time, the nurse should consult with the physician regarding initiation of tube feedings or TPN if no steps have been taken to do so. There is no disease process that benefits from starvation, and development or progression of nutritional deficits may contribute to complications (for example, decubitus ulcers, pulmonary or urinary tract infections, and sepsis, which prolong hospitalization, increase the costs of care, and may even result in death[64,67,69]).

Nutrition Teaching in Endocrine Alterations

Most nutrition teaching in the patient with endocrine alterations focuses on understanding of the diet of the diabetic

Table 10-9 Nutrition assessment of the patient with a hematoimmune disorder

Area of concern	History	Physical findings	Laboratory data
Protein-calorie malnutrition	Nutrient losses caused by malabsorption and diarrhea (AIDS) Increased needs caused by infection and fever Poor intake caused by: Anorexia (related to respiratory or other infections, emotional stress, medication side effects) Pain associated with eating (e.g., *Candida* esophagitis in the immunosuppressed patient) Dementia or CNS infections associated with AIDS	Recent weight loss Weight less than 90% of desirable Wasting of muscle and subcutaneous tissue Triceps skinfold <10th percentile*	Serum albumin <3.5 g/dl, or low transferrin or prealbumin Negative nitrogen balance Urinary creatinine <17 mg/kg (women) or 23 mg/kg (men)
DISORDERS OF MINERAL NUTRITURE			
Iron (Fe)	Blood loss Poor intake of meats, whole-grain or enriched breads and cereals, legumes because of: Anorexia Pain associated with eating	Pallor, blue sclerae Koilonychia Fatigue Tachycardia	Hct <37% (women) or 42% (men), hgb <12 g/dl (women) or 14 g/dl (men), low MCV, MCH, MCHC
Zinc (Zn)	Impaired absorption in diarrhea Poor intake of meats, whole grains, legumes because of: Anorexia Pain associated with eating	Hypogeusia, dysgeusia Alopecia Seborrheic dermatitis Impaired wound healing	Serum Zn <60 µg/dl
Selenium (Se)	Impaired absorption in diarrhea Poor intake of meats, fish, poultry	Congestive cardiomyopathy Muscle weakness Pallor, fatigue, tachycardia (anemia caused by RBC fragility)	Serum Se <0.08 µg/ml Presence of nucleated RBC, Howell-Jolly bodies, Heinz bodies (hemolytic anemia)

See Chapter 9 for further information regarding techniques of nutrition assessment and interpretation of findings.
Hct, hematocrit; hgb, hemoglobin; MCV, mean cell volume; MCH, mean cell hemoglobin; MCHC, mean cell hemoglobin concentration; RBC, red blood cell.
*6 mm for men and 14 mm for women.

patient and on achieving the desirable body weight. The underweight or overweight patient should be helped to understand the need for weight changes. For example, weight loss in the obese diabetic individual improves glucose tolerance and may reduce or eliminate the need for insulin. In addition, it usually has beneficial effects on blood pressure and serum cholesterol levels.

Diet instruction for the diabetic patient is usually carried out by the dietitian, but the nurse should be able to reinforce the information given. Among the most important concepts for the diabetic patient to understand are:

1. No planned meal or snack should ever be omitted, particularly if the patient is using insulin or an oral hypoglycemic agent.

2. Food exchanges should not be transferred from one meal to another. The planned exchanges should be eaten at regular times each day to avoid undue fluctuations in blood glucose.

3. No foods should be added to the diet, unless hypoglycemia occurs or unless the patient is engaging in vigorous physical exertion. The best way to know whether increased food is needed during exercise is to monitor blood glucose. Generally, no additional food is needed during light exercise (a leisurely walk or half-hour bicycle ride) if blood glucose is greater than 100 mg/dl. For moderate exercise, an extra 10 to 15 g of carbohydrate (one small apple or orange, or a slice of bread) may be needed before exercise if the blood glucose is near normal (100 to 180 mg/dl). Increased food intake is usually not needed if blood glucose is greater than 180 mg/dl. For strenuous exercise lasting 1 to 2 hours, when blood glucose is near normal, 25 to 50 g carbohydrate (for example, cottage cheese with rye wafers and fruit) will usually be needed before exercise.[63]

4. Emphasizing foods high in complex carbohydrate improves glucose tolerance and might promote gradual weight loss.

5. "Dietetic" and "diabetic" foods are unnecessary. Also, labels containing these words do not always mean that foods are unsweetened. They may be sweetened with fructose, sorbitol, or other absorbable sweeteners. The patient who wishes to use these products should read the label carefully to determine exactly what dietetic or diabetic means in this context. Some "dietetic" cookies contain more calories than the standard version of the product. Fruits canned in water or juice (with the juice drained before serving) are available in all supermarkets and are suitable for the diabetic patient.

6. Moderate exercise has many benefits, including increased insulin sensitivity and improved glucose tolerance, weight control, reduced blood cholesterol levels, and lowered blood pressure.[62,63] If the physician approves, the patient should be encouraged to begin an exercise program, gradually increasing the length and intensity of the exercise sessions. To be effective, exercise should be performed at least 4 days a week for 20 to 30 minutes at each session. Strenuous exercise and competitive jarring or bouncing activities can worsen retinopathy, nephropathy, and neuropathy associated with diabetes. For this reason, walking, bicycling, and swimming are preferable to racquetball, tennis, or rope skipping.[63]

NUTRITION AND HEMATOIMMUNE ALTERATIONS

Malnutrition has well-known adverse effects on hematoimmune function. Generalized protein-calorie malnutrition, for example, depresses cell-mediated immunity, secretory immunity, complement levels, and phagocyte activity.[75] Deficiencies of single nutrients—especially iron, zinc, selenium, folic acid, and vitamins B_{12}, B_6, C, and A—also impair immunological function.[72,73,75,77] Selenium depletion not only impairs fungicidal activity, creating a predisposition to candidiasis, but also increases the risk of neoplasm.[77,83] In the patient with an existing hematoimmune disorder, therefore, maintenance of adequate nutrition is essential to prevent additional immunological deficits.

Nutrition Assessment in Hematoimmune Alterations

Assessment of the patient with a hematoimmune disorder is summarized in Table 10-9. Unfortunately, generalized protein-calorie malnutrition is a common concomitant of the acquired immunodeficiency syndrome (AIDS). There are multiple etiological factors for the malnutrition. AIDS itself may be associated with a poorly understood enteropathy that causes diarrhea and malabsorption.[76,79] Furthermore, opportunistic gastrointestinal (GI) infections caused by various fungi, viruses, bacteria, and protozoans may cause diarrhea. *Cryptosporidium*, a particularly resistant protozoan, can cause intractable, profuse, watery diarrhea lasting for months.[81] Calorie and protein needs are elevated in AIDS, because metabolic rate and catabolism increase as a result of infection, fever, and malignancies such as lymphoma and Kaposi's sarcoma. At the same time, oral intake is frequently suppressed by emotional reactions to the personal, family, and financial stresses imposed by AIDS; oral and esophageal pain from lesions of Kaposi's sarcoma, herpes, candidiasis, and/or chemotherapy; nausea, vomiting, and anorexia associated with antibiotic therapy or chemotherapy for malignancies; and impaired motor ability, confusion, and dementia caused by AIDS encephalitis or opportunistic central nervous system infections. AIDS patients often have marked weight loss, hypoalbuminemia, and low levels of zinc, selenium, and other minerals.[71,77,78,80] Other hematoimmune disorders are less likely to be associated with such profound nutritional consequences.

Nutrition Intervention in Hematoimmune Alterations

Ideally, nutrition intervention in hematoimmune disorders can be achieved orally. TPN further increases the risk of infection in the immunosuppressed patient, and both TPN and tube feeding are more costly than oral feedings.

Promotion of adequate oral intake. As has already been discussed, oral intake may be severely reduced in the AIDS patient. Table 10-10 provides measures for improving intake.

Administration of nutrition support. Despite dietary modifications and encouragement, some patients may find consuming an adequate diet impossible. When tube feedings must be used, patients with stomatitis and esophagitis may

Table 10-10 Improving oral intake in the patient with AIDS

Problem	Suggested interventions
Anorexia	Offer small, frequent feedings. Save foods from the patient's tray for between-meal feedings or plan with the dietitian for regular snacks to be delivered. The patient may prefer to have snacks and supplemental beverages kept at the bedside so that they are available whenever desired.
	Discuss with the dietitian the possibility of using regular dishes and utensils, rather than disposable products (if isolation precautions are part of the institution's dietary policy for AIDS).* This decreases the patient's feelings of isolation, improves the appearance of the tray, and provides higher quality food at appropriate temperatures.[82]
	Encourage calorie-dense foods, e.g., shakes rather than fruit juice or soft drinks, buttered breads or potatoes with gravy rather than leafy vegetables, and pudding or yogurt rather than fresh fruit. Discourage drinking of water or other no-calorie beverages; keep calorie-containing fluids always available.
Oral and esophageal pain	Determine from the patient what seems to increase discomfort. Acidic foods such as orange or grapefruit juice, foods served at temperature extremes, highly spiced foods, and very coarse or fibrous foods are most likely to exacerbate mucositis.
	Suggest that the patient try pudding, custard, yogurt, gelatin, and canned fruits. Cool (not icy), smooth foods may be soothing.
	Discuss with the physician whether viscous lidocaine can be used to ease discomfort and encourage oral intake.
Nausea and vomiting	Find out from the patient which foods tend to worsen nausea and avoid offering these. Fatty foods and those with strong odors are often the worst offenders.
	Offer gelatin, sherbet, fruit ices, pudding, custard, and fruits. Cool foods may be tolerated better than hot ones.
	Serve small amounts frequently.
	Provide mouth care after emesis, and try to keep the environment as clean and odor free as possible.
Diarrhea	Encourage ample fluid intake. Keep calorie-containing beverages always available.
	Administer antidiarrheals as ordered.
	Consider the possibility of lactose (milk sugar) intolerance. Damage to the intestinal mucosa often decreases the level of lactase, the enzyme required for lactose digestion. Undigested lactose in the stool promotes osmotic diarrhea, bloating, and cramping. Many lactose-free liquid supplements are available; they can replace milk and milk-based supplements.
	Encourage low-fat foods if steatorrhea is present.
	Discuss with physician and dietitian the use of fiber-containing foods or supplements if the diarrhea is refractory to other interventions. Fruits, vegetables, and legumes provide "soluble" dietary fiber that may help to firm stools. Banana flakes and other fiber supplements are also available.

*AIDS has not been shown to be spread by food, food handlers, or dishes. Although the human immunodeficiency virus is found in saliva, it does not live long outside the body and should be inactivated by usual dishwashing procedures. See Conte JE: Ann Intern Med 105:730, 1986; and Resler SS: J Am Dietet Assoc 88:828, 1988.

complain of pain from the tube. To lessen the discomfort, the feeding tube should be the smallest size possible (usually 8 Fr in diameter), and the tube should be composed of a nonreactive material such as polyurethane or silicone rubber. Use of viscous lidocaine may also help to relieve discomfort.

The patient with diarrhea and malabsorption usually needs an elemental, or predigested, formula. These formulas contain medium-chain triglycerides, which are more readily digested than the long-chain triglycerides found in most foods and standard enteral formulas, and amino acids or peptides, rather than intact proteins. The patient with diarrhea usually tolerates continuous feedings better than intermittent feedings. Where diarrhea is refractory to treatment, administration of a fiber supplement may be beneficial in firming the stools.

Where enteral feedings are not tolerated, TPN may be appropriate. However, the question of whether aggressive nutrition support improves the patient's status enough to balance the risks and potential complications has not been answered.[78] When TPN is used, the nurse must be scrupulous in use of aseptic technique in order to avoid infection in the immunosuppressed patient.

Administration of vitamin-mineral supplements. Many patients with hematoimmune disorders require vitamin and mineral supplementation. Iron is especially important in the patient with anemia as a result of chronic disease or hemorrhagic losses. Iron, zinc, and selenium lost in diarrhea must be replaced in the patient with AIDS. The timing of delivery, as well as the foods administered concurrently, can significantly affect absorption of minerals, especially iron. Most minerals, including iron, are best absorbed when there are no other foods present in the stomach. However, patients may complain of gastric irritation when this is done. Giving the supplement at bedtime may minimize epigastric distress. Alternatively, supplements may be administered with acidic foods such as orange juice or with meats, both of which increase uptake. Coffee, tea, and milk impair absorption and should not be given at the same time as the supplement.

Nutrition Teaching in Hematoimmune Disorders

Nutrition teaching for the patient with AIDS should include the importance of good nutrition in maintaining strength and optimal functioning and in preventing additional deficits in immune function and wound healing. The patient should be discouraged from viewing nutrition itself as a panacea; its major role is in supportive care. Some patients may adopt food fads, such as consuming lecithin, orange juice, and butter mixtures or taking "megadose" vitamin supplements. These measures are not beneficial, and in a few cases they may be harmful (for example, when the vitamin supplements include dosages of fat-soluble vitamins that are several times the recommended dietary allowance, which could result in toxicity). The nurse should provide factual information about nutrition and avoid raising false hopes that nutrition can have any curative effects.

Consumption of an adequate diet. The AIDS patient should be encouraged to consume an adequate diet of regular foods, if at all possible. The guidelines in Table 10-10 and in the box on p. 108 can be shared with the patient and family, friends, or other caretakers. Frequent small feedings are essential if nutrient needs are to be met. Commercial supplements (lactose-free, if diarrhea seems to be worsened by milk intake) or nutritious shakes prepared from instant breakfast, ice cream, and cream are especially good sources of calories and nutrients for between-meal snacks.

Self-administration of vitamin-mineral supplements. When a supplement is indicated (for example, in the patient with iron deficiency as a result of posthemorrhagic anemia or in the AIDS patient with zinc deficiency), the nurse should ensure that the patient or caretaker understands the dosage and frequency of administration. Timing of the dosage and relationship of the supplement to food intake should also be explained. (See the previous section on nutrition intervention in hematoimmune alterations.)

Administration of tube feedings and TPN, if applicable. Home tube feeding and TPN is increasingly common among AIDS patients. When a patient is to be discharged on either of these nutrition support modalities, instruction should begin early in hospitalization. The patient (if possible) and some other responsible person such as a family member or friend, as well as home health nurses to be involved in the patient's care, should be thoroughly trained. Preparation for home tube feedings should include placing the feeding tube (if necessary), checking placement, irrigating the tube to maintain patency, obtaining or preparing the formula, administering the formula on the proper schedule, operating the enteral feeding pump (if applicable), and recognizing and coping with complications such as diarrhea, constipa-

tion, pulmonary aspiration, and clogging of the feeding tube. For patients receiving home TPN, instruction should include the rationale for and principles of aseptic technique, as well as performing catheter and dressing care, obtaining or preparing solutions, administering the solutions on the appropriate schedule, operating the infusion pump, and preventing, recognizing, and managing complications such as infection, catheter damage, hyperglycemia, and air embolus. Chapter 9 provides specific information about delivery of tube feedings and TPN and can be used as a basis for teaching the patient.

REFERENCES
Cardiovascular

1. American Heart Association: Dietary guidelines for healthy American adults, Dallas, 1986, The Association.
2. Bagatell CJ and Heymsfield SB: Effect of meal size on myocardial oxygen requirements: implications for postmyocardial infarction diet, Am J Clin Nutr 39:421, 1984.
3. Kaplan NM: Non-drug treatment of hypertension, Ann Int Med 102:359, 1985.
4. Kelsen SG: The effects of undernutrition on the respiratory muscles, Clin Chest Med 7:101, 1986.
5. Kinsella JE: Food components with potential therapeutic benefits: the n-3 polyunsaturated fatty acids of fish oils, Food Technol 40:89, 1986.
6. Kromhout D, Bosscheiter ED, and deLezenne Coulander C: The inverse relation between fish consumption and 20-year mortality from coronary heart disease, N Engl J Med 312:1205, 1985.
7. Myers MG and others: Caffeine as a possible cause of ventricular arrhythmias during the healing phase of acute myocardial infarction, Am J Cardiol 59:1024, 1987.
8. National Institutes of Health Consensus Development Conference: Lowering blood cholesterol to prevent heart disease, JAMA 253:2080, 1985.
9. National Cholesterol Education Program: Cholesterol Treatment Recommendations for Adults, Bethesda, Md, 1987, National Heart, Lung, and Blood Institute.
10. Nonpharmacological approaches to the control of high blood pressure: final report of the subcommittee on nonpharmacological therapy of the 1984 joint national committee on detection, evaluation, and treatment of high blood pressure, Hypertension 8:444, 1986.
11. Poindexter SM, Dear WE, and Dudrick SJ: Nutrition in congestive heart failure, Nutr Clin Prac 1:83, 1986.
12. Rock CL and Coulston AM: Weight-control approaches: a review by the California Dietetic Association, J Am Diet Assoc 88:44, 1988.
13. Schneider JR: Effects of caffeine ingestion on heart rate, blood pressure, myocardial oxygen consumption, and cardiac rhythm in acute myocardial infarction patients, Heart Lung 16:167, 1987.
14. Stevens J: Does dietary fiber affect food intake and body weight? J Am Diet Assoc 88:939, 1988.

Pulmonary

15. Flynn KT, Norton LC, and Fisher RL: Enteral tube feeding: indications, practices and outcomes, Image J Nurs Sch 19:16, 1987.
16. Goldstein SA, Thomashow B, and Askanazi J: Functional changes during nutritional repletion in patients with lung disease, Clin Chest Med 7:141, 1986.
17. Hageman JR and Hunt CE: Fat emulsions and lung function, Clin Chest Med 7:69, 1986.
18. Metheney NA, Eisenberg P, and Spies M: Aspiration pneumonia in patients fed through nasoenteral tubes, Heart Lung 15:256, 1986.
19. Sahebjami H: Nutrition and the pulmonary parenchyma, Clin Chest Med 7:111, 1986.

20. Shanbhogue RLK and others: The nutritional management of a patient on long-term mechanical ventilation, Nutr Clin Prac 2:23, 1987.

21. Taylor TT: A comparison of two methods of nasogastric tube feedings, J Neurosurg Nurs 14:49, 1982.

22. Treloar DM and Stechmiller J: Pulmonary aspiration in tube-fed patients with artificial airways, Heart Lung 13:667, 1984.

Neurological

23. Bauer RC: Interference of oral phenytoin absorption by continuous nasogastric feedings, Neurology 32:570, 1982.

24. Clifton GL, Robertson CS, and Constant CF: Enteral hyperalimentation in head injury, J Neurosurg 62:186, 1985.

25. Cox SAR and others: Energy expenditure after spinal cord injury: an evaluation of stable rehabilitating patients, J Trauma 25:419, 1985.

26. Hausmann D and others: Effects of steroid on nitrogen loss and plasma amino acid profiles after head injury, J Parent Ent Nutr 11:10S, 1987.

27. Kiver KF and others: Pre- and post-pyloric enteral feeding: analysis of safety and complications, J Parent Ent Nutr 8:95, 1984.

28. Lander V and others: Enteral feeding during barbiturate coma, Nutr Clin Prac 2:56, 1987.

29. Metheney NM, Eisenberg P, and Spies M: Aspiration pneumonia in patients fed through nasoenteral tubes, Heart Lung 15:256, 1986.

30. Metheny N, Eisenberg P, and McSweeney M: Effect of feeding tube properties and three irrigants on clogging rates, Nurs Res 37:165, 1988.

31. Norton J and others: Intolerance to enteral feeding in brain injured patients: possible mechanisms, J Parent Ent Nutr 11:10S, 1987.

32. Ott L and others: Does nutritional support affect outcome from severe head injury: a reexamination, J Parent Ent Nutr 11:10S, 1987.

33. Ott L, Young B, and McClain C: The metabolic response to brain injury, J Parent Ent Nutr 11:488, 1987.

34. Rapp RP and others: The favorable effect of early parenteral feeding on survival in head-injured patients, J Neurosurg 58:906, 1983.

35. Saklad JJ, Graves RH, and Sharp WP: Interaction of oral phenytoin with enteral feedings, J Parent Ent Nutr 10:322, 1986.

36. Saltzberg D and others: Pulmonary aspiration during nasogastric (NG) feeding, J Parent Ent Nutr 11:20S, 1987.

37. Shizgal HM and others: Body composition in quadriplegic patients, J Parent Ent Nutr 10:364, 1986.

Renal

38. Brenner MB, Meyer TW, and Hostetter TH: Dietary protein intake and the progressive nature of kidney disease: the role of hemodynamically mediated glomerular injury in the pathogenesis of progressive glomerular sclerosis in aging, renal ablation and intrinsic renal disease, N Engl J Med 307:652, 1982.

39. Feinstein EI: Total parenteral nutritional support of patients with acute renal failure, Nutr Clin Prac 3:9, 1988.

40. Freund HR and others: The effect of different intravenous nutritional regimens on renal function during acute renal failure in the rat, J Parent Ent Nutr 11:556, 1987.

41. Gleghorn EE and others: Observations of vitamin A toxicity in three patients with renal failure receiving parenteral alimentation, Am J Clin Nutr 44:107, 1986.

42. Johnson KS, Hendricks DG, and Wyse BW: Vitamin A and vitamin E status of hemodialysis patients, Dial Transplan 12:477, 1983.

43. Koo WWK and others: Aluminum in parenteral nutrition solution—sources and possible alternatives, J Parent Ent Nutr 10:591, 1986.

44. Kopple JD and Blumenkrantz MJ: Nutritional requirements for patients undergoing continuous ambulatory peritoneal dialysis, Kidney Int 16(suppl):S295, 1983.

45. Lucas PA and others: The risks and benefits of a low protein–essential amino acid–keto acid diet, Kidney Int 29:995, 1986.

46. Maschio G and others: Effects of dietary protein and phosphorus restriction on the progression of early renal failure, Kidney Int 22:371, 1982.

47. Mitch WE and others: The effect of a ketoacid–amino acid supplement to a restricted diet on the progression of chronic renal failure, N Engl J Med 311:623, 1984.

48. Seagraves A and others: Net protein catabolic rate after kidney transplantation: impact of corticosteroid immunosuppression, J Parent Ent Nutr 10:453, 1986.

49. Twardowski ZJ and Nolph KD: Blood purification in acute renal failure, Ann Int Med 100:447, 1984.

Gastrointestinal

50. American Society for Parenteral and Enteral Nutrition Board of Directors: Guidelines for the use of enteral nutrition in the adult patient, J Parent Ent Nutr 11:435, 1987.

51. Beyer PL and Frankenfield DC: Enteral nutrition in extreme short bowel, Nutr Clin Prac 2:60, 1987.

52. Bristol JB and Williamson RCN: Nutrition, operations, and intestinal adaptation, J Parent Ent Nutr 12:299, 1988.

53. Cerra FB and others: Disease-specific amino acid infusion (F080) in hepatic encephalopathy: a prospective, randomized, double-blind, controlled trial, J Parent Ent Nutr 9:288, 1985.

54. Cowan GSM Jr, Luther RW, and Sykes TR: Short bowel syndrome: causes and clinical consequences, Nutr Supp Serv 4:25, 1984.

55. Gulledge AD and others: Psychosocial issues of home parenteral and enteral nutrition, Nutr Clin Prac 2:183, 1987.

56. Hiyama DT and Fischer JE: Nutritional support in hepatic failure: current thought in practice, Nutr Clin Prac 3:96, 1988.

57. Lerebours E and others: Comparison of the effects of continuous and cyclic nocturnal parenteral nutrition on energy expenditure and protein metabolism, J Parent Ent Nutr 12:360, 1988.

58. Millikan WJ Jr and Hooks MA: Nutritional support in hepatic failure: clinical controversies, Nutr Clin Prac 3:94, 1988.

59. Wahren JJ and others: Is intravenous administration of branched chain amino acids effective in the treatment of hepatic encephalopathy? A multicenter study, Hepatology 3:475, 1983.

Endocrine

60. Anderson JW: High fiber diets for obese diabetic men on insulin therapy: short-term and long-term effects. In Vahouny GV, editor: Dietary fiber and obesity, New York, 1985, Alan R Liss.

61. Anderson JW and others: Dietary fiber and diabetes: a comprehensive review and practical application, J Am Diet Assoc 87:1189, 1987.

62. Bogardus C and others: Effects of physical training and diet therapy on carbohydrate metabolism in patients with glucose intolerance and non–insulin dependent diabetes, Diabetes 33:311, 1984.

63. Franz MJ: Exercise and the management of diabetes mellitus, J Am Diet Assoc 87:872, 1987.

64. Holmes R and others: Serum albumin (SA): a predictor of pressure sores, J Parent Ent Nutr 11:4S, 1987.

65. Krotkiewski M: Effect of guar gum on body weight, hunger ratings and metabolism in obese subjects, Br J Nutr 52:97, 1984.

66. Phillips ML: Enteral nutrition support in diabetes mellitus, Nutr Clin Prac 2:152, 1987.

67. Reilly JJ and others: Economic impact of malnutrition: a model system for hospitalized patients, J Parent Ent Nutr 12:371, 1988.

68. Stevens J: Does dietary fiber affect food intake and body weight? J Am Diet Assoc 88:939, 1988.

69. Warnold I and Lundhold K: Clinical significance of preoperative nutritional status in 215 noncancer patients, Ann Surg 199:299, 1984.

70. Wilmhurst P and Crawley JCW: The measure of gastric transit time using 24-Na and the effects of energy content and guar gum on gastric emptying and satiety, Br J Nutr 44:1, 1980.

Hematoimmune

71. Antonecchia P and others: Reduced cardiac selenium content in AIDS, J Parent Ent Nutr 12:7S, 1988.

72. Beisel WR and others: Single-nutrient effects on immunologic functions, JAMA 245:53, 1981.

73. Brock JH and Mainou-Fowler T: Iron and immunity, Proc Nutr Soc 45:305, 1986.

74. Conte JE: Infection with human immunodeficiency virus in the hospital: epidemiology, infection control, and biosafety considerations, Ann Intern Med 105:730, 1986.

75. Cunningham-Rundles S: Effects of nutritional status on immunologic function, Am J Clin Nutr 35:1202, 1982.

76. Dworkin B and others: Gastrointestinal manifestations of the acquired immunodeficiency syndrome: a review of 22 cases, Am J Gastroenterol 80:774, 1985.

77. Dworkin BM and others: Selenium deficiency in the acquired immunodeficiency syndrome, J Parent Ent Nutr 10:405, 1986.

78. Garcia ME, Collins CL, and Mansell PWA: The acquired immune deficiency syndrome, Nutr Clin Prac 2:108, 1987.

79. Kotler DP and others: Enteropathy associated with the acquired immunodeficiency syndrome, Ann Intern Med 101:421, 1984.

80. Kotler DP, Wang J, and Pierson RN: Body composition studies in patients with the acquired immunodeficiency syndrome, Am J Clin Nutr 42:1255, 1985.

81. Modigliani R and others: Diarrhea and malabsorption in acquired immune deficiency syndrome: a study of four cases with special emphasis on opportunistic protozoan infestations, Gut 26:179, 1984.

82. Resler SS: Nutrition care of AIDS patients, J Am Diet Assoc 88:828, 1988.

83. Salonen JT and others: Risk of cancer in relation to serum concentrations of selenium and vitamins A and E: matched case control analysis of prospective data, Br Med J 290:417, 1985.

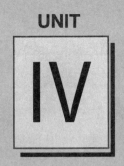

UNIT

IV

CARDIOVASCULAR ALTERATIONS

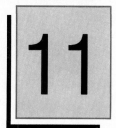

Cardiovascular Anatomy and Physiology

CHAPTER OBJECTIVES

- *Identify and briefly describe the physiology of the normal anatomical structures of the heart and blood vessels.*
- *Discuss the ionic and electrical basis of the resting membrane potential and the phases of the action potential.*
- *Discuss the role of calcium and the contractile proteins in excitation-contraction coupling.*
- *Trace the normal sequence of depolarization through the cardiac conduction system.*
- *Identify the determinants of cardiac output.*
- *Describe the nervous system control of the heart and blood vessels.*

The study of the structure and function of the heart and circulatory system will enhance the working knowledge in any area of critical care. This chapter provides the critical care nurse with concepts that will enable the delivery of more thorough and comprehensive nursing care. It is hoped that the information presented here will not only enlighten but also inspire further study and thought.

ANATOMY

Discussion of the structure of the heart and blood vessels will begin on a macroscopic level and progress to the cellular and molecular level.

Macroscopic Structure

Structures of the heart. The heart is situated in the anterior thoracic cavity, just behind the sternum (Fig. 11-1). Posterior to the heart are several structures, including the esophagus, aorta, vena cava, and vertebral column. The position of the heart is such that the right ventricle constitutes the majority of the inferior (or diaphragmatic) and anterior surfaces, and the left ventricle makes up the anterolateral and posterior surfaces. The broader side (base) of the heart is superior and the tip (apex) is inferior. The base of the heart includes not only the superior portion of the heart itself, but also the roots of the aorta, vena cava, and pulmonary vessels.

Size and weight of the heart. The average human heart is about the size of the clenched fist of that individual. In the adult, this averages 12 cm in length and 8 to 9 cm in breadth at the broadest part. In adult men, the weight of the heart averages 310 g, and that of women averages 255 g. Although there are no significant differences in ventricular wall thickness between men and women, mean values of heart weights increase in women between the third and tenth decades of life. In general, body weight appears to be a better predictor of normal heart weight than is body surface area or height.[17]

Layers of the heart. There are four distinct layers of the heart. The heart and roots of the great vessels are surrounded by a fibrous sac called the *pericardium,* also known as the parietal pericardium. The pericardium functions to hold the heart in a fixed position, as well as to provide a physical barrier to infection. The *epicardium* is tightly adhered to the heart and base of the great vessels and is sometimes referred to as the visceral pericardium. Together, the pericardium and epicardium form a sac around the heart. This sac normally contains a very small amount of pericardial fluid (approximately 10 ml) that serves as a lubricant between the pericardium and the epicardium. The pericardium is very noncompliant to rapid increases in cardiac size or amount of fluid in the sac. For example, blood or serum can abnormally collect in this sac, as in cardiac tamponade or pericardial effusion. If the fluid collection in the sac impinges on ventricular filling, ventricular ejection, or coronary artery perfusion, a clinical emergency may exist that would necessitate removal of the excess pericardial fluid to restore cardiac function.

Next is the thick muscular layer, the *myocardium,* or midwall. This layer includes all of the atrial and ventricular muscle fibers necessary for contraction. The fibers of the myocardium are not organized along a single plane throughout the thickness of the ventricular wall, but they have a distinct arrangement such that the force of contraction is most efficient in ejecting blood toward the outflow tracts in a wringing motion (Fig. 11-2, *A* and *B*).

133

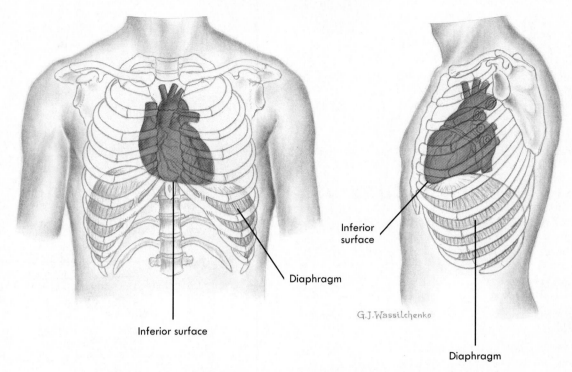

Fig. 11-1 Anatomic location of the heart within the thoracic cavity.

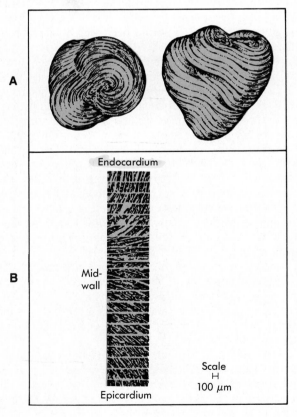

Fig. 11-2 Macroscopic and microscopic structure of the ventricular musculature. **A,** Spiral musculature of the ventricular walls. **B,** Sequence of photomicrographs showing fiber angles in successive sections taken from the middle of the free wall of the left ventricle from a heart in systole. The figer angle changes at various depths in the heart wall. Compare with **A** to obtain a concept of nonparallel forces generated during ventricular systole. (**B** from Streeter DD, Jr and others: Circ Res 24:339, 1969. Reprinted with permission of the American Heart Association, Inc.)

The innermost layer is the *endocardium,* which is a thin layer of endothelium and connective tissue lining the heart. The endothelial lining is continuous with the blood vessels and includes intracardiac structures such as the papillary muscles and valves. Disruption in the endothelium as a result of surgery, trauma, or congenital abnormality can predispose the area to infection. This infective endocarditis is a devastating disease that, if left untreated, can lead to massive valve damage or sepsis, and death.

Cardiac chambers. The human heart has four chambers—the left and right atria and the left and right ventricles. The atria, or auricles, are thin walled and normally low-pressure chambers. They function to receive blood from the vena cava and pulmonary arteries and to pump blood into their respective ventricles. Atrial contraction (also called "atrial kick") contributes about 30% to ventricular filling, while the other 70% occurs passively during diastole. The ventricles are the main pumping forces of the heart. The right ventricle is approximately 3 mm thick, while the left ventricle is 10 to 13 mm thick (Fig. 11-3). The right ventricle pumps blood into the low-pressured pulmonary circulation, which has a normal mean pressure of about 15 mm Hg. It is the left ventricle that must generate tremendous force to eject blood into the aorta (normal mean pressure about 100 mm Hg). Because of left ventricular thickness and the great force it must generate, the left ventricle is considered the major pump of the heart.

Cardiac valves. Cardiac valves are flexible fibrous tissue and are thinly covered by endocardium. The structure of the valves allows blood to flow in only one direction. The opening and closing of the valves is essentially passive and depends on pressure gradients on both sides of the valve.

There are four cardiac valves, all of which are essential to proper cardiovascular function. The two atrioventricular (AV) valves, so named for their location, are the *tricuspid* (three cusps) valve and the *mitral* (two cusps) valve. The AV valves prevent backflow of blood into the atria during ventricular contraction. The *chordae tendineae* and *papillary muscles,* which attach to the tricuspid and mitral valves, give the valves stability and prevent valve leaflet eversion

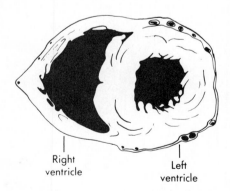

Fig. 11-3 A transverse section of the ventricles of the adult heart. The right ventricle forms the greater part of the anterior surface of the heart, and the wall of the left ventricle is three times as thick as the wall of the right ventricle. (From Quaal S: Comprehensive intra-aortic balloon pumping, St Louis, 1984, The CV Mosby Co.)

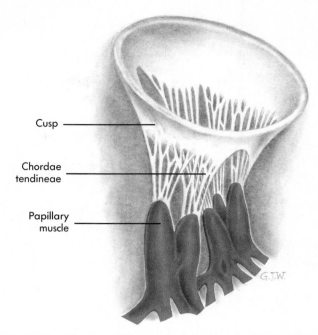

Cusp

Chordae tendineae

Papillary muscle

Fig. 11-4 Diagram of the mitral valve and the relationships of the cusps, chordae tendineae, and the papillary muscles.

during systole (Fig. 11-4). Papillary muscles, located in the apical area of the endocardium, derive their blood supply from the coronary arteries. Each papillary muscle gives rise to approximately four to ten main chordae that divide into finer and finer cords as they approach the valve leaflets. The chordae tendineae are basically avascular structures covered by a thin layer of endocardium. A dysfunction of the chordae tendineae or of a papillary muscle can cause incomplete closure of an AV valve, which can result in a murmur. For example, following an acute myocardial infarction (AMI), the papillary muscles may be at risk for rupture as a result of inadequate blood supply from the coronary circulation. When a papillary muscle in the left ventricle ruptures, the mitral valve leaflets do not close completely. Clinically, this situation can cause a mitral regurgitation murmur that can potentially worsen the pulmonary congestion and lower cardiac output.

The semilunar valves, the *pulmonic* and *aortic* valves, each have three main cuplike cusps (Fig. 11-5). These valves separate the ventricles from their respective outflow arteries (see Table 11-1 for summary). During ventricular systole, the semilunar valves open, allowing blood to flow out of the ventricles. As systole ends and the pressure in the outflow arteries exceeds that of the ventricles, the semilunar valves close, thus preventing blood regurgitation back into the ventricles (Fig. 11-6).

The conduction system. The history of the discovery of the conduction system dates back to 1845, when Purkinje wrote a classic paper describing ventricular conductive cells. Recently, breakthroughs in electrophysiology have advanced not only clinical cardiology but also have entered the cardiac surgery arena.[25,26] Despite these advances and the well-characterized nature of the cardiac conduction system, there are still many concepts in the area of impulse

Fig. 11-5 Diagram of the aortic valve and the cuplike cusps.

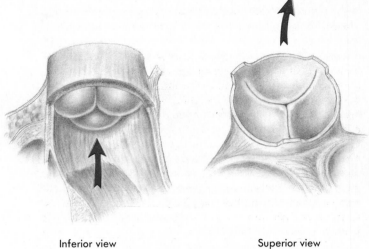

Inferior view   Superior view

Table 11-1 Summary of the cardiac valves and their locations

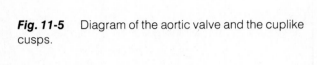

Valve	Type	Situated between
Tricuspid	AV	Right atrium, right ventricle
Pulmonic	SL	Right ventricle, pulmonary artery
Mitral	AV	Left atrium, left ventricle
Aortic	SL	Left ventricle, aorta

AV, atrioventricular; SL, semilunar.

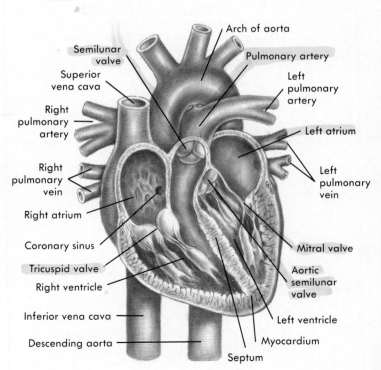

Fig. 11-6 Crossectional view of the heart. Note the position of the four cardiac valves. (From Thompson JM and others: Clinical nursing, ed 2, St Louis, 1989, The CV Mosby Co.)

propagation that require further emphasis.[9,30] This section will discuss the three main areas of impulse propagation and conduction—the SA node, the AV node, and the His/Purkinje fibers.

The sinoatrial node. The sinoatrial (SA) node is considered the natural pacemaker of the heart because it has the highest degree of automaticity or intrinsic heart rate (Table 11-2). The node is usually a spindle-shaped structure located near the mouth of the superior vena cava, on the posterior aspect of the right atrium. There is some normal variability in the position and shape of the node. The SA node contains basically two types of cells, the specialized pacemaker cells found in the node center and the border zone cells. Both the pacemaker cells and the border zone cells have inherent depolarization capabilities (they automatically depolarize 60 to 100 times per minute). It is the cells in the nodal center that are responsible for the actual pacemaking of the heart. The fibers in the border zone cells also have intrinsic pacemaker properties, but depolarization is depressed by the surrounding atrial tissue.[6]

Once the center nodal cells have depolarized, the impulse is conducted through the nodal border zone toward the atrium. Atrial depolarization occurs both cell to cell and also through four specialized conduction pathways that exit the SA node (Fig. 11-7, *A*). These conduction pathways are Bachman's bundle, which is directed to the left atrium, and three internodal pathways that are directed to the AV node.

Impulse conduction

Table 11-2 Intrinsic pacemaker rates of cardiac conduction tissue

Location	Rate (beats/min)
SA node *Sinoatrial node*	60-100
AV node	40-60
Purkinje fibers	15-40

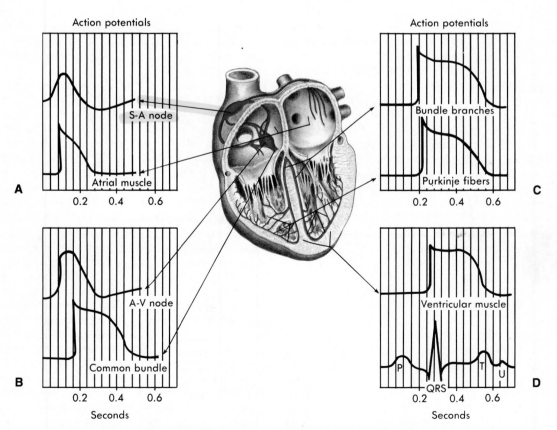

Fig. 11-7 Heart with normal conduction pathways and transmembrane action potentials of **A,** SA node and atrial muscle, **B,** AV node, **C,** bundle branches, and **D,** ventricular muscle. (From Thompson JM and others: Clinical nursing, ed 2, St Louis, 1989, The CV Mosby Co.)

The atrioventricular node. The atrioventricular (AV) node is located posteriorly on the right side of the interatrial septum. Because the atria and ventricles are separated by nonconductive tissue, all electrical impulses initiated in the atria will be conducted to the ventricles solely via the AV node. Although the AV node also possesses pacemaker cells, the intrinsic rhythmicity is less than that of the SA node (Table 11-2). So, as an impulse from the SA node arrives at the AV node, the AV node will be depolarized (Fig. 11-7, *B*) resetting its own pacemaker potential. This prevents the AV node from initiating its own pacemaker impulse that would compete with the SA node.

As the depolarization impulse from the SA node arrives at the AV node, a slight conduction delay occurs through the AV node. This delay is a result of the inherent properties of the nodal structures that cause a slowing of conduction velocity. The purpose of this delay is to allow adequate time for optimal ventricular filling from atrial contraction. If there was no electrical delay, the mechanical event of atrial contraction would not have sufficient time to add to ventricular filling. This would lower end-diastolic ventricular volume and potentially lead to lowered cardiac output. The AV nodal delay also functions as a protection mechanism for the ventricles. As a result of the slowed conduction velocity through the AV node, conduction is thus time dependent and hence limits the contraction frequency of the ventricles. For example, when there is an abnormal number of electrical impulses bombarding the AV node during atrial flutter or atrial fibrillation, the AV nodal delay limits the number of impulses that move through to the ventricles. Without this delay, the ventricles would receive each atrial impulse, and the heart would quickly decompensate.

Another property described in the AV node is that of retrograde (backward) conduction. This means that an electrical impulse that is initiated in or below the AV node can be conducted in a backward fashion. When this happens, the propagation time is generally longer than that of antegrade (forward) conduction. This may manifest itself in a variety of heart and conduction disease conditions, as well as in the postoperative recovery period after certain cardiac surgical procedures. In this instance, the coordinated efforts of atria and ventricles are diminished or lost, resulting in lack of atrial kick to ventricular filling. Detection of this condition is made by the electrocardiogram (ECG).

Bundle of His and Purkinje fibers. Electrical impulses are conducted in the ventricles through the bundle of His and the Purkinje fibers (Fig. 11-7, *C*). The bundle of His fibers runs through the subendocardium down the right side of the interventricular septum. About 12 mm from the AV node, the bundle of His divides into the right and left bundle branches. The right bundle branch continues down the right side of the interventricular septum toward the right apex. The left bundle branch is thicker than the right and takes off from the bundle of His at almost a right angle. It then traverses the septum to the subendocardial surface of the left interventricular wall, where it divides into a thin anterior and a thick posterior branch. Functionally, when one of the left branches is blocked, it is referred to as a hemiblock. All of the bundle branches are subject to conduction defects (bundle branch blocks) and give rise to characteristic changes in the electrocardiogram.

The right bundle branch and the two divisions of the left bundle branch eventually divide into the Purkinje fibers. These divide many times, terminating in the subendocardial surface of both ventricles. The Purkinje fibers have the fastest conduction velocity of all heart tissue. Ventricular muscle depolarizion follows (Fig. 11-7, *D*).

Coronary blood supply. The coronary circulation consists of those vessels which supply the heart structures with oxygenated blood (coronary arteries) and then return the blood to the general circulation (coronary veins). The right and left coronary arteries arise at the base of the aorta immediately after the aortic valve (Fig. 11-8). After leaving the base of the aorta, the coronary arteries traverse along the outside of the heart in the natural grooves (sulci). To perfuse the thick heart muscle, branches from these main arteries arise at acute angles, penetrating the muscular wall and eventually feeding the endocardium (Fig. 11-9).

The *right coronary artery* (RCA) serves the right atrium and the right ventricle in most people. In over half the population, it also is the usual blood supply for the SA and AV nodes. The *left coronary artery* (also referred to as the "widow maker," because occlusion of this main vessel usually results in immediate death) divides into two large arteries, the *left anterior descending* (LAD) and the *circumflex*. These vessels serve the left atria and most of the left ventricle (Fig. 11-10). There is a huge spectrum of variation in the disposition of coronary arteries. The term "dominant" coronary artery was introduced in 1940. The *dominant coronary artery* is that artery which traverses the posterior interventricular sulcus and supplies the posterior part of the ventricular septum and often part of the posterolateral wall of the left ventricle.[1]

After blood passes through the coronary capillaries, the majority of it is returned to the right atrium via the coronary veins, exiting via the coronary sinus. In addition, the *thebesian vessels* are small veins that connect capillary beds directly with the cardiac chambers and also communicate with cardiac veins and other thebesian veins. However, some of the blood returns directly to the chambers via vascular communications of irregular endothelium-lined sinuses within the muscular structure. These veins that drain into the left ventricle would therefore add unoxygenated blood to the freshly oxygenated blood. When unoxygenated blood mixes with freshly oxygenated blood in the left ventricle, it is called a *physiological shunt*. An example of a normal shunt is the previously mentioned situation in which unoxygenated blood from the myocardium drains into the left ventricle. An example of an abnormal shunt is an opening in the ventricular septum, called a ventricular septal defect (VSD), which allows large amounts of venous blood from the right ventricle to mix with the freshly oxygenated blood in the left ventricle.

Several clinical situations merit a brief discussion here. During ventricular contraction, there is no blood flow to the cardiac tissue. Coronary artery circulation is highest during early diastole, after the aortic valve has closed. During an episode of tachycardia, diastolic time is greatly diminished, hence coronary perfusion time is diminished. This offers a possible explanation for compromised coronary blood flow

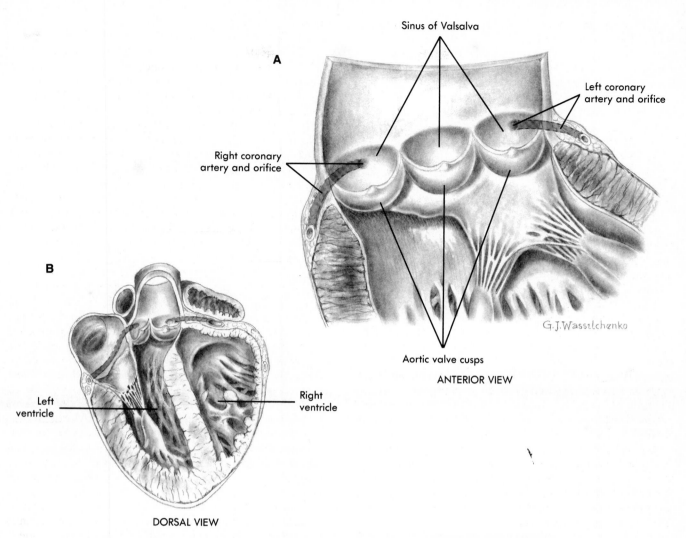

Fig. 11-8 Illustration of the proximity of the right and left coronary arteries to the aortic valve and the sinus of Valsalva.

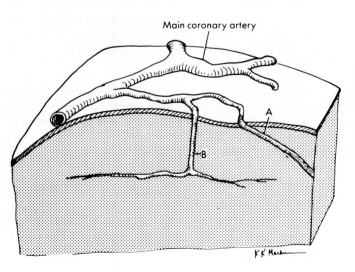

Fig. 11-9 Intramyocardial distribution of coronary arteries. **A,** Epicardial arteries arise at acute angles from main coronary vessels to supply epicardial surface of the heart. **B,** Smaller vessels branch at oblique angles from main coronary vessels that penetrate deeper into the myocardium and endocardium (intramural arteries). (From Quaal S: Comprehensive intra-aortic balloon pumping, St Louis, 1984, The CV Mosby Co.)

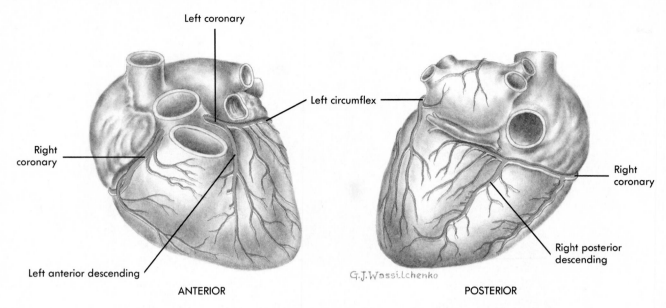

Fig. 11-10 Anterior and posterior views of the coronary artery circulation.

during times of rapid heart rate. Conversely, during brady-cardia, there is prolonged diastole. However, coronary in-flow may also be compromised as a result of the lack of adequate pressure and aortic recoil in late diastole to perfuse the myocardium.[18]

The systemic circulation. If the purpose of the heart is to generate enough pressure to pump the blood, then it is the function of the vascular structures to act as conduits to carry vital oxygen and nutrients to each cell and also to carry away waste products. Also of primary importance is the ability to exchange those nutrients and waste products at the cellular level. The vascular system not only acts as a conducting system for the blood, it also acts as a control mechanism for the pressure in the heart and vessels. So, it is actually the complex interplay between the heart and the blood vessels that maintains adequate pressure and velocity within this system for optimal functioning.

The arterial system. Arteries are constructed of three lay-ers (Fig. 11-11). The innermost layer, or the *intima,* is a thin lining of endothelium and a small amount of elastic tissue. This smooth lining decreases resistance to blood flow and minimizes the chance for platelet aggregation. The *media,* or middle layer, is made up of smooth muscle and elastic tissue. This muscular layer acts to change the lumen diameter when necessary. The *adventitia,* which is the out-ermost layer, is largely a connective tissue coat and functions to add strength and shape to the vessels.

The intima and the adventitia layers remain relatively constant in the vascular system, while the elastin and smooth muscle in the media change proportions, depending on the type of vessel. The aorta contains the greatest amount of elastic tissue, necessary because of the sudden shifts in pressure created by the left ventricle. The arterioles, or smaller arteries, and precapillary sphincters have more smooth muscle than the larger arteries, and aorta, because they function to change the luminal diameter when

regulating blood pressure and blood flow to the tissues (Fig. 11-12).

Blood flow and blood pressure. The pulsatile nature of arterial flow is caused by intermittent cardiac ejection and the stretch of the ascending aorta. The pressure wave ini-tiated by left ventricular ejection (Fig. 11-13) travels con-siderably faster than the blood itself. Thus when an examiner palpates a pulse, it is this propagation of the pressure wave that is perceived.

In the normal arterial system, the blood flow is called laminar, or streamlined, as the fluid moves in one direction. However, there are small differences in the linear velocities within a blood vessel. The layer of blood immediately ad-jacent to the vessel wall moves relatively slowly because of the friction caused as it comes in contact with the mo-tionless blood vessel wall. Similarly, the fluid more central in the lumen travels more rapidly. The most central blood travels at the highest velocity (Fig. 11-14). Clinical impli-cations include conditions in which the vessel wall has an abnormality, such as a small clot or plaque deposit. This disruption in the streamlined flow can set up eddy currents that may predispose the area to platelet aggregation and thus enlargement of the abnormality.

Blood pressure (BP) measurement has several compo-nents. The systolic blood pressure (SBP) represents the ven-tricular volume ejection and the response of the arterial system to that ejection. The diastolic value (DBP) indicates the ventricular resting state of the arterial system. The pulse pressure is the difference between the SBP and DBP. The mean arterial pressure (MAP) is the mean value of the area under the BP curve (Fig. 11-15). BP may be measured several ways. Direct measurement is accomplished by means of a catheter inserted into a large artery. The more common indirect method is by means of a stethoscope and sphygmomanometer (Fig. 11-16). Fig. 11-17 graphically summarizes blood pressures in various portions of the sys-temic circulatory system.

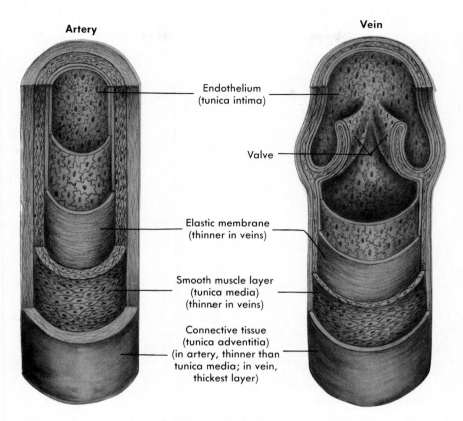

Artery

Vein

Endothelium
(tunica intima)

Valve

Elastic membrane
(thinner in veins)

Smooth muscle layer
(tunica media)
(thinner in veins)

Connective tissue
(tunica adventitia)
(in artery, thinner than
tunica media; in vein,
thickest layer)

Fig. 11-11 Cross section of an artery and vein showing the three layers: tunica intima, tunica media, and tunica adventitia. Note the difference in wall thickness between the artery and the vein and the lack of valves within the artery. (From Thompson JM and others: Clinical nursing, ed 2, St Louis, 1989, The CV Mosby Co.)

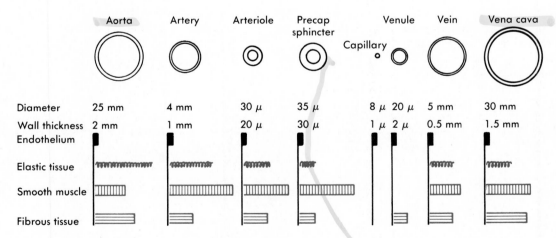

	Aorta	Artery	Arteriole	Precap sphincter	Capillary	Venule	Vein	Vena cava
Diameter	25 mm	4 mm	30 μ	35 μ	8 μ	20 μ	5 mm	30 mm
Wall thickness	2 mm	1 mm	20 μ	30 μ	1 μ	2 μ	0.5 mm	1.5 mm
Endothelium								
Elastic tissue								
Smooth muscle								
Fibrous tissue								

Fig. 11-12 Internal diameter, wall thickness, and relative amounts of the principal components of the vessel circulatory system. Cross sections of the vessels are not drawn to scale because of the huge range from aorta to vena cava to capillaries. (From Berne RM and Levy MN: Cardiovascular physiology, ed 5, St Louis, 1986, The CV Mosby Co.)

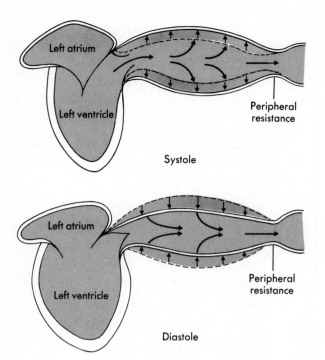

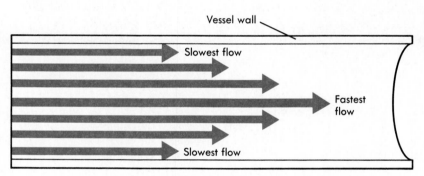

Fig. 11-13 Elastic and recoil properties of the aorta. (From Berne Rm and Levy MN: Cardiovascular physiology, ed 5, St Louis, 1986, The CV Mosby Co.)

Fig. 11-14 Illustration of laminar flow in an artery.

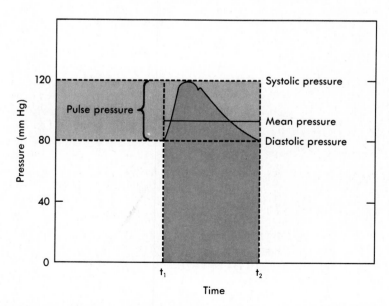

Fig. 11-15 Arterial systolic, diastolic, pulse, and mean pressures. (From Berne RM and Levy MN: Cardiovascular physiology, ed 5, St Louis, 1986, The CV Mosby Co.)

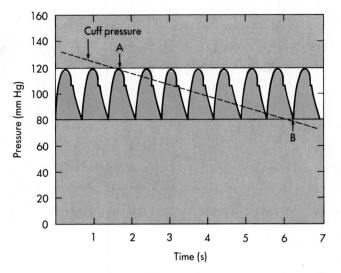

Fig. 11-16 Principles of blood pressure measurements with a sphygmomanometer. The oblique line represents pressure in the inflatable bag in the cuff. At cuff pressures greater than the systolic pressure (to the left of *A*), no blood progresses beyond the cuff and no sounds can be detected below the cuff with the stethoscope. At cuff pressures between the systolic and diastolic levels (between *A* and *B*), spurts of blood traverse the arteries under the cuff and produce Korotkoff's sounds. At cuff pressures below the diastolic pressure (to the right of *B*), arterial flow past the region of the cuff is continuous and no sounds are audible. (From Berne RM and Levy MN: Cardiovascular physiology, ed 5, St Louis, 1986, The CV Mosby Co.)

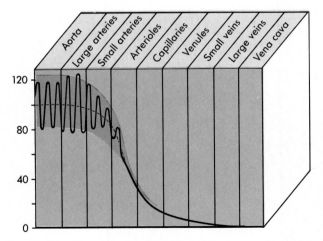

Fig. 11-17 Blood pressures in the different portions of the systemic circulatory system.

Vascular resistance is a reflection of arteriolar tone. The large amount of smooth muscle in the arterioles allows for relaxation or contraction of these vessels and causes changes in resistance and redistribution of blood flow. The values of systemic vascular resistance (SVR) and pulmonary vascular resistance (PVR) are based on calculations from other hemodynamic parameters (see Table 13-24 for formulas for normal values for SVR, PVR, and MAP).

Precapillary sphincters and the microcirculation. Where present, the precapillary sphincters are small cuffs of smooth muscle that control blood flow at the junction of the arterioles and the capillaries. The precapillary sphincters function to allow selective blood flow into capillary beds, depending on their contractile state. The precapillary sphincters are not innervated by the autonomic nervous system as are the arterioles; rather, they respond to local or circulating vasoactive agents. This means that they do not have direct nervous connection to sympathetic input but will respond to circulating epinephrine released by the adrenal gland.

As the blood reaches the capillary level, the pulsatile nature of arterial flow is dampened. Even though the diameter of a capillary is less than that of the arteriole, the pressure and flow velocity in the capillary bed is relatively low as a result of the branching nature and large cross-sectional area of the capillary bed (Fig. 11-18). The capillary consists of a single cell layer of endothelium and is devoid of muscle or elastin. Hence, diffusion of solutes into and out of the capillary is not impeded by mechanical barriers. Thus the capillaries normally retain large structures such as red blood cells but are permeable to smaller solutes such as electrolytes. Although true capillaries do not contain smooth muscle, there is evidence that the endothelium can change its shape and may even secrete substances that do influence smooth muscle in other vessels. Also, different capillary beds have greater permeability than others (for example, liver), and some sites along the same capillary have greater permeability (venous versus arterial end).

The venous system. As the blood leaves the capillary system, it passes through the venules and into the veins. Both venules and veins contain elastic tissue, smooth muscle, and fibrous tissue (Fig. 11-12). The veins, however, contain a greater percentage of smooth muscle and fibrous tissue in order to accommodate the large venous volume and demands for reserve capacity. The majority of circulating blood is contained in the veins that are referred to as *capacitance vessels* (Fig. 11-19). Approximately 60% of the total blood volume is found in the veins and is hemodynamically "inactive," meaning that this blood volume does not directly contribute to blood pressure and other hemodynamic parameters. This enables the body to tap into a ready reserve during times of need. For example, when a person changes from a supine to a sitting position, approximately 7 to 10 ml blood/kg of body weight is pooled in the legs. Cardiac output decreases about 25%, but arterial BP is maintained by reflex vasoconstriction. Thus the primary function of capacitance vessels under reflex control is to redistribute the blood to or from the heart to maintain optimum cardiac filling pressures. In human beings, these reservoirs are greatest in the splanchnic bed (liver and intestines).[13]

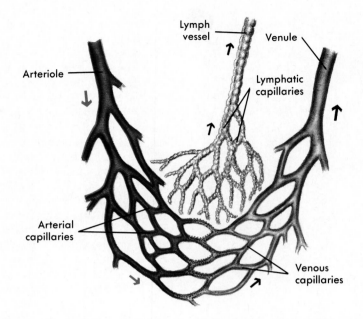

Fig. 11-18 The microcirculation. Note the branching nature and large cross-sectional area of the capillary bed. (From Thompson JM and others: Clinical nursing, ed 2, St Louis, 1989, The CV Mosby Co.)

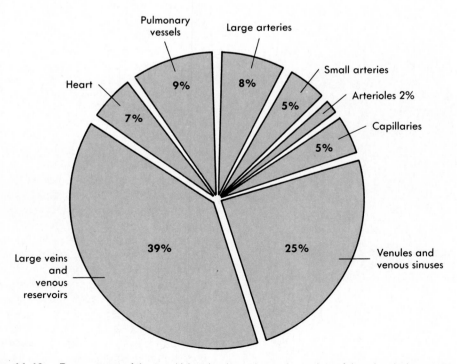

Fig. 11-19 Percentage of the total blood volume in each portion of the circulation system.

Microscopic Structure

To understand and appreciate the unique pumping ability of the heart, attention must be given to the cardiac cell structure and function. This section will review the anatomical mechanisms responsible for the contractile process in cardiac muscle cells.

Cardiac fibers. Cardiac muscle fibers are typically found in a latticework arrangement. The fiber cells (myofibrils) divide and then rejoin and then separate again, but they retain distinct cellular walls and possess a single nucleus.

This differs greatly from skeletal muscle, in which the cells have fused together to form a fiber, and have many nuclei.

In general, cardiac myofibrils run on a longitudinal axis, and the fibers appear striped, or striated. When viewed under an electron microscope, these striations are actually the contractile proteins (Fig. 11-20). The areas separating each myocardial cell from its neighbor are called *intercalated discs*, which are continuous with the *sarcolemma*, or cell membrane. At the point where a longitudinal branch of the cell meets another cell branch is the tight junction (or *gap*

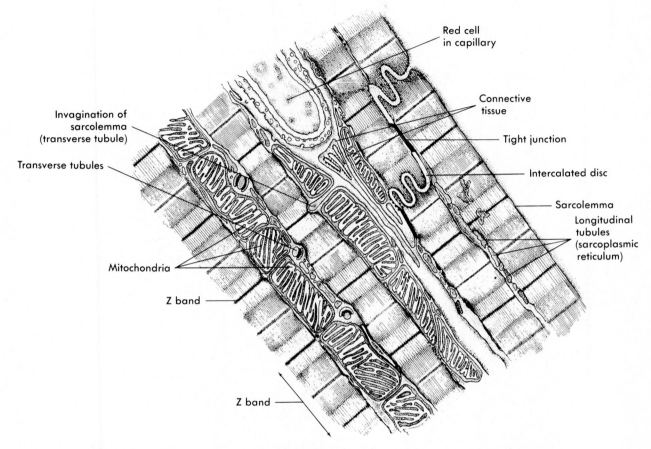

Fig. 11-20 Diagram of an electron micrograph of cardiac muscle showing the large numbers of mitochondria, the intercalated disks with tight junctions, the transverse tubules, and the longitudinal tubules (also known as the sarcoplasmic reticulum). (Approximately × 30,000) (From Berne RM and Levy MN: Cardiovascular physiology, ed 5, St Louis, 1986, The CV Mosby Co.)

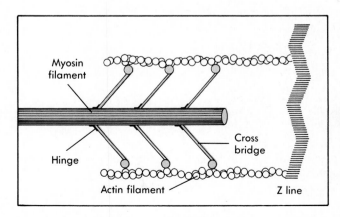
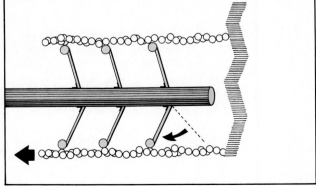

Fig. 11-21 Actin and myosin filaments and cross-bridges responsible for cell contraction.

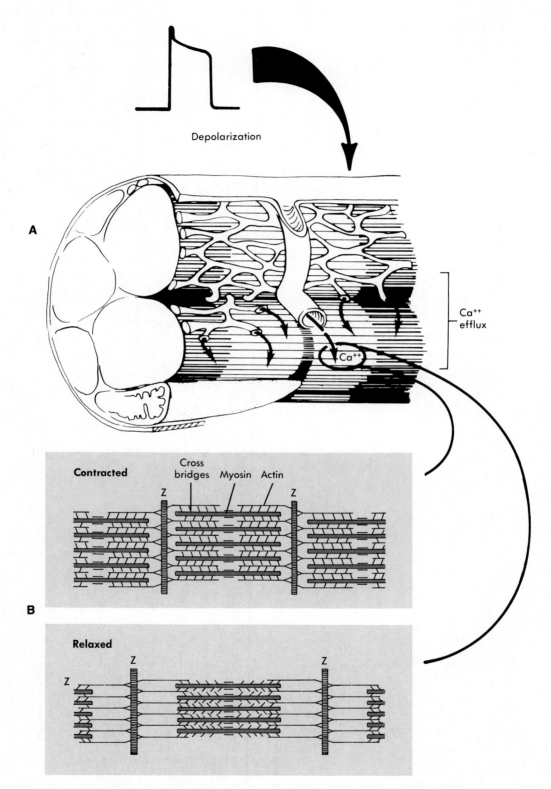

Depolarization

Ca++ efflux

Ca++

Contracted

Cross bridges Myosin Actin

Z Z

B

Relaxed

Z Z

Z

Fig. 11-22 **A,** Depolarization of a myocardial cell causes release of calcium from the sarcoplasmic reticulum and the transverse tubules. **B,** Calcium release allows for the cross-bridges on the myosin filaments to attach to the actin filaments to effect cell contraction. (From Quaal S: Comprehensive intra-aortic balloon pumping, St Louis, 1984, The CV Mosby Co.)

junction), which offers much less of an impedance to electrical flow than the sarcolemma. Because of this, depolarization will occur from one cell to another with relative ease.[11] Also, the cardiac muscle is a *functional syncytium,* in which depolarization started in any cardiac cell will quickly be spread to all of the heart.

Cardiac cells. Intracellularly, each cardiac cell contains two types of contractile proteins, *actin* and *myosin.* These proteins abound in the cell in organized longitudinal arrangements. When visualized by electronmicroscopy, the myosin filaments appear thick, whereas the almost double amounts of actin filaments appear thin. The actin filaments are connected to the Z bands on one end, leaving the other end free to interact with the myosin crossbridges. In the resting muscle cell, the actin and myosin partially overlap. The ends of the myosin filament that overlap with the actin have tiny projections (Fig. 11-21). For contraction to occur, these projections interact with the actin to form crossbridges (Fig. 11-21). The portion of the muscle fiber between two Z bands is called a *sarcomere.* In a normal resting state, the sarcomere is about 2.0 to 2.2 μm. Another extremely important intracellular structure necessary for successful contraction is the *sarcoplasmic reticulum* (SR). Calcium ions are stored in the SR and released for use following depolarization (Fig. 11-22, *A* and *B*). Deep invaginations into the sarcomere are called *transverse tubules,* or T-tubules. The T-tubules are essentially an extension of the cell membrane and thus function to conduct depolarization to structures deep within the cytoplasm, such as the SR. The cardiac cells abound with *mitochondria,* which contain respiratory enzymes necessary for oxidative phosphorylation. This enables the cell to keep up with the tremendous energy requirements of the repetitive contraction.

The importance of these precise and complex anatomical structures is evidenced in several clinical conditions. For example, chronic cardiomyopathy is a disease of the myocardium that most frequently results from viral, alcoholic, or idiopathic causes. The ventricular dilation commonly associated with this condition leads to poor approximation of the actin and myosin filaments. This results in decreased contraction at the microscopic level that is manifested by impaired myocardial contractility, low cardiac output, and increased diastolic volume. Eventually, biventricular heart failure may result.

PHYSIOLOGY

The study of the electrical and mechanical properties of cardiac tissue has fascinated scientists for more than 100 years. These properties include excitability, conductivity, automaticity, rhythmicity, contractility, and refractoriness. The following section will relate these concepts specifically to cardiac cells (see Table 11-3).

Electrical Activity

Transmembrane potentials. Electrical potentials across cell membranes are present in essentially all cells of the body. Some cells, such as nerve and muscle cells, are specialized for conduction of electrical impulses along their membranes. This electrical potential, or transmembrane potential, refers to the relative electrical difference between

Table 11-3 Definitions of terms related to cardiac tissue function

Term	Definition
Excitability	The ability of a cell or tissue to depolarize in response to a given stimulus
Conductivity	The ability of cardiac cells to transmit a stimulus from cell to cell
Automaticity	The ability of certain cells to spontaneously depolarize ("pacemaker potential")
Rhythmicity	Automaticity generated at a regular rate
Contractility	The ability of the cardiac myofibrils to shorten in length in response to an electrical stimulus (depolarization)
Refractoriness	The state of a cell or tissue during repolarization when the cell or tissue either cannot depolarize regardless of the intensity of the stimulus, or requires a much greater stimulus than is normally required

the interior of a cell and that of the fluid surrounding the cell. Ionic channels are pores in cell membranes that allow passage of specific ions at specific times or signals. Transmembrane potentials and ionic channels are extremely important in myocardial cells, because they form the basis for electrical impulse conduction and muscular contraction.[22]

Resting membrane potential. In a myocardial cell, the normal resting membrane potential (RMP) is approximately -80 to -90 mV. This means that the interior of the cell is relatively negative compared with the exterior medium when the cell is at rest. The relative negativity of the cell interior is created by an uneven distribution of positively charged ions and negatively charged ions. Hence there are relatively more of the positively charged ions outside of the cell than there are inside.

When the cell is at rest, the intracellular potassium (K^+) is very high, and sodium (Na^+) is low. Conversely, the extracellular K^+ is relatively low, compared with a high concentration of Na^+ (see Table 11-4). Like Na^+, calcium (Ca^{++}) also has a much higher concentration outside the cell. These large differences in individual ion concentrations are responsible for the *chemical gradients,* that is, the tendency of a ion to move from the area of higher concentration to the area of lower concentration. However, there is also an *electrical gradient,* in which the positively charged ions will move to the area of relative negativity. For example, the chemical gradient of K^+ is to move out of the cell, since the intracellular concentration is so much higher than the outside medium. But, as a result of the relative negativity inside the cell, the electrical gradient will work to retain the positively charged K^+ ion. An important factor influencing both gradients is *membrane permeability,* or the selectivity of the membrane to ionic movements. Even at rest, there is some slight movement of ions across the cell membrane. For example, the cell membrane is approximately 50 times more permeable to K^+ than it is to Na^+. Because K^+ movement out of the cell will create more negativity inside the cell, potassium is therefore the most important ion for maintaining the negative RMP.[7]

Phases of the action potential. In a myocardial cell, when there is a sudden increase in the permeability of the membrane to Na^+, there follows a rapid sequence of events that lasts a fraction of a second. This sequence of events is termed *depolarization.* The graphic representation of depolarization is the *action potential,* or AP (Fig. 11-23). As the membrane is depolarized, Na^+ begins to enter the cell, thus causing the interior of the cell to become more positive. At about -65 mV, the membrane reaches *threshold,* the point at which the inward Na^+ current overcomes the efflux of K^+. This is accomplished by means of the fast Na^+ channels. With the fast Na^+ channels open, the inward rush

of Na^+ is extremely rapid and briefly causes the inside of the cell to become slightly more positive than the outside of the cell. This is known as phase 0 of the AP and is reflected in the overshoot of the AP where the charge is $+20$ to $+30$ mV.

When the rapid influx of Na^+ is terminated, a brief period of partial repolarization occurs (phase 1 of the AP). This is followed by phase 2, or the plateau. During this phase, another set of channels, the slow Na^+ and Ca^{++} channels, open and allow the influx of Ca^{++} and Na^+. Also during phase 2, K^+ tends to diffuse out of the cell, balancing the slow inward flux of Na^+ and Ca^{++}, thereby maintaining the plateau of the AP. The Ca^{++} entering the cell at this phase causes cardiac contraction, which will be described later in this chapter. The inward flux of Ca^{++} during this phase can be influenced by many factors.[24,28] For example, agents such as verapamil, nifedipine, and diltiazem inhibit the inward Ca^{++} current and thus are known as calcium channel blockers.

Phase 3 of the AP is the final repolarization phase, and depends upon two processes. The first is the inactivation of the slow channels, thereby preventing further influx of Ca^{++} and Na^+. The other is the continued efflux of K^+ out of the cell. Both of these processes will cause the intracellular environment to become more negative, thereby reestablishing the RMP. Phase 4 of the AP is the return to RMP. The excess Na^+ that entered the cell during depolarization is now removed from the cell in exchange for K^+ by means of the Na^+ and K^+ pump. This mechanism returns the intracellular concentrations of Na^+ and K^+ to the levels

Table 11-4 The approximate extracellular and intracellular concentrations of K^+, Na^+, and Ca^{++} in a resting myocardial cell

Ion	Extracellular concentration (mM/L)	Intracellular concentration (mM/L)
K^+	4	135
Na^+	145	10
Ca^{++}	2	0.0001

From Berne and Levy: Cardiovascular physiology, ed 5, St. Louis, 1986, The CV Mosby Co.

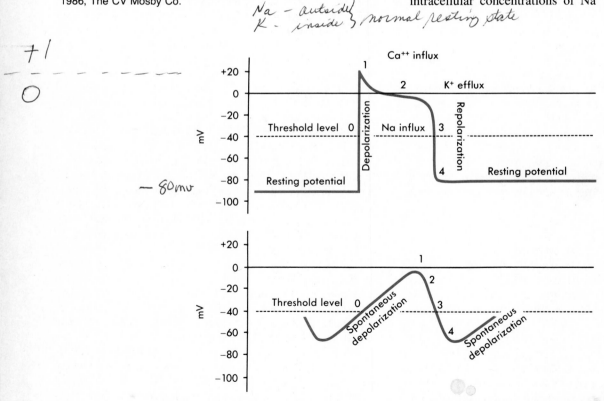

Fig. 11-23 Cardiac action potentials. **A,** Action potential phases 0 to 4 of a nonpacemaker cell. **B,** Action potential of a pacemaker cell. (From Thompson JM and others: Clinical nursing, ed 2, St Louis, 1989, The CV Mosby Co.)

Ca — property of contractility

Table 11-5 Summary of phases 0 through 4 of a cardiac cell AP

Phase	Description	Ionic movement	Mechanisms
0	Upstroke	Na$^+$ into cell	Fast channels open
1	Overshoot		Fast channels close
2	Plateau	Na$^+$, Ca^{++} into cell, K$^+$ out	Slow channels open
3	Repolarization	K$^+$ out of cell	Slow channels close
4	RMP	Na$^+$ out, K$^+$ in	Na$^+$/K$^+$ pump

STARTS
P generated in atrial muscle
QRS complex generated
initiation of repolarization
AP isoelectric
T wave - rapid repolarization
resting membrane potential

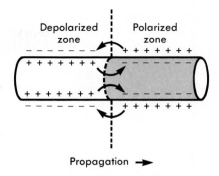

Fig. 11-24 Schematic representation of the propagation of an action potential along a cell membrane.

Depolarized zone / Polarized zone

Propagation →

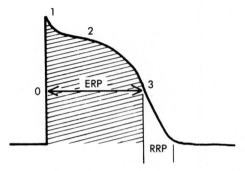

Fig. 11-25 The two parts of the refractory period. The effective (absolute) refractory period (ERP) extends from phase 0 to approximately −50 mV in phase 3. The remainder of the action potential is the relative refractory period (RRP). (From Conover MB: Understanding electrocardiography: arrhythmias and the 12 lead ECG, ed 4, St Louis, 1984, The CV Mosby Co.)

prior to depolarization and is essential for normal ionic balance[29] (see Table 11-5 for summary).

Fiber conduction and excitability. Propagation of an AP along a cardiac fiber occurs as a result of ionic shifts discussed previously. As a local section of the cell becomes depolarized, reaches threshold, and completely depolarizes, it affects the adjacent area of the cell and begins depolarization in that area. Thus the AP propagates down the fiber in a wavelike fashion (Fig. 11-24). This is somewhat analogous to a trail of gunpowder. When the gunpowder is lit at one end, a small area ignites, burns, and then ignites the area of gunpowder immediately adjacent, and so on.

The time from the beginning of the AP until the time when the fiber can accept another AP is called the *effective* or *absolute refractory period*. During this period, the cell cannot be depolarized regardless of the amount or intensity of the stimulus. This period lasts from the beginning of depolarization to approximately −50 mV during phase 3. Immediately following the absolute refractory period is the *relative refractory period*. At this time, the cell is not fully repolarized, but could depolarize with a strong enough stimulus (Fig. 11-25). This period lasts from approximately −50 mV during phase 3 to when the cell returns to RMP. At phase 4, the cell is fully repolarized and is again at RMP, ready to respond to the next stimulus.

Pacemaker versus nonpacemaker action potentials. The action potential as just discussed is representative of the depolarization of nonpacemaker myocardial cells. The AP generated by a Purkinje fiber is similar to that of a ventricular myocardial cell, except that phase 2 is usually more prolonged in the Purkinje fiber. Atrial myocardial cells exhibit a shortened plateau (phase 2) as compared with ventricular cells.

The pacemaker cells of the SA node have an AP that is very different from that of a myocardial or Purkinje cell. In the SA node, the RMP is less, at about −65 mV. And, rather than a RMP that remains constant, the cells slowly depolarize at a steady rate until threshold is reached (Fig. 11-23, *B*). Because there are no fast Na$^+$ channels in the pacemaker cells, the SA node AP has a different configuration from that of a myocardial cell and is referred to as

the slow response. The lack of a true RMP is largely the result of a steady Na$^+$ influx through the slow channels. This mechanism explains how the cells can spontaneously depolarize (automaticity). It also provides the basis for understanding alterations in the pacemaker cells. The frequency of the pacemaker cell discharge may be altered by a change in the rate of depolarization (changing the slope of phase 4), changing the level of the threshold, or raising or lowering the RMP.

Mechanical Activity

Excitation-contraction coupling. The electrical activity discussed in the previous section is the basis for mechanical contraction. As the myocardial cell is depolarized, specifically during phase 2 of the AP, some Ca^{++} enters the cytoplasm through the cell membrane via special Ca^{++} channels. The majority of Ca^{++} enters the cytoplasm from stores in the sarcoplasmic reticulum (SR).[19] The cytoplasmic Ca^{++} then binds with troponin and tropomyosin, molecules that are present on the actin filaments, resulting in contraction. Occurring throughout the myocardium, the result is myocardial contraction. Once contraction has occurred,

Ca^{++} is taken back up into the SR and the cytoplasmic concentration of Ca^{++} falls leading to muscular relaxation. Both contraction and relaxation are active processes because they require adenosine triphosphate (ATP) and because the Ca^{++} is removed from the cell by way of a Na^+/Ca^{++} pump. The role of this pump is not fully established, but it clearly contributes to intracellular Ca^{++} regulation during diastole.[14,21] The question of increased contractility is also not completely elucidated. Variations in strength of contraction may involve recruitment of more or fewer crossbridges, or a change in the Ca^{++} binding properties of the contractile proteins. There is also probably an increase in Ca^{++} sensitivity as the muscle fiber is stretched.[32] But, the role of Ca^{++} is much more complex than is presented here, because it involves not only the mechanical events in the cell, but also several metabolic and regulatory processes.[27]

The Cardiac Cycle

The cardiac cycle refers to one complete mechanical cycle of the heart beat, beginning with ventricular contraction and ending with ventricular relaxation.

Ventricular systole. As the ventricles are depolarized, the septum and papillary muscles tense first. This provides a stable outflow tract and competent AV valves. The ventricles begin to tense (endocardium to epicardium), causing a rise in pressure. When the intraventricular pressure exceeds that of the intraatrial pressure, the mitral and tricuspid valves close. This stage is known as *isovolumic contraction,* because, even though the ventricular muscle is tensing, the ventricular volume does not change. As the ventricular tension increases, the intraventricular pressures exceed those of the aorta and pulmonary arteries, causing the aortic and pulmonic valves to open. The blood ejected from the ventricles is called the *stroke volume.* Usually more than half of the total ventricular blood volume is ejected; the blood that remains in the ventricles is the *residual* or *end-systolic volume.* The *ejection fraction* is the ratio of the stroke volume ejected from the left ventricle per beat to the volume of blood in the left ventricle at the end of diastole (left ventricular end-diastolic volume). It is expressed as a percent, normal being at least greater than 50%. Both ejection fraction and LVEDV are widely used clinically as indices of contractility and cardiac function.

Ventricular diastole. Following ventricular systole is ventricular diastole. The first phase is *isovolumic relaxation,* which occurs between closure of the semilunar (aortic and pulmonic) valves and the opening of the AV (mitral and tricuspid) valves. Immediately following is the rapid filling phase, in which the AV valves open and the majority of the ventricular filling occurs. The next phase is ventricular diastasis or a reduced ventricular filling period. This is passive flow of blood from the periphery and pulmonary vasculature into the ventricles. The last part of ventricular diastole, known as atrial kick, provides approximately 30% of total ventricular filling. With this, the cycle is complete and begins once again with systole (Fig. 11-26).

Interplay of the Heart and Vessels: Cardiac Output

Cardiac output (CO) is defined as the volume of blood ejected from the heart over 1 minute. Therefore the determinants of CO are heart rate (HR) in beats per minute and stroke volume (SV) in milliliters per beat. The equation is as follows:

$$CO = HR \times SV$$

CO is normally expressed in liters per minute (L/min). The normal CO in the human adult is approximately 4 to 6 L/min. Cardiac index (CI) is the CO divided by the individual's estimated body surface area, expressed in square meters (m^2). The normal range for CI is 2.5 to 4.5 $L/min/m^2$. Changes in either the SV or HR can change the CO. However, all three parameters must be individually assessed. For example, for a person with an HR of 72 and SV of 70 ml,

$$CO = 72 \text{ (beats/min)} \times 70 \text{ (ml/beat)} = 5.040 \text{ L/min}$$

If, however, the parameters change to an HR of 140 and SV of 40 ml,

$$CO = 140 \text{ (beats/min)} \times 40 \text{ (ml/beat)} = 5.600 \text{ L/min}$$

Clearly, although the latter CO is greater, it does not reflect improved cardiac status. Rather, it could mean that cardiac decompensation is imminent. Although HR is influenced by many neurochemical factors to be discussed in the next section, this section will focus on the components of the SV (Fig. 11-27). These are preload, afterload, and contractility.

Preload. The concept of preload was introduced in the early 1900s when Ernest Starling described his findings in an isolated dog heart preparation. Starling found that as he increased the volume infused into a denervated heart, the cardiac output increased. And as the volume increased, so did the CO, until it reached a point at which further infusion actually caused the CO to decrease. This is now known as Starling's law of the heart, and it is graphically described as the Starling curve (Fig. 11-28). It can best be described on a molecular basis, using as a foundation the discussion of the actin and myosin crossbridges in the myofibril. As the diastolic volume increases, it stretches the actin and myosin molecules in their resting state. As contraction occurs, the contractility increases as a result of the increased stretch. However, if the stretch is excessive and causes the actin and myosin to be stretched beyond their crossbridging limits (that is, greater than 2.2 μm), contractility will decrease. This is the basis for the Starling curve. With the advent of critical care units and sophisticated monitoring, this principle has grown to great significance in clinical practice. For example, after a myocardial infarction (MI), the ability of the left ventricle to pump may be impaired. It is desirable to optimize the contractility of the remaining viable heart muscle by "stretching" it with added volume. But if the intravascular volume exceeds the stretch limit, cardiac output will diminish.

Preload, then, is a function of the volume of blood presented to the left ventricle and also the compliance (the ability of the ventricle to stretch) of the ventricles at the end of diastole. It has been described as left ventricular end-diastolic pressure (LVEDP). Factors affecting the volume aspect include venous return, total blood volume, and atrial kick. Factors affecting the compliance of the ventricles are

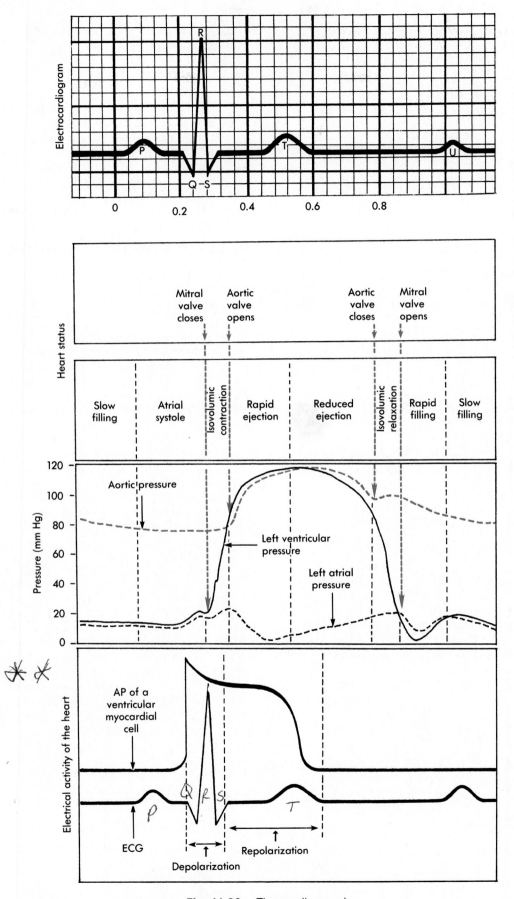

Fig. 11-26 The cardiac cycle.

Intraaortic Balloon Pump

RESEARCH ABSTRACT
Comparison of cardiac output in supine and lateral positions

Doering L and Dracup K: Nurs Res 37(2):114, 1988.

PURPOSE

The purpose of this study was to compare cardiac output determinations obtained by the thermodilution method in supine positions with those obtained in the right and left lateral positions.

FRAMEWORK

Frequent supine positioning has potentially adverse effects, such as interrupted sleep, increased pain and discomfort after surgery, compromised respiratory function, and skin integrity impairment. Nurses face a dilemma in clinical decision making when they attempt to balance the need for repeated cardiac output measurements with the potentially deleterious effects of frequent supine positioning.

METHODS

A total sample of 51 adult patients, aged 40 to 75 years, who underwent cardiac surgery with the use of a pump-oxygenator in a large western medical center were selected for the study. Patients were assigned by coin toss to one of two positions: supine-right-left or supine-left-right. Measurement of backrest angles was standardized at bed frame level; a 20 degree backrest angle was maintained for all three positions. Measurement of lateral angles was standardized at shoulder level, and patients were rotated laterally to 45 degrees for both side-lying positions. Patients were studied at three periods: 4 to 24 hours after surgery when the central venous pressure was greater than or equal to 5 cm water, at least 1 hour after fluid volume expansion, and at least 2 hours after administration of diuretics. After the first position was achieved, a waiting period of 15 minutes was observed. Two cardiac output measurements were taken in rapid succession using 10 ml iced saline injected into the proximal port of the pulmonary artery catheter. A manual technique was used and completed in less than 4 seconds, and the two measurements were averaged. The same procedure was repeated for the second and third positions, with the entire procedure lasting an average of 55 minutes.

RESULTS

Mean cardiac output was significantly different in the three positions at the p = .03 level. This difference resulted from changes in stroke volume, p = .004, rather than changes in heart rate, p = .12. The largest variation occurred between cardiac outputs measured in the supine position and those measured in the left lateral position. Patients at greatest risk for variations in cardiac output with lateral postural change were those with a cardiac index less than 2.3 L/min/m², those who had undergone surgery less than 12 hours before, and those receiving either vasoactive drugs or mechanical ventilation. Though statistically significant, mean output measures in each position did not differ greatly.

IMPLICATIONS

The results indicate that postural variation in cardiac output occurs and may be clinically important in cardiac surgical patients during the early postoperative period. Postural changes from supine to side-lying result in more significant hemodynamic alterations than do backrest changes in the supine position. Based on the study results, consistent measurement in a supine position is recommended. The nurse clinician should consider patients whose previous cardiac index has been below 2.3 L/min/m², those who have undergone surgery less than 12 hours before, and those who are receiving either vasoactive drugs or mechanical ventilation to be at greatest risk for variations in cardiac output with lateral postural change.

— *inotropic*
procanamide

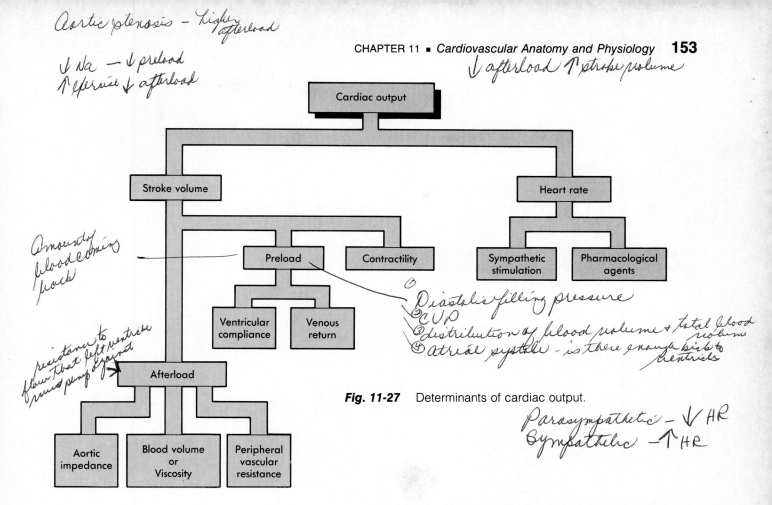

Handwritten annotations: Aortic stenosis – higher afterload; ↓ Na → ↓ preload; ↑ exercise ↓ afterload; ↓ afterload ↑ stroke volume; Amount of blood coming back; resistance to flow that left ventricle must pump against; Diastolic filling pressure; CVP; Distribution of blood volume + total blood volume; atrial systole – is there enough kick to ventricles; Parasympathetic – ↓ HR; Sympathetic – ↑ HR

Fig. 11-27 Determinants of cardiac output.

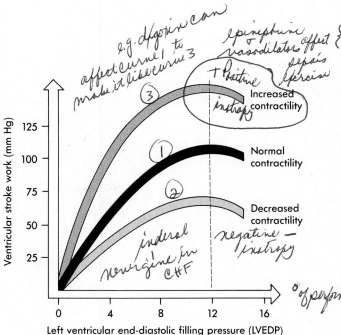

Handwritten annotations: e.g. digoxin can affect curve 1 to make it like curve 3; epinephrine + vasodilators affect sepsis exercise; ↑ Positive inotropy; inderal nervigine in CHF; negative inotropy; of performance; ↑ inotropic epi dig isuprel dopamine dobutamine; depresses contractility

Fig. 11-28 Starling's curve. As the left ventricular end-diastolic pressure (LVED) increases, so does ventricular stroke work or contractility. When left ventricular filling pressure exceeds a maximum point, contractility and cardiac output diminish.

the stiffness and thickness of the muscular wall. Preload is best measured hemodynamically as the pulmonary artery wedge pressure (see the section on hemodynamic monitoring).

Afterload. Afterload can be defined as the ventricular wall tension or stress during systolic ejection. An increase in afterload usually means an increase in the work of the heart. Afterload is increased by factors that oppose ejection. Examples of increased afterload would include aortic impedance (high diastolic aortic pressure, aortic stenosis), septal hypertrophy (obstruction in the outflow tract), vasoconstriction (increased systemic vascular resistance), and increased blood volume or viscosity. Therapeutic management to decrease afterload is done to decrease the work of the heart, thereby decreasing the myocardial oxygen demand.

An increase in afterload can evoke a type of autoregulation in which the ventricle adapts to changes in filling pressure without a continued increase in resting fiber length (the Anrep effect). For example, when peripheral vascular resistance increases abruptly during vasoconstriction, ventricular diastolic pressure rises temporarily until the ventricle reaches a new equilibrium level of pressure.

Contractility. Contractility refers to the heart's contractile force. It is also referred to as *inotropy* (literally, *ino* = strength and *tropy* = enhancing), which can be positive (stronger contraction) or negative (weaker contraction). As previously discussed, contractility can be increased by the Starling mechanism and by the sympathetic nervous system. It can be greatly affected by pharmacological agents, particularly those which mimic the sympathetic nervous system (sympathomimetic, adrenergics).

Handwritten annotations: HYPOXIA; METABOLIC ACIDOSIS; HYPERCAPNIA

Contractility may also be altered by a variety of other physiological phenomena. One such mechanism is the staircase or treppe phenomenon, which occurs when cardiac muscle contracts rapidly following a period of normal rate. During this tachycardia, the force of contraction progressively increases until a new steady state is reached. In addition, situations that cause an increase in the cytoplasmic Ca^{++} may result in positive inotropy. An example of this is the drug digoxin. Digoxin inhibits the Na^+/K^+ pump, which causes a slight rise in the intracellular Na^+. This rise in turn slows the Na^+/Ca^{++} pump that is responsible for removing the cytoplasmic Ca^{++} during diastole. The impaired Na^+/Ca^{++} pump causes a slight increase in cytoplasmic Ca^{++}, which is the basis for the increased inotropic properties of digoxin.

Regulation of the Heart Beat

Nervous control. The parasympathetic nervous system (PNS) and the sympathetic nervous system (SNS) are normally both active to create a balance between maintenance and fight-or-flight cardiovascular functions, respectively. Table 11-6 summarizes the effects on the heart of these divisions of the autonomic nervous system.

Parasympathetic fibers are mostly concentrated near the SA and AV conduction tissue. Specifically, this involves the right and left vagus nerve (Fig. 11-29). Stimulation of the vagus nerve produces bradycardia as a result of hyperpolarization of phase 4 of the AP, which causes the slope to take a longer time to reach threshold. There is also a concomitant decrease in sympathetic tone. Thus adjustments can be made by changes in both the PNS and the SNS or, under certain conditions, selective changes in one.

Sympathetic nerve fibers parallel the coronary circulation to some degree before the fibers penetrate the myocardium. The right and left sympathetic chains probably have slightly different effects on the myocardium. It appears that the right chain has more effect on acceleration properties, whereas the left chain has a greater influence on contractility.

Intrinsic regulation. Supplementing the nervous control are several reflexes that serve as feedback mechanisms to the brain. These reflexes work to maintain even blood flow and perfusion.

The *baroreceptors,* or pressure sensors, are located in the aortic arch and the carotid sinuses. They are more sensitive to wall changes (wall strain) in these areas than to the absolute pressure. As the receptors sense a change in wall conformation, usually as a result of a decrease or increase in pressure, the autonomic nervous system is activated to either raise or lower the heart rate, respectively. For example, a drop in blood pressure will alter the baroreceptor input to the vasomotor center in the medulla, causing a reflex tachycardia. Evidence also suggests that the baroreflex initiates changes in vascular capacity to alter cardiac output according to need.[12] Clinically, this would be evidenced not only by a reflex tachycardia in response to a decreased BP, but also venoconstriction in order to increase blood return to the heart and augment stroke volume. In the opposite situation, an elevated arterial pressure causes the baroreceptors to reset their sensitivity in a way that increases the

Table 11-6 Summary of the effects of the parasympathetic and sympathetic nervous systems on the heart

Function	Parasympathetic	Sympathetic
Automaticity	Decrease	Increase
Contractility	Decrease	Increase
Conduction velocity	Decrease	Increase
Chronotropy (rate)	Decrease	Increase

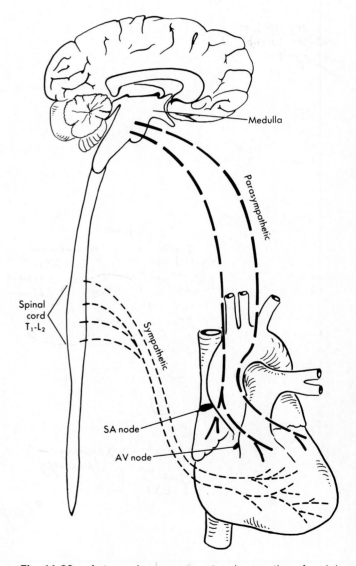

Fig. 11-29 Autonomic nervous system innervation of nodal tissue and myocardium by parasympathetic vagus nerve fibers and sympathetic chains. (From Quaal S: Comprehensive intra-aortic balloon pumping, St Louis, 1984, The CV Mosby Co.)

threshold pressure necessary for baroreceptor activation. This helps to explain why hypertension is not controlled by the baroreceptor response.[8]

The arterial *chemoreceptors,* or aortic bodies, are located in the bifurcation of the aortic arch. They possess a rich capillary blood supply and extensive innervation of the PNS. Their main function is to signal changes in oxygen tension (usually less than 80), a drop in pH below 7.40, or a carbon dioxide tension greater than 40. Stimulation of the chemoreceptors normally causes an increase in respiratory rate and depth.

The *Bainbridge reflex* is attributed to receptors in the right atrium. When the pressure in the right atrium raises sufficiently to stimulate these receptors, it causes a reflex tachycardia. The purpose of this reflex is probably to protect the right side of the heart from an overload state and to quickly equalize filling pressures of the right and left sides of the heart.

A recently described control mechanism is known as the *atrial natriuretic factor* (ANF). It was described in rats in 1981[10] and is now known to be present in all mammalian atria. It is a hormone secreted by the atria in response to increases in atrial pressure. This hormone causes Na^+ and water to be excreted by the kidneys and is also a potent vasodilator. Thus the body rids itself of excess extracellular volume and increases the capacity of the veins to restore total body blood volume. It is possible that ANF is the opposite regulatory mechanism countering the renin-angiotensin system, because the renin-angiotensin system works to conserve Na^+ and water and raise blood pressure[4,5] (Fig. 11-30).

Other reflexes involve the respiratory cycle and its effect on heart rate and stroke volume. Normally the heart rate varies slightly with the respiratory cycle. The heart usually accelerates on inspiration and decelerates with exhalation. Also, left ventricular stroke volume decreases during normal inspiration. There may be so many contributing factors to these phenomena that a single explanation would be inadequate. Possible contributors may include normal fluctuations in sympathetic and vagal tone during respiration, changes in intrathoracic pressure involving increased venous return and the Bainbridge reflex, stretch receptors in the lungs, interactions between the respiratory and cardiac centers in the medulla, increased capacity of the pulmonary vessels during lung inflation, decreased left ventricular compliance resulting from increased right ventricular return, increased impedance to left ventricular outflow related to the pleural pressure changes, or neural reflex mechanisms that are independent of mechanical influences.[2,3] Thus many complex hemodynamic changes occur throughout the respiratory cycle. Consideration must also be given to underlying lung and cardiac disease, intravascular volume status, respiratory rate, and added effects of mechanical ventilation.

Control of Peripheral Circulation

Intrinsic control. Intrinsic or local control of the peripheral circulation is most influential at the arteriolar level. The arterioles are the major *resistance vessels* because of the amount of smooth muscle in the vessel walls. Although the vascular smooth muscle differs in arrangement and amount in different organ beds, it is still subject to many influences. Since the smooth muscle is normaly under dual influence between the vasodilator and vasoconstriction mechanisms, the arteriole has the potential for either increasing or decreasing its lumen substantially. There are several local factors that influence this balance. One is pharmacological stimuli, such as locally released catecholamines, histamine, acetylcholine, serotonin, angiotensin, adenosine, and prostaglandins. These can be initiated by a variety of mechanisms such as tissue injury, hypoxemia, or hormones. Other factors that influence circulation locally are temperature and carbon dioxide.

Extrinsic control. Extrinsic control is mediated by several mechanisms of the central nervous system. The first is that of the autonomic nervous system, and the second that of the vascular reflexes, as previously discussed.

The autonomic nervous system exerts dual antagonistic control over most organ systems via the sympathetic and parasympathetic fibers.[16,20] The vasoconstrictor region in the medulla is normally tonically active. Experimentally, the neuronal activity of this region is essential for maintenance

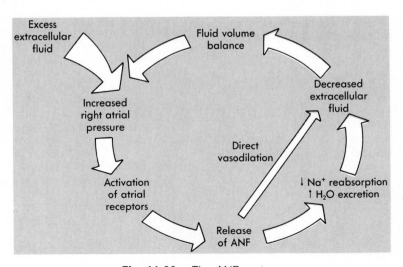

Fig. 11-30 The ANF system.

Table 11-7 Regions in the medulla affecting cardiovascular activity

Region	Activity
Dorsal lateral medulla (pressor region)	Vasoconstriction Cardiac acceleration Enhanced contractility
Ventromedial medulla (depressor region)	Direct spinal inhibition Inhibition of the pressor region

of arterial BP and heart rate. Stimulation causes increases in mean arterial pressure and heart rate by enhancing sympathetic outflow and possibly inhibiting PNS outflow.[31] The sympathetic outflow targets the resistance vessels, causing vasoconstriction. Inhibition of these areas causes the opposite effect, or vasodilation. Sympathetic fibers causing vasoconstriction supply the arteries, arterioles, and veins. However, the capacitance vessels (veins) are probably more responsive to sympathetic stimulation, but the effects are not as readily observed as are those on the arterial side. Table 11-7 summarizes the sympathetic receptors, including location and effects of stimulation.

Control of peripheral circulation is a combination of intrinsic and extrinsic mechanisms.[15] Additional influences include emotions, temperature, and humoral substances.[23]

SUMMARY

The human heart consists of four chambers, the left ventricle being the main pump force. The cardiac valves open and close as a result of pressure gradients. The electrical and mechanical activities of cardiac tissue depend on many ions, specialized structures, and energy expenditure. Myocardial cells have intracellular contractile proteins that enable the heart to contract as a whole. Determinants of cardiac output include preload, afterload, and contractility. The heart beat and peripheral circulation are controlled by several intrinsic and extrinsic mechanisms. Through these complex structures and functions, the heart and blood vessels are able to maintain optimal fluid flow balance throughout the body.

REFERENCES

1. Allwork S: The applied anatomy of the arterial blood supply to the heart in man, J Anat 153:1, 1987.
2. Ashton J and Cassidy S: Reflex depression of cardiovascular function during lung inflation, J Appl Physiol 58(1):137, 1985.
3. Biondi J, Schulman D, and Matthay R: Effects of mechanical ventilation on right and left ventricular function, Clin Chest Med 9(1):55, 1988.
4. Blaine E: Emergence of a new cardiovascular control system: atrial natriuretic factor, Clin Exp Hypertens 7(5-6):835, 1985.
5. Blaine E: Role of atriopeptin in blood pressure regulation, Am J Med Sci 295(4):293, 1988.
6. Bonke F and others: Impulse propagation from the SA-node to the ventricles, Experientia 43:1044, 1987.
7. Carmeliet E and others: Potassium currents in cardiac cells, Experientia 43:1175, 1987.
8. Chapleau M, Hajduczok G, and Abboud F: Mechanisms of resetting of arterial baroreceptors: an overview, Am J Med Sci 295(4):327, 1988.
9. Cranefield P: The conduction of the cardiac impulse 1951-1986, Experientia 43:1040, 1987.
10. deBold AJ and others: A rapid and potent natriuretic response to intravenous injection of atrial myocardial extract in rats, Life Sci 28:89, 1981.
11. Deleze J: Cell-to-cell communication in the heart: structure-function correlations, Experientia 43:1068, 1987.
12. Greene A and Shoukas A: Changes in canine cardiac function and venous return curves by the carotid baroreflex, Am J Physiol 251(part 2):H283, 1986.
13. Greenway C and Lautt W: Blood volume, the venous system, preload, and cardiac output, Can J Physiol Pharmacol 64(4):383, 1986.
14. Horackova M: Transmembrane calcium transport and the activation of cardiac contraction, Can J Physiol Pharmacol 62:874, 1984.
15. Jacob J and others: Studies on neural and humoral contributions to arterial pressure lability, Am J Med Sci 295(4):341, 1988.
16. Julius S: The blood pressure seeking properties of the central nervous system, J Hypertens 6(3):177, 1988.
17. Kitzman DW: Age-related changes in normal human hearts during the first 10 decades of life. Part II (maturity): a quantitative anatomic study of 765 specimens from subjects 20 to 99 years old, Mayo Clin Proc 63:137, 1988.
18. Klocke FJ and others: Coronary pressure-flow relationships, Circ Res 56:310, 1985.
19. Langer G: The role of calcium at the sarcolemma in the control of myocardial contractility, Can J Physiol Pharmacol 65:627, 1987.
20. Levy MN: Cardiac sympathetic-parasympathetic interactions, Fed Proc 43:2596, 1984.
21. Noble D: Experimental and theoretical work on excitation and excitation-contraction coupling in the heart, Experientia 43:1146, 1987.
22. Pelzer D and Trautwein W: Currents through ionic channels in multicellular cardiac tissue and single heart cells, Experientia 43:1153, 1987.
23. Reis D and Ledoux J: Some central neural mechanisms governing resting and behaviorally coupled control of blood pressure, Circulation 76(suppl I):2, 1987.
24. Reuter J: Calcium channel modulation by beta-adrenergic neurotransmitters in the heart, Experientia 43:1173, 1987.
25. Rosen M: The links between basic and clinical cardiac electrophysiology, Circulation 77(2):251, 1988.
26. Sealy W: Morphology of the conduction system and arrhythmia surgery, PACE 11:362, 1988.
27. Shamoo AE and Ambudkar IS: Regulation of calcium transport in cardiac cells, Can J Physiol Pharmacol 62:9, 1984.
28. Tsien R, Hess P, and Nilius B: Cardiac calcium currents at the level of single channels, Experientia 43:1169, 1987.
29. Vassalle M: Contribution of the Na^+/K^+-pump to the membrane potential, Experientia 43:1135, 1987.
30. Weidmann S: Cardiac cellular electrophysiology: past and present, Experientia 43:133, 1987.
31. Willette R and others: Cardiovascular control by cholinergic mechanisms in the rostral ventrolateral medulla, J Pharmacol Exp Ther 231(2):457, 1984.
32. Winegrad S: Regulation of cardiac contractile proteins, Circ Res 55:565, 1984.

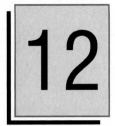

Cardiovascular Clinical Assessment

CHAPTER OBJECTIVES

- *Locate on the precordium and describe the normal size and physiology of the apical impulse.*
- *Describe the appearance of a patient in cardiac failure using the technique of inspection.*
- *Locate the cardiac auscultation areas of the precordium.*
- *Verbalize the difference between the first and second heart sounds according to anatomical cause and the auscultation areas where each sound is best heard.*
- *Define and explain the significance of physiological and paradoxical splitting of the second heart sound, ventricular and atrial gallops, and systolic and diastolic murmurs.*
- *Use the technique of palpation to thoroughly assess the vascular system.*
- *Describe the murmurs that may occur after a myocardial infarction.*

Hippocrates observed: "By opposites opposites are cured." While his aphorism suggests a belief in natural harmony or balance more than an empirical observation of effective medical practice, there is one sense in which it is relevant to the latter. In the systematic observation and recording of abnormal appearance or atypical behavior exhibited by a patient, a health professional gathers valuable information by which such "opposites are cured." If this is generally true of the profession as a whole, it is of critical importance in the care of the cardiovascular patient.

The purpose of this chapter is to demonstrate how the techniques of inspection, palpation, percussion, and auscultation are implemented in the monitoring of cardiovascular patients. In discussing each technique, this chapter will suggest the respective cardiac and vascular data to be collected. Noninvasive assessment of the cardiovascular system provides easily attainable and valuable data on cardiac and vascular status and on any immediate localized or systemic response to treatment. This information, combined with the cardiovascular history and the data from any hemodynamic monitoring equipment, will guide patient treatment and preserve the "excellence of care" reputation that the critical care units have established.

What this chapter cannot so readily convey is the professional challenge offered by—and commensurate personal satisfaction derived from—becoming proficient with these techniques. The reward will be the patient who does not succumb to acute cardiac failure because an S_3 was detected early in his course or the patient who does not have a pulmonary embolus because her thrombophlebitis was treated successfully after being discovered on a routine midshift vascular examination.

HISTORY

The patient history (see the box on p. 158) is important for providing data that contribute to the cardiovascular diagnosis and the treatment plan.

The patient's presenting symptoms or complaints should direct the history-taking part of the assessment. Each symptom should be further explored with the questions detailed in Table 12-1. For example, the vague complaint of *chest pain* can become "classic angina" when the patient is more specific (for example, ". . . a midchest pressure that radiates into my jaw and makes me short of breath when I walk more than a block—if I sit down, it goes away in about 5 minutes"). Other symptoms that may be indicative of cardiovascular problems are listed in the box on p. 158 under "common cardiovascular symptoms" and should be inquired about even if the patient does not complain of them.

The box lists the other parts of the patient history with specific cardiovascular information that should be solicited in each category. The past medical history, current medication usage, and cardiac studies that may have been done in the past are useful in determining cause and treatment of the current medical problem. Taking the time to obtain this information may prevent repetitive tests or ineffective therapy. Cardiac rehabilitation will be focused on the risk factor variables and personal lifestyle choices (patient profile) that place the patient at continued risk for cardiovascular disease.

PHYSICAL EXAMINATION
Inspection

The degree to which the body proclaims its condition is surprisingly explicit. To the educated observer, skin color, body posture, facial expression, and so on speak volumes

DATA COLLECTION FOR CARDIOVASCULAR HISTORY

COMMON CARDIOVASCULAR SYMPTOMS

Chest pains
Palpitations
Dyspnea
Cough
Nocturia
Edema
Dizziness/syncope
Claudication

PATIENT PROFILE

Personal habits
    Use of tea, coffee, alcohol, recreational drugs, over-the-
    counter drug use, smoking, exercise, and dietary habits
Lifestyle pattern
    Working, relaxing, coping
Recent life changes
    Within the past 6 months
Emotional state
    Evidence of psychological stress, worry, anxiety
Perception of illness and its meaning for the future

RISK FACTORS

Sex/age
Family history
Hypertension
Diabetes mellitus
Obesity
Smoking history
High serum cholesterol
Sedentary lifestyle

FAMILY HISTORY

Coronary artery disease
Myocardial infarction
Hypertension
Stroke
Diabetes mellitus
Lipid disorders

CARDIAC STUDIES IN PAST

Cardiac catheterization
Cardiac ultrasound
ECG
Exercise tolerance test
Myocardial imaging with radiographic isotopes
Percutaneous transluminal coronary angioplasty
Valvuloplasty

PAST MEDICAL HISTORY

Childhood
    Murmurs, cyanosis, streptococcal infections, rheumatic
    fever
Adult
    Heart failure, coronary artery disease, heart valve dis-
    ease, mitral valve prolapse, myocardial infarction, pe-
    ripheral vascular disease, diabetes mellitus, hyperten-
    sion, hyperlipidemia, dysrythmias, murmurs, endocar-
    ditis, psychiatric illnesses
Allergies
    Especially to radiographic contrast agents or iodine
Surgical history
    Coronary artery bypass grafting, valve replacement, pe-
    ripheral vascular bypasses or repairs

CURRENT MEDICATION USAGE

Digitalis
Diuretics
Potassium
Antidysrhythmics
Beta blockers
Calcium channel blockers
Nitrates
Antihypertensives
Anticoagulants

---

in the absence of a single word from the patient.

Inspection of the cardiovascular system centers on the patient's general appearance—face, extremities, neck, thorax, and abdomen. While experience will eventually allow one to inspect the patient in a more spontaneous, less compartmentalized fashion, attending to each area suggested ensures the comprehensiveness of the inspection.

General appearance and face. The weight in proportion to the height is assessed for obesity (a cardiac risk factor) or cachexia (which can be present in chronic congestive heart failure). The face is observed for the color of the skin (cyanotic, pale, or jaundice) and expressions of apprehen-

sion and pain. Body posture can indicate the amount of effort it takes to breathe or the position of comfort the patient chooses (for example, needing to sit upright can result from congestive heart failure, and leaning forward may be the least painful position with pericarditis).[1] The patient should be observed for diaphoresis, confusion, or lethargy, each of which could indicate hypotension or low cardiac output. It is important at this point to systematically inspect the skin, lips, mucous membranes, and conjunctiva for pallor or cyanosis and for signs indicating an alteration in fluid or nutritional status. The box on p. 159 summarizes the necessary information to obtain from the initial inspection of the patient.

Table 12-1 Clarification of symptoms by asking specific questions

Determine	Typical question
Location, radiation	Where is it? Does it move or stay in one place?
Quality	What's it like?
Quantity	How severe is it? How frequent? How long does it last?
Chronology	When did it begin? How has it progressed?
Aggravating and alleviating factors	What are you doing when it occurs? What do you do to get rid of it?
Associated findings	Are there any other symptoms you feel at the same time?
Treatment sought and effect	Have you seen a doctor in the past for this same problem? What was the treatment?

INSPECTION OF THE CARDIOVASCULAR SYSTEM
General appearance and face

GENERAL APPEARANCE
Weight
Nutritional status
Position of comfort
Color of skin

FACE
Expression
Emotional state
Presence of diaphoresis
Color of lips
Color of mucous membranes
Color of conjunctiva

INSPECTION OF THE CARDIOVASCULAR SYSTEM
Extremities

Nailbed color
Nailbed clubbing
Skin color
Skin condition
Hair distribution
Presence of edema
Presence of varicosities
Comparison of circumferences

Extremities. The nailbeds should be inspected for cyanosis and clubbing. Central cyanosis is a bluish discoloration of the skin, lips, circumoral area, mucous membranes, and nailbeds. It indicates a decreased oxygen saturation of the circulating hemoglobin molecule and may occur as a result of right-to-left intracardiac shunting, impaired pulmonary function, or hypoxia from any cause.[1] Peripheral cyanosis indicates reduction of peripheral blood flow as a result of vascular disease or decreased cardiac output and is usually seen in the nailbeds or the tip of the nose.[1]

Clubbing of the nailbeds is associated with central cyanosis as a sign of chronic oxygen deficiency. Clubbing is evaluated by assessing the angle between the nail and the nail base, which is normally less than 180 degrees. A flattened angle (equaling 180 degrees) with a springy or spongy nail base is "early" clubbing, and an angle greater than 180 degrees with a swollen nail base is "late" clubbing (see Fig. 18-1).

The extremities yield multiple signs of vascular disease. The parameters to be assessed are hair distribution (sparse or lacking), skin condition (dry, scaly, cracked, or shiny), temperature (cool or warm), color (pale, dusky, or hyperpigmented), and the presence of edema. With arterial insufficiency there is pallor when the legs are elevated and rubor when the legs are dependent. With venous thrombosis the color of the extremity may be dusky, and the circumference of the affected calf or thigh may be slightly larger compared with the other extremity. The lower extremities should be inspected for varicosities that may predispose a patient to develop thrombophlebitis and/or require special venous radiographic studies if the patient were to need coronary artery bypass grafting. The box above lists the specific information to be obtained by inspecting the extremities.

External jugular vein. Normally, in the upright position (sitting erect), the jugular veins are nondistended. Jugular venous distention (JVD) occurs when central venous pressure is elevated. The procedure for assessing JVD is as follows. With the patient reclined at a 30- to 45-degree angle, the examiner stands on the patient's right side and turns the patient's head slightly toward the left. If the jugular vein is not visible, light finger pressure is applied across the sternocleidomastoid muscle, just above and parallel to the clavicle. This will fill the external jugular vein by ob-

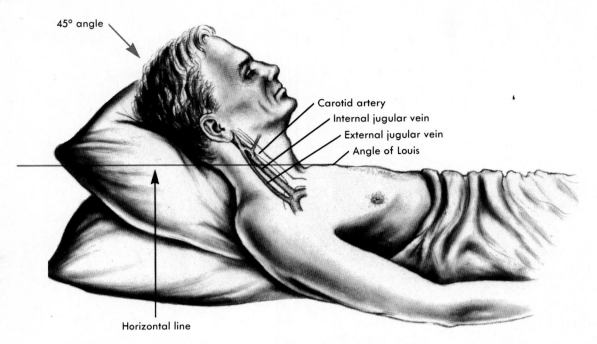

Fig. 12-1 Position of the internal and external jugular veins. (From Thompson JM and others: Clinical nursing, St Louis, 1986, The CV Mosby Co.)

structing flow. Once the location of the vein has been identified, the pressure is released and the presence of JVD is assessed. Because inhalation decreases venous pressure, JVD should be assessed at the end of exhalation. Any fullness in the vein extending more than 3 cm above the sternal angle is evidence of increased venous pressure.[2] Generally speaking, the higher the sitting angle of the patient when JVD is discovered, the higher the central venous pressure. This finding is reported by including the angle of the head of the bed at the time JVD was evaluated (that is, "presence of JVD with head of bed elevated to 45 degrees").

Internal jugular vein. The fluid column of the internal jugular vein is also used to estimate the amount of central venous pressure (in centimeters). This vein lies anterior to the external jugular at the level of the clavicle (Fig. 12-1) and follows a parallel path with the carotid and the trachea. The highest point of pulsation in this vein is observed during exhalation. The vertical distance between this pulsation, which is at the top of the fluid level, and the sternal angle is estimated in centimeters (Fig. 12-2). This number is then added to 5 cm for an estimation of central venous pressure. The 5 cm is the approximate distance of the sternal angle above the level of the right atrium. The degree of elevation of the patient is included in reporting this finding (that is, "central venous pressure estimated at 13 cm, using the internal jugular vein pulsation, with the head of the bed elevated 45 degrees").[2]

Hepatojugular reflex. Right-sided cardiac failure is one cause of elevated central venous pressure. To further assess for right-sided heart failure, one must assess for the presence of a hepatojugular reflex in the internal jugular vein. This is accomplished by observing the pulsation of the internal jugular as pressure is firmly applied over the right upper

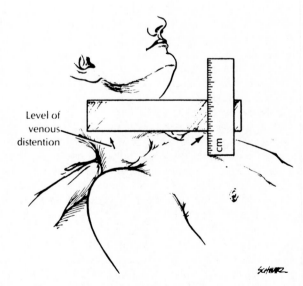

Fig. 12-2 Measurement of jugular venous pressure. The arrows indicate the height of the jugular venous presure in centimeters. (from Malasanos L, and others: Health assessment, ed 3, St Louis, 1986, The CV Mosby Co.)

quadrant of the patient's abdomen for 30 seconds. The normal response is a slight rise in the fluid level of the internal jugular vein followed by a prompt return to normal. If there is a greater than 1 cm sustained rise in the fluid level or amount of distension in the vein, the test is considered positive. This test is accurate because pressure on the abdomen causes increased venous return to the right atrium, which, if failing, cannot pump away the extra volume of blood.[2] If the patient tenses up or holds his or her breath during this procedure, a false positive may be elicited, because these maneuvers (tensing and breath holding) may increase venous return.

Thorax and abdomen. The next and final areas of inspection are the thorax and the abdomen. Both the anterior and posterior thorax should be assessed for skeletal deformities (for example, pectus excavatum, straight back) that may displace the heart and cause systolic murmurs.[1] The skin on the chest wall and the abdomen should be checked for scars, bruises, wounds, and pacemaker implants. Respiratory rate, pattern, and effort should also be observed and recorded.

Thoracic reference points. The thoracic cage is divided with imaginary vertical lines (sternal, midclavicular, and axillary, vertebral, scapular), and the intercostal spaces (ICS) are divided with horizontal lines, to serve as reference points in locating or describing cardiac findings (Figs. 12-3A, 12-3B, and 12-3C). The ribs are numbered from 1 (the first rib below the clavicle) to 12. The intercostal space between each rib is numbered the same as the rib that lies above it. The second rib is the easiest to locate because it is attached to the sternum at the angle of Louis. This angle (also called the sternal angle) is the bony ridge on the sternum that lies approximately 2 inches below the sternal notch

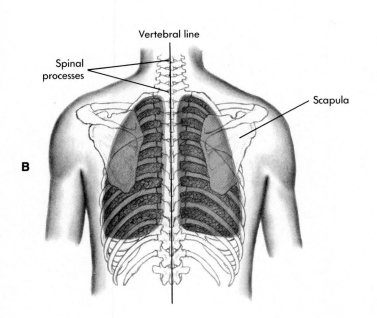

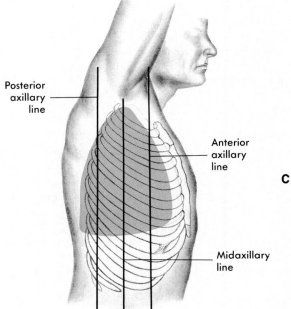

Fig. 12-3 **A,** Thoracic landmarks: anterior thorax. **B,** Thoracic landmarks: posterior thorax. **C,** Thoracic landmarks: right lateral thorax.

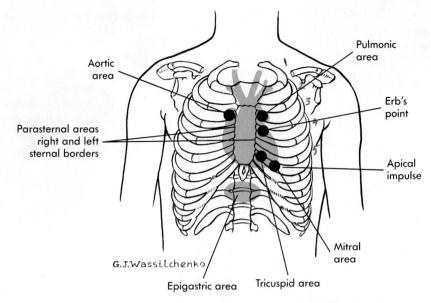

Aortic area

Pulmonic area

Erb's point

Parasternal areas right and left sternal borders

Apical impulse

Mitral area

G.J.Wassilchenko

Epigastric area   Tricuspid area

Fig. 12-4   Thoracic palpation and auscultation points.

(Fig. 12-3A). Once the second rib has been located, it can be used as a reference point to count off the other ribs and intercostal spaces.

Apical impulse. The anterior thorax must also be inspected for the apical impulse, sometimes referred to as the point of maximal impulse (PMI). The apical impulse occurs as the left ventricle contracts during systole and rotates forward causing the left ventricular apex to hit the chest wall. The impulse is a quick, localized (2 × 2 cm), outward movement normally located just lateral to the left midclavicular line at the fifth intercostal space in the adult patient (Fig. 12-4). The apical impulse is the only normal pulsation visualized on the chest wall, and, if visible, the location, size, and character should be noted. The rest of the anterior thorax should be inspected for abnormal pulsations that can indicate cardiac enlargement (that is, a visible pulsation in the left parasternal region suggests right ventricular enlargement). The abdomen is also inspected for normal pulsations of the aorta, frequently seen in the epigastric area (Fig. 12-4). To summarize the thoracic and abdominal areas of inspection refer to the box at right.

Palpation

Palpation is a technique that utilizes the sense of touch. The finger tips are sensitive to pressure, the backs of the fingers are sensitive to temperature, and the base of the fingers on the palmar side, as well as the lateral edge of the palm, are sensitive to pressure and vibrations. Palpation is done with a light touch and an unhurried, relaxed approach. Palpation is used to assess pulsations in the extremities, neck, thorax, and abdomen. Palpation is also used to assess the presence and amount of edema, the temperature of the skin, and capillary refill. The information obtained with palpation reinforces data collected with inspection and is especially important for the assessment of the vascular system.

INSPECTION OF THE CARDIOVASCULAR SYSTEM

Thorax and abdomen

THORAX

Skeletal deformities
Skin condition (scars, bruises, wounds)
Presence of pacemaker generator
Apical impulse
Abnormal pulsations

ABDOMEN

Skin conditions (scars, bruises, wounds)
Abdominal aortic pulsation

Arterial pulsations. There are seven major arterial areas that are assessed for pulse palpation. The examination must include bilateral assessment of the carotid, brachial, radial, ulnar, popliteal, dorsalis pedis, and posterior tibial arteries. The extremity pulses are assessed separately and compared bilaterally to check consistency. Pulse volume is graded on a scale of 0 to 4+.

Upper extremities. The radial and the brachial arteries are palpated for pulse quality in the upper extremities. These same arteries are also often punctured or cannulated for arterial blood gas specimens. It is imperative to frequently assess the pulse quality when the artery is cannulated, as well as the color, temperature, and pulse quality distal to the cannulated site. Occlusion of arterial blood flow would be reflected by the absence of a pulse and/or coolness and pallor of the distal extremity.

Allen test. Before a radial artery is punctured or cannulated, the Allen test should be done to assess adequate blood flow to the hand through the ulnar artery. The Allen test is performed as follows: (1) The patient is requested to make a tight fist to squeeze the blood out of his or her hand. (2) The brachial artery is compressed with firm thumb pressure by the examiner. (3) The patient is requested to open the hand, palm side up, while the brachial artery is still occluded. (4) The time it takes for the color to return to the hand is noted. If the ulnar artery is patent, the color will return within 3 seconds. Delayed color return (a "failed" Allen test), implies that the ulnar artery is occluded; therefore the radial artery is the only source of blood flow to the hand and should not be punctured or cannulated.

Capillary refill. Capillary refill assessment is a maneuver done on the nailbeds to evaluate arterial circulation to the extremity. The nailbed should be compressed to produce blanching, and release of the pressure should result in a return of blood flow and nail color in less than 3 seconds. The severity of arterial insufficiency is directly proportional to the amount of time necessary to reestablish flow and color.

Lower extremities. The lower extremity pulses are the most difficult to locate—the popliteal pulses perhaps being the most elusive. The popliteal pulses are found behind the knee, deep in the popliteal fossa, just lateral of the midline. The knee should be bent slightly to gain easier access to this area. The posterior tibial pulses are just behind the medial malleolus, and the dorsalis pedis pulses are on the dorsal areas of the feet, usually just lateral to the extensor tendon of the great toe. The lightest touch, with at least three fingertips, and systematic movement across the top of the foot will help to locate the dorsalis pedis. The dorsalis pedis pulses and the posterior tibial pulses may be congenitally absent, but their presence is not entirely ruled out until they are checked with the patient's extremity in the dependent position.

Edema. Edema is fluid accumulated in the extravascular spaces of the body, such as the abdomen and the dependent tissues of the legs and sacrum. The amount of edema is quantified by pressing the skin of the feet, ankles, and shins against the underlying bone. If there is an impression left in the tissue when the thumb is removed, it is called "pitting

---

LEGAL REVIEW

Patient care assessment in the critical care unit

CASE EXAMPLE: *Belmon v. St. Francis Cabrini Hospital,* 427 So.2d 541 (1983)

Alice Belmon was admitted through the emergency room (ER) to the critical care unit with a diagnosis of possible pulmonary embolism. In the ER, she received an immediate dose of 7500 unit bolus of heparin. She received heparin by continuous IV drip in the critical care unit, totaling 2000 units/hour. The critical care nurse observed Mrs. Belmon throughout the night, taking her blood pressure (BP) regularly. At 5 AM a medical technician took a blood sample from the patient's right arm. At 7:30 AM the arm began to hurt and showed swelling and discoloration. Mrs. Belmon and her husband complained to the critical care nurse about her arm. The nurse's notes contained BP readings. Mrs. Belmon's partial thromboplastin time (PTT) was 180 seconds, the maximum reading on the laboratory monitor.

At noon the patient's physician arrived and discovered a large hematoma on the patient's upper right arm, underneath the BP cuff. The patient's arm was wrapped and elevated, and the physician ordered that the heparin therapy be decreased by one half. At 2 PM the physician ordered the heparin therapy discontinued.

In this case the hospital was sued for the nurse's negligence under the principle of *respondeat superior,* making an employer liable for an employee's negligent acts. The allegation the plaintiff presented was that the nurse's failure to investigate the patient's complaints and her inaction

permitted the patient's injury to reach serious proportions before a physician was called and that the nurse failed to recognize and respond properly to signs of hemorrhage.

The plaintiff presented an expert nurse witness who testified that the nurse's duty of care to the patient increased as the PTT value increased. The hospital-defendant argued that this was improper testimony because it exceeded the nurse's expertise and invaded the physician's field of practice. The court did not accept this argument, stating that the expert nurse's testimony was proper because it stated the nursing standard of care at issue. In addition, the court said even if the nurse expert's opinion was discarded, there was other medical testimony to support a finding of liability.

In particular, the plaintiff had also presented a physician expert who testified that the patient experienced "blood pressure cuff trauma" and that the nurse should have properly investigated the patient's complaint of pain by looking under the BP cuff. The expert testified that hemorrhage is a substantial risk with heparin therapy and that the venipuncture and BP cuff added to the risk. He said he'd expect a critical care nurse to call him immediately if such a patient had pain, swelling, or bleeding.

The hospital was found liable for the nurse's negligence. The nurse breached a standard of care that led to and was the proximate cause of the patient's injuries, including pain, suffering, and longer hospital stay. The plaintiff was awarded $58,000 by the jury.

PALPATION OF THE CARDIOVASCULAR SYSTEM
Upper and lower extremities

UPPER EXTREMITIES

Brachial pulses
Radial pulses
Temperature
Capillary refill

LOWER EXTREMITIES

Popliteal pulses
Posterior tibial pulses
Dorsalis pedis pulses
Edema of feet, ankles, shins
Presence of phlebitis

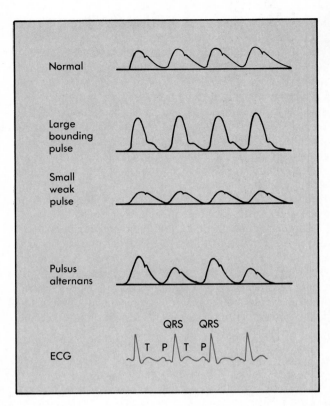

Fig. 12-5 The carotid pulse wave in relation to heart sounds and the ECG.

edema," and the depth, if quantified, should be recorded in millimeters. A patient with congestive heart failure may gain 10 pounds or more of excess fluid before "pitting" is noted. Liver or renal failure and venous insufficiency with venous stasis can also cause edema in the lower extremities.

Thrombophlebitis. The veins of the lower extremities are assessed with palpation, specifically for thrombophlebitis, which is an inflammation of the vein with thrombus formation that predisposes a patient to pulmonary emboli and chronic venous insufficiency. By squeezing or pressing the calves against the tibia, pain or tenderness or increased firmness or tension in the muscle may be elicited. These signs suggest phlebitis and should alert the examiner to check other parameters that may aid the diagnosis, such as comparing leg circumferences, checking for increased heat in the extremity or for unexplained fever or tachycardia. There is also Homan's sign, which in the company of the other signs can assist the diagnosing of phlebitis.[2] To elicit Homan's sign, the patient's knee should be flexed, and the examiner should forcefully and abruptly dorsiflex the patient's foot. The sign is positive when there is reported pain in the popliteal region and the calf. The box above lists the important points of palpation for upper and lower extremities.

Carotid pulses. The carotid pulses are assessed by palpation for cardiac rate and rhythm and also for the amplitude and contour of the pulsation. Normally there is a swift upstroke to this pulse, with a slight rounded plateau at its peak and a gradual descent (Fig. 12-5). With an increased pulse pressure, such as that which occurs with hyperdynamic states such as fever, anxiety, hyperthyroidism, anemia, and exercise, the carotid pulse is large and, "bounding," and the descending portion of the wave is as rapid as the upstroke. Aortic insufficiency can also cause this type of waveform because of the rapid runoff of blood through the incompetent valve. Decreased cardiac output (aortic stenosis or heart failure) or hypotension will create a small wave with an upstroke as gradual as the descent. If the carotid pulse is regular and alternates between large and small waves

with every other wave being small, it is called *pulsus alternans*. Pulsus alternans is evidence of left-sided heart failure (see Fig. 12-5).

If blood flow through the carotid arteries is compromised at all by arteriosclerosis or plaques, palpation could easily cause total occlusion; thus only one carotid artery at a time should be palpated. Also, they should be palpated in the lower half of the neck, well below the level of the carotid bodies, which, when stimulated, cause a decrease in heart rate.

Thorax. The chest wall should be palpated for the apical impulse described previously. Its location, size, amplitude, and duration should be recorded. An enlarged left ventricle (left ventricular hypertrophy) is suspected when the apical impulse is enlarged (>2 cm) and is displaced laterally. When the apical impulse is difficult to locate, the patient can be turned to the left lateral decubitus position. This facilitates palpation of the impulse because the left ventricle is against the chest wall in the left lateral position. While this makes palpation of the apical impulse easier, it may also distort the placement and size of the impulse—limitations the examiner must consider. Once the apical impulse has been examined, the entire precordium (the chest area overlying the heart and great vessels) must be assessed for other pulsations. The precordial areas are labeled according to the underlying anatomy (Fig. 12-4). Each area should be palpated in an orderly fashion.

The terminology used to communicate palpatory findings should describe as accurately as possible the sensation the examiner feels. Generally speaking, accepted terminology

PALPATION OF THE CARDIOVASCULAR SYSTEM
Neck, precordium, and abdomen

NECK
Carotid pulses

PRECORDIUM
Apical impulse
Other chest pulsations (lifts, thrusts, heaves, thrills)

ABDOMEN
Femoral pulses
Abdominal aortic pulse

refers to "thrusts" as localized and "heaves" or "lifts" as more diffuse movements. For example, right ventricular enlargement can cause a left parasternal "heave," and cor pulmonale, with both right atrial and right ventricular enlargement, can cause a sternal "lift." Left ventricular hypertrophy usually causes an apical "thrust" as previously described. The paradoxical movement or "heave" associated with ventricular aneurysm at the apex is often first detected by palpation. "Thrills" are vibrations that feel like a cat's purr and are associated with loud murmurs. Palpation of a thrill in the aortic area may indicate aortic stenosis or hypertension.

Description of location, amplitude, duration, direction (inward or outward), distribution (localized or diffuse), and timing in the cardiac cycle (systole or diastole) are helpful for determining the cause of a pulsation.

Abdomen. The abdomen is palpated for the pulsations of the femoral arteries and the abdominal aortic artery. The femoral arteries are palpated by pressing deeply into the groin beneath the inguinal ligament, about midway between the anterior superior iliac spine and the symphysis pubis on both the right and left sides.

The aortic pulsation is normally located in the epigastric area (Fig. 12-4) and can be felt as a forward movement by using firm fingertip pressure above the umbilicus. If the pulsation is prominent, diffuse, or extends in the midline below the umbilicus, it may indicate an abdominal aneurysm. Refer to the box above for specifics of palpation of the neck, precordium, and abdomen.

Percussion

Percussion may be used in the cardiac physical assessment to outline the left cardiac border. The apical impulse, however, located by inspection and palpation, is more reliable in determining the size of the left ventricle and is more quickly assessed.

Auscultation

Auscultation is used for blood pressure measurement, detection of carotid and femoral bruits, and assessment of normal and abnormal heart sounds and murmurs. There are many good articles available for detailed study of heart sounds and murmurs.[1-3,7,9] The information given here will introduce the normal heart sounds and the ventricular filling sounds. Murmurs will be presented in the broad categories of systolic and diastolic occurrence. The murmurs most commonly occurring subsequent to a myocardial infarction will be discussed in more detail. The extracardiac murmur of the pericardial friction rub will also be discussed, because it often occurs in the critical care setting and can be easily treated when properly identified.

Vasculature. The carotid and femoral arteries should be auscultated for bruits. A bruit is an extracardiac vascular sound resulting from either: (1) blood-flow through a tortuous or a partially occluded vessel or (2) from increased blood flow through a normal vessel. The sound is a high-pitched "sh-sh" sound that vacillates in volume with systole and diastole. Because the diaphragm of the stethoscope is usually too big to auscultate the carotid or femoral areas comfortably, the bell, pressed firmly enough into the skin to create a seal, will act as a good substitute. The skin, then, becomes a diaphragm and will transmit the high-pitched sound of the bruit. Light but firm pressure is the key when using the bell of the stethoscope to create a diaphragm.

Heart. Auscultation of the heart can be the most challenging part of the cardiac physical examination. To summarize the advice given by most authors, the examiner must (1) discipline herself or himself to auscultate systematically across the precordium, (2) visualize the cardiac anatomy under each point of auscultation, expecting to hear the physiologically associated sounds, (3) memorize the cardiac cycle to enhance ability to hear the abnormal sounds, and (4) practice, practice, practice.

First and second heart sounds (S_1 and S_2). Normal heart sounds are referred to as "sound one" (S_1) and "sound two" (S_2). S_1 is produced by the rapid deceleration of blood flow when the atrioventricular (mitral and tricuspid) valves close at the beginning of systole. S_2 is heard at the end of systole when the semilunar (aortic and pulmonic) valves reach closure. The actual sounds are caused, not by the valve leaflets touching each other when they close, but by the vibrations created by the abrupt interruption of retrograde blood flow against the closed, tensed valve leaflets.[9] Both sounds are high pitched and heard best with the diaphragm of the stethoscope. Each sound is loudest in an auscultation area located "downstream" from the actual valvular component of the sound (Fig. 12-6). For example, S_2, which is associated with aortic and pulmonary valve closure can be heard best at the base of the heart, at the second ICS to the right and left of the sternum, in the areas labeled aortic and pulmonic. This is true because these areas overlie a section of vasculature "downstream" from the valves and in the same direction that sound travels. S_1 associated with closure of the mitral and tricuspid valves is heard best in the mitral and tricuspid areas. S_1 occurs immediately before the carotid upstroke. To identify it, if the heart rate is over 80 bpm, it may be helpful to simultaneously palpate the carotid artery pulsation while auscultating in the tricuspid or mitral area.

Both S_1 and S_2 are split sounds (Fig. 12-7) because of

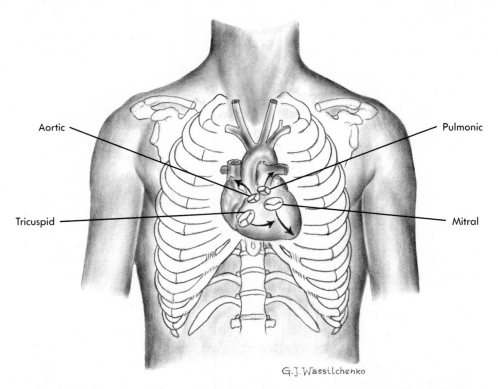

G.J.Wassilchenko

Fig. 12-6 Transmission of heart sounds to the thorax and their relationship to the anatomical position of the heart valves.

asynchronous left and right ventricular contraction. When there are no ventricular conduction blocks, the left side of the heart contracts milliseconds before the right. The left-sided heart valves, mitral and aortic, are the first heard components of each sound and are usually the loudest. The splits are best heard in the areas overlying the quieter components, the tricuspid and pulmonic valves. The S_2 is more obviously split, and the audible distance between the aortic and pulmonary components is increased with inhalation. This respiratory variation is called physiological splitting and occurs because inspiration causes changes in pulmonary vascular impedence and in systemic and pulmonary venous return. These changes result in a lengthening of right ventricular ejection time and a corresponding shortening of left ventricular ejection time.[9] All the components of the split sounds will be high pitched and best heard with the diaphragm of the stethoscope. This information should help to differentiate the normal split sound from the ventricular filling sounds that may indicate pathology. See Table 12-2 for detailed characteristics of the normal heart sounds.

An advanced skill in auscultation is determining whether the S_1 or S_2 is louder or softer than normal. The intensity of the sounds vary with dysrhythmias, hyperdynamic cardiac states, and the physical condition of the valves. Independent study, as well as practice and experience, will prepare the novice to detect abnormal auscultation of S_1 and S_2.

Third and fourth heart sounds (S_3 and S_4). The abnormal heart sounds are labeled "sound three" (S_3) and "sound four" (S_4) and are referred to as "gallops" when auscultated during tachycardia. They are ventricular filling sounds, occurring during diastole, and are low pitched. One can differentiate between right and left ventricular gallops by location. Left ventricular S_3 and S_4 are heard best with the bell of the stethoscope positioned lightly over the apical impulse with the patient in the left lateral decubitus position, and right ventricular gallops are heard best at the left lower sternal border (LLSB). They are rhythmic (like horses cantering) and have mimetic sounds as listed in Table 12-3. The sound of the S_3 is similar to that of a stone dropping into water at the bottom of a well—dull and "thuddy." The S_4 occurs at the end of diastole when the ventricle is full and is associated with the atrial contraction (kick). It is a hollow, snappy sound, as if the noncompliant ventricle cannot accept anymore volume unless it flows in hard and fast. The presence of an S_3 is normal in persons less than age 40 because of rapid filling of the ventricle and the motion it causes in the young healthy heart.[7]

It is important to remember that both S_3 and S_4 are diastolic sounds. If extra sounds are heard, they can best be labeled as systolic or diastolic by using the "inching technique."[2] This means the aortic area, where S_2 is loudest, would be auscultated first, then the stethoscope would be "inched" across the pericardium toward the mitral area where S_1 is loudest. It can then be determined whether the extra sound(s) is coming before S_2 (systolic event) or after S_2 (diastolic event). Once the timing is ascertained, the pitch should be assessed (high pitched would be a split S_1 or S_2, low pitched would be an S_3 or S_4). A useful test to differentiate between splits and ventricular filling sounds is to

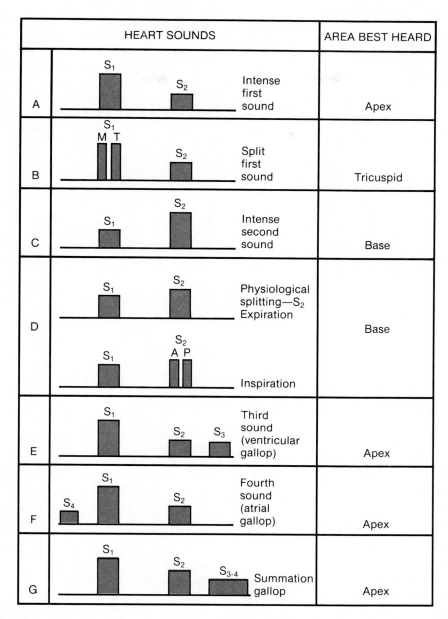

HEART SOUNDS		AREA BEST HEARD
A	S_1 S_2 — Intense first sound	Apex
B	S_1 M T S_2 — Split first sound	Tricuspid
C	S_1 S_2 — Intense second sound	Base
D	S_1 S_2 — Physiological splitting—S_2 Expiration	Base
	S_1 S_2 A P — Inspiration	
E	S_1 S_2 S_3 — Third sound (ventricular gallop)	Apex
F	S_4 S_1 S_2 — Fourth sound (atrial gallop)	Apex
G	S_1 S_2 S_{3-4} — Summation gallop	Apex

Fig. 12-7 Characteristics of normal and abnormal heart sounds and the auscultatory area where each is best heard.

Table 12-2 ▪ Characteristics of heart sounds one (S_1) and two (S_2)

S_1	S_2
High pitched	High pitched
Loudest in mitral area (apex)	Loudest in aortic area (base)
Normal split <20 msec	Normal split <30 msec
Split heard best in tricuspid area	Split heard best in pulmonic area
Important to differentiate between split S_1 and S_4	↑ Split with inhalation
Occurs immediately before carotid upstroke	↓ Split with exhalation

listen with the bell of the stethoscope. The bell is pressed down during auscultation, turning it into a diaphragm that accentuates only high-pitched sounds. If the extra sounds disappear, they may have been low pitched S_3 or S_4.

Murmurs. Heart murmurs are prolonged extra sounds that occur during systole or diastole. The sounds are vibrations caused by turbulent blood flow through the cardiac chambers. As indicated in the box on p. 168, not all murmurs are caused by cardiac valvular disease. Some murmurs are caused by a high rate of blood flow through the ventricle as with fever, anemia, and exercise (high output states), and other murmurs may be caused by structural defects such as patent foramen ovale (opening in the septum between the right and left atria). Murmurs are characterized by their

Table 12-3 Characteristics of heart sounds three (S_3) and four (S_4)

S_3	S_4
PHYSIOLOGICAL CAUSES	**PHYSIOLOGICAL CAUSES**
Related to diastolic motion and rapid filling of ventricles in early diastole	Related to diastolic motion and ventricular dilitation with atrial contraction in late diastole
Can be normal in children and young adults (<40 yr)	May occur with or without cardiac decompensation
PATHOLOGICAL CAUSES	**PATHOLOGICAL CAUSES**
Ventricular dysfunction with an increase in end systolic volume (MI, congestive heart failure, valvular disease, systemic or pulmonary hypertension)	Ventricular hypertrophy with a decrease in ventricular compliance (CAD, systemic hypertension, cardiomyopathy, aortic or pulmonary stenosis, ↑ in intensity with acute MI or angina)
Hyperdynamic states (anemia, thyrotoxicosis, mitral or tricuspid regurgitation)	Acute valvular regurgitation
	Hyperkinetic states (anemia, thyrotoxicosis, arteriovenous fistula)
RHYTHMIC WORD ASSOCIATION	**RHYTHMIC WORD ASSOCIATION**
Ken....tuck..y S_1 S_2 S_3	Ten...nes.....see S_4 S_1 S_2
SYNONYMS	**SYNONYMS**
Ventricular gallop Protodiastolic gallop	Atrial gallop Presystolic gallop

---

CAUSES OF CARDIAC MURMURS

- An increased rate of flow through cardiac structures
- Blood flow across a partial obstruction or irregularity
- Shunting of blood through an abnormal passage from high → low pressure
- Backflow across an incompetent valve

---

timing (systolic/diastolic), location and radiation, quality (blowing, grating, harsh), pitch (high or low), and intensity (loudness graded on a scale of I to VI, the higher the number, the louder the murmur). Tables 12-4 and 12-5 describe the most common murmurs in terms of these characteristics.

In children or adolescents, systolic "high flow" murmurs are common and are a result of vigorous ventricular contraction. These murmurs have a low-medium pitch (heard best with the bell of the stethoscope), grade I to II intensity, and a blowing quality. They are often heard best in the tricuspid area and do not radiate.

When auscultating murmurs, it is again helpful to visualize the cardiac anatomy, specifically the location of the heart valves and the direction of sound transmission with valve closure and murmur. Generally the systolic valvular murmurs will radiate downstream from the valve that is narrowed (stenotic), and the diastolic valvular murmurs, indicating a backflow of blood through an incompetent valve, will be auscultated best directly over the area of the valve (Fig. 12-6).

Murmurs associated with myocardial infarction. At the bedside, the nurse is often the first person to auscultate a murmur. The holosystolic or pansystolic murmurs that can occur in the acute myocardial infarction period are good examples. The auscultation of a new, high-pitched, holosystolic, blowing murmur at the cardiac apex heralds mitral valve regurgitation secondary to papillary muscle dysfunction. This murmur may be soft (I/VI or II/VI) and occur only during ischemic episodes when the papillary muscle contractility is impaired, but its presence is associated with persistent pain, heart failure, and higher mortality.[4] If the murmur is loud (V/VI or VI/VI), harsh, and radiating in all directions from the apex, the papillary muscle or chordae tendineae may have ruptured. This is an emergency situation requiring immediate medical and often surgical intervention.

Ventricular septal defect, or rupture, is another emergency situation. It creates the same type of harsh, holosystolic murmur, loudest along the left sternal border. The clinical picture associated with both the papillary muscle rupture and the ventricular septal defect is that of acute heart failure and cardiogenic shock. Immediate diagnosis and treatment is necessary to prevent deaths.

Pericardial friction rub. A pericardial friction rub is a sound that can occur within the first week of a myocardial infarction and/or cardiac surgery and is secondary to pericarditis. It is a "to-and-fro," scratchy sound that corresponds with cardiac motion within the pericardial sac (that is, ventricular systole, ventricular diastole, and atrial systole), so it can be both a systolic and diastolic sound. It is high pitched and best auscultated at Erb's point (the third ICS to the left of the sternum; see Fig. 12-4). It is often associated with chest pain and it is important to differentiate pericarditis from myocardial ischemia. The detection of the pericardial friction rub can assist in the proper diagnosis and treatment. The box on p. 170 reviews where sounds are best heard on the specific areas of the precordium.

Table 12-4 Characteristics of some systolic murmurs

Defect	Timing in the cardiac cycle	Pitch, intensity, quality	Location, radiation
Mitral regurgitation	S₁ S₂	High Harsh Blowing	Mitral area May radiate to axilla
Tricuspid regurgitation	S₁ S₂	High Often faint, but varies Blowing	Tricuspid RLSB, apex, LLSB, epigastric areas Little radiation
Ventricular septal defect	S₁ S₂	High Loud Blowing	Left sternal border
Aortic stenosis	S₁ S₂	Chhhh hh Medium Rough, harsh	Aortic area to suprasternal notch, right side of neck, apex
Pulmonary stenosis	S₁ S₂	Low to medium Loud Harsh, grinding	Pulmonic area No radiation

RLSB, right lower sternal border; LLSB, left lower sternal border.

Table 12-5 Characteristics of some diastolic murmurs

Defect	Timing in the cardiac cycle	Pitch, intensity, quality	Location, radiation
Mitral stenosis	Atrial kick S₂ S₁	Low Quiet to loud with thrill Rough rumble	Mitral area Usually no radiation
Tricuspid stenosis	Atrial kick S₂ S₁	Medium Quiet, louder with inspiration Rumble	Tricuspid area or epigastrim Little radiation
Aortic regurgitation	S₂ S₁	High Faint to medium Blowing	Aortic area to LLSB and aorta Erb's point
Pulmonic regurgitation	S₂ S₁	Medium Faint Blowing	Pulmonic area No radiation

LLSB, left lower sternal border.

AUSCULTATION OF THE CARDIOVASCULAR SYSTEM
Precordium

AORTIC AREA

S_2 loud
Aortic systolic murmur

PULMONIC AREA

S_2 loud and split with inhalation
Pulmonic valve murmurs

ERB'S POINT

S_2 split with inhalation
Aortic diastolic murmur
Pericardial friction rub

TRICUSPID AREA

S_1 split
Right ventricular S_3 and S_4
Tricuspid valve murmurs
Murmur of ventricular septal defect

MITRAL AREA

S_1 loud
Left ventricular S_3 and S_4
Mitral valve murmurs

REFERENCES

1. Braunwald E, editor: Heart disease: a textbook of cardiovascular medicine, ed 2, Philadelphia, 1984, WB Saunders Co.
2. Hurst J, editor-in-chief: The heart, arteries, and veins, ed 6, New York, 1986, McGraw-Hill Book Co.
3. Leonard JJ and others: Examination of the heart. Part four. Auscultation, Dallas, 1974, American Heart Association.
4. Maisel AS and others: The murmur of papillary muscle dysfunction in acute myocardial infarction: clinical features and prognostic implications, Am Heart J 112(4):705, 1986.
5. Malasanos L and others: Health assessment, St Louis, 1986, The CV Mosby Co.
6. Phipps WJ, Long BC, and Woods NF: Medical-surgical nursing: concepts and clinical practice, St Louis, 1987, The CV Mosby Co.
7. Reddy PS, Salerni R, and Shaver JA: Normal and abnormal heart sounds in cardiac diagnosis. Part II. Diastolic sounds, Curr Prob Cardiol 10(4):1, 1985.
8. Seidel HM and others: Mosby's guide to physical assessment, St Louis, 1987, The CV Mosby Co.
9. Shaver JA, Salerni R, and Reddy PS: Normal and abnormal heart sounds in cardiac diagnosis. Part I. Systolic sounds, Curr Prob Cardiol 10(3):1, 1985.
10. Thompson JM and others: Clinical nursing, ed 2, St Louis, 1989, The CV Mosby Co.

CHAPTER

13

Cardiovascular Laboratory Assessment and Diagnostic Procedures

CHAPTER OBJECTIVES

- *Describe the electrocardiographic changes that occur with hypokalemia and hyperkalemia.*
- *List important aspects of the normal chest radiograph with which the critical care nurse should be familiar.*
- *Describe proper placement of the electrodes for cardiac monitor leads II, MCL₁, and MCL₆ and for the 12-lead electrocardiograph.*
- *Explain the three methods for determining cardiac rate from an electrocardiogram.*
- *Explain the important electrocardiographic findings, assessment aspects, and nursing actions for each of the dysrhythmias described in the chapter.*
- *State the expected nursing actions for elevations in the central venous pressure and the pulmonary artery pressure and the pathologies responsible for these elevations.*

Information needed for assessment of the cardiovascular patient's status can be obtained through laboratory studies of blood serum. Accurate interpretation of these laboratory studies, along with the clinical picture, enables the critical care team to diagnose, treat, and assess the response to therapeutic interventions.

Laboratory studies of blood serum are performed to assess (1) other organ systems that reflect or secondarily affect cardiac status, (2) electrolyte levels that directly affect cardiac function, (3) enzyme levels that may reflect myocardial infarction, and (4) hematological status for determination of anemia or infection that may be a cause of cardiac disease or coagulation problems.

GENERAL CHEMISTRY STUDIES

The routine chemistry studies performed in most hospital laboratories when a patient is admitted give information about glucose metabolism, kidney function, liver function, and electrolyte concentrations. The presence of increased glucose during a fasting state (serum drawn 12 hours after ingestion of last food or drink) may indicate diabetes mellitus, which is believed to accelerate atherosclerosis. Renal failure, assessed by determining increased levels of urea nitrogen and creatinine, may cause electrolyte imbalances of potassium and calcium, which affect cardiac conduction and contractility. Abnormal liver function tests may alert the medical team to liver dysfunction caused by failure of the right side of the heart that is not clinically evident. Liver function indices seen on the chemistry report include alkaline phosphatase, bilirubin, aspartate aminotransferase (AST), and alanine aminotransferase (ALT). "Normal" laboratory values vary from institution to institution but should be readily available to the staff.

Potassium

During depolarization and repolarization of nerve and muscle fiber, potassium and sodium exchange occurs intracellularly and extracellularly. Thus both an excess or a deficiency of potassium can alter cardiac muscle function. Too much potassium (hyperkalemia) will decrease the rate of ventricular depolarization, shorten repolarization, and also depress atrioventricular (A-V) conduction. As the serum levels of potassium rise from the normal of 3.5 to 5.5 mEq/L, evidence of the above phenomena can be seen on the electrocardiogram (ECG) (Fig. 13-1). Tall, peaked T waves are usually, although not uniquely, associated with early hyperkalemia, followed by widening of the QRS complex and prolongation of the P wave and PR interval. If serum potassium levels rise above 10 to 14 mEq/L, depressed A-V conduction (Fig. 13-2) will lead to cardiac standstill or ventricular fibrillation. Coexisting low serum sodium, calcium, or pH levels potentiate the cardiac effects of hyperkalemia.

Low serum potassium (hypokalemia), commonly caused by gastrointestinal losses, diuretic therapy with insufficient replacement, and chronic steroid therapy, is also reflected by the ECG (Fig. 13-3). Myocardial conduction is impaired,

171

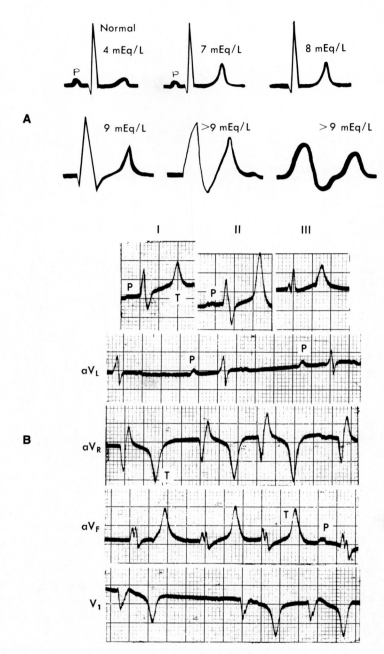

Fig. 13-1 Effects of hyperkalemia. **A,** The earliest electrocardiogram (ECG) change with hyperkalemia is peaking (tenting) of the T wave. With progressive increases in serum potassium, the QRS complexes widen, P waves disappear, and, finally, ventricular fibrillation develops. These changes do not necessarily occur with a specific serum potassium level. For example, some patients can have a normal ECG with a potassium level of 7 mEq/L, whereas other patients will have ventricular fibrillation at 9 mEq/L or less. **B,** Note the peaked T waves, widened QRS complexes, and prolonged PR intervals. Intermittently, a junctional rhythm is present with no P waves. (From Goldberger AL and Goldberger E: Clinical electrocardiography: a simplified approach, ed 3, St Louis, 1986, The CV Mosby Co.)

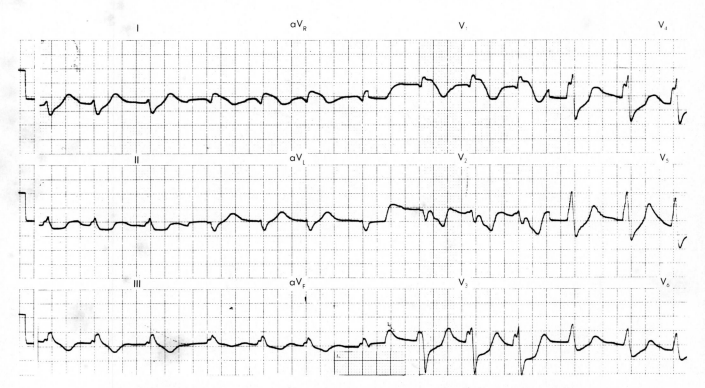

Fig. 13-2   Marked hyperkalemia. The potassium concentration is 8.5 mEq/L. Note the absence of P waves and the bizzare QRS complexes. (From Goldberger AL and Goldberger E: Clinical electrocardiography: a simplified approach, ed 3, St Louis, 1986, The CV Mosby Co.)

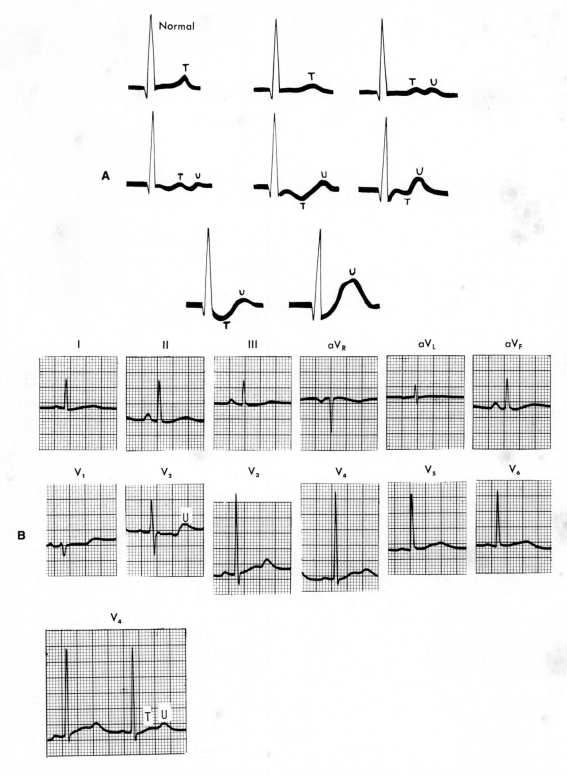

Fig. 13-3 Hypokalemia. **A,** Variable ECG patterns, ranging from slight T wave flattening to the appearance of prominent U waves, sometimes with ST segment depressions or T wave inversions, may be seen with hypokalemia. These patterns are not directly related to the specific level of serum potassium. **B,** Serum potassium level is 2.2 mEq/L. Notice the prominent U waves. (From Goldberger AL and Goldberger E: Clinical electrocardiography: a simplified approach, ed 3, St Louis, 1986, The CV Mosby Co.)

and ventricular repolarization is prolonged as evidenced by a prominent U wave. The U wave is not totally unique to hypokalemia, but its presence should alert the nurse to check the potassium serum level. Another ECG indicator of hypokalemia is the sudden occurrence of supraventricular and ventricular dysrhythmias. They result from the prolonged repolarization phase and can be evident in most patients with serum potassium levels below 2.6 mEq/L.[33] These rhythm disturbances are reversible with potassium replacement.

Calcium

Maintaining a normal serum calcium level is important because of its affect on myocardial contractility and cardiac excitability. The normal serum level ranges from 9 to 11 mg/dl. Increased amounts (hypercalcemia) strengthen contractility and shorten ventricular repolarization. The ECG demonstrates this shortened repolarization with a shortened QT interval. Low serum calcium (hypocalcemia) has the opposite effect on the myocardium. The ECG shows a prolonged QT interval. Below a level of 6 mg/dl, QT prolongation is common, proportional to the amount of hypocalcemia, and reversed with infusion of calcium.[25] Calcium levels are disrupted by tumors of the bone and lung, endocrine disorders, excessive intake or deficiency of vitamin D, intestinal malabsorption of calcium, kidney failure, and pancreatitis.

Cardiac Enzymes

Cardiac enzymes are proteins that are released from irreversibly damaged tissue cells. The enzymes released by damaged myocardial tissue include creatine phosphokinase (CPK), asparate aminotransferase (AST), and lactate dehydrogenase (LDH). Other organs, when damaged or necrotic, will emit these same enzymes. Therefore, when measured as a whole, the enzymes are not cardiac specific. Each enzyme, however, can be broken into its component parts, labeled isoenzymes, and the serum level of these cardiac-specific components will yield information of diagnostic value for cardiac disease. The typical sequence of appearance of each of the three enzymes and their isoenzymes is listed in Table 13-1.

Both CPK and LDH have isoenzymes that are cardiac specific. CPK has three isoenzymes composed of varying amounts of M (muscle) and B (brain) subunits. The brain and gastrointestinal tract contain high concentrations of CPK-BB; skeletal muscle and myocardium contain CPK-MM. Myocardial cells contain the CPK-MB isoenzyme that is only minimally found in any other tissue and appears in the serum only subsequent to myocardial cell death. CPK-MB is, at present, the most specific and sensitive serum index for diagnosing myocardial infarction in patients evaluated within 24 hours of onset of chest pain.[44] It can be used to estimate infarct size.[33] Serial samples should be drawn during admission and 12 and 24 hours after admission to help establish or rule out the diagnosis of myocardial infarction. The serum specimens must be kept on ice if more than 2 hours will elapse between the draw and assay time because time and heat will reduce the MB fraction.

LDH is composed of five isoenzymes (LDH_1, LDH_2, LDH_3, LDH_4, LDH_5), and myocardial cells contain a majority of LDH_1 and LDH_2. Normal serum levels of LDH contain varying amounts of all five isoenzymes, with LDH_2 the dominant fraction, followed by LDH_1, LDH_3, LDH_4, and LDH_5 in that order. When myocardial infarction occurs, both the LDH_1 and the LDH_2 levels rise, and the LDH_1:LDH_2 ratio becomes greater than 1 (normally it is less than 1). In other words, the normal situation wherein LDH_2 levels are greater than LDH_1 levels is reversed. LDH_1 greater than LDH_2 can be diagnostic, especially if the patient is initially seen more than 24 hours after onset of symptoms and the CPK-MB isoenzyme peak is missed. The LDH_1:LDH_2 ratio can flip back and forth, making it important to collect more than one specimen over time. False rises in LDH_1 can occur with hemolysis of red blood cells, so care must be taken in collecting the serum specimen.

Isoenzymes are also available for AST in the forms of myochondrial AST (m-AST) and cytosolic AST (c-AST), but their usefulness in clinical diagnosis or prognosis of myocardial infarction is undecided at present.[1,44] The fact that total and isoenzymatic (m-AST) levels of AST are higher in the presence of left-ventricular failure may make it very valuable in determining prognosis, in terms of mortality, after myocardial infarction.[1]

It cannot be overemphasized that all of these enzymes are found in multiple other tissues and are released by these tissues in times of stress or tissue damage.[25,33,43,58] Therefore a diagnosis of myocardial infarction can be determined only after assessing the ECG changes and clinical signs and symptoms, as well as the serum enzyme levels.

Table 13-1 Cardiac enzyme serum levels associated with myocardial infarction

Cardiac enzymes	Elevation (hours)	Peak (hours)	Duration (days)
Creatine phosphokinase (CPK)	4-8	12-24	3-4
Creatine phosphokinase-MB (CPK-MB)	4-8	12-20	2-3
Lactate dehydrogenase (LDH)	12-48	72-144	8-14
LDH_1:LDH_2 (normally ≤1)	12-14 (LDH_1:LDH_2 > 1)	72-144	14
Aspartate aminotransferase (AST)	6-12	18-48	3-4

HEMATOLOGICAL STUDIES

Hematological laboratory studies that are routinely ordered for the management of patients with altered cardiovascular status are red blood cell (RBC or erythrocyte) level, hemoglobin (Hb) level, hematocrit (Hct) level, erythrocyte sedimentation rate (ESR), white blood cell (WBC or leukocyte) level, and coagulation tests.

Red Blood Cells

The normal amount of RBCs varies with age, sex, environmental temperature, altitude, and exercise. Males produce 4.5 to 6 million RBCs per cubic millimeter, whereas the normal level for females is 4 to 5.5 million per cubic millimeter. The major function of RBCs is to carry hemoglobin (Hb), which transports and releases oxygen to the tissues of the body. Hb levels range from 14 to 18 g/dl in males and from 12 to 16 g/dl in females. Hematocrit (Hct) is the volume percentage of RBCs in whole blood—40% to 54% for males and 38% to 48% for females. When the serum level of total RBCs falls, it is logical also to see a fall in Hb and Hct. Anemia, a hematological disorder of insufficient amounts of RBCs (and concurrently, decreased Hb and Hct) can cause an increase in cardiac workload, cardiac dilation, and eventually cardiac failure. An increase in the amount of RBCs (polycythemia) also results in increased levels of Hb and Hct and often occurs as a response to tissue hypoxia.

The erythrocyte sedimentation rate (ESR) is a measurement of how quickly RBCs separate from plasma in 1 hour. With injury (for example, myocardial infarction), inflammation (for example, endocarditis), or pregnancy, RBCs have a higher content of globulin and fibrinogin levels, which cause faster precipitation and increase the sedimentation rate. Congestive heart failure can decrease the ESR because of associated decreased levels of serum fibrinogen.

White Blood Cells

Most inflammatory processes such as rheumatic fever, endocarditis, and myocardial infarction (producing necrotic tissue within the heart muscle) are reflected in an increased WBC level. The normal level of serum leukocytes for both sexes is 5000 to 10,000 per cubic millimeter.

BLOOD COAGULATION STUDIES

The coagulation studies usually ordered, prothrombin time (PT) and partial thromboplastin time (PTT), will determine serum clotting effectiveness. A patient who has stasis of blood (for example, with atrial fibrillation or prolonged bed rest) or who has a history of thrombosis is at risk for developing a thrombus. Heparin or oral anticoagulating drugs may be administered to prevent clot formation or extension of a clot, and coagulation studies will be ordered to guide dosage of these drugs. The therapeutic prolongation of clotting time for either one of these tests is approximately 2 times the normal.

CHEST RADIOGRAPHY
Basic Principles and Technique

Chest radiography is the oldest noninvasive method for visualizing images of the heart, yet it remains a frequently used and valuable diagnostic tool. Information about cardiac anatomy and physiology can be obtained with ease and safety at a relatively low cost. In the critical care unit, the nurse may be the first person to view the chest radiograph of an acutely ill patient. Nurses also have an important role in influencing the quality of the film through proper positioning and instruction of the patient. For these reasons, it is vital that critical care nurses gain a basic understanding of chest x-ray techniques and interpretation as it applies to the cardiovascular system.

Tissue densities. As x-rays travel through the chest from the emitting tube to the film plate, they are absorbed to a varying degree by the tissues through which they pass (Table 13-2). Very dense tissue such as bone will absorb almost all the x-rays, leaving the film unexposed, or white. The heart, aorta, pulmonary vessels, and the blood they contain are moderately dense structures, appearing as grey areas on the x-ray film. These vascular structures are surrounded by air-filled lung that allows the greatest penetration of x-rays, resulting in fully exposed (black) areas on the film.[7] Thoracic structures can be studied best by examining their borders. Two structures with the same density, when located next to each other, will have no visible border. If a structure is located next to a contrasting density (for example, vascular structures next to an air-filled lung), even subtle changes in size and shape can be seen.

Standard positions. Ideally, the chest radiograph is taken in the x-ray department with the patient in an upright position, the film exposed during a deep, sustained inhalation, and the x-ray tube aimed horizontally 6 feet from the film. This is a posterior-anterior (PA) film, since the beam traverses the patient from posterior to anterior. To understand why distance is important, place your hand between a light source (preferably a light bulb) and a piece of paper so that a shadow is cast. Try moving the light bulb closer, then farther away from your hand. As the light bulb is moved farther away, the shadow becomes smaller and sharper, with less distortion. In addition, the closer your hand is to the paper, the clearer the shadow becomes. In this illustration, the x-ray tube acts as the light bulb, providing the source of radiation. The film plate is the "paper" on which the shadow is cast.

Since most patients in critical care units are too ill to go to the x-ray department, chest radiographs are routinely obtained by using portable x-ray machines, with the patient either sitting upright or lying supine, depending on the patient's clinical condition and the judgment of the nurse. In both cases, the film plate is placed behind the patient's back

Table 13-2 X-ray densities of intrathoracic structures

Metal or bone (white)	Fluid (grey)	Air (black)
Ribs, clavicle, sternum, spine	Blood	Lung
Calcium deposits	Heart	
Surgical wires or clips	Veins	
Prosthetic valves	Arteries	
Pacemaker wires	Edema	

and an anterior-posterior (AP) projection is used, in which the x-ray beam enters from the front of the chest. In the supine film the x-ray tube can be only approximately 36 inches from the patient's chest because of ceiling height and x-ray equipment construction, resulting in an inferior quality film from a diagnostic standpoint, since the images of the heart and great vessels are somewhat magnified and not as sharply defined. Whenever possible, the upright (AP) film is preferred to the supine because it is quicker, it shows more of the lung since the diaphragm is lower, and the images are sharper and less magnified.

A deep, sustained inhalation is important. During exhalation, the lungs appear to cloud and the heart appears larger, possibly leading to an erroneous diagnosis of congestive heart failure. Alert patients will be encouraged by the radiology technician to take in a deep breath and hold it while the exposure is taken. With patients receiving mechanical ventilatory support, the exposure must be timed to coincide with maximal inhalation. Some patients will simply be unable to maintain a sustained inhalation on command, resulting in a distorted cardiac shadow and poor visualization of the lung fields. For this reason it is important to be able to compare and contrast serial chest films before determining that progress or deterioration has occurred.

Cardiac Radiographic Findings

Diagnosis from cardiac x-ray film is twofold; it involves observation of anatomical structures and observation of the pulmonary vascular bed to infer physiological data. Anatomical considerations center around elevation of the size and shape of cardiac chambers and great vessels, as well as valve calcifications, if present. Physiological observations are related to specific x-ray findings that suggest changes in pulmonary venous pressure, pulmonary artery pressure, or changes in pulmonary blood flow.

Enlargement of the heart and great vessels. There are four major factors that can cause enlargement of the heart and great vessels (Table 13-3). One is pressure overload, which results from obstruction of outflow and can be either a gradual or a sudden process.

Chronic systemic hypertension is an excellent clinical example of gradual pressure overload. The left ventricle tends to hypertrophy without significant dilation of the chamber. Ventricular wall thickness may increase two to

Table 13-3 Factors affecting enlargement of the heart and great vessels

Physiological factor	Clinical correlation
Pressure overload	
Gradual onset	Chronic hypertension
Sudden onset	Massive pulmonary emboli
Volume overload	Congestive heart failure
Abnormal tissue	
Cardiac muscle	Cardiomyopathies
Vascular wall	Aortic aneurysm
Poststenotic dilation	Pulmonic or aortic valve stenosis

three times its original mass at the expense of internal cavity volume rather than increase in external size. Since most of the enlargement is internal, the severity of the problem does not correlate well with x-ray findings of only mild ventricular enlargement. The chest radiograph fails to detect left-ventricular hypertrophy in hypertensive patients approximately 50% of the time,[15] although it is still useful in following serial changes. The atria can also experience hypertrophy because of gradual pressure overload, but because atrial wall are thin, dilation will occur as well, resulting in external enlargement and visualization on the x-ray film.

If the pressure overload is of sudden onset, there will not be time for hypertrophy to develop, and the result primarily will be chamber dilation. A clinical example of sudden pressure overload is massive pulmonary emboli; high pulmonary pressures that result from obstruction (emboli) of pulmonary blood flow will cause marked right-ventricular dilation, which can be seen on x-ray film.

A second factor resulting in heart and great vessel enlargement is volume overload, which results in dilation of all structures involved, usually without hypertrophy. The most common clinical example is congestive heart failure. The severity of the volume overload usually correlates well with the severity of chamber enlargement as seen on the chest radiograph.

An abnormal cardiac muscle or vascular wall can also be responsible for cardiac enlargement seen on chest x-ray film. Cardiomyopathies are examples of abnormal cardiac muscle. Hypertrophic cardiomyopathy involves extreme wall thickening with little or no dilation and only mild external enlargement. Congestive cardiomyopathy, on the other hand, results in moderate-to-severe dilation, often with a very thin muscle wall and marked cardiac enlargement on x-ray film. A thoracic aortic aneurysm is an example of a vascular wall abnormality that results in enlargement of the aorta.

Poststenotic dilation applies only to arteries. It occurs because of turbulent flow distal to an obstruction. Clinical examples include pulmonic valve stenosis, resulting in dilation of the trunk of the pulmonary artery, and aortic valve stenosis, resulting in dilation of the middle ascending aorta.

Assessment of chamber enlargement. Two basic principles apply to the assessment of cardiac enlargement through chest x-ray film: (1) in general, each chamber enlarges in a direction away from the remainder of the heart, and (2) if a particular chamber enlarges enough to come into contact with a rigid structure such as the spine or sternum, further enlargement will cause displacement and rotation of the entire heart.

Cardiothoracic ratio. Estimation of the cardiothoracic ratio (often abbreviated CT ratio) is a technique used to measure overall heart size, with some limitations (Fig. 13-4). It is done with a frontal view (AP or PA). The maximal cardiac diameter is measured and compared against the maximal thoracic diameter measured to the inner border of the ribs. The CT ratio is considered abnormal if the cardiac diameter is greater than 50% of the total thoracic diameter.[7] It is most sensitive in detecting left-ventricular enlargement, since the left ventricle enlarges toward the left chest wall. It is best to compare serial films, using the CT ratio to

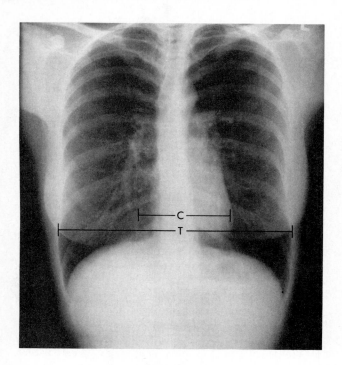

Fig. 13-4 Cardiothoracic (CT) ratio, a technique for estimating heart size on a PA chest film. Normally the cardiac diameter is 50% or less of the thoracic diameter when measured during full inhalation. *C*, Maximal cardiac diameter, *T*, maximal thoracic diameter measured to the inside of the ribs.

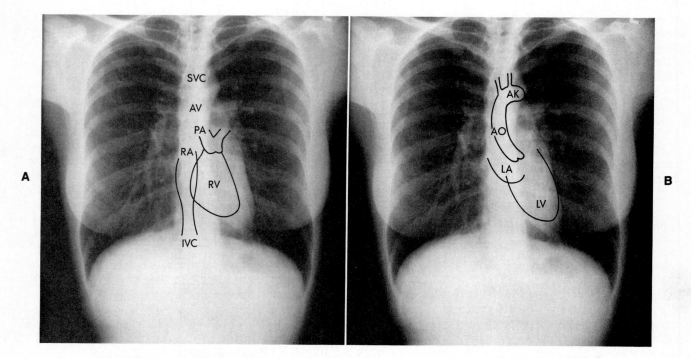

Fig. 13-5 Location of cardiac structures on a PA chest film. *AV*, Azygos vein, *SVC*, superior vena cava, *PA*, pulmonary artery, *RA*, right atrium, *RV*, right ventricle, *IVC*, inferior vena cava, *AO*, aorta, *AK*, aortic knob, *LA*, left atrium, *LV*, left ventricle.

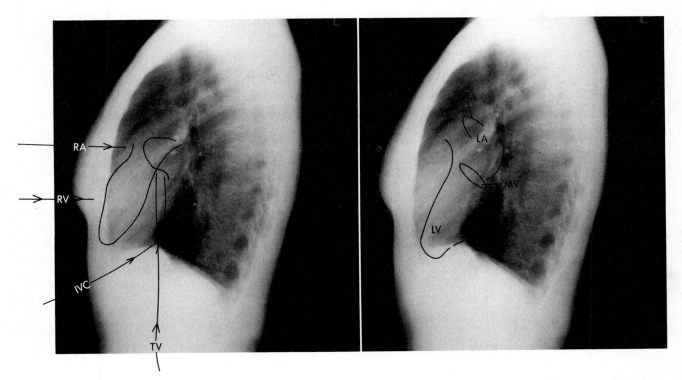

Fig. 13-6 Location of cardiac structures on a lateral chest film. *RV*, Right ventricle, *RA*, right atrium, *IVC*, inferior vena cava, *TV*, tricuspid valve, *LV*, left ventricle, *MV*, mitral valve, *LA*, left atrium, *LAA*, left-atrial appendage.

follow the progression of enlargement. One of the limitations of the CT ratio is that it may remain within normal limits in the presence of mild-to-moderate right-ventricular or left-atrial enlargement. The right ventricle initially enlarges anteriorly toward the sternum, and the left atrium initially enlarges posteriorly toward the spine, and neither enlargement could be visualized in a frontal view of the chest. In 70% of cases, heart size can be correctly determined from the chest film, either by evidence of specific chamber enlargement or by the CT ratio.[14]

In the frontal view of the chest, the right atrium composes the border of the right side of the heart, and the left ventricle represents the border of the left side (Fig. 13-5). Enlargement of either of these chambers could be seen and localized from this view. In the lateral view of the chest (Fig. 13-6), the anterior border of the heart is formed by the right ventricle, which normally does not touch the sternum. Contact with the sternum would indicate right-ventricular enlargement. The upper posterior border of the heart is formed by the left atrium, but it is poorly visible on x-ray film because of relatively little contact with lung tissue. The lower, more visible portion of the posterior border is composed of the left ventricle.

Use of the chest radiograph to determine specific chamber enlargement is not as accurate as the estimation of overall heart size.[40] The superior vena cava forms the upper right border of the mediastinum on the frontal view. Since only the right border is defined (the left border blends in with the opacity of the rest of the mediastinal structures), the size of the superior vena cava cannot be measured accurately by chest x-ray film. The inferior vena cava is seen best in the lateral view. The posterior border is visible from where it leaves the diaphragm to where it enters the pericardial sac. The thoracic aorta lies within the mediastinum and is not clearly visible on either PA or lateral films if normal. When enlarged, the thoracic aorta rises out of the mediastinum and into contact with lung tissue, making it easier to visualize.

Pericardial effusions can sometimes be visible on a chest radiograph. A pericardial effusion will cause the entire outline of the heart to enlarge symmetrically. Occasionally, the separation of layers of epicardial fat from layers of extrapericardial fat by fluid can be seen on a lateral view just anterior to the right ventricle. Normally, this separation should be no greater than 2 mm; if it is greater, a pericardial effusion exists.[22] However, other noninvasive procedures such as echocardiography are much more specific in diagnosing and quantifying pericardial effusions.

Interpretation of Pulmonary Vascular Patterns

Under normal conditions the pulmonary arteries and veins are sharply defined, with a gradual decrease in blood vessel diameter from the center of the lungs to the periphery.

Pulmonary artery hypertension exists when pulmonary artery pressures are elevated because of obstruction at the pulmonary arteriolar level. This condition is seen clinically in patients who have chronic obstructive pulmonary disease and in those who have had multiple pulmonary emboli. The major vascular change visible on chest radiograph is dilation of the main pulmonary artery and its central hilar branches. The degree of dilation of the pulmonary arteries seen on x-ray film correlates closely with the degree and duration of pressure elevation; in addition, peripheral vessels may appear decreased in size, and, if chronic, tortuosity of lobar and segmental arterial branches occurs.

Pulmonary venous hypertension actually represents high pressures throughout the pulmonary circulation, beginning in the left atrium, being transmitted backward across the pulmonary veins, pulmonary capillaries, and pulmonary arteries, and resulting in right-ventricular systolic hypertension. This entire sequence is caused by increased resistance to flow in the left side of the heart, either at the level of the mitral valve, as in mitral stenosis, or secondary to left-ventricular failure.

Pulmonary venous pressure can be measured directly by a balloon-tipped pulmonary artery catheter wedged in the pulmonary capillary bed. As pulmonary venous congestion develops, pulmonary artery wedge pressure (PAWP) can be estimated from the venous markings on the chest x-ray film (Table 13-4).[46] Normal PAWP is 5 to 10 mm Hg. As the PAWP rises to 10 to 15 mm Hg, venous blood flow is redistributed so that upper and lower lung fields are perfused equally. Blood vessels in the apex of the lung, which were previously collapsed, now open as pressure within the vascular bed exceeds alveolar pressure.

With a further rise in PAWP to 15 to 20 mm Hg, upper lung fields are actually better perfused than lower lung fields. On the chest x-ray film pulmonary arteries and veins in dependent parts of the lung become smaller because of several factors, including pressure-mediated vasospasm, but perivascular edema plays the major role.[18] When venous pressure, which is highest in the lower lobes of the lung because of gravity, exceeds plasma oncotic pressure (normally 20 to 25 mm Hg), fluid leaves the vascular bed and enters the interstitial space, causing edema. The edema surrounds and compresses arterioles and capillaries, increasing resistance to flow and decreasing size.

At PAWP of 25 to 35 mm Hg, edema of the interlobular

septa occurs and can be seen on chest x-ray film. Known as *Kerley-B lines,* these fine, straight, linear shadows occur at right angles to the pleura and are approximately 1 to 2 cm long. They first appear in the dependent basilar area of the lung. The main pulmonary artery and hilar branches increase in size because of the elevation of pressure. As edema increases, clear definition of the hilar branches is lost, and there is a faint, ill-defined increase in density around the hilum known as perihilar haze. Finally, as the PAWP exceeds 35 mm Hg, frank pulmonary edema ensues. The chest radiograph demonstrates these fluid-filled alveoli as diffuse infiltrates in the perihilar region.

The chest radiograph often continues to show evidence of pulmonary edema even after treatment has been initiated and pulmonary artery pressures have returned to normal. A recent study[56] found that radiographic evidence of pulmonary edema correlated very closely with extravascular lung water, measured by an indicator-dilution method. This extravascular water takes time to return to the vascular bed where it is and be removed, which probably accounts for the time lag seen between the return of the PA pressures to normal and the clearing on the x-ray film. X-ray findings and extravascular lung water usually return to normal within 2 days if the onset was acute or within 5 days if it was caused by an exacerbation of chronic heart failure.

Sometimes, coexisting conditions such as pneumonia or atelectasis render the chest radiograph less helpful in determining the extent of pulmonary edema. A different study[20] found that, although the chest x-ray film was useful in determining the presence of overt pulmonary edema, it was not as accurate ($r = 0.1$; $p > 0.05$) in detecting modest changes in the amount of extravascular lung water in critically ill patients with coexisting lung disease when using films obtained by portable machines with the patient supine. The limitations built into this study by including patients with coexisting lung disease and using portable-machine films from the supine position naturally lead to difficulties in assessing pulmonary edema. Unfortunately, that is often the reality of clinical practice.

ELECTROCARDIOGRAPHY

Electrocardiography is a very complex subject, about which much literature has been written and to which entire books have been devoted—and justifiably so. A detailed evaluation of a 12-lead electrocardiogram (ECG) can provide a wealth of cardiac diagnostic information and often provides the basis on which other definitive diagnostic tests are selected. This section provides a general understanding of dysrhythmias commonly encountered in clinical practice and a sound basis for understanding the value of the many clinical applications of electrocardiography.

Basic Principles

The ECG records electrical changes in heart muscle. It does not record mechanical contraction, which usually immediately follows electrical depolarization. However, a condition known as electromechanical dissociation occasionally occurs in which the heart is mechanically at a standstill while rhythmic electrical impulses

Table 13-4 Chest x-ray estimation of PAWP

Pulmonary artery wedge pressure (mm Hg)	Chest x-ray findings
5-10	Normal
10-15	Equal perfusion of upper and lower lung fields
15-20	Upper lung perfusion > lower lung perfusion
20-25	Interstitial edema in lower lobes
25-35	Kerley-B lines; increased size of main pulmonary artery and hilar branches; perihilar haze
>35	Diffuse perihilar infiltrates

continue to be generated and then recorded on the ECG.

A review of the cardiac action potential illustrates electrical changes that occur (see Fig. 11-23, *A*). During phase 0 *(depolarization)*, the electrical potential changes very rapidly from a baseline of -90 mV to $+20$ mV. Since this is a significant electrical change, it appears on the ECG. Phase 1 and 2 represent an electrical plateau, during which time excitation-contraction coupling occurs. Since there is no significant electrical change at this time, nothing shows on the ECG. During phase 3 *(repolarization)*, the electrical potential again changes, this time a little more slowly, from 0 mV back to -90 mV. This is another major electrical event, and it is reflected on the ECG. Phase 4 represents a resting period, during which chemical balance is restored by the sodium pump, but since positively charged ions are exchanged on a one-for-one basis, there is no electrical activity, and no visible change occurs on the ECG tracing.

Electrocardiographic leads. All electrocardiographs use a system of one or more *leads*. A lead consists of three electrodes, a positive electrode, a negative electrode and a ground electrode. The function of the ground electrode is to prevent the display of background electrical interference on the ECG tracing. Leads do not transmit any electricity to the patient, they just sense and record it.

The positive electrode on the skin acts as a camera. If the wave of depolarization travels toward the positive electrode, an upward stroke, or *positive deflection*, is written on the ECG paper (Fig. 13-7, *A*). If the wave of depolarization travels away from the positive electrode, a downward line, or *negative deflection*, will be recorded on the ECG (Fig. 13-7, *B*). A biphasic complex occurs when depolarization moves perpendicular to the positive electrode (Fig. 13-7, *C*). The size of the muscle mass also has an effect, with the larger muscle mass having a greater influence on the tracing.

The wave of ventricular depolarization in the healthy heart travels from right to left and head to toe. The appearance of the waveforms on the ECG will vary, depending on the location of the positive electrode. The standard 12-lead ECG provides a picture of electrical activity in the heart from the 12 different positions of the positive electrodes.

A 12-lead ECG consists of six standard limb leads and six chest leads (Fig. 13-8, *A*, *B*, and *C*). The limb leads are obtained by placing electrodes on all four extremities. The exact location on the extremities does not matter, as long as skin contact is good and bone is avoided. The ma-

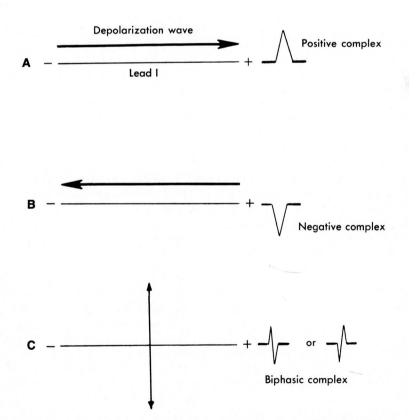

Fig. 13-7 Three basic laws of electrocardiography. **A,** Flow of depolarization toward the positive electrode results in a positive deflection on the ECG. **B,** Flow of depolarization away from the positive electrode results in a negative deflection on the ECG. **C,** Flow of depolarization perpendicular to the positive electrode results in a biphasic deflection on the ECG. These three basic laws apply to both the P wave and the QRS complex. (From Goldberger AL and Goldberger E: Clinical electrocardiography: a simplified approach, ed 3, St Louis, 1986, The CV Mosby Co.)

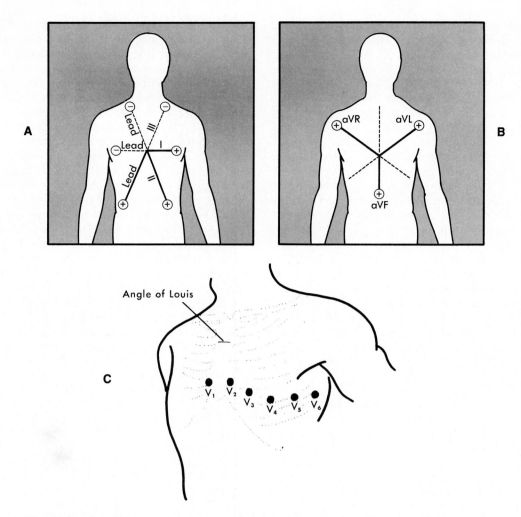

Fig. 13-8 **A,** Limb leads I, II, and III. Leads are actually located on the extremities. Illustrated are the angles from which these leads view the heart. **B,** Lead placement for augmented limb leads aVR, aVL, and aVF. These are unipolar leads that use the calculated center of the heart as their negative electrode. **C,** Lead placement for the chest electrodes: V_1, fourth intercostal space at the right sternal border; V_2, fourth intercostal space at the left sternal border; V_3, equidistant between V_2 and V_4; V_4, fifth intercostal space at the left midclavicular line; V_5, anterior axillary line and same horizontal level as V_4; V_6, midaxillary line and same horizontal level as V_4. (**C** from Goldberger AL and Goldberger E: Clinical electrocardiography: a simplified approach, ed 3, St Louis, 1986, The CV Mosby Co.)

chine will interpret all extremity signals as coming from the connection of the extremity to the torso, that is, the shoulder or groin.

Leads I, II, and III are bipolar limb leads in that they consist of a positive and a negative electrode. The other three limb leads are labeled aVR, aVL, and aVF, representing augmented vector right, left, and foot. These unipolar leads consist only of a positive electrode, with the negative electrode calculated within the machine at roughly the center of the heart. Under these circumstances the ECG tracing would ordinarily be very small, so the machine enhances, or *augments*, it. The term *vector* refers to directional force.

The precordial chest leads are labeled "V" leads and are distributed in an arch around the left chest. They are useful for viewing electrical forces traveling from right to left or front to back but are not helpful in evaluating vertical forces in the heart. For an accurate interpretation, all 12 leads must be taken into consideration.

Baseline distortion. It is important that the tracing have a flat baseline, which is that portion of the tracing that is between the various waveforms. Two forms of artifact can distort the baseline: 60-cycle interference and muscular movement. Sixty-cycle interference (Fig. 13-9, *A*) results from leakage of electrical current somewhere within the system and appears as a generalized thickening of the baseline. It can usually be resolved by ensuring that all electrical equipment at the bedside is well grounded. Occasionally, it may be necessary to unplug one piece of equipment at a time until the offending device is found. Muscular move-

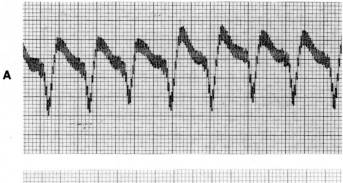

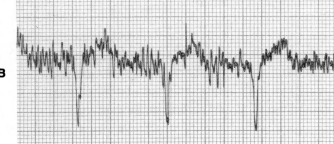

Fig. 13-9 **A,** Artifact—60-cycle interference. **B,** Artifact—muscular movement.

ment (Fig. 13-9, *B*) is displayed as a coarse, erratic disturbance of the baseline. In most cases, asking the patient to lie quietly while the ECG is being run is sufficient. If movement is caused by shivering or seizure activity, it is best to wait until the activity subsides before obtaining the 12-lead ECG. If tremor is caused by Parkinson's disease or other neuromuscular disorders, a resolution may not be possible. It should be remembered that the artifact will have an adverse effect on the accurate interpretation of the tracing.

Twelve-Lead ECG Analysis

Specialized ECG paper. ECG paper records the speed and magnitude of electrical impulses on a grid composed of small and large boxes (Fig. 13-10). There are five small boxes in every large box. At a standard paper speed of 25 mm/second, one small box (1 mm) is equivalent to 0.04 second, and one large box (5 mm) represents 0.20 second. Distances along the horizontal axis represent speed and are stated in seconds rather than in millimeters or number of boxes. The vertical axis represents magnitude or strength of force. At standard calibration, one small box equals 0.1 mV, and one large box equals 0.5 mV. It is important to look for the standardization mark, which is usually located at the beginning of the tracing (Fig. 13-11, *A*). The mark indicates 1 mV and at standard calibration should go up two large boxes. Twelve-lead ECGs are sometimes run at different calibrations. If, at standard calibration, some complexes are so tall they run off the paper, the tracing should be repeated at half standard (Fig. 13-11, *B*), and the calibration mark will only rise one large box. If all of the complexes on a standard tracing are very small, it may be repeated at double standard, with the calibration mark going

up four large boxes (Fig. 13-11, *C*). In any case, the calibration must be clearly marked on the tracing, since some diagnostic conclusions are based on the magnitude of specific portions of the ECG complex.

Waveforms. The meaning and duration of waveforms and intervals follow (Fig. 13-12). The P wave represents atrial depolarization. The QRS complex respresents ventricular depolarization, corresponding to phase 0 of the ventricular action potential. It is referred to as a complex because it can actually consist of several different waves, depending on the placement of the positive electrode and the direction of the spread of electrical activity in the heart. Basically, the letter Q is used to describe an *initial* negative deflection; in other words, only if the first deflection from the baseline is negative will it be labeled a Q wave. The letter R applies to any positive deflection. If there are two positive deflections in one QRS complex, the second is labeled R′ (read "R prime") and is commonly seen in lead V₁ in right bundle branch block. The letter S refers to any subsequent negative deflections. Any combination of these deflections can occur and is collectively called the QRS complex (Fig. 13-13). The QRS duration is normally 0.10 second (2½ small boxes) or less.

The T wave represents ventricular repolarization, corresponding to phase 3 of the ventricular action potential. The onset of the QRS to approximately the midpoint or peak of the T wave represents an absolute refractory period, during which the heart muscle cannot respond to another stimulus no matter how strong that stimulus might be (Fig. 13-14). From the midpoint of the T wave to the end of the T wave, the heart muscle is in the relative refractory period. The heart muscle has not yet fully recovered, but it could be depolarized again if a strong enough stimulus were received. This can be a particularly dangerous time for ectopy to occur.

Intervals between waveforms. Intervals between waveforms are also evaluated (Fig. 13-15). The PR interval is measured from the beginning of the P wave to the beginning of the QRS complex. Normally, the PR interval is 0.12 to 0.20 second in length and represents the time between sinus node discharge and the beginning of ventricular depolarization. Since most of this time period results from delay of the impulse in the A-V node, the PR interval is an indicator of A-V nodal function.

The portion of the wave that extends from the end of the QRS to the beginning of the T wave is labeled the ST segment. Its duration is not measured. Instead, its shape and location are evaluated. The ST segment should be flat and at the same level as the isoelectric baseline. Elevation or depression is expressed in millimeters and may indicate ischemia. The QT interval is measured from the beginning of the QRS complex to the end of the T wave and indicates the total time interval from the onset of depolarization to the completion of repolarization. At normal heart rates, the QT interval should be less than half of the RR interval (measured from one QRS complex to the next). However, the normal value of a QT interval is very dependent on heart rate. The most accurate method for evaluating a QT interval is to look up its normal value at the specific heart rate on a chart. Table 13-5 is an abridged form of such a chart,

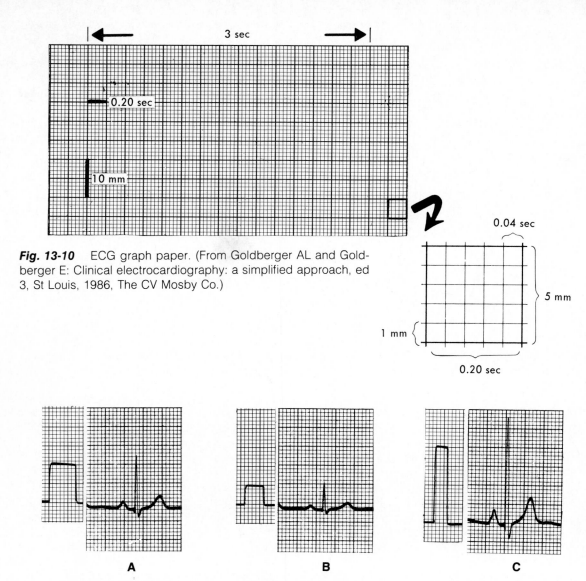

Fig. 13-10 ECG graph paper. (From Goldberger AL and Goldberger E: Clinical electrocardiography: a simplified approach, ed 3, St Louis, 1986, The CV Mosby Co.)

A   B   C

Fig. 13-11 **A,** Standardization mark. Before beginning the ECG, the machine must be calibrated so that the standardization mark is 10 mm tall. ECG can also be set at half standardization, **B,** or at twice normal standardization, **C**. (From Goldberger AL and Goldberger E: Clinical electrocardiography: a simplified approach, ed 3, St Louis, 1986, The CV Mosby Co.)

Fig. 13-12 Normal ECG waveforms. P wave represents atrial depolarization, QRS represents ventricular depolarization, and T wave represents ventricular repolarization. (From Conover MB: Understanding electrocardiography: arrhythmias and the 12-lead ECG, ed 5, St Louis, 1988, The CV Mosby Co.)

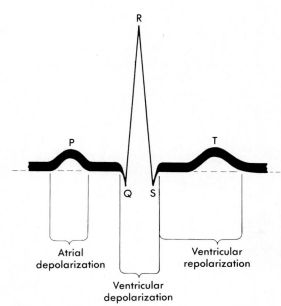

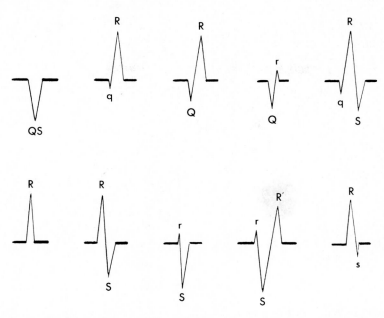

Fig. 13-13 Examples of various QRS complexes. Note that small deflections are represented with lowercase letters and large deflections are labeled with uppercase letters. (From Goldberger AL and Goldberger E: Clinical electrocardiography: a simplified approach, ed 3, St Louis, 1986, The CV Mosby Co.)

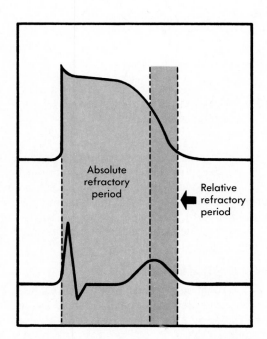

Fig. 13-14 Absolute and relative refractory periods correlated with the cardiac muscle's action potential and with an ECG tracing.

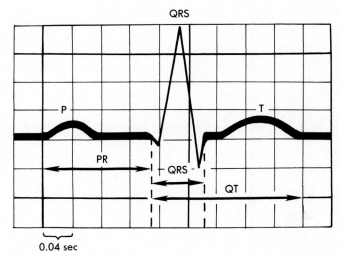

Fig. 13-15 ECG intervals. The PR interval corresponds to the spread of depolarization through the atria and the subsequent delay in the A-V node. The ST segment corresponds to phase 2 of the action potential, during which time the heart muscle is completely depolarized and contraction normally occurs. The QT interval is measured form the beginning of the QRS complex to the end of the T wave and represents the time from initial depolarization of the ventricles to the end of repolarization. (From Conover MB: Understanding electrocardiography: arrhythmias and the 12-lead ECG, ed 5, St Louis, 1988, The CV Mosby Co.)

Table 13-5   QT interval. Upper limits of normal

Measured RR Interval (sec)	Heart Rate (per min)	QT Interval Upper Normal Limits (sec)
1.50	40	0.50
1.20	50	0.45
1.00	60	0.42
0.86	70	0.40
0.80	75	0.38
0.75	80	0.37
0.67	90	0.35
0.60	100	0.34
0.50	120	0.31
0.40	150	0.25

From Goldberger AL and Goldberger E: Clinical electrocardiography: a simplified approach, ed 3, St. Louis, 1986, The CV Mosby Co.

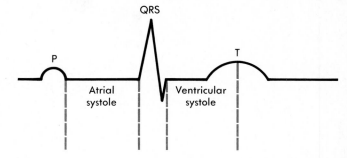

Fig. 13-16   Correlation of the ECG with the events of the cardiac cycle. Atrial systole immediately follows atrial depolarization, and ventricular systole immediately follows ventricular depolarization.

provided to illustrate the wide variability of the normal QT interval. The QT interval is also affected by drugs, most notably quinidine.

Although the ECG only records electrical events, it is helpful to understand the correlation of these intervals to the physiological events of the cardiac cycle. Immediately after the P wave and during the PR interval, atrial systole occurs. Similarly, ventricular systole begins immediately after the QRS complex and continues until approximately the midpoint of the T wave (Fig. 13-16).

Ventricular axis. Electrical impulses spread through cardiac muscle tissue in many directions at once when the ventricular muscle is depolarized. All of these individual forces can be averaged to describe the overall direction that current is traveling, which is called the *mean vector*. The mean vector can be plotted on a circular graph known as the hexaxial reference system (Fig. 13-17), and a degree can be assigned to it. This degree represents the ventricular axis.

Normal range for ventricular axis varies slightly, but it is approximately −30 to +110 degrees. Right axis deviation is present if the axis falls between +110 degrees and +180 degrees. Left axis deviation is present if the axis falls between −30 and −90 degrees. If the axis plots in the upper left portion of the circle, it is called an indeterminate axis and can happen only if the wave of depolarization starts in the bottom of the ventricle and spreads upward toward the atria. Clinically, this can be seen in beats of ventricular origin such as premature ventricular contractions (PVCs) and some pacemaker-initiated beats. To determine the frontal plane ventricular axis, the six limb leads are examined to find the lead with the smallest QRS complex or the most equiphasic (equal portions above and below the baseline) one if no complex is clearly the smallest. In Figure 13-18, lead aVF is the smallest. Next, using the hexaxial reference system (see Fig. 13-17), the lead is found that is perpendicular to the one that had the smallest complex. For example, perpendicular to lead aVF is lead I, so the mean vector lies parallel with lead I. The third step is to determine if the QRS complex is positive or negative in the lead of the mean vector (in this case, I). If the QRS is positive, the

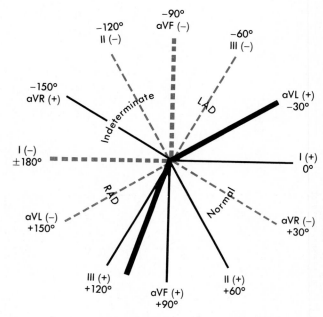

Fig. 13-17   Hexaxial reference system. *RAD,* Right axis deviation, *LAD,* left axis deviation.

mean vector is pointing toward the positive electrode. If the QRS is negative, the mean vector is pointing away from the positive electrode. In Figure 13-18, the QRS is positive. The positive pole of lead I is at the right midpoint of the hexaxial reference system and corresponds to a numerical degree of zero, which is normal. These steps are reviewed in the box on p. 187.

Cardiac Monitor Lead Analysis

During continuous cardiac monitoring, adhesive pregelled electrodes are used to obtain an ECG tracing that is similar to one lead of a 12-lead ECG. At a minimum, this requires three electrodes: one positive, one negative, and one ground. In some clinical areas, five electrodes are used, either to monitor two leads simultaneously or to allow selection of several different leads at any time through a lead selector switch on the monitor. Three leads, II, MCL$_1$, and MCL$_6$, are commonly used for continuous monitoring, although others may also be used.

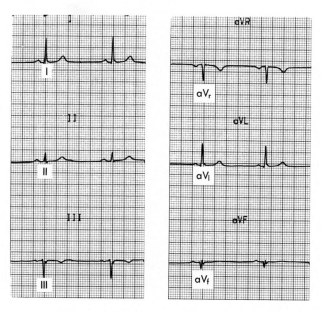

Fig. 13-18 Limb leads of normal ECG illustrating normal axis of 0 degrees.

STEPS IN DETERMINING AXIS

1. Find the most isoelectric limb lead.
2. Using the hexaxial reference system, find the lead that is perpendicular to the one identified in step 1.
3. Determine whether the QRS is positive or negative in the perpendicular lead.
4. Look at the corresponding positive or negative pole of the perpendicular lead on the hexaxial reference system.
5. The degree listed on the hexaxial reference system is the axis.

Lead II. On a standard 12-lead ECG, lead II is formed by a positive electrode attached to the left leg, a negative electrode attached to the right arm, and a ground electrode on the right leg. It is not practical to connect electrodes to the arms and legs during continuous monitoring, but the general placement remains the same. The positive electrode is placed on the lower left torso, the negative electrode is placed on the right shoulder, and the ground electrode is usually placed on the left shoulder (Fig. 13-19). The location of the ground is not significant. In most patients, this lead displays in a waveform that is predominantly upright (Fig. 13-20). For this reason, it has been a popular monitoring lead. P waves are usually easy to identify in lead II. However, it is difficult to identify right bundle branch block (RBBB) and left bundle branch block (LBBB) in this lead,

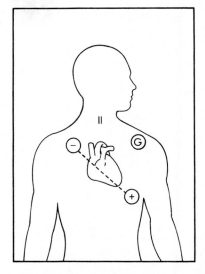

Fig. 13-19 Electrode placement for monitoring lead II.

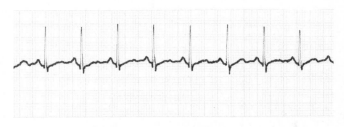

Fig. 13-20 Typical ECG tracing in lead II.

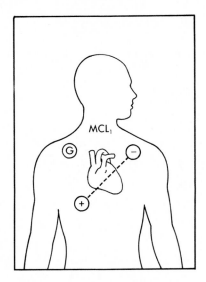

Fig. 13-21 Electrode placement for monitoring in lead MCL₁.

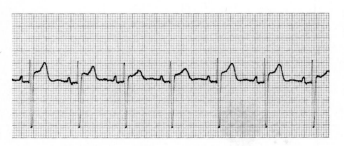

Fig. 13-22 Typical ECG tracing in lead MCL₁.

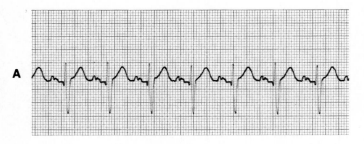

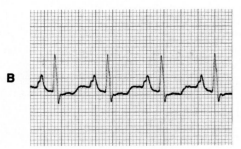

Fig. 13-23 Atrial hypertrophy. **A,** In left-atrial hypertrophy the P wave is broad and notched and is sometimes called P-mitrale since it is often associated with mitral valve disease. **B,** In right-atrial hypertrophy the P wave is tall and peaked and is sometimes called P-pulmonale since it is often associated with pulmonary disease.

since this is a vertical lead and does not clearly display changes in horizontal conduction.

Lead MCL₁. Identification of an RBBB pattern is important in continuous cardiac monitoring, not only for diagnosing a new conduction defect, but also for verifying placement of a pacemaker wire, differentiating between ventricular tachycardia and supraventricular tachycardia with aberrant conduction, and determining whether PVCs are originating in the right or left ventricle. Lead MCL₁ meets this need.

"MCL₁" stands for "modified chest lead one." It is equivalent to a V₁ lead on a 12-lead ECG. The tracings are similar but not identical. In both, the positive electrode is at the fourth intercostal space just to the right of the sternum. With V₁ the ECG machine calculates the negative electrode at the center of the heart, whereas with MCL₁ the negative electrode is located just below the left shoulder. With MCL₁ the ground electrode is usually placed on the right shoulder (Fig. 13-21). Since the positive electrode is to the right of the heart and most of the electrical activity in the heart is directed toward the left ventricle, the QRS complex in lead MCL₁ will normally be negative (Fig. 13-22). Any abnormal activity directed toward the right ventricle such as in RBBB will result in an upright QRS complex, often in an RSR′ pattern.

Lead MCL₆. An alternative to lead MCL₁ is lead MCL₆. This is a modified V₆, with the positive electrode located in the V₆ position (left fifth intercostal space, midaxillary line). The negative electrode is placed below the left shoulder, and the ground can be placed below the right shoulder. Lead MCL₆ is also an adequate lead for monitoring interventricular conduction changes.

Hypertrophy

Cardiac chamber enlargement can be suspected or diagnosed using the 12-lead ECG because muscle size will influence the ECG tracing. Atrial hypertrophy is identified by the size and shape of the P waves and is usually seen best in lead II. Wide m-shaped P waves are seen in left-atrial hypertrophy and are called *P-mitrale,* since left atrial hypertrophy is often caused by mitral stenosis (Fig. 13-23, *A*). Tall, peaked P waves occur in right-atrial hypertrophy and are referred to as *P-pulmonale,* since this condition is often the result of chronic pulmonary disease (Fig. 13-23, *B*.

Ventricular hypertrophy is basically an increase in the size and muscle mass of one or both ventricles. Since a larger muscle is being depolarized, a greater amount of electrical activity is recorded on the ECG during depolarization. In ventricular hypertrophy, specific changes occur in the QRS complex.[41] Upright QRS complexes become taller, and negative QRS complexes become even more negative. Often the QRS becomes slightly wider, since it takes longer to depolarize a larger muscle. The QRS axis often shifts toward the enlarged ventricle, since a greater portion of the total electrical activity of the heart occurs there.

Because normal heart size varies from one individual to the next, certain criteria have been developed to evaluate ventricular hypertrophy (Table 13-6). Note that there are separate criteria for right-ventricular hypertrophy and left-ventricular hypertrophy.

Table 13-6   Criteria for evaluating ventricular hypertrophy

Left ventricle	Right ventricle

Presence of any one of the following:
  S wave in V_1, + R wave in V_5 or V_6 >35 mm
  Left-atrial abnormality (broad, notched P waves)
  Intrinsic deflection (initial R or Q wave) in lead V_5 or V_6 ≥0.05 sec in duration
Note: sensitivity 57%-66%; specificity 85%-93%
	Presence of any one of the following:
	  R:S ratio in lead V_5 or V_6 ≤1
	  S wave in V_5 or V_6 ≥7 mm
	Right axis deviation > +90 degrees
	P pulmonale
	Note: sensitivity 18%-43%; specificity 83%-95%

Ischemia and Infarction

Ischemia occurs when the delivery of oxygen to the tissues is insufficient to meet metabolic demand. Cardiac ischemia can be the result of a sudden decrease in supply such as when coronary artery spasm occurs or can be the result of a sudden increase in demand such as exercise. Ischemia is by nature a transient process. Either the balance of supply and demand is restored and the muscle tissue recovers or the imbalance becomes so great that the tissue can no longer survive and it becomes necrotic. Many nursing and medical interventions are directed toward saving as much ischemic tissue as possible. Infarction refers to the actual death and disintegration of muscle cells and their eventual replacement by scar tissue. Once infarction has occurred, that process cannot be reversed.

Both ischemia and infarction cause changes in the way cardiac muscle cells respond to electrical stimuli, and these changes can usually be seen in a 12-lead ECG tracing. Ischemic changes can sometimes be seen on a single monitored lead, but they are not diagnostic. If a change is noted in a monitored lead and ischemia is suspected, a 12-lead ECG must be obtained to verify the presence and location of the ischemia.

The ECG changes that result from myocardial ischemia involve transient ST segment and T wave abnormalities. In general, if the positive electrode lies directly over the ischemic area, ST segment elevation will be seen and will indicate a localized total reduction of blood flow and transmural ischemia. If the reduction of blood flow is more diffuse and some normal muscle tissue remains between the ischemic area and the positive electrode, ST segment depression will be recorded.[55] When ischemia is not complete, it is most likely because of the involvement of the subendocardial muscle layer. In subendocardial ischemia, the ischemic area is closest to the inner cavity wall of the heart, and there is a layer of normal muscle tissue left surrounding it (Fig. 13-24). ST segment depression would result, since the positive electrode is separated from the ischemic area by normal tissue. T waves most commonly flatten or become inverted, in part because of the influence of the depressed ST segment "dragging" them down. Occasionally, T waves that were inverted on a normal 12-lead ECG become suddenly upright on a tracing obtained during an ischemic episode. Essentially, a baseline ECG must be available for comparison, and any change in ST segment or T waves from that baseline is significant.

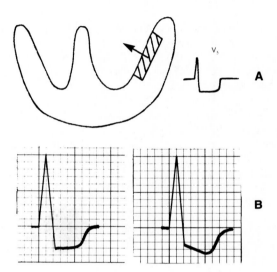

Fig. 13-24 **A,** Acute subendocardial ischemia. The electrical forces *(arrow)* responsible fore the ST segment are deviated toward the inner layer of the heart, causing ST depression in lead V_5, which faces the outer surface of the heart. **B,** Subendocardial ischemia producing ST segment depression. (From Goldberger AL and Goldberger E: Clinical electrocardiography: a simplified approach, ed 3, St Louis, 1986, The CV Mosby Co.)

Infarction involves actual necrosis of muscle cells with eventual formation of scar tissue. These cells can no longer be depolarized when an impulse reaches them. If the infarction involves the epicardial (outer) layer of the heart muscle or the entire thickness of the heart wall, the QRS complex will change. Abnormal Q waves will develop in the leads overlying the affected area. Occasionally, the entire QRS complex just becomes smaller, without actual development of Q waves. If only the subendocardial layer of the heart muscle is infarcted, abnormal Q waves will not develop. In fact, there may be no change in the QRS complex. The diagnosis is then dependent on CPK-MB or LDH_1 isoenzyme results. Chest pain, total CPK elevation, and ischemic ECG changes are nondiagnostic by themselves. Initially, it was thought that non-Q-wave infarctions were relatively benign compared to Q-wave or transmural infarctions. However, recent studies indicate that, although initial mortality and morbidity are less in patients with non-

Q-wave infarction, these patients are very vulnerable to reinfarction. Morbidity and mortality at the end of 2 years is the same for either group.[52]

The location of the infarction can be roughly determined by noting the specific leads in which the ST segment and T wave changes are seen (Table 13-7). As a general guideline, the more leads that are involved, the larger the infarct. However, this guideline applies most accurately to anterior wall infarctions. When compared to serum enzyme (CPK-MB) results, ECG estimates of the size of anterior wall infarctions correlated well with enzyme estimates. The same is not true of inferior wall infarcts, probably because of right-ventricular involvement, which is difficult to assess on a 12-lead ECG.[23]

The relative age of the infarction can also be estimated. When blood flow in a coronary artery is occluded, the entire area of heart muscle normally perfused by that artery becomes ischemic. Collateral arterioles exist, which overlap and supply the perimeter of this area, and may prevent necrosis of some of the affected tissue. At the center of the ischemic area, collateral blood flow is minimal or does not exist at all. Within a few hours, this tissue begins to necrose, or die. On the ECG tracing, this process is illustrated as follows. Within minutes of the onset of infarction, ST segment elevation occurs in the leads directly overlying the affected heart wall. This ST segment elevation will persist for several days, gradually becoming less severe. Meanwhile, usually within 4 to 24 hours from the onset of the infarction, abnormal Q waves begin to develop in the affected leads, and T waves begin to invert. The ST segments become isoelectric again in several days or weeks, and the

T wave becomes symmetrical and deeply inverted in the affected leads. Occasionally, these T wave changes do not ever resolve. Usually, however, the T waves return to normal within several months. The Q waves usually persist for the remainder of the patient's life. Table 13-8 summarizes the timing of these changes.

Ventricular Conduction Defects

Intraventricular conduction defects are the result of an abnormal pathway of conduction through the ventricles. Normally, conduction spreads from the A-V node to the bundle of His and from there down the right and left bundle branches. The right bundle branch is long and thin and terminates in a mass of Purkinje fibers, which spread the wave of depolarization to the surrounding right-ventricular muscle. The left bundle branch divides after only a short distance into the left anterior fascicle, the left posterior fascicle, and the left septal fibers (Fig. 13-25). Each of these fascicles causes depolarization of separate areas of the left ventricle. If any part of the conduction system fails, the muscle cells in that area will still be depolarized, but not as quickly. Depolarization must then spread from cell to cell, a slower process than activation through specialized conduction pathways.

On the ECG, intraventricular conduction defects cause a widening of the QRS because of the slower spread of depolarization. The affected muscle tissue begins the slower cell-to-cell depolarization just as the other areas in the ventricle are almost finished. This later depolarization is then tacked onto the end of the normal QRS, making it prolonged and altering its shape.

Any part of the conduction system can be affected. The term *bundle branch block* refers to complete interruption of conduction through either the right bundle or the entire left bundle branch. In complete right or left bundle branch block, the QRS will always be 0.12 second or longer in duration. When only one fascicle of the left bundle branch is blocked, the QRS duration will be within normal limits, although usually more prolonged than before the conduction disturbance occurred.

Right and left bundle branch block. The chest leads are the most useful in identifying complete right and left bundle branch blocks. Specifically, V_1 and V_6 are the best leads from which to identify forces traveling in a horizontal direction, because they are located on the right and left sides of the heart, respectively. Figure 13-26 illustrates the normal sequence of ventricular activation and the usual shape of the QRS complex in V_1 and V_6.

In complete right bundle branch block (Fig. 13-27), the right ventricle is not activated through the rapid conduction system. Rather, it must be activated slowly, from one cell to the next. Electrical forces, not counterbalanced by opposing forces on the left, will be traveling toward the right at the end of the ventricular activation. The septum is depolarized first, in a normal manner from left to right. Next the wave of depolarization spreads through the left ventricle and is recorded in lead V_1 as a negative deflection. The final portion of the QRS complex is upright, indicating final forces traveling toward the right. This represents right-ventricular depolarization that occurs after left-ventricular

Table 13-7 Location of ECG changes during myocardial infarction

Location of infarction	Leads involved
Anterior wall	I, aVL, V_{2-4}
Inferior wall	II, III, aVF
Ventricular septum	V_{1-2}
Lateral wall	V_{4-6}, I, aVL
True posterior wall	Mirror-image changes in V_{1-3}

Table 13-8 Timing of ECG changes during myocardial infarction

Timing	Change
Immediate	ST segment evaluation in leads over the area of infarction
Within a few hours	Giant upright T waves
Several hours to 2 weeks	ST segment normalizes; T waves invert symmetrically
Several hours to days; usually remain for life	Q waves or reduced R-wave voltage

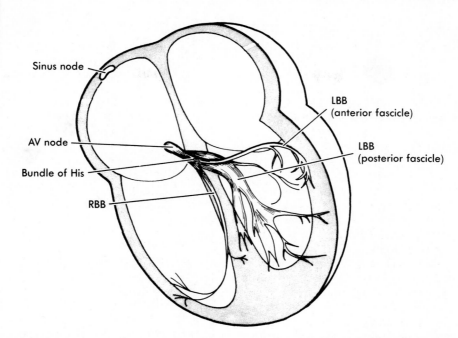

Fig. 13-25 Cardiac conduction system. (From Conover MB: Understanding electrocardiography: arrhythmias and the 12-lead ECG, ed 5, St Louis, 1988, The CV Mosby Co.)

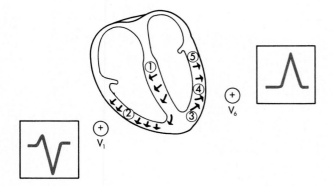

Fig. 13-26 Sequence of ventricular depolarization.

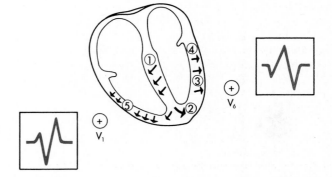

Fig. 13-27 Sequence of ventricular depolarization when right bundle branch block is present.

depolarization is nearly complete. In lead V_6, the positive electrode is on the left side of the chest, so the waveforms are reversed. The final forces of the QRS are negative, since they are traveling toward the right and away from the positive electrode of V_6. Note that the final negative deflection in V_6 is smaller than the final upright deflection in lead V_1, because the positive electrode in V_6 is at a greater distance from the right ventricle.

In complete left bundle branch block (Fig. 13-28), the conduction through the left ventricle must spread from cell to cell. Since a portion of the common left bundle normally initiates depolarization of the septum, the septum also will be depolarized in an abnormal direction, from right to left. In lead V_1 this will be recorded as an initial negative deflection. Next, the right ventricle will be depolarized, seen as a small upright notch in the QRS as the forces travel briefly toward the positive electrode of V_1. Sometimes this notch will be absent. The sequence of events has not

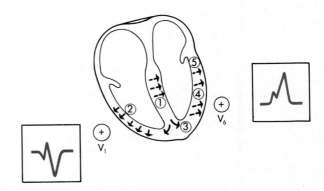

Fig. 13-28 Sequence of ventricular depolarization when left bundle branch block is present.

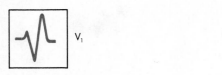

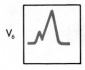

Fig. 13-29 ECG complex in right bundle branch block. Note the final upright forces in V₁ and final negative deflection in V₆.

Fig. 13-30 ECG complex in left bundle branch block. Note the final negative deflection in V₁ and the upright deflection in V₆.

changed, but the left ventricle is already beginning to be depolarized cell to cell and may offset the rightward forces of right-ventricular depolarization. The final forces travel toward the left as the left ventricle is being depolarized. The left ventricle is a very large muscle mass, so these final forces will be large and wide. In lead V₁ the final deflection will be a deep negative deflection (S wave), whereas in lead V₆ these final forces will inscribe a tall upright deflection (R wave).

In summary, a bundle branch block exists when the QRS complex is wider than 0.12 second (and the complex did not originate in the ventricles such as does a PVC). To determine which bundle branch is blocked, examine the last part of the QRS just before it returns to the baseline in leads V₁ and V₆. If upright in V₁ and negative in V₆, a right bundle branch block exists (Fig. 13-29). If negative in V₁ and upright in V₆, a left bundle branch block is present (Fig. 13-30).

Hemiblocks. Hemiblocks involve conduction failure of only part of the left bundle branch. In left-anterior fascicular block (also called left-anterior hemiblock), left-ventricular depolarization begins in the left-posterior fascicle and spreads anteriorly through Purkinje fibers distal to the block. The QRS is only slightly prolonged, up to 0.02 second longer than the patient's previous QRS. However, the axis changes dramatically and becomes more negative than −30 degrees (left axis deviation).[57] There are other causes of left axis deviation that must be ruled out before a clinical diagnosis of left-anterior hemiblock can be made (see box, "Causes of Left Axis Deviation"). In left-posterior fascicular block (also called left-posterior hemiblock), the anterior portion of the left ventricle is depolarized first. Conduction then spreads slowly to the right, inferiorly and posteriorly. Once again the QRS is slightly prolonged. The axis then swings entirely the other direction and becomes greater than +110 degrees (right axis deviation). Other causes of right axis deviation must be ruled out before a clinical diagnosis of left-posterior hemiblock can be made (see box, "Causes of Right Axis Deviation").

Bifascicular block. Blockage of any two branches of the ventricular conduction system constitutes bifascicular block. Any combination of these conduction disturbances can occur and can evolve into complete heart block. Development of right bundle branch block with left-anterior fascicular block occurs in approximately 5% of patients with acute myocardial infarction, as does left bundle branch block. Only 1% of patients experiencing myocardial infarction develops right bundle branch block in combination with left-posterior fascicular block, probably because the left-posterior fascicle is short and thick and has a dual blood supply from the left-

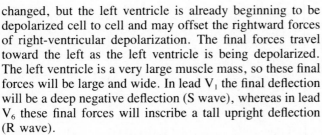

CAUSES OF LEFT AXIS DEVIATION

Normal variation
Mechanical shifts: exhalation, high diaphragm caused by pregnancy, ascites, or abdominal tumor
Left-anterior hemiblock
Left-ventricular hypertrophy
Pulmonary emphysema (uncommon)
Wolff-Parkinson-White syndrome
Hyperkalemia
Cardiomyopathy

CAUSES OF RIGHT AXIS DEVIATION

Normal variation
Mechanical shifts: inhalation, emphysema
Left-posterior hemiblock
Right-ventricular hypertrophy
Lateral wall myocardial infarction
Right bundle branch block
Dextrocardia

anterior descending and right-posterior descending coronary arteries.

Bifascicular block that develops during an acute myocardial infarction warrants placement of a temporary pacemaker in case complete heart block develops. When bifascicular block occurs in other patient populations, use of a pacemaker can be avoided if the patient is asymptomatic. However, most bifascicular block eventually progresses to complete heart block.

Dysrhythmia Interpretation

A dysrhythmia is any disturbance in the normal cardiac conduction pathway. Dysrhythmias can be detected on a 12-lead ECG, but very often they occur only sporadically. For this reason patients in a critical care unit are monitored continuously, using a single lead, and rhythm strips are recorded routinely, as well as any time there is a change in the patient's rhythm. A systematic approach to evaluation of a rhythm strip is introduced first in this section, followed by specific criteria for common dysrhythmias encountered in clinical practice.

Heart rate determination. The first thing to assess when evaluating a rhythm strip is the ventricular rate. Regardless of the dysrhythmia involved, the ventricular rate holds the key to whether or not the patient will be able to tolerate the dysrhythmia, that is, maintain adequate blood pressure, cardiac output, and mentation. If the ventricular rate is consistently >200 or <30, emergency measures must be started to correct the rate. A detailed analysis of the underlying rhythm disturbance can proceed later when the immediate crisis is over. There are three methods for calculating rate:

1. Number of RR intervals in 6 seconds times 10 (Fig. 13-31).
2. Number of large boxes between QRS complexes divided into 300 (Fig. 13-32).
3. Number of small boxes between QRS complexes divided into 1500 (Fig. 13-33).

In the healthy heart, the atrial rate and the ventricular rate are the same. However, in many dysrhythmias the atrial and ventricular rates are different; thus both must be calculated. To find the atrial rate, the PP interval, instead of the RR interval, is used in one of the three methods listed above for determining rate.

The choice of method for calculating the heart rate depends on the regularity of the rhythm. If the rhythm is irregular, the first method (RRs in 6 seconds × 10) is used. If the rhythm is regular, it is more accurate to use the second or third method. The second method can be easier to use when two consecutive R waves fall exactly on dark lines, and it provides a rapid estimate of rate. The third method is recommended when both R waves do not fall exactly on dark lines.

Rhythm determination. The term *rhythm* refers to the regularity with which the P waves or R waves occur. Calipers assist in determining rhythm. One point of the calipers is placed on the beginning of one R wave, while the other point is placed on the very next R wave. Leaving the calipers "set" at this interval, each succeeding RR interval is checked to be sure it is the same width.

In describing the rhythm, three terms are used. If the rhythm is *regular,* the RR intervals are the same, ±10%.

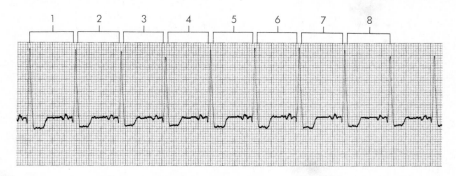

Fig. 13-31   Rate method number 1: number of RR intervals in 6 seconds multiplied by 10 (for example, 8 × 10 = 80/min).

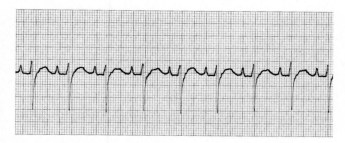

Fig. 13-32   Rate method number 2: number of large boxes between QRS complexes divided into 300 (for example, 300 ÷ 3 = 100/min).

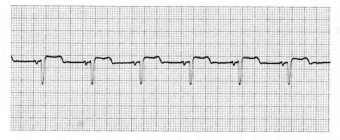

Fig. 13-33   Rate method number 3: number of small boxes between QRS complexes divided into 1500 (for example, 1500 ÷ 20 = 75/min).

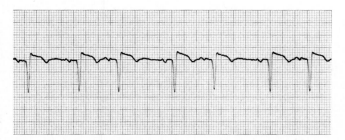

Fig. 13-34   Rhythm—irregular but with a constant pattern, every other beat is premature.

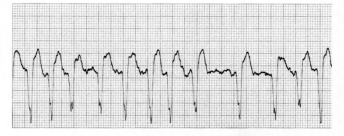

Fig. 13-35   Rhythm—irregularly irregular with no constant pattern.

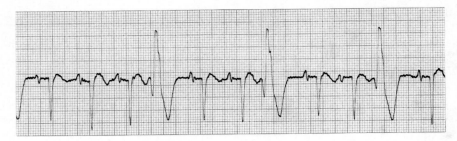

Fig. 13-36 QRS duration illustrating both normal and abnormal intervals. The narrow QRS complexes measure 0.08 seconds, which is normal. The wide QRS complexes measure 0.20 second and are caused by ventricular ectopy.

For example, if there are 20 small boxes in an RR interval, an R wave could be off by two small boxes, but the rhythm would still be considered regular.

If the rhythm is *regularly irregular,* the RR intervals are not the same, but there is some sort of pattern involved, which could be grouping, rhythmical speeding up and slowing down, or any other consistent pattern (Fig. 13-34).

If the rhythm is *irregularly irregular,* the RR intervals are not the same, and no pattern can be found (Fig. 13-35).

P-wave evaluation. The P wave should be analyzed by answering the following questions. First, is the P wave present or absent? Second, is it related to the QRS? Hopefully, there will be one P wave in front of every QRS. Sometimes there may be two, three, or four P waves in front of every QRS. If this pattern is consistent, the P wave and QRS are still related, although not on a 1:1 basis.

PR interval evaluation. The duration of the PR interval, which normally is 0.12 to 0.20 second, is measured first. Next, all PR intervals on the strip are checked to be sure they are the same duration as the original interval.

QRS evaluation. The entire ECG strip must be evaluated to ascertain that the QRS complexes are the same shape and width. The normal QRS duration is 0.06 to 0.10 second. If there is more than one QRS shape on the strip, each QRS must be measured (Fig. 13-36).

Sinus Rhythms

The cardiac cycle begins when an impulse originates in the sinus node (see Fig. 13-25). As the wave of depolarization spreads through the atria, a P wave is inscribed on the ECG. The impulse is delayed briefly in the A-V node, which corresponds to the PR interval on the ECG. After leaving the A-V node, the wave of depolarization spreads rapidly through the bundle of His and the bundle branches and causes ventricular depolarization, which is recorded as a QRS complex by the ECG. Contraction immediately follows depolarization. Contraction is terminated by repolarization, which is demonstrated as a T wave on the ECG.

Normal sinus rhythm. If all of the above events occur in their normal sequence with normal rates and intervals, the patient is in normal sinus rhythm. Specifically, the following are the criteria for normal sinus rhythm:

1. Rate. The intrinsic rate of the sinus node is 60 to 100 beats per minute. *Intrinsic rate* is the normal rate at which a pacemaker site in the heart will depolarize automatically with no outside influences such as drugs, fever, or exercise. In normal sinus rhythm, the rate must be whatever is "normal" for the sinus node, that is, 60 to 100 beats per minute.
2. Rhythm. The rhythm must be regular, plus or minus 10% (see "Rhythm Determination," p. 193).
3. P wave. P waves must be present, and one and only one must preceed every QRS complex.
4. PR interval. This interval is measured from the beginning of the P wave to the beginning of the QRS complex and represents delay in the A-V node. In normal sinus rhythm the PR interval is 0.12 to 0.20 second.
5. QRS. Size and shape does not matter in this complex, since it is dependent on lead placement and gain adjustments on the monitor. However, all QRS complexes should look alike. If conduction through the ventricles is normal, the QRS duration will be 0.06 second to 0.10 second. Figure 13-37 is an example of normal sinus rhythm in both leads II and MCL$_1$.

Sinus bradycardia. Sinus bradycardia meets all of the criteria for normal sinus rhythm except that the rate is less than 60 (Table 13-9). It is normally seen in well-trained

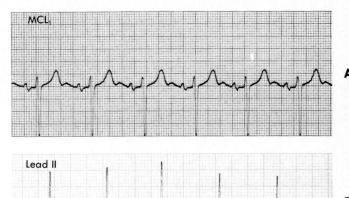

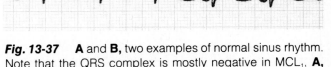

Fig. 13-37 **A** and **B,** two examples of normal sinus rhythm. Note that the QRS complex is mostly negative in MCL$_1$, **A,** and is caused by the location of the positive electrode in each of these leads.

Table 13-9 Sinus rhythms

Parameters	Normal sinus rhythm	Sinus bradycardia	Sinus tachycardia	Sinus dysrhythmia
Rate	60-100/min	<60/min	>100/min	Variable
Rhythm	Regular	Regular	Regular	Irregular; respiratory variation
P wave	Present, with one per QRS	Present, with one per QRS	Present, with one per QRS	Present, with one per QRS
PR interval	0.12-0.20 sec and constant	0.12-0.20 sec and constant	0.12-0.20 sec and constant	0.12-0.20 sec and constant
QRS	0.06-0.10 sec	0.06-0.10 sec	0.06-0.10 sec	0.06-0.10 sec

athletes at rest or in many other individuals during sleep. Other conditions in which sinus bradycardia occurs include vagal stimulation, increased intracranial pressure, drug therapy with digoxin or beta blockers, and ischemia of the sinus node caused by an acute inferior wall myocardial infarction. Sinus bradycardia is generally not treated unless the patient displays symptoms of hypoperfusion such as hypotension, dizziness, chest pain, or changes in level of consciousness.

Sinus tachycardia. Sinus tachycardia meets all the criteria for normal sinus rhythm except that the rate is greater than 100 beats per minute (see Table 13-9). Rates may be as high as 180 to 200 beats per minute in healthy young adults with strenuous exercise. However, in the critical care setting, bed rest has been prescribed for most patients. It is wise to be skeptical of any "sinus tachycardia" with a rate greater than 150 and to search for a triggering focus other than the sinus node. For example, atrial flutter waves might be difficult to see at first glance because of baseline distortion caused by the high ventricular rate (Fig. 13-38).

Sinus tachycardia can be caused by a wide variety of factors such as exercise, emotion, pain, fever, hemorrhage, shock, and congestive heart failure. Many drugs used in critical care can also cause sinus tachycardia, and common culprits are aminophylline, dopamine, beta stimulants such as epinephrine, hydralazine, and overzealous use of atropine. Tachycardia is detrimental to anyone with ischemic heart disease because it decreases time for ventricular filling, decreases stroke volume, and thus compromises cardiac output. Additionally, tachycardia will increase heart work and myocardial oxygen demand while decreasing oxygen supply by decreasing coronary artery filling time.

If the cause (for example, fever or pain) of the tachycardia can be determined, the cause should be treated rather than trying to treat the heart rate directly. Several drugs are available to decrease the heart rate, and both calcium channel blockers and beta blockers are widely used for this purpose. However, a word of caution is warranted here. Cardiac output is determined by heart rate and stroke volume. If an injured heart can no longer maintain an adequate stroke volume, heart rate can be increased to maintain cardiac output and supply an adequate blood flow to vital body tissues. If a drug is administered to force the sinus node to slow, severe and relatively immediate heart failure can result. The sinus node is controlled by many neural and humoral influences in the body, and the rate is set to try to

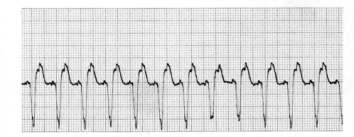

Fig. 13-38 Sinus tachycardia? In fact, this is atrial flutter with 2:1 conduction. Note how difficult it is to see the extra flutter waves that are hidden in the QRS complexes.

meet the perceived demands; thus a close examination of the reason for the tachycardia is mandatory before treatment decisions are made.

Sinus arrhythmia. Sinus arrhythmia meets all of the criteria for normal sinus rhythm except that the rhythm is irregular (see Table 13-9). Usually this irregularity coincides with the respiratory pattern; heart rate increases with inhalation and decreases with exhalation. Sinus dysrhythmia frequently occurs in children, and the incidence decreases with age. No treatment is required. To avoid being misled by other rhythm disturbances, all P waves should be examined closely to be sure that they are all the same shape and that the PR intervals are all constant.

Atrial Dysrhythmias

Atrial dysrhythmias originate from an ectopic focus in the atria, somewhere other than the sinus node. The ectopic impulse occurs prematurely before the normal sinus impulse is due to occur. Usually, the premature P wave initiates a normal QRS complex. However, some exceptions do occur. The early P wave usually looks different than the sinus P wave and often is inverted. The PR interval may be longer, shorter, or the same as the PR interval of a sinus beat.

Premature atrial contractions. Premature atrial contractions (PACs) are isolated, early beats from an ectopic focus in the atria. The underlying rhythm is usually sinus. The regular sinus rhythm is interrupted by an early, abnormally shaped P wave. If the impulse arrives in the A-V node after the A-V node is fully repolarized, it will be conducted to the ventricles. If the ventricles are also fully repolarized, conduction through them will be normal and a normal QRS

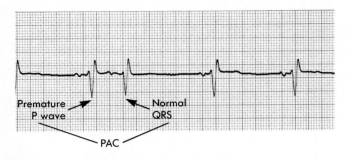

Fig. 13-39 Normally conducted premature atrial contraction (PAC). The early P wave is indicated by the arrow, and the QRS that follows is of normal shape and duration.

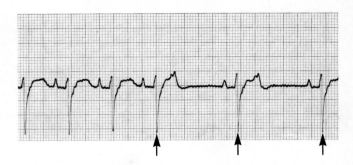

Fig. 13-40 Nonconducted (blocked) PACs. The early P waves are indicated by arrows. Note how they distort the T waves, making them appear peaked compared to the normal T waves seen after the third and fourth QRS complexes.

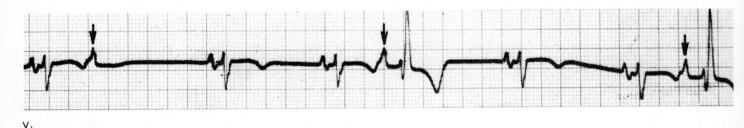

V₁

Fig. 13-41 Right bundle branch block aberration following a PAC. (From Andreoli K and others: Comprehensive cardiac care, ed 6, St. Louis, 1987, The CV Mosby Co.

will be recorded on the ECG (Fig. 13-39).

Sometimes, the ectopic P wave arrives so early that the A-V node is still in its absolute refractory period. In this case, the wave of depolarization will not move past the A-V node, and no QRS will follow. All that will be seen on the ECG is an early, abnormal P wave followed by a pause until the next sinus P wave occurs (Fig. 13-40). This is called a nonconducted PAC. Usually these P waves are so early that they are superimposed on the T wave of the previous beat, making them somewhat difficult to find. The pause that follows will still be clearly seen. Whenever an unexpected pause occurs in a rhythm, the T wave preceding the pause should be examined very carefully, comparing it to other T waves on the same strip and looking for distortions that may reveal a hidden, early P wave.

Occasionally, the early ectopic P wave can be conducted through the A-V node, but part of this conduction pathway through the ventricles is blocked. Since the right bundle branch normally has the longest refractory period, it is usually the right bundle branch that is still blocked when the early impulse arrives. On the ECG, this will appear as an early, abnormal P wave, followed by an abnormally wide QRS, usually with a shape consistent with right bundle branch block (Fig. 13-41). Conduction through the ventricles that is different from normal is termed aberrant. Consequently, these early, abnormally conducted PACs are called aberrantly conducted PACs.

PACs can occur in normal individuals. They are accentuated by emotional disturbances, nicotine, tea, caffeine, and digitalis. Mitral valve prolapse is associated with an increased frequency of atrial dysrhythmias. Congestive heart failure can also cause PACs. As atrial pressure begins to rise, the atrial walls are stretched, causing irritability of atrial cells and the occurrence of PACs.

Paroxysmal atrial tachycardia. "Paroxysmal" means starting and stopping abruptly. Paroxysmal atrial tachycardia (PAT) refers to the sudden interruption of sinus rhythm by an atrial ectopic focus that fires repetitively at a rate of 150 to 250 times per minute and eventually stops as suddenly as it began. The rhythm of the PAT is perfectly regular, because the same irritable ectopic focus in the atria is initiating each beat. P waves are present and abnormally shaped, although they may be difficult to identify because they often blend in with the previous T wave because of the rapid rate. It is most helpful if the beginning of the PAT run is captured and recorded on ECG paper, because the early, abnormal P wave is often easiest to identify in front of the first beat of the run. The PR interval should be the same for each cycle in the run, but it will probably be different from the PR interval of the patient's own normal sinus rhythm. Just as with PACs, the QRS complex is usually normal, because once the impulse passes through the A-V node, conduction through the ventricles follows the usual pathway (Table 13-10). However, aberrant conduction, usually in the form of right bundle branch block, can occur. It will cause a wide QRS complex and difficulty differentiating this relatively benign dysrhythmia from its more serious counterpart, ventricular tachycardia. Table 13-11 offers some guidelines for differentiating aberrant conduction from ventricular ectopy. Sometimes, because of refractoriness in

Table 13-10   Atrial dysrhythmias

Parameter	Paroxysmal atrial tachycardia	Multifocal atrial tachycardia	Atrial flutter	Atrial fibrillation
Rate				
Atrial	150-250/min	100-160/min	250-350/min	>350/min (unable to count it)
Ventricular	Same or less	Same	Half or less	100-180/min (uncontrolled); <100/min (controlled)
Rhythm	Regular	Irregular	Atrial—regular; ventricular—may or may not be regular	Irregularly irregular
P wave	Present; abnormally shaped	Present; three or more different shapes	F waves	F waves
PR interval	May be normal or prolonged	Variable	Conduction ratio: flutter waves per QRS	Absent
QRS	0.06-0.10 sec	0.06-0.10 sec	0.06-0.10 sec	0.06-0.10 sec

Table 13-11   Factors to consider in differentiating between ventricular tachycardia and supraventricular tachycardia with aberrant conduction

ECG observations	Aberrant conduction versus ventricular tachycardia
Heart rate	>170/min favors aberrant conduction 130-170/min favors ventricular tachycardia >220/min favors conduction over an accessory pathway
A-V dissociation	Favors ventricular ectopy
Ventricular rhythm	Tends to be regular in ventricular tachycardia
QRS width	>0.14 sec favors ventricular ectopy unless there is preexisting bundle branch block
QRS axis	Left axis deviation favors ventricular origin
QRS shape	Monophasic R or qR in V_1 favors ventricular ectopy rSR′ in V_1 favors aberration RSr′ in V_1 (first peak taller than the second) seen only in ventricular tachycardia Concordant precordial pattern (entirely upright or entirely negative QRS from V_1-V_6) seen only in ventricular tachycardia QS or QR in V_6 favors ventricular origin

Modified from Conover M and Marriott H: Advanced concepts in arrhythmias, St. Louis, 1983, The CV Mosby Co.

the A-V node, not all of the ectopic P waves are conducted to the ventricles. Usually, at least every other P wave conducts a QRS, but occasionally the conduction ratio may drop to three P waves for every QRS.

PAT has essentially the same causal factors as PACs. PAT has greater clinical significance, especially if it is sustained for any length of time, because it occurs at such a rapid rate. As stressed previously in the discussion of sinus tachycardia, rapid rates decrease ventricular filling time, increase myocardial oxygen consumption, and decrease oxygen supply. Congestive heart failure, angina, or even myocardial infarction can result. PAT usually responds rapidly to medical treatment, which may include the use of direct or indirect vagal maneuvers, intravenous calcium channel blocking agents, or electrical cardioversion.

Multifocal atrial tachycardia. Multifocal atrial tachycardia, sometimes referred to as chaotic atrial tachycardia, occurs when there are numerous irritable atrial foci that intermittently fire and generate an impulse. The atrial rate is greater than 100 beats per minute but generally does not exceed 160. The distinguishing feature on the ECG is that there are at least three different P wave shapes, indicating at least three different irritable foci. This is most commonly seen in elderly patients with chronic obstructive pulmonary disease. Unfortunately, this dysrhythmia is usually refractory to any treatment.

Atrial flutter. Atrial flutter is believed caused by a steady circular pathway through which the wave of depolarization is continually moving. The loop is sufficiently large (or conduction through it sufficiently slow) that the current fails to find the cells in front of it in a refractory state. As a consequence, the current continually perpetuates itself. The atrial rate in atrial flutter is 250 to 350 beats per minute and is most often at 300 (see Table 13-10). At this rate, separate distinction of individual P waves is lost, and they blend together in a saw-tooth pattern (Fig. 13-42). In this state, P waves are more appropriately called F waves (flutter waves). Fortunately, the A-V node does not allow conduc-

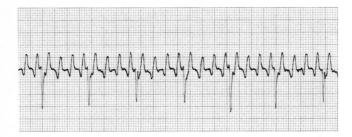

Fig. 13-42 Atrial flutter with 4:1 A-V conduction. The atrial rate is 330 beats per minute. Note the sawtooth appearance of the flutter waves.

A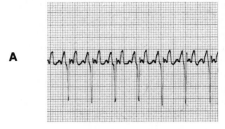

B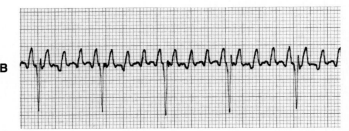

Fig. 13-43 Initial strip, **A,** shows atrial flutter with 2:1 conduction through the A-V node. During carotid sinus massage, **B,** the conduction rate is increased, more clearly revealing the flutter waves.

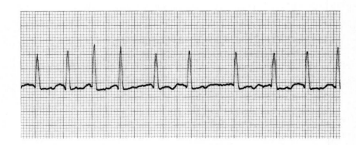

Fig. 13-44 Atrial fibrillation. Note the irregularly irregular ventricular rhythm.

tion of all these impulses to the ventricles. When evaluating the rate of atrial flutter, both atrial and ventricular rates must be calculated.

The atrial rhythm will be perfectly regular, since the circuit is always the same length and therefore always requires the same amount of time to complete. The ventricular rhythm will be regular if the same number of flutter waves occur between each QRS complex—in other words, if the degree of block at the A-V node remains constant. Sometimes the refractoriness in the A-V node changes from beat to beat, resulting in an irregular ventricular response. When describing atrial flutter, "PR interval" no longer applies; instead, it is a "conduction ratio," such as 3:1 or 4:1, that is used. Thus in normal sinus rhythm, measuring the PR interval allows evaluation of the speed of conduction through the A-V node; in atrial flutter, the number of flutter waves that bombard the A-V node before one is allowed to pass through to the ventricles is a measure of A-V nodal conduction. Once the impulse has passed the A-V node, conduction through the ventricles is unaltered. The QRS duration should remain normal or at least the same as it was in normal sinus rhythm.

The major key to the clinical significance of atrial flutter is the ventricular response rate. If the atrial rate is 300 and the A-V conduction ratio is 4:1, the ventricular response rate would be 75 beats per minute and should be well tolerated. If, on the other hand, the atrial rate is 300 but the A-V conduction ratio is 2:1, the corresponding ventricular rate of 150 may cause angina, congestive heart failure, or other signs of cardiac decompensation. An atrial rate of 250 with a 1:1 A-V conduction ratio would yield a ventricular response rate of 250, and emergency measures would be needed to decrease the ventricular rate.

Sometimes it is difficult to identify the flutter waves, especially if the conduction ratio is 2:1. Vagal maneuvers are useful to increase briefly the refractory period of the A-V node and allow better visualization of the flutter waves (Fig. 13-43). Only rarely will vagal maneuvers terminate atrial flutter. Usually atrial flutter can be converted back to sinus rhythm with the use of pharmacological agents or cardioversion. If an adequate ventricular rate is all that is desired, administering a maintenance dose of digoxin will usually suffice.

Atrial fibrillation. When numerous sites in the atria fire spontaneously and rapidly, an organized spread of depolarization can no longer take place, and atrial fibrillation results

(Fig. 13-44). Small sections of atrial muscle are activated individually, resulting in quivering of the atrial muscle without effective contraction. The ECG tracing in atrial fibrillation is characterized by an uneven baseline without clearly defined P waves and an irregularly irregular ventricular rhythm. The QRS complex is usually normal, since the pathway through the ventricles is unchanged once the impulse leaves the A-V node. The A-V node acts as a filter to protect the ventricles from the 350 to 500 sporadic atrial impulses that are occurring each minute (see Table 13-10). In addition, the A-V node itself does not receive all of the atrial impulses. When the atrial muscle tissue immediately surrounding the A-V node is in a refractory state, impulses generated in other areas of the atria are not able to reach the A-V node, helping to explain the wide variation in RR intervals during atrial fibrillation.

A normal A-V node will conduct impulses to the ventricles at a rate of 100 to 180 times per minute. This rapid rate is not desirable, and a major therapeutic goal is to reduce the ventricular response rate to below 100 beats per minute. There are two ways to approach this goal: (1) convert the atrial fibrillation back to sinus rhythm or (2) allow the atrial fibrillation to exist and use pharmacological measures to control the ventricular response rate.

Electrical cardioversion may be successful in converting the rhythm to sinus if attempted within a few days or weeks of the onset of atrial fibrillation. Its success is less likely if the atrial fibrillation has existed for a long time. Cardioversion also carries with it the threat of precipitating emboli. During atrial fibrillation the atria do not contract; hence, blood may pool in areas of the atrial walls. This pooling can promote thrombus formation (mural thrombi) within the atria. If cardioversion is successful and normal sinus rhythm is restored, the atria will again contract forcibly and, if thrombus formation has occurred, send clots traveling through the pulmonary or systemic circulation. To prevent this, patients often receive anticoagulation therapy for several days or weeks before electrical cardioversion.

Digoxin is the most common chronically used drug to control ventricular response rate. The dosage is adjusted to keep the ventricular rate between 60 and 100 beats per minute. Other drugs that can be used include calcium channel blockers and beta blockers.

Junctional Dysrhythmias

Only certain areas of the A-V node have the property of automaticity. The entire area around the A-V node is collectively called the junction; hence, impulses generated there are called junctional. After an ectopic impulse arises in the junction, it spreads in two directions at once. One wave of depolarization spreads upward into the atria and depolarizes them, causing the recording of a P wave on the ECG. At the same time, another wave of depolarization spreads downward into the ventricles through the normal conduction pathway, resulting in a normal QRS complex. Depending on timing, the P wave may be seen in front of the QRS but with a short PR interval, the P wave may be obscured entirely by the QRS, or the P wave may immediately follow the QRS. When atrial depolarization begins in the junction, the wave of depolarization spreads from the bottom of the atria upward, causing inversion of the P wave in lead II.

Premature junctional contraction. If only a single ectopic impulse originates in the junction, it is simply called a premature junctional contraction. On the ECG, the rhythm would be regular from the sinus node except for one early QRS complex of normal shape and duration. The P wave could be entirely absent. If a P wave could be found, it would very closely precede or follow the QRS. In lead II, the P wave would appear inverted (having a negative deflection), because the atria are being depolarized from the A-V node upward, which is the opposite direction from the wave of depolarization that occurs when triggered by the sinus node. If the P wave appeared before the QRS, the PR interval would be less than 0.12 second. Premature junctional contractions have virtually the same clinical significance as PACs. However, if the patient is receiving digoxin, digitalis toxicity should at least be suspected. Although digoxin slows conduction through the A-V node, it also increases automaticity in that area.

Junctional escape rhythm. Sometimes, the junction becomes the dominant pacemaker of the heart (Table 13-12). Normally, the intrinsic rate of the junction is 40 to 60 beats per minute. Since the intrinsic rate of the sinus node is 60 to 100 beats per minute, under normal conditions the junction never has a chance to "escape" and depolarize the heart. However, if the sinus node fails, the junctional impulses will be able to depolarize completely and to pace the heart. This is called a junctional escape rhythm and is a protective measure to prevent asystole in the event of sinus node failure. Generally, a junctional escape rhythm is well tolerated, although efforts should be directed toward restoring sinus rhythm. Sometimes a pacemaker is inserted as a protective measure in the event that the junction also fails.

Junctional tachycardia and accelerated junctional rhythm. A junctional rhythm can also occur at a higher rate (see Table 13-12). As with sinus rhythm, the term *tachycardia* is reserved for rates grater than 100 per minute; thus junctional tachycardia is a junctional rhythm, usually regular, at a rate greater than 100. But what if the junctional rate is greater than 60 and less than 100 (faster than the intrinsic rate of the junction, yet not fast enough to be considered a tachycardia)? The phrase *accelerated junctional rhythm* applies to this situation. Accelerated junctional rhythm is usually well tolerated by the patient, mainly because the heart rate is within a reasonable range. Junctional tachycardia may not be tolerated as well, depending on the rate and the patient's underlying cardiac reserve. Once again, digitalis toxicity should be strongly suspected, since digoxin enhances automaticity of the A-V node. If digitalis toxicity is present, the only treatment is to withhold digoxin until the dysrhythmia resolves.

Ventricular Dysrhythmias

Ventricular dysrhythmias result from an ectopic focus in any portion of the ventricular myocardium. The usual conduction pathway through the ventricles is not used, and the wave of depolarization must spread from cell to cell. As a

---

Table 13-12 Junctional rhythms

Parameter	Junctional escape rhythm	Accelerated junctional rhythm	Junctional tachycardia
Rate	40-60/min	60-100/min	>100/min
Rhythm	Regular	Regular	Regular
P waves	May be present or absent; inverted in lead II	May be present or absent; inverted in lead II	May be present or absent; inverted in lead II
PR interval	<0.12 sec	<0.12 sec	<0.12 sec
QRS	0.06-0.10 sec	0.06-0.10 sec	0.06-0.10 sec

result, the QRS complex is prolonged and is always greater than 0.12 second. It is the width of the QRS, not the height, that is important in diagnosing ventricular ectopy.

Premature ventricular contractions. A single ectopic impulse originating in the ventricles is called a premature ventricular contraction (PVC). Some PVCs are very small in height but remain wider than 0.12 second. If in doubt, a different lead should be evaluated. The shape of the QRS will vary, depending on the location of the ectopic focus. If the ectopic focus is in the right ventricle, the impulse will spread from right to left, and the QRS will resemble a left bundle branch block pattern, since the left ventricle is the last to be depolarized. In MCL₁, this would be a wide, negative QRS (Fig. 13-45, *A*). If the ectopic focus is in the left-ventricular free wall, the wave of depolarization will spread from left to right (Fig. 13-45, *B*).

Since the ectopic focus could be any cell in the ventricle, the QRS might take an unlimited number of shapes or patterns. If all of the ventricular ectopic beats look the same in a particular lead, they are called unifocal, which means that they probably all result from the same irritable focus (Fig. 13-46). Conversely, if the ventricular ectopics are of various shapes in the same lead, they are called multifocal (Fig. 13-47). Multifocal ventricular ectopics are more serious than unifocal ventricular ectopics because they indicate a greater area of irritable myocardial tissue and are more likely to deteriorate into ventricular tachycardia or fibrillation. In general, ventricular dysrhythmias have more serious implications than atrial or junctional dysrhythmias and occur only rarely in healthy individuals.

A PVC originates in a ventricular cell that has become abnormally permeable to sodium, usually as a result of damage of one kind or another. Because of this new permeability to sodium, the cell reaches depolarization threshold before an impulse is received from the sinus node. Once depolarization threshold is reached, the cell automatically depolarizes, thus beginning total ventricular depolarization. Ordinarily, the ventricular impulse does not conduct back through the A-V node; hence, the sinus node is not disturbed and continues to depolarize the atria, resulting in a normal P wave. Conduction, however, will not proceed into the ventricles if they are in a refractory state. The next sinus beat, assuming there is no further ventricular ectopy, will conduct normally through the A-V node and into the ventricles.

Compensatory pause. If the interval from the last normal QRS preceding the PVC to the one following it is exactly equal to two complete cardiac cycles (Fig. 13-48), a compensatory pause is present. It does not usually occur in PACs or premature junctional contraction, so when present it is somewhat diagnostic of ventricular ectopy. If the normal sinus P wave that occurs immediately after the PVC finds the ventricles sufficiently recovered to accept another impulse, a normal QRS will result, and the PVC is sandwiched between two normal beats (Fig. 13-49). This PVC is referred to as *interpolated*, meaning "between." Interpolated PVCs usually occur when either the PVC is very early or the normal sinus rate is relatively slow.

Occasionally, the ventricular impulse spreads backward across the A-V node to depolarize the atria. When this

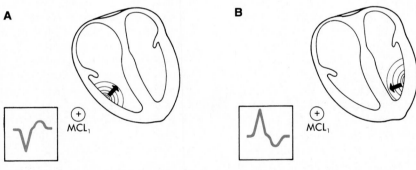

Fig. 13-45 **A,** Right-ventricular premature ventricular contraction (PVC). The spread of depolarization is from right to left, away from the positive electrode in lead MCL₁, resulting in a wide, negative QRS complex. **B,** Left-ventricular PVC. The spread of depolarization is from left to right, toward the positive electrode in lead MCL₁. The QRS complex will be wide and upright.

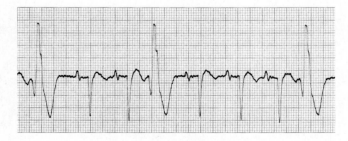

Fig. 13-46 Unifocal PVCs.

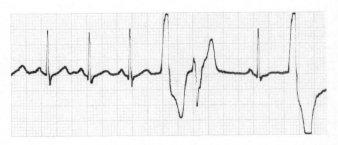

Fig. 13-47 Multifocal PVCs.

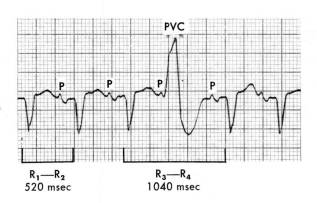

R₁—R₂
520 msec

R₃—R₄
1040 msec

Fig. 13-48 Some PVCs cause a fully compensatory pause—the interval between the two sinus beats that surround the PVC (R₃ and R₄ in this case) is exactly two times the normal interval between sinus beats (R₁ and R₂). Notice that the P waves come on time except that the third P wave is interrupted by the PVC and therefore does not conduct normally through the A-V junction. The next (fourth) P wave also comes on time. The fact that the sinus node continues to pace despite the PVC results in the fully compensatory pause. (From Goldberger AL and Goldberger E: Clinical electrocardiography: a simplified approach, ed 3, St Louis, 1986, The CV Mosby Co.)

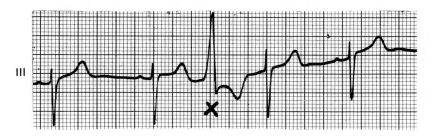

Fig. 13-49 Sometimes a PVC *(X)* will fall between two normal QRS complexes without disturbing the rhythm. This is called an interpolated PVC. Note that the RR interval between sinus beats remains unchanged. (From Goldberger AL and Goldberger E: Clinical electrocardiography: a simplified approach, ed 3, St Louis, 1986, The CV Mosby Co.)

occurs, the sinus node is reset, and there is not a full compensatory pause.

Describing ventricular ectopy. PVCs can develop concurrently with any supraventricular dysrhythmia. Therefore it is not sufficient to describe a patient's rhythm as "frequent PVCs" or even "frequent unifocal PVCs." The underlying rhythm must always be described first, for example, "sinus bradycardia with frequent unifocal PVCs" or "atrial fibrillation with occasional multifocal PVCs." Timing of PVCs can also be described. When a PVC follows each normal beat, *ventricular bigeminy* is present (Fig. 13-50). If a PVC follows every two normal beats, it would be called *ventricular trigeminy*.

The timing of PVCs can be important, especially if myocardial ischemia is present. The relative refractory period, represented on the ECG by the last half of the T wave, is a particularly vulnerable time for ectopy to occur because repolarization is not yet complete. Repolarization is even more delayed in ischemic tissue so that various portions of the ventricular muscle are not repolarized simultaneously. If a PVC occurs at this critical point when only a part of the muscle is repolarized, individual segments of muscle can depolarize separately from each other, resulting in ventricular fibrillation. This is called the *R-on-T phenomenon* (Fig. 13-51).

Two PVCs in a row are described as a couplet, and three PVCs in a row can be called either a triplet or a three-beat run of ventricular tachycardia. More than three PVCs in a row are considered ventricular tachycardia, but it is still

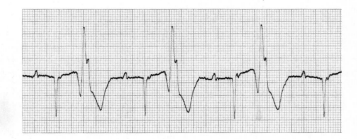

Fig. 13-50 Ventricular bigeminy.

useful to state how many beats of ventricular tachycardia occurred if the run was short, that is, less than 20 beats.

Causes of PVCs. There are many causes of PVCs. They have been known to occur, although rarely, in healthy individuals with no evidence of heart disease. The critical care nurse has an important role in identifying factors that may be causing or at least contributing to the occurrence of PVCs. Acute ischemia is the most dangerous cause of ventricular ectopy. Ischemia causes cell membrane permeability to change, giving rise to early depolarization and the initiation of ectopic impulses. PVCs that occur during acute ischemia must be immediately and effectively treated with appropriate antidysrhythmic drugs. Sometimes antidysrhythmic drugs are given prophylactically when an acute ischemic event is suspected.

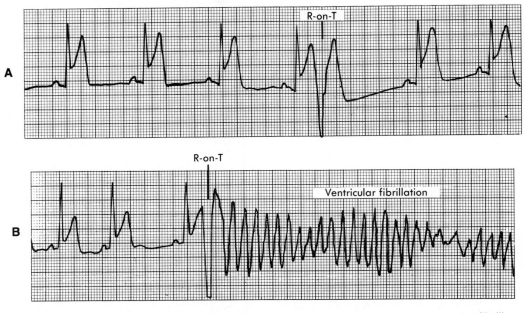

Fig. 13-51 **A,** R-on-T phenomenon. **B,** R-on-T phenomenon causing ventricular fibrillation. (From Conover MB: Understanding electrocardiography: arrhythmias and the 12-lead ECG, ed 5, St Louis, 1988, The CV Mosby Co.)

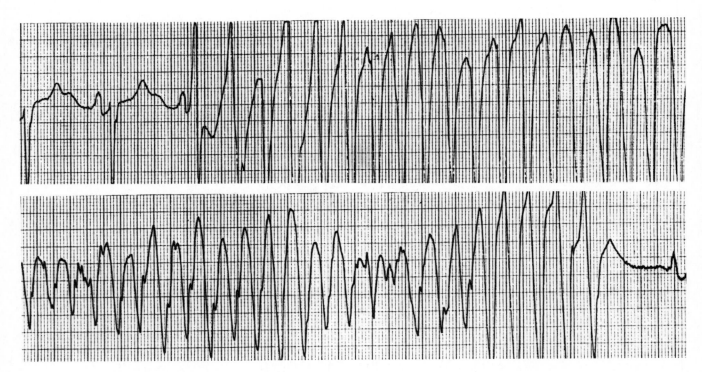

Fig. 13-52 Torsade de pointes. (From Andreoli and others: Comprehensive cardiac care, ed 6, St Louis, 1987, The CV Mosby Co.)

Metabolic abnormalities are frequent causes of the development of PVCs. Hypokalemia, hypoxemia, and acidosis predispose the cell membrane to instability and may cause ventricular ectopy. Treatment should be directed toward identifying the metabolic disturbance and correcting it. Arterial blood gas values and serum potassium level should be obtained if no recent results are available. The ability of oxygen and potassium values to change very rapidly in a critically ill patient must not be underestimated. If PVCs develop during suctioning of an intubated patient, a few additional breaths of 100% oxygen usually will be sufficient to restore adequate oxygenation and eliminate the ventricular ectopy.

Certain drugs can cause ventricular ectopy. Digitalis toxicity is often accompanied by PVCs, which are somewhat resistant to conventional antidysrhythmic therapy. Quinidine can prolong the QT interval to such an extent that a characteristic form of ventricular tachycardia, *torsade de pointes,* develops[59] (Fig. 13-52). In this dysrhythmia the ventricular tachycardia is very rapid, and the QRS complexes appear to twist in a spiral pattern around the baseline. Clinically, torsade de pointes is poorly tolerated because of the extremely rapid rate. If not terminated, death will result. Fortunately, torsade de pointes often stops spontaneously, although the patient may experience a syncopal episode at the time of the dysrhythmia.[5]

Any form of heart disease can lead to the development of ventricular ectopy. Patients with cardiomyopathy or ventricular aneurysms can have chronic severe ventricular ectopy, which may prove to be refractory to any antidysrhythmic agent. Invasive procedures such as insertion of a Swan-Ganz catheter or cardiac catheterization can cause PVCs by mechanically irritating the ventricular muscle. In these situations the ectopy will resolve with removal of the catheter. If the catheter must remain, a onetime bolus of lidocaine can be used as a precaution against the development of a life-threatening dysrhythmia.

Treatment of PVCs. Not all ventricular ectopy requires treatment. In individuals without underlying heart disease, PVCs do not represent an increased risk for sudden death and are considered benign. If the patient is complaining of palpitations, therapy initially includes reassurance and elimination of factors such as caffeine or alcohol ingestion, emotional stress, and sympathomimetic drugs that increase ventricular irritability. If symptoms continue, antidysrhythmic drugs may be used, although no change in mortality has been demonstrated when ventricular ectopy is suppressed under these circumstances.[47]

For patients with acute myocardial ischemia, aggressive treatment of any ventricular ectopy is required. Sometimes intravenous lidocaine is used prophylactically for patients with acute myocardial infarction even in the absence of PVCs. When ventricular ectopy does occur, intravenous lidocaine should be administered until the ectopy is suppressed. If sustained ventricular tachycardia occurs, the patient should be rapidly evaluated for hemodynamic compromise. If the patient is still alert and arterial blood pressure remains adequate, lidocaine or procainamide (Pronestyl) can be given intravenously in an attempt to stop the ventricular tachycardia. Sometimes hemodynamic instability will require electrical conversion of this dysrhythmia. Every effort should be made not to perform electrical cardioversion on a patient who is still conscious.[30] If pharmacological therapy is unsuccessful, sedation should be provided before performing cardioversion.

Other forms of cardiac disease such as coronary artery disease, cardiomyopathy, and mitral valve prolapse can be associated with ventricular ectopy. With them, therapeutic goals are suppression of symptoms and reduction of mortality. Antidysrhythmic drugs are especially useful if complex forms of ventricular ectopy exist.

Patients who have already experienced sustained ventricular tachycardia or cardiac arrest are at especially high risk for sudden death, whether or not underlying heart disease is present. An extensive workup of these patients is warranted, including cardiac catheterization and electrophysiological testing with programmed ventricular stimulation. Therapy is aimed at eliminating malignant ventricular ectopy and preventing recurrence of sustained ventricular tachycardia or ventricular fibrillation and may include treating the underlying cause, administering antidysrhythmic drugs, performing antidysrhythmic surgery, or implanting an antitachycardia pacemaker or a defibrillator.

Dangerous PVCs. Some types of PVCs have been associated with future development of ventricular tachycardia or ventricular fibrillation. They have been called "warning" dysrhythmias, "complex" dysrhythmias, and "malignant" ventricular ectopy. Basically, this category includes frequent PVCs (usually defined as greater than six per minute), multifocal PVCs, R-on-T phenomenon, couplets, and three or more beats of ventricular tachycardia. In the critical care setting, these warning dysrhythmias generally require treatment with antidysrhythmic drugs and a careful search for precipitating factors such as hypoxia, hypokalemia, or catheter irritation.

Pharmacological agents. In the critical care unit initial treatment of ventricular dysrhythmias usually involves administering intravenous (IV) medications. IV lidocaine is the first drug of choice and is given in a dose of 1 to 2 mg/kg bolus, followed by a continuous infusion of 1 to 4 mg per minute. Lidocaine is metabolized primarily by the liver, so caution must be exercised in patients with impaired liver function. Toxic effects may include drowsiness, slurred speech, hallucinations, and seizures.

If ventricular ectopy is not adequately controlled by lidocaine, procainamide can also be given intravenously. Procainamide is administered as a loading dose of 10 to 20 mg/kg during 20 to 40 minutes, followed by a continuous infusion of 1 to 4 mg per minute. The loading dose is given at a rate of 20 mg per minute until either the dysrhythmia is suppressed, significant hypotension occurs, the QRS complex widens by 50%, or the total loading dose has been administered.

Bretylium is given intravenously when lidocaine and/or procainamide has failed. It is especially effective when recurrent ventricular tachycardia or ventricular fibrillation is present. Bretylium raises the ventricular fibrillation threshold, making it less likely that ventricular fibrillation will occur and favorably affecting the success of defibrillation in patients already in ventricular fibrillation. Bretylium does not directly suppress spontaneous depolarization of Purkinje fibers (one cause of PVCs), so it is usually administered in combination with another antidysrhythmic such as lidocaine.

The method of administration of bretylium varies, depending on the clinical situation. In patients with ventricular fibrillation, 5 mg/kg of undiluted bretylium is administered by rapid IV bolus. Defibrillation is then attempted again. If defibrillation is unsuccessful, the dose may be increased to 10 mg/kg IV bolus. In patients with recurrent ventricular tachycardia, the loading dose of 5 mg/kg should be diluted and given slowly for 8 to 10 minutes. Nausea and vomiting may occur in the conscious patient if bretylium is administered too rapidly. An initial rise in heart rate and blood pressure should be expected because of the release of norephinephrine from nerve endings. This rise is followed by postural hypotension, which is best controlled by maintaining the patient in the supine position and administering IV

fluids as necessary. Because of its effect on adrenergic nerve endings, patients receiving bretylium are extremely sensitive to catecholamines. For this reason, vasopressors, if used, must be administered in lower doses and with caution.

Numerous oral antidysrhythmic agents are available for long-term control of ventricular dysrhythmias. They can be divided into four general categories based on mechanism of action (Table 13-13). Since each of these drugs works in a different way, one drug may be effective when another one has failed. If a particular agent is effective but produces intolerable side effects, another drug in the same class can be substituted, often proving just as effective without the side effects.

Some antidysrhythmic drugs also have a prodysrhythmic effect, meaning that they can actually precipitate recurrent ventricular tachycardia. Patients with preexisting malignant ventricular dysrhythmias are at highest risk for developing drug-induced ventricular tachycardia and should be hospitalized and continuously monitored when antidysrhythmic therapy is initiated with these drugs. The most notable agents that have this effect are encainide and flecainide.

Idioventricular rhythm. At times an ectopic focus in the ventricle can become the dominant pacemaker of the heart (Table 13-14). If both the sinus node and the A-V junction fail, the ventricles will depolarize at their own intrinsic rate of 20 to 40 times per minute. This is called an idioventricular rhythm and is protective in nature. Rather than trying to abolish the ventricular beats, the aim of treatment is to increase the effective heart rate and reestablish a higher pacing site such as the sinus node or A-V junction. Temporary pacemakers are often used to increase heart rate until the underlying problems that caused failure of the other pacing sites can be resolved.

An accelerated idioventricular rhythm occurs when a ventricular focus assumes control of the heart at a rate greater than its intrinsic rate of 40 per minute but less than 100 per minute. Although relatively benign in and of itself, this rhythm must be closely observed for any increase in rate or hemodynamic deterioration. Usually it is not treated if well tolerated.

Ventricular tachycardia. Ventricular tachycardia is caused by a ventricular pacing site's firing at a rate of 100 times or more per minute (Fig. 13-53). The complexes are wide, and the rhythm may be slightly irregular, often accelerating as the tachycardia continues (see Table 13-14). In most cases the sinus node is not affected, and it will continue to depolarize the atria on schedule. P waves can

Table 13-13 Classification of antidysrhythmic drugs

Class	Electrophysiological action	Examples
I	Membrane-stabilizing agents	
A	Moderate slowing of conduction	Quinidine
	Prolong repolarization	Procainamide
		Disopyramide
B	Shorten repolarization	Lidocaine
		Mexiletine
		Tocainide
		Phenytoin
C	Marked slowing of conduction	Encainide
		Flecainide
		Lorcainide
II	Beta-adrenergic blocking agents	Propranolol
		Atenolol
		Metoprolol
		Sotalol
III	Prolong repolarization	Amiodarone
		Sotalol
		Bretylium
IV	Calcium channel blockers	Verapamil
		Diltiazem

Modified from Platia E: Management of cardiac arrhythmias: the nonpharmacologic approach, Philadelphia, 1987, JB Lippincott Co.

Table 13-14 Ventricular rhythms

Parameter	Idioventricular rhythm	Accelerated idioventricular rhythm	Ventricular tachycardia
Rate	20-40/min	40-100/min	>100/min
Rhythm*	Usually regular	Usually regular	Usually regular
P waves	Absent or retrograde	Absent or retrograde	Absent or retrograde
PR interval	None	None	None
QRS	>0.12 sec	>0.12 sec	>0.12 sec

*See text for each type.

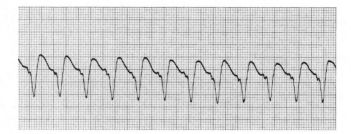

Fig. 13-53   Ventricular tachycardia.

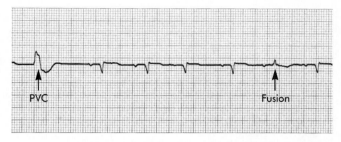

Fig. 13-54   Ventricular fusion beat *(arrows)*. The QRS duration is only 0.08 second, and the shape represents both the normal QRS and the previous PVC.

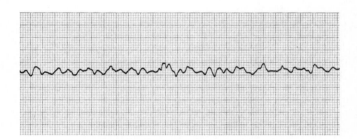

Fig. 13-55   Ventricular fibrillation.

sometimes be seen on the ECG tracing. They are not related to the QRS and may even conduct a normal impulse to the ventricles if their timing is just right. If the sinus impulse and the ventricular ectopic impulse meet in the middle of the ventricles, a fusion beat results. Fusion beats are narrower than the ventricular beats and look like a cross between the patient's sinus QRS and the ventricular QRS (Fig. 13-54). When present, P waves and fusion beats are helpful in verifying the diagnosis of ventricular tachycardia.

Ventricular tachycardia can occur acutely in a variety of clinical settings, including myocardial ischemia, digitalis toxicity, electrolyte disturbances, and an adverse reaction of certain antidysrhythmic drugs. Patients with chronic, severe heart disease such as cardiomyopathy or ventricular aneurysm may experience frequent episodes of ventricular tachycardia, which may be very difficult to treat even with the recent advances in antidysrhythmic drugs. Ventricular tachycardia is a serious dysrhythmia and must be treated quickly. Its rapid rate alone makes this dysrhythmia poorly tolerated. The benefit of the proper timing of atrial contraction, which would add volume to the ventricles just before contraction and enhance the force of contraction, is lost, thus greatly reducing cardiac output. The fall in cardiac output may cause the patient to lose consciousness. Finally, if not terminated quickly, ventricular tachycardia is very likely to degenerate into ventricular fibrillation and death.

Ventricular fibrillation. Ventricular fibrillation is the result of a rapid discharge of impulses from single or multiple foci in the ventricles, resulting in ventricles that are unable to respond completely and effectively. The ventricles merely quiver, and there is no forward flow of blood. Without forward flow, there will be no palpable pulse or audible apical heart tones. Clinically, ventricular fibrillation is indistinguishable from asystole (absence of electrical activity). On the ECG, ventricular fibrillation appears as a coarse wavy baseline (Fig. 13-55), whereas in asystole the baseline is flat.

Atrioventricular Conduction Disturbance

Normally, the sinoatrial (S-A) node triggers electrical depolarization in the heart. From there, the impulse travels through internodal tracts to the atrioventricular (A-V) node. The impulse is delayed in the A-V node to allow the atria to contract before the impulse is conducted to the bundle of His, bundle branches, and Purkinje fibers.

Clinically, the ability of the A-V node to conduct is evaluated by measuring the PR interval and the relationship of

P waves to QRS complexes (Table 13-15). The normal PR interval, measured from the beginning of the P wave to the beginning of the QRS complex, ranges from 0.12 to 0.20 second.

First degree A-V block. When all atrial impulses that should be conducted to the ventricles are conducted, but the PR interval is greater than 0.20 second, a condition known as first degree A-V block exists (Fig. 13-56). First degree A-V block is not clinically significant by itself, but in a patient with an acute myocardial infarction, it may be a forerunner of more severe conduction disturbances and deserves close monitoring.

Second degree A-V block. Second degree A-V block can be broadly defined as a condition in which one or more (but not all) atrial impulses that should be conducted fail to reach the ventricles. This very general description covers a wide variety of patterns with markedly variable clinical significance. Second degree A-V block can be divided into Mobitz type I (also known as Wenckebach), Mobitz type II, and high grade A-V blocks.

Mobitz type I. In Mobitz type I block, the A-V conduction time progressively lengthens until a P wave is not conducted. Mobitz I is caused by an abnormally long relative refractory period. The rate of conduction depends on the moment of impulse arrival: the earlier the impulse arrives in the A-V node, the longer it takes to conduct; the later it arrives, the shorter is the conduction time. Mobitz I second degree A-V block develops because each successive sinus impulse arrives earlier and earlier in the relative refractory period of the A-V node until one sinus impulse finally arrives during the absolute refractory period and fails to conduct.

Table 13-15   A-V block

Parameter	First degree	Second degree Mobitz I (Wenckebach)	Second degree Mobitz II	Third degree (complete)
PR interval	>0.20 second and constant	Increases with each consecutively conducted P wave	Constant	Varies randomly
P waves	1 P wave for each QRS	Intermittently not conducted, yielding more P waves than QRS complexes	Intermittently not conducted, yielding more P waves than QRS complexes	P waves independent and not related to QRS complexes
QRS	0.06-0.10 second	0.06-0.10 second	May be normal, but usually coexists with bundle branch block (>0.12)	0.06-0.10 second if junctional escape pacemaker activates the ventricles >0.12 if ventricular escape pacemaker activates the ventricles

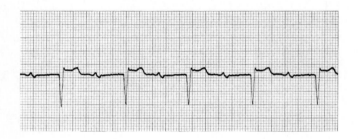

Fig. 13-56   First degree A-V block. The PR interval is prolonged to 0.44 second.

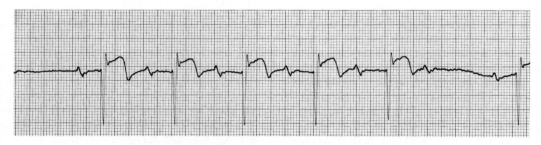

Fig. 13-57   Mobitz type I (Wenckebach) second degree A-V block. Note that the PR intervals gradually increase from 0.36 to 0.46 second until, finally, a P wave is not conducted to the ventricles.

On the ECG Mobitz type I A-V block can be distinguished by PR intervals that progressively lengthen until a P wave finally is not conducted and is therefore not followed by a QRS (Fig. 13-57). If four P waves are conducted to the ventricles and the fifth one is not, a 5:4 conduction ratio is present (five P waves to four QRS complexes). The PR interval lengthening is always greatest with the second beat of the cycle. The RR intervals become progressively shorter until the sinus P wave is not conducted. Following that pause, the cycle will repeat itself again. It is useful to look at the RP interval to determine the earliness of the sinus impulse arrival in the A-V node. The RP interval is measured from the beginning of the QRS to the beginning of the following P wave. As the RP interval decreases, the PR interval will increase, and vice versa. This phenomenon is known as *RP-PR reciprocity* and always indicates Mobitz type I block.[10]

In Mobitz type I block the actual anatomical site of the block is usually at the level of the A-V node itself. Usually, with an acute inferior wall infarction, the block is caused by ischemia and is transient. Still, the possibility of progression to a more serious conduction disturbance exists, warranting close observation and, occasionally, placement of a temporary pacemaker as a precautionary measure.

Mobitz type II. Mobitz type II block occurs in the presence of a long absolute refractory period with virtually no relative refractory period. This results in an "all or nothing" situation. Sinus P waves either will or will not be conducted. When conduction does occur, all PR intervals will be the same. There is no RP-PR reciprocity. Usually, Mobitz II indicates block below the A-V node, either in the His bundle or in both bundle branches. Most often, it occurs when one bundle branch is blocked and the other one is ischemic. Mobitz II block is more ominous clinically than Mobitz I

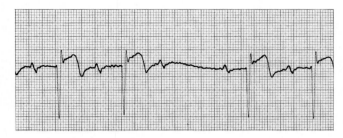

Fig. 13-58 Mobitz type II second degree A-V block. Note that the PR intervals remain constant.

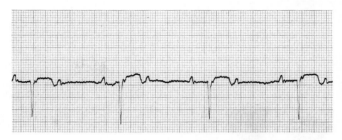

Fig. 13-59 2:1 A-V block. Since no two consecutive P waves are conducted, it is not possible to determine with certainty whether this is Mobitz I or Mobitz II second degree A-V block.

and often progresses to complete A-V block. On the ECG the PR interval is constant (Fig. 13-58). If consecutive P waves are conducted, the difference between Mobitz I and Mobitz II second degree A-V block is apparent: in Mobitz I the PR interval gradually lengthens until finally a P wave is not conducted or is missed; in Mobitz II the PR intervals remain exactly the same, but suddenly a normal P wave (not premature) fails to conduct.

Occasionally, only every other P wave is conducted through the A-V node (Fig. 13-59). This pattern could indicate either Mobitz I or II, since consecutive conduction of P waves, which would reveal either a lengthening or constant PR, does not occur. In Mobitz I the conduction ratios may have decreased from 4:3 to 3:2 to 2:1, yet the site and type of block has not changed. The change in conduction ratio may be caused by an increase in atrial rate, or it may change spontaneously.

In 2:1 conduction it is impossible to be certain whether the block is Mobitz type I or II from the surface ECG. If it occurs along with other Mobitz I ratios, it is probably still Mobitz I, and vice versa. If it is an isolated occurrence with no other strips for comparison, the QRS width and the PR interval offer valuable clues to the site of the block. In Mobitz I the QRS is usually normal, and the PR interval is prolonged. In Mobitz II the QRS is usually wide, and the PR interval is normal. Also, during an acute inferior myocardial infarction, type I 2:1 conduction is much more common than type II.[10]

High grade A-V block. High-grade or advanced A-V block is a form of second degree A-V block in which two or more consecutive atrial impulses fail to conduct through the A-V node. On the ECG several P waves will occur before each QRS, but the PR intervals of all of the P waves that are followed by a QRS will be the same. This is a very severe form of second degree A-V block that is often followed by complete heart block.

In making this diagnosis, two very important factors must be considered. First, the atrial rate must be reasonable— approximately 130 beats per minute or less. At high atrial rates, blocking of conduction at the level of the A-V node is normal; in fact, it is crucial to protect the ventricles from dangerously high rates. In atrial flutter, with an atrial rate of 300 per minute, there is often 4:1 conduction, which yields a ventricular response rate of 75 per minute. This is desirable and is not high-grade A-V block. Second, the

failure of conduction must be caused by the existing block itself and not by a junctional or ventricular escape beat, which fires first and prevents conduction. If the sinus rate is 50 per minute and a junctional focus is firing at a rate of 60 per minute, there will be many P waves that do not have an opportunity to conduct because they occur shortly after the junctional beat and find the A-V node or bundle branches still in the absolute refractory period. Marriott[36] has coined the term "block-acceleration dissociation" for this condition. It can occur during mild or nonexistent A-V block and yet can mimic complete A-V block if not examined closely.

Third degree A-V block. Third degree, or complete, A-V block is a condition in which no atrial impulses can conduct through the A-V node to cause ventricular depolarization. The opportunity for conduction is optimal, yet none occurs. Hopefully, a junctional or ventricular focus will depolarize spontaneously at its intrinsic rate of 20 to 40 beats per minute, and ventricular contraction will continue. If not, asystole occurs; there is no pulse, and death will result if intervention is not immediate.

On the ECG P waves will be present and usually occur at regular intervals. If a junctional focus is pacing the heart, normal QRSs will be present but will occur at a rate and timing interval totally independent of the P waves. The PR intervals will vary widely, since the P wave and QRS are not related to each other. If a ventricular focus is pacing the heart, the QRS complex will be wide and unrelated to the P waves (Fig. 13-60).

Clinically, the consequences of A-V block range from benign to life-threatening. First degree A-V block is seldom of immediate concern but bears close observation for progression of the conduction disturbance. Second degree Mobitz I (Wenckebach) is usually benign, especially during an acute ischemic episode. If hemodynamic compromise is present or deemed likely, a temporary pacemaker can be inserted prophylactically until the situation stabilizes or normal conduction is restored. Second degree Mobitz II is more serious and often precedes complete A-V block. Use of a temporary pacemaker is usually necessary, but its insertion can be elective if the patient remains hemodynamically stable. Complete heart block almost always requires use of a pacemaker. If the patient is hemodynamically unstable, an isoproterenol (Isuprel) drip or external pacemaker can be used to maintain an adequate ventricular rate until a temporary pacemaker can be inserted.

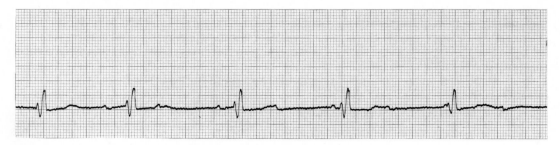

Fig. 13-60 Third degree (complete) heart block.

HOLTER MONITORING

Holter monitoring, also known as continuous ambulatory electrocardiography, is a technique that records the electrocardiogram (ECG) of patients while they perform their usual activities. The patient wears skin electrodes and carries a box very similar to a tape recorder, either with a shoulder strap or clipped to his belt or pocket. Usually the monitor is left on for 24 hours and then is returned to the hospital or clinic for reading. This is a totally noninvasive procedure with no immediate adverse effects.

When it was initially developed by Dr. Norman J. Holter more than 40 years ago, the equipment consisted of an 85-pound backpack with a short-range radio transmitter. The invention of the transistor in the 1950s reduced the recorder's weight to 6½ pounds, making it much more realistic for use on cardiac patients. As technology has improved, the recording devices have become even smaller so that at present a 4- × 6-inch recorder weighs less than 1 pound.

Indications

Holter monitors are widely used in a variety of clinical situations (see following box). Often transient symptoms

---

CLINICAL USES OF HOLTER MONITORING

Detection of supraventricular and ventricular dysrhythmias
  In patients at high risk for asymptomatic dysrhythmias
  For correlation of patient's symptoms with dysrhythmic occurrence
Detection of paroxysmal heart block
Evaluation of antidysrhythmic therapy
  Reveals decrease in frequency and/or severity of dysrhthmias with therapy
  Reveals increase in frequency and/or severity of dysrhythmias because of prodysrhythmic effect of some drugs
Detection of ST segment level or shape in patients with or without suspected ischemic heart disease
Evaluation of pacemaker function or dysfunction

Modified from Morganroth J: Ann Intern Med 102(1):73, 1985.

---

such as syncope, palpitations, or chest pain cannot be reproduced in the clinical or hospital setting, but through use of a Holter monitor designed to be worn in the patient's usual environment, documentation of dysrhythmias or ST segment changes can be correlated with symptoms. Patients with cardiac disease may be asymptomatic yet can have significant ventricular ectopy, which places them at a higher risk for sudden death. Holter monitors are useful in identifying these high-risk patients, quantifying the frequency of the dysrhythmias, and evaluating the response to antidysrhythmic agents once treatment has begun.

All Holter monitors record at least two leads, primarily to minimize inaccurate interpretation caused by artifact. Usually five electrodes are placed. Two of them are positive electrodes, corresponding approximately to the V_1 and V_5 positions on a standard 12-lead ECG. There are also two negative electrodes and one ground. Occasionally, additional electrodes are used to improve diagnostic capabilities. For example, a separate lead can be used to detect pacemaker spikes if the patient is being monitored for pacemaker dysfunction.[17] The skin electrodes are disposable, pregelled, and self-adhering. They should be kept dry—not because of any electrical danger, but to prevent their falling off before the recording is completed. If skin irritation or hypersensitivity occurs, it can usually be relieved with hydrocortisone cream. The recorder is battery powered and can use either a reel-to-reel or cassette magnetic tape. Reel-to-reel tapes have fewer technical problems and can provide a clearer recording, but cassette tapes are smaller and more convenient for the patient.

The use of Holter monitors is expected to increase significantly in the future. There is currently much interest in ambulatory monitoring for ST segment changes with or without chest pain. At present, these changes are not necessarily reliable indicators of ischemia. Nonischemic ST segment changes have been observed in some young people, people with mitral valve prolapse, and those with ST or T wave abnormalities on their baseline 12-lead ECG. In addition, studies on healthy individuals have shown that ST segments can vary with position and often correlate with autonomic changes such as eating, smoking, sleep, and defecation.[4] The use of multiple leads may decrease the risk of false-positive interpretations, and further clarification of the population groups in which this technique is not useful will add greatly to the reliability of Holter monitors in evaluation of ischemic heart disease.

Some dual-chamber pacemakers now have the ability to

transmit ECG tracings to an outside receiver, serving as a form of internal implantable Holter. In the near future, they may provide on-line diagnostic decisions, complete with early warning signals to alert the patient or physician to the problem.

Procedure

Many variations of Holter monitors exist, but at present they can be divided into three basic recording modes.[38] The first and most common is the continuous recording mode. In this mode the tape saves all of the ECG tracings for a given period of time, usually 8 to 24 hours. The tape can correlate time with the tracing and display the time that an event occurred when the tape is decoded. Most also have an event marker, which the patient can press to indicate the onset of symptoms or another event that may be important. The patient is asked to keep a diary of his or her activities, symptoms, and any medications that are taken.

When the tape is returned to the hospital or clinic for reading, a technician places it in a machine that displays the tracing for review. The tracing is run at a faster speed than normal, or it would take 24 hours to read a 24-hour recording, and the cost would be prohibitive. Usually the tape is run at 60 times normal speed, although various devices use speeds ranging from 30 to 480 times normal. Several techniques are used to aid the technician in interpretation of the tracing. One technique, audiovisual superimposition electrocardiographic presentation (AVSEP), places each QRS complex on top of the prior ones so that any that are abnormal stand out. R-to-R intervals are also measured by the machine, and a tone that varies in pitch, depending on the heart rate, is emitted. Using this system, a run of ventricular tachycardia would be both seen and heard by the technician.

Printed reports are also generated as the tape is read. Real-time printouts, at normal speed, can be run when any significant dysrhythmias are noted. A trend plot of heart rate, ST segment level, or number of ectopics can also be printed. Most decoding machines count ectopics automatically, but it is up to the operator to validate that the decoder is really counting ectopy and not artifact.

A second type of recording mode is the intermittent, or patient-activated, recording mode. In this mode, when the patient is having symptoms, he or she presses a button to initiate the recording manually. Some of the newer devices can transmit this recording telephonically to a diagnostic center. Advantages of this mode center around the ability to leave the recorder on the patient for longer periods of time. Patients with infrequent symptoms do not benefit from a 24-hour continuous recording if the symptoms do not occur during that time.[26] With the intermittent recorder mode, the device can be worn for up to 96 hours, and the patient can trigger active recording at the appropriate times. The disadvantage of this approach is that the ECG tracing just before the onset of symptoms will not be recorded, leaving the precipitating factors a mystery. Also, the patient must be able to trigger the device; if loss of consciousness occurs rapidly, this would not be possible, and the dysrhythmia would not be recorded. In addition, if the machine is used frequently by the patient in the initial hours of the recording or is left on by mistake, the memory may be full when an

important symptomatic event occurs, and no recording could be done.

Real-time analytical or event recording is the most recent recording mode development. A built-in computer analyzes the ECG as it is recorded and stores only abnormal patterns. The device weighs approximately twice as much as a standard Holter monitor because of the built-in computer. It also costs three to five times more, but this cost is offset by the decrease in man-hours needed for interpretation. This recording mode is very useful because the recorder can be used over a longer period of time (since the entire tracing is not stored) and interpretation is immediately available from the computer without needing an operator to decode it. Unfortunately, there are still some drawbacks. Accuracy is questionable since events the computer considered insignificant are not stored. This may be all right for general screening purposes but could be a problem if therapeutic decisions are based on the results. As with the patient-activated recorder, this device will no longer record when the memory is full. If for some reason the battery fails, all information can be lost.

Nursing Care

Nurses have a vital role in ensuring that patients receive maximal benefit from wearing a Holter monitor. A well-informed patient greatly enhances the quality of the recording.

Many patients' symptoms do not occur every day and may be missed during a random 24-hour recording. Often symptoms tend to occur in association with specific activities. The nurse should inquire about the types of activities that tend to provoke symptoms for a specific patient and encourage the patient to pursue those activities while wearing the monitor. In general, the patient should be encouraged to be as active as possible. Keeping an accurate diary of activities is important, since it allows correlation of an identified dysrhythmia with a specific activity or symptom. Examples of items that the patient should record include medications, meals, exercise, emotional stress, arguments, smoking, bowel movements, urination, sexual intercourse, and sleep periods. In addition, any symptoms such as palpitations, lightheadedness, or chest pressure should be recorded.

The only activities that are restricted while wearing a Holter monitor are those that would get the chest electrodes or monitor wet, eliminating swimming and taking a shower or tub bath. Sponge baths are permitted as long as the chest electrodes are avoided.

EXERCISE ELECTROCARDIOGRAPHY

Exercise places unique demands on the cardiovascular system. Systemic oxygen consumption increases markedly, requiring the heart to increase cardiac output to meet these demands. Myocardial contractility increases, resulting in greater stroke volume and systolic blood pressure. Heart rate is also increased as a result of circulating catecholamines. Normally, as heart rate and stroke volume rise, cardiac output is increased dramatically, and the tissue needs for oxygen are met. This enhanced myocardial performance is not without its price. Even at rest, the heart muscle extracts 70% of the oxygen available in the circulating blood.[8] When the myocardial demand for oxygen increases during exercise, coronary blood flow must increase to maintain an adequate oxygen supply. In patients with coronary artery disease, coronary blood flow is not able to increase sufficiently to provide the high metabolic needs of the myocardium during exercise, and ischemia will result.

Indications

Exercise tolerance testing, or stress testing, is clinically useful in several settings. It helps evaluate the presence, absence, or severity of coronary artery disease, both in patients with known coronary heart disease, as well as in those initially seen with chest pain of unclear origin. Stress testing can evaluate the functional capacity of patients with or without heart disease and can be done serially to evaluate the effectiveness of medical or surgical therapy.

Procedure

Originally exercise tests were conducted using a two-step platform that the patient climbed up and down repeatedly. This is called a Master's two-step exercise test and is still used in a few places because the cost of the equipment is minimal. The vast majority of exercise tests in the United States, however, are now performed using a treadmill on which both speed and slope can be varied. A number of protocols have been developed using a treadmill. All reach virtually the same end point, but they vary the speed with which they approach that end point. Two popular ones are the Bruce protocol, in which both grade and speed are varied every 3 minutes, and the Balke protocol, in which speed remains constant and grade is gradually increased every minute.

Regardless of the protocol used, the electrocardiogram (ECG) is printed at 1-minute intervals, as well as during any symptoms, visible ECG changes, or dysrhythmias. Blood pressure is also measured and recorded every minute.

The treadmill test is terminated whenever the patient requests that it be stopped, if symptoms such as chest pain, dyspnea, dizziness, or fatigue occur, if there are significant ECG changes or dysrhythmias, or if there is significant hypotension or hypertension. Blood pressure is expected to rise during exercise, but a systolic blood pressure >220 mm Hg or a diastolic blood pressure >110 mm Hg is considered high enough to stop the test.[8] If none of the above situations occur, the test is stopped when a desirable level, based on the patient's heart rate, is reached. A maximal stress test is one in which the predicted maximal heart rate for that patient is reached (Table 13-16). A goal of 85% to 90% of the predicted maximal heart rate is set for a submaximal test, and in most patients this level of exercise is sufficient to unmask any significant coronary artery disease.

A low-level stress test is sometimes performed before discharge from the hospital on patients who have suffered an acute myocardial infarction. In this case the heart rate is raised only to 120 or 130 beats per minute. Current results indicate that ST segment depression or elevation that occurs during the predischarge low-level stress test is a reliable indicator of additional myocardium at risk. However, exercise-induced angina or abnormal blood pressure re-

Table 13-16 Predicted maximal heart rates by age

Age	Maximal predicted heart rate
20	197
25	195
30	193
35	191
40	189
45	187
50	184
55	182
60	180
65	178
70	176
75	174
80	172
85	170

Modified from Chung E: Manual of exercise ECG testing, Stoneham, Mass, 1986, Butterworth Publisher.

sponses to exercise often do not appear during a low-level stress test, so a "normal" predischarge stress test must be followed later by a test closer to maximal level.[21]

Patient preparation. The exercise test can be performed on an outpatient or inpatient basis. In either case, a physician must be present to supervise the test directly. As with any diagnostic procedure with inherent risks, the patient must be fully informed and consent obtained. It would be ideal always to conduct the exercise test in the morning after an overnight fast, since, after eating, blood is diverted from the general circulation to the gastrointestinal tract, especially the stomach, to facilitate absorption of nutrients during the digestive process, making less blood available to the coronary and systemic circulation. Logistically, however, exercise tests must be performed throughout the day. Patients are advised to eat a light meal no closer than 3 hours before the test is scheduled. They should dress comfortably in light clothing and wear comfortable shoes for brisk walking or running.

A brief history and physical examination of the patient should be obtained before beginning the exercise test to identify any contraindications to performing the test and to document medications the patient is taking that might interfere with test results.

A 12-lead ECG is recorded at rest before beginning the exercise protocol, and another 12-lead ECG is usually recorded on completion of the test.

Various lead positions are used during the testing, depending on the number of leads that the equipment is able to monitor. Additional leads improve the accuracy of the test, since ischemia may be missed if there is not a lead monitoring that particular portion of the myocardial wall. Some institutions use a six-lead system, but most currently use three leads, usually II, V_3, and V_5. Lead II will detect ischemic changes in the inferior wall, lead V_3 will show ischemia in the anterior wall, and lead V_5 will reveal ischemia in the lateral wall. Skin preparation for electrode placement is of vital importance, since the recording will be meaningless if an electrode falls off during exercise. A blood pressure cuff is also placed on one arm to measure the blood pressure response to exercise.

Interpretation of results. Considerable controversy exists about interpretation criteria for exercise ECG. ST-segment depression, either horizontal or downsloping, of 1 mm or more during or after exercise is the most diagnostic of coronary artery disease. Other criteria that are strongly suggestive of a positive result are found in Table 13-17.

ST-segment elevation, although a rare finding, is usually indicative of myocardial wall motion abnormalities such as an aneurysm, especially in patients who have had a previous myocardial infarction, and may actually be a more serious finding than ST depression.[6]

The point at which the end of the QRS complex intersects with the baseline is known as the J point (Fig. 13-61, *A*). A certain amount of J-point depression (Fig. 13-61, *B*) is normal during exercise and is only considered indicative of ischemia if it is upsloping, greater than 2 mm below baseline, and greater than 0.08 second in duration.

Ventricular dysrhythmias are common in healthy individuals, especially at high levels of exercise. If they occur frequently at low levels or are multifocal or grouped, underlying heart disease is usually present.

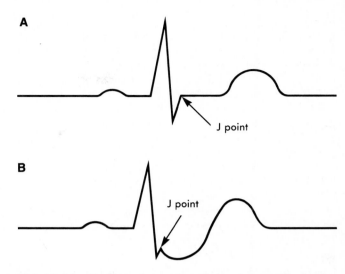

Fig. 13-61 **A,** Normal position of the J point. **B,** J-point depression.

Hypotension during exercise is defined as a drop in blood pressure of more than 10 mm Hg. Care must be taken to differentiate clinically significant hypotension from the physiologically normal drop in blood pressure that occurs during the first stage of exercise in an anxious patient. Pretest anxiety results in the release of excess catecholamines, which cause the blood pressure to rise before the test is begun. As exercise begins and the large blood vessels in the leg muscles dilate to increase blood flow, this elevated blood pressure will fall to normal. As exercise continues, however, an appropriate rise in systolic pressure should be expected. If the blood pressure falls as exercise increases, especially if accompanied by angina, ST-segment changes, or a drop in heart rate, the patient usually has severe three-vessel disease, global ischemia, and myocardial dysfunction.

Many dysrhythmias and ECG changes during exercise are insignificant (see the following box). Hyperventilation can also cause ST-segment depression as a result of changes in vasomotor tone, and when this occurs, it is actually ev-

Table 13-17 Criteria for positive exercise ECG test

Definitely positive	Strongly suggestive
Horizontal ST-segment depression of 1 mm or more during or after exercise	Horizontal or downsloping ST-segment depression of <1 mm during or after exercise
Downsloping ST-segment depression of 1 mm or more during or after exercise	Upsloping ST-segment depression of 2 mm or more beyond 0.08 sec from J point during or after exercise
	Horizontal or upsloping ST-segment elevation of 1 mm or more during or after exercise
	ST-segment sagging 1 mm or more during or after exercise
	Hypotension
	Inverted U wave
	Frequent premature ventricular contractions (PVCs), multifocal PVCs, grouped PVCs, ventricular tachycardia provoked by mild exercise (70% or less of maximal heart rate)
	Exercise-induced typical angina S₃, S₄, or heart murmur

INSIGNIFICANT EXERCISE ECG CHANGES

Occasional unifocal premature ventricular contractions (PVCs)
Atrial or junctional tachycardias
First degree or Wenckebach A-V block
Bundle branch block or hemiblock
Alteration of T wave shape
Alteration of P wave shape
J-point ST depression less than 2 mm
QT interval change
Prominent U waves

idence against coronary artery disease. To rule out hyperventilation as a potential cause of ST-segment depression, the ECG tracing should be recorded during a brief period of hyperventilation before the test is begun.

Many drugs can influence the results of an exercise ECG test. Two of the most important groups are digitalis-related preparations and beta blockers. Digitalis causes ST-segment depression at rest, which is accentuated with exercise, leading to a greater-than-average number of false-positive stress test results. In general, ST-segment depression of 4 to 5 mm almost always indicates ischemia. For those patients who experience mild ST-segment depression during exercise and who are also on digitalis, exercise test results will be inconclusive. Beta blockers have the opposite effect. Since beta blockers decrease heart rate, blood pressure, and vascular response to circulating catecholamines, these drugs also blunt the normal response to exercise. Consequently, patients on beta blockers can usually exercise longer and have less ST-segment depression, increasing the likelihood of a false-negative test result. Whenever possible, beta blockers are withdrawn for 2 days before the scheduled exercise test. The decision to withdraw the patient from beta blocker therapy should be made only after careful evaluation of the patient's clinical status, current dose of beta blockers, and the original reason for therapy.

Unfortunately, both false-positive and false-negative exercise ECG interpretations occur. False-positive results are high in asymptomatic healthy individuals. The incidence of false-positive results is especially high in asymptomatic middle-aged women. As discussed previously, hyperventilation can cause false ST-segment depression, as can mitral valve prolapse syndrome, Wolff-Parkinson-White syndrome, and digitalis therapy.

False-negative results may be caused by early termination of the test for other reasons such as fatigue or claudication before the level of imbalance between oxygen supply and myocardial demand is reached. Overly strict diagnostic criteria can cause real disease to be missed. The lead system used can result in certain areas of the myocardium not being represented, and ischemia in those areas will be missed. Antianginal drug therapy can also mask ischemia. False-negative results become less likely as the extent of disease increases (Table 13-18).

Recent advances in test interpretation. Recently, work has been done using the ST segment/heart rate slope to improve accuracy of the exercise tolerance test.[28] This technique normalizes the amount of ST-segment depression during exercise for changes in heart rate. The specificity reported with this technique is greater than 90%, with a sensitivity of 91%. This method also claims the ability to separate patients into categories of one-vessel, two-vessel, and three-vessel coronary artery disease. Since this is a relatively new approach to exercise ECG interpretation, more research is needed to determine in which patient populations this method is reliable and in which groups it is not.

If a false-positive or false-negative result is suspected, exercise testing can be combined with thallium imaging for more definitive results.

Complications and contraindications. Complications

Table 13-18 Correlation of positive exercise ECG tests with location of coronary artery disease

Location of obstruction (>75% stenosis)	Incidence of positive exercise tolerance testing (%)
Single-vessel disease	
Right coronary artery	44
Left circumflex artery	44
Left anterior descending artery	77
Two-vessel disease	91
Three-vessel disease	100

From Chung K: Manual of exercise ECG testing, Stoneham, Mass, 1986, Butterworth Publishers.

are rare during exercise testing, but they do occur. The mortality rate is 0.01% (1:10,000). Morbidity is 0.02% (2.4:10,000) and includes such adverse outcomes as myocardial infarction, cardiac arrest, and sustained ventricular tachycardia.[8] Cardiopulmonary resuscitation equipment must be readily available whenever exercise testing is done.

Contraindications to exercise testing can be divided into cardiac and noncardiac problems. Cardiac contraindications include acute myocardial infarction, acute congestive heart failure, cardiogenic shock, unstable angina (as opposed to stable angina), severe aortic stenosis, and digitalis toxicity with its inherent increased risk of life-threatening dysrhythmias. Noncardiac contraindications include fever, acute illness such as hepatitis, renal failure, or pneumonia, pulmonary emboli, or severe physical disability.

Nursing Care

Many patients are anxious about undergoing exercise testing, and the anxiety is often multifactorial. Patients without known heart disease may be afraid that they will "fail" the test, find they have heart disease, and perhaps need open heart surgery. If the patient generally follows a sedentary lifestyle, anxiety may be caused by the fear of "collapsing" on the treadmill or spending several days recovering from exhaustion. Some are afraid that they will be forced to go beyond their endurance. Often, low-level exercise testing is performed before discharge on patients who have been hospitalized for an acute myocardial infarction. These patients may be afraid that the strain on their heart is too great or that they will die during the test.

Proper patient teaching can do much to allay these fears. In addition to describing the procedure itself, the nurse should instruct the patient to fast for 3 hours before the test, refrain from smoking for at least 2 hours before the test, and wear comfortable shoes and loose-fitting clothes. The patient should be reassured that his or her heart will be monitored closely during the test and a physician will be standing by. Although the patient will be encouraged to continue as long as possible, the test will be stopped at the patient's request for symptoms such as fatigue, shortness of breath, or leg cramps. In addition, the staff will stop the test for significant ECG changes, blood pressure changes, or development of angina. The patient should also be told that the diagnostic value of the test is based on the maximal heart rate achieved, not on the length of time that he or she is able to remain on the treadmill. A well-trained athlete might be able to stay on the treadmill for 15 minutes, whereas an elderly or sedentary person may only last 3 to 5 minutes; yet if 85% of the predicted maximal heart rate is achieved, both tests will have been equally diagnostic.

After the exercise test is completed, the patient will be assisted into a supine position. The ECG, pulse rate, and blood pressure will be monitored for at least 10 more minutes to detect dysrhythmias or signs of ischemia. The patient should be instructed to rest for the next 30 to 60 minutes after release from the exercise laboratory. Hot showers should be avoided for 3 to 4 hours to prevent development of orthostatic hypotension.

The nurse performing the test must be certain that emergency medications and a defibrillator are available in the test area and should be familiar with their use.

VECTORCARDIOGRAPHY
Indications

The main advantage of vectorcardiography is that the spread of depolarization through the ventricles can be analyzed very accurately. When this analysis is performed by comptuer, myocardial infarction can be detected more accurately than is possible from a standard 12-lead electrocardiogram (ECG) alone.[11] Vectorcardiograms are also useful in the diagnosis of ventricular hypertrophies and conduction defects such as bundle branch block and hemiblocks.

Procedure

The heart, like any other organ in the body, is three dimensional. As electrical events occur in the myocardium, the current flows simultaneously in many directions. The standard 12-lead ECG records only a single axis, or direction of current flow, in any one lead. Specifically, each positive electrode senses electrical activity either coming toward or traveling away from it. Current traveling toward the positive electrode results in a positive or upright deflection from baseline. Current traveling away from the positive electrode transcribes a negative or downward deflection.

More information about the pathway of electrical activity in the heart could be obtained from recording the electrical events in two perpendicular axes simultaneously. Vectorcardiography does this by recording loops on an oscilloscope screen. Three planes can be recorded, and each plane is composed of two axes. The frontal plane loop represents electrical activity in the right-to-left (X) axis and the head-to-foot (Y) axis. The sagittal plane loop visualizes the head-to-foot (Y) axis and the anterior-posterior (Z) axis. The horizontal loop represents the right-to-left (X) axis and the anterior-posterior (Z) axis. Actually, using any two planes provides information about all three axes, but it is helpful to use the third plane to check the accuracy of the other two.

For several reasons it is difficult to record accurately the electrical activity in the heart from body surface electrodes. The heart is not centrally located in the chest, and the human torso resembles a cylinder rather than a sphere. This means that various electrodes, no matter how carefully placed, will always be at varying distances from the heart. To make matters worse, body tissues differ in their ability to conduct electricity. Standard 12-lead electrocardiography ignores these problems. The hexaxial reference system, commonly used to plot axis from a 12-lead ECG, assumes that the heart is at the center of the chest with all electrodes equidistant from it, but this is not a valid assumption. To compensate as much as possible for these deficiencies, "corrected" orthogonal lead systems have been developed for recording vectorcardiograms. None of these lead systems is perfect. The Frank and Schmitt systems are most popular at present, but many different ones exist, resulting in a lack of standardization.[27]

In the Frank system seven electrodes are placed at specific locations. A beam, interrupted at a rate of 500 cycles per second, is displayed on an oscilloscope. The result is a series of dashes, each with a head and tail to indicate the direction that the beam is traveling. Each loop is superimposed on top of the previous loop. A sudden change in conduction such as occurs with a premature ventricular contraction is readily apparent since the "ectopic" loop does not match previous loops.

The complete cardiac cycle is represented on the vectorcardiogram by three loops, which correspond to the familiar wave forms on the standard ECG. Depolarization of the atria results in a small "P" loop. The "QRS" loop represents ventricular depolarization and is much larger. Ventricular repolarization inscribes a "T" loop, which is smaller than the QRS loop but larger than the P loop, similar to the conventional ECG. Intervals during which there is no electrical activity (for example, the PR interval, ST segment, and TP interval on the standard ECG) will cause the beam to remain stationary and will not be seen on the vectorcardiogram, thus severely limiting the value of vectorcardiography in dysrhythmia interpretation.

Despite the improved accuracy of vectorcardiography, it is rarely used clinically for several reasons. There is no standard lead system as yet, criteria for "normal" loops has not been completely established, and the equipment is expensive, especially if a computer is used for interpretation. Lead placement is awkward for continuous monitoring, and there is no printout of the loops for documentation— photographs must be taken if a permanent record is desired. At present, vectorcardiography is most useful as a teaching tool and as an aid to understanding the intricacies of the standard 12-lead ECG.

Nursing Care

The procedure for obtaining a vectorcardiogram is very similar to the procedure for obtaining a 12-lead ECG. The patient should be told that additional electrodes will be placed, including some on his or her back. The electrodes will remain in place only while the recording is taken. The procedure does not cause any discomfort. The patient should relax and lie still, since any muscle movement can interfere with the quality of the recording.

PHONOCARDIOGRAPHY
Indications

With practice, normal heart sounds can be heard quite clearly with a stethoscope, but low frequency sounds such as an S_4 or a soft murmur can be more difficult to identify, especially if the patient has a tachycardia. Abnormal sounds may be too rapid or subtle for discernment by the senses. A sound recording, or phonocardiogram, permits accurate timing of sounds and events and can reveal information about underlying hemodynamic events that is not obtainable through the physical examination alone. For example, the width of an S_2 split can be used as an index of severity in pulmonic stenosis.[62] The phonocardiogram can point out abnormalities of valve function or wall structure (such as idiopathic hypertrophic subaortic stenosis) and can actually improve results from subsequent cardiac catheterization by targeting specific areas for closer study.

Another advantage of a phonocardiogram over simple auscultation is that it provides a permanent, objective record of events. Subsequent comparisons can be made to evaluate progression of valvular dysfunction or to measure the degree of improvement after therapeutic interventions.

Phonocardiography can be combined with echocardiography to yield more information than either technique alone. The echocardiogram provides a time-frame reference for the phonocardiogram, allowing identification of sound components by their relationship to certain defined valvular motions (Fig. 13-62). At the same time, the phonocardiogram provides reference points for the echocardiogram, which improves the timing of certain phases of the cardiac cycle. The second heart sound, which represents the end of systole, is used most often in this regard. In aortic stenosis, the marked leaflet distortion prevents accurate estimates of the severity of obstruction by echocardiography alone. The phonocardiogram can provide an independent assessment of severity and can also follow the serial progression of the stenosis to help determine proper timing of intervention.

Several studies have been done using the phonocardiogram to correlate electrical and mechanical events in the heart. Inferences are then made regarding left-ventricular

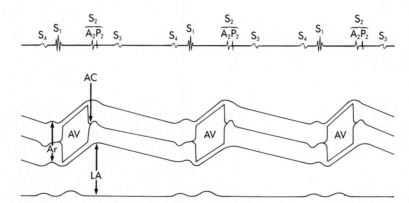

Fig. 13-62 Schematic drawing of a phonocardiogram and an echocardiogram at the aortic valve performed simultaneously; the sounds can be correlated with the actual valve motion. *Ar,* Aortic root, *AV,* aortic valve in open position, *LA,* left atrium, *AC,* aortic valve in closed position.

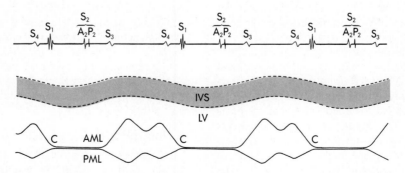

Fig. 13-63 Schematic drawing of a phonocardiogram and an echocardiogram at the mitral valve performed simultaneously. The C point on the echocardiogram occurs with the closing of the mitral valve and represents the onset of systole. The aortic component of the second heart sound (A_2) occurs with the closing of the aortic valve and represents the end of systole. *AML,* Anterior mitral leaflet, *PML,* posterior mitral leaflet, *C,* closure of the mitral valve, *LV,* left ventricle, *IVS,* interventricular septum.

filling pressures and hemodynamics. The C point represents mitral valve closure on the echocardiogram and corresponds to the onset of systole (Fig. 13-63). The aortic component of the second sound on the phonocardiogram represents the end of systole. The distance between these two points indicates the duration of systole and can be used to estimate left-atrial pressures noninvasively. This technique can be used clinically to determine which patient needs invasive pulmonary artery pressure monitoring. It can also replace pulmonary artery pressure monitoring in these patients for whom a high degree of accuracy is not critical.

Another technique that is being evaluated is continuous electrocardiogram (ECG) and phonocardiogram recording in critically ill patients. The distance from the R wave on the ECG to S_1 on the phonocardiogram is measured and recorded, as is the distance from the R wave to S_2. The proposed theory is that the time from electrical stimulation to mechanical activation will lengthen with myocardial dysfunction and an impending crisis will be detected sooner with this method than with current hemodynamic monitoring, which relies on rising pressures after ventricular failure has already begun.[60]

By far the greatest value of phonocardiography at present is as a tool for teaching auscultation. After studying a phonocardiographic recording of a patient's heart sounds, students can return to the bedside and visualize each sound in their mind's eye. With practice, the ability to separate distinct sounds and quantify murmurs improves. Eventually, expert bedside auscultation replaces the need for the phonocardiogram except in rare instances.

Procedure

Phonocardiography is the graphic display on paper of the sounds that occur in the heart and great vessels. The sounds are recorded from a transducer placed on the surface of the chest wall. The recording corresponds to the sounds heard during cardiac auscultation with a stethoscope.

Nursing Care

Patient teaching is important in relieving anxiety and eliciting cooperation. A quiet environment is desirable for proper recording of a phonocardiogram, since the equipment is very sensitive to sound waves. Several small microphones are placed on the patient's chest. In males, small areas of the chest may need to be shaved to improve skin contact with the microphones. The procedure is not uncomfortable and is usually completed in less than 20 minutes. When combined with echocardiography, which is often the case, the entire procedure may take as long as 45 minutes to 1 hour.

ECHOCARDIOGRAPHY
Indications

Echocardiography is used to detect cardiac abnormalities such as mitral valve stenosis and regurgitation, prolapse of mitral valve leaflets, aortic stenosis and insufficiency, idiopathic hypertrophic subaortic stenosis, atrial septal defects, and pericardial effusions. Recent developments also allow detection of wall-motion abnormalities, estimation of

ejection fraction and pulmonary artery pressures, and identification of intracardiac myomas. In the future, echocardiography may be able to detect and quantify coronary artery disease.

Procedure

Echocardiography uses waves of ultrasound to obtain and display images of cardiac structures. Normal human hearing occurs at a sound frequency of 20 to 20,000 cycles per second (hertz). Ultrasound uses sound frequencies greater than 20,000 hertz (Hz). When used to image cardiac structures, the best results are achieved using 1.5 to 5 million hertz (mHz). Usually 2.25 mHz are used with adults to allow optimal depth penetration, whereas 3 to 5 mHz are used in pediatrics to provide a clearer image of the smaller structures.[38]

While the test is performed, the patient is in either a supine, left-lateral, or semi-Fowler's position. Which position is used depends on the patient's clinical condition and on which position provides the best view of the structures examined. A transducer is placed on the skin, with lubricant between the transducer and the skin to improve contact and reduce artifact. The active element in the transducer is a piezoelectric crystal. *Piezoelectric* refers to the ability to transform electrical energy into mechanical (in this case, sound) energy, and vice versa. The transducer emits ultrasound waves and receives a signal from the reflected sound waves. Periods of sound transmission alternate with periods of sound reception.

Ultrasonic waves do not travel through air very well, and they are unable to penetrate very dense structures such as bone; hence, in adults, the transducer is usually placed in the third or fourth intercostal space to the left of the sternum, since at that point the pericardium is in direct contact with the chest wall and the ultrasonic waves are not obstructed by either air or bone. Other positions are sometimes used if the standard location does not provide adequate visualization of the cardiac structures.

Ultrasound is reflected best at interfaces between tissues that have different densities. In the heart these are the blood, cardiac valves, myocardium, and pericardium. Since all these structures differ in density, their borders can be seen on the echocardiogram. In one type of echocardiography, a thin beam of ultrasound is directed through the heart (Fig. 13-64). Each interface is represented by a dot, and when recorded over time (like an ECG), each dot becomes a line on an oscilloscope. A strip-chart recording can be made of this tracing as the heart beats. Since this is a recording of heart motion over time, this technique is called an *M-mode* (motion-mode) echocardiogram. A typical M-mode echo is shown in Fig. 13-65.

M-mode echocardiogram. The M-mode echocardiogram is particularly useful for measuring cardiac wall thickness and chamber size, evaluating valve motion, and assessing contractile motion of certain portions of the heart wall. It provides a good view of the anterior interventricular septum, the left-ventricular posterior wall from the base to the midportion, the aortic and mitral valves, and the left atrium. Areas that cannot be studied include the apex, lateral or free wall segments, and the true posterior and inferior wall of

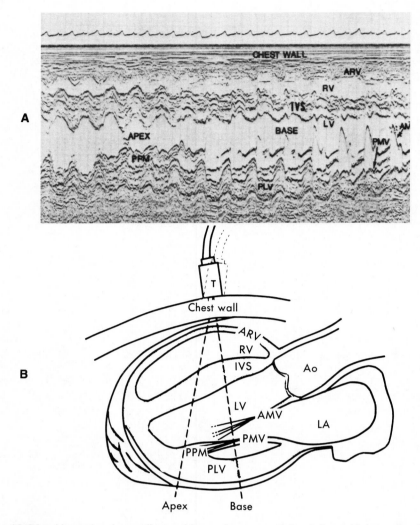

Fig. 13-64 Normal echocardiographic sector scan of the left ventricle and schematic presentation of the cardiac structures traversed by two echo beams. During ejection, the left septal and left posterior ventricular wall echos move toward the center of the ventricular cavity. *AMV*, Anterior mitral valve leaflet, *AO*, aorta, *ARV*, anterior right ventricular wall, *IVS*, interventricular septum, *LA*, left atrium, *LV*, left ventricle, *PLV*, posterior left ventricular wall, *PMV*, posterior mitral valve leaflet, *RV*, right ventricle, *PPM*, posterior papillary muscle, *T*, transducer. (From Corya BC: Cardiovasc Clin 2:113, 1975.)

the left ventricle. Since all portions of the ventricular wall cannot be examined, it is difficult to determine the size of dyskinetic areas using this technique. Aneurysms are also hard to diagnose, depending on their location. If the heart muscle is contracting uniformly throughout, estimates of left-ventricular function are quite accurate. However, if wall-motion abnormalities exist, this estimate of cardiac output will be unreliable. Estimates of left-ventricular size and function are also unreliable if significant aortic regurgitation is present. Since this is a one-dimensional technique, spatial relationships between structures cannot be appreciated.

Two-dimensional echocardiogram. Other techniques have been developed over the past several years to improve

the accuracy of echocardiograms. One popular technique is the two-dimensional (2-D) echocardiogram. It uses numerous crystals in the transducer to create a cross-sectional imaging plane. Sections of the heart are then viewed from a number of different angles (Fig. 13-66). The picture is displayed on an oscilloscope, and photographs are taken to serve as a permanent record. Since there are no timing markers built into this technique, it is less accurate in measuring stroke volume when the rhythm is irregular and in detecting constrictive pericarditis and tamponade.[38] In many other ways it is superior to the M-mode echocardiogram. The 2-D echocardiogram provides better quantification of valvular stenosis and a greater ability to detect ventricular aneurysms. Because a whole "slice" of the heart is seen at

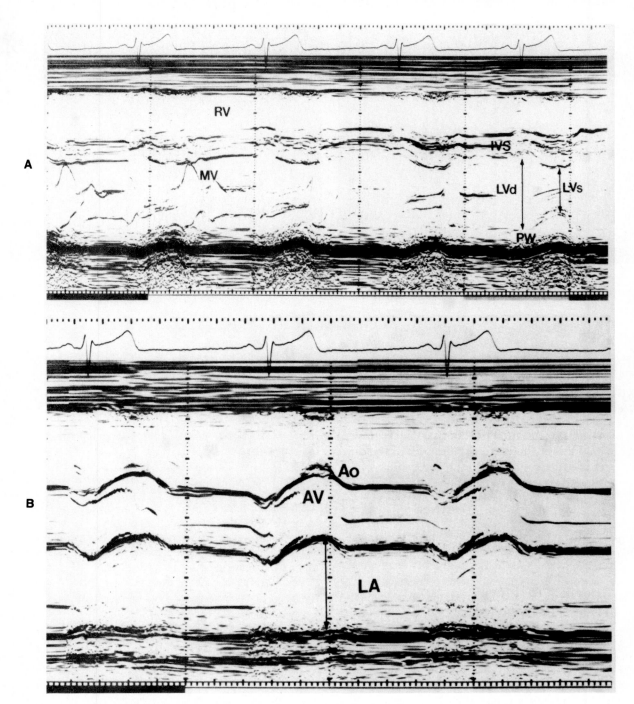

Fig. 13-65 **A,** M-mode echocardiogram. The M-shaped wave in the center is made by movement of the mitral valve. **B,** Normal M-mode echocardiogram at the level of the aorta *(Ao),* aortic valve *(AV)* leaflets, and left atrium *(LA). IVS,* interventricular septum, *LVd,* left ventricular diastolic dimensions, *LVs,* left ventricular systolic dimensions, *PW,* posterior wall, *RV,* right ventricle, *MV,* mitral valve. (From Andreoli K and others: Comprehensive cardiac care, ed 6, St Louis, 1987, The CV Mosby Co.)

once, the location of various structures in relationship to the rest of the heart is better appreciated, and the size of dyskinetic wall segments can be determined.

Several studies have shown that wall-motion abnormalities can be detected in nearly all patients within 4 hours after an acute myocardial infarction and the extent of muscle dysfunction is highly predictive of later complications.[45] When wall-motion abnormalities exceed 20% of the size of the left ventricle, there is a substantial rise in in-hospital complications.[29] Based on this information, the performance

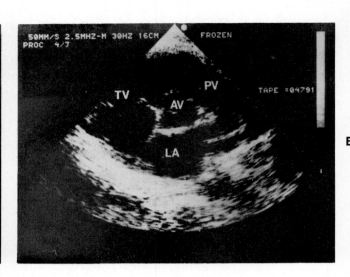

Fig. 13-66 2-D echocardiogram. Note that several sections of the heart can be viewed at one time, and it is easier to see the relationship of the chambers to one another. Abbreviations are as in Figure 13-65, plus *RA*, right atrium, *TV*, tricuspid valve, *LV*, left ventricle. (From Andreoli K and others: Comprehensive cardiac care, ed 6, St Louis, 1987, The CV Mosby Co.)

of an echocardiogram on all patients being evaluated for chest pain could help identify those patients who are likely to have had a myocardial infarction or who are at risk for complications and could benefit from admission to a coronary care unit.

Before the development of echocardiography, intracardiac myomas could be found only with angiography. M-mode echocardiograms could identify some intracardiac masses but could not define them clearly enough to differentiate myomas from clots or vegetations. Currently, the 2-D echocardiogram is able to locate and identify intracardiac masses and differentiate myomas from other causes of an intracardiac mass.

Doppler echocardiography. Doppler echocardiography provides a special kind of echocardiogram that assesses blood flow. It uses a pulsed or continuous wave of ultrasound that records frequency shifts of reflected sound waves, showing velocity and direction of blood flow relative to the transducer. Doppler echocardiography is especially useful in patients with valvular heart disease. Both regurgitation and stenosis can be detected and estimates made of their severity. When compared to cardiac catheterization results, Doppler echocardiography has been shown to predict accurately the pressure gradient across the affected valve.[51] When multiple valves are involved, the Doppler technique can clarify the extent of damage to the individual valves. Prosthetic valve function can also be evaluated, although this is best done in combination with phonocardiography since dysrhythmias or conduction disturbances can produce motion patterns that could mimic valve malfunction on the echocardiogram alone.[37] Other uses for Doppler echocardiography include evaluation of congenital anomalies, especially shunts and atresias, measurement of volume flow, and assessment of cardiac output. By measuring flow velocity in the right-ventricular outflow tract, mean pulmonary artery pressure can be estimated with a high degree of reliability.[40]

Recently, Doppler signals have become available in color. Known as color flow mapping or imaging, this technique analyzes Doppler signals from multiple intracardiac sites simultaneously. The Doppler tracing for each site is displayed in a color-coded format superimposed on a real-time 2-D echocardiographic image. Flow toward the transducer is displayed in one color, while flow away from the transducer is displayed in a contrasting color. The brightness of the color is varied to signify varying flow velocities.

Research is being conducted to determine if echocardiography can be used to detect lesions in the coronary arteries. Contrast dye can be injected into the coronary arteries while the echocardiogram is being done, revealing underperfused areas. This technique is still under investigation. Even without contrast, high-intensity echocardiograms can identify lesions in the walls of the left main and left anterior descending coronary arteries when significant obstruction is present. Compared to findings on cardiac catheterization, this technique yields 98% sensitivity and 67% specificity.[50] This could become a practical means of screening patients for left main coronary artery disease.

Nursing Care

The echocardiograph can be brought to the bedside if necessary, but whenever possible the patient should be transported to the echocardiography laboratory. The room will be somewhat dark to improve the visual clarity of the images displayed on the screen. Lubricant is placed on the patient's chest, and a transducer is placed in various positions to visualize cardiac and valvular structures. The procedure is not uncomfortable, but it may be tiresome for certain patients because of the length of the procedure, which is usually 30 to 60 minutes.

NUCLEAR MAGNETIC RESONANCE

Nuclear magnetic resonance (NMR) is a noninvasive imaging technique that can obtain specific biochemical information from body tissue without the use of ionizing radiation. The procedure does not present any known hazard to living cells. In many respects, the image created is superior to both x-ray film and ultrasonography because bone does not interfere with magnetic resonance imaging.

Indications

Currently, cardiac magnetic resonance imaging can provide information about tissue integrity, wall-motion abnormalities and aneurysms, ejection fraction,[63] cardiac output, and patency of proximal coronary arteries.[48] In a recent study of 22 patients, the ejection fraction calculated from magnetic resonance imaging had an excellent linear correlation with the ejection fraction determined by left-ventricular angiography ($r = 0.95$).[61] At present, however, the drawbacks to magnetic resonance imaging outweigh its advantages for most patients (Table 13-19), and it is currently not competitive with echocardiography and angiography.

Blood that is actively flowing does not emit a magnetic resonance signal; thus it provides a natural dark contrast material in the lumen of proximal coronary arteries. As a result, abnormalities of lumen size such as narrowing, which may provide evidence of obstruction, can be visualized.[48]

Procedure

The method by which NMR scanning is performed is quite complex, but the basic concept is fairly simple. Certain atoms within molecules act as tiny bar magnets with north and south poles. The nuclei spin around this axis like a spinning top. Under normal conditions these small atomic magnets are arranged at random. If a patient is placed within a strong magnetic field, many of the nuclei line up in the same direction as the magnetic force. When a radio frequency wave is sent, some of the nuclei absorb this energy, causing them to fall out of alignment and wobble like a gyroscope that is winding down. This "wobbling" out of alignment is termed *resonance*. The process of returning to alignment with the magnetic field after the radio frequency signal is turned off is called *relaxation*. These energy changes can be detected and recorded by the scanner.

Each type of atom has its own unique resonance and relaxation pattern. The easiest one to record at present is the hydrogen ion, although other atoms such as phosphorus, sodium, and carbon are also being studied. Since there are two hydrogen ions per molecule of water, magnetic resonance imaging is especially sensitive to changes in tissue water content. Myocardial ischemic injury results in predictable increases in regional myocardial water content,[9] allowing differentiation between normal and ischemic tissue. Infarction leading to myocardial scarring will result in tissue with a decreased water content, which can be identified on a magnetic resonance scan as an area of decreased signal intensity.

Magnetic resonance imaging works well for structures that have little or no motion such as the brain. Cardiac applications have been limited because of the constant motion of the heart. In an attempt to overcome this limitation, various gating or slicing techniques have been used in attempts to time the images at exact phases of the cardiac cycle. The gating can be timed from the R wave of the ECG or from the arterial pulse tracing.[48] Either method is satisfactory as long as the patient is in normal sinus rhythm. With any irregularity of the rhythm, the gating technique becomes much less helpful.

Nursing Care

Magnetic resonance imaging is actually a very safe procedure. The main hazard is related to the presence of other metal substances in the environment. Since the magnetism used is approximately 40,000 times stronger than the magnetic field of the earth, metal objects such as intravenous (IV) poles or oxygen tanks can become projectiles if they come close enough to the magnet's pull. To avoid this, adequate security around the scanner is important, and many facilities use a metal detector to screen for metal objects on all people entering the area.

Many patients have implanted metallic devices that have caused concern in the past. Laakman and others[31] tested 236 patients who had metallic implants and developed some guidelines about which implants are safe and which are not

Table 13-19 Advantages and limitations of cardiac nuclear magnetic resonance imaging

Advantages	Limitations
Entirely noninvasive	Time-consuming
Does not involve ionizing radiation	Accurate gating limited to patients in normal sinus rhythm
Provides images in multiple planes with uniformly good resolution	Not widely available
	Expensive
Provides information about tissue characterization and blood flow	Cannot be used on critically ill patients because of access and equipment problems

From Stratemeier E and others: Ejection fraction determination by MR imaging: comparison with LV angiography, Radiology 158:775, 1986.

Table 13-20 Metallic implants in nuclear magnetic resonance imaging

Safe	Unsafe
Metallic orthopedic devices	Cardiac pacemaker
Surgical wires	Other electrical stimulating devices
Surgical clips	Aneurysm clips
Skin staples	Unknown types of metal implants in potentially dangerous areas of the body
Central nervous system shunting devices	
Tantalum mesh	

From Laakman R and others: Imaging in patients with metallic implants, Radiology 157:711, 1985.

(Table 13-20). Basically, wearing a cardiac pacemaker is not safe because it may turn off or switch modes when exposed to a strong external magnetic field. Aneurysm clips are composed of ferromagnetic materials and could experience significant torque when exposed to the magnetic field.

BEDSIDE HEMODYNAMIC MONITORING

Invasive hemodynamic monitoring has become one of the major skill areas necessary for the critical care nurse. Using invasive catheters and sophisticated monitors, the nurse evaluates a patient's cardiac function, circulating blood volume, and physiological response to treatment. Often, the inexperienced clinician in critical care, feeling overwhelmed by all of the machines, focuses intently on the numbers these monitors produce, but with experience, the critical care nurse concentrates on the patient and follows hemodynamic trends.[2] Knowledge of hemodynamic monitoring will assist the clinician in developing decision-making skills to move beyond recording vital signs to interpretation and

Table 13-21 Integration of nursing and medical diagnosis: alteration in cardiac output

Nursing diagnostic label	Pathophysiology	Impact on hemodynamic function	Medical diagnosis
Decreased cardiac output	Acute heart muscle damage	Decreased contractility Increased preload Decreased or increased heart rate	Acute myocardial infarction
	Chronic heart muscle damage	Decreased contractility Increased preload Decreased or increased heart rate	Aortic or mitral valve disease Cardiomyopathy (dilated)

	Decreased venous return and compression of heart chambers	Decreased preload
		Decreased contractility
		Equalization of intracardiac pressures
			Cardiac tamponade
			  Trauma
			  Aortic dissection into the pericardium
			  After open heart surgery
			  Effusion (pericardial)
			  Cardiomyopathy (restrictive)

	Increased left-ventricular workload with increased systemic vascular resistance	Increased afterload	Hypothermia after cardiopulmonary bypass/open heart surgery Septic shock (late) Coarctation of the aorta
	Increased left-ventricular workload with normal systemic vascular resistance	Increased contractility Normal systemic vascular resistance	Aortic stenosis Cardiomyopathy (hypertrophic)
	Increased right-ventricular workload	Increased pulmonary vascular resistance	Idiopathic pulmonary hypertension Chronic obstructive pulmonary disease Congenital heart disease (with right-to-left shunt)

	Decreased circulating blood volume	Decreased preload
		Increased heart rate
		Increased afterload
			Bleeding
			  Traumatic injury
			  After surgery
			  Coagulopathy
			  Internal bleeding (occult)

		Decreased heart rate	Bradycardia
			  Three degree heart block
			  Idioventricular rhythm
			  Myocardial infarction

	Decreased diastolic filling time with decreased stroke volume	Increased heart rate
		Decreased preload
			Tachycardia
			  Paroxysmal atrial tachycardia
			  Ventricular tachycardia

	Loss of heart rhythm	Cardiac arrest	Ventricular tachycardia Ventricular fibrillation Asystole
Increased cardiac output	Vasodilation	Decreased afterload Decreased preload Increased heart rate	Rewarming after open heart surgery Septic shock (early) Use of inotropic/vasodilator therapy

analysis of that information to formulate a nursing plan of care appropriate for the individual patient.

Indications for Hemodynamic Monitoring

The range of medical diagnoses for which hemodynamic monitoring can be used is enormous. All of these medical diagnoses are linked by two principal nursing diagnoses: (1) potential or actual alteration in cardiac output, and (2) potential or actual alteration in fluid volume. These nursing diagnoses are based on pathophysiological processes that alter one of the four hemodynamic mechanisms that support normal cardiovascular function: preload, afterload, heart rate, and contractility. These determinants were described in detail in the section in Chapter 11 covering cardiac anatomy and physiology. As described in Tables 13-21 and 13-22, diseases of the cardiovascular system can affect several different aspects of hemodynamic function. Medical treatment of alterations in cardiac output and fluid volume vary, based on the precipitating cause and medical diagnosis.

There are different levels of hemodynamic monitoring intensity, depending on the clinical needs of the patient. The simplest level includes monitoring heart rhythm, central venous pressure (CVP), and arterial blood pressure, a combination that is frequently used after uncomplicated general surgery or cardiac surgery. If the patient has a low cardiac output such as might occur subsequent to an acute myocardial infarction, a more intense level of surveillance may be necessary. It might include use of a thermodilution pulmonary artery catheter, which provides hemodynamic information that includes intracardiac pressures, direct measurement of cardiac output, and, if necessary, continuous measurement of pulmonary arterial oxygen saturation ($S\dot{v}O_2$). Another catheter used in critical care is the left-atrial pressure line, which may be used in selected patients after cardiac surgery.

Overview of Hemodynamic Monitoring Equipment

A hemodynamic monitoring system has three component parts: (1) the invasive catheter and tubing attached to the patient, (2) the transducer, which receives the physiologic signal from the catheter and converts it into electrical energy, and (3) the amplifier/recorder, which increases the volume of the electrical signal and displays it on an oscilloscope and on a digital scale read in millimeters of mercury (mm Hg).

Athough many different catheters are inserted to monitor hemodynamic pressures, all catheters are connected to similar equipment, which consists of a bag of 0.9% normal saline solution with 1 or 2 units of heparin per milliliter of the solution, a 300 mmHg pressure infusion cuff, intravenous (IV) tubing, three-way stopcocks, and an in-line flush device for both continuous and manual fluid infusion. The IV setup is designed to maintain catheter patency and to connect the invasive catheter to the transducer to avoid damping (flattening) of the waveform and resulting in inaccurate pressure readings. There are several types of transducers in clinical use, all of which provide the same information. The transducer may be fully disposable or reusable with a disposable sterile dome. Depending on the pressure being monitored, the setup may be modified as described in Table 13-23.

Calibration of Equipment

To ensure accurate hemodynamic pressure readings, two baseline measurements are necessary: (1) calibration of the system to atmospheric pressure, and (2) use of the phlebostatic axis for transducer height placement. To calibrate the equipment, the three-way stopcock nearest to the transducer is turned simultaneously to open the transducer to air (atmospheric pressure) and to close it to the patient and the

Table 13-22   Integration of nursing and medical diagnosis: alteration in fluid volume

Nursing diagnostic label	Pathophysiology	Impact on hemodynamic function	Medical diagnosis
Fluid volume deficit	Decreased circulating blood volume	Decreased preload Increased heart rate Increased afterload	Bleeding Traumatic injury After surgery Coagulopathy Internal bleeding (occult) Dehydration
	Vasodilation	Decreased preload Increased heart rate Decreased afterload	Rewarming after open heart surgery Septic shock (early)
Fluid volume excess	Increased intravascular and extravascular fluid Pulmonary and systemic edema	Increased preload Decreased contractility	Congestive heart failure Cardiogenic pulmonary edema Failure of right side of heart, causing pedal edema, ascites
	Increased intravascular and extravascular fluid Pulmonary edema	Normal preload and contractility	Noncardiogenic pulmonary edema or acute respiratory distress syndrome (ARDS)

Table 13-23 Special features required in different hemodynamic monitoring systems

Monitoring system	Special features	Rationale
Intraarterial blood pressure monitoring	In-line three-way stopcock	Many patients have an arterial line in situ, not only for hemodynamic monitoring, but also for withdrawal of laboratory studies such as arterial blood gases (ABGs), electrolytes, and coagulation studies.
	Continuous infusion containing heparin at 3 ml/hour; includes a manual fast-flush system	The continuous infusion containing heparin maintains catheter patency and prevents the formation of clots at the tip of the catheter that may throw off microemboli to the distal extremity. The manual system is used to quickly clear the tubing and catheter of blood to prevent clotting.
	Pressure cuff that will inflate to 300 mmHg placed around the heparin-containing bag of saline solution, which is used for the continuous flush system	Systemic blood pressure is one of the highest physiological pressures in the body. The pressure bag must be inflated higher than 200 mmHg, or blood will back into the tubing and produce damping of the waveform.
	High-pressure tubing between the catheter and the mercury transducer	Use of nondistensible high-pressure tubing ensures that the waveform and pressures are transmitted accurately without damping.
Central venous pressure (CVP) monitoring		
Using a mercury transducer	In-line three-way stopcock	Stopcock serves a dual function: (1) it isolates the mercury transducer when solutions are infusing, and (2) it isolates the intravenous (IV) solution when CVP measurements are being recorded. A second three-way stopcock may be added to the system if venous blood samples will be withdrawn.
Using a water manometer	High-pressure tubing between the catheter and the mercury transducer	Nondistensible high-pressure tubing ensures that the waveform and pressures are transmitted accurately without damping.
	In-line three-way stopcock	The in-line stopcock is pivital to obtaining accurate CVP measurements as described in Table 13-26. The stopcock is turned to (1) isolate the water manometer when solutions are infusing, (2) isolate the patient when the manometer is being filled with IV solution, and (3) isolate the IV solution when CVP measurements are being recorded. A second three-way stopcock may be added to the system if venous blood samples will be withdrawn.
	Continuous infusion of IV solutions	The water manometer system does not include an in-line flush device; therefore, to ensure patency of the CVP catheter, an IV solution must be continuously infused. Frequently, heparin at 1 unit/ml is added to the maintenance solution.
Left atrial pressure (LAP) monitoring	In-line air filter	Because of the position of the catheter in the left atrium, any air bubbles accidentally introduced could be carried to the cerebral circulation.
	Continuous in-line flush device; does not use manual fast-flush system	The LAP catheter is not flushed manually because to do so could force emboli from the tip of the catheter forward into the arterial system. If the waveform becomes damped, the catheter may be lying against the wall of the left atrium. The patient may be asked to cough or change positions as a noninvasive troubleshooting measure.

Table 13-23   Special features required in different hemodynamic monitoring systems—cont'd

Monitoring system	Special features	Rationale
	No in-line stopcocks or means of entering the system	Blood is not withdrawn from the LAP catheter because of the risk of air emboli or entry of particulate matter.
	Pressure cuff that will inflate to 300 mmHg placed around the bag of saline solution that contains heparin, which is used for the continuous flush system	Use of pressure cuff prevents blood's backing up into the tubing.
	High-pressure tubing between the catheter and the mercury transducer	Use of nondistensible high-pressure tubing ensures that the waveform and pressures are transmitted accurately without damping.
	Chest tubes left in place for 12 hours after the LAP catheter is removed	After the catheter is removed, there is increased risk of pericardial tamponade (bleeding into the cavity that surrounds the heart). Therefore the chest tubes are placed routinely after cardiac surgery and should be left in place for drainage.
Pulmonary artery (PA) pressure monitoring, pulmonary artery wedge pressure (PAWP) monitoring, and right atrial pressure (CVP) monitoring	In-line three-way stopcocks for both the PA and right atrial CVP catheters	The stopcock nearest to the right atrial catheter is used to (1) withdraw venous samples, (2) deliver the injectate volume for cardiac output measurement, and (3) infuse small volumes of drugs or fluids. The stopcock nearest to the PA catheter is used to withdraw mixed-venous blood samples to analyze oxygen saturation.
	For both the PA and CVP catheters, continuous in-line flush device with a manual fast-flush system	The continuous flush system decreases the risk of clots forming in the catheter and ensures catheter patency. The fast-flush system is used to clear the catheter after blood withdrawal.
	Pressure cuff that will inflate to 300 mm Hg placed around the bag of saline solution that contains heparin is used for the continuous flush system	Pressure cuff is used to prevent blood's backing up into the tubing.
	High-pressure tubing between the catheter and the mercury transducer	Use of nondistensible high-pressure tubing ensures that the waveform and pressures are transmitted accurately without damping.
	1-1.5 ml syringe to inflate the latex PAWP balloon to obtain the PAWP reading	The PAWP reading indicates left ventricular end diastolic pressure (LVEDP) and allows close monitoring of left-ventricular function. A small syringe is used to avoid overdistention and perforation of the balloon. If the balloon ruptures, the external balloon port should be covered and labeled as "ruptured" to avoid the introduction of air into the pulmonary artery.
	External cardiac output computer can be attached to the catheter to permit calculation of cardiac output in liters per minute (L/min)	Normal saline at a predetermined volume and temperature is injected into the right-atrial CVP stopcock. This injection is timed with end exhalation and the external computer to produce a numerical value in L/min of cardiac output. Although equipment malfunction is rare, it is important that the nurse check that the numerical cardiac output value is congruent with the patient's clinical condition.

Continued.

Table 13-23 Special features required in different hemodynamic monitoring systems—cont'd

Monitoring system	Special features	Rationale
	A mixed venous oxygen saturation (SvO_2) fiberoptic lumen may be incorporated into the PA catheter design. Continuous SvO_2 is displayed on an external bedside computer in percent and as a waveform.	The SvO_2 reading describes the balance between oxygen supply and metabolic demand. The fiberoptics measure SvO_2 from the tip of the PA catheter.
	Cardiac pacing capability may be added to the PA catheter design by two methods: (1) atrial and ventricular electrodes incorporated into the length of the catheter; and (2) passage of a transvenous electrode down a specialized right-ventricular port.	Certain critically ill patients who require a PA catheter may also require cardiac pacing.

flush system. The monitor is adjusted so that "0" is displayed, which equals atmospheric pressure. Then, using the monitor, the upper scale limit is calibrated while the system remains open to air. Standard scale limits for that monitor system are used. Finally, the stockcock is returned to its original position to visualize the waveform and hemodynamic pressures.

The phlebostatic axis is a physical reference point on the chest that is used as a baseline for consistent transducer height placement. To obtain the axis, a theoretical line is drawn from the fourth intercostal space where it joins the sternum to a midaxillary line on the side of the chest. This point approximates the level of the atria. If the transducer air-reference stopcock is level with this reference point, accurate hemodynamic pressure measurements can be obtained for most patients if the head of the bed is positioned up to 45 degrees.[33] If the transducer is placed *below* the phlebostatic axis, fluid in the system will weigh on the transducer and produce a false-high reading. If the transducer is placed *above* this atrial level, gravity and lack of fluid pressure will give an erroneously low reading. If several clinicians will be taking measurements, the reference point can be marked on the side of the patient's chest to ensure accurate measurements.

INTRAARTERIAL BLOOD PRESSURE MONITORING
Indications

Intraarterial blood pressure monitoring is indicated for any major medical or surgical condition that compromises cardiac output or fluid volume status as described in Tables 13-21 and 13-22. The system is designed for continuous measurement of three blood pressure parameters—systole, diastole, and mean arterial blood pressure (MAP). In addition, the direct arterial access is helpful in the management of patients with acute respiratory failure who require frequent arterial blood gas (ABG) measurements.

Catheters

The size of the catheter used is proportionate to the diameter of the cannulated artery. In small arteries such as the radial or dorsalis pedis a 20-gauge, 3.8- to 5.1-cm, nontapered Teflon catheter is most often used. If the larger femoral or axillary arteries are used, a 19- or 20-gauge, 16-cm, Teflon catheter is used. Teflon catheters are preferred because of their lower risk of causing thrombosis.[12]

The catheter insertion is usually percutaneous, although the technique varies with vessel size. Cannulas are most frequently inserted in the smaller arteries, using a "catheter-over-needle" unit in which the needle is used as a temporary guide for catheter placement. With this method, once the unit has been inserted into the artery, the needle is withdrawn, leaving the supple plastic cannula in place. Insertion of a cannula into a larger artery usually necessitates use of the Seldinger technique. This procedure involves (1) entry into the artery, using a needle, (2) passage of a supple guidewire through the needle into the artery, (3) removal of the needle, (4) passage of the catheter over the guidewire, and (5) removal of the guidewire, leaving the cannula in the artery. If a cannula cannot be inserted into the artery using percutaneous methods, an arterial cutdown may be performed. This procedure invovles a skin incision to expose the artery directly.

Insertion

Several major peripheral arteries are suitable for receiving a cannula and for long-term hemodynamic monitoring. The most frequently used site is the radial artery. If this artery is not available, the dorsalis pedis, femoral, axillary, or brachial arteries may be used. The major advantage of the radial artery is that collateral circulation to the hand is provided by the ulnar artery and palmar arch in most of the population; thus there are other avenues of circulation if the radial artery becomes blocked after catheter placement. Before radial artery cannulation, collateral circulation must be assessed, either by using the Doppler flowmeter or by the Allen test. In the Allen test the radial and ulnar arteries are compressed simultaneously. The patient is asked to clench and unclench the hand until it blanches. One of the arteries is then released, and the hand should immediately flush from that side. The same procedure is repeated for the remaining artery.

Nursing Care

Intraarterial blood pressure monitoring is designed for continuous assessment of arterial perfusion to the major organ systems of the body. Mean arterial pressure (MAP) is the clinical parameter most frequently used to assess perfusion because MAP represents perfusion pressure throughout the cardiac cycle. Because one third of the cardiac cycle is spent in systole and two thirds in diastole, the MAP calculation must reflect the greater amount of time spent in diastole. The MAP formula is explained in Table 13-24.

A MAP greater than 60 mm Hg is necessary to perfuse the coronary arteries, brain, and kidneys. A MAP between 70 and 90 mm Hg is ideal. Systolic and diastolic pressures are monitored in conjunction with the MAP as further guide to the accuracy of perfusion. Should cardiac output decrease, the body will compensate by constricting peripheral vessels to maintain the blood pressure. In this situation the MAP may remain constant, but the pulse pressure (difference between systolic and diastolic pressures) will narrow. The following examples explain this point:

Mr. A: BP, 90/70 MAP, 76 mm Hg
Mr. B: BP, 150/40 MAP, 76 mm Hg

Both of these patients have a perfusion pressure of 76 mm Hg, but clinically they are very different. Mr. A is peripherally vasoconstricted, as is demonstrated by the narrow pulse pressure (90/70). His skin is cool to touch, and he has weak peripheral pulses. Mr. B has a wide pulse pressure (150/40), warm skin, and normally palpable peripheral pulses. Thus nursing assessment of the patient with an arterial line includes comparison of clinical findings with arterial line readings, including perfusion pressure and MAP.

Another clinical example of this hemodynamic nursing assessment is seen in patient JW 1 day after his coronary artery bypass graft (CABG) surgery. JW has recently been weaned from low-dose dopamine (Intropin) and sodium nitroprusside and has received a diruetic (20 mg of furosemide IV). He has excreted 800 ml of urine during the last 2 hours. JW's MAP remains at 80 mm Hg, but his pulse pressure has narrowed from 120/60 to 100/70. His heart rate has increased from 90 beats per minute (bpm) to 110 bpm. This clinical situation is not uncommon after furosemide administration, but the narrowed pulse pressure and increased heart rate may indicate hypovolemia. The nurse caring for

JW is to monitor the *trend* of the MAP. If the MAP begins to decrease and JW shows signs of low cardiac output, JW's physician should be notified. In most nonemergency situations, following the trend of the arterial pressure is more valuable than an isolated measurement.

The nurse caring for the patient with an arterial line must be able to assess whether a low MAP, or narrowed perfusion pressure, represents decreased arterial perfusion or equipment malfunction. Assessment of the arterial waveform on the oscilloscope in combination with clinical assessment will yield the answer. If there are air bubbles, clots, or kinks in the system, the waveform will become damped or flattened, and the troubleshooting methods described in Table 13-25 can be implemented. If the line is unreliable or becomes dislodged, a cuff pressure can be used as a reserve system. There are slight differences between cuff and arterial pressures, but in the normovolemic patient differences of 5 to 10 mm Hg do not affect clinical management. If the patient has a low cardiac output or is in shock, the cuff pressure will be unreliable because of vasoconstriction, and an arterial line should be inserted.

Arterial Pressure Waveform Interpretation

The arterial pressure waveform represents the ejection phase of left-ventricular systole and is shown in Fig. 11-26. As the aortic valve opens, blood is ejected from the left ventricle and is recorded as an increase of pressure in the arterial system. The highest point recorded is called systole. Following peak ejection (systole) there is a decrease in force and a drop of pressure. A notch (the dicrotic notch) may be visible on the downstroke of this arterial waveform, representing closure of the aortic valve. The dicrotic notch signifies the beginning of diastole. The remainder of the downstroke represents diastolic runoff of blood flow into the arterial tree. The lowest point recorded is called diastole. A normal arterial pressure tracing is described in Figure 13-67. Note that the arterial pressure tracing always follows the initiating QRS.

Specific problems with heart rhythm can translate into poor arterial perfusion if cardiac output falls. Poor perfusion may be seen as a single nonperfused beat following a premature ventricular contraction (PVC) (Fig. 13-68) or as multiple non-perfused beats. In ventricular bigeminy in which every second beat is poorly perfused (Fig. 13-69). A disorganized atrial baseline such as during atrial fibrillation creates a variable arterial pulse because of the differences in stroke volume between each beat (Fig. 13-70). These cases illustrate that when two beats are close together, the left ventricle does not have time to fill adequately and the second beat is poorly perfused or is not perfused. If a stethoscope is placed over the apex of the heart, the beat can be heard but cannot be felt as a radial pulse. A pulse deficit occurs when the apical heart rate and the peripheral pulse are not equal. To determine whether a pulse deficit is significant, it is necessary to evaluate the clinical impact on the patient and whether there is any change in MAP or pulse pressure. Generally the more nonperfused beats there are, the more serious the problem.

Text continued on p. 234.

Table 13-24 Hemodynamic pressures and calculated hemodynamic values

Hemodynamic pressure or value	Abbreviation	Definition and explanation	Normal range*	Formula
Mean arterial pressure	MAP	Average perfusion pressure created by arterial blood pressure during the complete cardiac cycle. The normal cardiac cycle is one third systole and two thirds diastole. These three components are divided by 3 to obtain the average perfusion pressure for the whole cardiac cycle.	70-90 mm Hg	$\dfrac{(\text{Diastolic} \times 2) + (\text{Systolic} \times 1)}{3}$
Central venous pressure	CVP	Pressure created by volume in the right side of the heart. When the tricuspid valve is open, the CVP reflects filling pressures in the right ventricle. Clinically, the CVP is often used as a guide to overall fluid balance.	2-4 mm Hg 3-8 cm water (H_2O)	$\dfrac{(\text{CVP diastolic} \times 2) + (\text{CVP systolic} \times 1)}{3}$
Left atrial pressure	LAP	Pressure created by volume in the left side of the heart. When the mitral valve is open, the LAP reflects filling pressures in the left ventricle. Clinically, the LAP is used after cardiac surgery to determine how well the left ventricle is ejecting its volume. In general, the higher the LAP, the lower is the ejection fraction from the left ventricle.	5-10 mm Hg	$\dfrac{(\text{LAP diastolic} \times 2) + (\text{LAP systolic} \times 1)}{3}$
Pulmonary artery pressure (systolic, diastolic, mean)	PAP, PA systolic (PAS), PA diastolic (PAD), PAP mean (PAP_M)	Pulsatile pressure in the pulmonary artery, measured by an indwelling catheter.	PAS 20-30 mm Hg PAD 5-10 mm Hg PAM 10-15 mm Hg PAP_M 5-12 mm Hg	$\dfrac{(\text{PAD} \times 2) + (\text{PAS} \times 1)}{3}$
Pulmonary capillary wedge pressure or pulmonary artery wedge pressure	PCW or PCWP or PAWP	Pressure created by volume in the left side of the heart. When the mitral valve is open, the PAWP reflects filling pressures in the pulmonary vasculature, and pressures in the left side of the heart are transmitted back to the catheter "wedged" into a small pulmonary arteriole.		

Term	Abbr.	Description	Normal Value	Formula
Cardiac output	CO	The amount of blood pumped out by a ventricle. Clinically, it can be measured using the thermodilution CO method, which calculates CO in liters per minute (L/min).	4-6 L/min (at rest)	Heart rate × Stroke volume
Cardiac index	CI	Cardiac output divided by body surface area (BSA), tailoring the CO to individual body size. A BSA conversion chart is necessary to calculate CI, which is considered more accurate than CO because it is individualized to height and weight. CI is measured in liters per minute per square meter BSA (L/min/m²).	2.5-4.0 L/min/m²	$\dfrac{CO}{BSA}$
Stroke volume	SV	Amount of blood ejected by the ventricle with each heart beat. Hemodynamic monitoring systems calculate SV by dividing cardiac output (CO in L/min) by the heart rate (HR) then multiplying the answer by 1000 to change liters to milliliters (ml).	60-70 ml	$\dfrac{CO}{HR} \times 1000$
Stroke volume index	SI	SV indexed to BSA.	40-50 ml/m²	$\dfrac{SV}{BSA}$
Systemic vascular resistance	SVR	Mean pressure difference across the systemic vascular bed, divided by blood flow. Clinically, SVR represents the resistance against which the left ventricle must pump to eject its volume. This resistance is created by the systemic arteries and arterioles. As SVR increases, cardiac output falls. SVR is measured in either units or dynes/sec/cm⁻⁵. If the number of units is multiplied by 80, the value is converted to dynes/sec/cm⁻⁵.	10-18 units or 800-1400 dynes/sec/cm⁻⁵	$\dfrac{MAP - CVP}{CO} = $ Units $\dfrac{MAP - CVP}{CO} \times 80 = $ Dynes/sec/cm⁻⁵
Systemic vascular resistance index	SVRI	SVR indexed to BSA.	2000-2400 dynes/sec/cm⁻⁵/m²	$\dfrac{MAP - CVP}{CI} \times 80 = $ Dynes/sec/cm⁻⁵/m²

Continued.

Table 13-24 Hemodynamic pressures and calculated hemodynamic values—cont'd

Hemodynamic pressure or value	Abbreviation	Definition and explanation	Normal range*	Formula
Pulmonary vascular resistance	PVR	Mean pressure difference across pulmonary vascular bed, divided by blood flow. Clinically, PVR represents the resistance against which the right ventricle must pump to eject its volume. This resistance is created by the pulmonary arteries and arterioles. As PVR increases, the output from the right ventricle decreases. PVR is measured in either units or dynes/sec/cm^{-5}. PVR is normally one-sixth of SVR.	1.2-3.0 units or 100-250 dynes/sec/cm^{-5}	$$\frac{\text{PAP mean} - \text{PAWP}}{\text{CO}} = \text{Units}$$
Pulmonary vascular resistance index	PVRI	PVR indexed to BSA.	225-315 dynes/sec/cm^{-5}/m^2	$$\frac{\text{PAP mean} - \text{PAWP}}{\text{CI}} \times 80 =$$ Dynes/sec/cm^{-5}/m^2
Left cardiac work index	LCWI	Amount of work the left ventricle does *each minute* when ejecting blood. The hemodynamic formula represents pressure generated (MAP) multiplied by volume pumped (CO); 0.0136 is a conversion factor to change mm Hg to kilogram-meter (kg-m). LCWI is always represented as an indexed volume (BSA chart). LCWI increases or decreases because of changes in either pressure (MAP) or volume pumped (CO).	3.4-4.2 kg-m/m^2	1. MAP $\times$ CO $\times$ 0.0136 = LCW 2. $\dfrac{\text{LCW}}{\text{BSA}}$ = LCWI
Left ventricular stroke work index	LVSWI	Amount of work the left ventricle performs with *each heartbeat*. The hemodynamic formula represents pressure generated (MAP) multiplied by volume pumped (SV); 0.0136 is	50-62 g-m/m^2	1. MAP $\times$ SV $\times$ 0.0136 = LVSW 2. $\dfrac{\text{LVSW}}{\text{BSA}}$ = LVSWI

		a conversion factor to change ml/mmHg to gram-meter (g-m). LVSWI is always represented as an indexed volume. LVSWI increases or decreases because of changes in either pressure (MAP) or volume pumped (SV).	
Right cardiac work index	RCWI	Amount of work the right ventricle performs *each minute* when ejecting blood. The hemodynamic formula represents pressure generated (PAP mean) multiplied by volume pumped (CO); 0.0136 is a conversion factor to change mm Hg to kilogram-meter (kg-m). RCWI is always represented as an indexed value (BSA chart). Similar to LCWI, the RCWI increases or decreases because of changes in either pressure (PAP mean) or volume pumped (CO).	0.54–0.66 kg-m/m²	1. PAP mean × CO × 0.0136 = RCW 2. $\dfrac{\text{RCW}}{\text{BSA}}$ = RCWI
Right ventricular stroke work index	RVSWI	Amount of work the right ventricle does *each heart beat*. The hemodynamic formula represents pressure generated (PAP mean) multiplied by volume pumped (SV); 0.0136 is a conversion factor to change mm Hg to gram-meter (g-m). RVSWI is always represented as an indexed value (BSA chart). Similar to LVSWI, the RVSWI increases or decreases because of changes in either pressure (PAP mean) or volume pumped (SV).	7.9–9.7 g-m/m²	1. PAP mean × SV × 0.0136 = RVSW 2. $\dfrac{\text{RVSW}}{\text{BSA}}$ = RVSWI

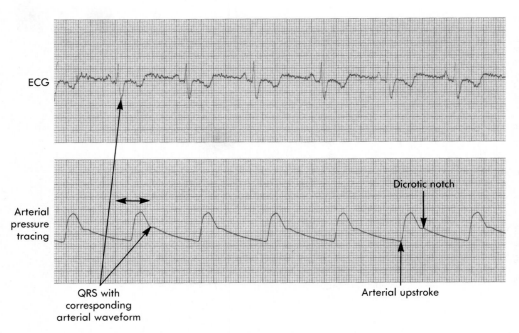

ECG

Arterial
pressure
tracing

Dicrotic notch

QRS with
corresponding
arterial waveform

Arterial upstroke

Fig. 13-67 Simultaneous ECG and arterial pressure tracing.

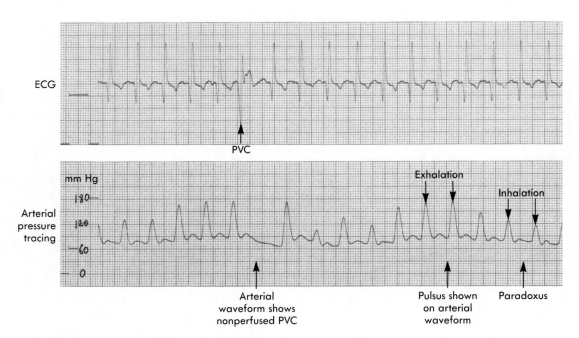

ECG

PVC

Arterial
pressure
tracing

mm Hg

180

120

60

0

Exhalation

Inhalation

Arterial
waveform shows
nonperfused PVC

Pulsus shown
on arterial
waveform

Paradoxus

Fig. 13-68 Simultaneous ECG and arterial pressure tracing shows normal arterial waveform with a nonperfused premature ventricular contraction (PVC). Arterial waveform also
shows evidence of pulsus paradoxus in a patient who is mechanically ventilated.

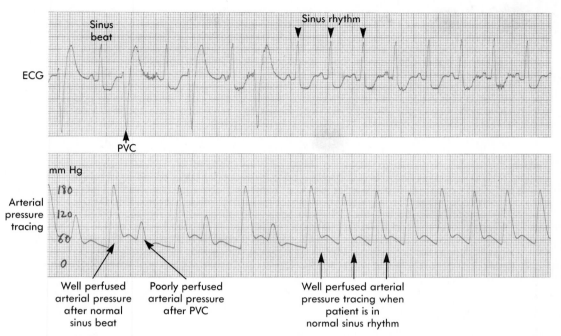

Fig. 13-69   Simultaneous ECG and arterial pressure tracing shows ventricular bigeminy in which each ventricular beat is poorly perfused on the arterial pressure waveform in the first part of the tracing. In the second half of the tracing, there is a well-perfused arterial pressure tracing as the patient converts to normal sinus rhythm.

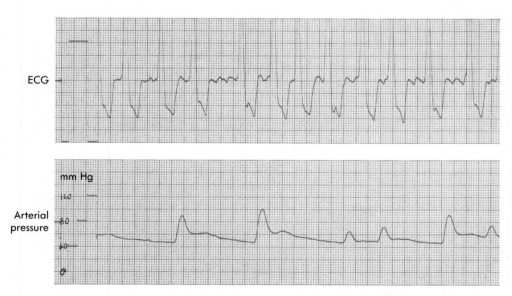

Fig. 13-70   Simultaneous ECG and arterial pressure tracing shows atrial fibrillation, which results in irregular atrial pulsations. They create differences in beat-to-beat ventricular upstroke volume, resulting in diminished or absent ventricular output as seen on the arterial waveform.

Table 13-25 Nursing measures to ensure patient safety and to troubleshoot problems with hemodynamic monitoring equipment

Problem	Prevention	Rationale	Troubleshooting
Damping of waveform	Provide continuous infusion of solution containing heparin through an in-line flush device (1 unit of heparin for each millimeter of flush solution).	To ensure that recorded pressures and waveform are accurate since a damped waveform gives inaccurate readings.	Before insertion, completely flush the line and/or catheter. In a line attached to a patient, back flush through the system to clear bubbles from tubing or transducer.
Clot formation at end of catheter	Provide continuous infusion of solution containing heparin through an in-line flush device (1 unit of heparin for each millimeter of flush solution).	Any foreign object placed in the body can cause local activation of the patient's coagulation system as a normal defense mechanism. The clots that are formed may be dangerous if they break off and travel to other parts of the body.	If a clot in the catheter is suspected because of a damped waveform or resistance to forward flush of the system, gently aspirate the line using a small syringe inserted into the proximal stopcock. Then flush the line again once the clot is removed and inspect the waveform. It should return to a normal pattern.
Hemorrhage	Use Luer-lock (screw) connections in line setup. Close and cap stopcocks when not in use.	A loose connection or open stopcock will create a low-pressure sump effect, causing blood to back into the line and into the open air.	Once a blood leak is recognized, tighten all connections, flush the line, and estimate blood loss.
	Ensure that the catheter is either sutured or securely taped in position.	If a catheter is accidentally removed, the vessel can bleed profusely, especially with an arterial line or if the patient has abnormal coagulation factors resulting from heparin in the line or has hypertension.	If the catheter has been inadvertently removed, put pressure on the cannulation site. When bleeding has stopped, apply a sterile dressing, estimate blood loss, and inform the physician. If the patient is restless, an armboard may protect lines inserted in the arm.
Air emboli	Ensure that all air bubbles are purged from a new line setup before attachment to an indwelling catheter.	Air can be introduced at several times, including when central venous pressure (CVP) tubing comes apart, when a new line setup is attached, or when a new CVP or pulmonary artery (PA) line is inserted. During insertion of a CVP or PA line, the patient may be asked to hold his or her breath at specific times to prevent drawing air into the chest during inhalation.	Since it is impossible to get the air back once it has been introduced into the bloodstream, prevention is the best cure.
	Ensure that the drip chamber from the bag of flush solution is more than half full before using the in-line fast-flush system.	The in-line fast-flush devices are designed to permit clearing of blood from the line after withdrawal of blood samples.	If any air bubbles are noted, they must be vented through the in-line stopcocks, and the drip chamber must be filled.

Table 13-25 Nursing measures to ensure patient safety and to troubleshoot problems with hemodynamic monitoring equipment—cont'd

Problem	Prevention	Rationale	Troubleshooting
	Some sources recommend removing all air from the bag of flush solution before assembling the system.	If the chamber of the intravenous (IV) tubing is too low or empty, the rapid flow of fluid will create turbulance and cause flushing of air bubbles into the system and into the bloodstream.	The left atrial pressure (LAP) line setup is the only system that includes an air filter specifically to prevent air emboli.
Normal waveform with *low* digital pressures	Ensure that the system is calibrated to atmospheric pressure. Ensure that the transducer is placed at the level of the phlebostatic axis.	To provide a 0 baseline relative to atmospheric pressure. If the transducer has been placed *higher* than the phlebostatic level, gravity and the lack of hydrostatic pressure will produce a false *low* reading.	Recalibrate the equipment if transducer drift has occurred. Reposition the transducer at the level of the phlebostatic axis. Misplacement can occur if the patient moves from the bed to the chair or if the bed is placed in a Trendelenburg position.
Normal waveform with *high* digital pressure	Ensure that the system is calibrated to atmospheric pressure. Ensure that the transducer is placed at the level of the phlebostatic axis.	To provide a 0 baseline relative to atmospheric pressure. If the transducer has been placed *lower* than the phlebostatic level, the weight of hydrostatic pressure on the transducer will produce a false *high* reading.	Recalibrate the equipment if transducer drift has occurred. Reposition the transducer at the level of the phlebostatic axis. This situation can occur if the head of the bed was raised and the transducer was not repositioned. Some centers require attachment of the transducer to the patient's chest to avoid this problem.
Loss of waveform	Always have the hemodynamic waveform monitored so that changes or loss can be quickly noted.	The catheter may be kinked, or a stopcock may be turned off.	Check the line setup to ensure that all stopcocks are turned in the correct position and that there is not a kink in the tubing. Sometimes the catheter migrates against a vessel well, and having the patient change position will restore the waveform.
Infection	Change the bag of flush solution every 24 hours. Change the line setup and the disposable transducer every 72 hours. Change the catheter insertion site dressing every 24 hours, and inspect the cannulation site for signs of infections. Apply antiseptic ointment and a sterile dressing to the catheter site.	These recommendations are provided by the Center for Disease Control (CDC) and Maki and associates[35] and are based on research studies with hemodynamic monitoring equipment and on reports of infectious complications.	If local infection occurs, the catheter must be placed elsewhere by the physician, and the new insertion site must be dressed using antiseptic ointment and a sterile dressing. Sterile equipment must always be used, disposable equipment must not be reused, and nondisposable transducers must be sterilized after each patient usage. Hands should be washed before handling monitoring setup or dressings.

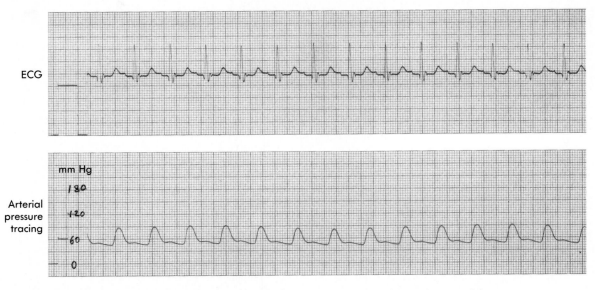

Fig. 13-71 Simultaneous ECG and arterial pressure tracing show a low arterial pressure waveform.

Pulsus paradoxus is a decrease of more than 10 mm Hg in the arterial waveform that occurs during inhalation (Fig. 13-68). It is caused by a fall in cardiac output as a result of increased negative intrathoracic pressure during inhalation. As pressure within the thorax falls, blood pools in the large veins of the lungs and thorax, and stroke volume is decreased. This can be seen on an arterial waveform in a patient with cardiac tamponade, pericardial effusion, or constrictive pericarditis. It commonly occurs in hypovolemic patients who are mechanically ventilated, using large tidal volumes (12 to 15 ml/kg), or in patients who are spontaneously breathing very deeply. In pulsus alternans, every other arterial pulsation is weak, and this sometimes occurs in patients with advanced left-ventricular failure. If the arterial monitor shows a low blood pressure, it is the responsibility of the nurse to determine whether it is a true patient problem or a problem with the equipment as described in Table 13-25.

A low arterial blood pressure waveform is shown in Fig. 13-71. In this case the digital readout correlated well with the patient's own cuff pressure, confirming that the patient was hypotensive. This arterial waveform is more rounded, without a dicrotic notch, when compared with the normal waveform in Fig. 13-67. A damped (flattened) arterial waveform is shown in Fig. 13-72. In this case the patient's cuff pressure was significantly higher than the digital readout, thus representing a problem with equipment. A damped waveform occurs when communication from the artery to the tranducer is interrupted and produces false values on the monitor and oscilloscope. Damping may be caused by a clot at the end of the catheter, by kinks in the catheter or tubing, or by air bubbles in the system. Troubleshooting techniques (see Table 13-25) are used to find the origin of the problem and to remove the cause of damping. If there is any doubt about the accuracy of the arterial waveform, a cuff blood pressure reading should be taken. As part of the routine nursing assessment, a cuff blood pressure should

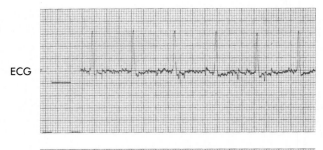

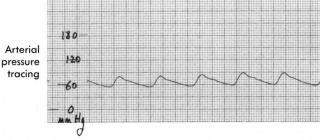

Fig. 13-72 Simultaneous ECG and arterial pressure tracing show a damped arterial pressure waveform.

be taken every shift and correlated with the intraarterial pressure.

CENTRAL VENOUS PRESSURE MONITORING
Indications

Central venous pressure (CVP) monitoring is indicated whenever a patient has an alteration in fluid volume (see Table 13-24). The CVP can be used as a guide in fluid volume replacement in hypovolemia and to assess the impact of diuresis after diuretic administration in the case of fluid overload. Additionally, when a major intravenous (IV) line is required for volume replacement, a central venous line is a good choice because large volumes of fluid can be easily delivered.

Catheters

Since many patients are awake and alert when a CVP catheter is inserted, a brief explanation about the procedure will minimize patient anxiety and gain cooperation during the insertion. This cooperation is important because it is a sterile procedure and because the supine or Trendelenburg position may not be comfortable for many patients.

CVP catheters are available as single-, double-, or triple-lumen infusion catheters, depending on the specific needs of the patient. The catheters are designed for placement by percutaneous injection after skin preparation and administration of a local anesthetic. The standard CVP kit contains sterile towels, a needle introducer, syringe, guidewire, and catheter. The Seldinger technique is the preferred method of placement in which the vein is located by using a needle and syringe. A guidewire is passed through the needle, the needle is removed, and the catheter is passed over the guidewire. Once the catheter is correctly placed at the level of the right atrium, the guidewire is removed. Finally, an IV setup is attached, and the catheter is sutured in place.

Insertion

The large veins of the upper thorax (subclavian or internal jugular) are most frequently used for percutaneous CVP line insertion. During insertion the patient may be placed in a Trendelenburg position. Placing the head in a dependent position causes the internal jugular veins in the neck to become more prominent, facilitating line placement. To minimize the risk of air embolus during the procedure, the patient may be asked to hold his or her breath any time the needle or catheter is open to air. After cannulation of the internal jugular or subclavian vein, a chest radiograph should be obtained to verify placement of the catheter and the absence of an iatrogenic pneumothorax. Other suitable insertion sites include the femoral and antecubital fossae veins. In the rare case that it is not possible to insert a CVP catheter percutaneously, a surgical cutdown may be performed.

Nursing Care

The CVP is used to measure the filling pressures of the right side of the heart. During diastole when the tricuspid valve is open and blood is flowing from the right atrium to the right ventricle, the CVP will accurately reflect right ventricular end diastolic pressure (RVEDP). The normal CVP is 2 to 5 mm Hg (3 to 8 cm H_2O).

A low CVP often occurs in the hypovolemic patient and suggests there is insufficient blood volume in the ventricle at end diastole to produce an adequate stroke volume. Thus, to maintain normal cardiac output, the heart rate must increase.* This increase produces the tachycardia frequently observed in hypovolemic states and increases myocardial oxygen demand. An elevated CVP occurs in cases of fluid overload. To circulate the excess blood volume the heart must greatly increase contractility to move a large volume of blood, again increasing the work load of the heart and increasing myocardial oxygen consumption.

The CVP is used in combination with the mean arterial pressure (MAP) and other clinical parameters to assess hemodynamic stability. In the hypovolemic patient, the CVP will fall before there is a significant fall in MAP because peripheral vasoconstriction will keep the MAP normal. Thus the CVP is an excellent early warning system for the patient who is bleeding, vasodilating, receiving diuretics, or rewarming after cardiac surgery. The CVP, however, is not a reliable indicator of left-ventricular dysfunction. Left-ventricular dysfunction, which can occur after an acute myocardial infarction, will increase filling pressures on the left side of the heart. The CVP, since it measures RVEDP, will remain normal until the increase in pressure from the left side is reflected back through the pulmonary vasculature to the right ventricle. In this situation a pulmonary artery catheter that measures pressures on the left side is the monitoring method of choice.

To take CVP measurements the clinician has a choice of two methods—either a mercury (mm Hg) system, using a transducer and a monitor, or a water (cm H_2O) manometer system. The procedure for taking a CVP reading with a water manometer is described in Table 13-26. If a patient changes from one system to the other, the CVP value will also change because mercury is heavier than water, and 1 mm Hg is equal to 1.36 cm H_2O. To convert water to mercury, the water value is divided by 1.36 ($H_2O \div 1.36$), and to convert mercury to water, the mercury value is multiplied by 1.36 (mm Hg × 1.36). To achieve accurate CVP measurements the phlebostatic axis should be used as a reference point on the body, and the transducer or water manometer zero should be level with this point. If the phlebostatic axis is used and the transducer or water manometer are correctly aligned, any head-of-bed position up to 45 degrees may be accurately used for CVP readings. Elevating the head of bed is especially helpful for the patient with respiratory or cardiac problems who will not tolerate a flat position.

The risk of air embolus, although uncommon, is always present for the patient with a central venous line in place. Air can enter during insertion through a disconnected or broken catheter or along the path of a removed CVP catheter. This is more likely if the patient is in an upright position because air can be pulled into the venous system with the increase in negative intrathoracic pressure during inhalation. If a large volume of air (200 to 300 cc) is infused rapidly, it may become trapped in the right-ventricular outflow tract, stopping blood flow from the right side of the heart to the lungs. The patient may experience respiratory distress and cardiovascular collapse. Treatment involves administering 100% oxygen and placing the patient on the left side with the head downward (left-lateral Trendelenburg position). This position displaces the air from the right-ventricular outflow tract to the apex of the heart where it can be either reabsorbed or aspirated. Precautions to prevent an air embolism in a CVP line include using only Luer-lock connections, avoiding long loops of IV tubing, and using screw caps on three-way stopcocks.

---

*Formula: heart rate times stroke volume equals cardiac output (HR × SV = CO). Thus any decrease in stroke volume must be balanced by an increase in heart rate to maintain cardiac output.

Table 13-26 Procedure for central venous pressure (CVP) measurement using a water manometer

Action	Rationale
1. With the three-way stopcock turned off to the plastic disposable manometer, check that the intravenous (IV) solution will run freely. If not, the catheter can be aspirated with a small syringe to verify that it is not clotted and then flushed for patency.	The catheter must be patent to ensure accurate CVP readings. If the IV solution runs freely, this is a good indication that the line is clear.
2. The zero level of the water manometer is placed at the plebostatic axis.	The phlebostatic axis provides a baseline for accurate CVP measurements at head-of-bed positions up to 45 degrees.
3. The three-way stopcock is turned off to the patient catheter and is opened between the IV solution and the water manometer. The IV solution is used to fill the water manometer to approximately 25 cm H_2O but not to overflow from the tube.	The water manometer is filled to a level higher than the patient's expected CVP measurement. It is not allowed to overflow to avoid contamination of the solution.
4. The three-way stopcock is turned off to the IV solution and is opened between the patient and the water manometer. The fluid in the manometer should fall rapidly and then stabilize. The fluid level should visibly fluctuate with each respiration.	If the zero level of the manometer is level with the phlebostatic axis, the point at which the fluid level stabilizes is the mean CVP measurement. The most common error in measurement is not placing the manometric zero at the phlebostatic axis.
5. The CVP reading should be taken at end-exhalation when the chest wall is seen to fall. The measurement should be recorded at the lowest point of the water meniscus.	In the spontaneously breathing patient intrathoracic pressure falls during inhalation and produces a false low reading if the CVP measurement is recorded during inhalation. In the intubated and ventilated patient, ventilator breathing will cause intrathoracic pressure to rise during inhalation, possibly producing a false-high reading if the measurement is recorded then. For these reasons, end-exhalation is the most stable and reliable point in the respiratory cycle at which to measure the CVP.
6. The three-way stopcock is returned to its original position so that IV solutions can be infused.	To guarantee line patency, the CVP catheter must always be perfused with IV solution. If the volume of infused solution per hour is small, it is advisable to add heparin (1 unit/1 ml) to prevent clot formation in the catheter. If the volume of infused solution is large, this addition is rarely necessary.

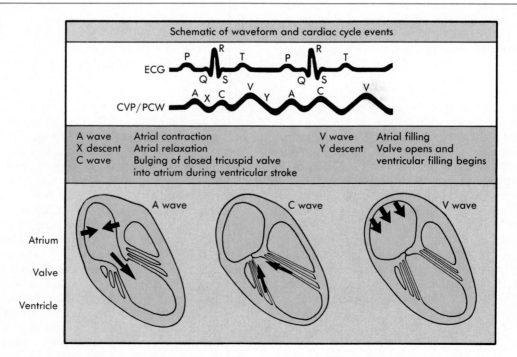

Fig. 13-73 Cardiac events that produce the CVP waveform with a, c, and v waves. A wave represents atrial contraction. X descent represents atrial relaxation. C wave represents the bulging of the closed tricuspid valve into the right atrium during ventricular systole. V wave represents atrial filling. Y descent represents opening of the tricuspid valve and filling of the ventricle.

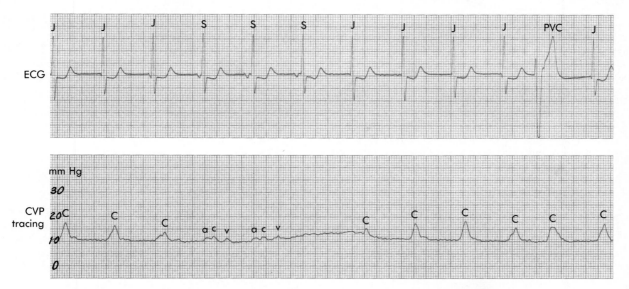

Fig. 13-74 Simultaneous ECG and CVP pressure tracing. The CVP waveform shows large cannon waves (c waves) corresponding to the junctional beats or premature ventricular contractions *(strip above)*. As the patient converts to sinus rhythm, the CVP waveform has a normal configuration. *J*, Junctional rhythm followed by cannon waves on CVP waveform, *PVC*, premature ventricular contraction followed by cannon wave on CVP, *S*, sinus rhythm followed by normal CVP tracing with a, c, and v waves, *C*, cannon waves on CVP tracing; *ac*, normal right atrial pressure tracing. See Fig. 13-73 for more explanation.

CVP Waveform Interpretation

The right-atrial (CVP) waveform has three positive deflections, called a, c, and v waves, that correspond to specific atrial events in the cardiac cycle (Fig. 13-73). The a wave reflects atrial contraction and follows the P wave seen on the electrocardiogram (ECG). The downslope of this wave is called the x descent and represents atrial relaxation. The c wave refelcts the closure of the tricuspid valve as it moves toward the right atrium in early ventricular contraction. The c wave is small and not always visible but corresponds to the QRS-T interval on the ECG. The v wave represents atrial filling and pressure increase against the closed tricuspid valve in early diastole. The downslope of the v wave is named the y descent and represents the fall in pressure as the tricuspid valve opens and blood flows from the right atrium to the right ventricle.

Certain heart rhythms can change the normal CVP waveform. In atrial fibrillation the CVP waveform has no recognizable pattern because of the disorganization of the atria. In a junctional rhythm or after a premature ventricular contraction (PVC), the atria are depolarized after the ventricles if there is retrograde conduction to the atria. This may be seen as a retrograde P wave on the ECG and as a large combined ac wave or cannon wave on the CVP waveform (Fig. 13-74). Pathological conditions such as advanced right-ventricular failure or tricuspid valve insufficiency allow backflow of blood from the right ventricle to the right atrium during ventricular contraction, producing large v waves on the right-atrial waveform.

LEFT-ATRIAL PRESSURE MONITORING
Indications

Left atrial pressure (LAP) monitoring is used in selected cases after major cardiac surgery. Until the advent of the pulmonary artery catheter in the 1970s, LAP monitoring was used to assess hemodynamics on the left side of the heart. Today it is not used for routine monitoring. However, it has been found clinically effective in the postoperative management of the cardiac surgery patient who has significant pulmonary hypertension. In this case, inotropic drugs are infused directly into the left side of the heart, while vasodilator drugs are infused into the right heart through a right-atrial catheter.[13] This technique optimizes pulmonary vasodilation and minimizes the vasoconstrictive effect of inotropic drugs on the hypertensive pulmonary bed. In addition, accurate left atrial pressures can be obtained.

Insertion

The LAP catheter is inserted into the left atrium during open heart surgery. The single-lumen catheter exits through the chest wall and is attached to a routine hemodynamic monitoring setup that contains an in-line air filter.

Nursing Care

The placement of the LAP catheter directly into the left atrium places the patient at particular risk for air or tissue emboli. Nursing care is planned to reduce these equipment-related risks. An in-line air filter is added to the flush system that contains heparin to reduce the risk of air emboli. If the waveform becomes damped, noninvasive methods of troubleshooting such as repositioning the patient are performed. The catheter is not manually flushed since to do so may increase the risk of emboli resulting from clot formation at the tip of the catheter. Some sources recommend gentle aspiration of the LAP catheter. If there is no blood return, the catheter should be removed. Pericardial tamponade is a potential complication of LAP catheter removal. Therefore mediastinal chest tubes should be left in position until after the catheter is discontinued. Because of these risks, the LAP catheter is rarely left in place for more than 48 hours.

LAP Waveform Interpretation

The LAP waveform consists of two positive deflections, which are termed the a and v waves. The a wave represents atrial contraction, and the v wave represents filling of the left atrium against a closed mitral valve. Normal LAP pressure ranges from 5 to 10 mm Hg and is elevated with mitral valve disease or severe heart failure on the left side.

PULMONARY ARTERY PRESSURE MONITORING
Indications

When specific hemodynamic and intracardiac data are required for diagnostic and treatment purposes, a thermodilution pulmonary artery (PA) catheter may be inserted. This catheter is used for diagnosis and evaluation of heart disease, shock states, and medical conditions that cause an alteration in cardiac output (see Table 13-21) or an alteration in fluid volume (see Table 13-22). In addition, the PA catheter is used to evaluate patient response to treatment as described in Table 13-27.

A significant advantage of the PA catheter over the previously described methods of monitoring is that it simultaneously assesses several hemodynamic parameters, including pulmonary artery systolic and diastolic pressures, the pulmonary artery mean pressure, and the pulmonary artery wedge pressure (PAWP) (see Table 13-24).

Although the PA catheter is inserted into the right side of the heart, it is used to measure pressures on the left side of the heart through the pulmonary artery wedge pressure (PAWP) and the pulmonary artery diastolic (PAD) pressure. This is possible because during ventricular diastole when the mitral valve is open, there is a clear pathway between the tip of the catheter and the left ventricle. In the absence of pulmonary hypertension, the pressure along this pathway (from catheter tip to left ventricle) is equal; thus the pressure that registers on the catheter tip is identical to the pressure registered within the left ventricle. The pressure recorded in the left ventricle is called left ventricular end-diastolic pressure (LVEDP).

Measurement and interpretation of LVEDP allow the clinician to make accurate judgments about a patient's cardiac status and fluid volume status. Diastole is the filling stage of the cardiac cycle so that the volume that has filled the left ventricle by end diastole represents the amount of blood available for ejection during systole. This left-ventricular volume is known as the preload. Although it is not possible to measure preload volume at the bedside, the pressure created by this volume can be measured using the PA catheter. Preload is equal to LVEDP as measured by the PAWP or left atrial pressure (LAP).

A significant relationship exists between LVEDP and myocardial dysfunction. As a general rule, the higher the LVEDP, the greater is the degree of myocardial dysfunction because the compromised ventricle is unable to eject all of the preload blood volume. A normal left-ventricular ejection fraction (EF) is 70%. The greater the degree of myocardial dysfunction, the lower is the EF and the higher the preload and LVEDP.

LVEDP can be measured by two methods using a PA catheter. The most accurate is to use the PAWP. When the small latex balloon is inflated and lodged in a pulmonary capillary, it occludes the vessel and blocks the pulmonary arterial pulsations. Thus the only pressure the catheter tip measures is the left atrial pressure, which is a reflection of LVEDP, because the mitral valve is open during diastole, but closed during systole; thus the PA catheter does not record left-ventricular systolic pressures. The second method is to use the pulmonary artery diastolic (PAD) pressure, because during diastole the PAD is equal to mean PAWP and LVEDP. However, if the patient has lung disease that has elevated the PA pressures independently from the cardiac pressures, the PAD will not accurately reflect function of the left side of the heart. Thus if there is a gradient between the PAWP and PAD pressure when the catheter is inserted, the patient may have significant lung disease. With pulmonary disease the PAD may be significantly higher than the PAWP (see Table 13-28, *C*). In failure of the left side of the heart, both the PAWP and the PAD pressure will be elevated and equal (see Table 13-27).

Stenosis of the mitral valve will alter the accuracy of PAWP and PAD pressures as parameters of left-ventricular function. In mitral valve stenosis left-atrial pressure and PAWP are increased, but these values are *not* reflective of LVEDP because a stenotic mitral valve decreases normal blood flow from the left atrium to the left ventricle, decreasing left-ventricular preload and consequently lowering LVEDP. Therefore a nonstenotic mitral valve is essential for accurate readings because a narrowed mitral valve will increase PAWP and PAD pressure in the presence of a normal LVEDP. If mitral regurgitation is present, the mean PAWP reading will be artificially elevated because of abnormal backflow of blood from the left ventricle to the left atrium during systole. Thus this PAWP reading may not be reflective of true LVEDP and is distinguished by very large v waves on the PAWP tracing (Table 13-28, *F*).

Catheters

The traditional PA catheter has four lumens for measurement of central venous pressure (CVP), PA pressures, PAWP, and cardiac output (Fig. 13-75, *A*). Catheters may have additional lumens, which can be used for intravenous (IV) infusion (Fig. 13-75, *B*) to measure continuous mixed venous oxygen saturation (Svo_2)[64] (Fig. 13-75, *C*), or to pace the heart using transvenous pacing electrodes (Fig. 13-75, *D* and *E*).

The PA catheter is 110 cm in length. The most frequently used size is No. 7 Fr, although 5 and 7.5 Fr sizes are available. Each of the four lumens exits into the heart at a

Table 13-27   Pulmonary artery catheters: selected indications for use and response to treatment

Diagnostic indications*	Possible cause	Associated clinical findings	Hemodynamic profile†	Treatment and expected response
Hypovolemic shock	Trauma Surgery Bleeding Burns Excessive diuresis	Cardiovascular (CV): sinus tachycardia, decreased blood pressure (BP) (systolic blood pressure [SBP] <90 mm Hg), weak peripheral pulses Pulmonary: lungs clear Renal: decreased urinary output Skin: normal skin temperature, no edema Neurological: variable	Low cardiac output (CO) Low cardiac index (CI) (<2.2 L/min/m²) High systemic vascular resistance (SVR) (>1600 dynes/sec/cm⁻⁵) Low pulmonary artery pressures (PAP) Low pulmonary artery wedge pressure (PAWP)	Treatment: fluid challenge Expected hemodynamic response: Decreased heart rate (HR) Increased BP Increased PA Increased PAWP, central venous pressure (CVP) Increased CO/CI Decreased SVR
Early septic shock	Sepsis	CV: sinus tachycardia, decreased BP (SBP <90 mm Hg), bounding peripheral pulses Pulmonary: lungs may be clear or congested, depending on the origin of the sepsis Renal: decreased urinary output Skin: warm and flushed Neurological: variable	High Co (>8 L/min) High CI Low SVR (<600 dynes/sec/cm⁻⁵) Low PAP Low PAWP Low CVP	Treatment: Intravenous (IV) fluid to maintain hemodynamic function Peripheral vasoconstricting agent (alpha) to increase SVR Antibiotics and laboratory cultures to find site of infection Expected hemodynamic response: Decreased HR Increased BP Increased PA pressures Increased PAWP/increased CVP Increased CO/CI Increased SVR
Advanced septic shock or multisystem failure shock	Sepsis Multisystem failure	CV: normal sinus rhythm or sinus tachycardia, decreased BP, weak peripheral pulses Pulmonary: lungs may be clear or congested, depending on the site of sepsis; acidosis based on arterial blood gas (ABG) values, may require mechanical ventilation Renal: decreased urinary output, may have increased blood urea nitrogen (BUN) and increased creatinine Skin: cool and mottled Neurological: variable, depending on fluid status and drugs used in treatment	Low CO Low CI (<2.2 L/min/m²) High SVR (>1600 dynes/sec/cm⁻⁵) High or low PAP High or low PAWP High or low CVP	Treatment: Vasodilators to decrease SVR Antibiotics Support of body systems as necessary (e.g., mechanical ventilation or hemodialysis) Expected hemodynamic response: Decreased HR Increased BP Normal PA/PAWP/CVP pressures Decreased SVR, decreased pulmonary vascular resistance Increased CO/CI

*Patients undergoing major vascular or cardiac surgery may also have a PA catheter in situ to follow the trend of CO/CI, SVR/PVR, and fluid status during the first 24 hours after surgery.

†See Table 13-24 for definitions and normal values of hemodynamic parameters listed in this table.

Continued.

Table 13-27 Pulmonary artery catheters: selected indications for use and response to treatment—cont'd

Diagnostic indications*	Possible cause	Associated clinical findings	Hemodynamic profile†	Treatment and expected response
Cardiogenic shock	Left-ventricular pump failure caused by acute myocardial infarction, severe mitral or aortic valve disease	CV: sinus tachycardia, possibly dysrhythmias, BP <90 mm Hg systolic, S_3 or S_4, weak peripheral pulses Pulmonary: lungs may have crackles or pulmonary edema Renal: decreased urinary output Skin: cool, pale, and moist Neurological: may have decreased mentation casued by low BP and CO	Low CO Low CI (<2.2 L/min/m²) High SVR (>1600 dynes/sec/cm⁻⁵) High PAP High PAWP (>15 mm Hg) High CVP Low stroke volume index (SI) Low left cardiac work index (LCWI) Low left-ventricular stroke work index (LVSWI)	Treatment: Inotropic drugs to increase left-ventricular contractility Vasodilators or intra-aortic balloon pump (IABP) to decrease afterload Diuretics to decrease preload Optimization of heart rate and control of dysrhythmias Expected hemodynamic response: Decreased HR Increased BP Decreased PAP Decreased PAWP Decreased CVP Decreased SVR Decreased PVR Increased CO/CI Increased SI Increased LCWI Increased LVSWI
Acute respiratory distress syndrome (ARDS) *or* noncardiogenic pulmonary edema	Trauma Sepsis Shock Inhaled toxins (smoke, chemicals, 100% oxygen) Aspiration of gastric contents Metabolic disorders	CV: sinus tachycardia, high or low BP, normal peripheral pulses Pulmonary: poor oxygenation and pulmonary edema, increased respiratory rate or need for mechanical ventilation Renal: increased or decreased urinary output Skin: normal temperature Neurological: anxiety or confusion associated with respiratory distress and poor oxygenation	Normal CO Normal CI Normal SVR Normal PAWP High PAP High PVR (>250 dynes/sec/cm⁻⁵) Low righ cardiac work index (RCWI) Low right-ventricular stroke work index (RVSWI)	Treatment: Eliminate cause of ARDS Support pulmonary function as necessary Expected hemodynamic resonse: Decreased HR Normal BP Decreased PAP Decreased PVR Increased RCWI Increased RVSWI Normal CO/CI Normal SVR

different point along the catheter length (see Fig. 13-75, *A*). The proximal (CVP) lumen is situated in the right atrium and is used for IV infusion, CVP measurement, withdrawal of venous blood samples, and injection of fluid for cardiac output determinations. The distal (PA) lumen is located at the end of the PA catheter and is situated in the pulmonary artery. It is used to record PA pressures and can be used for withdrawal of blood samples to measure SvO_2. The third lumen opens into a latex balloon at the end of the catheter that can be inflated with 0.8 to 1.5 cc of air. The balloon is inflated during catheter insertion once the catheter reaches the right atrium to assist in forward flow of the catheter and to minimize right-ventricular ectopy from the catheter tip. It is also inflated to obtain PAWP measurements when the

PA catheter is correctly positioned in the pulmonary artery. The fourth lumen is a thermistor used to measure changes in blood temperature. It is located 4 cm from the catheter tip and is used to measure thermodilution cardiac output. The connector end of the lumen is attached directly to the cardiac output computer.

If continuous SvO_2 will be measured, the catheter will have an additional fiberoptic lumen that exits at the tip of the catheter. If cardiac pacing will be used, two PA catheter methods are available. One type of catheter has three atrial (A) and two ventricular (V) pacing electrodes attached to the catheter so that when it is properly positioned, the patient can be connected to a pacemaker and A-V paced. The other catheter method uses a specific transvenous pacing wire that

Table 13-28   Clinical interpretation of pulmonary artery (PA) waveforms

PA pressure	Clinical interpretation	Waveform interpretation
Pulmonary artery systolic (PAS) pressure	PAS pressure reflects the systolic pressure in the pulmonary vasculature. See waveform A for normal waveform. It is elevated in pulmonary hypertension because of idiopathic causes, in some congential heart defects, and in lung disease.	
Pulmonary artery diastolic (PAD) pressure	In the patient with healthy lung vasculature, PAD pressure reflects left ventricular end diastolic pressure (LVEDP) as shown in waveform B. In the presence of lung disease or pulmonary hypertension, PAD pressure is *not* an accurate reflection of pulmonary artery wedge pressure (PAWP), as shown in waveform C.	
Mean pulmonary artery pressure (PAP mean or PAP$_M$)	PAP mean pressure is used in the calculation of pulmonary vascular resistance (PVR) and pulmonary vascular resistance index (PVRI) as described in Table 13-24. High mean pressures can be reflective of either cardiac or pulmonary disease. Low mean pressures are reflection of hypovolemia. See waveform D for PA mean placement.	
Pulmonary artery wedge pressure (PAWP) or pulmonary capillary wedge pressure (PCWP)	In the healthy patient, PAWP reflects blood in the left ventricle at end diastole (LVEDP). The normal PAWP waveform is a left-atrial waveform, as shown in waveform E. If a patient has mitral valve regurgitation, the v waves are larger than normal, increasing PAWP and possibly not reflecting true LVEDP, as shown in waveform F. PAWP is elevated in many cardiac disease states in which left-ventricular function is compromised. PAWP is low in hypovolemic states.	

passes down an additional catheter lumen and exits in the right ventricle if ventricular pacing is required.

Insertion

If a PA catheter is to be inserted into a patient who is awake, some brief explanations about the procedure are very helpful to ensure that the patient understands what is going to happen. The insertion techniques used for placement of a PA catheter are very similar to those described in the section on CVP line insertion. In addition, because the PA catheter will be positioned within the heart chambers and pulmonary artery on the right side of the heart, catheter passage is monitored, using either fluoroscopy (Fig. 13-76) or waveform analysis on the bedside monitor (see Table 13-28).

Before inserting the catheter into the vein, the physician, using sterile technique, will test the balloon for inflation and will flush the catheter with normal saline solution to remove any air. The PA catheter is then attached to the bedside hemodynamic line setup and monitor so that the waveforms can be visualized while the catheter is advanced through the right side of the heart (Fig. 13-77).

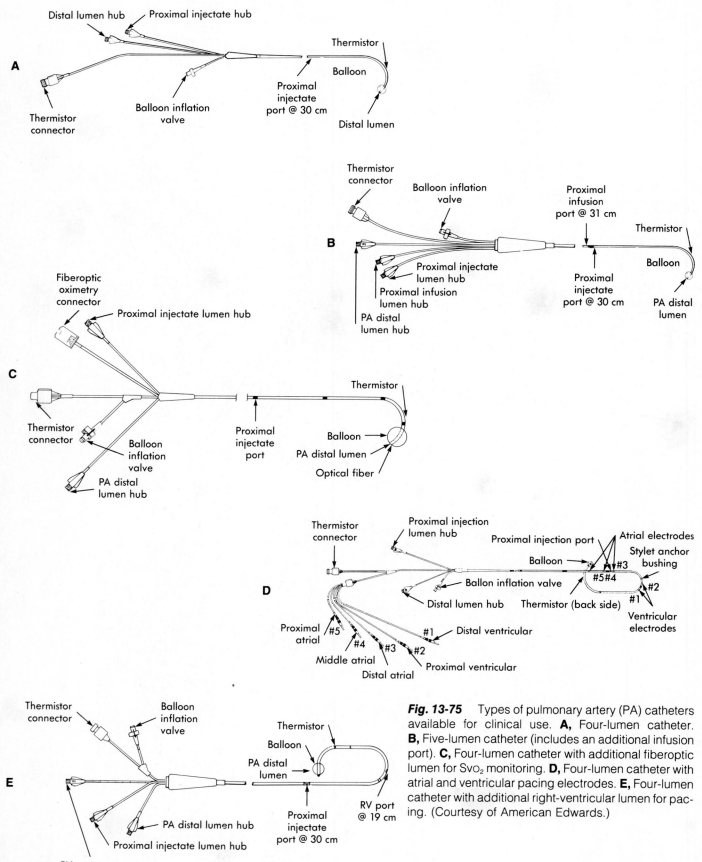

Fig. 13-75 Types of pulmonary artery (PA) catheters available for clinical use. **A,** Four-lumen catheter. **B,** Five-lumen catheter (includes an additional infusion port). **C,** Four-lumen catheter with additional fiberoptic lumen for SvO₂ monitoring. **D,** Four-lumen catheter with atrial and ventricular pacing electrodes. **E,** Four-lumen catheter with additional right-ventricular lumen for pacing. (Courtesy of American Edwards.)

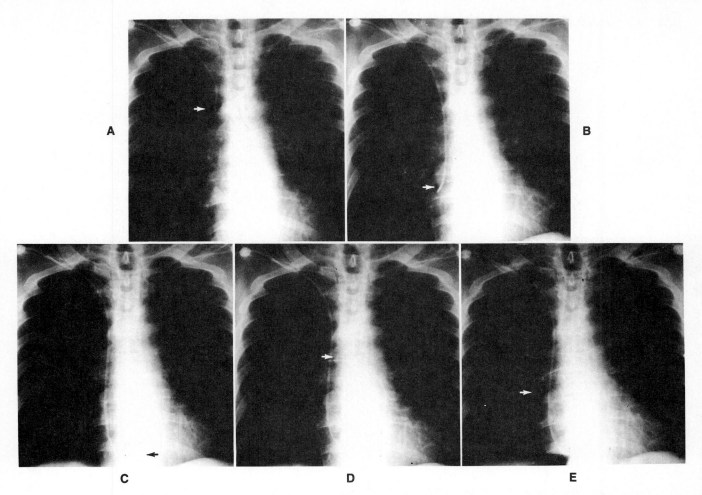

Fig. 13-76 **A,** Balloon-tipped catheter entering the thorax from the right basilic vein; the catheter tip is in the superior vena cava. **B,** Catheter tip is in the middle of the right atrium. **C,** Catheter tip is in the right ventricle. **D,** Catheter tip is in the pulmonary artery. **E,** Catheter tip is advanced to the PAWP position. (From Daily EK and Schroeder JS: Techniques in bedside hemodynamic monitoring, ed 3, St Louis, 1985, The CV Mosby Co.)

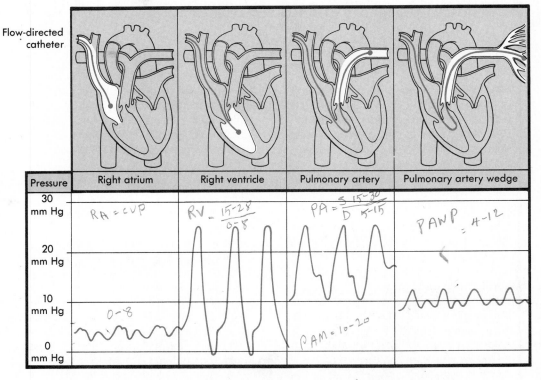

Fig. 13-77 PA catheter insertion with corresponding waveforms.

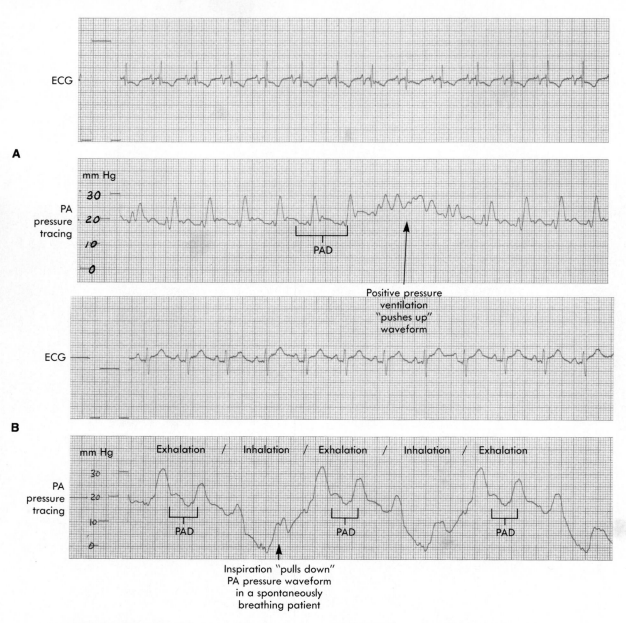

Fig. 13-78 PA waveforms that demonstrate the impact of ventilation of PA pressure readings. For accuracy, PA pressures should be read at end exhalation. **A,** Positive pressure ventilation: the increase in intrathoracic pressure during inhalation "pushes up" the PA pressure waveform, creating a false high reading. **B,** Spontaneous breathing: the decrease in intrathoracic pressure during normal inhalation "pulls down" the PA waveform, creating a false low reading.

Pulmonary Artery Waveform Interpretation

During insertion as the PA catheter is advanced into the right atrium, a right-atrial waveform should be visible on the monitor, with recognizable a, c, and v waves (see Fig. 13-77). The normal mean pressure in the right atrium is 2 to 5 mm Hg. Before passage through the tricuspid valve, the balloon at the tip of the catheter is inflated for two reasons: first, it cushions the pointed tip of the PA catheter so that if the tip comes into contact with the right ventricular wall, it will cause less myocardial irritability and conse-

quently fewer ventricular dysrhythmias; second, inflation of the balloon assists the catheter to float with the flow of blood from the right ventricle into the pulmonary artery. The right-ventricular waveform has a saw-toothed pattern and is pulsatile, with distinct systolic and diastolic pressures. Normal right-ventricular pressures are 20-30/0-5 mm Hg. Even with the balloon inflated, it is not uncommon for ventricular ectopy to occur at this time. All patients who have a PA catheter inserted must have simultaneous electrocardiographic monitoring, with defibrillator and emergency resuscitation equipment nearby.

As the catheter enters the pulmonary artery, the waveform again changes. The diastolic pressure rises. Normal PA systolic and diastolic pressures are 20-30/10 mm Hg. A dicrotic notch, visible on the downslope of the waveform, represents closure of the pulmonic valve.

While the balloon remains inflated, the catheter is advanced into the wedge position. Here, the waveform decreases in size and is nonpulsatile, reflective of a normal left-atrial tracing with a and v wave deflections. This is described as a wedge tracing because the balloon is "wedged" into a small pulmonary vessel (see Fig. 13-77). The balloon occludes the pulmonary vessel so that the PA lumen is only exposed to left atrial pressure and is protected from the pulsatile influence of a normal PA tracing. When the balloon is deflated, the catheter should spontaneously float back into the pulmonary artery. When the balloon is reinflated, the wedge tracing should be visible. The PAWP ranges from 4 to 12 mm Hg.

After insertion, the catheter is sutured to the skin, and a chest radiograph is taken to verify placement. If the catheter is advanced too far into the pulmonary bed, the patient is at risk for infarction of a segment of lung because the balloon will occlude blood flow to the area. If the catheter is not sufficiently advanced into the PA, it will not be useful for PAWP readings. The chest radiograph is also used to verify that the PA catheter has not looped or knotted in one of the cardiac chambers and to check for possible pneumothorax.

Nursing Care

When caring for a patient with a PA catheter, the PA tracing must be continuously monitored. A significant component of the nursing assessment involves evaluation of the PA waveform to ensure that the catheter has not migrated forward into the wedge position since a segment of lung can be infarcted if the catheter occludes an arteriole for a prolonged period. Other factors that affect PA measurement include head-of-bed position and lateral body position relative to transducer height placement, respiratory variation, and positive end-expiratory pressure (PEEP).[32] If the transducer is placed at the level of the phlebostatic axis, a head-of-bed position up to 45 degrees is appropriate for most patients in the supine position.[32] In the lateral position the fourth intercostal space and midsternum are suggested as the reference level.[32] All PA and PAWP tracings are subject to respiratory interference, especially if the patient is on a positive pressure volume-cycled ventilator. During inhalation the ventilator "pushes up" the PA tracing to produce an artificially high reading (Fig. 13-78, A). During spontaneous respiration, negative intrathoracic pressure "pulls down" the waveform and can produce an erroneously low measurement (Fig. 13-78, B). To minimize the impact of respiratory variation, the PAD should be read at end exhalation, which is the most stable point in the respiratory cycle. If the digital number fluctuates with respiration, a paper readout can be obtained to verify true PAD.

If PEEP greater than 10 cm H_2O is used, PAWP and PA pressure will be artificially elevated. Because of this impact of PEEP, patients were taken off the ventilator to record PA pressure measurements in the past. However, today it is believed that since patients remain on PEEP for treatment, they may remain on it during measurement of PA pressures. In this situation the trend of PA readings is more important than one individual measurement.

Use of PA catheters is not entirely risk free. Potential complications include ventricular dysrhythmias, rupture of a pulmonary artery, endocarditis, pulmonary artery thrombosis, embolus, or hemorrhage.[53]

Cardiac Output

The PA catheter measures cardiac output (CO), using the thermodilution method. This technique can be performed at the bedside and results in CO calculated in liters per minute. A known amount (5 or 10 ml) of iced or room temperature normal saline solution is injected into the proximal lumen of the catheter. The injectant exits into the right atrium and travels with the flow of blood past the thermistor (temperature sensor) at the distal end of the catheter. The thermodilution CO method uses the indicator-dilution principle, in which a known temperature is the indicator, and it, in turn, is based on the principle that the change in temperature over time is inversely proportional to blood flow.[27] Blood flow can be diagrammatically represented as a CO curve, on which temperature is plotted against time (Fig. 13-79, A). Many of the most recent hemodynamic monitors display this CO curve, which must then be interpreted to determine whether the CO injection is valid. The normal curve has a smooth upstroke, with a rounded peak and a gradually tapering downslope. If the curve has an uneven pattern, it may indicate faulty injection technique, and the CO measurement should be repeated. Patient movement or coughing will also alter the CO (Fig. 13-79, B).

Generally, three cardiac outputs that are within a 10% mean range are obtained and are averaged to calculate CO. To ensure accurate readings, the difference between injectant temperature and body temperature must be at least 10° to 12° C, and the injectant must be delivered within 4 seconds, with minimal handling of the syringe to prevent warming of the solution.[34] The injectant should always be delivered at the same point in the respiratory cycle; usually end exhalation is used.[32,34] Reliable CO measurements can be obtained with the head of bed elevated up to 20 degrees, with the patient in the supine or lateral position.[32,34]

Calculated Hemodynamic Profiles

For the patient with a thermodilution PA catheter in place, additional hemodynamic information can be calculated using routine vital signs, cardiac output, and body surface area. These measurements are calculated using specific formulas or are indexed to a patient's body size, using either the DuBois Body Surface Chart or the computer program associated with the new generation of hemodynamic monitors.[49]

The calculated hemodynamic profiles were described in Table 13-24. Clinical use of these profiles is described in two case studies. Case study 1 is a step-by-step interpretation of the hemodynamic profile to familiarize the reader with use of calculated values, and case study 2 uses only values indexed to body weight and illustrates the impact of treatment on these values over time (see the boxes on pp. 247 and 248).

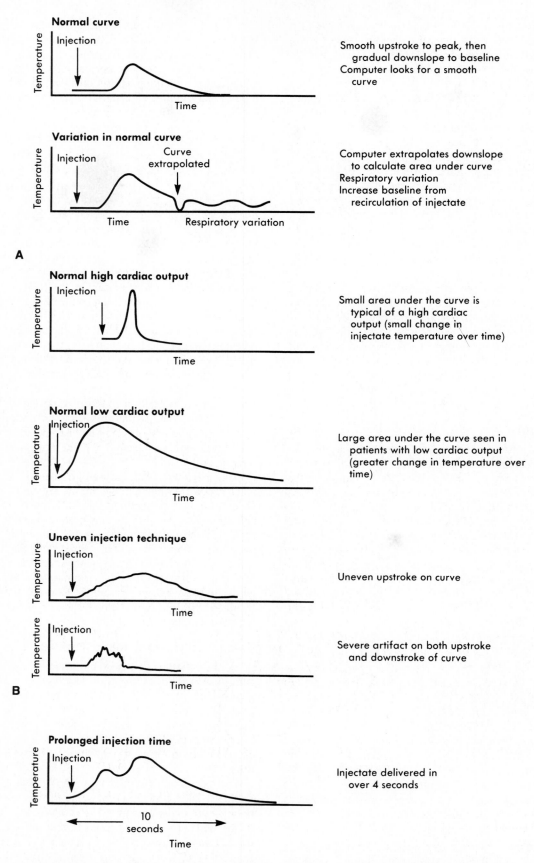

Normal curve

Smooth upstroke to peak, then gradual downslope to baseline
Computer looks for a smooth curve

Variation in normal curve

Computer extrapolates downslope to calculate area under curve
Respiratory variation
Increase baseline from recirculation of injectate

A

Normal high cardiac output

Small area under the curve is typical of a high cardiac output (small change in injectate temperature over time)

Normal low cardiac output

Large area under the curve seen in patients with low cardiac output (greater change in temperature over time)

Uneven injection technique

Uneven upstroke on curve

Severe artifact on both upstroke and downstroke of curve

B

Prolonged injection time

Injectate delivered in over 4 seconds

Fig. 13-79   A, Variations in the normal cardiac output curve. **B,** Abnormal cardiac output curves that will produce an erroneous cardiac output valve.

HEMODYNAMIC PROFILE: CASE STUDY I

Mr. SR has a medical history of cardiomyopathy and chronic obstructive pulmonary disease (COPD). He is admitted to a coronary care unit because of an exacerbation of his biventricular heart failure. He has been complaining of anginal pain and shortness of breath. His nursing diagnoses are decreased cardiac output and impaired gas exchange.

Height	163 cm	PAD	27 mm Hg	PVR	322 dynes/sec/cm^{-5}
Weight	79 kg	PAP$_M$	36 mm Hg	PVRI	612 dynes/sec/cm^{-5}/m²
Body surface		PAWP	26 mm Hg	LCW	2.1 kg-m
area (BSA)	1.9 m²	CVP	24 mm Hg	LCWI	1.1 kg-m/m²
HR	104 bpm	CO	2.48 L/min	LVSW	2.4 g-m
ABP		CI	1.31 L/min/m²	LVSWI	10.7 g-m/m²
Systolic	88 mm Hg	SV	23.8 ml	RCW	1.21 kg-m
Diastolic	51 mm Hg	SI	12.5 ml/m²	RCWI	0.64 kg-m/m²
MAP	63 mm Hg	SVR	1257 dynes/sec/cm^{-5}	RVSW	11.7 g-m
PAS	55 mm Hg	SVRI	2388 dynes/sec/cm^{-5}/m²	RVSWI	6.2 g-m/m²

ANALYSIS OF HEMODYNAMIC PROFILE*

Profile	*Analysis*
HR	Heart rate of 104 beats per minute (bpm) is above normal limits (normal, 60-100 bpm).
ABP (arterial blood pressure)	Narrow pulse pressure of 88/51 with a low mean arterial pressure (MAP) of 63 mm Hg (normal MAP, 65-90).
Pulmonary artery pressure	Pulmonary artery pressures are elevated (55/27 mm Hg), consistent with diagnosis of cardiomyopathy, failure of left side of the heart, and COPD (normal PA, 25/10 mm Hg).
PAWP (pulmonary artery wedge pressure)	Elevated PAWP (26 mm Hg), consistent with diagnosis of cardiomyopathy and failure of left side of heart (normal PAWP, 6-12 mm Hg).
CVP (central venous pressure)	Elevated CVP (24 mm Hg), consistent with diagnosis of cardiomyopathy, failure of right side of heart and COPD (normal CVP, 4-6 mm Hg).
CO (cardiac output) and CI (cardiac index)	Poor CO and CI (CO 2.48 L/min, CI 1.31 L/min/m²). Both values are below normal (normal CO, 4-6 L/min; normal CI, 2.2-4 L/min/m²).
SV (stroke volume) and SI (stroke volume index)	SV and SI are low (SV 23.8 ml, SI 12.5 ml/min/m²). These results would be anticipated from the low cardiac output (normal SV, 60-70 ml; normal SI, 40-50 ml/min/m²).
SVR (systemic vascular resistance) and SVRI (systemic vascular resistance index)	SVR and SVRI are at the upper normal range (SVR 1257 dynes/sec/cm^{-5}, SVRI 2388 dynes/sec/cm^{-5}/m²). These values are not contributing to the low cardiac output at this time (normal SVR, 800-1400 dynes/sec/cm^{-5}; normal SVRI, 2000-2400 dynes/sec/cm^{-5}/m²).
PVR (pulmonary vascular resistance) and PVRI (pulmonary vascular resistance index)	PVR and PVRI are elevated (PVR 322 dynes/sec/cm^{-5}, PVRI 612 dynes/sec/cm^{-5}/m²). High pulmonary vascular resistance may be contributing to the low cardiac output (normal PVR, 100-250 dynes/sec/cm^{-5}; normal PVRI, 225-315 dynes/sec/cm^{-5}/m²).
LCWI (left cardiac work index) and LVSWI (left-ventricular stroke work index)	Both LCWI and LVSWI are below normal (LCWI 1.1 kg-m/m², LVSWI 10.7 gm/m²), indicating left-ventricular myocardial damage may be present. This is consistent with SR's diagnosis of cardiomyopathy (normal LCWI, 3.4-4.2 kg-m/m²; normal LVSWI, 50-62 g-m/m²).
RCWI (right cardiac work index) and RVSWI (right-ventricular stroke work index)	RCWI is normal, but RVSWI is below normal (RCWI 0.64 kg-m/m², RVSWI 6.2 g-m/m²), indicating right-ventricular myocardial damage may be present. This is consistent with SR's diagnosis of cardiomyopathy and history of COPD (normal RCWI, 0.54-0.66 kg-m/m²; normal RVSWI, 7.9-9.7 g-m/m²).
Nursing impression:	The hemodynamic data confirms the nursing clinical diagnosis of poor cardiac output. The goal will be to improve CO within the limits of SR's myocardial dysfunction and COPD. As CO improves and PA pressures decrease, the patient will have less pulmonary congestion, which will improve alveolar gas exchange.

*Formulas and normal values for the hemodynamic values are in Table 13-24.

HEMODYNAMIC PROFILE: CASE STUDY 2

1. ADMISSION

Mrs. JL has been admitted to the critical care unit with pulmonary edema. She has a history of anterior wall myocardial infarction and severe chronic obstruction pulmonary disease (COPD).

Height	159 cm	MAP	106 mm Hg	SI	9.9 ml/m²
Weight	45.8 kg	PAS	53 mm Hg	SVRI	5351 dynes/sec/cm⁻⁵/m²
Body surface		PAD	27 mm Hg	PVRI	1046 dynes/sec/cm⁻⁵/m²
area (BSA)	1.40 m²	PAP$_M$	44 mm Hg	LCWI	1.9 kg-m/m²
HR	131 bpm	PAWP	27 mm Hg	LVSWI	14.3 gpm/m²
ABP		CVP	19 mm Hg	RCWI	0.78 kg-m/m²
Systolic	160 mm Hg	CO	1.82 L/min	RVSWI	5.9 gpm/m²
Diastolic	80 mm Hg	CI	1.3 L/min/m²		

Analysis of hemodynamic profile 1*

In the above hemodynamic profile, note the fast heart rate, high MAP, high pulmonary artery and CVP filling pressures, low CI, SI, LVSWI, and RVSWI, and high SVRI and PVRI. These values are consistent with a diagnosis of failure of the left side of the heart, causing pulmonary edema, that may lead to cardiogenic shock. Treatment focused on increasing the cardiac index by lowering SVRI and PVRI, using intravenous (IV) sodium nitroprusside and IV nitroglycerin in continuous infusion.

2. 3 HOURS LATER

Height	159 cm	MAP	83 mm Hg	SI	16.5 ml/m²
Weight	45.8 kg	PAS	41 mm Hg	SVRI	3088 dynes/sec/cm⁻⁵/m²
Body surface		PAD	26 mm Hg	PVRI	300 dynes/sec/cm⁻⁵/m²
area	1.40 m²	PAM	33 mm Hg	LCWI	2.1 kg-m/m²
(BSA)	113 bpm	PAWP	26 mm Hg	LVSWI	18.6 g-m/m²
HR		CVP	11 mm Hg	RCWI	0.84 kg-m/m²
ABP	104 mm Hg	CO	2.61 L/min	RVSWI	7.4 g-m/m²
Systolic	69 mm Hg	CI	1.86 L/min/m²		
Diastolic					

Analysis of hemodynamic profile 2

Results 3 hours later after sodium nitroprusside administration: note improving hemodynamics shown above as normal MAP and lower intracardiac filling pressures (PA and CVP). However, CI and SI remain low, and SVRI is above normal. Mrs. JL remains in severe left-ventricular failure because of her low CI.

3. THE NEXT DAY

Height	159 cm	MAP	75 mm Hg	SI	22.5 ml/m²
Weight	45.8 kg	PAS	31 mm Hg	SVRI	2423 dynes/sec/cm⁻⁵/m²
Body surface		PAD	15 mm Hg	PVRI	273 dynes/sec/cm⁻⁵/m²
area	1.40 m²	PAP$_M$	23 mm Hg	LCWI	2.4 kg-m/m²
(BSA)	104 bpm	PAWP	15 mm Hg	LVSWI	22.9 g-m/m²
HR		CVP	4 mm Hg	RCWI	0.74 kg-m/m²
ABP	111 mm Hg	CO	3.28 L/min	RVSWI	7.1 g-m/m²
Systolic	60 mm Hg	CI	2.34 L/min/m²		
Diastolic					

Analysis of hemodynamic profile 3

The following day Mrs. JL's hemodynamics have improved with continued use of sodium nitroprusside and nitroglycerin. CI is in the low-normal range, and SVRI and PVRI are in the high-normal range. LVSWI remains low, reflecting the patient's compromised left ventricle from the previous anterior wall myocardial infarction.

*See previous box for explanation of abbreviations, and see Table 13-24 for explanation of hemodynamic values.

CONTINUOUS MONITORING OF MIXED VENOUS OXYGEN SATURATION
Indications

Continuous monitoring of mixed venous oxygen saturation (SvO_2) is indicated for the patient who has the potential to develop an imbalance between oxygen supply and metabolic tissue demand. This includes the patient in a shock state and the patient with severe respiratory compromise such as adult respiratory distress syndrome (ARDS). Continuous SvO_2 monitoring is a relatively new clinical tool in critical care. It measures the balance achieved between arterial oxygen supply (SaO_2) and oxygen demand at the tissue level by sampling desaturated venous mixed blood from the pulmonary artery (SvO_2).[64] It is called mixed venous blood because it is a mixture of all of the venous blood saturations from many body tissues. Under normal conditions the cardiopulmonary system achieves a balance between oxygen supply and demand. The four factors that contribute to this balance include cardiac output (CO), hemoglobin (Hb), arterial oxygen saturation (SaO_2), and tissue metabolism (VO_2). Three of these factors (CO, Hb, and SaO_2) contribute to the *supply* of oxygen to the tissues. Tissue metabolism determines the quantity of oxygen extracted at tissue level or oxygen consumption, and creates the *demand* for oxygen.[16]

In addition to interpreting SvO_2, it is possible to calculate the amounts of oxygen that are provided by the cardiopulmonary system and the amount of oxygen consumed by the body tissues. These calculations are based on the principles of oxygen transport physiology and are the basis for calculation of SvO_2. These formulas are explained in greater detail in Table 13-29.

Catheters

In 1981 a fiberoptic pulmonary artery catheter was designed that continuously monitored SvO_2. The catheter contains the traditional four lumens plus a lumen containing optical fibers. The fiberoptics are attached to an optical module that is connected by a cable to a small bedside computer (Fig. 13-80). The optical module transmits a narrow band–width light. The light travels down one optical fiber, is reflected off the hemoglobin in the blood, and returns to the optical module through the second fiberoptic. The SvO_2 signal is averaged every 5 seconds and is recorded on a continuous display or printout.[64]

The catheter is calibrated before insertion into the patient by using a standard color reference system, which comes as part of the catheter package. Insertion technique and insertion sites are identical to those used for placement of a conventional pulmonary artery catheter. Waveform analysis and/or SvO_2 can be used for accurate placement. Once the catheter is inserted, recalibration is unnecessary unless the catheter becomes disconnected from the optical module. To calibrate when the catheter is inserted in a patient, a mixed venous blood sample must be withdrawn from the pulmonary artery lumen and sent to the laboratory for analysis of oxygen saturation (SvO_2). To obtain accurate results, the laboratory should use a "reflectance" technique similar to the principle used by the fiberoptic catheter.

Nursing Care

SvO_2 monitoring provides a continuous assessment of the balance between oxygen supply and oxygen demand for an individual patient. Nursing assessment includes evaluation of the SvO_2 value and evaluation of the four factors (SaO_2, CO, Hb, and VO_2) that maintain the oxygen supply–demand balance.

Normal SvO_2 is 75%. For most critically ill patients, an SvO_2 value between 60% and 80% is evidence of adequate balance between oxygen supply and demand. If the SvO_2 value changes by more than 10% and this change is maintained for more than 10 minutes, the nurse should determine which of the four factors is affecting SvO_2.

Assessment of arterial oxygen saturation. The change in SvO_2 may be caused by a change in SaO_2. If the SaO_2 is increased because supplemental oxygen is being given, the SvO_2 will also rise. If the SaO_2 is decreased, SvO_2 will fall. Decreased SaO_2 can be caused by any action or disease that reduces oxygen supply, including ARDS, endotracheal suctioning, removing a patient from the ventilator, or removal of an oxygen mask. Figure 13-81 shows a fall in SvO_2 after suctioning in a patient with ARDS. Transient decreases in SvO_2 related to a nursing action such as endotracheal suctioning are not usually a cause for concern. Some patients may be slow to resaturate up to the presuction level of SvO_2. In this case an appropriate nursing intervention is to wait until SvO_2 has again returned to baseline before initiating other nursing activities.

Assessment of cardiac output. A change in SvO_2 may also be caused by an alteration in cardiac output (CO). Four hemodynamic factors affect CO—preload, afterload, heart rate, and contractility. Changes in one or more of these individual factors will affect CO. Fig. 13-82 shows an improvement in a patient's SvO_2 from 70% to 80% after volume administration that increased preload (point A). A while later the patient's CO fell after a short run of ventricular tachycardia (point B). Any major loss of heart rate will drop CO. Alterations in contractility and afterload (systemic vascular resistance) also have the potential to alter CO.

Assessment of hemoglobin. Hemoglobin (Hb) is the transport mechanism for oxygen in the blood. When oxygen is bound to Hb, it is described as oxyhemoglobin (HbO_2). If the hemoglobin level falls as a result of bleeding or red cell destruction, the body maintains oxygen transport by increasing cardiac output and using oxygen reserves in the venous blood return. Therefore the body is able to compensate efficiently for anemia. In the healthy person hemoglobin must be extremely low before SvO_2 falls. However, in an anemic patient with a compromised cardiovascular system who is unable to adequately increase cardiac output, SvO_2 will decline as venous oxygen reserves are consumed by the body.

Assessment of oxygen consumption. Oxygen consumption (VO_2) describes the amount of oxygen the body tissues consume for normal function in 1 minute. If the body's metabolic demands increase because of exercise or increased metabolic rate, the body will increase cardiac output to augment oxygen supply and will also use reserve oxygen in the venous system. Normal oxygen delivery to

Table 13-29 Calculations and explanation of oxygen transport physiology

Name	Abbreviation	Formula	Normal value	Explanation
Arterial oxygen saturation	SaO_2	$\dfrac{HbO_2}{(Hb + HbO_2)} \times 100$	>96%	Hb, hemoglobin; HbO_2, oxyhemoglobin. The arterial oxygen saturation represents the amount of oxyhemoglobin (oxygen bound to hemoglobin) divided by the total hemoglobin. Normally 96% of oxygen is bound to hemoglobin.
Blood oxygen content	CaO_2 (arterial) CvO_2 (venous)	$(O_2$ dissolved$) + (O_2$ saturation$)$ $(PO_2 \times 0.0031) + (1.34 \times Hb \times SO_2)$	19-20 vol % 12-15 vol %	Blood oxygen (O_2) content represents the amount of oxygen dissolved in 100 ml of blood. It can be calculated for both arterial blood (CaO_2) and for venous blood (CvO_2) and is measured in volume percent (vol %). It is the combination of both dissolved O_2 (PaO_2) and O_2 saturation (SaO_2).
Blood oxygen transport		$CO \times CaO_2 \times 10$ (arterial) $CO \times CvO_2 \times 10$ (venous)	1000 ml/min 750 ml/min	Oxygen transport represents the amount of oxygen transported to or from the tissues each minute in milliliters (ml/min). Arterial O_2 transport is a measure of the O_2 delivered to the tissues. Venous O_2 transport reflects the venous return to the right side of the heart. Oxygen transport is calculated by multiplying the cardiac output (CO) by the oxygen content $(CaO_2$ or $CvO_2)$ and by the number 10. The difference between normal arterial and normal venous O_2 return represents oxygen consumption by the tissues.

Tissue oxygen consumption	$\dot{V}O_2$	250 ml/min	Arterial O_2 transport minus venous O_2 transport $(CO \times CaO_2 \times 10) - (CO \times CvO_2 \times 10)$	Oxygen consumption represents the amount of oxygen consumed by the tissues in 1 minute. To calculate VO_2, it is necessary to know both arterial oxygen transport and venous oxygen transport values, which are calculated in ml/min. The difference represents tissue oxygen consumption.
Arterial venous oxygen difference	A-VO_2 difference	3.0-5.5 vol %	Arterial O_2 content minus venous O_2 content $CaO_2 - CvO_2$	The arterial-venous oxygen difference represents the difference between the arterial oxygen content (CaO_2) and the venous oxygen content (CvO_2). Because CaO_2 and CvO_2 are measured in volume percent (vol %), A-VO_2 difference is also measured in vol %.
Mixed venous oxygen saturation	SvO_2	60%-80%	Arterial O_2 transport minus tissue consumption equals venous return $(CO \times CaO_2 \times 10) - VO_2$	Mixed venous oxygen saturation (SvO_2) represents the venous oxygen return that is bound (saturated) with hemoglobin. Saturation is measured in percent (%). The SvO_2 value is a function of the amount of oxygen delivered to the tissues minus the amount of oxygen consumed by the tissues (VO_2) in milliliters per minute. The higher the amount (ml) of oxygen in the venous return, the greater the hemoglobin saturation will be.

FIBEROPTIC CATHETER

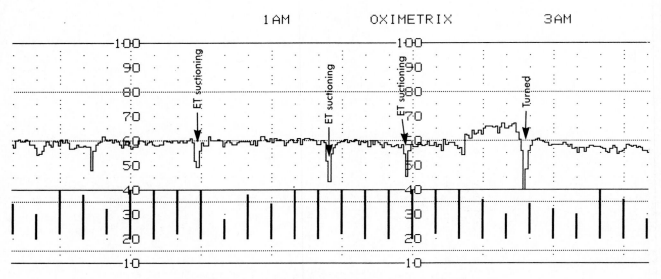

Fig. 13-80 Oximetric fiberoptic PA catheter and optical module. (Courtesy Abbott Critical Care and Control Systems, Mountain View, Calif.)

Fig. 13-81 Fall in Svo₂ during endotracheal suctioning.

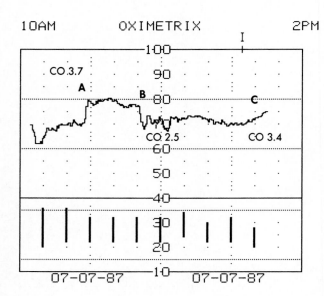

Fig. 13-82 Impact of changes in cardiac output (CO) on Svo₂ values. Point *A:* Just before point A, Svo₂ readings are low because CO and pulmonary artery pressures were low as a result of excessive diuresis. Infusion of 500 ml of colloid solution and 1000 ml of lactated Ringer's solution crystalloid increased the Svo₂ and improved the CO, which rose to 3.7 L/min. Point *B:* A short run of ventricular tachycardia caused the CO to fall to 2.5 L/min and decreased the Svo₂ value. Point *C:* The beginning of an upward trend in Svo₂ is related to administration of fluids and to improvement in CO and in filling pressures. CO is now 3.4 L/min. Graph represents a 4-hour printout; the space between each dotted line represents 20 minutes.

the tissues is 1000 ml of oxygen per minute. At rest a person might consume 250 ml of oxygen per minute, leaving a venous oxygen reserve of 750 ml of oxygen per minute (Table 13-30). Thus for the normal individual the combination of increased CO and utilization of considerable venous oxygen reserve provides adequate compensation for increased metabolic needs. However, for the critically ill patient with either cardiac or respiratory dysfunction, an increase in activity leading to increased oxygen consumption may overwhelm the cardiopulmonary system and oxygen reserves.

An example of the impact of increased oxygen consumption on SvO_2 is shown in the case study in the box on p. 254. Patient EH has just been admitted to the intensive care unit and is cold and shivering after cardiopulmonary bypass and cardiac surgery. At point A, the shivering has greatly increased EH's oxygen consumption. In addition, his CO is low, as is his arterial oxygen supply (because of compromised cardiovascular function). At point B, the shivering has stopped after sedation; consequently, his tissue oxygen consumption (VO_2) has decreased, and SvO_2 has increased. However, because of EH's compromised cardiovascular system, CO remains low with a low arterial oxygen transport. Thus the very low SvO_2 at point A is clearly caused by increased oxygen consumption in the presence of a compromised cardiovascular system.

Simple patient movements such as getting out of bed or being weighed on a bed scale can also decrease SvO_2, especially if the patient has cardiopulmonary dysfunction. In compromised patients it may take several minutes for resaturation (rise in SvO_2) to occur. In this situation the appropriate nursing action is to observe the patient clinically in conjunction with monitoring SvO_2 and to postpone additional maneuvers until the SvO_2 has returned to baseline.

Assessment of SvO_2. If SvO_2 is within the normal range (60% to 80%) and the patient is not clinically compromised, one can assume that oxygen supply and demand are balanced for that individual. The situation becomes out of balance when there is either a decrease in oxygen delivery because of changes in SaO_2, CO, or Hb or an increase in oxygen demand (increased VO_2). If SvO_2 falls below 60% and is sustained, the clinician must assume that oxygen supply is not equal to demand (see Table 13-29). It is helpful to assess the cause of decreased SvO_2 in a logical sequence that reflects knowledge of the meaning of the SvO_2 value: (1) to assess whether decreased SvO_2 is caused by decreased oxygen supply, verify the effectiveness of the ventilator or oxygen mask or check arterial oxygen saturation (SaO_2) by transcutaneous oximetry or from arterial blood gas values, (2) to assess cardiac function, perform a CO measurement, (3) to assess hemogobin (Hb), draw a blood sample for laboratory analysis, and (4) to assess whether decreased SvO_2 is the result

Table 13-30 Clinical interpretation of SvO_2 measurements

SvO_2 measurement	Physiological basis for change in SvO_2	Clinical diagnosis and rationale
High SvO_2 (80%-95%)	1. Increased oxygen supply	1. Patient receiving more oxygen than required by clinical condition
	2. Decreased oxygen demand	2. Anesthesia, which causes sedation and decreased muscle movement Hypothermia, which lowers metabolic demand (e.g., with cardiopulmonary bypass) Sepsis caused by decreased ability of tissues to use oxygen at a cellular level
Normal SvO_2 (60%-80%)	Normal oxygen supply and metabolic demand	Balanced oxygen supply and demand
Low SvO_2 (less than 60%)	Decreased oxygen supply caused by	
	Low hemoglobin (Hb)	Anemia or bleeding with compromised cardiopulmonary system
	Low arterial saturation (SaO_2)	Hypoxemia resulting from decreased oxygen supply or lung disease
	Low cardiac output	Cardiogenic shock caused by left-ventricular pump failure
	Increased oxygen consumption (VO_2)	Metabolic demand exceeds oxygen supply in conditions that increase muscle movement and increase metabolic rate, including physiological states such as shivering, seizures, and hyperthermia and nursing interventions such as obtaining bed-scale weight and turning.

HEMODYNAMIC PROFILE: CASE STUDY 3

EH has just been admitted to the cardiovascular intensive care unit after open heart surgery. At point A, he has an extremely low mixed venous oxygen saturation (SvO_2) of 40%. An SvO_2 below 40% indicates that the oxygen supply is not adequate to meet the demands of the body tissues, resulting in metabolic acidosis. To determine the reason for the low SvO_2 it is necessary to know the hemoglobin (Hb), the arterial oxygen saturation (SaO_2), the cardiac output (CO), and the tissue oxygen consumption (VO_2). EH's Hb value is 11.6 g/dl (normal male Hb, 13.5-18.0 g/dl), which is acceptable after major surgery; the SaO_2 is 99.6% (normal, >97%), which is high because this patient is receiving mechanical ventilation with 70% oxygen immediately after surgery; and the CO is low at 3.15 L/min (normal, 4-6 L/min). EH is receiving dopamine 5 μg/kg/min for his low cardiac output. He is shivering and cold because his body temperature is only 35.2° C after the surgery. Using the values described above, Hb 11.6 g/dl, SaO_2 99.6%, and CO 3.15 L/min), it is possible to calculate the VO_2 for EH.

$$\text{ARTERIAL SUPPLY} \qquad\qquad \text{VENOUS RETURN}$$
$$\text{CO}\ (PaO_2 \times 0.0031) + (1.34 \times Hb \times SaO_2)\ 10 - \text{CO}\ (PvO_2 \times 0.0031) + (1.34 \times Hb \times SvO_2)\ 10 = VO_2$$

(To calculate arterial oxygen supply, the oxygen in the venous return, VO_2, and the difference between the arterial and venous oxygen content (A-V O_2 difference), insert EH's values into the above formula).

ARTERIAL SUPPLY	VENOUS RETURN	VO_2	A-VO_2 difference
3.15(354 × 0.0031) + (1.34 × 11.6 × 0.99)10	− 3.15(20 × 0.0031) + (1.34 × 11.6 × 0.38)10		
3.15(1.0 + 15.3)10	3.15(0.06 + 5.90)10		
3.15(16.3)10	3.15(5.90)10		
505 ml/min	183 ml/min	= 322 ml/min	10.4 vol %

At point A the arterial oxygen supply to the tissues is 505 ml/min (normal, 1000 ml/min), whereas the oxygen returned in the venous blood is only 183 ml/min (normal, 750 ml/min). EH's VO_2 is elevated at 322 ml/min (normal, 250 ml/min). The clinical goals for this patient would be to (1) increase the cardiac output and (2) use sedation or muscle relaxants to decrease oxygen consumption by controlling the shivering. The difference betwen the oxygen content in the arterial and the venous blood (A-V O_2 difference) is very large at 10.4 vol % (normal, 3.5-5.0 vol %). These calculated values confirm the nursing diagnosis of altered tissue perfusion with a decreased cardiac output.

Two hours later, at point B, EH's SvO_2 has improved to a low normal value of 60%. Additional inotropic drugs have been administered. At this time the Hb is 10.8 g/dl, SaO_2 is 99.6%, and CO remains low at 3.3 L/min. Thus the improvement in SvO_2 has not been caused by a dramatic increase in cardiac output. When EH's oxygen consumption is calculated at point B, it becomes evident that the decrease in physical activity after sedation with morphine sulphate to reduce shivering has improved the SvO_2.

$$\text{ARTERIAL SUPPLY} \qquad\qquad \text{VENOUS RETURN}$$
$$\text{CO}\ (PaO_2 \times 0.0031) + (1.34 \times Hb \times SaO_2)\ 10 - \text{CO}\ (PvO_2 \times 0.0031) + (1.34 \times Hb \times SvO_2)\ 10 = VO_2$$

ARTERIAL SUPPLY	VENOUS RETURN	VO_2	A-VO_2 difference
3.3(266 × 0.0031) + (1.34 × 10.8 × 0.99)10	− 3.3(28 × 0.0031) + (1.34 × 10.8 × 0.60)10		
3.3(0.82 + 14.32)10	3.3(0.86 + 8.6)10		
3.3(15.1)10	3.3(9.4)10		
498 ml/min	300 ml/min	= 198 ml/min	5.7 vol %

At Point B, EH's arterial oxygen supply is still low at 498 ml/min and the oxygen in his mixed venous blood return remains low at 300 ml/min. VO_2 is now lower than normal (typical after sedation)—198 ml/min. At this time the A-VO_2 difference is almost within normal limits at 5.7 vol %. These findings are confirmed by the low-normal SvO_2 value of 60% at point B. This case study illustrates the point that tissue oxygen consumption (O_2 demand) can be as important as cardiac output and oxygenation (O_2 supply) in determining mixed venous oxygen saturation (SvO_2) in the patient with a compromised cardiovascular system.

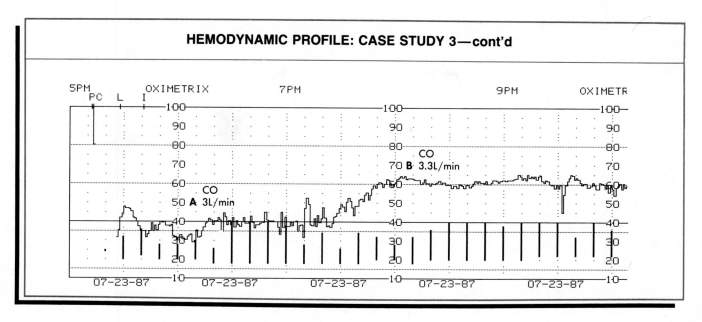

HEMODYNAMIC PROFILE: CASE STUDY 3—cont'd

of a recent patient movement (Vo$_2$) or a nursing action, clinically assess the patient.

If Svo$_2$ falls below 40%, the balance of oxygen supply and demand may not be adequate to meet tissue needs at the cellular level. The cells change from an aerobic to anaerobic mode of metabolism, which results in the production of lactic acid and is representative of a shock state in which cellular injury or cell death may result. At this point every attempt should be made to determine the cause of the low Svo$_2$ and to correct the oxygen supply–oxygen demand imbalance.

In certain clinical conditions Svo$_2$ may be increased above normal (>80%), including times of low oxygen demand (decreased Vo$_2$) such as during anesthesia and in certain cases of sepsis in which the tissue cells are unable to use the oxygen supplied to them and, as a consequence, venous oxygen reserve remains elevated and Svo$_2$ is higher than normal (see Table 13-29).

CARDIAC CATHETERIZATION AND CORONARY ARTERIOGRAPHY
Indications

Cardiac catheterization and coronary arteriography are routine diagnostic procedures for patients with known or suspected heart disease. Clinical indications for cardiac catheterization include myocardial ischemia, unstable angina, evolving myocardial infarction, congestive heart failure with a history that suggests coronary artery disease or valvular disease, and congenital heart disease. Cardiac catheterization is used both to confirm physical findings and to provide a baseline for medical or surgical therapy. During catheterization of the left side of the heart, hemodynamic pressure measurements are taken in the aortic root, the left ventricle, and the left atrium. Radiopaque contrast (dye) is used to visualize the left side of the heart (angiogram) and the coronary arteries (arteriogram). Catheterization of the right side of the heart is performed using a thermodilution pulmonary artery catheter. Information obtained includes hemodynamic pressure measurements in the right atrium, right ventricle, pulmonary artery, and pulmonary capillary

wedge and measurement of cardiac output, calculated hemodynamic values, oxygen saturations, and an angiogram of the right heart chambers using radiopaque contrast.

Procedure

Before the catheterization the patient will meet with the cardiologist to discuss the purpose, benefit, and risks of the study. For many patients, cardiac catheterization is the first major procedure after a diagnosis of possible cardiac disease. The patient is often very anxious and has many questions. It is important that both nursing and medical staff fully answer patients' questions about the catheterization experience.

The morning of the procedure the patient fasts except for ingesting prescribed cardiac medications. Light premedication is given before the patient goes to the catheterization laboratory. If there is a history of allergy, an antihistamine or corticosteroid may be administered to prevent an anaphylactic reaction to the radiopaque contrast. Throughout the cardiac catheterization the patient remains awake and alert. He or she is positioned on a hard table with a C- or U-shaped camera arm overhead or to the side. This arm can be moved to view the heart from several different angles. Cardiac catheterization catheters, available in a variety of designs and sizes, are placed in the groin area after the patient receives a local anesthetic. The choice of catheters is based on the cardiologist's experience and the diagnostic study required. The femoral artery is used to catheterize the left side of the heart, including the coronary arteries. The femoral vein is used to pass catheters to the right side of the heart. During the study the patient receives heparin systemically to reduce the risk of emboli. Many patients also receive nitroglycerin to control chest pain, particularly when the coronary arteries are full of contrast material during the coronary arteriographic procedure. At this time the patient may also experience bradycardia or hypotension. To move the contrast dye more quickly and minimize the vagal effect on heart rate and blood pressure, the patient may be asked to cough. If the bradycardia persists, atropine or, occasionally, a transvenous pacemaker may be used. If hypotension continues, intravenous (IV) fluids are administered as a bolus.

At the end of the study the heparin effect is reversed with Protamine. The catheters are then removed, and pressure is placed on the groin area until bleeding has stopped. After catheterization the patient remains flat for 6 hours. Nursing care involves care of the groin site, which is checked frequently for evidence of bleeding or hematoma. Pedal and posterior tibial pulses are assessed every 15 minutes for the first hour after the catheterization and every 30 minutes to 1 hour thereafter. The patient is encouraged to drink large amounts of clear liquids, and the IV fluid rate is increased to 100 ml/hour. The additional fluid is given for rehydration because the radiopaque contrast acts as an osmotic diuretic. Patients who have an elevated blood urea nitrogen (BUN) or creatinine before catheterization are at risk for renal failure from the dye. For these patients the quantity of contrast material is consciously limited to preserve kidney function. After the catheterization the cardiologist will meet with the patient and family to discuss the findings and plan of care.

RADIONUCLIDE STUDY: THALLIUM SCAN
Indications

The purpose of a thallium scan is to determine whether there is a perfusion defect in cardiac muscle.[3] It was developed as an adjunct to the exercise electrocardiogram (ECG) stress test. A thallium scan is indicated for the patient with chest pain and known or suspected coronary artery disease and for the patient with a left bundle branch block (LBBB) or a permanent pacemaker in whom an ECG stress test may be difficult to interpret.

A thallium scan combines the techniques of both cardiology and radiology. In cardiology coronary artery anatomy is important because regional myocardial blood supply is from specific coronary arteries and any blockage of an artery can lead to a discrete myocardial perfusion defect, meaning that the blood supply to this area is either decreased or absent. Although coronary arteriography will define the anatomy of the coronary arteries, it does not show whether the arteries perfuse the cardiac muscle. The radiology component involves the use of thallium 201 and a specialized perfusion scanning camera. Thallium 201 is a low energy radioactive isotope. It is an analogue of potassium and acts like potassium when injected into the bloodstream. Because thallium is similar to potassium, it is absorbed from the bloodstream by cardiac muscle cells as part of the sodium-potassium adenosine triphosphatase (ATPase) pump. Thallium uptake is dependent on two factors: (1) the patency of the coronary arteries and (2) the amount of healthy myocardium with a functional sodium-potassium ATPase pump. If an area of myocardium is infarcted (dead), it will not take up thallium. Once thallium has been injected, a specialized scintillation camera and computer system can detect the areas of thallium concentration (uptake).

Procedure

Before the thallium scan the patient should have the procedure fully explained, including a description of the equipment since it may be overwhelming to some patients. The patient is usually fasting because a thallium scan involves vigorous exercise. He or she should have a patent intravenous line inserted before the test. The thallium test takes place in a specialized laboratory that contains ECG monitoring equipment, cardiovascular exercise equipment (treadmill or stationary bicycle), and an Anger gamma scintillation camera. Once in the laboratory the patient is asked to exercise vigorously for up to 1 minute or longer or until angina or fatigue develops. At this point the thallium is injected into the bloodstream. After the injection the patient is asked to exercise vigorously for another minute to stress the heart and circulate the thallium. As soon as possible after exercise (within 10 minutes), the patient is asked to lie on the examination table for the first perfusion scan by the scintillation camera. The camera examines the heart from three angles, anterior, left anterior oblique, and left lateral oblique, to increase accuracy. On the camera screen the heart image looks like a circle with a hole. The myocardium appears, but the fluid-filled center does not. If no perfusion defect is seen, the test is complete for that patient. If a perfusion defect is noted, the patient will be asked to return for a repeat scan in 4 hours. A perfusion defect present 4 hours later means the area is infarcted. If the perfusion defect has taken up thallium since the first test (redistribution), the area is ischemic.

Occasionally, a patient who cannot tolerate a thallium/ECG stress test will have a pharmacological thallium test. In this case the patient is given dipyridamole (Persantine) to increase coronary artery blood flow, and the thallium test is then performed.

REFERENCES

1. Annoni G, Chirillo R, and Swannie D: Prognostic value of mitochondrial aspartate aminotransferase in acute myocardial infarctions, Clin Biochem 19(4):235, 1986.
2. Benner P: From novice to expert, Menlo Park, Cal, 1984, Addison-Wesley Publishing Co.
3. Bentley LJ: Radionuclide imaging techniques in the diagnosis and treatment of coronary heart disease, Focus Crit Care 14(6):27, 1987.
4. Berman D, Rozanski A, and Knoebel S: The detection of silent ischemia: cautions and precautions, Circulation 75(1):101, 1987.
5. Bhandari A, and Sheinman M: The long QT syndrome, Mod Conc Cardiovasc Dis 54(9):45, 1985.
6. Bruce R and others: ST segment elevation with exercise: a marker for poor ventricular function and poor prognosis, Circulation 77 (4):897, 1988.
7. Canobbio M: Chest x-ray film interpretation, Focus Crit Care 11(2):18, 1984.
8. Chung E: Manual of exercise ECG testing, New York, 1986, Yorke Medical Books.
9. Come P: Diagnostic cardiology: noninvasive imaging techniques, Philadelphia, 1985, JB Lippincott Co.
10. Conner R: The Wenckebach phenomenon, Heart Lung 16(5):506, 1987.
11. Cowan M and others: Comparative accuracy of computerized spatial vectorcardiography and standard electrocardiography for detection of myocardial infarction, J Electrocardiol 18(2):111, 1985.
12. Daily EK and Tilkian AG: Hemodynamic monitoring. In Tilkian AG and Daily EK, editors: Cardiovascular procedures, St Louis, 1986, The CV Mosby Co.
13. D'Ambra MN and others: Prostaglandin E, J Thorac Cardiovasc Surg 89(4): 567, 1985.

14. Davis J and others: A comparison of objective measurements on the chest roentgenogram as screening tests for right or left ventricular hypertrophy, Am J Cardiol 58(7):658, 1986.
15. Dunn F: Hypertensive heart disease in the patient with normal electrocardiogram and chest radiograph, J Cardiovasc Pharmacol (suppl 6):5870, 1984.
16. Fahey PJ: Continuous measurement of blood oxygen saturation in the high risk patient, Mountain View, Calif, 1985, Oximetric, Inc.
17. Famularo M and Kennedy H: Ambulatory electrocardiography to assess pacemaker function, Am Heart J 104:1086, 1982.
18. Francis G: Neurohumoral mechanisms involved in congestive heart failure, Am J Cardiol 55(2):15A, 1985.
19. Goldberger AL and Goldberger E: Clinical electrocardiography: a simplified approach, St Louis, 1986, The CV Mosby Co.
20. Halperin B and others: Evaluation of the portable chest roentgenogram for quantitating extravascular lung water in critically ill adults, Chest 88(5):649, 1985.
21. Handler C and Sowton E: Stress testing predischarge and 6 weeks after myocardial infarction to compare submaximal and maximal exercise predischarge and to assess the reproducibility of induced abnormalities, Int J Cardiol 9(2):173, 1985.
22. Heinsimer J and others: Supine cross-table lateral chest roentgenogram for the detection of pericardial effusion, JAMA 257(23):3266, 1987.
23. Hindman N and others: Relation between electrocardiographic and enzymatic methods of estimating acute myocardial infarct size, Am J Cardiol 58(1):31, 1986.
24. Hoffman I: Clinical vectorcardiography in adults, Am Heart J 100:239, 1980.
25. Hurst JW: The heart, arteries, and veins, ed 6, New York, 1986, McGraw-Hill Book Co.
26. Hysing J and Grendahl H: Ambulatory 24-hour ECG in patients with a history of syncope: a retrospective follow-up study over 2 years, Eur Heart J 6(2):120, 1985.
27. Kadota LT: Theory and application of thermodilution cardiac output measurement: a review, Heart Lung 14(6):605, 1985.
28. Kligfield P and others: Evaluation of coronary artery disease by an improved method of exercise electrocardiography: the ST segment/heart rate slope, Am Heart J 112(3):589, 1986.
29. Kloner R and Parisi A: Acute myocardial infarction: diagnostic and prognostic applications of two-dimensional echocardiography, Circulation 75(3):521, 1987.
30. Kowey P: The calamity of cardioversion of conscious patients, Am J Cardiol 61(13):1106, 1988.
31. Laakman R and others: Magnetic resonance imaging in patients with metallic implants, Radiology 157:711, 1985.
32. Laurent-Bopp D and Gardner PE: Clinical nursing research in cardiac care. In Kern L, editor: Cardiac critical care nursing, Rockville, Maryland, 1988, Aspen Publishers, Inc.
33. Lee TH and Goldman L: Serum enzyme assays in the diagnosis of acute myocardial infarction, Ann Intern Med 105(2):221, 1986.
34. Loveys BJ and Woods SL: Current recommendations for thermodilution cardiac output measures, Prog Cardiovasc Nurs 1(1):242, 1986.
35. Maki DG and others: Prospective study of replacing administration sets for intravenous therapy at 48- vs. 72-hour intervals, JAMA 258(13):1777, 1987.
36. Marriott HJL: AV block: an overdue overhaul, Emerg Med 13(6):85, 1981.
37. Missri J: Clinical Doppler echocardiography, New York, 1986, Yorke Medical Books.
38. Morganroth J: Ambulatory holter electrocardiography: choice of technologies and clinical uses, Ann Intern Med 102(1):73, 1985.
39. Morganroth J, Parisi A, and Pohost G: Noninvasive cardiac imaging, Chicago, 1983, Year Book Medical Publishers, Inc.
40. Murphay M and others: The reliability of the routine chest roentgenogram for determination of heart size based on specific ventricular chamber evaluation at post-mortem, Invest Radiol 20(1):21, 1985.
41. Murphy M and others: Reevaluation of ECG criteria for left, right and combined cardiac ventricular hypertrophy, Am J Cardiol 53:1140, 1984.
42. Musewe N and others: Validation of Doppler-derived pulmonary arterial pressure in patients with ductus arteriosus under different hemodynamic states, Circulation 76(5):1081, 1987.
43. Ng RHB and others: Increased activity of creatine kinase isoenzyme MB in a theophylline-intoxicated patient, Clin Chem 31(10):741, 1985.
44. Niblock AE and others: Changes in mass and catalytic activity concentrations of aspartate aminotransferase isoenzymes in serum after a myocardial infarction, Clin Chem 32(3):496, 1986.
45. Pandian N, Skorton D, and Kerber R: Role of echocardiography in myocardial ischemia and infarction, Mod Conc Cardiovasc Dis 53(4):19, 1984.
46. Pistolesi M and others: The chest roentgenogram in pulmonary edema, Clin Chest Med 6(3):315, 1985.
47. Platia E: Management of cardiac arrhythmias: the nonpharmacologic approach, Philadelphia, 1987, JB Lippincott Co.
48. Pohost G and Canby R: Nuclear magnetic resonance imaging: current applications and future prospects, Circulation 75(1):88, 1987.
49. Pollard D and Seliger E: An implementation of bedside physiological calculations, Waltham, GA, 1985, Hewlett Packard.
50. Presti C and others: Digital two-dimensional echocardiographic imaging of the proximal left anterior descending coronary artery, Am J Cardiol 60(6):1254, 1987.
51. Richards K: Doppler echocardiography in the diagnosis and quantification of valvular disease, Mod Conc Cardiovasc Dis 56(8):43, 1987.
52. Roberts R: Recognition, pathogenesis and management of non-Q-wave infarction, Mod Conc Cardiovasc Dis 56(4):17, 1987.
53. Robin ED: The cult of the Swan-Ganz catheter, Ann Intern Med 103:445, 1985.
54. Forrester JS and others: Filling pressures in the right and left sides of the heart in acute myocardial infarction, N Engl J Med 285(4):190, 1971.
55. Sclarovsky S and others: Unstable angina: the significance of ST segment elevation of depression in patients without evidence of increased myocardial oxygen demand, Am Heart J 112(3):459, 1986.
56. Slutsky R and Brown J: Chest radiographs in congestive heart failure: response to therapy in acute and chronic heart disease, Radiology 154(3):557, 1985.
57. Spodick D: Left axis deviation and left anterior fascicular block, Am J Cardiol 61(1):869, 1988.
58. Staubli M and others: Creatine kinase and creatine kinase MB in endurance runners and in patients with myocardial infarction, Eur J Applied Physiol 54(1):40, 1985.
59. Steger K, Remy J, and Krueger S: Drug-induced torsade des pointes: case report and implications for the critical care staff, Heart Lung 15(2):200, 1986.
60. Stodieck L and Luttges M: Relationships between the ECG and phonocardiogram: potential for improved heart monitoring, Biomed Sci Instrum 20:47, 1984.
61. Stratemeier E and others: Ejection fraction determination by magnetic resonance imaging: comparison with left ventricular angiography, Radiology 158:775, 1986.
62. Tavel M: Clinical phonocardiography and external pulse recording, Chicago, 1985, Year Book Medical Publishers, Inc.
63. Van Rossum A and others: Evaluation of magnetic resonance imaging for determination of left ventricular ejection fraction and comparison with angiography, Am J Cardiol 62(9):628, 1988.
64. White KM: Completing the hemodynamic picture Svo_2, Heart Lung 114(3):272, 1985.

14

Cardiovascular Disorders

CHAPTER OBJECTIVES

- *Describe the epidemiology and pathophysiology associated with coronary artery disease.*
- *Identify and describe the pathological significance of nonmodifiable, minor modifiable, and major modifiable risk factors for the development of coronary artery disease.*
- *List the electrocardiographic, hemodynamic, and physiological changes associated with myocardial infarction.*
- *List important aspects of the diagnosis and treatment of patients with congestive heart failure, cardiogenic shock, endocarditis, cardiomyopathy, valvular heart disease, hypovolemic shock, hypertensive crisis, and peripheral vascular disease.*
- *List important aspects in the nursing assessment and care of patients with myocardial infarction, congestive heart failure, cardiogenic shock, endocarditis, cardiomyopathy, valvular heart disease, hypovolemic shock, hypertensive crisis, and peripheral vascular disease.*

Cardiovascular disease remains the leading cause of mortality in the United States. It claims more than 900,000 lives annually and places a heavy emotional and financial burden on society.[40] In 1968 a massive public health campaign was initiated to increase people's awareness of the risk factors attributed to the development of coronary artery disease. Since that time, mortality has been steadily declining, and at least part of this positive effect is thought caused by changes in lifestyles.[35] This is an encouraging trend, but enthusiasm must be tempered by the knowledge that the population is aging and cardiovascular disease is a progressive, degenerative process that is most prevalent in the elderly.

CORONARY ARTERY DISEASE
Description

Coronary artery disease (CAD) is an insidious, progressive disease of the coronary arteries that results in their

---

CAUSES OF CORONARY ARTERY DISEASE

Atherosclerosis
Thrombosis
Spasm
Coronary dissection
Aneurysm formation

---

narrowing or complete occlusion. There are multiple causes for coronary artery narrowing (see the box above), but atherosclerosis is the most prevalent and affects the medium-sized arteries perfusing the heart, brain, kidneys, and extremities and the large arteries branching off the aorta. Atherosclerotic lesions may take different forms, depending on their anatomical location; the individual's age, genetic makeup, and physiological status; and the number of risk factors the individual manifests.

CAD has a long latent period. Fatty streaks appear within the aorta shortly after birth, but most individuals are not symptomatic until late middle age when they have coronary artery lesions that are greater than 75% (that is, 75% of the vessel lumen is occluded by atherosclerotic plaque).

Even though symptoms of atherosclerosis have been recognized in humans for thousands of years and lesions have been identified in mummies preserved from the fifteenth century BC,[40] the exact pathogenesis of atherosclerosis is not yet completely understood.

Etiology

Epidemiological and actuarial data collected during the past 40 years have demonstrated an association between specific risk factors and the development of CAD. One of the most important epidemiological studies is the Framingham Heart Study,[19,47] which began in 1948 and continues today with a second generation of subjects. Participants in this study have their blood cholesterol levels measured, their smoking and activity histories recorded, and blood pressure and electrocardiographic results checked on

CARDIAC RISK FACTORS

NONMODIFIABLE	MODIFIABLE
Age	**Major**
Sex	Elevated serum lipids
Family history	Hypertension
Race	Cigarette smoking
	Impaired glucose tolerance
	Diet high in saturated fat, cholesterol, and calories
	Minor
	Sedentary lifestyle
	Psychological stress
	Personality type

FOODS HIGH IN SATURATED FATS

Whole milk
Canned whole milk
Regular buttermilk
Whole milk yogurt
Dairy cream substitutes made with coconut or palm oil
All natural and processed cheeses unless made from skim milk
Poultry skin
Fried fish
Heavily marbled and fatty meats
   Brisket
   Ribs
   Prime rib
   Regular ground beef
   Cold cuts (e.g., bologna, salami, corned beef, pastrami)
   Bacon
   Sausage
   Hot dogs
Butter
Lard
Meat fat
Coconut and palm oil
Commercial bakery products (e.g., donuts, croissants) containing saturated fats (e.g., hydrogenated vegetable shortening, lard, coconut or palm oil)

a regular basis. As a result of this study and others like it, specific lifestyle habits have been identified that are associated with an increased probability of developing CAD. These lifestyle habits are referred to as coronary risk factors.[11,40,113] Several tools have been developed to assist the clinician in quickly and accurately identifying patients and populations at risk.[8]

Risk factors. The risk factors for development of CAD are age, sex, race, elevated serum cholesterol, elevated blood pressure, cigarette smoking, abnormal glucose tolerance, sedentary lifestyle, stress, and type A behavior pattern. These factors are further delineated into nonmodifiable and major and minor modifiable factors (see box above).

Nonmodifiable risk factors. CAD occurs approximately 10 years later in women than it does in men. After menopause, rates become the same for both sexes. Family history is another significant risk factor. An individual has a positive family history if a close blood relative has had a myocardial infarction or stroke before age 60 years. It is unclear whether the family history of CAD relates more to genetic predisposition or to family lifestyle habits. Since 1968 nonwhite populations of both sexes have had higher CAD mortality rates than white populations.[102]

Major modifiable risk factors

ELEVATED SERUM LIPIDS. Hyperlipidemia is a leading factor responsible for severe atherosclerosis. Cholesterol, triglycerides, and free fatty acids are all plasma lipids that are carried in the blood. Cholesterol is a steroid that is obtained endogenously by synthesis, especially in the liver, and exogenously from a diet high in saturated fats. The box at right lists foods that may contribute to elevated serum cholesterol. Fatty acids are classified according to their level of saturation with hydrogen. Saturated fats (for example, lard and butter) are unable to absorb more hydrogen and tend to be solid at room temperature. Unsaturated fats are able to absorb additional hydrogen and are usually in soft or liquid form at room temperature. Triglycerides consist of three fatty acids connected to a glycerol molecule.

Serum cholesterol levels below 200 mg/dl are associated with minimal risk of CAD, whereas levels >270 mg/dl carry a fourfold increase in the risk.[102] Cholesterol and triglycerides are transported in the blood by lipoprotein complexes, of which there are four major classes. These classes are distinguished by their protein density or by the percent of protein they carry.

High density implies a high protein content, whereas low density indicates a low protein content. The first of these lipoproteins, chylomicrons, are composed primarily of triglycerides. The second, very low density lipoproteins (VLDL), also known as B-lipoprotein, transport mainly triglycerides. The third, low density lipoproteins (LDL) are B-lipoproteins, which are metabolized from VLDL and carry 60% to 75% of the total plasma cholesterol. The fourth, high density lipoproteins (HDL), are composed of 50% protein, 25% phospholipid, 20% cholesterol, and 5% triglyceride. High density lipoproteins apparently clear cholesterol from the tissues and transport it to the liver. Children and premenopausal women often have an elevated HDL concentration, and both groups are considered low coronary risks. High density lipoprotein levels are thought to increase in response to increasing one's activity level and especially in response to aerobic exercises, weight loss, and cessation of cigarette smoking.[35]

HYPERTENSION. In the context of CAD, hypertension is the elevation of either systolic or diastolic pressure. Elevated systolic pressure is more predictive of risk, with levels consistently above 160 mm Hg of definite concern. The risk for developing CAD in the presence of hypertension is proportional to the degree of blood pressure elevation. Hypertension is thought a risk factor because it causes damage to the vessel's endothelium and disrupts the antithrombogenic and permeability barrier.

Predisposing factors for hypertension are increased dietary sodium, obesity, sedentary lifestyle, excessive alcohol intake, oral contraceptives, and other medical problems that may influence the intrinsic mediators of blood pressure—the renin-angiotensin-aldosterone system and the sympathetic nervous system.[37] Hypertension has a profound effect on the CAD risk profile in populations with elevated cholesterol levels (>160 mg/dl).

CIGARETTE SMOKING. Cigarette smoking is another major modifiable risk factor. Several studies have indicated that the risk of developing CAD is directly proportional to the number of cigarettes smoked per day.[35] Those at highest risk are women smokers who are also using oral contraceptives, young men who smoke in excess of three packs per day, and middle-aged men with elevated cholesterol levels. Recent studies reveal that more women are smoking than ever before and that more teenaged girls are starting to smoke than are teenaged boys.[112] Cigarette smoking unfavorably alters lipid levels, decreasing HDL levels and increasing LDL levels and triglyceride levels. Smoking results in cardiac electrical instability within cell membranes and impairs oxygen transport and use while increasing myocardial oxygen demand. Smoking is also thought to alter intimal endothelial permeability and to foster platelet agglutination. Fortunately, the damage from smoking is not unalterable, and after cessation the coronary risk falls rapidly, with a decrease of approximately 50% within 1 year.[8,11]

DIABETES MELLITUS. Diabetes mellitus is another potent risk factor. Women with diabetes mellitus are at greater risk for developing CAD than men with diabetes mellitus. Diabetes triples or quadruples a woman's risk, whereas a diabetic man's risk is increased by only 50%.[112] The younger the woman, the greater is her risk because diabetes negates the protective effect of estrogen.

The mechanism of how diabetes effects the coronary arteries is not well understood. However, it may alter platelet function or increase red blood cell adhesion. There is also a positive association between diabetes and hypertension, hypertriglyceridemia, and low levels of HDL. Diabetics also tend to be more susceptible to both macrovascular and microvascular disease.

OBESITY. Obesity apparently affects the coronary artery risk profile by enhancing an individual's susceptibility to developing other risk factors such as hypertension, impaired glucose tolerance, and hyperlipidemia, with increased LDL and decreased HDL levels. Obesity is also often associated with a sedentary lifestyle.

ORAL CONTRACEPTIVES. Oral contraceptives increase a woman's risk, especially after age 35, because oral contraceptives (1) alter blood coagulation, (2) alter platelet function, (3) alter fibinolytic activity, and (4) may inversely affect the integrity of vascular endothelium. This risk becomes significantly greater if the woman also smokes.

TYPE A PERSONALITY CHARACTERISTICS

Sense of time urgency
Hostility
Aggression
Ambition
Competitiveness
Impatience
Frustration

Minor modifiable risk factors

SEDENTARY LIFESTYLE. Evidence continues to accumulate that a sedentary lifestyle has an effect on the risk of developing CAD. A 20-year follow-up of 16,936 Harvard alumni demonstrated that those alumni who burned less than 2000 calories per week beyond their basal (minimal) level had a 64% higher risk for CAD.[73] A sedentary lifestyle is also associated with lower HDL levels, higher LDL levels, hypertension, obesity, increased glucose intolerance, and elevated triglycerides.[73]

STRESS AND PERSONALITY. Researchers have been studying the effects of stress and personality on cardiac risk. The breakdown of families, poverty, stressful life events, and limited social support are being studied as potential precipitating factors. Certain behavioral characteristics (see the box above) have been identified by Rosenman and Friedman[11,47] as associated with increased coronary risk. How stress or behavior influence the development of CAD is not well understood, but stress is associated with increased circulating catecholamines, which may precipitate hypertension, alteration in platelet function, increased fatty acid mobilization, and a resultant elevation of free fatty acids.[8]

In summary, there is a great deal still to be learned about atherosclerosis. One cannot pinpoint with absolute certainty the origins of atherosclerotic lesions. Further, researchers are uncertain why a risk factor in one individual may result in serious consequences but not be problematic for another individual. Studies have shown that CAD is a multifactorial disease, and the number of known risk factors increases the risk of developing the disease in an exponential rather than additive manner.[19,32]

Pathophysiology of CAD

Normal arterial walls are composed of three cellular layers: the intima, the innermost layer; the media, the middle layer; and the adventitia, the outermost layer (see Chapter 11, Fig. 11-11). The intima is the most susceptible to trauma; hence, most primary lesions occur there, whereas the lesions that occur in the media are associated with more severe disease.

Three key elements that result in luminal narrowing or occlusions have been identified. They include the following[40]:
1. Smooth muscle proliferation
2. Formation of a connective tissue matrix composed of collagen, elastic fibers, and proteoglycans

3. Accumulation of lipids

Stages of plaque development. Three stages of atherosclerotic plaque development have been identified (Fig. 14-1).[11,21,40] The first stage, *fatty streaks,* consists of broad-based lesions composed of lipid-laden macrophages and smooth muscle cells. Fatty streaks appear in the aorta soon after birth and at around age 15 begin to develop in the coronary arteries, usually at bifurcation points. Remarkably, fatty streaks appear in all populations, even those with a low incidence of coronary artery disease; therefore the role they play as precursors of more complex lesion is unclear.

The second stage, the *fibrous plaque phase,* is usually identified by the occurrence of "classic" atherosclerotic plaques. Fibrous plaques are progressive lesions that begin to appear in young adults in their middle twenties. Changes that occur within the intima of the fibrous plaque include the key elements mentioned previously—proliferation of smooth muscle cells, the development of a connective tissue matrix, and the accumulation of intracellular and extracellular lipids.

The third stage, the *advanced (complicated) lesion phase,* consists of lesions usually seen with advancing age. The fibrous plaque undergoes several changes: (1) it becomes vascularized, (2) the core becomes calcified, and (3) the surface may desegregate and ulcerate, possibly resulting in (4) hemorrhage and thromboembolic episodes. Furthermore, the media may develop aneurysmal changes resulting from the decrease in smooth muscle cells.

Pathogenesis of plaque development. There are multiple theories about atheroma (plaque) formation, three of which are discussed here.

Response to injury. The response-to-injury hypothesis holds that the endothelium sustains some type of injury (either chemical or mechanical). As a result, structural and/or functional changes take place. The endothelium has two primary functions—first as a permeability barrier and second to provide a thrombo-resistant smooth surface. Injury disrupts the permeability barrier, allowing interaction between elements in the blood such as between LDL and the wall of the vessel. The accompanying alteration in the thrombo-resistant surface may lead to platelet adherence, aggregation, and the release of platelet-derived growth factor, which is usually stored in the platelet.[82,83]

Monoclonal hypothesis. The monoclonal hypothesis put forth by Benditt and Benditt[4,5] proposes that each lesion has a common ancestral origin. Cell proliferation takes place because viruses or chemicals such as hydrocarbons or cholesterol alter the cellular genetic makeup, thereby producing a mutation. This mutation has a reproductive advantage over other cells and is able to reproduce at an enhanced rate. As a result the proliferating cells of an atherosclerotic plaque all stem from one mutated cell.

Thrombogenic hypothesis. The thrombogenic hypothesis, also known as the encrustation theory, relates closely to the injury hypothesis, which states that whenever there is endothelial injury, platelet agglutination and thrombus formation follow. Over time, platelet growth-promoting factor is released, resulting in proliferation of smooth muscle cells, which then become encased in connective tissue.[82] This is seen as the major mechanism for disease progression.[40]

Hemodynamic effect of CAD. The major hemodynamic effect of CAD is the disturbance in the delicate balance between myocardial oxygen supply and demand. The three major determinants of this balance are heart rate, myocardial contractility, and myocardial wall tension. In healthy coronary arteries, myocardial oxygen extraction is almost maximal at rest, but it can increase fivefold with an increase in heart rate, blood pressure, or ventricular contractility. This increase in oxygen extraction occurs because healthy vessels

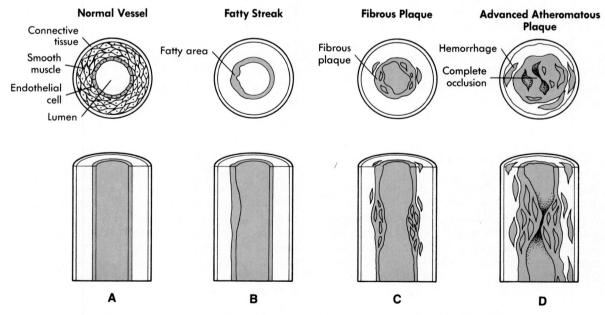

Fig. 14-1 The progression of atherosclerosis shown in both the longitudinal and the cross-sectional views. **A,** Normal vessel. **B,** First stage, fatty streaks. **C,** Second stage, fibrous plaque development. **D,** Third stage, advanced (complicated) lesions.

are able to vasodilate in response to tissue hypoxia when oxygen demand increases.[55]

Atherosclerosis alters the normal coronary artery's response to increased demand in two ways: (1) lesions that result in vessel-lumen occlusion of 75% or more restrict flow under resting conditions, and (2) the vessels becomes stiff and lose the ability to dilate. The result is decreased driving pressure beyond the site of the lesion and less oxygenated blood available to the myocardial cells perfused by that vessel.[55] As a result, the myocardium is forced to shift from aerobic metabolism to anaerobic metabolism, the consequences of which are (1) less efficient energy production, (2) lactic acid buildup, (3) intracellular hypokalemia, (4) intracellular acidosis, (5) intracellular hypernatremia, and (6) interference with the release of calcium from its storage sites in the sarcoplasmic reticulum.[11,40,55] The end result is left-ventricular dysfunction. This impaired left-ventricular function results in decreased fiber stretch and contractility, decreased stroke volume, increased left-ventricular end diastolic volume (LVEDV), and increased left-ventricular end diastolic pressure (LVEDP). Further, the impairment of the calcium mechanism causes incomplete ventricular relaxation. This, in combination with poor ventricular emptying, may increase the LVEDP even more. Tissue hypoxia or ischemia is the end result of this process.

Angina. Angina is the sensory response to a transient lack of oxygen in the myocardium. It is not a disease but rather a symptom of CAD. Angina has many characteristics (see the box at right), but the word itself was intended to describe a sensation of strangling in the breast, accompanied by anxiety or a fear of death. This description was first published by Dr. William Heberden in 1772, and it is still accurate.[11]

Anginal pain may occur anywhere in the chest, neck, arms, or back, but the most common location is the retrosternal region. The pain frequently radiates to the left arm but may also radiate to both arms, the mandible, and/or the neck (Fig. 14-2). Levine's sign, a clenched fist placed over the sternum, is frequently demonstrated when patients indicate the location of their discomfort.[11]

Angina is classified as stable, unstable, and variant.

Stable angina usually begins gradually and reaches maximal intensity during a matter of minutes before dissipating. It may be precipitated by activity, tachycardia, systemic hypertension, thyrotoxicosis, sympathomimetic drugs, systemic illness, or anemia. Correction of the precipitating event or the administration of vasodilators will usually result in the termination of the angina.[92]

Stable angina may be subdivided into *fixed threshold angina* or *varied threshold angina*. Fixed threshold angina is that which is predictable and caused by the same precipitating factors. It is usually the result of fixed lesions, with little acute vasoconstriction involved. Varied threshold angina is unpredictable. Patients may be able to walk two blocks pain free some days, whereas on other days they may need to stop after only one block. Although a fixed lesion may be present, there is also a dynamic component of coronary artery spasm present. These patients may also have more angina in the morning, since angiographic studies have shown smaller coronary arterial lumens in the morning

CHARACTERISTICS OF ANGINA PECTORIS

LOCATION

Beneath sternum, radiating to neck and jaw
Upper chest
Beneath sternum, radiating down left arm
Epigastric
Epigastric, radiating to neck, jaw, and arms
Neck and jaw
Left shoulder, inner aspect of both arms
Intrascapular

DURATION

0.5 to 30 minutes

QUALITY

Sensation of pressure or heavy weight on the chest
Feeling of tightness, like a vise
Visceral quality (deep, heavy, squeezing, aching)
Burning sensation
Shortness of breath, with feeling of suffocation
Most severe pain ever experienced

RADIATION

Medial aspect of left arm
Jaw
Left shoulder
Right arm

PRECIPITATING FACTORS

Exertion/exercise
Cold weather
Exercising after a large, heavy meal
Walking against the wind
Emotional upset
Fright, anger
Coitus

NITROGLYCERIN RELIEF

Usually within 45 seconds to 5 minutes of administration

hours than at other times of the day.[17]

Unstable angina is defined as a change in a previously established stable pattern or a new onset of severe angina. It is usually more intense than stable angina and is often described as pain rather than discomfort. Unstable angina can also be referred to as *preinfarction* or *crescendo angina, acute coronary insufficiency,* or *intermediate coronary syndrome.* It may be precipitated by the same events associated with stable angina or by (1) acceleration of atherosclerosis in multiple vessels, (2) left main coronary disease, (3) increase in localized platelet agglutination, (4) acute or chronic thrombosis, (5) plaque hemorrhage or fissure, or (6) acute vasoconstriction.[15,22]

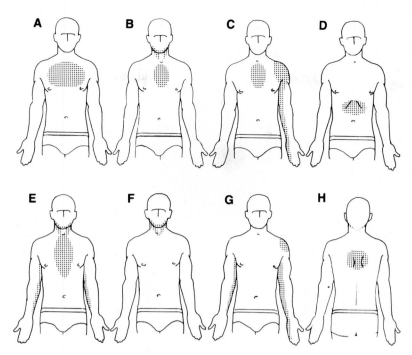

Fig. 14-2 Common sites for anginal pain. **A,** Upper chest. **B,** Beneath sternum radiating to neck and jaw. **C,** Beneath sternum radiating down left arm. **D,** Epigastric. **E,** Epigastric radiating to neck, jaw, and arms. **F,** Neck and jaw. **G,** Left shoulder, **H,** Intrascapular. (From Phipps WJ, Long BC, and Woods NF: Medical-surgical nursing: concepts and clinical practice, ed 3, St Louis, 1987, The CV Mosby Co.)

Unstable angina may occur after a myocardial infarction as the result of mechanical problems such as left-ventricular aneurysm, mitral regurgitation secondary to ruptured papillary muscles, ventricular septal defect, or global left-ventricular failure.[17] It is usually more intense, persists longer (up to 30 minutes), and may awaken patients from sleep.[11] The symptoms of unstable angina may only be partially relieved by rest or nitrates.

Variant, or *Prinzmetal's, angina* is defined as a reversible focal reduction in coronary artery diameter, leading to myocardial ischemia in the absence of preceding increases in myocardial oxygen consumption (mVo_2) as reflected in elevation of heart rate or blood pressure. It is thought the result of spasm with or without atherosclerotic lesion. Variant angina frequently occurs at rest and can also be cyclical, occurring at the same time everyday. It is usually associated with ST segment elevation and occasionally with transient abnormal Q waves.[11] Smoking tobacco and ingestion of alcohol and cocaine may also precipitate spasm.

Consequences of vasospasm include (1) a transient increase in myocardial oxygen demand over a fixed coronary reserve and (2) a transient decrease in myocardial oxygen supply.[40]

TREATMENT OF VARIANT ANGINA. Treatment of variant angina is aimed at decreasing the incidence of spasm and thereby reducing the risk of infarction or sudden death. Drugs of choice for the treatment of spasm are vasodilators such as nitroglycerin (either sublingual, paste, patch, or spray), isosorbide dinitrate, or calcium channel blockers such as nifedipine and diltiazem. If a patient has a fixed atherosclerotic lesion, coronary artery bypass surgery may be indicated. Percutaneous transluminal coronary angioplasty (PTCA) may be performed with selected patients as long as extreme care is taken not to induce spasm.

Treatment of CAD

The major goals of medical therapy for CAD are to increase coronary perfusion and decrease myocardial work. Medical management will depend on the frequency, severity, duration, and hemodynamic consequences of the angina. Pharmacological therapy may include nitrates, beta adrenergic blockers, and calcium channel antagonists. CAD risk factors such as hypertension or hyperlipidemia should be aggressively treated. A low-sodium, low-cholesterol diet may be recommended. Activity will be restricted until episodes of angina are controlled. If pain persists despite maximal pharmacological therapy and rest, an intraaortic balloon may be inserted to increase coronary artery perfusion pressure and reduce afterload.

Tachycardias will usually be treated with digoxin, calcium blockers, beta blockers, or antidysrhythmics. Hypertension will be treated with diuretics or afterload reducers. Anemia may be treated with blood transfusions or iron supplements. Coronary spasm may be treated with nitrates and/or calcium blockers.

The change from stable to unstable angina represents a serious problem. The patient is usually admitted to a hospital, and bed rest is prescribed. It is important that any identified precipitating problems be treated. If the anginal pain continues, cardiac catheterization, intraaortic balloon support, thrombolic therapy, PTCA, or surgery may be indicated.

Nursing Care

Nursing care of the patient admitted with angina focuses on continuous assessment and documentation of episodes of chest pain and on providing an environment that will help alleviate fear and anxiety and provide rest and security.

On admission, cardiac monitoring should be instituted, a 12-lead ECG obtained, and any ongoing pain controlled. Then a systematic, holistic nursing assessment should be performed, nursing diagnoses should be identified and ranked, and an individualized plan of care should be developed.

Complaints of chest pain must be evaluated quickly. Chest pain in the patient with known or suspected coronary disease may represent myocardial ischemia, which must be treated while it is still reversible. Assessment parameters should include documentation of the characteristics of the pain, the patient's heart rate and rhythm, the presence of ectopic beats or conduction defects, the patient's mentation, and the overall status of his or her tissue perfusion (that is, skin color, temperature, and pulses), and urine output.

Smith[95] identified 11 factors that must be taken into account when assessing chest pain. They include the following:

- Onset (either sudden or gradual)
- Precipitating factors (did visitors come or leave; was the patient up moving around?)
- Location (was it substernal; was it located in same area as previous pain?)
- Radiation (did it radiate to the jaw, neck, arm, or shoulder?)

- Quality (was it similar to previous anginal pain; was it less or worse?)
- Intensity (on a scale of 1 to 10, where would the patient rate it?)
- Duration (did it last seconds or minutes; how soon after onset did the patient call for help?)
- Relieving factors (what made it better—changing position, nitroglycerin, oxygen, the presence of the nurse?)
- Aggravating factors (did the environment, telephone calls, waiting for help worsen the pain?)
- Associated symptoms (was the pain accompanied by nausea, vomiting, diaphoresis or dyspnea?)
- Emotional response (how did the patient feel about the pain; was he or she anxious, fearful, angry?)

MYOCARDIAL INFARCTION

With the advent of coronary care units in the late 1960s, great strides have been made in the treatment and survival rate of patients with myocardial infarctions. However, today, almost 3 decades later, more than 500,000 people per year still die of acute myocardial infarctions, with about 30% dying before reaching the hospital.[81] Of those who do receive treatment, approximately 80% survive.[81]

Description

Myocardial infarction is the term used to describe irreversible cellular loss and myocardial necrosis secondary to an abrupt decrease or total cessation of coronary blood flow to a specific area of the myocardium. Infarction is more prevalent in the left ventricle, and occlusions are most likely to cause myocardial necrosis when occurring in vessels that have not developed collateral flow. Infarction also occurs with more frequency in individuals with multivessel occlusions.

Etiology

Atherosclerosis is responsible for the majority of myocardial infarctions because it causes luminal narrowing and reduced blood flow, resulting in decreased oxygen delivery to the myocardium. The three mechanisms that are primarily responsible for the reduction in oxygen delivery to the myocardium are (1) coronary artery thrombosis, (2) plaque fissure or hemorrhage, and (3) coronary artery spasm.

Coronary artery thrombi are now thought present in almost all acute occlusions. DeWood and others[21] found thrombus formation in 87% of patients who underwent cardiac catheterization within the first 4 hours after the onset of the symptoms of infarction. These thrombi, usually composed of platelets, fibrin, erythrocytes, and leukocytes, may be superimposed on a plaque or may align adjacent to a plaque. They release thromboxane A2, serotonin, and thrombin, all vasoconstricting substances that compound the vessel narrowing and set up a vicious cycle of recurrent occlusion.[35]

Scientists have not determined the cause of thrombus formation, but plaque fissure and/or hemorrhage are thought predisposing events.[11,21,40,64] Plaques are classified according to their composition. Hard plaques are heavily calcified and fibrotic, whereas soft plaques are composed of cholesterol

---

Nursing Diagnosis and Management
Coronary artery disease/angina

- Acute Pain related to transmission and perception of noxious stimuli secondary to myocardial ischemia, p. 594

- Activity Intolerance related to myocardial tissue perfusion alterations, p. 345

- Anxiety related to threat to biological, psychological, and/or social integrity, p. 852

- Knowledge Deficit: _____ (Specify) related to lack of previous exposure to information, p. 69

- Body Image Disturbance related to actual change in body function, p. 833

- Altered Sexuality Patterns related to fear of death during coitus, secondary to myocardial infarction, p. 863

RESEARCH ABSTRACT

Importance of nurse caring behaviors as perceived by patients after myocardial infarction

Cronin SN and Harrison B: Heart Lung 17(4):374, 1988.

PURPOSE

The purpose of this study was to identify coronary care unit (CCU) nursing behaviors perceived as indicators of caring by patients who have had a myocardial infarction.

FRAMEWORK

Effective caring promotes health and a higher level of wellness, and systematically designed caring interventions can enhance patients' coping abilities and help them deal with stress more effectively. The framework for this study is based on the concept of caring as defined by Watson, who identified 10 carative factors that nurses use as a basis for the caring process. Caring is defined as the process by which the nurse becomes responsive to another person as a unique individual, perceives the other's feelings, and sets that person apart from the ordinary. Nurse caring behaviors are those things that a nurse says or does that communicate caring to the patient.

METHODS

Patients who met the following criteria were nonrandomly selected from transitional care units of two acute care community hospitals: (1) diagnosis of myocardial infarction, (2) CCU stay of at least 24 hours and not more than 7 consecutive days, (3) transferred directly from CCU to transitional care unit, (4) ability to speak and understand English, and (5) physical and mental ability to participate in the study. Demographic information was obtained, and the subjects were asked an open-ended question about what the nurses in the CCU did or said that made them feel cared for by the nurses. Subjects were given a copy of the Caring Behaviors Assessment (CBA) instrument, which lists 61 nursing behaviors, ordered in seven subscales, that are congruent with Watson's carative factors and is scored on a five-point Likert-type scale.

RESULTS

A total of 22 subjects, from 35 to 83 years of age, participated in the study. All subjects were white and had at least a high school diploma, and the majority had retired from their employment before hospitalization. The average length of stay in the CCU was 3.59 days, and nine subjects had been in a CCU previously. An analysis of the relative importance of each identified behavior revealed that nursing actions that focused on the physical care and monitoring of patients were seen as most indicative of caring. Teaching activities were also perceived as significant, whereas extra, individualized aspects of care were viewed as less important in the critical care setting. No significant differences in perception were found on the basis of sex, age, education level, number of CCU admissions, or length of CCU stay. Content analysis of responses to the open-ended question revealed only two behaviors that were not included on the CBA: (1) "... are gentle with me," and (2) "are cheerful...."

IMPLICATIONS

Nurses must be aware that the development of a caring relationship may be enhanced if nursing care is provided calmly and expertly and the nurse appears in control of what is happening. In addition, high visibility of the nurse may heighten the patient's sense of security and well-being. Basic needs must be satisfied for the patient before attention can be given to a higher-order needs. Sensitivity on the part of the patients in this study to the environment and its perceived activities may have accounted for the lessened importance attributed to the individualized aspects of care. Nurses must be cognizant of postmyocardial infarction patients' needs for information about what has happened to them. Nursing behaviors identified in this study may be so basic to the perception of care that they are common to the experience, regardless of individual characteristics. Replication of this study to a larger and more diverse population is recommended, and investigations into the effects of caring on patient outcome should be undertaken.

---

esters and lipids. Coronary artery thrombosis has been associated with rupture or cracks of the plaques and release of the plaque material into the vascular lumen. Plaque rupture can induce thrombosis by (1) forming a platelet plug, (2) releasing tissue thromboplastin from the plaque material activating the clotting cascade, and (3) obstructing the vessel lumen with plaque components.

The role of coronary artery spasm in partial or complete coronary artery occlusion remains a mystery. Direct evidence has shown vasospasm is present, but it is not known whether this results from hyperactive smooth muscle or whether it is a secondary response related to a plaque rupture and the release of vasoactive substances.

Pathophysiology

Zones of infarction, ischemia, and injury. The area of cellular death and muscle necrosis in the myocardium is known as the *zone of infarction* (Fig. 14-3). On the electrocardiogram evidence of this zone is seen by pathological Q or QS waves, which reflect a lack of depolarization from

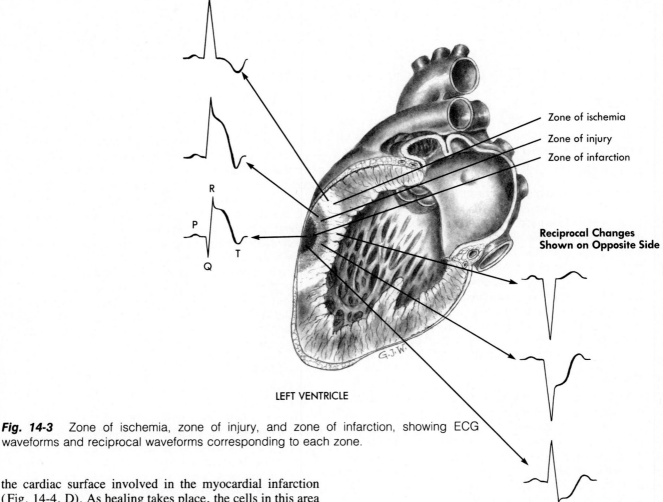

Fig. 14-3 Zone of ischemia, zone of injury, and zone of infarction, showing ECG waveforms and reciprocal waveforms corresponding to each zone.

the cardiac surface involved in the myocardial infarction (Fig. 14-4, D). As healing takes place, the cells in this area are replaced by scar tissue.

The infarcted zone is surrounded by injured but still potentially viable tissue in an area known as the *zone of injury*. (see Fig. 14-3). Cells in this area do not fully repolarize because of the deficient blood supply. This is recorded as elevation of the ST segment (Fig. 14-4, C).

The outer region, as illustrated in Figure 14-3, is the *zone of ischemia* and is composed of viable cells. Repolarization in this zone is impaired but is eventually restored to normal. Repolarization of the cells in this area is manifested as T wave inversion (Fig. 14-4, B). This region also is the apparent site of many of the dysrhythmias associated with an infarction because of the impaired repolarization.

During the first 6 weeks after an infarction, the myocardium itself undergoes many changes. Approximately 6 hours after the infarction, the muscle becomes distended, pale, and cyanotic. Over the next 2 days the myocardium becomes reddish purple, and an exudate may form on the epicardium. Leukocyte scavenger cells begin to infiltrate the muscle and carry away the necrotic debris, thereby thinning the necrotic wall. Approximately 3 to 4 weeks after the infarction, scar tissue begins to form, and the affected wall becomes whiter and thicker.[11]

Classification of infarctions. Myocardial infarctions are frequently classified according to their location on the myo-

cardial surface and the muscle layers affected. A *transmural infarction* involves all three muscle layers—the endocardium, the myocardium, and the epicardium (Fig. 14-5). Transmural infarctions, because they result in full-thickness necrosis, have a higher incidence of left-ventricular dysfunction. One method of determining left-ventricular function involves calculating the ejection fraction. Ejection fraction is the volume of blood ejected with each contraction. The normal ejection fraction ranges from 63% to 70% and can be calculated noninvasively at the bedside by the Gated Blood Pool Scan. In the early postinfarction period an ejection fraction of 40% or more indicates a good prognosis, whereas an ejection fraction of less than 40%, and certainly less than 30%, suggests a poor prognosis.[49]

The electrocardiographic changes produced by a transmural infarction demonstrate alteration in both myocardial depolarization (QRS complex) and repolarization (ST-T complex). The change in depolarization is represented by the appearance of new Q waves. These Q waves are deeper (one third to one fourth the height of the R wave) and wider than normal (0.04 seconds or longer in duration).

The changes in repolarization involve ST-T changes that occur in two phases, the acute and the evolving. The acute phase changes are manifested by ST segment elevation in

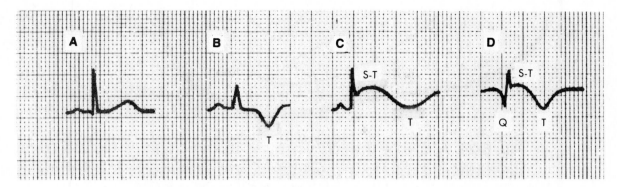

Fig. 14-4 ECG changes indicative of ischemia, injury, and infarction (necrosis) of the myocardium. **A,** Normal ECG. **B,** Ischemia indicated by inversion of the T wave. **C,** Ischemia and current of injury indicated by T wave inversion and ST segment elevation. The ST segment may be elevated above or depressed below the baseline, depending on whether the tracing is from a lead facing toward or away from the infarcted area and depending on whether epicardial or endocardial injury occurs. Epicardial injury causes ST elevation in leads facing the epicardium. **D,** Ischemia, injury, and myocardial necrosis. The Q wave indicates necrosis of the myocardium. (From Andreoli KG and others: Comprehensive cardiac care: a text for nurses, physicians, and other health practitioners, ed 6, St Louis, 1987, The CV Mosby Co.)

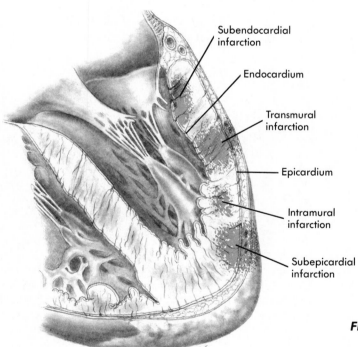

Subendocardial infarction

Endocardium

Transmural infarction

Epicardium

Intramural infarction

Subepicardial infarction

Fig. 14-5 Location of infarctions in the ventricular wall.

the leads overlying the involved surface, with reciprocal ST changes in the leads reflecting the opposite surface. This ST elevation may be preceded by hyperacute T waves. During the evolving phase the elevated ST segments and hyperacute T waves become deeply inverted T waves.

Nontransmural infarctions are classified as either subendocardial, involving the endocardium and the myocar-dium, or subepicardial, involving the myocardium and the epicardium (see Fig. 14-5).

Because the endocardium has a much higher oxygen need than the epicardium, subendocardial infarctions are the more common of the nontransmural infarctions. The most common electrocardiographic change seen with subendocardial ischemia is ST depression (Fig. 14-6). Generally, abnormal

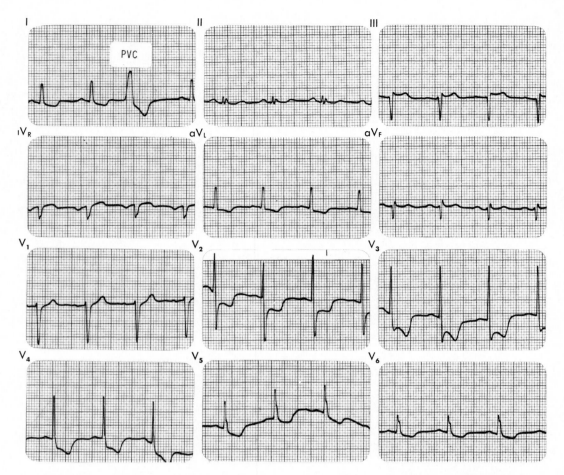

Fig. 14-6   Subendocardial infarction. Note the marked ST segment depressions, best seen in chest leads V_2 to V_5, consistent with subendocardial infarction. Slight ST segment elevations are seen in the reciprocal leads AVr and lead III. (From Goldberger AL and Goldberger E: Clinical electrocardiography: a simplified approach, St Louis, 1986, The CV Mosby Co.)

Q waves are not seen, and R wave progression is normal with a subendocardial infarction.

Location of myocardial infarctions. The location and extent of a myocardial infarction is dependent on (1) the site and severity of coronary artery narrowing, (2) the presence, site, and severity of coronary artery spasm, (3) the size of the vascular bed perfused by compromised vessels, (4) the extent of collateral vessels, and (5) the oxygen needs of the poorly perfused myocardium.[40]

The location of infarction can be determined by correlating the electrocardiographic (ECG) leads with Q waves and the ST segment–T wave abnormalities (Table 14-1). Infarction most commonly occurs in the left ventricle and the interventricular septum; however, close to 25% of all patients who sustain an inferior myocardial infarction have some right ventricular damage.[106] Although rare, atrial infarcts have also been reported.

When examining an ECG, it is essential that groups of leads, rather than one lead at a time, be evaluated. Correlating a group of leads that display ECG change with the

Table 14-1   Correlation between ECG leads, ventricular surface, and coronary arteries

ECG leads	Ventricular surface	Coronary artery
II, III, aVF	Inferior	Right coronary
I, aVL	Lateral	Left circumflex
V_2-V_4	Anterior	Left anterior descending
V_1, V_2	Septal	Left anterior descending
V_5, V_6	Apical	Left anterior descending
V_1, V_2 (reciprocal changes)	Posterior	Left circumflex

From Price SA and Wilson LM: Pathophysiology: clinical concepts of disease processes, ed 3, St Louis, 1986, The CV Mosby Co.

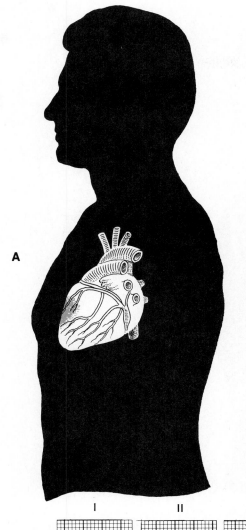

A

area of the heart reflected by the leads allows (1) identification of the location of the infarction and (2) anticipation of potential electrical or mechanical complications. Remembering that the right coronary artery (RCA) perfuses the SA node, the proximal bundle of His, and the AV node and that an inferior wall infarction results from RCA occlusion will make one alert to the conduction disturbances that are possible with an inferior wall myocardial infarction. Changes in the leads overlooking the anterior wall will alert the observer to the possibility of mechanical problems or pump failure.

The three ECG manifestations used to diagnose infarction and to pinpoint the area of damaged ventricle are inverted T waves, indicative of myocardial ischemia; ST segment elevation, indicative of myocardial injury; and pathological Q waves, indicative of cell death or infarction.

Anterior wall infarctions. Because the anterior surface is so large, it is often subdivided into anteroseptal, true anterior, and anterior-lateral sections.

Anteroseptal infarctions are usually a result of an occlusion of the left anterior descending coronary artery (LAD). Leads V_1 through V_4 reflect the electrical activity of the anteroseptal wall. On an ECG, a loss of septal depolarization is reflected as a loss of R wave progression in V_1 and V_2, leaving a QS complex. Q waves are seen in V_2 through V_4, and ST segment elevations and T wave inversions are seen in V_4 and V_5. Reciprocal changes are not usually seen with an anteroseptal myocardial infarction.

True anterior infarctions (Fig. 14-7, *A*) usually result from occlusion of the LAD and are seen on the ECG as loss of positive R progression in the chest leads (V_1 through V_6). ST segment elevation may be seen in leads V_1 through V_4,

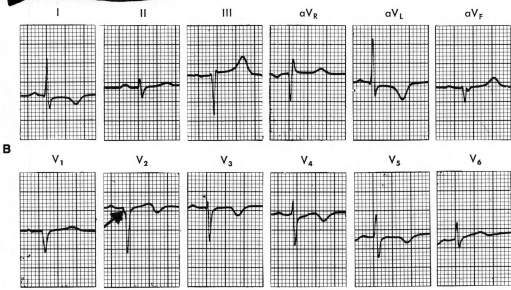

B

Fig. 14-7 **A,** Position of an anterior wall infarction. **B,** Anterior wall infarction. Note the QS complexes in leads V_1 and V_2, indicating anteroseptal infarction. There is also a characteristic notching (*arrow,* V_2) of the QS complex, often seen in infarctions. In addition, note the diffuse ischemic T wave inversions in leads I, aVI, and V_2 to V_5, indicating generalized anterior wall ischemia. (From Goldberger AL and Goldberger E: Clinical electrocardiography: a simplified approach, St Louis, 1986, The CV Mosby Co.)

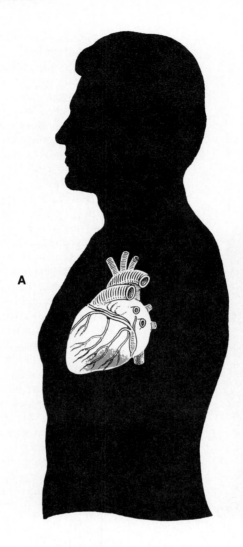

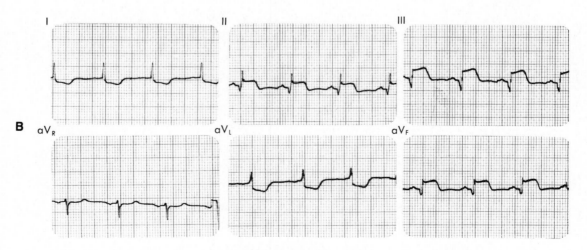

Fig. 14-8 **A,** Position of an inferior wall infarction. **B,** Acute inferior wall infarction. Note the ST elevations in leads II, III, and aVf with reciprocal ST depressions in leads I and aVl. Abnormal Q waves are also seen in leads II, III, and aVf. (From Goldberger AL and Goldberger E: Clinical electrocardiography: a simplified approach, St Louis, 1986, The CV Mosby Co.)

changes seen as tall R waves and ST segment depression in leads V_1 and V_2.

The location of an infarction may be very indicative of overall outcome. Anterior and anteroseptal infarctions, which result from occlusion of the LAD, are the least favorable types because of the serious left-ventricular dysfunction that results. Anterior wall infarctions are associated with twice the mortality of inferior wall infarctions.[14]

Assessment and Diagnosis

The definitive diagnosis of myocardial infarction is based on the patient's clinical signs and symptoms, electrocardiographic changes discussed in the previous section, and enzyme levels.

Clinical manifestations. The most common clinical manifestation of infarction is prolonged severe chest pain, which is frequently associated with nausea, vomiting, and diaphoresis. This pain generally lasts 30 minutes or more and is usually located in the substernal or left precordial area. Unlike angina, which is often described as a discomfort, the pain of infarction may be described as the most severe pain the individual has ever experienced. Descriptors used are "a heaviness," "like an elephant sitting on my chest," or a "viselike tightness." The pain may radiate to the back, the neck, the jaw, or the left arm, particularly down its ulnar aspect. Neither rest nor nitrates relieve the pain. See the following box for other commonly occurring clinical manifestations of infarction.

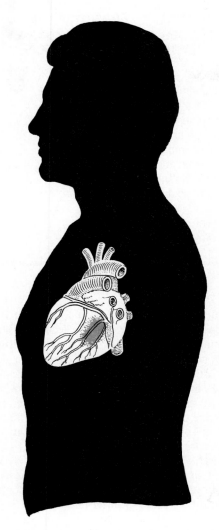

Fig. 14-9 Position of a posterior wall infarction.

and T wave inversion may occur in leads I, aVL, and V_3 to V_5 (Fig. 14-7, *B*).

Anteriorlateral infarction occurs as a result of occlusion of the circumflex coronary artery. On ECG, Q waves and ST-T wave changes are seen in leads I and aVL and in leads V_4, V_5, and V_6, which reflect lower lateral wall or left apical involvement. Reciprocal changes occur in the inferior leads II, III, and aVF.

Inferior wall infarctions. Inferior (diaphragmatic) infarctions (Fig. 14-8, *A*) occur with occlusion of the right coronary artery and are manifested by ECG changes in leads II, III, and aVF. Reciprocal changes occur in leads I and aVL (Fig. 14-8, *B*).

Posterior wall infarctions. Posterior infarctions (Fig. 14-9) occur with occlusion of the circumflex branch of the left coronary artery. Since the standard 12-lead ECG does not directly record activity on the posterior surface, a posterior wall myocardial infarction is documented by reciprocal

---

CLINICAL MANIFESTATIONS OF ACUTE MYOCARDIAL INFARCTION

Tachycardia with or without ectopi
Bradycardia
Normotensive or hypotensive
Tachypnea
Diminished heart sounds, especially S_1
If left-ventricular dysfunction present, may have S_3 and/or S_4
Systolic murmur
Pulmonary crackles
Pulmonary edema
Air hunger
Orthopnea
Frothy sputum
Decreased cardiac output
    Decreased urine output
    Decreased peripheral pulses
    Slow capillary refill
Restlessness
Confusion
Anxiety
Agitation
Denial
Anger

Enzyme manifestations. A complete discussion of the relationship of enzymes to diagnosis of myocardial infarction was presented in Chapter 13. The reader is referred to that chapter for review.

Complications of Myocardial Infarction

Unfortunately, many patients will have complications occurring either early or late in their postinfarction course (see following box). These complications may result from pumping or electrical dysfunctions. Pumping complications include congestive heart failure (CHF), pulmonary edema, and cardiogenic shock. Electrical dysfunctions include bradycardia, bundle branch blocks, and varying degrees of heart block.[42,85]

Dysrhythmias. Close to 95% of all patients who experience a myocardial infarction will have dysrhythmias.[88] There are many potential causes such as those included in the box at right, but ischemia of the pacemaker cells is the most common cause. Ischemia results in alterations in membrane excitability and in conduction and refractory periods, which in turn result in ST changes, enhanced automaticity, and reentry. Reentry is the reactivation of a tissue for the second time by the same impulse.

Sinus bradycardia (heart rate < 60) occurs in approximately 40% of all patients who sustain an acute myocardial infartion and is more prevalent with an inferior wall infarction.[97] Inferior wall myocardial infarctions are usually the result of a right coronary artery occlusion. The right coronary artery perfuses the SA and AV nodes in most people. Some bradycardia associated with an inferior wall myocardial infarction may be a compensatory response, since a slower heart rate will reduce myocardial oxygen demands. However, a slower heart rate increases the risk for ectopic foci. Sinus bradycardia is most frequently seen in the immediate postinfarction period.

Sinus tachycardia (heart rate > 100) most often occurs with anterior wall myocardial infarctions. Anterior infarctions impair the left-ventricular pumping ability, thereby reducing the ejection fraction and stroke volume. In an attempt to maintain cardiac output, the heart rate increases. Tachycardia must be corrected, not only because it greatly

---

CAUSES OF DYSRHYTHMIAS IN MYOCARDIAL INFARCTION

Tissue ischemia
Hypoxemia
Autonomic nervous system influences
Metabolic derangements
 Acid-base imbalances
Hemodynamic abnormalities
Drugs (especially digoxin toxicity)
Electrolyte imbalances (e.g., hypokalemia)
Fiber stretch
 Chamber dilation
 Cardiomyopathy

---

increases myocardial oxygen consumption, but because it shortens diastolic filling time, thereby decreasing stroke volume, systemic perfusion, and coronary artery filling.

Premature atrial contractions (PACs) occur in almost one half of all patients who sustain acute infarction.[11] PACs are most commonly caused by cell irritability resulting from distention of the left atrium secondary to increased left-ventricular end diastolic pressure and volume. The increase in volume and pressure of the left ventricle results from its poor contraction after the infarction.

Atrial fibrillation is a commonly seen atrial dysrhythmia associated with myocardial infarction and is more prevalent with an anterior wall infarction. It may occur spontaneously or be preceded by PACs or atrial flutter. With atrial fibrillation there is loss of atrial contraction, hence a loss of atrial kick and the extra stroke volume it carries. It is estimated that cardiac output can decrease by 30% when atrial kick is lost.[11] For this reason, atrial dysrhythmias are significant because of their ability to decrease cardiac output.

Within the first few hours after a myocardial infarction, almost all patients will have *premature ventricular contractions* (PVCs).[77] PVCs are usually controlled well by administering oxygen to reduce tissue hypoxia, correcting any acid-base imbalance, and administering intravenous lidocaine or other antidysrhythmic drugs.

PVCs and ventricular tachycardia occurring early (within the first few hours) in the postinfarction course are usually transient. However, when these same dysrhythmias occur late in the course, they tend to be associated with high hospital mortality, because they are usually related to the cumulative loss of myocardium.[77,106]

AV heart block most frequently follows an inferior wall myocardial infarction. Because the right coronary artery perfuses the AV node in 90% of the population, occlusion of it leads to ischemia and infarction of the cells of the AV node.

The major goal of therapy for any dysrhythmia is preservation of cardiac output and tissue perfusion. Medications must be used with caution, particularly those that increase the cardiac workload or depress myocardial function.

COMPLICATIONS OF MYOCARDIAL INFARCTION

Dysrhythmias
Ventricular aneurysms
Ventricular septal defect
Papillary muscle rupture
Pericarditis
Cardiac rupture
Sudden death
Congestive heart failure
Pulmonary edema
Cardiogenic shock

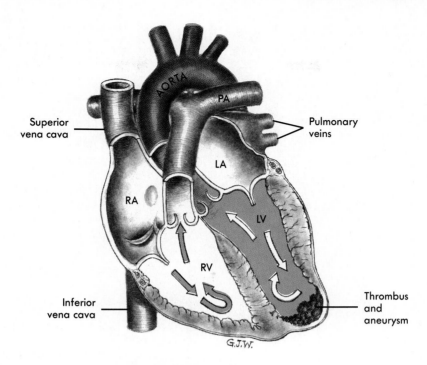

Fig. 14-10 Ventricular aneurysm.

Ventricular aneurysm. A ventricular aneurysm (Fig. 14-10) is a noncontractile, thinned left-ventricular wall, which results in a reduction of the stroke volume. It occurs in approximately 12% to 15% of patients who survive acute transmural infarction.[85] A ventricular aneurysm most frequently occurs in the apical area and may develop within hours, or it may develop and enlarge over a period of weeks. The most common complications of a ventricular aneurysm are congestive heart failure, ventricular tachycardias, and embolism. Treatment is usually directed towards management of these complications.

The prognosis depends on the size of the aneurysm, overall left-ventricular function, and the severity of coexisting coronary artery disease. Rupture of the aneurysm is very rare and usually only occurs if there is reinfarction of the border of the aneurysm.

Ventricular septal defect. When rupture of the ventricular septal wall (Fig. 14-11) occurs, it usually does so within the first week after the infarction.[11] This complication affects approximately 1% to 3% of the patients who sustain acute infarctions and is the result of severe multivessel disease, with a lack of blood flow to the septum.[11] The rupture is often followed by congestive heart failure and shock, the seriousness of which is dependent on the size of the defect.

Rupture of the septum is manifested by severe chest pain, syncope, hypotension, and sudden hemodynamic deterioration caused by shunting of blood from the left ventricle into the right ventricle through the septal opening. A new holosystolic murmur (accompanied by a thrill) can be auscultated and is best heard along the left sternal border. A definitive diagnosis of a ventricular septal defect (VSD) can be made at the bedside by using the pulmonary artery catheter. Blood samples drawn from both the distal pulmonary artery (PA) port and proximal central venous pressure (CVP) port will show an increase in oxygen saturation in the right ventricle (sampled from the CVP port) with a VSD. Normally, oxygen saturation in the right ventricle is 75%; with a VSD the saturation level will be increased to approximately 85%. The increase is the result of shunting of oxygenated blood from the left ventricle through the new defect into the right heart. This is documented as the P/S ratio, or the ratio of blood going to the pulmonary circulation versus blood going to the systemic circulation. It is written, for example, as P/S 2:1, which means for every liter of blood going into the systemic circulation, 2 L are going into the pulmonary circulation.

Since rupture of the septum is a medical and surgical emergency, patients must be stabilized with vasodilators and an intraaortic balloon pump to decrease afterload. The goal of afterload reduction in these patients is to decrease the amount of blood being shunted back to the right side of the heart and to increase the forward flow of blood to the systemic circulation. Mortality exceeds 80% with medical therapy alone; therefore the majority of patients require emergency surgery to close the ventricular septum.

The surgical approach is usually through the left ventricle and frequently through the infarction itself. The septum is patched with a knitted Dacron velour patch lined, if possible, with pericardium to make it immediately leakproof.[54] If pericardium is not used, there may be residual shunting until platelets and fibrin agglutinate along the patch to seal it.

Papillary muscle rupture. Papillary muscle rupture can occur when the myocardial infarction involves the area around the mitral valve. The papillary muscles function to keep the mitral valve closed tightly during ventricular systole. Infarction of the papillary muscles results in their in-

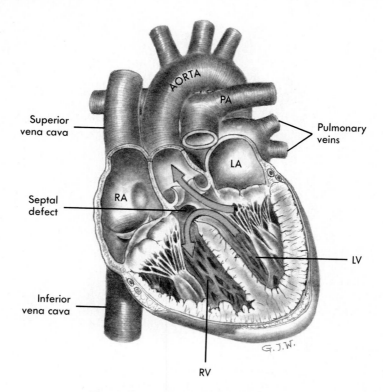

Fig. 14-11   Ventricular septal defect.

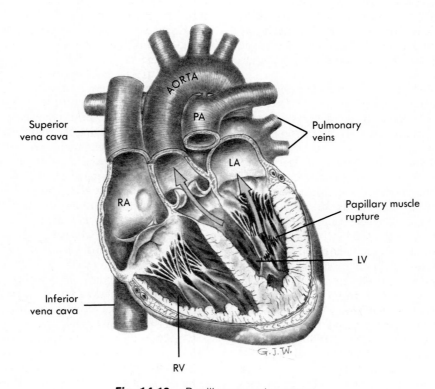

Fig. 14-12   Papillary muscle rupture.

ability to effect a mitral valve seal; consequently, blood is forced through the weakened mitral valve back into the lower-pressured left atrium during ventricular systole. The posterior-medial papillary muscle has a single blood supply; therefore it has an increased incidence of rupture as compared to the anterior-lateral muscle, which has a dual blood supply.

The rupture may be partial or complete. Complete rupture is catastrophic and precipitates severe acute mitral regurgitation, shock, and death. Partial rupture (Fig. 14-12) will also result in mitral regurgitation, but usually the condition can be stabilized with the intraaortic balloon pump and vasodilators before surgery, during which a mitral valve replacement will take place.

Pericarditis. Pericarditis is inflammation of the pericardial sac that occurs after acute myocardial infarction when the damage extends into the epicardial surface of the heart (as in transmural infarction). The damaged epicardium then becomes rough and tends to irritate and inflame the pericardium lying adjacent to it, precipitating the development of pericarditis.

Pain is the most common symptom of pericarditis, whereas the presence of a pericardial friction rub is the most common sign and is considered a clinical hallmark. Although the friction rub may not be audible at all times, it is best heard at the sternal border during inhalation and is described as a grating, scraping, or leathery scratching. Friction rubs often change from one examination to the next, thus complicating documentation. However, pericardial pain is aggravated by deep ventilations, change of position, swallowing, and coughing.

Narcotics do not provide the relief that aspirin, indomethacin and the nonsteroidal antiinflammatory drugs, dexamethasone or methylprednisolone, do. Long-term or high-dose steroids should be used with caution, because they may impede tissue healing and scar formation.

Cardiac rupture. Fifteen percent of deaths following myocardial infarction can be attributed to cardiac rupture,[85] which often occurs in older patients who have systemic hypertension during the acute phase of their infarctions. Rupture frequently occurs around the fifth postinfarction day when leukocyte scavenger cells are removing necrotic debris, thinning the myocardial wall.

The onset is usually sudden. Bleeding into the percardial sac results in tamponade, cardiogenic shock, electromechanical dissociation, and death. Survival is rare, and emergency pericardiocentesis is required to relieve the tamponade until a surgical repair can be attempted.

Sudden death. Death that occurs within 2 hours of onset of symptoms is classified as sudden. More than 1000 people per day in the United States are classified as having sudden death.[81] The majority are men aged 20 to 60 years. Many have had no prior symptoms of cardiac disease, although on autopsy nearly all have extensive multivessel coronary artery disease.[81]

The most common cause of sudden death is ventricular fibrillation. Precipitating factors include left-ventricular dysfunction, with an ejection fraction less than 30%, clinical diagnosis of congestive heart failure, and residual myocardial ischemia.

Two major therapeutic goals for the prevention of sudden death are the identification and treatment of high-risk patients. Survivors are usually placed on antidysrhythmics and overdrive pacing or, in some cases, may have an internal defibrillator unit implanted.

Treatment of Myocardial Infarction

The three principal goals of medical management for myocardial infarction are relief of pain, control of lethal dysrhythmias, and preservation of the myocardium.

The first 6 hours following the onset of chest pain constitute the crucial period for salvage of the myocardium. During this period it may be possible to achieve reperfusion of the infarcting myocardium with either intravenous or intracoronary thrombolysis, thrombolysis with percutaneous transluminal coronary angioplasty (PTCA), emergency PTCA, or emergency coronary artery bypass surgery (these therapies are discussed in Chapter 15). Studies have shown that myocardial tissue can be salvaged for at least 2 to 3 hours after the onset of symptoms, but in some patients this period may extend to 6 hours. Unfortunately, many people do not seek treatment until after this phase has passed.

Pain control is a priority since continued pain is a sign of ongoing ischemia, which places additional risk on noninfarcted myocardial tissue. Morphine remains the analgesic of choice, since it decreases anxiety, restlessness, autonomic nervous system activity, and preload, thereby decreasing myocardial oxygen demands.

Intravenous nitrates, beta-blocking agents, and calcium-channel antagonists may be instituted to reduce myocardial oxygen demand by decreasing both preload and afterload or by direct effect on the coronary circulation. Beta-blocking agents may reduce infarct size by decreasing sympathetic tone, thus decreasing afterload.

Oxygen is used for a minimum of 24 to 48 hours postinfarction to treat tissue hypoxia, which may be caused by left-ventricular failure.

Because ventricular dysrhythmias are most prevalent in the early postinfarction period, the patient is monitored for heart rate and rhythm. Most patients also begin receiving intravenous lidocaine during this period.

Many times a pulmonary artery catheter is inserted, which allows correlation of chamber pressures to heart rate, blood pressure, urine output, and cardiac output. Thus pharmacological and fluid replacement decisions can be based on concrete parameters of ventricular function.

To decrease cardiac work and myocardial oxygen consumption, bed rest with commode privileges is usually prescribed for the patient during the first 24 to 48 hours. Stool softeners are used to decrease the risk of constipation from analgesics and bed rest and to decrease the risk of straining.

For the first 24 hours the patient may be placed on a liquid or soft diet to decrease the risk of aspiration should cardiac arrest occur during this time. Furthermore, liquids and soft foods are nonirritating and easily digested; therefore myocardial oxygen consumption and basal metabolic rate may decrease.

Anticoagulants are sometimes used to decrease the incidence of embolic complications from deep-vein thrombosis and left-ventricular thrombi, especially while bed rest is prescribed for the patient. Antiplatelet agents may also be started to decrease release from platelets of thromboxane A2, which causes vasoconstriction and platelet aggregation. This therapy may be continued for an indefinite period of time since recent studies have documented the beneficial antiplatelet effect of prophylactic aspirin.[49]

Diagnostic studies that assess left-ventricular function (such as echocardiography and angiography) and studies that assess electrical function (such as 24-hour Holter monitoring and exercise stress testing) are all important in the decision-making process for risk assessment and both short-term and long-term management of the patient with acute myocardial infarction.

Nursing Care

The focus of the plan of care for the patient with a myocardial infarction must include (1) the recognition and treatment of potentially life-threatening complications, (2) the manipulation of the critical care environment so that it is therapeutic, and (3) the identification of the psychosocial impact of the infarction on the patient.

A considerable portion of time will be spent monitoring the patient for dysrhythmias and conduction defects and assessing vital signs for indications of shock, breath sounds for signs of pulmonary congestion, and heart sounds for abnormalities such as an S_3 or an S_4 or a murmur.

Medications must be administered as prescribed, followed by assessment for side effects or toxic responses. If the patient develops chest pain or dysrhythmias, it is important to record the onset in relation to the medication schedule. Sometimes medications must be given in smaller, more frequent doses to maintain a stable blood level and to avoid peaks and troughs in blood levels. If dysrhythmias continue, it is important to assess for noncardiac causes such as fever, anxiety, tissue hypoxia, position of the pulmonary wedge catheter, and acid-base or electrolyte disturbances.

During the time bed rest is prescribed for the patient, it is important that he or she is in an upright or semi-Fowler's position to foster better lung expansion, thereby decreasing the risk of atelectasis. An upright position will also decrease venous return, lower preload, and decrease cardiac work.

The nurse needs to control the critical care unit's environment to decrease noise, diminish sensory overload, and allow adequate rest periods.

CONGESTIVE HEART FAILURE

The most common cause of in-hospital mortality for patients with cardiac disease is congestive heart failure (CHF).[96] CHF is responsible for one third of the deaths of patients with an acute myocardial infarction. In 1983 it was estimated that 2.5 to 3 million Americans had been diagnosed with CHF and that the incidence would increase by approximately 400,000 new cases per year because of the aging of the population.[96] The heart failure rate is higher in men than in women for all age groups.

Description

Heart failure is a pathophysiological state in which an abnormality of cardiac function is responsible for the failure

---

Nursing Diagnosis and Management
Myocardial infarction and complications

- Acute Pain related to transmission and perception of noxious stimuli secondary to myocardial ischemia, p. 594
- Decreased Cardiac Output related to relative excess of preload and afterload secondary to impaired ventricular contractility, p. 335
- Decreased Cardiac Output related to supraventricular tachycardia, p. 334
- Decreased Cardiac Output related to ventricular tachycardia, p. 338
- Decreased Cardiac Output related to atrioventricular (AV) heart block, p. 336
- Activity Intolerance related to decreased cardiac output and/or myocardial tissue perfusion alterations, p. 345
- Sleep Pattern Disturbance related to fragmented sleep, p. 88
- Sensory-Perceptual Alterations related to sensory overload, sensory deprivation, and sleep pattern disturbance, p. 601
- Anxiety related to threat to biological, psychological, and/or social integrity, p. 852
- Ineffective Individual Coping related to situational crisis and personal vulnerability, p. 850
- Powerlessness related to illness-related regimen, p. 837
- Altered Role Performance related to physical incapacity to resume usual or valued role, p. 836
- Body Image Disturbance related to actual change in body function, p. 833
- Sexual Dysfunction related to activity intolerance secondary to myocardial infarction, p. 863
- Altered Sexuality Patterns related to fear of death during coitus secondary to myocardial infarction, p. 866
- Altered Health Maintenance related to lack of perceived threat to health, p. 67
- Knowledge Deficit: Activity Restrictions, Fluid Restrictions, Medication, Reportable Symptoms related to lack of previous exposure to information, p. 69.

of the heart to pump blood at a volume commensurate with venous return and/or with the requirements of the metabolizing tissues.[11,56,98] The basic function of the heart is to transfer blood coming into the ventricles from the lower pressure venous system into the higher pressure arterial system. Impaired cardiac function results in failure to empty the venous system and reduces delivery of blood to the pulmonary and arterial circulation—hence, heart failure.

Congestive heart failure (CHF) is circulatory overload secondary to heart failure and fluid overload secondary to activation of compensatory mechanisms.[74] In this section all references to heart failure relate to CHF.

Classifications of heart failure. Heart failure may be classified in various ways. However heart failure is classified, it is important to remember that the cardiac chambers do not function in isolation. For example, the ventricles have a common septal wall and are encircled and bound together by continuous muscle fibers; therefore any interruption or damage to one chamber will eventually affect both of the chambers.

Failure of right side of heart. Failure of the right side of the heart is defined as ineffective right-ventricular contractile function. Pure failure of the right side of the heart may result from an acute condition such as a pulmonary embolus or a right-ventricular infarction, but it is most commonly caused by failure of the left side of the heart or the backing up of blood behind the left ventricle. Its common manifestations are weakness, peripheral or sacral edema, jugular venous distention, hepatomegaly, jaundice, liver tenderness, and elevated central venous pressure. If peripheral perfusion is greatly compromised, cyanosis may be present. Gastrointestinal symptoms include anorexia, nausea, and a feeling of fullness.[61]

Failure of left side of heart. Failure of the left side of the heart is defined as a disturbance of the contractile function of the left ventricle, resulting in pulmonary congestion and edema and/or decreased cardiac output. It most frequently occurs in patients with left-ventricular infarctions, hypertension, and aortic and/or mitral valve disease. Over a period of time with progression of the disease state, the fluid accumulation behind the dysfunctional left ventricle will produce dysfunction of the right ventricle, resulting in failure of the right side of the heart and its manifestations.

Forward heart failure. Forward failure is defined as inadequate delivery of blood into the arterial system. It occurs when systemic resistance (afterload) is increased, producing decreased flow of blood out of the ventricles. This decrease results in a reduced cardiac output and hypoperfusion of vital organs. Forward failure frequently occurs with aortic stenosis or systemic hypertension.

Backward failure. Backward failure is defined as failure of the ventricle to empty. This results in an accumulation of fluid and an elevation of pressure in all the chambers and in the venous system behind the affected ventricle. It frequently occurs in conditions that result in a decreased systolic ejection such as myocardial infarction and cardiomyopathy. When the left ventricle pumps ineffectively, blood pools within the chamber, and left ventricular end-diastolic pressure (LVEDP) increases. As the mitral valve opens, the increased LVEDP results in increased atrial pressure, which

is then transmitted back into the pulmonary circuit. The net effect is an increase in both the pressure and the fluid within and behind the affected ventricle.

Acute versus chronic heart failure. Acute versus chronic failure refers to the rapidity with which the syndrome develops, the presence and activation of compensatory mechanisms, and the presence or absence of fluid accumulation in the interstitial space. Any condition that results in a sudden drop in cardiac output will also result in the manifestations of acute heart failure. Chronic failure results when more gradual ventricular dysfunction occurs, allowing the development of compensatory mechanisms such as ventricular hypertrophy; thus the manifestations of failure will not be sudden. Chronic failure may be abruptly exacerbated by the onset of dysrhythmias or by acute ischemia, causing the individual to display the manifestations of acute failure. In summary, acute heart failure has a sudden onset, with no compensatory mechanisms. Chronic failure has a progressive onset, with symptoms that may be suppressed by medication, diet, and low activity level. However, the chronic state can be exacerbated to acute failure by sudden illness or by cessation of medications.

Low-ventricular versus high-ventricular output failure. Low ventricular output failure is defined as a low-ventricular output state that can be caused by infarction, hypotension, cardiomyopathy, or hemorrhage. Classic signs and symptoms are those of decreased peripheral perfusion such as weak or diminished pulses, cool, pale extremities, and peripheral cyanosis. High-ventricular output failure occurs in conditions that increase the cardiac output such as thyrotoxicosis, anemia, and pregnancy. Peripherally, the pulse is strong, and the extremities are warm and pink.[11]

Functional classification. The New York Heart Association developed a method of classifying patients with heart disease based on the activity level that initiates the onset of symptoms. The abbreviated functional classification is as follows:

Class I: Normal daily activity does not initiate symptoms.

Class II: Normal daily activities initiate onset of symptoms, but symptoms subside with rest.

Class III: Minimal activity initiates symptoms. Patients are usually symptom free at rest.

Class IV: Any type of activity initiates symptoms, and symptoms are present at rest.

Etiology

The elderly, men, the hypertensive, individuals with coronary artery disease, smokers, diabetics, and individuals with elevated cholesterol levels have been identified by the Framingham study as having high CHF risk profiles.[11,74,79,86,96] Many precipitating causes of CHF are listed in the box on p. 278.

A common precipitating cause is reduction or cessation of cardiac therapy, either pharmacological or dietary. Patients with heart disease are usually on multiple medications and may, at one time or another, question the financial burden or, when asymptomatic, the need to continue therapy. Reduction or cessation of some therapy such as di-

---

PRECIPITATING CAUSES OF CHF

Reduction or cessation of medication
Dysrhythmias
Systemic infection
Pulmonary embolism
Physical, environmental, and emotional stress
Pericarditis, myocarditis, and endocarditis
High-ventricular output states
Development of serious systemic illness
Administration of a cardiac depressant or salt-retaining
    drug
Development of a second form of heart disease

---

uretics usually results in sodium and water retention, which may precipitate CHF.

Dysrhythmias are another major precipitating or aggravating factor. Tachycardias reduce diastolic filling time, thereby decreasing stroke volume. They also increase myocardial oxygen demand and, by decreasing diastolic filling time, may precipitate angina. Atrial dysrhythmias may decrease cardiac output by approximately 30% through loss of the "atrial kick." Ventricular conduction defects, which result in loss of ventricular synchrony during ventricular contraction, also decrease stroke volume, thereby decreasing overall perfusion.[76]

Viral and bacterial infections and environmental, emotional, or physical stress that increases myocardial oxygen demands can precipitate heart failure. Other precipitating factors such as bacterial endocarditis, myocarditis, and inflammation decrease ventricular contractility. A noncardiac illness or a second form of heart disease such as left-ventricular failure secondary to a myocardial infarction in a patient with chronic hypertension and left-ventricular hypertrophy may cause ischemia, which will lead to decreased contractility and CHF.

Pathophysiology

The two major determinants of cardiac output are heart rate and stroke volume; thus anything that affects one or both will affect cardiac output. Stroke volume, the volume of blood ejected with each systole, is dependent on three factors: (1) preload—the degree of fiber stretch at the end of diastole; (2) contractility—the change in the force of contraction; and (3) afterload–the pressure the ventricle must generate for ejection to occur. These three factors are the principal determinants of mechanical performance of the heart.

When the heart begins to fail and the cardiac output is no longer sufficient to meet the metabolic needs of the tissues, three major compensatory mechanisms are activated: the adrenergic system, the renin-angiotensin-aldosterone system, and the development of ventricular hypertrophy. These compensatory mechanisms maintain adequate perfusion pressure and enhance cardiac output by the ma-

nipulation of one or more of five factors: (1) heart rate, (2) stroke volume, (3) preload, (4) contractility, and (5) afterload.

The adrenergic compensatory mechanism is a result of increased sympathetic activity, which stimulates the release of catecholamines and increases the levels of circulating catecholamines, especially epinephrine.[29,30] The increase in circulating catecholamines results in peripheral vasoconstriction, which leads to shunting of blood from nonvital organs such as the kidneys and skin to vital organs such as the heart and brain.[29,30] This, in turn, increases venous return, which increases preload.

Activation of the renin-angiotensin-aldosterone system results in constriction of the renal arterioles, decreasing the glomerular filtration rate and increasing the reabsorption of sodium from the proximal and distal tubules, which promotes fluid retention. Fluid retention is also augmented by the diminished hepatic metabolism of aldosterone secondary to systemic venous congestion and diminished hepatic perfusion. Severe heart failure will increase the antidiuretic hormone level, enhancing the retention of water.

The final compensatory mechanism is the increase in ventricular wall thickness known as ventricular hypertrophy. An increase in systolic wall stress leads to replication of sarcomeres in parallel, which increases ventricular wall thickness in an arrangement known as concentric hypertrophy. An increase in volume or volume overload leads to replication of sarcomeres in series, resulting in fiber elongation and chamber enlargement known as eccentric hypertrophy. Myocardial hypertrophy increases the force of contraction. Therefore hypertrophy helps the ventricle overcome an increase in afterload.

In summary, the compensatory mechanisms may sustain cardiac function, especially at rest, but over a period of time may worsen the degree of failure as the retention of sodium and water leads to overdistention of the ventricles and a consequent decrease in the force of ventricular contraction.

Tachycardia may eventually become a negative factor because it increases myocardial oxygen demand while shortening coronary artery perfusion. This imbalance can lead to myocardial ischemia, which may decrease ventricular contraction, reduce ventricular filling, and necessitate a higher filling pressure. The end result may be both forward and backward failure.

Assessment and Diagnosis

The clinical manifestations of CHF result from tissue hypoperfusion and organ congestion.[107] Symptoms can be cardiac or noncardiac in origin. Signs and symptoms are frequently described according to the form of failure; that is, forward failure is manifested by fatigue and weakness, whereas backward failure is manifested by pulmonary congestion and edema. Failure of the right side of the heart manifests as systemic venous congestion and peripheral edema, whereas failure of the left side results in pulmonary venous congestion and pulmonary edema (Table 14-2).

The severity of signs and symptoms progresses as heart failure worsens. Initially signs and symptoms appear only with exertion, but eventually occur at rest.

Dyspnea, which is labored breathing and is frequently

Table 14-2   Signs and symptoms of failure of right and left sides of heart

Left-ventricular failure		Right-ventricular failure	
Signs	**Symptoms**	**Signs**	**Symptoms**
Tachypnea	Fatigue	Peripheral edema	Weakness
Tachycardia	Dyspnea	Hepatomegaly	Anorexia
Cough	Orthopnea	Splenomegaly	Indigestion
Bibasilar crackles	Paroxysmal noctural dyspnea	Hepatojugular reflux	Weight gain
Gallop rhythms (S_3 and S_4)	Nocturia	Ascites	Mental changes
Increased pulmonary artery pressures		Jugular venous distention	
Hemoptysis		Increased central venous pressure	
Cyanosis		Pulmonary hypertension	
Pulmonary edema			

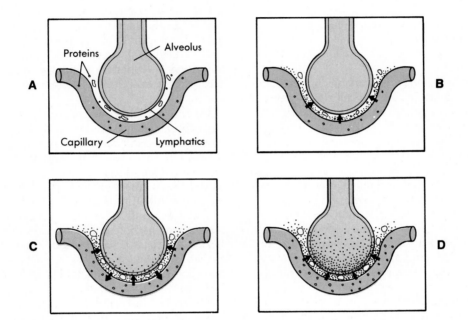

Fig. 14-13   As pulmonary edema progresses, it inhibits oxygen and carbon dioxide exchange at the alveolar capillary interface. **A,** Normal relationship. **B,** Increased pulmonary capillary hydrostatic pressure causes fluid to move from the vascular space into the pulmonary interstitial space. **C,** Lymphatic flow increases in an attempt to pull fluid back into the vascular or lymphatic space. **D,** Failure of lymphatic flow and worsening of left heart failure results in further movement of fluid into the interstitial space and into the alveoli.

described by patients as shortness of breath, results from pulmonary vascular congestion and decreased lung compliance. Dyspnea may then progress to orthopnea (difficulty breathing when supine) because of an increase in venous return (preload) that occurs in the supine position. Paroxysmal nocturnal dyspnea is a severe form of orthopnea in which the patient awakens from sleep gasping for air. Other respiratory symptoms include cardiac asthma (dyspnea with wheezing), a nonproductive cough, and pulmonary crackles progressing to the gurgling sounds of pulmonary edema.

Pulmonary edema. Pulmonary edema (Fig. 14-13) inhibits gas exchange by impairing the diffusion pathway between the alveolus and the capillary. Pulmonary edema is caused by increased left-atrial and left-ventricular pressure and results in an excessive accumulation of serous or serosanguineous fluid in the interstitial spaces and alveoli of the lungs. The most common causes are left-ventricular failure resulting from acute myocardial infarction, acute myocardial ischemia, tight mitral stenosis, or rupture of chordae tendineae and severe aortic regurgitation or aortic stenosis.[35]

There are two stages in the formation of pulmonary edema. Stage I is characterized by interstitial edema, engorgement of the perivascular and peribronchial spaces, and increased lymphatic flow. Stage II is characterized by alveolar edema resulting from fluid moving into the alveoli from the interstitium. Eventually, blood plasma moves into the alveoli faster than the lymphatic system can clear it, interfering with diffusion of oxygen, depressing the arterial partial pressure of oxygen (PaO_2), and leading to tissue hypoxia. The sensation of suffocation that can occur at this time intensifies the patient's fright and elevates heart rate, further restricting ventricular filling. Increased discomfort and work of breathing place an additional load on the heart, and cardiac function becomes further depressed.

With acute onset, patients are often extremely breathless and anxious. They expectorate pink, frothy liquid, causing them to feel as if they are drowning. They may sit bolt upright, gasp for breath, or thrash about. The respiratory rate is elevated, and the use of accessory muscles of ventilation becomes apparent by observation of nasal flaring and bulging neck muscles. Respirations are characterized by loud inspiratory and expiratory gurgling sounds. Diaphoresis is profuse, and the skin is usually cold, ashen, and cyanotic, reflecting low cardiac output, increased sympathetic stimulation, peripheral vasoconstriction, and desaturation of arterial blood.

Arterial blood gas values may be variable. In the early stage of pulmonary edema, respiratory alkalosis may be present because of hyperventilation. However, as the pulmonary edema progresses and as gas exchange becomes impaired, respiratory acidosis and hypoxemia will ensue. Laboratory studies may also document elevated liver function, bilirubin, liver enzymes, serum glutamic-oxaloacetic transaminase (SGOT), and serum glutamic-pyruvic transaminase (SGPT). Elevated blood urea nitrogen (BUN) and creatinine levels reflect renal hypoperfusion. Urine output will be low, and urine will be concentrated, with low urine sodium and high urine osmolarity levels because of dilutional hyponatremia. The serum potassium level may vary, depending on the overall state of renal function and aggressiveness of diuresis.

The chest radiograph usually confirms an enlarged cardiac silhouette, pulmonary venous congestion, and interstitial edema. The interstitial edema markings or chest radiograph are frequently referred to as Kerley-B lines.[110]

Treatment

The goals of management of heart failure are threefold: (1) to identify and correct precipitating causes, (2) to relieve symptoms, and (3) to enhance cardiac performance.

In the acute phase the patient will usually have a pulmonary artery catheter in place so that left-ventricular function can be followed closely. Diuretics are administered to decrease preload. The intraaortic balloon pump and vasodilators such as sodium nitroprusside and intravenous nitroglycerin may be required to decrease afterload. Digitalis and positive inotropic agents such as dopamine or dobutamine may be administered to increase ventricular contractility. If the patient develops pulmonary edema, morphine and diuretics will be used to remove excess fluid, to facilitate peripheral dilation, and to decrease anxiety.

Hemodialysis or continuous arterial-venous hemofiltration with or without dialysis may be required to control sodium and water retention.

Nursing Care

The focus of the plan of care for a patient with CHF must include interventions that will decrease cardiac work, optimize cardiac function, and promote emotional and physical rest.

During periods of breathlessness, activity must be restricted; bed rest is usually prescribed for the patient, who is positioned with the head of the bed elevated to allow maximal lung expansion. The arms must be supported on pillows so there is no undue stress placed on the shoulder muscles. The legs may be placed in a dependent position to encourage venous pooling, thereby decreasing venous return.

Breath sounds should be auscultated frequently to determine adequacy of respiratory effort and to assess for onset or worsening of congestion. Oxygen through a nasal cannula may be administered to relieve dyspnea, blood should be evaluated, and diuretics or vasodilators may be administered. If the patient is not hypotensive, morphine may be administered to decrease hyperventilation and anxiety. If the patient's ventilatory status worsens, the nurse must be prepared for endotracheal intubation and mechanical ventilation.

Patients in CHF require aggressive pharmacological therapy. The nurse must know the action, side effects, therapeutic levels, and toxic effects of the diuretics, the positive inotropic agents used to increase ventricular contractility, and vasodilators used to decrease preload. The patient's hemodynamic response to these agents, as well as to diuretic therapy and fluid restrictions, must be closely monitored.

The patient's ECG must be evaluated for any dysrhythmias that may be present or may develop as a result of drug toxicity or electrolyte imbalance. Patients in heart failure are prone to digoxin toxicity secondary to decreased renal perfusion, as well as to electrolyte (most frequently, sodium and potassium) imbalances.

The patient in heart failure may be prone to skin breakdown resulting from immobility, bed rest, inadequate nutrition, edema, and decreased perfusion to the skin and subcutaneous tissue. Frequent position changes and padding of dependent areas and bony prominences may be helpful.

Patients in failure frequently experience decreased appetite; therefore small, frequent meals may be more appropriate than the standard three large meals. Food should be as tasty as possible; their favorite foods, as well as food from home, may be worked into their diet as long as the foods are compatible with nutritional restrictions.

Another major nursing function is to maintain an environment that fosters physical and emotional rest. The nurse needs to assess the patient's understanding of conservation of energy in planning activities and to collaborate with the patient in organizing the day's schedule. Rest periods must be carefully planned and adhered to, while independence within his or her activity prescription is fostered. The patient's vital signs should be recorded before an activity is begun, immediately on completion of the activity, and 5 minutes after completion. Signs of activity intolerance (that is, dyspnea, fatigue, sustained increase in pulse, and onset of dysrhythmias) must be documented and reported to the

---

Nursing Diagnosis and Management
Acute congestive heart failure and pulmonary edema

- Impaired Gas Exchange related to ventilation-perfusion inequality secondary to pulmonary vascular congestion, p. 487

- Decreased Cardiac Output related to relative excess of preload and afterload secondary to impaired ventricular contractility, p. 335

- Activity Intolerance related to decreased cardiac output, p. 345

- Potential Impaired Skin Integrity risk factors: reduced mobility, poor subcutaneous tissue support (peripheral and sacral edema), p. 725

- Potential for Infection risk factors: invasive monitoring devices, p. 720

- Sensory-Perceptual Alterations related to sensory overload, sensory deprivation, and sleep pattern disturbance, p. 601

- Anxiety related to threat to biological, psychological, and/or social integrity, p. 852

- Ineffective Individual Coping related to situational crisis and personal vulnerability, p. 850

- Sleep Pattern Disturbance related to circadian desynchronization, p. 89

- Knowledge Deficit: Medications, Fluid Restrictions, Activity Restrictions, Diet, Reportable Symptoms related to lack of previous exposure to information, p. 69

---

physician. Activity should must be gradually increased in a step-wise fashion.

CARDIOGENIC SHOCK

Whenever there is loss of more than 40% of functional myocardium, a clinical syndrome manifested by decreased perfusion, hypotension, decreased or absent urine output, obtundation, sweating, pallor, and tachycardia occurs. Close to 20% of patients sustaining an anterior myocardial infarction will develop this syndrome—cardiogenic shock.[36,47]

Etiology

The most common cause of cardiogenic shock is extensive left-ventricular dysfunction resulting from an acute myocardial infarction with or without associated complications. Examples of complications that may result in cardiogenic shock include papillary muscle rupture, left-ventricular free wall rupture, acute ventricular septal defect (VSD), end

stage cardiomyopathy, severe valvular dysfunction, myocardial contusion, cardiac tamponade, left-atrial myxoma, and thrombus and/or a massive pulmonary embolus.

Stages of Cardiogenic Shock

Four stages of cardiogenic shock have been identified (Table 14-3). The first, the initial stage, is identified when the cardiac output begins to decrease in the absence of clinical symptoms.

The second stage, the compensatory stage, is a period wherein the cardiac output is decreased and early clinical signs and symptoms are evident. Most early manifestations result from cellular alterations as the body attempts to maintain homeostasis. During this period sympathetic and hormonal compensatory mechanisms are activated. Sympathetic compensation results in an increase in heart rate and in the force of ventricular contraction.

Activation of the hormonal compensatory response, resulting in secretion of renin-angiotensin, occurs as a result of the decreased perfusion of blood to the kidneys. The release of this potent arterial and venous hormone is an attempt to raise the declining cardiac output. The adrenal

---

Nursing Diagnosis and Management
Chronic congestive heart failure

- Impaired Gas Exchange related to ventilation-perfusion inequality secondary to pulmonary vascular congestion, p. 487

- Decreased Cardiac Output related to relative excess of preload and afterload secondary to impaired ventricular contractility, p. 335

- Activity Intolerance related to decreased cardiac output, p. 345

- Activity Intolerance related to postural hypotension secondary to prolonged immobility, vasodilator therapy, p. 344

- Potential Impaired Skin Integrity risk factors: reduced mobility, poor subcutaneous tissue support (peripheral and sacral edema), p. 725

- Anxiety related to threat to biological, psychological, and/or social integrity, p. 852

- Sleep Pattern Disturbance related to fragmented sleep secondary to paroxysmal nocturnal dyspnea, p. 88

- Noncompliance: Medications, Fluid Restrictions, Activity Restrictions, Diet related to knowledge deficit and/or lack of resources, p. 68

- Altered Health Maintenance related to lack of perceived threat to health, p. 67

Table 14-3 Stages of shock

Stage	Definition	Signs and symptoms
Initial	Cardiac output decreased in absence of symptoms	Decreased cardiac output
Compensatory	Attempt by body's compensatory mechanisms, mediated by the sympathetic nervous system, to increase cardiac output	Sinus tachycardia Elevated pulmonary artery wedge pressure readings; PAW > 18-20 mmHg Cool palm, clammy skin Decreased urinary output, usually <20 ml/hr Decreased urinary sodium; increased urinary osmolarity Rapid, deep ventilations, respiratory alkalosis Altered level of consciousness Decreased bowel sounds Hyperglycemia Hypernatemia
Progressive	Compensatory mechanisms no longer helpful but now perpetuate shock cycle	Severe peripheral vasoconstriction Decreased oxygen delivery to cells Anaerobic metaboism Metabolic acidosis Sinus tachycardia, weak pulse Chest pain, palpitations Nausea, vomiting, anorexia Rapid, shallow ventilations Elevated pulmonary artery pressure readings
Refractory	Irreversible stage; signs and symptoms not changed by therapy	Cardiac failure (severely decreased cardiac output) Elevated pulmonary artery pressure readings Acidosis Alterations in blood clotting Inadequate cerebral perfusion Cardiac and respiratory arrest Death

cortex is also stimulated to intensify the release of aldosterone, leading to increased reabsorption of sodium. The result is more water reabsorption and an increase in total fluid volume with which to enhance venous return and cardiac output.

The hormonal response also includes the release of ACTH from the anterior pituitary, resulting in glycogenolysis and rising blood sugar.

Stage III is the progressive stage. If the shock state is not reversed by this time, the compensatory mechanisms become debilitating. Although initially enhancing arterial blood pressure and major organ tissue perfusion, the effect generated by the compensatory mechanisms or the myocardium now becomes deleterious because of the increased cardiac work and oxygen demand. During the progressive stage as the cardiovascular system decompensates, toxic substances such as enzymes, lactate, intracellular ions, and vasoactive substances are released. There is a reduction in ATP and an increase in anaerobic metabolism, which eventually will lead to metabolic acidosis.

At the same time capillary dysfunction becomes apparent as the acidotic state allows leakage of blood out of the capillary bed. Edema develops when fluid shifts out of the capillaries into the tissues or interstitial space. The decrease

in intravascular volume may result in increased blood viscosity.

Because of sustained vasoconstriction in the periphery, the fingers, toes, tip of the nose, and ear lobes will be cold and pulseless.

Stage IV is the refractory stage. At this point the shock state is irreversible to any form of therapy.

Clinical Manifestions

Cardiogenic shock is a multisystem disease. The cardiac injury tends to be progressive and interrelated so that decreasing function adversely affects the other body systems.[7] Clinical manifestations depend on the severity of the shock state and the patient's underlying medical status. Furthermore, some clinical manifestations are related to decreased tissue perfusion and/or to the effect of the compensatory mechanisms.

Hemodynamics. The patient will be hypotensive with a systolic pressure of less than 90 mm Hg or, in a previously hypertensive patient, with a 30 to 60 mm Hg decrease. A compensatory tachycardia, resulting from increased levels of circulating catecholamines, increased sympathetic tone, decreased parasympathetic activity, and an increase in the metabolic demands of the tissues will be present. The central venous pressure will be elevated, and the central veins may be distended. Pulmonary artery pressures will be elevated.

Renal. The patient will become progressively oliguric secondary to decreased renal perfusion. Diuretics will have little or no effect.

Respiratory. Rapid shallow ventilations will be present. On auscultation, crackles and rhonchi will be heard. Endotracheal intubation and mechanical ventilation will become necessary as the cardiogenic shock worsens and as ventilatory failure develops.

Gastrointestinal. Initially, bowel sounds may be hypoactive or hyperactive. However, as perfusion decreases, peristalsis will decrease, and bowel sounds will not be auscultated.

Neurological. The patient in cardiogenic shock becomes more obtunded as the condition worsens. In the late stages, severe mental obtundation will be present.

Skin. The skin will appear cool, pale, and diaphoretic. As the shock state progresses, the skin will become mottled and cyanotic secondary to increased oxygen extraction and venous sludging of blood in the capillaries.

Hematological. As the shock state progresses, abnormalities in blood clotting become apparent. Cell aggregation frequently occurs and may be the precursor to the development of disseminated intravascular coagulation (DIC).

Treatment

Therapies are directed toward reducing infarct size, improving coronary and systemic perfusion, decreasing myocardial oxygen consumption, controlling heart rate, and increasing ventricular contractility. These goals may be accomplished by using venovasodilators to decrease preload and arterial vasodilators to decrease afterload. The intraaortic balloon pump is used for afterload reduction, whereas positive inotropic agents are used to increase ventricular contractility. Care must be taken to maintain an adequate perfusion pressure when using vasodilators. Inotropic agents must be used cautiously so that myocardial V_{O_2} is not increased excessively. Pulmonary artery wedge pressures (PAW) or pulmonary artery diastolic pressures (PAD) should be used to guide the administration of pharmacological agents.

Oxygenation must be supported to keep the Pa_{O_2} above 80 mm Hg. If ventilatory failure ensures (arterial partial pressure of carbon dioxide [Pa_{CO_2}] above 50 mm Hg in a previously normocapnic patient), endotracheal intubation and mechanical ventilation will be necessary.

Nursing Care

The focus of nursing care for the patient in cardiogenic shock is the continuous assessment of tissue and organ perfusion.

Patients experiencing cardiogenic shock will have an arterial line, pulmonary artery catheter, urinary drainage catheter, and, frequently, an intraaortic balloon pump. During the acute phase, these patients require frequent assessment of left-ventricular function as manifested by their pulmonary artery pressure, pulmonary artery wedge pressure, cardiac output, urine output, skin color and temperature, presence or absence of peripheral pulses, level of

---

Nursing Diagnosis and Management
Cardiogenic shock

■ Decreased Cardiac Output related to relative excess of preload and afterload secondary to impaired ventricular contractility, p. 335

■ Potential for Altered Peripheral Tissue Perfusion Risk Factor: vasopressor therapy, p. 341

■ Potential for Infection risk factor: invasive monitoring devices, p. 346

■ Potential for Aspiration risk factors: endotracheal tube, situation hindering elevation of upper body, reduced level of consciousness, p. 489

■ Ineffective Airway Clearance related to impaired cough secondary to loss of glottic closure with cuffed endotracheal tube, p. 476

■ Sleep Pattern Disturbance related to circadian desynchronization, p. 89

■ Sensory-Perceptual Alterations related to sensory overload, sensory deprivation, sleep pattern disturbance, p. 601

■ Body Image Disturbance related to functional dependence on life-sustaining technology, p. 834

■ Anxiety related to biological, psychological, and/or social integrity, p. 852.

---

mentation, and presence or absence of bowel sounds.

To support the patient, sympathomimetic drugs, diuretics, vasodilators, and antidysrhythmics should be administered as ordered. Since fluids are frequently restricted, care must be taken in mixing and administering medications. Infusion pumps should always be used and a precise record of intake and output maintained.

Changes in mentation will occur secondary to decreased cerebral perfusion or to tissue hypoxia. Oxygen is administered, and arterial blood gas values are closely monitored. Respiratory assessment for pulmonary congestion is performed hourly or more often to assess the need for ventilatory support.

Patients in cardiogenic shock are sometimes confused and restless. Safety precautions must be taken to protect them, as well as to maintain the security of invasive catheters and tubes. Reassurance and careful and frequently repeated explanations by the nurse may help avert the use of restraints. Nurses must also strive to maintain as calm and quiet an environment as the patient's acuity will allow.

It is important to maintain the patient in a positive nitrogen balance; most often, this is accomplished with hyperalimentation or tube feedings. If the patient is receiving parenteral intake, bowel sounds must be auscultated every shift because shock may precipitate intestinal ischemia. Care must also be taken to see that the patient does not aspirate.

The skin integrity of patients in shock may be compromised secondary to their low perfusion state. Therefore use of heel and elbow protectors and of water, air, or other special mattresses, frequent turning, and performance of passive range of motion activities are important.

ENDOCARDITIS
Description

Infection by a microorganism of a platelet-fibrin vegetation on the endothelial surface of the heart results in infective endocarditis. It is a relatively uncommon disorder, which is seen more frequently in men than women. In a study of 582 persons with infective endocarditis conducted by the Royal College of Physicians Research Unit, 137 had preexisting rheumatic heart disease, 108 had congenital heart disease, 145 had other cardiac abnormalities, chiefly mitral valve prolapse and calcific aortic valve disease, and 97 had prosthetic valves.[3] One-hundred and thirty-eight had suffered previous attacks of infective endocarditis. The remaining 183 patients had no known previous cardiac history. Major predisposing factors are listed in the box below; however, no predisposing factor can be identified in 20% to 40% of patients with this disease.[3]

Pathophysiology

The disease may be classified as acute and subacute. Acute infection develops on normal valves, progresses rapidly, causes severe destruction, and may be fatal if the patient is not treated. Subacute infection occurs on damaged heart valves and progresses much more slowly, and the outcome is usually positive with treatment. Survival may be possible even without treatment. The term subacute *bacterial* endocarditis (SBE) is not always accurate because, although most infections are bacterial, some are caused by yeast or fungus. It is much more useful to classify the disease according to causative microorganism.[70]

Etiology

The development of endocarditis is dependent on two factors: (1) there must be a susceptible lesion in the vascular endothelium, and (2) there must be an organism to establish an infection.[4] The source of the organism may be unknown, or it may be traced to any type of invasive procedure such as a biopsy, cannulation of the veins or arteries, urogenital procedures (especially if the patient has a urinary tract infection), dental work, or intravenous drug use.[53] Almost any bacteria or fungus can infect a susceptible site. In Western Europe and North America, streptococci and staphylococci account for approximately 90% of all endocarditis.

Endocarditis begins after the onset of bacteremia and the colonization of thrombotic vegetation.[3] The bacteria is then encased in a platelet and fibrin shell, which protects it from destruction by phagocytic neutrophils, leading to a zone of localized agranulocytosis. It is because of this extensive protective mechanism and its ability to restrict the body's normal response to infection that antibiotic therapy must be so intensive and extensive.[23,70]

Clinical Manifestations

See the following box for the signs and symptoms of endocarditis. A positive blood culture is usually necessary for a definitive diagnosis.

Treatment

Treatment requires prolonged parenteral therapy with adequate doses of bactericidal antibiotics.[23,48,53] An increasing number of patients are being discharged home to continue their parenteral therapy. Home patients should be followed closely to assess for acute valvular incompetence or acute onset of prosthetic valve dehiscence with accompanying cardiac failure, which will require emergency cardiac surgery.[48,108,111]

PREDISPOSING FACTORS IN ENDOCARDITIS

Rheumatic heart disease
Congenital heart disease
Mitral valve prolapse
Marfan's syndrome
Idiopathic hypertropic subaortic stenosis
Peripheral arteriovenous fistulas
Indwelling intravenous or intraarterial catheters
Cardiac and prosthetic valve surgery
Prosthetic aortic grafts
Degenerative heart disease
Alcoholism
Chronic hemodialysis
Intravenous drug abuse
Syphilitic aortic disease
Immunosuppression
Severe burns

SIGNS AND SYMPTOMS OF ENDOCARDITIS

Fever
Splenomegaly
Hematuria
Petechiae
Cardiac murmurs
Easy fatigability
Osler nodes (small raised tender areas most commonly found in pads of fingers and toes)
Splenic hemorrhages
Roth's spots (round or oval spots consisting of coagulated fibrin; seen in the retina and leads to hemorrhage)

Nursing Care

The focus of nursing care for patients with infective endocarditis is resolution of infection, prevention of or early identification of complications, and preventive teaching.

Endocarditis requires a long course, usually 6 weeks, of intravenous antibiotics. During this time the patient must be continuously assessed for any signs of worsening or reoccurrence of the infection. The patient's temperature must be monitored closely and any elevation reported to the physician. The patient also must be monitored for subtle signs of infection such as malaise, weakness, easy fatigability, and night sweats.

Antibiotics must be administered as ordered and the patient assessed for signs and symptoms of side effects and drug toxicity. Intravenous access may become a problem, and the patency and integrity of the line must be assessed before and immediately after each antibiotic dose.

The nurse must be alert for signs and symptoms of heart failure secondary to worsening valve dysfunction. Therefore the cardiovascular assessment should include the auscultation of heart sounds for the presence of or change in cardiac murmur.

A patient with infective endocarditis is also at risk for embolic events, either cerebral or pulmonary. Therefore level of consciousness, any visual changes, or headache should be documented. Any shortness of breath or chest pain with hemoptysis must also be reported.

The patient must have adequate nutrition. Often small, frequent meals, which include favorite foods from home, are required. Obtaining daily weights is important until his or her weight stabilizes; then the daily weight is used in fluid management, and weekly weights are used for checking body weight.

During the most critical period bed rest is prescribed for the patient. He or she requires range-of-motion exercises to maintain muscle tone and frequent turning and repositioning to prevent skin breakdown. Support and diversional activity are also important at this time, because depression related to a prolonged hospital stay commonly occurs.

As the patient recovers, he or she needs to know what signs and symptoms to report to the physician, how to take an oral temperature, activities that place him or her at risk for recurrence, and the necessity of letting other health care providers (for example, dentist, podiatrist) know of the history of endocarditis. Before discharge from the hospital, the patient should carry a Medic Alert bracelet or emergency identification card.

CARDIOMYOPATHY
Description

Cardiomyopathies are diseases of the heart muscle and are classified as primary or secondary. Primary, or idiopathic, cardiomyopathy is defined as heart muscle disease of unknown cause, although both viral infections and autoimmunity are suspected causes. In recent years, with more widespread use of percutaneous endomyocardial biopsy, many patients originally diagnosed with idiopathic cardiomyopathy have been found to have active lymphocytic myocarditis.[50] Treatment of idiopathic cardiomyopathy is not curative but is directed toward controlling symptoms. Treatment includes a decrease in activity, restriction of sodium intake, administration of diuretics, positive inotropic agents, vasodilators, and antidysrhythmics, and administration of oxygen during periods of acute exacerbations of heart failure; ultimately, cardiac transplantation may be the patient's only hope for survival.

Secondary cardiomyopathy is defined as heart muscle disease secondary to some other systemic disease such as coronary artery disease, valvular disease, or severe hypertension.[1,40]

Pathophysiology

Cardiomyopathies are further classified into three main categories based on abnormalities of structure and function. These categories include hypertrophic, restrictive, and congestive cardiomyopathy.

Hypertrophic cardiomyopathy. Hypertrophic cardiomyopathy is a genetically transmitted autosomal dominant trait, which frequently appears in relatives who may be asymptomatic. It is characterized by left-ventricular hypertrophy and bizarre cellular hypertrophy of the upper-ventricular septum, which may or may not result in outflow tract obstruction (Fig. 14-14). Frequently, septal hypertrophy pulls the papillary muscle out of alignment, resulting in altered function of the anterior leaflet of the mitral valve and mitral regurgitation. The myocardial muscle becomes stiff and less compliant, resulting in increased resistance to blood entering the left atrium and an increase in diastolic filling pressures.

The most common symptom is exertional dyspnea related to elevated left-ventricular diastolic pressure and increased wall stiffness, resulting in a decreased cardiac output. Syncope or "graying out" spells are also common because of the inability to increase the cardiac output with exertion.

Treatment is aimed at relaxing the ventricle and decreasing obstruction of the outflow tract. Most frequently used therapies are beta blockers and calcium channel blockers.[46,62] It must be clearly stated in the patient's record that

---

> ## Nursing Diagnosis and Management
> ### *Endocarditis*
>
> ▪ Activity Intolerance related to decreased cardiac output secondary to valvular dysfunction, p. 345.
>
> ▪ Potential for Infection risk factor: invasive lines, p. 720.
>
> ▪ Knowledge Deficit: Home Intravenous Medication Regimen related to lack of previous exposure to information, p. 69.
>
> ▪ Altered Health Maintenance related to lack of perceived threat to health, p. 67.

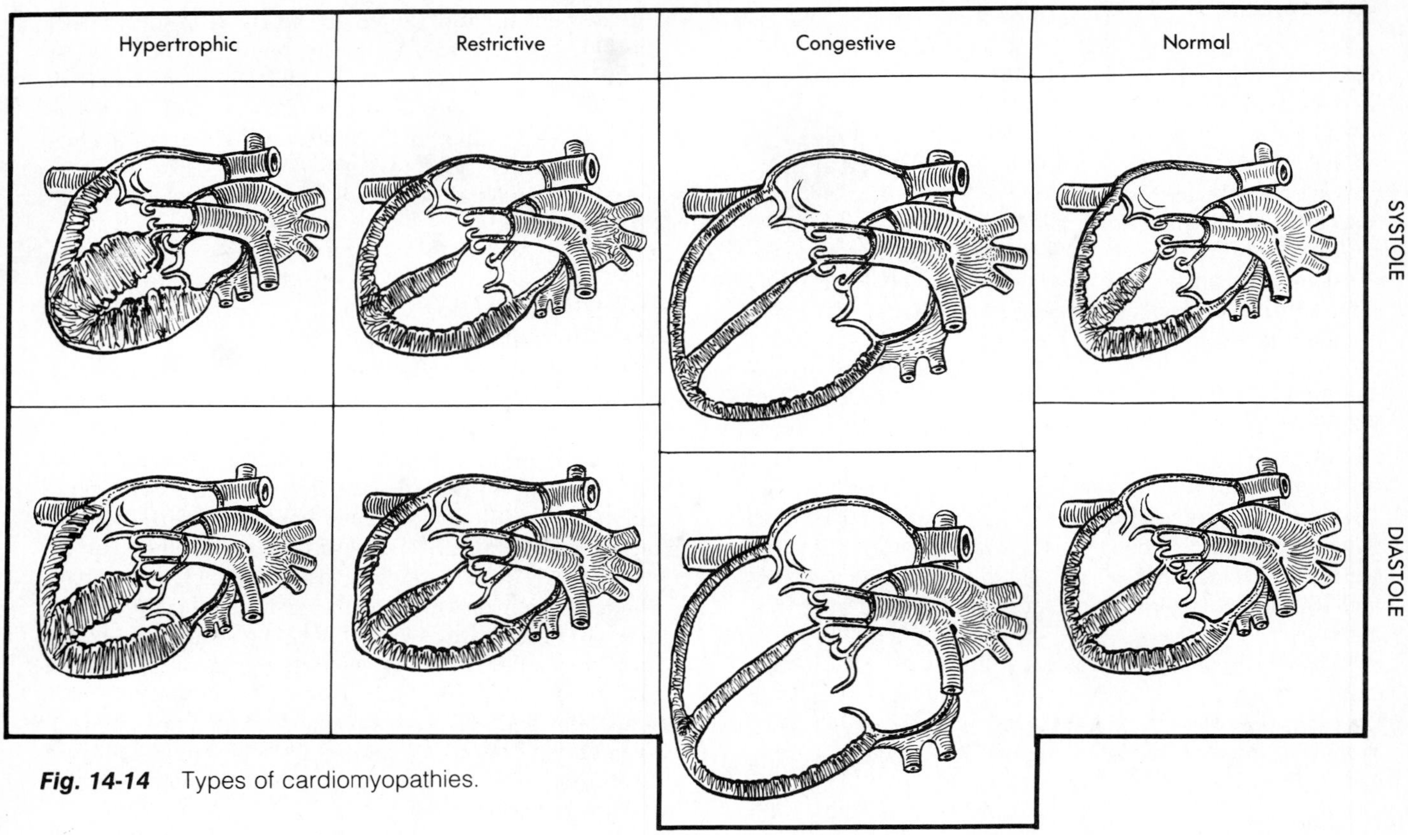

Hypertrophic	Restrictive	Congestive	Normal	

Fig. 14-14 Types of cardiomyopathies.

positive inotropic drugs should not be administered because of their propensity to increase ventricular contractility, thereby increasing outflow tract obstruction.

Congestive cardiomyopathy. Congestive (dilated) cardiomyopathy is characterized by grossly dilated ventricles without muscle hypertrophy (see Fig. 14-14). The muscle fibers contract poorly, resulting in global left-ventricular dysfunction, low cardiac output, atrial and ventricular dysrhythmias, pooling of blood, leading to embolic episodes, and eventually refractory congestive heart failure and premature death.

Restrictive cardiomyopathy. Restrictive cardiomyopathy (see Fig. 14-14) is the least common form of cardiomyopathy and is characterized by abnormal diastolic function. This cardiomyopathy results in ventricular-wall rigidity as a direct conseqeunce of wall fibrosis. The overall effect is to obstruct ventricular filling. Restrictive cardiomyopathy may be misdiagnosed as constrictive pericarditis.

Backward heart failure, low cardiac output, dyspnea, orthopnea, and liver engorgement are the most common signs and symptoms of restrictive cardiomyopathy. Treatment is directed toward the improvement of pump function, the removal of excess fluid, and administration of a low sodium diet.

Nursing Care

Many of the nursing interventions for the patient with cardiomyopathy are similar to those for the patient with congestive heart failure. Patients must be monitored for

---

Nursing Diagnosis and Management
Cardiomyopathy

- Decreased Cardiac Output related to relative excess of preload and afterload secondary to impaired ventricular contractility, p. 335.

- Activity Intolerance related to knowledge deficit of energy-saving techniques, p. 34.

- Activity Intolerance related to decreased cardiac output, p. 345.

- Anxiety related to threat to biological, psychological, and/or social integrity, p. 852.

- Powerlessness related to illness-related regimen, p. 837.

- Powerlessness related to physical deterioration despite compliance, p. 838.

- Hopelessness related to perceptions of failing or deteriorating physical condition, p. 839.

- Sensory-perceptual alterations related to sensory overload, sensory deprivation, and sleep pattern disturbance, p. 601.

signs or symptoms of worsening heart failure, that is, tissue edema, increased ventricular filling pressures, or neck vein engorgement, pulmonary congestion, weight gain, increased fatigue, and onset of gallop rhythms. Diuretics, medications to increase contractility, calcium channel or beta blockers, and vasodilators to reduce preload should be administered as ordered and the patient's response to them assessed. Obtaining daily weights, maintenance of fluid restriction if ordered, and maintenance of accurate intake and output records are important. Patients with cardiomyopathy are prone to digoxin toxicity related to decreased excretion of the drug secondary to a decreased glomerular filtration rate.

Nursing interventions should also be directed at maintaining the patient's current level of conditioning and toward collaborating with the physical therapist to maintain and, hopefully, improve the patient's functional level. Activity plans need to reflect energy conservation; therefore activities should be clustered and include frequent rest periods.

The patient's understanding of his or her illness and his or her coping mechanisms and support systems must be assessed. Patients and families need to know what support services are available.

VALVULAR HEART DISEASE
Description

Valvular heart disease is a cardiac dysfunction produced by structural and/or functional abnormalities of single or multiple cardiac valves. The result is alteration in blood flow across the valve.

There are two types of lesions, *stenotic* and *regurgitant.* Valvular stenosis results in impeded flow across the valve, and valvular regurgitation results in bidirectional flow of blood across the valve. Valvular dysfunction affects overall cardiac function by increasing pressure work with stenotic lesions and by increasing volume work with regurgitant lesions. In an attempt to compensate for these dysfunctions, the myocardium will either dilate to accommodate an increased volume or hypertrophy to increase contractility to maintain forward flow.[99]

In the past it was believed that almost all valvular lesions were rheumatic in origin; that is, damage was a direct result of group A beta-hemolytic streptococcal pharyngitis. In the United States and much of Western Europe, rheumatic disease continues to be a major cause of stenotic lesions but not of regurgitant lesions (see following box).[108]

CAUSES OF VALVULAR HEART DISEASE

Rheumatic fever
Infective endocarditis
Inborn defects of connective tissue
Dysfunction or ruptures of the papillary muscles
Congenital malformations

Mitral valve dysfunction. *Mitral valve stenosis* (Table 14-4) is a progressive narrowing of the mitral valve orifice from 4 to 6 cm to less than 1.5 cm. This narrowing is usually the result of acute rheumatic valvulitis, which results in diffuse leaflet thickening or fibrotic thickening of the margins of closure. The diffuse leaflet fibrosis and fusion of one or both commissures contributes to reduced leaflet mobility. The chordae tendineae may also be thickened, shortened, and fused, further contributing to the stenotic mitral orifice. As a result, the mitral valve is no longer able to open and close passively in response to chamber pressure changes; therefore blood flow across the valve is impeded.

Symptoms do not usually appear until the valve orifice is narrowed to 1.5 cm.[99] Early symptoms reflect failure of the left side of the heart, but as the dysfunction progresses, bilateral heart failure will be evidenced. Once the valve orifice narrows to 1.5 cm, left-atrial pressure increases in an attempt to force blood through the narrowed valve. This increase in pressure is followed by left-atrial dilation, which distorts the myocardial fibers, resulting in multiple ectopic atrial beats and the potential onset of atrial fibrillation. Atrial fibrillation will further decrease the cardiac output and exacerbate the symptoms of heart failure and decreased perfusion. This combination of increased pressure and volume leads to pulmonary congestion, which may progress from mild congestion to pulmonary edema. As excess blood fills the pulmonary vasculature, the pulmonary vascular resistance increases, resulting in extra work by the right ventricle causing right-ventricular hypertrophy. Because the right ventricle is ill-suited to function as a pump under these circumstances, the right side of the heart will eventually fail, leading to systemic engorgement of demonstrated by jugular venous distention, ascites, and peripheral edema. Failure of the right side of the heart may be compounded by functional tricuspid regurgitation secondary to the high pressure and volume on the right side.

Mitral valve regurgitation (see Table 14-4) can be secondary to rheumatic disease or it can be caused by endocarditis, papillary muscle dysfunction, or a number of other causes. In mitral valve regurgitation the valve annulus, leaflets, commissures, chordae tendineae, and papillary muscles may all be dysfunctional, or the dysfunction may be isolated to just one component of the valve. The primary effects of mitral valve regurgitation result in thickening and retraction of a portion of the leaflet.

Mitral valve regurgitation results in retrograde flow of blood into the left atrium with each ventricular contraction. The left atrium dilates to accommodate this additional volume, whereas the left ventricle hypertrophies as it tries to maintain forward flow and an adequate stroke volume. Mitral valve regurgitation tends to beget mitral valve regurgitation in that, as the volume and dimensions increase, the regurgitation worsens.[99] Once the left ventricle fails, the pulmonary venous pressure increases, leading to pulmonary congestion, increased pulmonary artery pressure, and right-ventricular enlargement.

Acute mitral valve regurgitation occuring secondary to papillary muscle rupture is a medical emergency that is not tolerated without aggressive medical therapy and, usually, surgical replacement of the mitral valve. The patient's con-

Table 14-4 Valvular dysfunction

Pathophysiology	Signs/symptoms	Physical signs
MITRAL VALVE STENOSIS		
Left atrium must generate more pressure to propel blood beyond the lesion Rise in left-atrial pressure and volume reflected retrograde into pulmonary vessels Right-ventricular hypertrophy Right-ventricular failure	Dyspnea on exertion Fatigue and weakness Pronounced respiratory symptoms—orthopnea, paroxysmal nocturnal dyspnea Mild hemoptysis with bronchial capillary rupture Susceptibility to pulmonary infections	Chest radiograph—pulmonary congestion, redistribution of blood flow to upper lobes Electrocardiogram (ECG)—atrial fibrillation and other atrial dysrhythmias Auscultation—diastolic murmur, accentuated S_1, opening snap Catherization—elevated pressure, gradient across valve; increased left-atrial pressure, pulmonary artery wedge, pulmonary artery pressure; low cardiac output
MITRAL VALVE REGURGITATION		
Left-ventricular dilation and hypertrophy Left-atrial dilation and hypertrophy	Weakness and fatigue Exertional dyspnea Palpitations Severe symptoms precipitated by left-ventricular failure, with consequent low output and pulmonary congestion	Chest radiograph—left-atrial and left-ventricular enlargement, variable pulmonary congestion ECG—P-mitrale, left-ventricular hypertrophy, atrial fibrillation Auscultation—murmur throughout systole Catherization—opacification of lefta-trium during left-ventricular injection, V waves, increased left-atrial and left-ventricular pressures Variable elevations of pulmonary pressures
AORTIC VALVE STENOSIS		
Left-ventricular hypertrophy Progressive failure of ventricular emptying Pulmonary congestion Failure of right side of heart, with systemic venous congestion Sudden death	Exertional dyspnea Exercise intolerance Syncope Angina Congestive heart failure (left-ventricular failure)	Chest radiograph—poststenotic aortic dilation, calcification ECG—left-ventricular hypertrophy Auscultation—systolic ejection murmur Catherization—significant pressure gradient, increased left ventricular end diastolic pressure
AORTIC VALVE REGURGITATION		
Increased volume load imposed on left ventricle Left-ventricular dilation and hypertrophy	Fatigue Dyspnea on exertion Palpitations	Chest radiograph—boot-shaped elongation of cardiac apex ECG—left-ventricular hypertrophy Auscultation—diastolic murmur Catherization —opacification of left ventricle during aortic injection Peripheral signs—hyperdynamic myocardial action and low peripheral resistance

Table 14-4 Valvular dysfunction—cont'd

Pathophysiology	Signs/symptoms	Physical signs
TRICUSPID VALVE STENOSIS		
Right atrium must generate higher pressure to eject blood beyond the lesion Right-atrial dilation Systemic venous engorgement Increased venous pressures	Venous distention Peripheral edema Ascites Hepatic engorgement Anorexia	Chest radiograph—right-atrial enlargement ECG—right-atrial enlargement (P pulmonale) Auscultation—diastolic murmur Catherization—elevated right-atrial pressure with large a waves; pressure gradient across the tripcuspid valve
TRICUSPID VALVE REGURGITATION		
Right-ventricular hypertrophy and dilation	Decreased cardiac output Neck vein distention Hepatic engorgement Ascites Edema Pleural effusions	Chest radiograph—right-atrial and ventricular enlargement. ECG—right-ventricular hypertrophy and right-atrial enlargement, atrial fibrillation Auscultation—murmur throughout systole Catheterization—elevated right-atrial pressure and V waves

dition must be stabilized with aggressive medical therapy, which frequently includes use of an intraaortic balloon pump. Once the patient has stabilized, he or she is taken to surgery for surgical replacement of the incompetent valve.

Aortic valve dysfunction. *Aortic valve stenosis* (see Table 14-4) can occur secondary to aging, calcification of a congential bicuspid valve, or rheumatic valvulitis. Irrespective of its cause, the effect is to impede ejection of blood from the left ventricle into the aorta, resulting in increased left-ventricular systolic pressure, left-ventricular hypertrophy, and eventually, at end-stage disease, left-ventricular dilation. Additionally, when the increase in volume and pressure is communicated back to the atrial and pulmonary vasculature, the result is an increase in left-atrial pressure and volume, pulmonary venous pressure, and pulmonary congestion. In rare cases, if left untreated, right-ventricular failure may develop. An incidence of sudden death is associated with aortic valve stenosis and usually occurs during exertion when demand acutely outstrips the heart's ability to provide an adequate cardiac output.

Aortic valve regurgitation (see Table 14-4) can occur secondary to rheumatic fever, systemic hypertension, Marfan's syndrome, syphilis, rheumatoid arthritis, or discrete subaortic stenosis. Aortic valve regurgitation results in reflux of blood back into the left ventricle during ventricular diastole. To accommodate this extra volume, the left ventricle dilates. Over a period of time, however, the left ventricle hypertrophies in an attempt to empty more completely and to meet the needs of the peripheral circulation.

Tricuspid valve dysfunction. *Tricuspid valve stenosis* (see Table 14-4) is rarely an isolated lesion and usually occurs in conjunction with mitral and/or aortic disease. Its

origin is most often rheumatic fever. Tricuspid valve stenosis increases the pressure work of the usually low-pressure right atrium, resulting in right-atrial hypertrophy. Additionally, the right atrium dilates in an attempt to accommodate the residual right-atrial volume and the incoming venous return. As a result, systemic venous congestion occurs, the consequences of which include jugular venous congestion, liver failure, hepatomegaly, ascites, and peripheral edema.

Tricuspid valve regurgitation (see Table 14-4) usually occurs secondary to advanced failure of the left side of the heart or severe pulmonary hypertension.

Pulmonary valve dysfunction. *Pulmonary valve disease* is most often related to congenital anomalies and produces failure of the right side of the heart. If untreated, it can result in severe irreversible pulmonary vascular changes.

Mixed valvular lesions. Many people will have mixed lesions, that is, an element of both stenosis and regurgitation. Mixed lesions can accentuate a condition the way aortic stenosis and aortic regurgitation do when they both increase left-ventricular volume and pressure and thereby multiply the degree of left-ventricular work. On the other hand, mitral valve stenosis and aortic valve stenosis protect the left ventricle from the strain produced by aortic valve stenosis alone. Mitral valve stenosis, by decreasing forward flow from the left atrium to the left ventricle, reduces the residual volume in the left ventricle because of the aortic valve stenosis.[31,46]

Nursing Care

The focus of care for the patient with valvular heart disease is to assess the patient's functional activity level and fluid volume status and to monitor for signs of heart failure, syncope, or anginal pain.

Nursing Diagnosis and Management
Valvular heart disease

- Decreased Cardiac Output related to relative excess of preload and afterload, p. 335.

- Activity Intolerance related to decreased cardiac output, p. 345.

- Activity Intolerance related to postural hypotension secondary to prolonged immobility, vasodilator therapy, p. 344.

- Potential for Altered Peripheral Tissue Perfusion risk factor: vasopressor therapy, p. 341.

- Body Image Disturbance related to actual change in body function, p. 833.

Patients with valvular heart disease frequently have decreased cardiac output because of decreased forward flow secondary to obstruction of flow through a stenotic valve or because of bidirectional flow across an incompetent valve. Positive inotropic and afterload-reducing agents should be administered as ordered and their effect carefully assessed and documented.

Vital signs should be assessed frequently, and if the patient has indwelling catheters, hemodynamic parameters should also be assessed.

Activities should be carefully planned to provide adequate rest periods to prevent fatigue.

Fluid status should be assessed by auscultating breath and heart sounds. The appearance of pulmonary crackles or an S_3 may be indicative of fluid-volume overload. The jugular vein should be assessed for signs of increased distention, and diuretics and vasodilators should be administered as ordered. The patient should be weighed daily and the intake and output accurately monitored.

Activities that precipitate anginal pain must be clearly documented. The patient may require oxygen and pain medication to treat the discomfort. Decreasing his or her anxiety may also lessen the discomfort.

Patient teaching should include information related to (1) any diet and/or fluid restrictions, (2) actions and side effects of the medications, (3) the need to check with the primary care physician before undergoing any invasive procedures such as dental work, and (4) when to call the physician about a change in condition.

HYPOVOLEMIC SHOCK
Description

Hypovolemic shock is the most commonly occurring of the shock states. It results from reduction of the circulating blood volume, leading to an inability of the circulation to meet the body's metabolic needs.

Etiology

Hypovolemic shock may result from either direct or indirect volume loss. Direct volume losses result from hemorrhage, severe diarrhea and/or vomiting, massive diuresis, and loss of plasma from skin lesions or burns.[68]

Indirect volume loss frequently results from sequestering of fluids into another body space because of an alteration in capillary permeability or a fall in colloidal osmotic pressure. Indirect loss frequently occurs with cirrhosis, hemorrhagic pancreatitis, long-bone fracture, severe sodium depletion, ruptured spleen, addisonian crisis, or hypopituitarism.

Pathophysiology

The loss of intravascular volume leads to decreased venous return (preload), decreased cardiac filling pressures, decreased stroke volume, decreased cardiac output, and ultimately, decreased tissue perfusion. Once this spiral begins and the body's compensatory mechanisms, mediated by the sympathetic nervous system, are activated, vasoconstriction occurs, the renin-aldosterone system is activated, and antidiuretic hormone is secreted.

Hypovolemic shock may be classified as mild, moderate, or severe, depending on the estimated fluid loss.[7]

Assessment and Diagnosis

The clinical manifestations of shock depend on the severity of fluid loss. Mild shock is defined as a volume loss of approximately 10% to 25% or 500 to 1200 ml of fluid. In this stage the patient may be hypotensive and slightly tachycardic.

Moderate hypovolemic shock results from a fluid loss of approximately 25% to 35% or 1200 to 1800 ml of fluid. At this time a marked decrease in blood pressure and cardiac output follow. Clinical manifestations include severe arterial vasoconstriction, diminished blood flow to the kidneys, gastrointestinal tract, and liver, development of a rapid, thready pulse, diaphoresis, decreased urine output, and increasing anxiety and restlessness.

A fluid loss of 35% to 50% or 1800 to 2500 ml results in severe shock causing the patient to be severely hypotensive, with marked peripheral vasoconstriction, marked diaphoresis, obtundation, and anuria.

Treatment

The major goal of therapy is to restore and maintain tissue perfusion and to correct the underlying physiological abnormality. This is accomplished by replacing intravascular volume with either a crystalloid (for example, Ringer's lactate or other balanced electrolyte solution) or a colloid (that is, blood or blood components) solution or a combination of both. Initially, the lost volume is replaced quickly through one to three large peripheral intravenous catheters until the shock state is corrected or there is evidence of fluid overload. Autotransfusion, the collection and administration of the patient's own blood, may be used for trauma injuries. A Pneumatic Anti-Shock Garment (PASG) may also be used for a patient in profound shock as a means of increasing venous return, and vasopressors may be used to maintain perfusion pressure as the fluid resuscitation continues.

Nursing Diagnosis and Management
Hypovolemic shock

- Fluid Volume Deficit related to active blood loss, p. 668.

- Potential for Altered Peripheral Tissue Perfusion risk factor: vasopressor therapy, p. 341.

- Potential for Infection risk factor: invasive monitoring devices, p. 346.

- Potential for Aspiration risk factors: endotracheal tube, situation hindering elevation of upper body, reduced level of consciousness, p. 489.

- Ineffective Airway Clearance related to impaired cough secondary to loss of glottic closure with cuffed endotracheal tube, p. 476.

- Sleep Pattern Disturbance related to circadian desynchronization, p. 89.

- Sensory-Perceptual Alterations related to sensory overload, sensory deprivation, sleep pattern disturbance, p. 601.

Nursing Care

The focus of nursing care for the patient in hypovolemic shock is to assess overall perfusion status, administer fluids as ordered, assess pulmonary and renal status, and observe for signs or symptoms of fluid overload.

Patients in shock may have pulmonary artery catheters, central venous catheters, and/or arterial lines in place, depending on the severity and the cause of the shock and their preshock medical history. The patient in shock requires frequent documentation of hemodynamic response to therapy and assessment of renal status, pulmonary function, and mentation.

Patients are positioned with their legs elevated, trunk flat, and head and shoulders elevated higher than the chest to increase venous return.[68]

HYPERTENSIVE CRISIS
Description

Hypertensive crisis represents a clinical situation in which hypertension is associated with irreversible vital organ damage or a threat to life over a short period of time. The critical factor in hypertensive crisis is the accelerated rise of the blood pressure, which results in complications occurring over a period of hours or days rather than days to weeks.[67] A diastolic pressure greater than 130 mm Hg is usually labeled as severe hypertension.

Etiology

The overall incidence of hypertensive crisis is less than 1% of known hypertensives. It is usually precipitated by noncompliance with medical therapy and/or diet or inadequate treatment. Hypertensive crisis may be detected in patients with no previous history of the condition.

In patients with no previous history of hypertension, common causes of crisis include (1) acute or chronic renal disease, (2) acute central nervous system (CNS) events, (3) drug-induced hypertension (for example, from ingestion of contraceptives), and (4) the ingestion of tyramine-containing foods or beverages (for example, beer or cheese) during treatment with monoamine oxidase inhibitors (MAOI). In addition, a state like that of catecholamine excess may follow the abrupt cessation of clonidine and guanabenz.[67]

Pathophysiology

The exact mechanism of hypertensive crisis is not known, but it is characterized by fibrinoid necrosis of the arterioles.

Assessment and Diagnosis

Hypertensive crisis is manifested by CNS compromise (headache, papilledema, coma), cardiovascular compromise

Table 14-5 Hypertensive emergencies

Emergencies	Examples of causes
CARDIOVASCULAR COMPROMISE	
Chest pain	Unstable angina, myocardial infarction, aortic dissection
Congestive heart failure	Myocardial infarction, severe hypertension, pheochromocytoma (very rare)
Hypertension after vascular surgery	Aortic aneurysmectomy, carotid endarterectomy, coronary artery bypass grafting
CENTRAL NERVOUS SYSTEM (CNS) COMPROMISE	
Papilledema	Increased intracranial pressure—mass lesion
	Malignant hypertension—any cause
Headache, agitation, lethargy, confusion	Hypertensive encephalopathy—any cause, subarachnoid hemorrhage, cerebrovascular accident (CVA)
Coma	CVA, advanced hypertensive encephalopathy, trauma, tumor
Seizures	Advanced hypertensive encephalopathy, CNS tumor, eclampsia, CVA (less common)
Focal neurological deficit	CVA, CNS tumor, hypertensive encephalopathy
ACUTE RENAL FAILURE	Malignant hypertension, vasculitis, scleroderma, glomerulonephritis
HISTORY CONSISTENT WITH CATECHOLAMINE EXCESS	
Pheochromocytoma, MAOI in combination with certain drugs and foods, clonidine and guanabenz withdrawal	

Modified from McRae RP and Liebson PR: Med Clin North Am 70(4):749, 1986.

(angina, myocardial infarction), acute renal failure, and a history consistent with catecholamine excess. Table 14-5 lists clinical findings that suggest hypertensive emergencies and gives examples of causes.

Treatment

Hypertensive crisis necessitates admitting the patient to a critical care unit where antihypertensive therapy can be administered parenterally and blood pressure monitored continuously using an arterial line. Frequently used medications include furosemide, sodium nitroprusside, diazoxide, trimethaphan camsylate, and labetalol.

Clonidine administered in hourly doses of 0.1 to 0.2 mg lowers severe hypertension. Other parenteral drugs that apparently are effective during crisis are guanabenz, minoxidil, oral nifedipine, and captopril. A loop diuretic and beta blocker are usually used concurrently to prevent reflex tachycardia and fluid retention, both of which may increase the blood pressure.[57,67]

It is important to remember that cerebral hypoperfusion can occur if mean blood pressure is lowered too rapidly. During the first 24 hours of treatment, it has been recommended that mean arterial pressure be decreased by no more than 20% to 30%.[67]

Nursing Care

The focus of nursing care for the patient with hypertensive crisis is to return the blood pressure to the desired range and then to identify the factors that resulted in this life-threatening condition.

During the acute phase the patient must be closely observed for signs and symptoms of cardiac or neurological compromise such as cardiovascular collapse, ischemia, dysrhythmias, mental confusion, stupor, seizures, or coma.

Antihypertensives should be administered as ordered and the blood pressure closely monitored. If potent vasodilators such as nitroprusside are being used, they should be infused through an infusion pump, and an arterial line should be placed in the patient.

While obtaining the health history, the nurse needs to identify risk factors and also clarify any misconceptions the patient may have regarding hypertension and its treatment.

Prognosis

Hypertensive crisis with current therapy is associated with a 25% mortality at 1 year and 50% at 5 years. Most common

causes of death are uremia, myocardial infarction, heart failure, and cerebrovascular accident.

PERIPHERAL VASCULAR DISEASE

Atherosclerosis is the most common cause of peripheral vascular disease. Alterations can occur in either the venous or arterial systems, with most occurring in the vessels of the lower extremities. Risk factors associated with peripheral vascular disease are the same as those for coronary artery disease.

Arterial Disease

Occlusive arterial disease. There are two major causes of occlusive arterial disease. The first is *arteriosclerosis obliterans,* a consequence of atherosclerosis. These lesions tend to occur at the origin or bifurcations of a vessel. The aortoiliac vessels, femoropopliteal vessels, and popliteal-tibial vessels are the most common sites for atherogenesis.

The second major cause of occlusive arterial disease is *thromboangiitis obliterans* (Buerger's disease), an occlusion caused by inflammation and thrombosis. Thrombi may originate in the left side of the heart as a consequence of atrial fibrillation or mitral stenosis. Thrombogensis also occurs at the site of artherosclerotic plaque. Arterial occlusion obstructs blood flow to the distal extremity.

Assessment and diagnosis. Intermittent claudication (cramping, aching pain during ambulation) is usually the first symptom of occlusive disease. This pain is relieved by rest, but as the disease progresses, the pain develops during rest. Relief may be obtained by placing the extremity in a dependent position. The site of the pain is usually indicative of location of the lesion. Arterial pulses may be diminished, transiently present (vessel spasm), or absent distal to the site of occlusion.

Postural changes result in changes in skin color. With extremity elevation, the limb becomes pale. Dependency of the extremity yields a rubor or purplish discoloration.

Atrophic tissue changes include thickening of the nails and drying of the skin. Hair loss is common on the lower leg, dorsum of the feet, and toes. A temperature gradient is usually present as a line of demarcation between areas that are well perfused and those that are poorly perfused. There may also be wasting of muscle, as well as of soft tissue. As the disease progresses, it may result in ulcerations and gangrene.

Acute occlusions usually are initially seen with sudden onset of severe pain, loss of pulses, collapse of superficial veins, coldness and pallor, and impaired motor and sensory function.

Treatment. Medical therapy is geared toward controlling or eliminating risk factors, providing good foot care, and suggesting alterations in lifestyle to promote rest and pain relief. Therapy may also include the use of anticoagulants, vasodilators, or antiplatelet drugs. If the above-listed therapies do not produce positive results, the patient may be a candidate for angioplasty.

Surgical therapy may be required if symptoms become disabling or threaten limb viability. Surgical procedures and the purpose of each include the following: (1) arterial re-

---

Nursing Diagnosis and Management
Hypertensive crisis

- Anxiety related to threat to biological, psychological, and/or social integrity, p. 852.
- Altered Cerebral Tissue Perfusion related to increased intracranial pressure secondary to hemorrhage, p. 581.

construction—to restore unimpeded flow and to redirect blood flow around the site of occlusion, (2) endarterectomy—to remove discrete plaque, and (3) lumbar sympathectomy—to decrease sympathetic tone and increase peripheral vasodilation. Severe occlusions may necessitate limb or partial limb amputation.

Nursing care. The focus of nursing care for the patient with arterial insufficiency is to increase the arterial blood supply, decrease venous pooling, promote vasodilation, maintain tissue integrity, treat tissue hypoxia, and provide patient teaching.

The arterial blood supply may be increased by maintaining the extremity in a neutral (flat) or dependent position, encouraging ambulation (walking but not standing) as ordered, and performing active range-of-motion exercises when bed rest has been prescribed for the patient.

To decrease venous pooling, the patient should not sit or stand for long periods of time. If pooling does occur, the legs should be elevated to a neutral position. Walking should be encouraged.

The patient can promote vasodilation by keeping the extremity warm, ceasing smoking, and stopping the use of other vasoconstricting substances such as caffeine. The legs should not be crossed when sitting or lying flat, and anything that constricts blood flow such as socks with tight-fitting elastic tops or garters should be avoided.

Nursing interventions intended to preserve tissue integrity include (1) performing special foot care, which includes washing and carefully drying the feet each day, (2) having the patient wear cotton or wool stockings that are not mended and are seamless, and (3) having him or her wear protective footwear (that is, a soft, flexible leather shoe with a closed toe and a high toebox whenever out of bed. Sandals, thongs, elastic bands over the instep, and pressure on the dorsum of the foot from tied laces should be avoided. Skin color, temperature, and elasticity should be checked. Adhesive tape should not be applied directly to the skin. Any

ulcerations should be promptly identified and treated. The patient should be encouraged to have a well-balanced diet to maintain tissue integrity and foster wound healing.[24,38]

Tissue hypoxia may be treated by increasing blood flow to the extremity by walking or performing range-of-motion exercises. Tissue hypoxia is painful, and analgesics should be administered to allow the patient to achieve a comfort level that will foster his or her cooperation in ambulating.

Aneurysmal arterial disease
Description. An aneurysm is a localized dilation of the arterial wall that results in an alteration in vessel shape and blood flow. Figure 14-15 displays the four types of aneurysms.

Etiology. The majority (90%) of patients who are initially seen with an aneurysm have a history of systemic hyper-

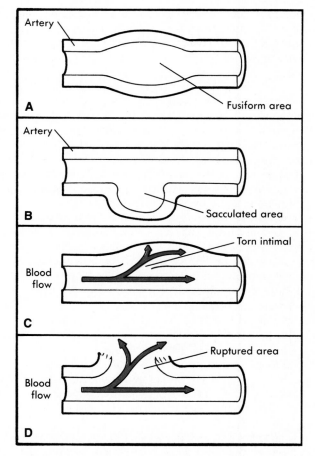

Fig. 14-15 Four basic types of aneurysms. **A,** Fusiform aneurysm, in which an entire segment of an artery is dilated, thus taking on a spindle or bulbous shape. Fusiform aneurysms occur most often in the abdominal aorta secondary to atherosclerosis. **B,** Sacculated aneurysm, which involves only one side of an artery and is usually located in the ascending aorta. **C,** Dissecting aneurysm, which occurs because of a tear in the intima, resulting in the shunting of blood between the intima and media of a vessel. **D,** Pseudoaneurysm, which results from a ruptured artery.

tension. Other causes of aneurysm include (1) atherosclerotic changes in the thoracic and abdominal aorta, (2) blunt trauma (deceleration injury), (3) cystic medial necrosis (Marfan's syndrome), (4) pregnancy, and (5) iatrogenic injury or dissection. Blunt trauma can cause rupture of the intimal and medial layers of the descending aorta at the ligamentum arteriosum. Increased blood volume and hypertension contribute to rupture of the aorta during pregnancy. Iatrogenic injuries may occur as a result of the use of instruments during arteriography, cardiopulmonary bypass, intraaortic balloon procedures, and aortic surgery.

Pathophysiology. Medial degeneration is the most common pathology of aneurysm formation. Medial degeneration occurs as a normal part of the aging process and as a complication of Marfan's syndrome (Erdheim's cystic medial necrosis).

The ascending aorta and the aortic arch are the sites of the greatest hemodynamic stress and are also the most frequent sites of arterial dissection. Extensive medial degeneration frequently occurs in hypertensive patients and is a major contributing factor to aneurysmal risk.

Assessment and diagnosis. For many years a person may be asymptomatic or the aneurysm may be detected during routine abdominal examination as a palpable, pulsatile mass located in the umbilical region of the abdomen to the left of midline. A thoracic aneurysm may be identified on a routine chest x-ray film. However, patients with an acute dissection or rupture will be initially seen with sudden onset of sharp, ripping, or tearing pain located in the anterior chest, epigastric area, shoulders, or back.

Cardiovascular symptoms include severe hypertension, acute neurological deficits, fleeting peripheral pulses, and a new murmur indicative of aortic insufficiency.

Treatment. An aneurysm less than 4 cm in size can be managed medically with frequent monitoring of blood pressure and ultrasound testing to document any changes in size of the aneurysm. The patient will be encouraged to lose weight if obesity is a factor, and blood pressure will be carefully monitored and hypertension treated to decrease hemodynamic stress on the site. An aneurysm greater than 6 cm is usually treated surgically (see box at right).

Aortic dissection

Description. An aortic dissection occurs when there is separation of the vascular layers by a column of blood. This creates a false lumen, which communicates with the true lumen through a tear in the intima. This separation extends along the length of the vessel rather than coursing around the circumference.

Classification of dissections. The site of the aortic dissection is most commonly described according to the DeBakey classification system. Type I dissections extend from just above the aortic valve to the iliac bifurcation. Type II dissections are limited to the ascending aorta and are most frequently seen with Marfan's syndrome. Type III dissections begin in the descending aorta distal to the left subclavian artery and extend distally to the aortic bifurcation. Another classification used by Dr. Shumway from Stanford University groups types I and II together as type A, or ascending, dissection and labels type III as type B, or descending, dissection.[22]

INDICATIONS FOR ANEURYSM SURGERY
Aneurysm greater than 5 cm Aneurysm progressively increasing in size Impending rupture Symptoms resulting from cerebral or coronary ischemia Pericardial tamponade Uncontrollable pain Aortic insufficiency

---

Assessment and diagnosis. The classic clinical manifestation is the sudden onset of intense, severe, tearing pain, which may be localized initially in the chest, abdomen, or back. As dissection extends, pain radiates to the back or distally toward the lower extremities.

Another cardiovascular sign may be a new murmur of aortic regurgitation if the dissection moves retrograde, extending back to the aortic valve. At this time the coronary arteries may be at risk, putting the patient in jeopardy of sustaining a myocardial infarction. Signs of shock may quickly develop with this type of lesion.

Patients usually exhibit severe hypertension and loss of peripheral pulses, and they may demonstrate acute neurological deficits, which include syncope, altered level of consciousness, varying levels of paresthesia and paralysis, or possibly a cerebrovascular accident. Gastrointestinal symptoms include acute abdominal pain, melena, and hyperactive bowel sounds.

Renal symptoms include oliguria and hematuria. These symptoms usually occur with dissections causing hypotension and those involving the renal arteries.

The location of the dissection may be established by the site of pain. A distal dissection is usually accompanied by chest pain, which radiates to the back, abdomen, or legs. Central chest pain is indicative of an ascending dissection.[22]

Treatment. Medical management involves controlling hypertension and pain. Progression of the dissection is evaluated by the patient's report of worsening or new pain.

Surgical procedures include resection of the affected areas, followed by graft placement, repair or replacement of the aortic valve, and restoration of blood flow to major branches of the aorta.

Nursing care. The focus of nursing care for the patient with an aortic dissection is to maintain the blood pressure within prescribed parameters, stabilize the patient hemodynamically, and control the pain.

The cardiovascular status should be assessed hourly, including monitoring blood pressure in both arms, checking peripheral pulses bilaterally, auscultating for an aortic murmur, and monitoring the ECG for ischemic changes and/or dysrhythmias. Patients usually require an arterial line and are on potent vasodilators.

The patient's neurovascular status is also assessed hourly. Included in this assessment should be documentation of the presence and distribution of pain, pallor, paresthesia, paralysis, and pulselessness.

A quiet, nonstimulating environment is maintained to decrease stress, which can lead to increased levels of circulating catecholamines and consequent increases in heart rate and blood pressure. Analgesics are also useful in decreasing anxiety and increasing comfort. Since analgesics can mask the pain of further dissection, they are administered judiciously.

Venous Disease

Description. Venous disease occurs when there is alteration in the integrity of veins, resulting in decreased venous return or thrombosis.

Thrombolic venous disease. The most common form of venous disease is usually manifested as thrombophlebitis. Thrombophlebitis is the formation of a thrombus, accompanied by inflammation, pain, tenderness, and redness at the site. The incidence is greatest in the lower-extremity vessels, especially the saphenous, femoral, and popliteal veins. Thrombophlebitis can occur in either deep or superficial vessels and in upper- or lower-extremity vessels.

Etiology and pathophysiology. Stasis of blood, endothelial injury, and hypercoagulability of blood are referred to as Virchow's triad. Usually two of the three conditions must be present for thrombosis to occur.

Superficial thromboses. Superficial thromboses are characterized by cordlike veins that are readily palpable. The area surrounding the affected vessel will often be tender to palpation, erythematous, and warm. The most common cause of superficial thromboses of the arms is intravenous therapy.

TREATMENT. Patients with superficial thromboses do not usually require anticoagulation therapy, and bed rest may be prescribed until the extremity is less tender and ambulation can be considered. Warm compresses may be used, along with elastic stockings. Superficial thromboses are usually not precursors of more serious conditions.

Deep vein thrombophlebitis. Obstruction of blood flow can occur within a deep vessel of the pelvis or lower extremity. This markedly increases the patient's risk of pulmonary embolism and long-term disability resulting from chronic venous insufficiency.

ASSESSMENT AND DIAGNOSIS. Development of deep-vein thrombosis may be very insidious. It occurs as a result of edema, causes of which include increased intravascular volume and increased intravascular pooling of blood. Pain is described as an aching or throbbing sensation, which worsens with ambulation. A positive Homan's sign, which is pain on dorsiflexion of the foot, heightens the suspicion of a deep vein thrombosis. Other manifestations include increased tissue turgor with swelling, increased skin temperature, dilation of superficial veins, and mottling and cyanosis caused by stagnant flow.

Treatment. Major therapeutic emphasis is placed on prophylaxis. The patient is confined to bed rest, along with elevation of the limb, anticoagulation therapy, and local applications of moist heat. Analgesics are prescribed to reduce discomfort. Measurement of both the affected calf and thigh should be done once a day. The measurement site should be marked on the extremity. Patients receiving anticoagulation therapy require careful assessment for bleeding tendencies, including obtaining frequent bleeding studies, testing stool and urine for occult blood, and inspecting gums for bleeding. Once the patient begins to ambulate, full-length, custom-fitted elastic stockings should be ordered. Complaints of or observation of dyspnea or chest pain must be evaluated secondary to risk of pulmonary embolism.

Most patients will be managed medically with anticoagulants, but those at high risk for pulmonary embolism (that is, cancer patients, patients with bleeding disorders, or patients who have a spinal cord injury, or who are comatose) may require surgical intervention. Possible procedures include venous thrombectomy, femoral vein interruption, inferior vena cava interruption, insertion of filtering devices, thrombolytic therapy, angioplasty, and laser treatment.

Chronic venous insufficiency. Chronic venous insufficiency is produced by extensive deep vein thrombosis with resultant venous valve insufficiency. It is usually precipitated by chronic venous stasis and elevation of venous pressures, resulting in stretching and weakening of the valves. Over a period of time, this condition may lead to the development of stasis ulcers.

Nursing care. The focus of care for the patient with venous disease is to increase blood flow and to prevent complications from deep vein thrombosis or anticoagulant therapy.

During the acute phase, self-care activities should be limited and bed rest maintained. The affected limb should be elevated above the level of the right atrium to decrease edema and venous stasis. Range-of-motion exercises should be performed with the unaffected leg. The patient should be instructed to avoid use of the knee gatch because elevation of the knee impedes venous return. Warm, moist compresses may be applied as ordered, and calf and/or thigh measurements should be obtained daily. Thigh-high or knee-high elastic stockings that have been custom fitted or Ace wraps should be applied as ordered. The patient with a deep vein thrombosis should be closely monitored for signs of pulmonary embolism, and the patient should be instructed to report immediately any chest pain, dyspnea, or tachypnea. Once the patient is ambulatory, he or she should be encouraged to walk but not to sit or stand for long periods of time. When sitting in a chair, low elevation of the affected extremity should be maintained.

Anticoagulant therapy should be monitored by obtaining daily coagulation values. Bleeding should be treated promptly. Stools should be checked for occult blood. Mechanical trauma should be avoided (for example, the patient should use an electric razor, soft toothbrush, and unobstructed walkway).

RESEARCH ABSTRACT

Evaluation of bruises and areas of induration after two techniques of subcutaneous heparin injection

Woolridge JB and Jackson JG: Heart Lung 17(5):476, 1988.

PURPOSE

The purpose of this study was to evaluate bruises, induration, or both that occurred after use of two techniques of subcutaneous heparin injection in current use by nurses.

FRAMEWORK

The subcutaneous administration of the anticoagulant heparin is a frequently performed nursing intervention. Bruising (discoloration) and induration (hardening) occur after some, but not all, such injections. Not only does the patient experience the physical discomfort and the psychological impact of visible body trauma, but bruising and induration limit possible sites for future injections. Administration technique is frequently cited as a possible cause of bruising and induration. Based on a review of the literature and investigators' experiences, four variables were selected for evaluation in this study: (1) syringe size, (2) use of an air bubble in the syringe, (3) change of needles after drawing heparin into the syringe, and (4) type of material placed over the site after injection.

METHODS

Fifty hospitalized adult medical-surgical patients over the age of 18 years who received 5000 units of heparin every 12 hours and who had normal platelet counts, no known clotting disorders, and adequate abdominal surface for administration were selected. The investigators randomly selected one of two administration techniques and administered the prescribed heparin. Twenty-four hours later the same investigator gave the subject a second injection, using the other technique. Fifty-two hours after each injection, an investigator unaware of which technique was used evaluated each injection site.

RESULTS

To compare the site of bruises and indurations, the data were analyzed by the Mann-Whitney U-Wilcoxon rank sum test, which demonstrated a 0.003 level of signficiance for bruises and a 0.02 level of significance for induration. To compare the number of subjects in whom bruises and indurations developed, the data were analyzed by the chi-square test, which showed a 0.0458 level of significance for induration but only a 0.1371 level of signifiance for bruising. Men had smaller bruises than women, regardless of age, and younger women had smaller bruises. There were only 10 indurated areas resulting from all injections, but the pattern for size according to age and sex was similar.

IMPLICATIONS

It was concluded for this sample that the technique using a 3-ml syringe with a 25-gauge, ⅝ inch needle, a change of needle after drawing medication into the syringe, an air bubble, and a dry sponge after administration resulted in fewer areas of induration. Administering subcutaneous heparin in a way that minimizes local trauma will reduce patient discomfort and preserve body surface for future injections. Although one technique was found more effective, future studies must be done to determine whether any one of the four variables investigated in this study made the difference.

REFERENCES

1. Abelmann WH: Classification and natural history of primary myocardial disease, Prog Cardiovasc Dis 27(2):73, 1984.
2. Anderson UK: Mitral valve prolapse: a diagnosis for primary nursing intervention, J Cardiovasc Nurs 1(3):41, 1987.
3. Bayless R and others: Incidence, mortality and prevention of infective endocarditis, J R Coll Physicians Lond 20(1):12, 1986.
4. Benditt E: The origin of atherosclerosis, Sci Am 236:74, 1977.
5. Benditt EP and Benditt JM: Evidence for a monoclonal origin of human atherosclerotic plaques, Proc Natl Acad Sci 70:1753, 1973.
6. Bigger JT and others: Prognosis after recovery from acute myocardial infarction, Annu Rev Med 35:127, 1984.
7. Billhardt RA and Rosenbush SW: Cardiogenic and hypovolemic shock, Med Clin North Am 70(4):853, 1986.
8. Blessey R: Epidemiology, risk factors, and pathophysiology of ischemic heart disease, Phys Ther 65(12):1796, 1985.
9. Bondestam E and others: Pain assessment by patients and nurses in the early phase of acute MI, J Adv Nurs 12(6):677, 1987.
10. Bondy B: An overview of arterial disease, J Cardiovasc Nurs 1(2):1, 1987.
11. Braunwald E, editor: Heart disease, ed 3, Philadelphia, 1988, WB Saunders Co.
12. Bressack MA and Raffin TA: Importance of venous return, venous resistance and mean circulatory pressure in the physiology and management of shock, Chest 92(5):906, 1987.
13. Burke LE: Nursing grand rounds: risk-factor modification in the prevention of coronary heart disease, J Cardiovasc Nurs 1(4):67, 1987.
14. Bush DE and Healy B: Management of a patient recovering from myocardial infarction: a decision tree, Adv Intern Med 31:469, 1986.
15. Cohn JM: Management of acute myocardial infarction, Am J Med 77:67, 1984.
16. Condini MA: Management of acute myocardial infarction, Med Clin North Am 70(4):769, 1986.
17. Conti CR: Unstable angina before and after infarction: thoughts on pathogenesis and therapeutic strategies, Heart Lung 15(4):361, 1986.
18. Cox JL and others: Laser-assisted angioplasty treating peripheral vascular disease, AORN J 46(5):835, 1987.
19. Dawber TR and others: Epidemiological approaches to heart disease: the Framingham study, Am J Public Health 41:279, 1951.
20. Deans KW and Hartshorn JC: Cardiovascular pharmacology: nitrates in the treatment of coronary artery disease, J Cardiovasc Nurs 1(1):81, 1986.
21. DeWood MA and others: Prevalence of total coronary occlusion during the early hours of transmural MI, N Engl J Med 303:897, 1980.
22. Dixon MB: Acute aortic dissection, J Cardiovasc Nurs 1(2):24, 1987.
23. Donabedian H and Freimer EH: Pathogenesis and treatment of endocarditis, Am J Med 78(6A):127, 1985.
24. Doyle JE: Treatment modalities in peripheral vascular disease, Nurs Clin North Am 21(2):241, 1986.
25. Eberts A: Advances in the pharmacologic management of angina pectoris, J Cardiovasc Nurs 1(1):15, 1986.
26. Epstein SE and Palmeri ST: Mechanisms contributing to precipitation of unstable angina and acute myocardial infarction: implications regarding therapy, Am J Cardiol 54(10):1245, 1984.
27. Ferguson RK and others: Clinical applications of angiotensin-converting enzyme inhibitors, Am J Med 77(4):690, 1984.
28. Fozzard HA and Makielski JC: The electrophysiology of acute myocardial ischemia, Annu Rev Med 36:275, 1985.
29. Francis GS: Neurohumoral mechanisms involved in congestive heart failure, Am J Cardiol 55(2):15A, 1985.
30. Francis GS and Cohn JN: The autonomic nervous system in congestive heart failure, Annu Rev Med 37:235, 1986.
31. Gillum RF and others: Decline in coronary heart disease mortality. Old questions and new facts, Am J Med 76(6):1055, 1984.
32. Glueck CJ: Role of risk factor management in progression and regression of coronary and femoral artery atherosclerosis, Am J Cardiol 57(14):35G, 1986.
33. Goldberg RJ and others: Long-term anticoagulant therapy after acute myocardial infarction, Am Heart J 109(3):616, 1985.
34. Goldberg RJ and others: The role of anticoagulant therapy in acute myocardial infarction, Am Heart J 108(5):1387, 1984.
35. Goldman L and Cook EF: The decline in ischemic heart disease mortality rates. An analysis of the comparative effects of medical interventions and changes in lifestyle, Ann Intern Med 101(6):825, 1984.
36. Handler CE: Cardiogenic shock, Postgrad Med J 61(718):705, 1985.
37. Hansson L and Lundin S: Hypertension and coronary heart disease: cause and consequence or associated diseases? Am J Med 76(2A):41, 1984.
38. Herman J: Nursing assessment and nursing diagnosis in patients with peripheral vascular disease, Nurs Clin North Am 21(2):219, 1986.
39. Hjalmarson A: Early intervention with a beta-blocking drug after acute myocardial infarction, Am J Cardiol 54(11):11E, 1984.
40. Hurst W, editor: The heart, ed 6, New York, 1986, McGraw-Hill Book Co.
41. Irwin S: Clinical manifestations and assessment of ischemic heart disease, Phys Ther 65(12):1806, 1985.
42. Jaffe AS: Complications of acute myocardial infarction, Cardiovasc Clin 2(1):79, 1984.
43. Jarzemsky P: Nursing care of the patient with dilated cardiomyopathy, Crit Care Nurs 6(2):10, 1986.
44. Jeffries PR and Whelan SK: Cardiogenic shock: current management, Crit Care Nurs 11(1):48, 1988.
45. Johnson J: Valvular heart disease in the elderly, J Cardiovasc Nurs 1(2):72, 1987.
46. Josephson MA and Singh BN: Use of calcium antagonists in ventricular dysfunction, Am J Cardiol 55(3):81B, 1985.
47. Kannel WB and others: A general cardiovascular risk profile: The Framingham Study, Am J Cardiol 38:46, 1976.
48. Kaye D: Prophylaxis for infective endocarditis: an update, Ann Intern Med 104(3):419, 1986.
49. Kelly DT: Clinical decisions in patients following myocardial infarction, Curr Probl Cardiol 10(11):1, 1985.
50. Kereiakes DJ and Parmley WW: Myocarditis and cardiomyopathy, Am Heart J 108(5):1318, 1984.
51. Kern LS: Advances in the surgical treatment of coronary artery disease, J Cardiovasc Nurs 1(1):1, 1986.
52. King K and Harkness JL: Infective endocarditis in the 1980s. Part 1. Etiology and diagnosis, Med J Aust 144(10):536, 1986.
53. King K and Harkness JL: Infective endocarditis in the 1980s. Part 2. Treatment and management, Med J Aust 144(11):588, 1986.
54. Kirklin JW and Barratt-Boyes BG: Cardiac surgery, New York, 1986, John Wiley & Sons, Inc.
55. Kjekshus JK: The coronary circulation in normal and ischemic hearts, Scand J Clin Lab Invest 173:9, 1984.
56. Klamerus KJ: Current concepts in clinical therapeutics: congestive heart failure, Clin Pharm 5(6):481, 1986.
57. Kochar MS and Woods KD: Hypertension control for nurses and other health professionals, ed 2, New York, 1985, Springer-Verlag Publishing Co.
58. Lanoue AS, Snyder BA, and Galan KM: Percutaneous transluminal coronary angioplasty: nonoperative treatment of coronary artery disease, J Cardiovasc Nurs 1(1):30, 1986.
59. Levy RI: Changing perspectives in the prevention of coronary artery disease, Am J Cardiol 57(14):17G, 1986.
60. Lewis VC: Monitoring the patient with acute myocardial infarction, Nurs Clin North Am 22(1):15, 1987.
61. Mancini DM and others: Central and peripheral components of cardiac failure, Am J Med 80(2B):2, 1986.

62. Mancini DM and others: Inotropic drugs for the treatment of heart failure, J Clin Pharmacol 25(7):540, 1985.

63. Mancini DM and others: Intravenous use of amrinone for the treatment of the failing heart, Am J Cardiol 56(3):8B, 1985.

64. Maseri A and others: Pathophysiology of coronary occlusion in acute infarction, Circulation 73(2):233, 1986.

65. Massie B: Updated diagnosis and management of congestive heart failure, Geriatrics 41(3):30, 1986.

66. McKool K: Facilitating smoking cessation, J Cardiovas Nurs 1(4):28, 1987.

67. McRae RP and Liebson PR: Hypertensive crisis, Med Clin North Am 70(4):749, 1986.

68. Meyers KA and Hickey MK: Nursing management of hypovolemic shock, Crit Care Nurs 11(1):57, 1988.

69. Nowakowski JF: Use of cardiac enzymes in the evaluation of acute chest pain, Ann Emerg Med 15(3):354, 1986.

70. Oikawa JH and Kaye D: Endocarditis: epidemiology, pathophysiology, management, and prophylaxis, Cardiovasc Clin 16(2):335, 1986.

71. Opie LH: Drugs and the heart four years on, Lancet 1(8375):496, 1984.

72. Owens-Jones S and Hopp L: Viral myocarditis, Focus Crit Care 15(1):25, 1988.

73. Paffenbarger RS and others: Physical activity as an index of heart attack risk in college alumni, Am J Epidemiol 108:161, 1978.

74. Parmley WW: Pathophysiology of congestive heart failure, Am J Cardiol 55:9A, 1985.

75. Pearle DL: Nifedipine in acute myocardial infarction, Am J Cardiol 54(11):21E, 1984.

76. Pitt B: Evaluation of the patient with congestive heart failure and ventricular arrhythmias, Am J Cardiol 57(3):19B, 1986.

77. Pratt CM and others: The clinical significance of ventricular arrhythmias after myocardial infarction, Cardiol Clin 2(1):3, 1984.

78. Quaal SJ: Thrombolytic therapy: an overview, J Cardiovasc Nurs 1(1):45, 1986.

79. Remme WJ: Congestive heart failure—pathophysiology and medical treatment, J Cardiovasc Pharmacol 8(suppl 1):36, 1986.

80. Renlund DG and Gerstenblith G: Angina: current approaches to diagnosis, drug therapy, and surgical referral, Geriatrics 41(1):35, 1986.

81. Rosenthal ME and others: Sudden cardiac death following acute myocardial infarction, Am Heart J 109(4):865, 1985.

82. Ross R and Glomset J: Atherosclerosis and the arterial smooth muscle cell, Science 180:1332, 1973.

83. Ross R and Glomset JA: The pathogenesis of atherosclerosis, Part I, N Engl J Med 295(7):369, 1976.

84. Ross R and Glomset JA: The pathogenesis of atherosclerosis, Part II, N Engl J Med 295(8):420, 1976.

85. Rude RE: Acute myocardial infarction and its complications, Cardiol Clin 2(2):163, 1984.

86. Ruggie N: Congestive heart failure, Med Clin North Am 70(4):829, 1986.

87. Ryan P: Strategies for motivating life-style change, J Cardiovasc Nurs 1(4):54, 1987.

88. Sasyniuk BI: Symposium on the management of ventricular dysrhythmias. Concept of reentry versus automaticity, Am J Cardiol 54(2):1A, 1984.

89. Schakenbach LH: Physiologic dynamics of acquired valvular heart disease, J Cardiovasc Nurs 1(3):1, 1987.

90. Schroeder JS: Combination therapy with isosorbide dinitrate: current status and the future, Am Heart J 110(1):284, 1985.

91. Scrima DA: Infective endocarditis: nursing considerations, Crit Care Nurse 7(2):47, 1987.

92. Silverman KJ and Grossman W: Angina pectoris. Natural history and strategies for evaluation and management, N Engl J Med 310(26):1712, 1984.

93. Smilack JD and Horn VP: Acute infective endocarditis, Cardiol Clin 2(2):201, 1984.

94. Smith A: Physiology, diagnosis, and life-style modifications for hyperlipidemia, J Cardiovasc Nurs 1(4):15, 1987.

95. Smith CE: Assessing chest pain, Nursing 88 18(5):52, May 1988.

96. Smith WM: Epidemiology of congestive heart failure, Am J Cardiol 55:3A, 1985.

97. Sobel BE: Early intervention in acute myocardial infarction: one center's perspective, Am J Cardiol 54(11):2E, 1984.

98. Srebro J and Karliner JS: Congestive heart failure, Curr Probl Cardiol 23(6):301, 1986.

99. Stapleton JF: Natural history of chronic valvular disease, Cardiovasc Clin 16(2):105, 1986.

100. Streff MM: Exercise in the prevention of coronary artery disease, J Cardiovasc Nurs 1(4):42, 1987.

101. Stuart EM and others: Nonpharmacologic treatment of hypertension: a multiple-risk-factor approach, J Cardiovasc Nurs 1(4):1, 1987.

102. Superko HR and others: Coronary heart disease and risk factor modification. Is there a threshold? Am J Med 78(5):826, 1985.

103. Sutton FJ: Vasodilator therapy, Am J Med 80(2B):54, 1986.

104. Turner J: Nursing interventions in patients with peripheral vascular disease, Nurs Clin North Am 21(2):233, 1986.

105. Tyroler HA: Cholesterol and cardiovascular disease. An overview of Lipid Research Clinics (LRC) epidemiologic studies as background for the LRC Coronary Primary Prevention Trial, Am J Cardiol 54(5):14C, 1984.

106. Wagner GS: Arrhythmias in acute myocardial infarction, Med Clin North Am 68(4):1001, 1984.

107. Wagner MM: Pathophysiology related to peripheral vascular disease, Nurs Clin North Am 21(2):195, 1986.

108. Waller BF: Rheumatic and nonrheumatic conditions producing valvular heart disease, Cardiovasc Clin 16(2):3, 1986.

109. Warbinek E and others: Peripheral arterial occlusive disease: nursing assessment and standard care plans, Part 2, Cardiovasc Nurse 22(2):6, 1986.

110. Weber KT and others: Advances in the evaluation and management of chronic cardiac failure, Chest 85(2):253, 1984.

111. Weinstein L: Life-threatening complications of infective endocarditis and their management, Arch Intern Med 146(5):953, 1986.

112. Wenger NK: Coronary disease in women, Annu Rev Med 36:285, 1985.

113. Wilhelmsen L: Risk factors for coronary heart disease in perspective. European intervention trials, Am J Med 76(2A):37, 1984.

15

Cardiovascular Therapeutic Management

CHAPTER OBJECTIVES

- *Discuss the prevention, identification, and management of pacemaker malfunction.*
- *Describe the immediate postoperative medical and nursing management of the adult cardiac surgical patient.*
- *Summarize the nursing interventions pertinent to the patient undergoing percutaneous transluminal coronary angioplasty.*
- *Describe the role of the critical care nurse during and following the administration of thrombolytic therapy.*
- *Identify the major nursing implications related to the administration of antidysrhythmic and vasoactive drug therapy.*

TEMPORARY PACEMAKERS

Pacemakers are electronic devices that can be used to initiate the heartbeat when the heart's intrinsic electrical system is unable to effectively generate a rate adequate to support cardiac output. Pacemakers can be used temporarily, either supportively or prophylactically, until the condition responsible for the rate or conduction disturbance (actual or potential) has resolved. Pacemakers can also be used on a permanent basis if the patient's condition persists despite adequate therapy. The use of temporary pacemakers as a diagnostic tool is also gaining in popularity.[18,37]

This section will emphasize temporary pacemakers because the critical care nurse will most often encounter these in critical care areas where the attending nurse is charged with the responsibility of preventing, assessing, and managing pacemaker malfunctions. References will be made to permanent pacemakers where appropriate.

Indications

The clinical indications for instituting temporary pacemaker therapy are similar regardless of the cause of the rhythm disturbance necessitating the placement of a pacemaker (see the box at right). Such causes range from drug

---

INDICATIONS FOR TEMPORARY PACING

Bradydysrhythmias
  Sinus bradycardia and arrest
  Sick sinus syndrome
  Heart blocks
Tachydysrhythmias
  Supraventricular
  Ventricular
Permanent pacemaker failure
Support of cardiac output
  Status following cardiac surgery
Diagnostic studies
  Electrophysiology studies (EPS)
  Atrial electrograms (AEG)

---

toxicities and electrolyte imbalances to sequelae related to acute myocardial infarction or cardiac surgery.

Dysrhythmias that are unresponsive to drug therapy and result in compromised hemodynamic status are a definite indication for pacemaker therapy. The goal of therapy in the case of bradydysrhythmia is to increase the ventricular rate and thus enhance cardiac output. Alternately, "overdrive" pacing can be used to decrease the rate of a rapid supraventricular or ventricular rhythm. This rapid pacing of the heart, or overdrive pacing, functions either to prevent the "breakthrough" ectopics that can result from a slow rate or "capture" an ectopic focus and allow the natural pacemaker to regain control.

Following cardiac surgery, temporary pacing can be used to improve a transiently depressed, rate-dependent cardiac output. In addition, conduction disturbances that can occur following valvular surgery can be managed effectively with temporary pacing.[64]

Several diagnostic uses for temporary pacing have evolved over the past several years. Electrophysiology studies (EPS) use special pacing electrodes to induce dysrhythmias in patients with recurrent symptomatic dysrhythmias.[37,41] This allows the physician to closely evaluate the particular dysrhythmia and determine appropriate therapy.

The atrial electrogram (AEG) is simply an amplified recording of atrial activity that can be obtained through the use of atrial pacing wires and a standard electrocardiogram (ECG) machine.[18] It is often used after cardiac surgery to facilitate the diagnosis of supraventricular dysrhythmias in patients with temporary atrial epicardial electrodes already in place.[58]

The Pacemaker System

A pacemaker system is a simple electrical circuit consisting of a pulse generator and a pacing lead (an insulated electrical wire) with either one or two electrodes. The pulse generator is designed to generate an electrical current that travels through the pacing lead and exits through an electrode (exposed portion of the wire) that is in direct contact with the heart. This electrical current initiates a myocardial depolarization. The current then seeks to return by one of several ways to the pulse generator to complete the circuit.

The power source for a temporary external pulse generator is the standard alkaline or mercury battery. Implanted permanent pacemaker batteries are now either nuclear powered or, as is more often the case, long-lived lithium cells.

The pacing lead used for temporary pacing may be bipolar or unipolar. The bipolar lead used in transvenous pacing has two electrodes in close proximity. The distal, or negative, electrode is at the tip of the pacing lead and is in direct contact with the heart. Approximately 1 cm above the negative electrode is a positive electrode. The negative electrode is attached to the negative terminal, and the positive electrode is attached to the positive terminal of the pulse generator, either directly or via a bridging cable (Fig. 15-1).

The bipolar epicardial lead system used for temporary pacing following cardiac surgical procedures has two separate insulated wires (one negative and one positive electrode) loosely secured with sutures to the cardiac chamber to be paced and attached to the pulse generator as just described.[22]

In both cases, the current will flow from the negative terminal of the pulse generator down the pacing lead to the

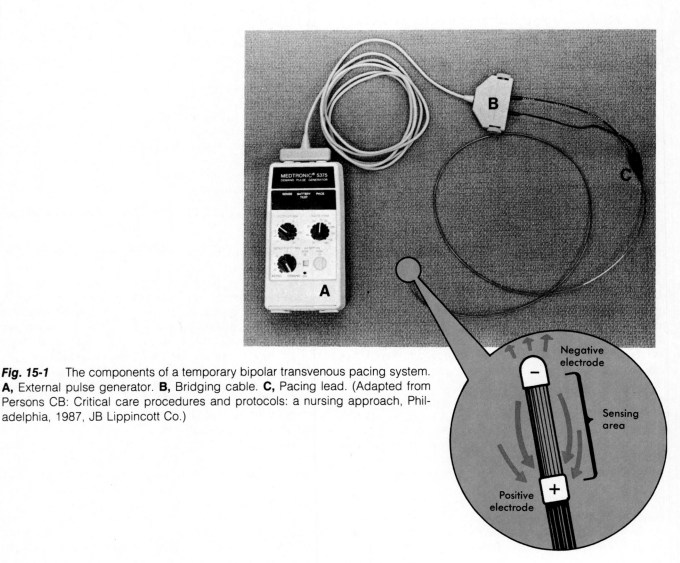

Fig. 15-1 The components of a temporary bipolar transvenous pacing system. **A,** External pulse generator. **B,** Bridging cable. **C,** Pacing lead. (Adapted from Persons CB: Critical care procedures and protocols: a nursing approach, Philadelphia, 1987, JB Lippincott Co.)

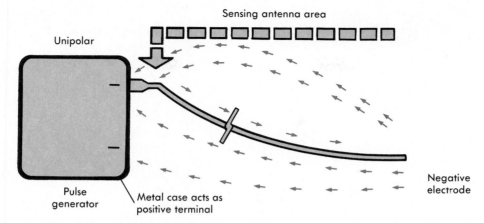

Fig. 15-2 The components of a permanent unipolar transvenous pacing system.

negative electrode and into the heart. The current is then picked up by the positive electrode and flows back up the lead to the positive terminal of the pulse generator.

A unipolar pacing system has only one electrode (a negative electrode) making contact with the heart. In the case of a permanent pacemaker, the positive electrode can be created by the metallic casing of the subcutaneously implanted pulse generator (Fig. 15-2). Or as is the case with a unipolar epicardial lead system, the positive electrode can be formed by a piece of surgical steel wire sewn into the subcutaneous tissue of the chest.[22]

Because the unipolar pacing system has a wide sensing area as a result of the relatively large distance between the negative and positive electrodes, it has better sensing capabilities than a bipolar system. However, this makes the unipolar system more susceptible to electromagnetic interference (EMI) or stray electrical impulses from the heart itself or from the critical care environment such as intravenous infusion pumps that can adversely affect pacemaker function.[40]

Pacing Routes

Several routes are available for temporary cardiac pacing (see the box at right). Permanent pacing is usually accomplished transvenously, although in situations in which a thoracotomy is otherwise indicated, such as cardiac surgery, the physician may elect to insert permanent epicardial pacing wires.

Transcutaneous cardiac pacing is enjoying a revival of sorts, after having been abandoned many years ago because of the painful muscle contractions and soft tissue burns it caused.[45] Transcutaneous cardiac pacing involves the use of two skin electrodes, one placed anteriorly and the other posteriorly on the chest, connected to an external pulse generator (Fig. 15-3). It is a rapid, noninvasive procedure that nurses can perform in the emergency setting and has been gaining in popularity since improved technology has helped to minimize the problems associated with it.

Transthoracic pacing is also an emergency procedure that involves the insertion of a pacing wire into the ventricle through a needle inserted through the chest wall. However, this is an invasive procedure associated with serious com-

---

ROUTES FOR TEMPORARY PACING

Transcutaneous

Emergency pacing is achieved by depolarizing the heart through the chest by means of two large skin electrodes.

Transthoracic

A pacing wire is inserted emergently by threading it through a transthoracic needle into the right ventricle.

Epicardial

Pacing electrodes are sewn to the epicardium during cardiac surgery.

Transvenous (endocardial)

The pacing electrode is advanced through a vein into the right atrium, right ventricle, or both.

---

plications such as pneumothorax and cardiac tamponade.[2]

The insertion of temporary epicardial pacing wires has become a routine procedure during most cardiac surgical cases. Ventricular, and in many cases atrial, pacing wires are loosely sewn to the epicardium. The terminal pins of these wires are pulled through the skin before closing the chest. If both chambers have pacing wires attached, the atrial wires exit subcostally to the right of the sternum and the ventricular wires exit in the same region but to the left of the sternum.[22] These wires can be removed by gentle traction at the skin surface with minimal risk of bleeding.

Temporary transvenous endocardial pacing is accomplished by advancing a pacing electrode wire through a vein, often the subclavian or internal jugular, into the right atrium or right ventricle. Insertion can be facilitated either through direct visualization with fluoroscopy or by the use of the standard electrocardiogram. Electrode placement can be accomplished electrocardiographically by attaching the distal

A 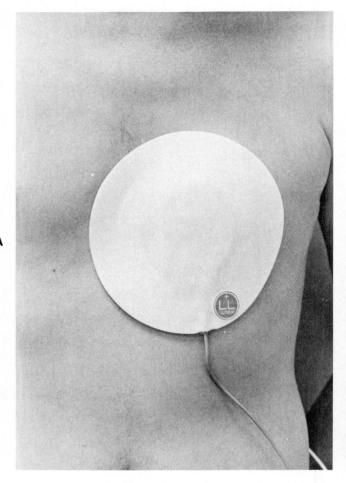 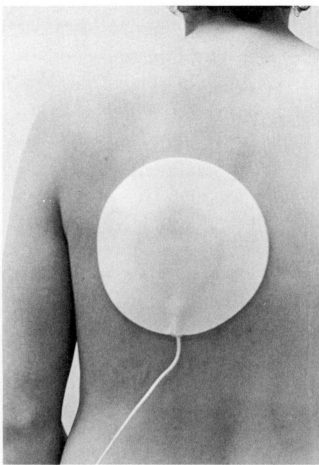 B

Fig. 15-3 Placement of transcutaneous pacing electrodes. (From Persons CB: Critical care procedures and protocols: a nursing approach, Philadelphia, 1987, JB Lippincott Co.)

electrode of the pacing catheter to the V lead of a properly grounded ECG machine via an alligator clamp. With the limb leads attached and the lead selector switch set on V, the distal electrode serves as an exploring electrode that will display various intracardiac ECG patterns verifying proper advancement and placement of the electrode.

Inter-Society Commission for Heart Disease Classification Code

In the 1960s, pacemaker terminology was limited to "fixed-rate" and "demand" pacing, followed by the introduction of "AV sequential" pacing in the early 1970s. Although these terms are still useful today for understanding pacemaker function (see the box at right), the continued expansion of functional capabilities of pulse generators made it necessary to develop a more precise classification system. Therefore, in 1974, the Inter-Society Commission for Heart Disease (ICHD) adopted a three-letter code for describing the various pacing modalities available. Although the code was later revised by adding two more letters to include increased programming characteristics and anti-

---

PACEMAKER TERMINOLOGY

Fixed-rate (asynchronous)

Delivers a pacing stimulus at a set (fixed) rate regardless of the occurrence of spontaneous myocardial depolarizations.

Demand (synchronous)

Delivers a pacing stimulus only when the heart's intrinsic pacemaker fails to function at a predetermined rate; the pacing stimulus will either be inhibited or triggered into the QRS complex when the intrinsic pacemaker functions.

AV sequential (dual-chamber pacing)

Delivers a pacing stimulus to both the atrium and ventricle in proper sequence with sufficient AV delay to permit adequate ventricular filling.

Table 15-1 ICHD classification code

Chamber(s) paced	Chamber(s) sensed	Mode of response	Programmable functions	Antitachycardia function
V—ventricle	V—ventricle	T—triggered	P—programmable (rate and output)	B—bursts
A—atrium	A—atrium	I—inhibited	M—multiprogrammable	N—normal rate competition
D—double (both A and V)	D—double	D—double (ventricular inhibited; atrial triggered)	O—none	S—scanning
	O—none	O—none R—reverse	O—none	E—external control

Parsonnet V, Furman S, and Smyth N: A revised code for pacemaker identification, PACE 4:401, 1981.

Table 15-2 Descriptions of pulse generators

Pulse Generator	Description
AOO	Atrial fixed rate
	Atrial pacing, no sensing
VOO	Ventricular fixed rate
	Ventricular pacing, no sensing
DOO	AV sequential fixed rate
	Atrial and ventricular pacing, no sensing
VVI	Ventricular demand
	Ventricular pacing, ventricular sensing, inhibited response to sensing
VVT	Ventricular demand
	Ventricular pacing, ventricular sensing, triggered response to sensing
AAI	Atrial demand
	Atrial pacing, atrial sensing, inhibited response to sensing
AAT	Atrial demand
	Atrial pacing, atrial sensing, triggered response to sensing
VAT	AV synchronous
	Ventricular pacing, atrial sensing, triggered response to sensing (The ventricular pacing stimulus will fire at a set time following sensing of a spontaneous atrial depolarization.)
DVI	AV sequential
	Atrial and ventricular pacing, ventricular sensing, inhibited response to sensing (Both atrial and ventricular pacing is inhibited if spontaneous ventricular depolarization is sensed; if no spontaneous ventricular activity is sensed, then the atrial and ventricle will be paced sequentially.)
VDD	Atrial synchronous, ventricular inhibited
	Ventricular pacing, atrial and ventricular sensing, inhibited response to sensing in the ventricle and triggered response to sensing in the atrium
DDD	Universal
	Both chambers are sensed and paced, inhibited response to sensing in the ventricle and triggered response to sensing in the atria

tachycardia functions, the original three-letter code remains adequate to describe basic pacemaker function.[44] (See Table 15-1 for revised five-letter code.)

The original code is based on three categories, each represented by a letter. The first letter refers to the cardiac chamber that is paced. The second letter designates which chamber is sensed, while the third letter indicates the response to the sensed event. For example, a VVI pacemaker will pace the ventricle if the pacemaker fails to sense an intrinsic ventricular depolarization. However, sensing of a spontaneous ventricular depolarization will inhibit ventricular pacing. On the other hand, a VAT pacemaker will pace the ventricle at a fixed time following the sensing of a spontaneous atrial depolarization, that is, ventricular pacing is triggered by sensing of an atrial event. (See Table 15-2 for description of all types of pacemakers.)

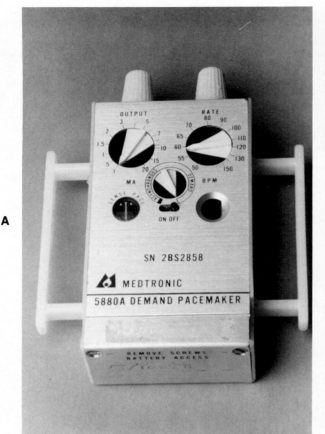
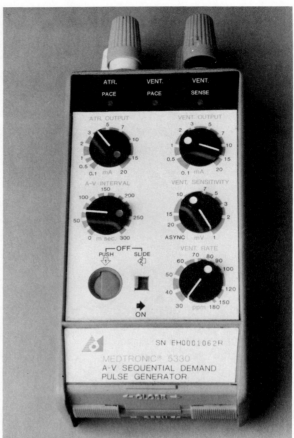

Fig. 15-4 External demand pulse generator **(A)** and AV sequential pulse generator **(B)**.

Pacemaker Settings

The controls on all external temporary pulse generators are similar, and their function should be thoroughly understood so that pacing can be initiated quickly in an emergency situation and troubleshooting can be facilitated should problems with the pacemaker arise.

The rate control (Fig. 15-4) regulates the number of impulses that can be delivered to the heart per minute. The rate setting will vary depending on the physiological needs of the patient, but in general will be maintained between 60 and 80 beats/min. Pacing rates for overdrive suppression of tachydysrhythmias may greatly exceed these values. If the pacemaker is operating in the AV sequential mode, the ventricular rate control will also regulate the atrial rate.

The output dial regulates the amount of electrical current (measured in milliamperers or mA) that is delivered to the heart to initiate depolarization. The point at which depolarization occurs is termed *threshold* and is indicated by a myocardial response to the pacing stimulus (capture). Threshold can be determined by gradually decreasing the output from 20 mA until 1:1 capture is lost. The output setting is then slowly increased until 1:1 capture is reestablished; this threshold to pace should be less than 1.0 mA with a properly positioned pacing electrode. However, the output should be set two to three times higher than threshold,

since thresholds tend to fluctuate. There will be separate output controls for both the atrium and the ventricle when an AV sequential pulse generator is utilized.

The sensitivity control regulates the ability of the pacemaker to detect the heart's intrinsic electrical activity. If the sensitivity is turned all the way up, that is, a setting of 1 mV millivolts (mV), the pacemaker is maximally sensitive and will be able to respond to even low-amplitude electrical signals coming from the heart. On the other hand, turning the sensitivity all the way down (adjusting the dial to a setting of 20 mV or to area labeled "async") will result in the inability of the pacemaker to sense any intrinsic electrical activity and cause the pacemaker to function at a fixed rate. The sensitivity control is usually set at 6 mV. There is a sense indicator (often a light) on the pulse generator that will signal each time intrinsic cardiac electrical activity is sensed. A pulse generator may be designed to sense atrial or ventricular activity or both. The pacemaker's sensing ability is evaluated by observing for a change in pacing rhythm in response to spontaneous depolarizations. (See the section on pacemaker malfunctions for sensing problems.)

The AV interval control (only available on AV sequential pacers) regulates the time interval between the atrial and ventricular pacing stimuli. Proper adjustment of this interval to between 150 to 250 msec preserves AV synchrony in order to maximize ventricular stroke volume and enhance cardiac output.

Finally, an on/off switch is provided with a safety feature that prevents the accidental termination of pacing.

Pacing Artifacts

All patients with temporary pacemakers should have continuous ECG monitoring. The pacing artifact is the spike that is seen on the ECG tracing as the pacing stimulus is delivered to the heart. A P wave should be visible following the pacing artifact if the atrium is being paced (Fig. 15-5, *A*). Similarly, a QRS complex should follow a ventricular

pacing artifact (Fig. 15-5, *B*). A pacing artifact will precede both the P wave and the QRS complex with dual chamber pacing (Fig. 15-5, *C*).

Not all paced beats look alike. For example, the artifact produced by a unipolar pacing electrode is larger than that produced by a bipolar lead (Fig. 15-6). Furthermore, the QRS complex of paced beats will appear different, depending on the location of the pacing electrode. If the pacing electrode is positioned in the right ventricle, an LBBB pattern will be displayed on the ECG. On the other hand, an RBBB pattern will be visible if the pacing stimulus originates from the left ventricle.

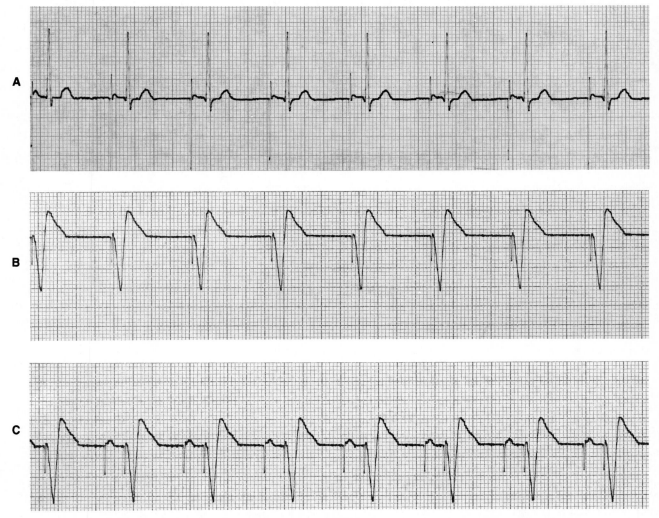

Fig. 15-5 **A,** Atrial pacing. **B,** Ventricular pacing. **C,** Dual chamber pacing. (From Seidel JC: *Basic electrocardiography: a modular approach,* St Louis, 1986, The CV Mosby Co.)

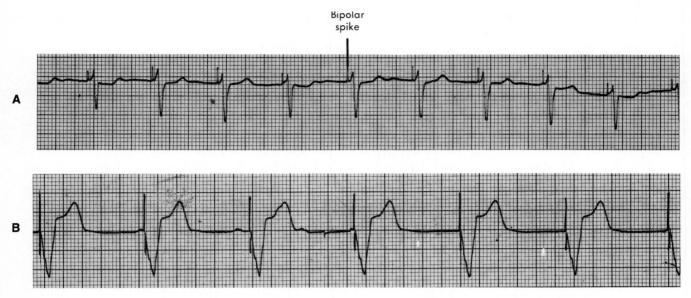

Fig. 15-6 **A,** Bipolar pacing artifact. **B,** Unipolar pacing artifact. (From Conover MB: Understanding electrocardiography, ed 4, St Louis, 1984, The CV Mosby Co.)

Pacemaker Malfunctions

The majority of pacemaker malfunctions can be broken down into abnormalities of either pacing or sensing.

Problems with pacing can involve the failure of the pacemaker to deliver the following: the pacing stimulus, a pacing stimulus that depolarizes the heart, or the correct number of pacing stimuli per minute.

Failure of the pacemaker to deliver the pacing stimulus will result in the disappearance of the pacing artifact, even though the patient's intrinsic rate is less than the set rate on the pacer (Fig. 15-7). This can occur either intermittently or continuously and can be attributed to failure of the pulse generator or its battery, a loose connection between the various components of the pacemaker system, broken lead wires, or stimulus inhibition as a result of EMI. Tightening connections, replacing the batteries or the pulse generator itself, or removing the source of EMI may restore pacemaker function.

If the pacing stimulus fires but fails to initiate a myocardial depolarization, a pacing artifact will be present but will not be followed by the expected P wave or QRS complex, depending on the chamber being paced (Fig. 15-8). This "loss of capture" can most often be attributed to either displacement of the pacing electrode or to an increase in threshold (electrical stimulus necessary to elicit a myocardial depolarization) as a result of drugs, metabolic disorders, electrolyte imbalances, and fibrosis or myocardial ischemia at the site of electrode placement.[43] Repositioning the patient to the left side or increasing the output (mA) may elicit capture.

Pacing can also occur at inappropriate rates. For example, impending battery failure can result in a gradual decrease in paced rate or "rate drift." Another phenomenon, commonly referred to "runaway pacemaker," will result in firing of the pacemaker stimulus at rates greater than the set rate. This malfunction is universally caused by failure of the pulse generator's circuitry necessitating replacement.

Sensing abnormalities include both failure to sense and oversensing. Failure to sense is the inability of the pacemaker to sense spontaneous myocardial depolarizations. This will result in competition between paced complexes and the heart's intrinsic rhythm. This malfunction can be demonstrated on the ECG by pacing artifacts that follow too closely behind spontaneous QRS complexes (Fig. 15-9). "R on T" phenomenon is a real danger with this type of pacer aberration; therefore the nurse must act quickly to determine the cause. Often the cause can be attributed to inadequate wave amplitude (or height of the P or R wave). If this is the case, the situation can be promptly remedied by increasing the sensitivity (moving the sensitivity dial toward its lowest setting). Other possible causes include lead displacement or fracture, pulse generator failure, or EMI-precipitated asynchronous pacing.

Oversensing results from the inappropriate sensing of extraneous electrical signals leading to unnecessary triggering or inhibiting of stimulus output, depending on the pacer mode. The source of these electrical signals can range from the presence of tall, peaked T waves to EMI in the critical care environment. Since the majority of temporary pulse generators currently in use today are ventricular inhibited, oversensing will result in unexplained pauses in the ECG tracing as the extraneous signals are sensed and inhibit ventricular pacing. Often, simply moving the sensitivity dial toward 20 mV will stop the pauses.

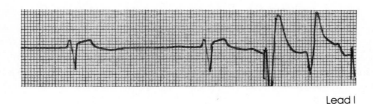

Fig. 15-7   Intermittent failure to pace. (From Seidel JC: Basic electrocardiography: a modular approach, St Louis, 1986, The CV Mosby Co.)

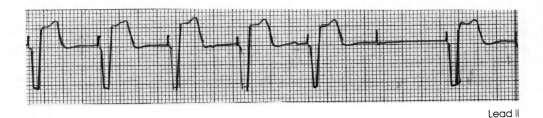

Fig. 15-8   Intermittent loss of caputure. (From Seidel JC: Basic electrocardiography: a modular approach, St Louis, 1986, The CV Mosby Co.)

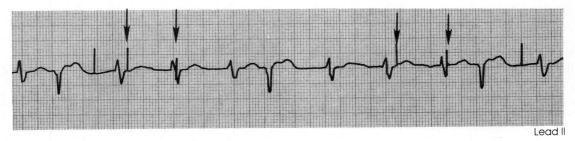

Fig. 15-9   Failure to sense. (From Seidel JC: Basic electrocardiography: a modular approach, St Louis, 1986, The CV Mosby Co.)

Nursing Care

There are a myriad of nursing responsibilities associated with the care of a patient who has a temporary pacemaker, but four major areas should be emphasized: surveillance for complications, protection against microshock, prevention of pacemaker malfunction, and patient teaching.

Infection at the lead insertion site is one complication associated with pacemakers. The site(s) should be carefully inspected for purulent drainage, erythema, or edema, and the patient should be monitored for signs of systemic infection. Site care should be performed according to the institution's policy and procedure. Although most infections remain localized, endocarditis can occur in patients with endocardial pacing leads. A less frequent complication associated with transvenous pacing is myocardial perforation, which can result in rhythmic hiccoughs or cardiac tamponade.

Because the pacing electrode is in intimate contact with the heart, special care must be taken while handling the external components of the pacing system to avoid conducting stray electrical current from other equipment. Even a small amount of stray current could precipitate a lethal tachycardia. The possibility of "microshock" can be minimized by wearing rubber gloves when handling the pacing wires and by properly insulating terminal pins of pacing wires when they are not in use. The latter can be accomplished either by using caps provided by the manufacturer or improvising with a needle cover or section of disposable rubber glove. The wires should then be taped securely to the patient's chest to avoid accidental electrode displacement. Additional safety measures include using a nonelectric or a properly grounded electric bed, keeping all electrical equipment away from the bed, and permitting the use of only rechargeable electric razors.[52]

Continuous ECG monitoring is essential to facilitate prompt recognition of and appropriate intervention for pacemaker malfunction. But there is much the nurse can do to prevent pacing abnormalities.

As previously mentioned, the temporary pacing lead and bridging cable should be properly secured to the body with tape to prevent the accidental displacement of the electrode, which can result in failure to pace or sense. The external pulse generator can be secured to the patient's waist with a strap or placed in a telemetry bag for the mobile patient. For the patient on bed rest, suspending the pulse generator with twill tape from an IV pole mounted overhead on the ceiling will not only prevent tension on the lead while moving the patient (given adequate length of bridging cable) but will also alleviate the possibility of accidental dropping of the pulse generator.

The nurse should be aware of all sources of EMI which, within the critical care environment, could interfere with the pacemaker's function. Sources of EMI in the clinical area include electrocautery, defibrillation current, radiation therapy, magnetic resonance imaging devices, and transcutaneous electrical nerve stimulation (TENS) units.[52] In most cases, if EMI is suspected of precipitating pacemaker malfunction, converting to the asynchronous mode (fixed-rate) will maintain pacing until the cause of the EMI can be removed. If the patient requires defibrillation, the pulse generator should be temporarily turned off during delivery of the shock to prevent possible damage to the pacemaker circuitry.

Finally, the nurse should inspect for loose connections between lead and pulse generator on a regular basis. In addition, there should always be replacement batteries and pulse generators available on the unit. Although the battery has an anticipated life span of 1 month, it is probably sound practice to change the battery if the pacemaker has been operating continually for several days. The pulse generator should always be labeled with the date that the battery was replaced.

Patient teaching for the client with a temporary pacemaker should emphasize the same areas of prevention that the nurse must address in her or his care. The patient should be instructed not to handle any exposed portion of the lead wire and to notify the nurse should the dressing over the insertion site become soiled or dislodged. The patient should also be advised not to use any electric devices brought in from home that could interfere with pacemaker functioning. Furthermore, patients with temporary transvenous pacemakers need to be taught to restrict movement of the affected extremity to prevent lead displacement.

Summary

The recent introduction of physiological pacing (DDD), which is both rate responsive (atrial sensing allows for increases in heart rate with exercise) and AV synchronous, and the development of physiological sensors that will permit pacemaker autoregulation to maintain optimal physiological function, demonstrates the complexities of present-day pacemaker technology.[39] The aforegoing discussion has been an introduction to the basic concepts of temporary pacemaker therapy. However, it is essential that the nurse who cares for patients with either permanent or temporary pacemakers be intimately familiar with even the most sophisticated modes of pacemaker function. Only by keeping "pace" with current technology can the nurse accurately interpret pacer function and thereby safely and effectively care for these patients.

CARDIAC SURGERY

The nursing care of the cardiac surgical patient is a demanding yet exciting job requiring the talents of an experienced team of critical care nurses. The following discussion introduces basic cardiac surgical techniques and principles of cardiopulmonary bypass and highlights the key points about postoperative care of the adult patient who requires either valve replacement or coronary revascularization.

Coronary Artery Bypass Surgery

Since its introduction nearly 2 decades ago, coronary artery bypass surgery has been proved both safe and effective in relieving medically uncontrolled angina pectoris in the majority of patients. However, with improved medical management of coronary artery disease (CAD), much debate has been generated regarding the efficacy of medical versus surgical therapy of CAD. One of several large randomized trials attempting to address this issue, the Coronary Artery Surgery Study (CASS), found no statistical difference in survival between medical and surgical patients with mild to moderate angina or in patients who have no symptoms following myocardial infarction.[31] However, the data do suggest that coronary artery bypass grafting (CABG) may improve survival in selected patients with reduced ventricular function who have double or triple vessel disease.[31] The combined results of CASS and other large randomized trials continue to support the view that CABG affords dramatic symptomatic improvement and an improved quality of life.[31]

Myocardial revascularization involves the use of a conduit or channel designed to bypass an occluded coronary artery. Currently, the two most successful conduits are the sa-

---

Nursing Diagnosis and Management
Temporary pacemakers

Decreased Cardiac Output related to atrioventricular heart block, p. 336

Potential for Infection related to invasive monitoring devices, p. 346

Knowledge Deficit: Position Restrictions related to lack of previous exposure to information, p. 69

Body Image Disturbance related to functional dependence on life-sustaining technology, p. 834

Self-Esteem Disturbance related to feelings of guilt over physical deterioration, p. 835

Powerlessness related to health care environment or illness-related regimen, p. 837

Anxiety related to threat to biological, psychological, and/or social integrity, p. 852

RESEARCH ABSTRACT

Effect of nitroglycerin ointment placement on the severity of headache and flushing in patients with cardiac disease

Riegel B, Heywood G, and Jackson W: Heart Lung 17(4):426, 1988.

PURPOSE

The purpose of this study was to determine whether the severity of headache and flushing caused by nitroglycerin (NTG) ointment as measured by self-report with a visual analogue scale (VAS) differed among three body sites in hospitalized patients with cardiac disease. An additional purpose was to determine whether the severity of headache and flushing changed when the subsequent dose of NTG ointment was moved to a different site compared with the previous site.

FRAMEWORK

The vasodilatory effects of NTG cause the side effects associated with the drug. Vasodilation in the cerebral circulation causes headaches, and dilation of the cutaneous vessels may result in the sensation of flushing. Side effects are thought to be a function of the blood levels of the drug. Absorption of the drug through the skin is variable and dependent on a variety of factors. The research was based on the conceptual framework of Roy. The patient with cardiac disease who has side effects from a medication is in need of nursing care to assist with adaptation. The patient who adapts to a treatment may adhere better to that plan.

METHODS

A convenience sample from all patients on a postcoronary care unit of a southern California hospital who had NTG as a new drug within the last 3 days and who were receiving it routinely were selected. Data on headache and flushing were obtained from patients by use of a VAS on which patients were to designate the amount of headache and flushing on a 100 mm continuous line. Application of the drug and data collection were done by volunteers from the nursing staff on the unit after an educational session in which the study and procedure was explained. A repeated-measures design was used. Each subject had the dose applied to the upper arm, midsternum, and iliac crest at 4- to 6-hour intervals. Doses between ½ and 1½ inches of ointment varied among patients but remained consistent for each patient during the study. The sequence of doses was determined by a table of random numbers. Patients were asked to complete the VAS approximately 30 minutes after NTG was applied, and the scales were then retrieved by the nurse before the next NTG administration. Data on extraneous and potentially intervening variables were collected and included: age, sex, race, activity level, diagnosis, previous exposure to NTG, days of the present NTG regimen, concurrent medications, and estimated percent of body fat.

RESULTS

Of the 56 patients who agreed to participate in the study, 46 completed all three testing sites. Data were analyzed from all patients regardless of the number of testing sites completed and reanalyzed with only those who completed all three sites. No significant difference in the severity of side effects was found when the three sites were compared by multivariate analysis of variance with repeated measures. Overall, side effects of NTG ointment were minimal in this sample. Severity of headache and flushing were not affected by any of the extraneous or intervening variables, and those who reported headache did not experience any decrease over time.

IMPLICATIONS

The results of this study suggest that the common nursing intervention of teaching patients that NTG side effects can be minimized by placing the drug at an alternative site may not be effective. Administration of minor analgesics may blunt the headache associated with NTG ointment. Suggestions for future research include replication of this study under more controlled conditions, perhaps with normal subjects in a laboratory setting. Reports of headache and flushing should be elicited more than one time after drug application, and use of another tool to collect data in the clinical setting may be beneficial.

RESEARCH ABSTRACT

Comparison of two types of communication methods used after cardiac surgery with patients with endotracheal tubes

Stovsky B, Rudy E, and Dragonette P: Heart Lung 17(28):281, 1988.

PURPOSE

The purpose of this study was to compare two types of communication methods (planned and unplanned) for effectiveness in communication in the early postoperative intubation period in patients who have had cardiac surgery.

FRAMEWORK

Even though most patients undergoing cardiac surgery have endotracheal tubes in place only a short time, they may become anxious because of lack of control, dependency, and a sense of unimportance. The nurse is challenged by the difficulty in interpreting the patient's behavior and clinical symptoms without benefit of oral communication. Unplanned, spontaneous communication was defined as communication that is not planned and is not carried out by a specific method. The nurse's creativity, judgment, and spontaneity determine the method used, such as lipreading, using hand gestures, writing, or asking yes and no questions. Planned communication consisted of use of a picture board with words, which was called a communication board.

METHODS

A total convenience sample of 40 patients undergoing open heart surgery who participated in preoperative teaching were studied. The control group (n = 20) relied on the experience and creativity of the nurse to provide a method of postoperative communication. The experimental group (n = 20) was introduced to a communication board before surgery and used the board during the postoperative intubation period. After discharge from the intensive care unit, each patient completed an open-ended patient interview, a patient satisfaction questionnaire, and a visual analogue scale to assess satisfaction with communication.

RESULTS

An independent t test indicated that a planned method of communication does significantly increase patient satisfaction in the early postoperative intubation period (t = 2.09, p = 0.05, n = 35). Content analyses of the patient interviews further supported this finding. Validity of the patient satisfaction questionnaire was supported by a high correlation (r = 0.70) with results from the visual analogue scale. Nurse satisfaction with communication during intubation was analyzed by use of a nurse satisfaction questionnaire and open-ended questions that were completed by the nurse after caring for patients in this study. A dependent t test (t = 1.25, not significant, n = 20) and content analyses indicated that planned communication did not increase nurse satisfaction; however, it did add to the repertoire of methods that nurses currently use in trying to communicate with their patients.

IMPLICATIONS

On the basis of the results of this study, the following recommendations were made. Patients who will undergo mechanical ventilation after surgery should be instructed on specific communication techniques before surgery. The communication techniques taught before surgery should be available to all patients who have endotrachael tubes after surgery. A communication board is considered as a supplement to other methods of communication currently being used. Nurses need to identify the communication methods most useful for individual patients and integrate them into the written care plan. Nurses can facilitate communication by providing patient's eyeglasses, removing any ophthalmic ointment or petroleum jelly from the patient's eyes after surgery, and, when using a communication board, placing the board in an optimal position for the patient to see. Further research on the usefulness of various communication methods for patients with both short-term and long-term mechanical ventilation is recommended.

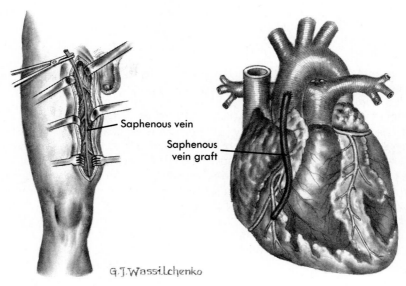

Fig. 15-10   Saphenous vein graft.

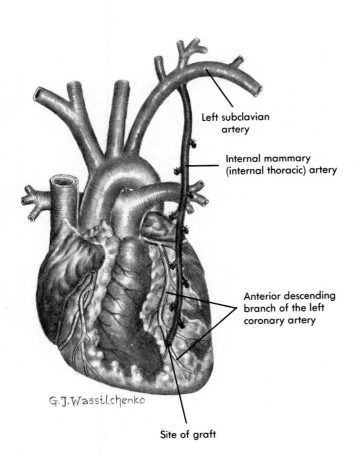

Fig. 15-11   Internal mammary artery graft.

phenous vein graft (SVG) and the internal mammary artery (IMA) graft.[29] SVG involves the anastomosis of an excised portion of the saphenous vein proximally to the aorta and distally to the coronary artery below the obstruction (Fig. 15-10). The IMA, which remains attached to its origin at the subclavian artery, is swung down and anastomosed distally to the coronary artery (Fig. 15-11). Although only recently introduced, the IMA graft is gaining in popularity because it has demonstrated both short-term and long-term patency rates superior to those of the SVG.[35]

Valvular Surgery

Valvular disease results in various hemodynamic dysfunctions that can usually be managed medically so long as the patient remains asymptomatic. There is reluctance to surgically intervene early in the course of the disease because of the surgical risks and long-term complications associated with prosthetic valve replacement. However, this must be weighed against the possibility of irreversible deterioration in left ventricular function that may develop during the compensated asymptomatic phase.

There are two categories of prosthetic valves: mechanical and biological or tissue valves. Mechanical valves are made from combinations of metal alloys, pyrolite carbon, and dacron (Fig. 15-12). Their construction renders them highly durable, but all patients will require anticoagulation to reduce the incidence of thromboembolism. The biological or tissue valves, usually constructed from animal cardiac tissue, offer the patient freedom from therapeutic anticoagulation as a result of their low thrombogenicity (Fig. 15-13). However, their durability is limited by their tendency toward early calcification. (See the box on p. 314 for a description of various valvular prostheses.)

The choice of a valvular prosthesis depends on many factors. For example, because mechanical valves are more durable, they may be chosen over a tissue valve for a young person who has a relatively long life span ahead. Similarly,

Product liability is the area of law that recognizes that a manufacturer, wholesaler, or retail dealer has a responsibility to the user or consumer of a product. *Product liability* is a broad term that applies to situations in which an individual has been harmed by a product. Liability can be based on statements about the nature or quality of a product, such as warranties, express or implied. *Negligence* is another area of product liability wherein the defendant (that is, manufacturer, wholesaler, or retailer) is liable to a plaintiff (for example, a patient) if a duty of due care is breached and injury results. The duty of due care includes proper design, handling, and functioning of a product. Everyone involved in the chain of commercial distribution owes an obligation of due care to each person foreseeably endangered by a defective product.

Critical care nurses administer a wide variety of products, including medical devices, drugs, and equipment. Therefore they have unique legal duties in this regard. For example, equipment needs maintenance and checking for proper working condition *before* use in patient care. Standards of care, including quality assurance and risk management strategies, dictate that steps be taken to protect patients and workers alike from faulty equipment. However, if the product defect is not detectable by a user (for example, a critical care nurse), the manufacturer will probably be held liable for injuries resulting from the defect.

Another product liability theory is *strict liability* or *absolute liability in tort*. In this theory, a plaintiff may recover from any commercial supplier who places a product on the market that is in a defective condition so as to be unreasonably dangerous. Liability applies even though the manufacturer exercised all possible due care in preparing and selling the product in question. The gist of the lawsuit based on strict product liability is that the defendant sold a product that contained a defect, rendering it unreasonably dangerous, and the plaintiff was injured by it. The defect may be a manufacturing error, a design that is unreasonably dangerous, or a failure to warn the user of the product's hazards.

In *Phelps v. Sherwood Medical Industries,* 836 F.2d 296 (7th Cir. 1987), a patient brought a strict product liability suit against the manufacturer of an allegedly defective heart catheter, which broke when a nurse was attempting to remove it, resulting in a portion of the catheter remaining inside the patient's heart. During a single coronary artery bypass operation, the surgeon inserted a catheter into the left atrium of the patient's heart to monitor his postoperative condition. The catheter was held in place by a "purse-string" suture and followed a path to the left atrial cavity.

After surgery the nurse encountered some resistance in attempting to remove the catheter. The catheter broke, and a portion remained inside the patient's heart. She contacted the surgeon, whose partner was on call. She later testified at trial that had she known the catheter was sutured to the pulmonary vein, she would not have tried to remove it.

The surgeon contended that the manufacturer was liable, because the catheter broke when the nurse attempted to remove it. He alleged that the product was defective because of its inability to stretch before separating and that the manufacturer failed to warn of this potential hazard. The manufacturer produced evidence showing that the label on the catheter's container stated that the catheter was not to be removed while its needle was in place.

The surgeon then contended that the manufacturer's duty to warn about hazards extended to the nurse and that the manufacturer's failure to warn the nurse caused the injury. The manufacturer responded that it had the duty to warn only the surgeon, who, as a learned intermediary, should then have passed on any potential dangers of catheter use to the nurse and patient.

The court applied Indiana law in affirming the jury's finding that the manufacturer was not liable. To establish the manufacturer's liability, the patient was required to demonstrate that the manufacturer sold a defective product that was unreasonably dangerous to any user (any individual who uses or consumes the product or any other person who, while acting for or on behalf of the injured party, was in possession and control of the product in question).

The court noted that the catheter in this case could be sold only to physicians who then receive the label warning and therefore are the "users" of the product. The court held that the physician, as the learned intermediary, intervened and affected the manufacturer's duty to warn users of potential dangers. Citing cases involving drug manufacturers, the court noted that the manufacturer has an initial duty to warn of risks by alerting doctors, who then determine whether to prescribe the drug. The court held that this "learned intermediary" exception has equal application to cases concerning medical devices, such as catheters. It is incumbent on the physician who knows the risks and benefits of this kind of catheter usage to warn the patient (and in this case, the nurse too).

Additionally, a manufacturer may defend itself against liability if its product is misused or substantially changed by the plaintiff. In this case, the manufacturer presented evidence that its catheter was designed for general and variable therapeutic purposes but not specifically for the kind of use to which the surgeon put it in open-heart surgery. The manufacturer asserted that its catheter was substantially changed by being connected to a heart with a purse-string suture and that this method and routing of the catheter increased the likelihood of a malfunction, such as the separation of the catheter's tubing on an attempted removal. Weighing the evidence, the jury determined that the surgeon sutured the catheter in a manner not intended by the manufacturer and that the catheter had undergone substantial change from the time it left the manufacturer's hands to the time of its separation.

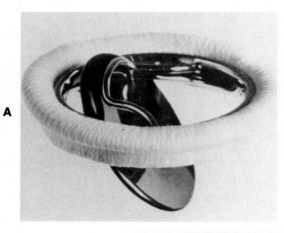
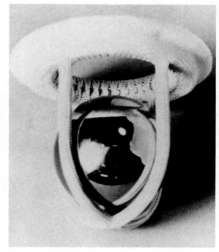
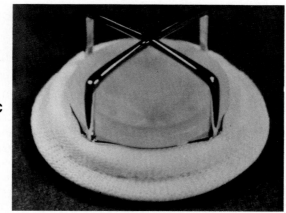

Fig. 15-12   A, The Bjork-Shiley tilting disc valve with pyrolytic-carbon disc, stellite cage, and Teflon cloth sewing ring. The valve opens to 60 degrees. **B,** Starr-Edwards caged-ball valve model 6320 with completely cloth-covered stellite cage and hollow stellite ball with specific gravity close to that of blood. **C,** The Starr-Edwards caged-disc mitral valve, model 6520 with polyethylene disc, stellite cage, and sewing ring composed of Teflon and polypropylene cloth. The disc contains a thin titanium ring for fluroscopic analysis of disc motion. (From Eagle K and others: The practice of cardiology, ed 2, Boston, 1989, Little Brown & Co.)

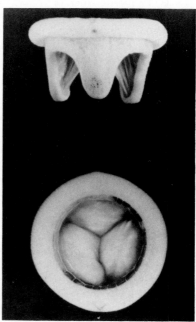

Fig. 15-13   Hancock II porcine aortic valve is chemically treated to retard calcification. The flexible Delrin stent and sewing ring are covered in Dacron cloth. (From Eagle K and others: The practice of cardiology, ed 2, Boston, 1989, Little Brown & Co.)

CLASSIFICATION OF PROSTHETIC CARDIAC VALVES

MECHANICAL VALVES

Tilting-disk: a free-floating lens-shaped disk mounted onto a circular sewing ring
  Bjork-Shiley
  Omniscience (Lillehei-Kaster)
  Medtronic-Hall (Hall-Kaster)
Caged-ball: a ball moves freely within a three- or four-sided metallic cage mounted on a circular sewing ring
  Starr-Edwards
Bileaflet: two semicircular leaflets, mounted on a circular sewing ring, that open centrally
  St. Jude Medical

BIOLOGICAL TISSUE VALVES (BIOPROSTHESES)

Porcine heterograft: a porcine aortic valve mounted on a semiflexible stent and preserved with glutaraldehyde
  Hancock
  Carpentier-Edwards
Bovine pericardial heterograft: bovine pericardium fashioned into three identical cusps that are then mounted on a cloth-covered frame
  Ionescu-Shiley

---

a bioprosthesis may be chosen for an older patient (older than 65 years of age), because although the valve has a reduced longevity, the patient has a decreased life expectancy. For patients with medical contraindications to anticoagulation or patients whose past compliance with drug therapy has been questionable, a tissue valve should be selected. Technical considerations such as the size of the annulus (or anatomic ring in which the valve sits) can also influence the choice of valve (a bioprosthesis may be too big for a small aortic root).[6]

Cardiopulmonary Bypass

Cardiopulmonary bypass (CPB) is a mechanical means of circulating and oxygenating a patient's blood while diverting most of the circulation from the heart and lungs during cardiac surgical procedures.[66] The extracorporeal circuit consists of cannulas that drain off venous blood, an oxygenator that oxygenates the blood by one of several methods, and a pump head that pumps the arterialized blood back to the aorta through a single cannula. The patient is systemically heparinized before initiation of bypass to prevent clotting within the bypass circuit.

Systemic hypothermia during bypass can reduce tissue oxygen requirements to 50% of normal, which affords the major organs additional protection from ischemic injury.[66] Lowering the body temperature to about 28° C (82.4° F) is accomplished through a heat exchanger incorporated into the pump. The blood is warmed back up to normal body temperature before bypass is discontinued.

The technique of hemodilution is also used to enhance tissue oxygenation by improving blood flow through the systemic and pulmonary microcirculation during bypass. Hemodilution refers to the dilution of autologous (patient's own) blood with the isotonic crystalloid solution used to prime the pump. Capillary perfusion is enhanced by hemodilution, because the reduced viscosity (stickiness) of the blood decreases both resistance to flow through the capillaries and the possibility of microthrombi formation. At the

Table 15-3 Physiological effects of CPB

Effects	Causes
Intravascular fluid deficit (hypotension)	Third spacing
	Postoperative diuresis
	Sudden vasodilation (drugs, rewarming)
Third spacing (weight gain, edema)	Decreased plasma protein concentration
	Increased capillary permeability
Myocardial depression (decreased cardiac output)	Hypothermia
	Increased systemic vascular resistance
	Prolonged pump run
	Preexisting heart disease
	Inadequate myocardial protection
Coagulopathy (bleeding)	Systemic heparinization
	Mechanical trauma to platelets
	Depressed release of clotting factors from liver as a result of hypothermia
Pulmonary dysfunction (decreased lung mechanics and impaired gas exchange)	Decreased surfactant production
	Pulmonary microemboli
	Interstitial fluid accumulation in lungs
Hemolysis (hemoglobinuria)	Red blood cells damaged in pump circuit
Hyperglycemia (rise in serum glucose)	Decreased insulin release
	Stimulation of glycogenolysis
Hypokalemia (low serum potassium)	Intracellular shifts during bypass
	Postoperative diuresis secondary to hemodilution
Neurological dysfunction (decreased level of consciousness, motor/sensory deficits)	Inadequate cerebral perfusion
	Microemboli to brain (air, plaque fragments, fat globules)
Hypertension (transient rise in blood pressure)	Catecholamine release and systemic hypothermia causing vasoconstriction

completion of CPB, the large quantities of "pump blood" that remain in the bypass circuit can be collected and used for initial postoperative volume replacement.

Recently, in response to findings that the low cardiac output syndrome often seen postoperatively might be a result of intraoperative myocardial ischemia or necrosis, efforts have been directed toward providing additional protection to the myocardium during bypass. At present, rapidly stopping the heart in diastole by perfusing the coronary arteries with a cold potassium cardioplegic ("heart-paralyzing") agent is the vehicle of choice for intraoperative myocardial protection. Cardioplegic solution is reinfused at regular intervals during bypass to keep the heart cold and still, which minimizes myocardial oxygen requirements.

Numerous clinical sequelae can result from CPB[66] (Table 15-3). Knowledge of these physiological effects will allow the nurse to anticipate problems and intervene appropriately.

Postoperative Management

Cardiovascular support. Postoperative cardiovascular support is often indicated because of a low output state resulting from preexisting heart disease, prolonged pump run, and/or inadequate myocardial protection.[66] Cardiac output can be maximized by adjustments in cardiac rate, preload, afterload, and contractility.

In the presence of low cardiac output, the heart rate can be appropriately regulated by means of temporary pacing or drug therapy. Temporary epicardial pacing is usually instituted when the adult cardiac surgical patient's heart rate drops below 80 beats/min.[17] In the case of tachycardia, intravenous verapamil has proved quite effective when used to slow supraventricular rhythms with a ventricular response that exceed 110 beats/min. Since ventricular ectopy can result from hypokalemia, serum potassium levels are maintained in the high normal range (4.5 to 5.0 mEq/L) to provide some margin for error.

In the majority of patients, reduced preload is the cause of low postoperative cardiac output. If a left atrial line has been inserted during surgery, monitoring left atrial pressures (LAP) can provide a more convenient and accurate guide to left ventricular preload than can the monitoring of the pulmonary capillary wedge pressure (PCWP).[59] To enhance preload, volume is usually administered in the form of colloid or packed red cells. It is not uncommon for cardiac

---

Nursing Diagnosis and Management
Status post open heart surgery

Decreased Cardiac Output related to hemopericardium secondary to open heart surgery, p. 336

Decreased Cardiac Output related to supraventricular tachycardia, p. 334

Decreased Cardiac Output related to atrioventricular heart block, p. 336

Decreased Cardiac Output related to ventricular tachycardia, p. 338

Decreased Cardiac Output related to decreased preload secondary to mechanical ventilation with or without PEEP, p. 335

Decreased Cardiac Output related to relative excess of preload and afterload secondary to impaired ventricular contractility, p. 335

Fluid Volume Deficit related to active blood loss, p. 668

Potential for Altered Peripheral Tissue Perfusion risk factor: vasopressor therapy, p. 341

Potential For Aspiration risk factors: endotracheal tube, gastrointestinal tube, depressed cough and gag reflexes secondary to anesthesia, decreased gasrointestinal motility secondary to an anesthesia, situation hindering elevation of upper body, p. 489

Ineffective Airway Clearance related to impaired cough secondary to loss of glottic closure with cuffed endotracheal tube, p. 476

Ineffective Airway Clearance related to thoracic pain, p. 477

Ineffective Breathing Pattern related to thoracic pain, p. 483

Acute Pain related to transmission and perception of noxious stimuli secondary to leg and/or sternotomy incision, p. 594

Potential for Infection risk factor: invasive monitoring devices, p. 346

Activity Intolerance related to postural hypotension secondary to immobility, narcotics, vasodilator therapy, p. 344

Sensory-Perceptual Alterations related to sensory overload, sensory deprivation, sleep pattern disturbance, p. 601

Sleep Pattern Disturbance related to circadian desynchronization, p. 89

Knowledge Deficit: Postoperative Exercise Regimen, Fluid Restrictions, Medication, Wound Care, Reportable Symptoms related to lack of previous exposure to information, p. 69

Body Image Disturbance related to actual change in body structure, function, and appearance, p. 833

Altered Sexuality Patterns related to fear of death during coitus secondary to myocardial infarction, p. 866

surgical patients to be most stable hemodynamically when filling pressures (LAP or PCWP) are in the range of 18 to 20 mm Hg (normally 4 to 12 mm Hg).[59]

Partly as a result of the peripheral vasoconstrictive effects of hypothermia, many cardiac surgical patients will demonstrate postoperative hypertension. Although transient, postoperative hypertension can precipitate or exacerbate bleeding from the mediastinal chest tubes. In addition, the high systemic vascular resistance (afterload) resulting from the intense vasoconstriction can cause deterioration of cardiac performance. Therefore, vasodilator therapy with intravenous nitroprusside is often used to reduce afterload that will control hypertension and improve cardiac output.

If these adjustments in heart rate, preload, and afterload fail to produce significant improvement in cardiac output, contractility can be enhanced with positive inotropic support or intraaortic balloon pumping, thus augmenting circulation.

Nursing care. Hypothermia can contribute to depressed myocardial contractility in the cardiac surgical patient. While hyperthermia blankets are used to warm the patient, care should be taken to remove the blankets promptly when the temperature reaches 98.4° F to prevent subsequent excessive temperature elevations.[48]

Control of bleeding. Postoperative bleeding from the mediastinal chest tubes can be caused by inadequate hemostasis, disruption of suture lines, or coagulopathy associated with CPB.[66] Bleeding is more likely to occur with IMA grafts as a result of the extensive chest wall dissection required to free the IMA.[25,29] If bleeding in excess of 150 ml/hr occurs early in the postoperative period, clotting factors (fresh-frozen plasma and platelets) and additional protamine (used to reverse the effects of heparin) may be administered along with prompt blood replacement. Recently, autotransfusion devices, which facilitate the collection and reinfusion of shed mediastinal blood, have become widely available.

The use of prophylactic positive end-expiratory pressure (PEEP) in conjunction with mechanical ventilation may be helpful in controlling bleeding in some cases by increasing intrathoracic pressure enough to tamponade oozing mediastinal blood vessels.[3] Rewarming the patient will reverse the depressed manufacture and release of clotting factors that result from hypothermia. However, persistent mediastinal bleeding, usually in excess of 500 ml in 1 hour or 400 ml/hr for 2 consecutive hours, despite normalization of clotting studies, is an indication for reexploration of the surgical site.

Nursing care. Chest tube stripping, done to maintain patency of the tubes, is controversial because the high negative pressure generated by routine methods of stripping is believed to result in tissue damage that can contribute to bleeding.[24] However, this risk must be carefully weighed against the very real danger of cardiac tamponade if blood is not effectively drained from around the heart. Therefore chest tube stripping is frequently advocated in instances of postoperative bleeding. However, the technique of milking the chest tubes may be advisable for routine postoperative care because this technique generates less negative pressure and decreases the risk of bleeding.[24]

Pulmonary care. Most cardiac surgery patients remain intubated overnight to facilitate lung expansion and optimize gas exchange. This is particularly advantageous for IMA bypass patients who tend to be more prone to postoperative pulmonary complications, such as atelectasis and pleural effusions, because the pleural space is entered during surgery.[25,29] IMA bypass surgery is also associated with more postoperative pain than is SVG surgery.[29] This postoperative chest pain can lead to shallow breathing, which if not corrected will aggravate atelectasis. Some patients who have underlying pulmonary disease related to long-term valvular dysfunction may require longer periods of mechanical ventilation. However, most patients will be successfully weaned from the ventilator within 8 to 12 hours after surgery.

Neurological complications. The transient neurological dysfunction often seen in cardiac surgical patients can probably be attributed to decreased cerebral perfusion and to cerebral microemboli, both related to the pump run. Compounding these are the environmental factors such as sensory deprivation and sensory overload associated with being in a critical care unit.[6] "Postcardiotomy psychosis" has been used to describe this postoperative syndrome that may initially be seen as only a mild impairment of orientation but may progress to agitation, hallucinations, and paranoid delusions.[47]

Nursing care. Patients and family members need to be reassured that postcardiotomy psychosis is a temporary phenomenon that will resolve quickly. Meanwhile, every effort should be made to keep the patient informed of all that is going on in the surroundings so that unfamiliar sights, sounds, and smells are not overwhelming and confusing. Painful stimuli should be kept to a minimum, and meaningful stimuli such as touching should be encouraged. Nursing care should be organized to maximize optimal sleep patterns.

Infection. Postoperative fever is fairly common following CPB. However, persistent temperature elevation above 101° F should be investigated. Sternal wound infections and infective endocarditis are the most devastating infectious complications, but leg wound infection, pneumonia, and urinary tract infection can also occur.[21]

Renal involvement. Hemolysis caused by trauma to the red blood cells in the extracorporeal circuit results in hemoglobinuria, which can damage renal tubules. Therefore small amounts of furosemide (Lasix) will usually be given to promote urine flow if the urine output is low (less than 25 to 30 ml/hr) and "pink-tinged."

Recent Advances in Cardiac Surgery

Coronary endarterectomy is currently enjoying a modest revival as an adjunct to bypass procedures in patients with diffuse or small vessel disease.[29] Laser technology has paved the way for investigation into intraoperative coronary laser recanalization. The introduction of heart transplantation has generated much excitement and anticipation for patients who suffer from otherwise untreatable heart disease.

Although future trends in the surgical management of cardiac disease are difficult to predict, the critical care nurse must continue to be prepared to meet the challenge of providing a high level of nursing care at the bedside. A solid knowledge base and keen assessment skills are prerequisite for the accurate anticipation of problems and prompt intervention necessary to stabilize the patient and prevent the occurrence of life-threatening complications.

PERCUTANEOUS TRANSLUMINAL CORONARY ANGIOPLASTY

Percutaneous transluminal coronary angioplasty (PTCA) involves the use of a balloon-tipped catheter that when advanced through an atherosclerotic coronary lesion (atheroma) can be intermittently inflated for the purpose of dilating the stenotic area and improving blood flow through it (Fig. 15-14). The mechanism of dilation was originally thought to be plaque compression that resulted in the immediate expression of plaque contents or its redistribution within the vessel wall. However, it is now believed that the stretching of the vessel wall as a result of high balloon inflation pressures results in fracture of the plaque that enlarges the vessel lumen.[65] PTCA provides an alternative to both traditional medical management of atheriosclerotic heart disease and coronary artery bypass surgery, as well as a valuable adjunct to thrombolytic therapy in terms of reducing a severe stenosis that persists following thrombolysis.[68]

Indications for PTCA

Indications for PTCA have been considerably broadened since the initial application of this therapeutic technique. Whereas once only patients with single-vessel disease were considered for PTCA, now patients with multivessel disease, even those who have previously undergone saphenous vein grafting, may be eligible for this procedure (see the box at right).

The restrictions regarding the characteristics of the lesion have also been loosened with improved technology. Left main coronary lesions have been successfully dilated. Also, no longer is the presence of an eccentric, moderately cal-

cified, or nonproximal lesion an absolute contraindication to PTCA. Furthermore, it is now even possible to traverse and dilate a totally occluded vessel.[36]

However, the most significant advancement has been the lifting of the requirement that only patients with disabling angina unresponsive to medical therapy be considered for PTCA. Clinical indications for PTCA have been expanded to include chronic stable angina, angina following coronary artery bypass grafting (CABG), both recent-onset as well as postinfarction unstable angina, and in acute myocardial infarction alone or in conjunction with thrombolytic agents.[33] Even patients who are asymptomatic but demonstrate evidence of ischemia during exercise testing (positive treadmill) may be considered as candidates for elective PTCA.[65]

TRADITIONAL ELIGIBILITY CRITERIA FOR PTCA

Single vessel disease exclusive of left main lesions
Characteristics of the lesion
    Concentric
    Noncalcified
    Proximal
    Discrete (less than 1 cm length)
    No total occlusions
History of disease
    Short history of angina (less than 1 year)
    Inadequate control on medications
Normal ventricular function
Not in the setting of acute myocardial infarction
Must be a candidate for CABG

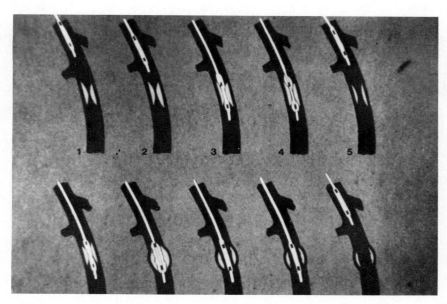

Fig. 15-14   Balloon compression of an atherosclerotic lesion. (From Andreoli KG and others: Comprehensive cardiac care, ed 6, St Louis, 1987, The CV Mosby Co.)

Most institutions still require that the patient preparing to undergo PTCA be a candidate for coronary bypass surgery.[20] Complications such as acute coronary occlusion may arise during angioplasty that result in intractable angina necessitating immediate aortocoronary bypass grafting. Therefore it is the responsibility of the nurse to provide the patient with some preoperative instruction before PTCA.

Procedure

PTCA is performed in the cardiac catheterization laboratory by means of fluoroscopy. Introducer sheaths are commonly inserted percutaneously into the femoral artery and vein. The venous sheath can be used to perform a right heart catheterization with a Swan-Ganz catheter and/or to insert a pacing catheter. A catheter with pacing capabilities may be indicated if dilation of the right coronary artery or circumflex artery is anticipated because the blood supply to the conduction system of the heart may be interrupted, thus requiring emergency pacing.[33] The pacing catheter will also serve as an anatomical landmark for locating the lesions to be dilated. The patient is systemically heparinized to prevent clots from forming on or in any of the catheters. A special guiding catheter designed to engage the coronary ostia is inserted through the arterial sheath and advanced in retrograde manner through the aorta. Nitroglycerin or calcium channel blockers may be given at this time to prevent coronary artery spasm and maximize coronary vasodilation during the procedure. A guidewire is then advanced down the coronary artery and negotiated across the occluding atheroma. The balloon catheter is advanced over this guidewire and positioned across the lesion. The balloon is inflated and deflated repetitively (each inflation not to exceed 90 seconds) until evidence of dilation is demonstrated on angiogram[33] (Fig. 15-15).

The patient is transferred to the coronary care unit for overnight care and observation. The introducer sheaths are left in place for several reasons. First, the intravenous infusion of heparin is continued for 6 to 24 hours following PTCA to prevent clot formation on the roughened endothelium at the site of dilation.[33,65] Therefore removal of the sheaths during this time would predispose to bleeding. Second, it allows for rapid vascular access should redilation become necessary. However, the arterial sheath must be attached to a continuous heparinized saline flush, and intravenous fluids must be infused through the venous sheath to maintain luminal patency. If the patient's postangioplasty course is uneventful, the sheaths are usually removed within 24 hours.

Complications. As stated earlier, serious complications can result from angioplasty that will necessitate emergency CABG surgery. These complications include persistent coronary artery spasm, myocardial infarction, and acute coronary occlusion.[12] Other complications that can occur in the period immediately after angioplasty include bleeding and hematoma formation at the site of vascular cannulation, compromised blood flow to the involved extremity, allergic reaction to radiopaque contrast dye, dysrhythmias, and vasovagal response (hypotension, bradycardia, and diaphoresis) during manipulation or removal of introducer sheaths. Restenosis can occur up to 6 months after angioplasty; however, this late complication is typically amenable to repeat angioplasty. The mechanism involved in restenosis remains unclear, but it is thought to be related to platelet deposition and thrombus formation.[33] For this reason, patients are started on a regimen of antiplatelet drugs, for example, a combination of aspirin and dipyridamole.

Nursing Care

The nursing care of the patient following angioplasty focuses on accurate assessment and prompt intervention. The nurse is in the unique position at the bedside to continuously monitor for signs of potential problems and take quick and appropriate action to minimize the deleterious effects of complications related to angioplasty.

It is essential that the nurse assess the patient for recurrent angina. Angina during angioplasty is an expected occur-

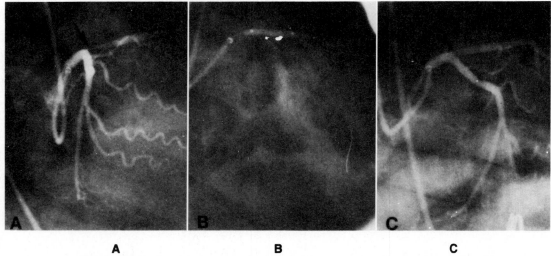

A   **B**   **C**

Fig. 15-15 Coronary arteriograms during PTCA. Arrows denote the lesion before dilation **(A)**, with the balloon inflated **(B)**, and after dilation **(C)**. (From Andreoli KG and others: Comprehensive cardiac care, ed 6, St Louis, 1987, The CV Mosby Co.)

rence at the time of balloon inflation. It is a result of the temporary interruption of blood flow through the involved artery. However, it should subside with deflation or removal of the balloon and/or the administration of nitroglycerin. Angina following PTCA may be a result of transient coronary vasospasm or it may herald a more serious complication. In any case, the nurse must act quickly to assess for signs and symptoms of myocardial ischemia and initiate appropriate interventions as indicated. (See Chapter 14 on the care of the patient with acute myocardial infarction.) The physician will usually order intravenous nitroglycerin to be titrated to alleviate chest pain. Continued angina despite maximal vasodilator therapy usually rules out transient coronary vasospasm as the source of ischemic pain, and redilation and/or emergency coronary artery bypass surgery must be considered.

Bleeding or hematoma at the sheath insertion site may occur while the sheath is in place or after its removal as a result of the effects of heparin. The nurse must monitor for bleeding or swelling at the puncture site as well as frequently assess for adequacy of circulation to the involved extremity. The nurse should also assess the patient for back pains, which might indicate retroperitoneal bleeding from oozing puncture sites. The patient should be instructed to keep the involved leg straight and not to elevate the head of the bed any more than 45 degrees while the sheath is in place (to prevent dislodgement) and for several hours after its removal (to prevent bleeding). Following sheath removal, direct pressure should be applied to the puncture site for 15 to 30 minutes; a sandbag may be ordered if the former is inadequate for hemostasis. Patients are usually allowed to resume ambulation 6 to 8 hours later, depending on institutional protocol. Excessive bleeding or hematoma formation can become a very serious problem, since it may result in hypotension and/or compromised blood flow to the involved extremity, thus necessitating surgical intervention in rare cases.[65]

Typically, patients undergoing elective angioplasty are hospitalized for only a few days. Because PTCA is only a palliative procedure, these patients need education in risk factor modification. Because of abbreviated hospital stay, the nurse often has insufficient time to do more than identify the offending risk factors and initiate basic instruction. Patients should be referred to local cardiac rehabilitation centers for more extensive teaching and follow-up to facilitate understanding and compliance with the therapeutic regimen.

Another teaching need that must be addressed is the patient's knowledge deficit related to discharge medications. As stated earlier, patients are frequently sent home on antiplatelet drugs as well as a nitrate such as a nitroglycerin preparation or isosorbide to promote vasodilation. Additionally, if the patient has demonstrated evidence of a vasospastic component to the disease, calcium channel blockers will be prescribed. It is essential that the patient clearly understand the rationale for therapy as well as potential side effects of each drug.

Summary

PTCA was originally introduced as an invasive but non-surgical alternative for patients requiring coronary revas-cularization. It has now been demonstrated to be an effective adjunct to thrombolytic therapy in acute myocardial infarction.[68] Its use has also been demonstrated in patients with recurrent angina following coronary artery bypass surgery with successful dilation of native coronary arteries, saphenous vein grafts, and, recently, internal mammary artery grafts.[14,65] Currently, clinical trials are underway in which laser energy is used to recanalize obstructed coronary arteries.[19] Other recent developments include stent devices that could be left in the coronary artery to prevent acute occlusion or restenosis and atherectomy catheters designed to remove the plaque with rotating cutting tips.

Improving technology has rapidly expanded the options available to patients with coronary artery disease (CAD). However, research needs to be generated to determine which therapeutic approach or combinations of approaches will ultimately lead to an improved quality and quantity of life for the patient with CAD.

THROMBOLYTIC THERAPY

Thrombolytic therapy offers a promising new approach for the patient experiencing acute myocardial infarction (AMI). Before the introduction of streptokinase as a thrombolytic agent, the medical management of AMI focused on decreasing myocardial oxygen demands in an effort to minimize myocardial necrosis and thus preserve ventricular function. Recently, however, efforts to limit the size of infarction have been directed toward the timely reperfusion of the jeopardized myocardium. The use of thrombolytic therapy to accomplish this is predicated on the prevailing theory that the terminal event in the majority of transmural infarctions is a fresh thrombus superimposed on a high-grade coronary lesion.[46] The administration of a thrombolytic agent will result in the lysis of the acute thrombus, thus recanalizing the obstructed coronary artery and restoring blood flow to the affected myocardium.

Thrombolytic Agents

Streptokinase. Streptokinase (SK) is a thrombolytic agent derived from beta-hemolytic streptococci, which, when combined with plasminogen, catalyzes the conversion of plasminogen to plasmin, the enzyme responsible for clot dissolution in the body.[53] SK can be administered either intravenously or by an intracoronary approach necessitating cardiac catheterization. The efficacy of both routes has been established, and both have been used in clinical practice.[62] However, because of the significant lag time between onset of symptoms and the initiation of intracoronary SK, the intracoronary route is now considered obsolete.[9,62,68]

The three major problems associated with the use of SK are its systemic lytic effects coupled with a long half-life, its potential antigenic effects if readministered, and hypotension. Because the anticoagulant action of streptokinase is indiscriminate (non-clot specific) and prolonged (half-life 10 to 18 minutes), bleeding is a common complication that should be carefully monitored for during the 12 hours immediately following administration[68] (see the box on p. 320). In addition, because streptokinase is a bacterial protein, it is strongly antigenic and can produce a variety of allergic reactions, including anaphylaxis, especially when

---

SIGNS OF INADEQUATE HEMOSTASIS RELATED TO THROMBOLYTIC THERAPY

Bleeding or hematoma at puncture sites
Hematuria, hematemesis, hemoptysis, melena, epistaxis
Bruising or petechiae (pinpoint hemorrhages)
Flank ecchymoses with complaints of low back pain (suggestive of retroperitoneal bleeding)
Gingival bleeding
Change in neurological status (intracranial bleeding)
Deterioration in vital signs, decreased hematocrit values (internal bleeding)

POSSIBLE ALLERGIC MANIFESTATIONS RELATED TO STREPTOKINASE THERAPY

Anaphylaxis
Urticaria
Itching
Nausea
Flushing
Fever
Chills

---

administered to a patient who has either received SK therapy previously or had a recent streptococcal infection. It is necessary to be familiar with the possible allergic manifestations (see the box above), as well as cognizant of the fact that as a result of delayed antibody formation, symptoms may develop several days after infusion.[46] Hypotension is sometimes associated with the rapid administration of SK.[62] This fall in blood pressure will usually respond to volume replacement but occasionally will require vasopressor support.

Urokinase. Urokinase (UK) is an enzymatic protein secreted by the parenchyma of the human kidney. Its thrombolytic effect results from the direct activation of plasminogen to form plasmin. This differs from streptokinase, which must first form a complex with plasminogen to activate plasmin to dissolve the clot[53] (Fig. 15-16). UK is also non-clot-specific (activates circulating, non-clot-bound plasminogen as well as clot-bound plasminogen) but has a shorter half-life than SK.[68] Although a systemic lytic state may also be produced, its administration is associated with fewer bleeding complications.[49] Because urokinase is produced by the kidney, it is nonantigenic and thus well suited for use if subsequent thrombolytic therapy is indicated. However, it is currently difficult and expensive to produce, precluding extensive clinical use.

Tissue Plasminogen Activator. The most exciting advance in thrombolytic therapy is the recent approval by the FDA (November, 1987) of a newly available agent, tissue plasminogen activator (t-PA).[67] Marketed under the name Activase, t-PA is a naturally occurring enzyme (thus nonantigenic) that is clot specific and has a very short half-life (3 to 5 minutes).[32] It converts plasminogen to plasmin after binding to the fibrin-containing clot. This clot specificity results in an increased concentration and activity of plasmin at the site of the clot where it is needed[9] (Fig. 15-17). It was hoped that this characteristic of t-PA would prevent the induction of a systemic lytic state that occurs with SK therapy. However, the results of recent studies comparing the adverse effects of SK and t-PA show similar incidences of bleeding following administration.[61] Nonetheless, the intravenous administration of t-PA appears to be superior to intravenous streptokinase in terms of efficacy (recanalization of the affected coronary artery).[32]

Successful gene cloning has made sufficient quantities of t-PA available for clinical use.[11] This same DNA technology, however, has resulted in a prohibitive cost. The manufacturer of t-PA, Genentech, Inc., has recently begun to investigate ways of offsetting the cost to facilitate more widespread clinical use of the drug.

Eligibility Criteria

Certain criteria have been developed, based on research findings, to determine the patient population that would most likely benefit from the administration of thrombolytic therapy. In general, patients with recent onset of chest pain (less than 6 hours' duration) may be selected to receive thrombolytic therapy. Research suggests that the earlier the treatment is instituted, the higher the likelihood of successful reperfusion.[28] Chest pain persisting longer than 6 hours is probably indicative of completed transmural infarction, and therefore no benefit would be gained from thrombolysis.

Patients with persistent ST segment elevation despite sublingual nitroglycerin or nifedipine, indicative of impending transmural infarction, are considered candidates for therapy. Patients with abnormal Q waves should not be excluded from therapy, because it is not necessarily evidence of a completed infarction.

Other common criteria for the use of thrombolytic therapy are included in the box below.

SELECTION CRITERIA

Less than 6 hours from onset of chest pain
ST segment elevation on ECG
Ischemic chest pain of 30 minutes' duration
Chest pain unresponsive to sublingual nitroglycerine or nifedipine
Less than 75 years of age
No conditions that might predispose to hemorrhage

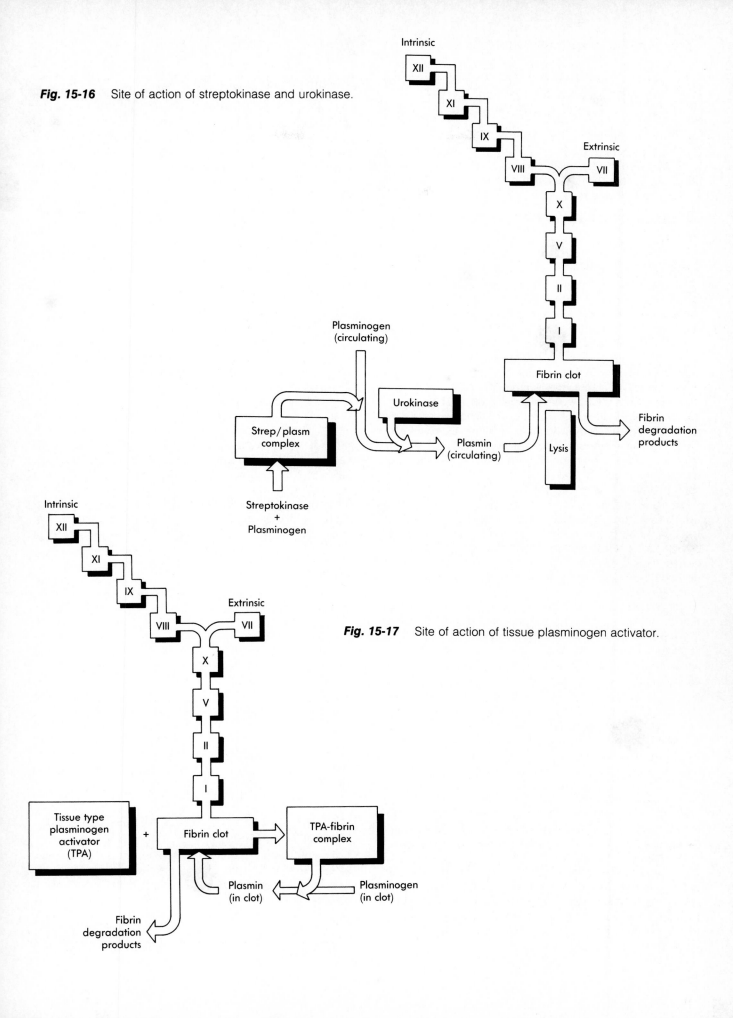

Fig. 15-16 Site of action of streptokinase and urokinase.

Fig. 15-17 Site of action of tissue plasminogen activator.

NONINVASIVE EVIDENCE OF REPERFUSION

Cessation of chest pain
Reperfusion dysrhythmias primarily ventricular
Return of elevated ST segments to baseline
Early and marked peaking of creatine kinase

Evidence of Reperfusion

Several phenomenon can be observed following the reperfusion of an artery that has been completely occluded by a thrombus (see the box above). Initially, there is an abrupt cessation of ischemic chest pain as blood flow is restored. Another reliable indicator of reperfusion is the appearance of various "reperfusion" dysrhythmias. Accelerated idioventricular rhythm (AIVR) is the most common reperfusion dysrhythmia, but premature ventricular contractions, bradycardias, heart block, ventricular tachycardia, and, rarely, ventricular fibrillation may also occur.[57] The reason for the occurrence of these dysrhythmias remains unclear. However, vigilant monitoring of the patient's ECG is essential because a stable condition may rapidly deteriorate when recanalization occurs, and dysrhythmias should be treated appropriately.

Another noninvasive marker of recanalization is the rapid resolution of the previously elevated S-T segments indicating restoration of blood flow to previously ischemic myocardial tissue. However, the unexplained and accelerated development of abnormal Q waves following thrombolysis may indicate exacerbation of injury and requires further investigation.

The serum concentration of creatine kinase (formerly creatine phosphokinase) rises rapidly and markedly following reperfusion of the ischemic myocardium.[9] This phenomenon is termed "washout," because it is thought to be a result of the rapid readmission into the circulation of creatine kinase, an enzyme released by damaged myocardial cells, following restoration of blood flow to previously unperfused areas of the heart.

Recognition of these noninvasive markers of recanalization is essential for documenting the patient's response to thrombolytic therapy.

Administration

Streptokinase. Intravenous streptokinase, although not as effective in terms of recanalization as intracoronary streptokinase, has the advantage of being more practical in that it can be administered more rapidly following the onset of symptoms.[49] Therefore SK is now routinely administered intravenously, (even though this route of administration has not yet been approved by the Food and Drug Administration). The recommended dosage is 1,500,000 IU of streptokinase administered intravenously over 30 to 60 minutes to achieve clot lysis. The patient is then heparinized to prevent early rethrombosis.

Tissue Plasminogen Activator. Tissue plasminogen activator was approved specifically for intravenous administration. The total dose of t-PA is 100 mg, 60 mg of which is administered over 1 hour to rapidly recanalize the infarct-related coronary artery. The remaining 40 mg is given over the next 2 hours, followed by a heparin drip to maintain patency of the recanalized artery and prevent rethrombosis.

Nursing Care

The most common complication related to thrombolysis is bleeding, not only as a result of the thrombolytic therapy itself but also because the patients routinely receive anticoagulation therapy for several days to minimize the possibility of rethrombosis. Therefore, the nurse must continually monitor for signs and symptoms of bleeding (refer to the box on p. 320 listing signs of inadequate hemostasis related to thrombolytic therapy). Mild gingival bleeding and oozing around venipuncture sites is common and therefore not to be considered worrisome.[42] Should serious bleeding occur, such as intracranial or internal bleeding, all fibrinolytic and heparin therapy should be discontinued, and appropriate volume expanders and/or coagulation factors should be administered.

In addition to accurate assessment of the patient for the evidence of bleeding, the nurse should also intervene appropriately to prevent possible bleeding episodes. The nurse should avoid nonessential handling of the patient, keep injections to a minimum, and remember to keep additional pressure on injection, venipuncture, and particularly arterial puncture sites. Antacids can be given prophylactically, especially if the patient complains of gastric discomfort. The patient should be cautioned against vigorous toothbrushing and told to refrain from using straight-edge razors.

Summary

Thrombolytic therapy has been determined to be successful in the majority of cases in terms of reopening occluded coronary arteries in the setting of acute myocardial infarction. This results in the salvage of myocardium by limiting infarct size, thus preserving left ventricular function and significantly reducing morbidity and mortality.

However, residual coronary stenosis resulting from the atherosclerotic process remains even after successful thrombolysis. This residual coronary stenosis can result in rethrombosis. Therefore thrombolytic therapy is recognized as an emergency procedure to restore patency until more definitive therapy can be initiated to effectively reduce the degree of stenosis (PTCA) or to bypass the offending occlusion (coronary artery bypass surgery).

MECHANICAL CIRCULATORY ASSIST DEVICES
Intraaortic Balloon Pump

The intraaortic balloon pump (IABP) is currently the most widely employed temporary mechanical circulatory assist device used to support failing circulation[8,16] (see the box on p. 323). Its therapeutic effects are based on the hemodynamic principles of diastolic augmentation and afterload reduction.

The most commonly used intraaortic balloon consists of

COMMON INDICATIONS FOR THE USE OF IABP

Left ventricular failure after cardiac surgery
Unstable angina refractory to medications
Recurrent angina following AMI
Complications of AMI
    Cardiogenic shock
    Papillary muscle dysfunction/rupture with mitral regurgitation
    Ventricular septal defect
    Refractory ventricular dysrhythmias

a single sausage-shaped polyurethane balloon that is wrapped around the distal end of a vascular catheter and positioned in the descending thoracic aorta just distal to the take-off of the left subclavian artery. The second generation of intraaortic balloon catheters is more flexible and can be wrapped to a smaller diameter than their predecessors and therefore can be inserted into the femoral artery percutaneously rather than surgically.[8] When attached to a bedside pumping console and properly synchronized to the patient's ECG pattern, the intraaortic balloon will inflate during diastole and deflate just before systole.

Initially, as the balloon is inflated in diastole concurrent with aortic valve closure, the blood in the aortic arch above the level of the balloon will be displaced retrograde (backward) toward the aortic root, augmenting diastolic coronary arterial blood flow and increasing myocardial oxygen supply (Fig. 15-18, *A*). The blood volume in the aorta below the level of the balloon will be propelled forward toward the peripheral vascular system, which may enhance renal perfusion. Subsequently, the deflation of the balloon just before the opening of the aortic valve creates a potential space or vacuum toward which blood will flow unimpeded during systole (Fig. 15-18, *B*). This decreased resistance to left

A

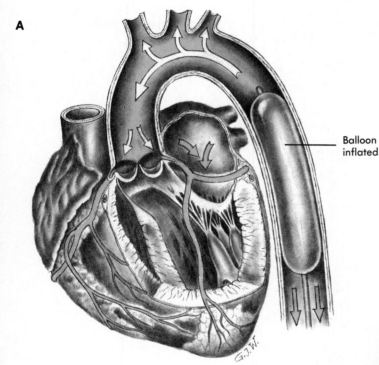

Balloon
inflated

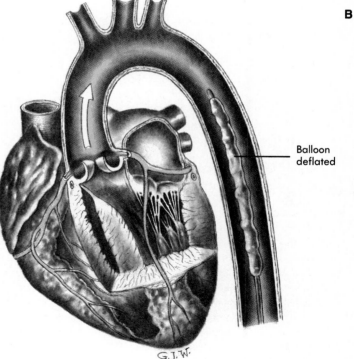

B

Balloon
deflated

Fig. 15-18 Mechanisms of action of intraaortic balloon pump. **A,** Diastolic balloon inflation augments coronary blood flow. **B,** Systolic balloon deflation decreases afterload.

ventricular ejection, or decreased afterload, will facilitate ventricular emptying and reduce myocardial oxygen demands. The overall physiological effect of IABP therapy is an improvement in the balance between myocardial oxygen supply and demand.[27] Contraindications to balloon pumping include aortic aneurysm, aortic valve insufficiency, and severe peripheral vascular disease.

Although the actual management of the pumping console and its timing functions are usually delegated to specially trained personnel on the unit, there are several important nursing responsibilities related to the care of the patient on the intraaortic balloon pump.

The ECG and arterial pressure tracing should be constantly monitored to verify the timing and effect of balloon counterpulsations (Fig. 15-19). Dysrhythmias can adversely affect the timing of balloon inflation and deflation, thus rhythm disturbances must be detected and treated promptly.[8] In addition, balloon deflation can be accidentally triggered by pacemaker spikes that are mistaken for R waves. The resulting early deflation is not dangerous, but, since it limits effective afterload reduction, an ECG lead that minimizes the pacing spike should be selected. Mean arterial pressure should be maintained at about 80 mm Hg with adequate pumping.

A major complication of IABP is ischemia of the involved limb secondary to occlusion of the femoral artery either by the catheter itself or by emboli from thrombus formation on the balloon. Consequently, the presence and quality of peripheral pulses distal to the catheter insertion site should be frequently assessed along with color, temperature, and capillary refill of the involved extremity. A doppler may be required if pulses are difficult to palpate on the cannulated extremity. Signs of diminished perfusion must be reported immediately.

In addition, the balloon catheter may migrate proximally, occluding the left subclavian artery or distally compromising renal circulation. Therefore careful assessment of the left radial pulse and urinary output is essential. Measures to avoid accidental displacement of the balloon catheter include keeping the patient on complete bedrest with the head of the bed elevated no more than 30 degrees and preventing any flexion of the involved hip.

The patient should be log rolled from side to side every 2 hours to maintain skin integrity and to prevent pulmonary atelectasis. The presence of the balloon pump should never be a deterrent to appropriate pulmonary toilet. Thrombocytopenia may occur as a result of mechanical destruction of the platelets by the pumping action of the balloon. Therefore platelet counts should be closely monitored, and the patient watched for evidence of bleeding. Since the groin insertion site is at high risk for contamination, a daily regimen of aseptic dressing changes with betadine should be adhered to closely.

Finally, the psychological needs of the patient must not

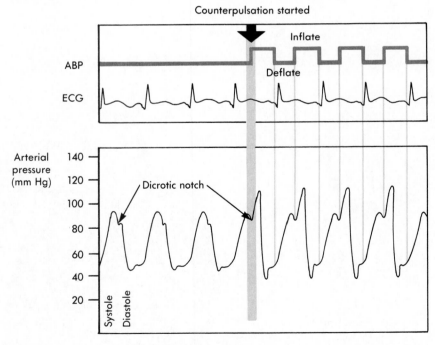

Fig. 15-19 The timing and effect of balloon counterpulsations. Timing is adjusted by synchronizing balloon inflation with the dicrotic knotch on the arterial waveform resulting in an elevated diastolic pressure. Inflation continues until the next R wave serves as a stimulus for balloon deflation. The arterial waveform will exhibit a reduced systolic pressure during counterpulsation. (From Guzzetta CE and Dossey BM: Cardiovascular nursing: bodymind tapestry, St Louis, 1984, The CV Mosby Co.)

be overlooked. Sleep deprivation is not at all uncommon, partly a result of the continuous nursing care requirements of the patient but also related to the noise level in the unit, including the sounds made by the balloon pumping device. In addition, these patients universally experience anxiety related to fear of not recovering and loss of control because of forced immobility.

Weaning from the ballon pump should be considered when the patient has been hemodynamically stable with no or only minimal pharmacological support. The weaning procedure consists of slowly decreasing the pumping frequency from every beat down to every eighth beat as tolerated.[27] The IABP should remain at this minimal pumping ratio (or in a flutter mode) until its removal, to prevent thrombus formation on the balloon surface. Dependence on the balloon for over 48 hours, indicative of severe cardiac dysfunction, is usually associated with a poor prognosis.[27]

External Counterpulsation

External counterpulsation (ECP) is a noninvasive method of diastolic augmentation in which the lower extremities are used as the pumping chambers. The system consists of two tapered, rigid cylinders that enclose the legs from ankle to thigh[55] (Fig. 15-20). Between the leg and the rigid outer housing is a water-filled bag that obliterates the remaining space to form an airtight seal. Water is then pumped in and out of the bag in synchrony with the ECG to apply alter-

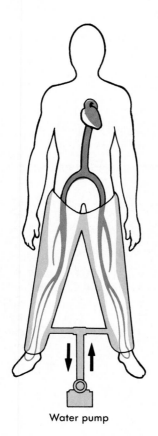

Water pump

Fig. 15-20 External counterpulsation (ECP).

nating positive and negative pressure to veins and arteries within the legs. During diastole, inflation of the bag forces both venous and arterial blood back toward the heart, increasing preload and coronary filling, respectively. Negative pressure can be generated during systolic deflation to produce a vacuum effect similar to that seen with IABP that decreases afterload.

Compromised lower extremity circulation is the major complication associated with ECP. Patients will frequently complain of pain, muscular cramping, and numbness and tingling in the lower extremities that in some cases may necessitate discontinuance of therapy. Prolonged periods of pumping should be interrupted for brief periods when possible to provide skin care and passive range of motion.

Indications for ECP are similar to those for IABP, with the obvious exceptions of patients who have undergone coronary revascularization with saphenous vein grafts.

Ventricular Assist Devices

The ventricular assist device (VAD) is indicated for patients who, despite aggressive medical therapy, cannot be weaned from cardiopulmonary bypass because of persistent ventricular failure with cardiogenic shock.[38] VAD application in refractory cardiogenic shock following AMI and in patients whose condition is deteriorating while awaiting cardiac transplantation is currently being studied.[26]

The basic premise underlying the use of VAD following an acute myocardial infarction or after cardiac surgery is that myocardial function will improve if the heart is given time to rest and recover. This is accomplished by diverting a moderate amount of systemic blood flow (25% to 50%) around the failing ventricle by means of an extracorporeal pump.[7]

The left ventricular assist device (L-VAD) is used most commonly because LV failure occurs more frequently than RV failure.[7] Surgically placed cannulas in the left atrium and aorta are attached to an external pump device by connecting tubing (Fig. 15-21). Both cannulae exit the skin either through the sternal incision or through separate chest incisions.[38] Blood is diverted from the left atrium via the atrial cannula into the pumping device, which then pumps the blood out to the systemic circulation by way of the aortic cannula. A flow rate of between 1 and 5 L/min is used to maintain adequate cardiac output while decreasing the left ventricular workload.[7]

Weaning proceeds after several days by gradually decreasing flow rates to allow the patient's ventricle to contribute more to total blood flow.

Patients on the VAD are routinely anticoagulated to prevent clotting in the extracorporeal circuit. Activated clotting times (ACT) are usually maintained between 100 and 150 seconds with heparin, so the patient must be closely monitored for bleeding diathesis.[7]

These patients are also extraordinarily prone to infection because of the multiple portals of entry (invasive lines and, in some cases, open sternal incision); every precaution must be taken to prevent unnecessary exposure to organisms, and the patient should be closely monitored for signs and symptoms of infection.[7]

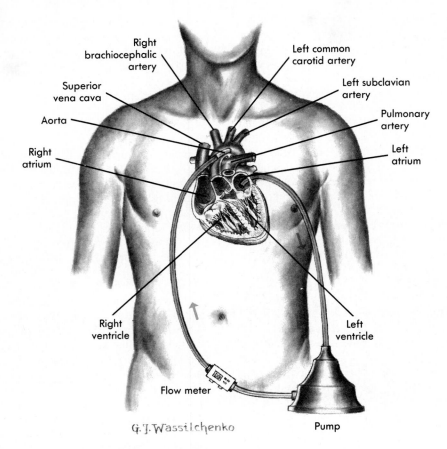

Right brachiocephalic artery
Superior vena cava
Aorta
Right atrium
Left common carotid artery
Left subclavian artery
Pulmonary artery
Left atrium
Right ventricle
Left ventricle
Flow meter
Pump
G. J. Wassilchenko

Fig. 15-21   Left ventricular assist device (L-VAD).

THE EFFECTS OF CARDIOVASCULAR DRUGS
Antidysrhythmic Drugs

Classification. Antidysrhythmic drugs can be grouped into four categories based on their electrophysiological effects on the heart (Table 15-4). Knowledge of the cardiac action potential is prerequisite to the understanding of the mechanism of action of most antidysrhythmic agents (Fig. 15-22).

Drugs used to treat "irritable" dysrhythmias function primarily by prolonging the duration of the action potential and refractory period. The effect is to decrease the possibility of premature discharges from ectopic foci.

Class I drugs prolong the absolute (effective) refractory period by depressing the rate of inward sodium current during phase 0 of the action potential. In addition, these drugs act to depress automaticity by slowing the rate of spontaneous phase 4 depolarization of pacemaker cells.[60]

Class I drugs can be further subdivided into three groups based on the intensity of the effects on phase 0 depolarization as well as on the duration of phase 3 repolarization.[23] Class IA agents have a moderate depressant effect on phase 0 depolarization. Drugs in this class will also greatly prolong phase 3 repolarization seen as a prolonged Q-T interval on the ECG. Class IB agents have very little effect on phase 0 of the action potential and actually shorten phase 3 repolarization (shorter Q-T interval). These drugs have less effect on cardiac conduction than other agents. Class IC

Table 15-4   Classification of antidysrhythmics

Class	Agent
IA*	Quinidine
	Disopyramide
	Procainamide
IB	Lidocaine
	Phenytoin
	Tocainide
	Mexiletine
IC*	Encainide
	Flecainide
	Lorcainide
II	Propranolol
III	Bretylium
	Amiodarone
IV	Verapamil

*Possesses anticholinergic properties.

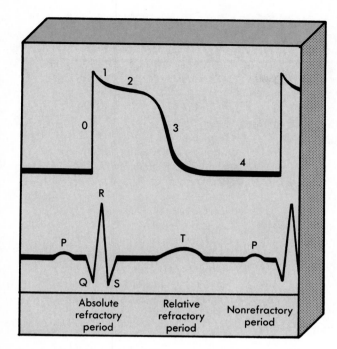

Fig. 15-22 The phases of the cardiac action potential and their relationship to the heart's refractory periods. *Phase 0*, depolarization—rapid influx of sodium. *Phase 1*, rapid repolarization—rapid eflux of potassium ions and decreased sodium conductance. *Phase 2*, plateau—slow influx of sodium and calcium ions. *Phase 3*, repolarization—continued eflux of potassium ions. *Phase 4*, resting phase—restoration of ionic balance by sodium and potassium pumps.

Table 15-5 Classification of beta adrenergic blockers

Cardioselective	Noncardioselective
Atenolol	Propranolol
Metoprolol	Timolol
Acebutolol	Nadolol
	Pindolol
	Labetalol

Table 15-6 Selected cardiovascular and pulmonary effects of adrenergic receptor stimulation

Receptor	Effects
Alpha	Vasoconstriction of peripheral arterioles
Beta₁	Increased myocardial contractility
	Increased heart rate
	Increased AV conduction
Beta₂	Vasodilation of peripheral arterioles
	Bronchodilation

agents will markedly prolong depolarization but have little effect on repolarization time. The new drugs of this antidysrhythmic group essentially abolish dysrhythmias but are also associated with dangerous side effects.

Class I antidysrhythmics are also categorized as local anesthetics and can be further subdivided into two groups based on their autonomic properties: local anesthetic agents with anticholinergic effects and those without anticholinergic activity[10] (Table 15-4). This knowledge can assist the nurse in predicting certain side effects associated with the use of these drugs; for example, some common anticholinergic effects include increased heart rate, dry mouth, urinary retention, and constipation.

Class II antidysrhythmics, or the beta-adrenergic receptor blocking agents, act by blocking the catecholamine effect on the heart, thus slowing phase 4 depolarization of the action potential and decreasing automaticity.[60] Drugs in this class can be further subdivided into cardioselective (those that selectively block only cardiac beta-1 receptors) and noncardioselective (those that block both beta₁ and beta₂ receptors) beta blockers (Table 15-5).[15] Therefore knowledge of the effects of adrenergic receptor stimulation will allow for the anticipation of not only therapeutic responses but also the adverse effects of these drugs (Table 15-6). For example, bronchospasm can be precipitated by noncardioselective beta blockers in patients with COPD as a result

of the blocking effects on beta₂ receptors in the lungs. Interestingly, of all the beta blockers currently approved for use, only propranolol is indicated for the treatment of dysrhythmias. Other uses for beta blocks include treatment of angina and hypertension, and, more recently, reduction of the risk of cardiovascular death in survivors of AMI.[5, 51]

Class III agents exert antidysrhythmic effect by markedly prolonging the repolarization phase of the action potential, thereby increasing the effective refractory period and decreasing the potential for premature impulses.[60] There are currently two antidysrhythmic agents in this class—bretylium and amiodarone.

Class IV antidysrhythmics are commonly referred to as calcium antagonists or calcium channel blockers, because they inhibit the flow of calcium ions through slow channels in both cardiac and vascular smooth muscle, resulting in a decreased force of cardiac contraction and vasodilation, respectively. The primary electrophysiological effect is to depress phase 4 depolarization of the action potential especially in nodal tissue, thus slowing impulse generation.[30,60] Of the three calcium antagonists currently approved for use in the United States, only verapamil is indicated as an antidysrhythmic. The others (nifedipine and diltiazem) are effective in treating angina pectoris, especially that associated with coronary vasospasm.[63]

Administration. Antidysrhythmics are a diverse category of pharmacological agents used to terminate and/or prevent an array of cardiac dysrhythmias. The classes of drugs referred to in the preceding discussion are indicated for the management of tachydysrhythmias of both supraventricular and ventricular origin. Certain other agents are available to treat cardiac rhythm disturbances. For example, atropine and isoproterenol are useful in the management of certain

Table 15-7 Pharmacology of selected antidysrhythmics

Drug	Indications	Dosage	Major side effects
Lidocaine	Ventricular ectopy; PVC prophylaxis in AMI	50-100 mg bolus followed by continuous infusion of 1-4 mg/min	CNS toxicity
Procainamide	Ventricular ectopy resistant to lidocaine	50 mg IV every 5 min up to 1 g followed by infusion of 1-4 mg/min	Hypotension GI effects Widening of QRS and QT interval Drug-induced lupus syndrome
Propranolol	Supraventricular tachycardia	1-3 mg IV every 5 min not to exceed 0.1 mg/kg	Bradycardia Heart failure Heart block
Amiodarone	Life-threatening ventricular dysrhythmias	5-10 mg/kg slowly IV followed by an infusion of 10 mg/kg/d for 3-5 days	Corneal deposits Slate-grey or bluish skin Photosensitivity Pulmonary fibrosis Thyroid dysfunction
Bretylium	Refractory ventricular fibrillation	5 mg/kg IV bolus followed by 10 mg/kg doses repeated at 15-30 min intervals for total of 30 mg/kg	Initially: hypertension, tachycardia, PVCs
	Ventricular tachycardia (second-line agent)	500 mg in 50 ml 5% dextrose in water to infuse over 8-10 min then continuous infusion at 1-2 mg/min	Subsequently: hypotension, bradycardia, nausea and vomiting
Verapamil	Supraventricular tachycardia	5-10 mg IV over 2 min followed 10 mg in 30 min if needed	Heart failure AV block Bradycardia Dizziness Peripheral edema

bradydysrhythmias by virtue of their ability to increase sinus node firing and AV conduction. Digoxin, when used to suppress supraventricular dysrhythmias in certain cases, differs from most other antidysrhythmics in that it is a positive inotropic agent.

It is incumbent upon the critical care nurse to be familiar with the dosages, clinical indications, and potential side effects of the most common intravenously administered antidysrhythmic agents (Table 15-7). However, new antidysrhythmic agents are continually being developed, tested, and marketed, charging the nurse with the additional responsibility of keeping abreast of technology through current journals.

General knowledge of *characteristics common to most* antidysrhythmic agents is essential in anticipating side effects of these drugs. For example, care must be taken to avoid rapid intravenous administration of antidysrhythmics, because marked hypotension can occur related to the myocardial depressant and/or vasodilatory effects of many agents. Myocardial depression extends to the conduction system as well, so that the patient should be closely monitored for the appearance or progression of AV block.

A paradox associated with the administration of many antidysrhythmics is the arrhythmogenic effect they may generate, especially at higher doses. For example, quinidine, procainamide, disopyramide, and amiodarone administra-

tion have been associated with "torsades de pointes," a very serious ventricular dysrhythmia.[13,34,54,56]

CNS depressant effects can occur at higher plasma levels as well. Therefore patients requiring prolonged continuous intravenous infusions of these drugs should be continually observed for neurological symptoms ranging from drowsiness to seizures. Other common side effects include various gastrointestinal disturbances and occasional hypersensitivity reactions.

Since many of these agents are metabolized by the liver and/or excreted in the urine, caution must be exercised when administering these drugs to patients with hepatic or renal dysfunction. Plasma levels should be closely monitored in these patients to ensure maximum therapeutic effect while avoiding toxic reactions. In addition, the prevalence and potential severity of adverse effects from these drugs in the elderly population require vigilant nursing surveillance.

It is not unusual to infuse several antidysrhythmic agents concurrently, especially if attempting to taper one off while instituting another. In addition, these agents are often given intravenously with other emergency drugs in the critical care setting. Therefore it is essential that the nurse be aware of potential incompatibilities that can affect drug effectiveness. Many pharmaceutical companies provide large incompatibility charts that should be posted in a convenient location on the unit.

Inotropic Agents

Inotropic drugs are those that enhance cardiac contractility and are therefore effective in the treatment of pump failure. Digitalis has been a mainstay therapy for long-term congestive failure for years. However, it has limited use as an inotropic agent in the emergency cardiac setting.[1] The three inotropic drugs most frequently utilized to combat acute pump failure are dopamine, dobutamine, and amrinone.

Dopamine hydrocholoride (Intropin) is one of the most widely used drugs in the management of shock states. It is a chemical precursor of norepinephrine which, in addition to both alpha and beta adrenergic receptor stimulating effects, can combine with specialized "dopaminergic" receptors in the renal and mesenteric blood vessels. The actions of this drug are entirely dose related.[1] At low intravenous doses of 1 to 2 μg/kg/min, dopamine will stimulate dopaminergic receptors causing renal and mesenteric vasodilation. The resultant increase in renal perfusion will increase urinary output. Moderate doses (2 to 10 μg/kg/min) of dopamine will result in the stimulation of beta-1 receptors that will improve myocardial contractility and thus increase cardiac output. At dosages greater than 10 μg/kg/min, dopamine will cause alpha adrenergic–mediated peripheral vasoconstriction, which will increase blood pressure through elevation of peripheral resistance, often resulting in the loss of both beta-adrenergic and dopaminergic effects.

Dobutamine hydrochloride (Dobutrex) is a synthetic catecholamine that has predominently beta₁ adrenergic effects. Dobutamine is more effective than dopamine in increasing myocardial contractility with less risk of drug-induced tachycardia. It also has some peripheral vasodilatory effects. However, it lacks the dopaminergic effects associated with the administration of dopamine. The usual dosage range is 2.5 to 10 μg/kg/min as a continuous intravenous infusion.[1]

Amrinone lactate (Inocor) is a member of a relatively new class of nonadrenergic positive inotropic agents that also has some vasodilator activity.[50] The mechanism by which amrinone increases myocardial contractility and cardiac output is unclear, but its hemodynamic effects are similar to those of dobutamine.[4] Continuous intravenous infusion for severe congestive heart failure is titrated between 5 and 10 μg/kg/min according to the patient's response.[1] Thrombocytopenia has been associated with its administration, making it necessary to observe the patient for hemorrhagic complications such as bruising or excessive oozing from puncture sites.[4]

All patients receiving positive inotropic support should be closely observed for tachycardias, dysrhythmias, and complaints of ischemic chest pain that can result from increased myocardial oxygen demands.

Vasodilators

Vasodilators are pharmacological agents that improve cardiac output by either decreasing cardiac filling pressures (preload) or reducing the resistance against which the heart has to pump (afterload) or both. This is accomplished by direct relaxation of vascular smooth muscle.[15] The two most frequently used "unloading" agents in the treatment of acute pump failure are intravenous nitroprusside and nitroglycerin.

Sodium nitroprusside (Nipride) is a potent, rapidly acting venous and arterial vasodilator that is effective in the management of pump failure by reducing preload and afterload. Since blood pressure is reduced in response to the vasodilation, nitroprusside is also effective in the management of hypertensive crisis. Nitroprusside is often used to manage postoperative hypertension often seen immediately following cardiac surgical procedures. The usual intravenous infusion rate is 1 to 10 μg/kg/min.[1] However, excessive, prolonged nitroprusside administration can result in thiocyanate toxicity, therefore blood levels should be monitored (normal serum thiocyanate level is 5 to 10 mg/dl), and the patient should be assessed for blurred vision, delirium, and tinnitus.[50]

The simultaneous administration of dopamine and nitroprusside has been successful in the treatment of pump failure, even in AMI. The combination of the unloading effects of the nitroprusside with the positive inotropic effects of dopamine can significantly improve cardiac output.

Intravenous nitroglycerin (Tridil) is most often utilized in the critical care setting for pump failure, unstable angina, and for recurrent angina during AMI. Although nitroglycerin causes both venous and arterial vasodilation, it has a more profound effect on the venous capacitance vessels, reducing cardiac filling pressures and relieving pulmonary congestion and decreasing cardiac workload and oxygen consumption. The mechanism by which nitroglycerin relieves angina is less clear. However, its use in relieving ischemic cardiac pain complicated by congestive failure has been clearly demonstrated. The initial dose is 10 μg/min; however, it can be titrated up to a maximum of 500 μg/min for effect.[1] The most significant side effects are hypotension, especially in hypovolemic patients, and headache, which can sometimes be severe.

Vasopressors

Vasopressors are drugs that mediate peripheral vasoconstriction through alpha adrenergic receptor stimulating properties. Vasoconstriction increases peripheral vascular resistance and elevates blood pressure. Several of these drugs (epinephrine and norepinephrine) also have beta₁ receptor stimulating properties. However, these drugs are no longer widely used in patients with pump failure, because newer drugs such as dopamine and dobutamine are, in most instances, as effective in increasing cardiac output with fewer troublesome side effects. Occasionally, vasopressors will be used to induce vasoconstriction in low cardiac output states to maintain tissue perfusion pressure. For example, phenylephrine hydrochloride (Neo-Synephrine) or norepinephrine (Levophed) is often administered as a continuous intravenous infusion to increase peripheral vascular resistance in the warm phase of septic shock.

Other Drugs

Morphine sulfate is a narcotic analgesic that is particularly useful in relieving the pain associated with AMI and in the management of cardiogenic pulmonary edema. Its profound venodilator effect increases pooling of blood in the periphery, which decreases venous return to the heart, thereby relieving pulmonary congestion. Morphine is also a mild arterial vasodilator that will reduce afterload, thereby decreasing myocardial oxygen requirements. Since the major side effects of morphine administrations are hypotension and respiratory depression, it should be administered slowly and in small 2 to 5 mg increments intravenously.[1]

Diuretics are frequently administered intravenously in the acute setting to stimulate a rapid diuresis in acute pulmonary edema or fluid volume overload. Furosemide (Lasix) and ethacrynic acid (Edecrin), the most commonly used diuretics for this purpose, inhibit the reabsorption of sodium in the proximal and distal renal tubules as well as the loop of Henle and are therefore often referred to as "loop" diuretics. Hypokalemia is a very serious side effect of this type of diruetic therapy that can be associated with tachycardia in the cardiac patient. Patients will often be given supplemental potassium chloride intravenously before administration of the diuretic if serum potassium levels are less than 4.0 mEq/L.

Although the administration of sodium bicarbonate is not considered as efficacious in cardiac arrest situations as it once was, it is nonetheless a valuable adjunct to adequate alveolar ventilation in maintaining acid-base balance. When indicated, sodium bicarbonate is usually administered as an intravenous bolus with an initial dose of 1 mEq/kg (which would be about the equivalent of one ampule or Bristojet [Bristol Meyers] for an average adult).[1] The side effect of metabolic alkalosis can be avoided by basing any subsequent dosing on the results obtained from arterial blood gas analyses.

Because the overall goal of pharmacological intervention in shock is to improve tissue perfusion and oxygen delivery to the cells, oxygen therapy should be considered an essential cardiovascular drug. Administration of oxygen will increase arterial oxygen tension and hemoglobin saturation in the presence of adequate ventilation and improve tissue oxygenation when circulation is maintained. Oxygen should also be administered any time myocardial ischemia is suspected.

REFERENCES

1. American Heart Association: Standards for cardiopulmonary resuscitation and emergency cardiac care, JAMA 255:2905, 1986.
2. American Heart Association: Textbook of advanced cardiac life support, Dallas, 1987, The Association.
3. Banasik JL and Tyler ML: The effect of prophylactic positive end-expiratory pressure on mediastinal bleeding after coronary revascularization surgery, Heart Lung 15:43, 1986.
4. Barr S: Inocor, Crit Care Nurs 5:64, 1985.
5. Bassan MM, Oded S, and Eliakim A: Improved prognosis during long-term treatment with beta-blockers after myocardial infarction: analysis of randomized trials and pooling of results, Heart Lung 13:164, 1984.
6. Bonchek LI: Basis for selecting a valve prosthesis, Cardiovasc Clin 17:107, 1987.
7. Brannon PHB and Towner SB: Ventricular failure: new therapy using the mechanical assist device, Crit Care Nurs 6:70, 1986.
8. Bregman D and Kaskel P: Advances in percutaneous intraaortic balloon pumping, Crit Care Clin 2:221, 1986.
9. Brewer CC and Markis JE: Streptokinase and tissue plasminogen activator in acute myocardial infarction, Heart Lung 15:552, 1986.
10. Catalano JT: Antiarrhythmic medications classified by their autonomic properties, Crit Care Nurse 6:44, 1986.
11. Collen D and others: Coronary thrombolysis with recombinant human tissue-type plasminogen activator: a prospective, randomized placebo-controlled trial, Circulation 70:1012, 1984.
12. Cowley MJ and others: Acute coronary events associated with percutaneous transluminal coronary angioplasty, Am J Cardiol 53:12C, 1984.
13. DeAngelis R: Amiodarone, Crit Care Nurse 6:12, 1986.
14. Dorros G and others: Percutaneous transluminal coronary angioplasty in patients with prior coronary artery bypass grafting, J Thorac Cardiovasc Surg 87:17, 1984.
15. Eberts MA: Advances in the pharmacologic management of angina pectoris, J Cardiovasc Nurs 1:15, 1986.
16. Fenton M: Intra-aortic balloon pump therapy, Crit Care Nurse 5:54, 1985.
17. Finkelmeier BA and O'Mara SR: Temporary pacing in the cardiac surgical patient, Crit Care Nurse 4:108, 1984.
18. Finkelmeier BA and Salinger MH: The atrial electrogram: its diagnostic use following cardiac surgery, Crit Care Nurse 4:42, 1984.
19. Fox J: Laser coronary angioplasty, J Cardiovasc Nurs 1:57, 1986.
20. Gershan JA and Jirika MK: Percutaneous transluminal coronary angioplasty: implications for nursing, Focus Crit Care 11:28, 1984.
21. Gurevich I: Infectious complications after open heart surgery, Heart Lung 13:472, 1984.
22. Haywood DL: Temporary A-V sequential pacing using an epicardial lead system, Crit Care Nurse 5:21, 1985.
23. Huang SK and Marcus FI: Antiarrhythmic drug therapy of ventricular arrhythmias, Current Probl Cardiol 11:1, 1986.
24. Isaacson JJ, George LT, and Brewer MJ: The effect of chest tube manipulation on mediastinal drainage, Heart Lung 15:601, 1986.
25. Jansen KJ and McFadden PM: Postoperative nursing management in patients undergoing myocardial revascularization with internal mammary artery bypass, Heart Lung 15:48, 1986.
26. Jorge E, Pae WE, and Pierce WS: Left heart and biventricular bypass, Crit Care Clin 2:267, 1986.
27. Jorge E and Pierce WS: Mechanical support or replacement of the heart, Cardiovasc Clin 17:361, 1987.
28. Kennedy JW and others: Acute myocardial infarction treated with intracoronary streptokinase: a report of the society for cardiac angiography, Am J Cardiol 55:871, 1985.
29. Kern LS: Advances in the surgical treatment of coronary artery disease, J Cardiovasc Nurs 1:1, 1986.
30. Kienzle MG and others: Antiarrhythmic drug therapy for sustained ventricular tachycardia, Heart Lung 13:614, 1984.
31. Killip T: Coronary bypass surgery—where we stand today, Drug Therap 14:71, 1984.
32. Kline EM: Recombinant tissue-type plasminogen activator in acute myocardial infarction: role of the critical care nurse, Heart Lung 16:779, 1987.
33. Lanoue AS, Snyder BA, and Galen KM: Percutaneous transluminal coronary angioplasty: nonoperative treatment of coronary artery disease, J Cardiovasc Nurs 1:30, 1986.
34. Lasater MG: Torsades des pointes etiology and treatment, Focus Crit Care 13:17, 1986.
35. Loop FD and others: Influence of the internal-mammary-artery graft on 10 year survival and other cardiac events, N Engl J Med 314:1, 1986.
36. Meier B and Gruentzig A: Learning curve for PTCA: skills, technology on patient selection, Am J Cardiol 53:65C, 1984.
37. Mercer ME: The electrophysiology study: a nursing concern, Crit Care Nurse 7:58, 1987.
38. Mulford E: Nursing perspectives for the patient receiving post-operative ventricular assistance in the critical care unit, Heart Lung 16:246, 1987.
39. Mullet K: State of the art in neurostimulation, PACE 10:162, 1987.
40. Murdock DK and others: Pacemaker malfunction: fact or artifact?, Heart Lung 15:150, 1986.
41. Nieminski KE, Kay RH, and Rubin DA: Current concepts and management of the sick sinus syndrome, Heart Lung 13:675, 1984.

42. Ong YC and Wescott BL: Intravenous fibrolytic therapy in a community hospital, Focus Crit Care 5:30, 1986.

43. Parker MM and Lemberg L: Pacemaker update 1984. Part I. Introduction to electrocardiographic analysis of pacing function and site, Heart Lung 13:315, 1984.

44. Parsonnet V, Furman S, and Smyth N: A revised code for pacemaker identification, PACE 4:401, 1981.

45. Persons CB: Transcutaneous pacing - meeting the challenge, Focus Crit Care 14:13, 1987.

46. Quaal SJ: Thrombolytic therapy: an overview, J Cardiovasc Nurs 1:45, 1986.

47. Quinless FW, Cassese M, and Atherton N: The effect of selected preoperative, intraoperative, and postoperative variables on the development of postpericardiotomy psychosis in patients undergoing open heart surgery, Heart Lung 14:334, 1985.

48. Rafalowski MM: Relationship of core temperature at time of blanket removal to subsequent core temperature in patients immediately after coronary artery bypass, Heart Lung 16:9, 1987.

49. Relman AS: Intravenous thrombolysis in acute myocardial infarction, N Engl J Med 312:915, 1985.

50. Rice V: Shock management. Part II. Pharmacologic intervention, Crit Care Nurse 5:42, 1985.

51. Rotmensch HH, Vlasses PH, and Ferguson RK: Prophylactic use of beta-adrenergic blockage in survivors of myocardial infarction, Heart Lung 13:366, 1984.

52. Sager DP: Current facts on pacemaker electromagnetic interference and their application to clinical care, Heart Lung 16:211, 1987.

53. Sipperly ME: Thrombolytic therapy update, Crit Care Nurs 5:30, 1985.

54. Smith A: Amiodarone: clinical considerations, Focus Crit Care 11:30, 1984.

55. Soroff HS, Hui J, and Giron F: Current status of external counterpulsation, Crit Care Clin 2:277, 1986.

56. Steger KE, Remy J, and Krueger S: Drug-induced torsades des pointes: case report and implications for critical care staff, Heart Lung 15:200, 1986.

57. Strauss E and Rudy EB: Tissue-plasminogen activator: a new drug for reperfusion therapy, Crit Care Nurse 6:30, 1986.

58. Sulzbach LM: The use of temporary atrial wire electrodes to record atrial electrograms in patients who had cardiac surgery, Heart Lung 14:540, 1985.

59. Taylor T: Monitoring left atrial pressure in the open-heart surgical patient, Crit Care Nurse 6:62, 1986.

60. Thielbar S: Antiarrhythmic drug therapy: an overview, Crit Care Q 7:21, 1984.

61. TIMI Study Group: The thrombolysis in myocardial infarction (TIMI) trials: phase I finding, N Engl Med 312:932, 1985.

62. Topol EJ: Clinical use of streptokinase and urokinase therapy for acute myocardial infarction, Heart Lung 16:760, 1987.

63. Touloukian JE: Calcium channel blocking agents: physiologic basis of nursing interventions, Heart Lung 14:342, 1985.

64. Vitello-Cicciu JM and others: Profile of patients requiring the use of epicardial pacing wires after coronary artery bypass surgery, Heart Lung 16:301, 1987.

65. Vlietstra RE and Holmes DR: Percutaneous transluminal coronary angioplasty, J Cardiac Surg 3:56, 1988.

66. Weiland AP and Walker WE: Physiologic principles and clinical sequelae of cardiopulmonary bypass, Heart Lung 15:34, 1986.

67. Wescott BL: Tissue plasminogen activator: a new advancement in fibrinolytic therapy, Focus Crit Care 13:22, 1986.

68. Zwerner PL and Gore JM: Thrombolytic therapy in acute myocardial infarction, J Intens Care Med 1:302, 1986.

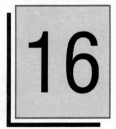

CHAPTER

Cardiovascular Care Plans

THEORETICAL BASIS AND MANAGEMENT

CHAPTER OBJECTIVES

- *Discuss the theoretical concepts related to decreased cardiac output.*
- *Identify and describe nursing interventions that are essential in the treatment of decreased cardiac output.*
- *Discuss the theoretical concepts related to tissue perfusion.*
- *Identify and describe nursing interventions that are essential in the treatment of alterations in tissue perfusion.*
- *Discuss the theoretical concepts related to activity intolerance.*
- *Identify and describe nursing interventions that are essential in the treatment of activity intolerance.*

THEORETICAL CONCEPTS OF DECREASED CARDIAC OUTPUT

Cardiac output is an important measure of the functional ability of the heart. The heart is a pump. If the blood supply to the heart is sufficient, a healthy heart will generally produce enough output to meet the body's metabolic needs. When the pump is damaged, cardiac output may drop and a form of failure ensues. Determining cardiac output is a way of measuring how well the heart is performing.

Cardiac output (CO) is defined as the amount of blood ejected by the ventricles during a one-minute period. The formula for determining CO is as follows:

$$CO = HR \times SV$$

Normal (N) = Heart rate (HR) (60-100 beats/min) × Stroke volume (SV) (60-130 ml) = 4-6 L/min (at rest)

Stroke volume (SV) is the amount of blood ejected by the ventricle each time it contracts. The formula for calculating SV is:

$$SV = \frac{CO\ in\ ml/min}{HR\ in\ beats/min}$$

The portion of blood ejected by the ventricle with each contraction is known as the ejection fraction. N = 60% to 75%; therefore 60% to 75% of total end diastolic volume is ejected with each systole. The amount of blood left in the ventricle at the end of systole is known as the end systolic volume. Decreased ventricular function results in lower ejection fractions and increased end systolic volumes.[23] Since normal CO for an individual is based on body size, a more accurate measure of ventricular function is the cardiac index (CI). The formula for determining CI is:

$$CI = \frac{CO\ in\ L/min}{Body\ surface\ area\ in\ square\ meters}$$

$$N = 2.5\text{-}4.0\ L/min/m^2$$

Nomograms are available to help determine CI, based on height and weight.

$$CO = HR \times SV$$

Preload Contractility Afterload

Many factors can alter CO, such as an increased or decreased heart rate or changes in stroke volume. Stroke volume is determined by preload, afterload, and contractility.

Determinants of Stroke Volume

Preload. Preload is the volume of blood in the ventricles at the end of diastole and is determined by the amount and distribution of intravascular volume, venous return, and atrial contraction. It is preload that determines the initial stretch on the ventricles. Preload of the right ventricle is measured by the central venous pressure (CVP), N = 0 to 6 mm Hg, and preload of the left ventricle by the pulmonary capillary wedge pressure (PCWP), N = 6 to 12 mm Hg.

Preload can be altered by inadequate intravascular volume caused by severe vomiting, diarrhea, hemorrhage, diuresis, or third spacing (fluid leaving the intravascular space

332

through leaky capillaries and moving into the interstitial spaces). Because these conditions lessen intravascular fluid, preload will drop. Preload will also decrease when vasodilation occurs and blood pools in the extremities such as in sepsis and neurogenic or anaphylactic shock. Left ventricular preload may decrease following damage to the right side of the heart. Myocardial infarction, cor pulmonale, or a pulmonary embolus may result in less blood being injected into the pulmonary artery and therefore the ventricle.

Increased intrathoracic pressure also may decrease venous return to the right ventricle. During normal inhalation, intrathoracic pressure falls slightly, allowing for blood return to the right side of the heart. When this negative pressure is lost during inhalation, as with mechanical ventilation and high inspiratory pressures, high levels of positive end-expiratory pressure (PEEP), or continuous positive airway pressure (CPAP), the venous return decreases. Tension pneumothorax decreases venous return for the same reason.[24]

In cardiac tamponade or constrictive pericarditis, the heart is surrounded by either fluid or a scarred pericardium. Increased pressure surrounding the heart decreases normal diastolic dimensions. Subsequently, pressure equalizes in all four heart chambers. Blood flow through the heart is normally maintained when enough pressure is built up in one chamber to push open the valve and force blood into the next chamber. With tamponade or constrictive pericarditis, the pressure in all four chambers equalizes and backs up into the chamber offering least resistance. CVP must increase for flow to continue. With the rise in right atrial pressure, venous return decreases and CO decreases.[25]

Afterload. Afterload is the pressure the ventricles must pump against to eject blood. The degree of afterload depends on the condition of the semilunar valves, the patency of the outflow tracts, and resistance in the pulmonary and systemic circulation. Left ventricular afterload is dependent upon aortic valve condition and the resistance of the systemic circulation. Constricted blood vessels increase afterload, and dilated blood vessels decrease afterload.

Afterload becomes a critical factor in conditions in which left ventricular function is impaired, such as in congestive heart failure, cardiomyopathy, or myocardial infarction. Because these conditions impair ventricular contraction, CO can fall to a level at which sympathetic nervous stimulation triggers peripheral arterioconstriction. This, unfortunately, increases afterload, further worsening the situation. If the weakened ventricle cannot overcome the high afterload, CO will drop further.

The reverse situation can be seen in septic shock in which blood vessel dilation reduces afterload and increases cardiac output. The formula to determine left ventricular (LV) afterload is as follows:

Systemic vascular resistance (SVR) = mean arterial pressure (MAP) in mm Hg − central venous pressure (CVP) in mm Hg × 80 divided by the cardiac output (CO) in liters per minute.

$$SVR = \frac{MAP \ mm \ Hg - CVP \ mm \ Hg}{CO \ in \ LPM} \times 80$$

$$N = 800 - 1400 \ dynes/sec/cm^{-5}$$

$$Mean \ arterial \ pressure = \frac{systolic \ BP - diastolic \ BP}{3}$$

added to the diastolic BP

$$MAP = \frac{SBP - DBP}{3} + DBP$$

The right ventricular afterload depends on the condition of the pulmonic valve and the resistance in the pulmonary circulation. Chronic pulmonary disease can result in a constricted pulmonary vascular bed that will increase right ventricular afterload.

Pulmonary vascular resistance (PVR) = pulmonary artery (PA) mean in mm Hg − pulmonary capillary wedge pressure in mm Hg (PCWP) divided by the CO in liters per minute.

$$PVR = \frac{PAP \ mean - PCWP}{CO \ liters/minute} \times 80$$
$$N \times 100 = 250 \ dynes/sec/cm^{-5}$$

Contractility. The contractility or the inotropic state of the heart is the shortening ability of cardiac muscle fibers that determine the pumping ability of the heart. The basic principle of contractility is the Frank-Starling law of the heart, which states: The more the cardiac muscle fibers are stretched during diastole, the stronger the next contraction will be. This is true within limits. Fibers can be stretched only so far before they lose resiliency and the ability to return to prestretched levels. Therefore increased preload in a healthy heart will increase cardiac output. Increased preload in a heart that has lost its elasticity may result in elevated central venous and pulmonary artery pressures and decreased cardiac output.[30] The sympathetic nervous system exerts a positive inotropic effect on the heart, whereas the parasympathetic nervous system has a negative inotropic effect. Therefore drugs used to treat decreased contractility such as occurs in left ventricular failure have a positive inotropic effect. Drugs that decrease contractility have a negative inotropic effect and block action of the sympathetic nervous system or the action of calcium.

Heart rate. An additional determinant of CO is the heart rate (HR). The autonomic nervous system largely controls the heart rate in response to metabolic demands. Stimulation of the parasympathetic nervous system decreases heart rate, whereas sympathetic stimulation increases heart rate.

The HR can normally increase from a resting level of 60 to 100 beats/min to approximately 180 beats/min through sympathetic stimulation. Rates higher than this are not useful for increasing CO, because the decreased diastolic filling time will eventually result in decreased stroke volume. Thus supraventricular tachycardia can increase CO up to a point, after which it will decrease CO. Heart rate usually rises secondary to metabolic demands, such as increased exercise, fear, pain, stress, hyperthermia, congestive heart failure, or infection. Generally, the cause of the increased rate is treated, not the rate itself, unless it is higher than 150 beats/min.

It is unusual for a sinus tachycardia to result in syncope, unless the rate is extremely rapid or there is underlying heart disease. (CO may, however, at a heart rate of 120 to 140 beats/min, decrease enough to cause symptoms in older, nonathletic persons with heart disease.)[23] An additional determinant of preload is atrial contraction. Normally atrial contraction constitutes 25% to 30% of the preload. Loss of atrial kick, such as in atrial fibrillation, can decrease stroke volume 10% to 30%. Atrial fibrillation decreases CO by three mechanisms: (1) ineffective atrial contraction, (2) a rapid ventricular response that decreases ventricular filling time, and (3) a slow ventricular response that may not produce adequate CO to meet the body's oxygen needs. Atrial flutter can decrease CO for the same reasons.

Junctional rhythms can decrease cardiac output secondary to a slow rate and inappropriately timed contractions. With heart blocks, the hemodynamic effect is determined by the rate. In third-degree heart block, output is usually decreased because of the slow rate and loss of atrioventricular synchronous contractions. Premature ventricular contractions that are infrequent usually cause no problems, except in the case of myocardial infarction, when they may lead to ventricular tachycardia or fibrillation. The latter decreases CO secondary to decreased ventricular filling time.[6]

To determine measures necessary to optimize cardiac output, heart rate, preload, afterload, and contractility must be considered. Any of these parameters can be altered to increase output.

Decreased Cardiac Output related to supraventricular tachycardia

DEFINING CHARACTERISTICS

- Sudden drop in blood pressure
- Atrial and/or ventricular rate > 100
- Decreased mentation
- Decreased urine output
- Chest pain
- Dyspnea

OUTCOME CRITERIA

- Systolic blood pressure is > 100.
- Mean arterial pressure (MAP) is > 80.
- Ventricular rate is < 100.
- Sensorium is intact.
- Urine output is > 30 ml/hr.

NURSING INTERVENTIONS *AND RATIONALE*

1. Continue to monitor the assessment parameters listed under "Defining Characteristics."
2. Carefully distinguish supraventricular tachycardia from ventricular tachycardia. Monitoring the patient in lead MCL_1 *may assist in distinguishing ventricular ectopy from aberrancy.*
3. Follow critical care emergency standing orders regarding the administration of supraventricular antidysrhythmic agents, such as verapamil, quinidine, procainamide, propranolol, edrophonium, digoxin, and phenylephrine.
4. Consider positioning patient supine *to increase preload.*
5. Identify precipitating factors when possible, such as emotional stress, caffeine, nicotine, and sympathomimetic drugs and intervene to reduce or eliminate their effect.
6. Assess apical-radial pulse *to identify deficits indica-*

ting nonperfused beats. Monitor amplitude of peripheral pulses *to ascertain perfusion to extremities.*
7. Monitor arterial blood pressure *to determine symptomatic decompensation.*
8. With physician collaboration, consider carotid sinus massage or Valsalva maneuver, *thereby increasing vagal tone.*
9. Anticipate possibility of synchronized cardioversion or overdrive pacing.
10. For atrial fibrillation that is either spontaneously, pharmacologically, or electrically converted, monitor for signs of cerebral, pulmonary, and/or peripheral thromboembolization as a result of liberation of mural thrombi.
11. If patient is hypoxemic, or if dysrhythmia is suspected to be a result of or exacerbated by ischemia, administer oxygen observing the following principles:
    - Without physician collaboration, liter flow should be no greater than 2 L/min via nasal prongs in patients whose pulmonary history is either unknown or reveals a pattern of chronic CO_2 retention. *Administration of oxygen at concentrations higher than 2 L/min via nasal prongs may induce CO_2 narcosis in patients who chronically retain CO_2.*
    - Oxygen should be administered with the goal of achieving a PaO_2 no greater than 95 mm Hg *to avoid toxic concentrations of oxygen.*
    - Observe caution when administering oxygen at an FIO_2 greater than 40% *in view of the higher risk for oxygen toxicity.*
12. Assess serum electrolyte levels, especially potassium and calcium, because *increased or decreased electrolyte levels may exacerbate the dysrhythmia or may impair treatment of the dysrhythmia.*

Decreased Cardiac Output related to relative excess* of preload and afterload secondary to impaired ventricular contractility

DEFINING CHARACTERISTICS

- Systolic blood pressure (SBP) < 100
- Mean arterial pressure (MAP) < 80
- Change in mentation
- Decreased urine output
- Cardiac index < 2.5
- Pulmonary artery wedge pressure (PAWP) > 15
- Pulmonary artery diastolic (PADP) pressure > 15
- Bibasilar fluid crackles
- Faint peripheral pulses
- Ventricular gallop rhythm (S₃)
- Skin cool, pale, moist
- Activity intolerance

OUTCOME CRITERIA

- Cardiac index is 2.5-4.0.
- SBP is > 90.
- MAP is > 80.
- PAWP and PADP are < 15.

NURSING INTERVENTIONS *AND RATIONALE*

The following interventions reduce preload

1. Continue to monitor the assessment parameters listed under "Defining Characteristics."
2. Implement fluid restriction.
3. Double concentrate intravenous drug drips when possible *to decrease the amount of volume infused to the patient.*
4. Position patient with extremities dependent *to pool blood in the extremities, thus decreasing preload.*

5. With physician collaboration, administer diuretics.
6. Titrate venous vasodilators and inotropic drips, per protocol, to desired SBP, MAP, PAWP, and/or PADP. Withhold and/or change drip rate when SBP, MAP, PAWP, and/or PADP begin to drop.

The following interventions reduce afterload

1. Intervene to reduce anxiety and *thereby limit catecholamine release:* administer intravenous MSO₄ per protocol and titrate to MAP or SBP, relaxation techniques, imagery (See care plan on Anxiety, Chapter 48).
2. Titrate arterial vasodilator drips to attain desired SBP, PAWP, and/or PADP. Change drip rate when SBP, PAWP, and/or PADP stabilize or begin to drop.
3. Anticipate possibility of intraaortic balloon pumping.

The following interventions reduce myocardial oxygen consumption

1. Absolute bed rest *to decrease metabolic demand.*
2. Consider slackening activity restrictions if such restrictions precipitate anxiety. *Anxiety stimulates the sympathetic outpouring of catecholamines and thereby increases myocardial oxygen consumption.*
3. *Ensure that patient and family understand routine of critical care unit and explain all care given to patient to increase patient comfort level and to decrease catecholamine release associated with fear of being in an unknown environment.*

Relative excess of preload and afterload refers not to an actual increase in these volumes, but rather to the inability of the ventricle to handle normal volumes because of impaired ventricular function. Therefore the normal volumes become "excessive" to the poorly functioning ventricle.

Decreased Cardiac Output related to decreased preload secondary to mechanical ventilation with or without PEEP

DEFINING CHARACTERISTICS

- Sudden drop in SBP, PAWP, or PADP corresponding to the application of mechanical ventilation or PEEP, or changes in tidal volume delivery or level of PEEP.

OUTCOME CRITERIA

- SBP is > 90, MAP is > 80.
- PAWP, PAD are > 6.

NURSING INTERVENTIONS *AND RATIONALE*

1. Continue to monitor the assessment parameters listed under "Defining Characteristics."

2. Monitor vital organ perfusion (through assessment of urine output and mentation, for example) carefully, because *some degree of reduction in cardiac output will coexist with the successful application of mechanical ventilation and/or PEEP.*
3. Position patient supine *to increase preload and therefore cardiac output.*
4. With physician collaboration, consider increasing the administration of parenteral fluids to achieve ideal preload. *(The ideal preload may be that which existed before the application of mechanical ventilation and/or PEEP).*

Decreased Cardiac Output related to atrioventricular (AV) heart block

DEFINING CHARACTERISTICS

- Systolic blood pressure < 100
- Mean arterial pressure (MAP) < 80
- Ventricular rate < 60
- Decreased mentation or syncope
- Decreased urine output

OUTCOME CRITERIA

- Systolic blood pressure is > 90.
- MAP is > 80.
- Ventricular rate is > 60.
- The patient is awake and responsive.
- Urine output is > 30 ml/hr.

NURSING INTERVENTIONS *AND RATIONALE*

First-degree AV Block

1. Continue to monitor the assessment parameters listed under "Defining Characteristics."
2. Monitor closely, measuring P-R intervals *to determine further prolongation, which would suggest progression of heart block.*
3. With physician collaboration, consider withholding supraventricular antidysrhythmic agents such as digitalis, quinidine, beta blocking agents, and calcium channel blockers.

Second-Degree AV Block—Mobitz I (Wenckebach pattern)

1. Continue to monitor the assessment parameters listed under "Defining Characteristics."
2. Monitor for symptomatic decompensation resulting from slow ventricular rate (rare).
3. While symptomatic, position patient supine *to increase preload and therefore cardiac output.*

4. Monitor for progression to complete heart block.
5. With physician collaboration, consider withholding digitalis.
6. Eliminate sources of vagal stimulation. *Vagal stimulation increases the delay in conduction at the AV node.*

Second-Degree AV Block—Mobitz II

1. Continue to monitor the assessment parameters listed under "Defining Characteristics."
2. Monitor closely for symptomatic decompensation as a result of slow ventricular rate (common).
3. While symptomatic, position patient supine *to increase preload and therefore cardiac output.*
4. Monitor for progression of existing block, such as 2:1, 3:1, 4:1 conduction and for progression to complete heart block.
5. Follow critical care emergency standing orders regarding the administration of positive chronotropic agents, such as atropine, or isoproterenol.
6. Anticipate possibility of pacemaker insertion.

Third-Degree (Complete) AV Block

1. Continue to monitor the assessment parameters listed under "Defining Characteristics."
2. Monitor closely for symptomatic decompensation resulting from slow ventricular rate (common).
3. While symptomatic, position patient supine *to increase preload and therefore cardiac output.*
4. Follow critical care emergency standing orders regarding the administration of isoproterenol.
5. Anticipate the necessity of pacemaker insertion or use of external pacemaker (for example, Pace-Aid).

Decreased Cardiac Output related to hemopericardium secondary to open heart surgery

DEFINING CHARACTERISTICS

- Cardiac output < 5
- Cardiac index < 2.5
- Elevated PAWP, PADP, or CVP
- Narrowed pulse pressure
- Pulsus paradoxus
- Muffled heart sounds
- Distended neck veins
- Decreasing SBP or MAP
- Tachycardia
- Enlarged cardiac silhouette on chest film

OUTCOME CRITERIA

- Cardiac output is > 5.
- Cardiac index is > 2.5.
- PAWP, PADP, CVP are reduced to baseline.
- Crisp heart sounds are heard.
- SBP is > 100, MAP is > 80.

- Heart rate is reduced to baseline.
- Cardiac silhouette is reduced to baseline.

NURSING INTERVENTIONS *AND RATIONALE*

1. Continue to monitor the assessment parameters outlined under "Defining Characteristics."
2. Monitor mediastinal tube drainage for sudden cessation and/or increase. *Either event is to be considered highly suggestive of impending cardiac tamponade.*
3. Milk mediastinal tubes per protocol *to ensure continual patency.*
4. Titrate vasodilator drips *to keep SBP below level at which graft(s) or anastomoses may leak or tear (usually SBP kept < 150).*
5. Anticipate the necessity of either bedside pericardiocentesis or return to surgery.

Decreased Cardiac Output related to decreased preload secondary to fluid volume deficit

DEFINING CHARACTERISTICS

- CO < 5
- CI < 2.5
- PAWP, PADP, CVP less than normal or less than baseline
- Tachycardia
- Narrowed pulse pressure
- SBP < 100
- Mean arterial pressure (MAP) < 80
- Urine < 30/hr
- Skin pale, cool, moist
- Apprehensiveness

OUTCOME CRITERIA

- CO is > 5.
- CI is > 2.5.
- PAWP, PADP, CVP are normal or back to baseline level.
- Pulse is normal or back to baseline.
- SBP is > 90.
- MAP is > 80.
- Urine is > 30/hr.

NURSING INTERVENTIONS *AND RATIONALE*

For Active Blood Loss

1. Continue to monitor the assessment parameters listed under "Defining Characteristics." Additionally, a serum lactate level > 3 mosm is felt to represent cellular perfusion failure at its earliest stage.
2. Secure airway and administer oxygen.
3. Position patient supine with legs elevated *to increase preload and therefore cardiac output.* Avoid Trendelenburg's position because *this position causes abdominal viscera to exert pressure against the diaphragm, thereby limiting diaphragmatic descent and inhalation.* Consider low Fowler's position with legs elevated for patients with head injury *to avoid increases in intracranial pressure.*
4. For fluid repletion use the 3:1 rule, replacing 3 parts of fluid for every unit of blood lost.
5. Administer solutions using the fluid challenge technique: infuse precise amounts of fluid (usually 5 to 20 ml/min) over 10-minutes periods and monitor cardiac loading pressures serially to determine successful challenging. If the PAWP or PADP elevates more than 7 mm Hg above beginning level, the infusion should be stopped. If the PAWP or PADP rises only to 3 mm Hg above baseline, or falls, another fluid challenge should be given.

6. Assess for signs and symptoms of fluid overload once fluid replacement has begun. These may include elevations above normal of PAP or CVP levels, pulmonary crackles, or dyspnea.
7. Replete fluids first before considering use of vasopressors since *vasopressors increase myocardial oxygen consumption out of proportion to the reestablishment of coronary perfusion in the early phases of treatment.*
8. When blood available or indicated, replace with fresh packed red cells and fresh-frozen plasma *to keep clotting factors intact.*
9. Move or reposition patient minimally *to decrease or limit tissue oxygen demands.*
10. Evaluate patient's anxiety level and intervene via patient education or sedation *to decrease tissue oxygen demands.*
11. Be alert to the possibility of development of adult respiratory distress syndrome (ARDS) and/or disseminated intravascular coagulation (DIC) in the ensuing 72 hours.

For Dehydration

1. Continue to monitor the assessment parameters listed under "Defining Characteristics."
2. Position patient supine with legs elevated *to increase preload and therefore cardiac output.* Avoid Trendelenburg's position, because this position causes abdominal viscera to exert pressure against the diaphragm thereby limiting diaphragmatic descent and inhalation. Consider low Fowler's position with legs elevated for patients with head injury to *avoid increases in intracranial pressure.*
3. Calculate the patient's 24-hour fluid requirements per BSA and replete with the appropriate electrolyte solution.
4. Administer solutions using the fluid challenge technique: infuse precise amounts of fluid (usually 5 to 20 ml/min) over 10-minute periods and monitor cardiac loading pressure serially to determine successful challenging. If the PAWP or PADP elevates more than 7 mm Hg above beginning level, the infusion should be stopped. If the PAWP or PADP rises only to 3 mm Hg above baseline, or falls, another fluid challenge should be given.
5. Assess for signs and symptoms of fluid overload once fluid replacement has begun. These may include, elevations of PAP or CVP to above normal levels, pulmonary crackles, or dyspnea.
6. Replete fluids first before considering use of vasopressors *since vasopressors increase myocardial oxygen consumption out of proportion to the re-establishment of coronary perfusion in the early phase of treatment.*

Decreased Cardiac Output related to ventricular tachycardia

DEFINING CHARACTERISTICS

- Sudden drop in blood pressure
- Syncope
- Loss of consciousness
- Faint or absent peripheral pulses

OUTCOME CRITERIA

- Systolic blood pressure is > 90.
- Mean arterial pressure (MAP) is > 70.
- The patient is awake and responsive.
- Peripheral pulses are palpable.

NURSING INTERVENTIONS *AND RATIONALE*

1. Continue to monitor the assessment parameters listed under "Defining Characteristics."
2. Carefully distinguish ventricular tachycardia from supraventricular tachycardia. Monitoring the patient in lead MCL_1 *may assist in distinguishing ventricular ectopy from aberrancy.*
3. Monitor and treat the "warning dysrhythmias" (that is, >6 premature ventricular contractions [PVCs] per minute, multifocal PVCs, R on T phenomenon, couplets, bursts of ventricular tachycardia, bigeminy, trigeminy).
4. Assess serum electrolyte levels, especially potassium *as increased or decreased electrolyte levels may exacerbate the dysrhythmia or may impair treatment of the dysrhythmia.*
5. Follow critical care emergency standing orders regarding the administration of ventricular antidysrhythmic agents, such as lidocaine, bretylium, and procainamide.
6. For asymptomatic ventricular tachycardia, treat with lidocaine. For symptomatic ventricular tachycardia, treat with synchronized cardioversion. For pulseless ventricular tachycardia, treat as ventricular fibrillation and defibrillate. (See ACLS algorithms in Appendix B.)
7. Position patient supine *to increase preload.*
8. Anticipate possibility that sporadic ventricular dysrhythmias may progress to ventricular tachycardia or ventricular fibrillation and be prepared to treat with implementation of synchronized cardioversion and defibrillation, respectively.
9. Anticipate possibility of cardiac standstill and activation of resuscitation protocol.
10. When safe rhythm is reestablished, carefully assess for femoral and carotid pulsations *to rule out electromechanical dissociation.*
11. Identify precipitating factors when possible, such as hypoxia, electrolyte abnormalities, drug toxicity (especially amrinone, digitalis, quinidine, disopyramide, procainamide, phenothiazines, tricyclic and tetracyclic antidepressants), or recent MI, and intervene to reduce or eliminate their effect.

Decreased Cardiac Output related to decreased preload secondary to septicemia

DEFINING CHARACTERISTICS

- Tachycardia > 100
- Skin dry, warm, flushed (early stage); cold, clammy, cyanotic (late stage)
- CO, CI, elevated (early stage); CO, CI, decreased (late stage)
- PA pressures decreased (early stage), elevated (late stage)
- SBP, MAP, less than normal or baseline (early); profound hypotension (late stage)
- Urine output < 30 ml/hr

OUTCOME CRITERIA

- Heart rate is normal or back to baseline.
- CO is > 5, CI is > 2.5, SBP is > 90, MAP is > 80.
- Urine output > 30 ml/hr.

NURSING INTERVENTIONS *AND RATIONALE*

1. Continue to monitor the assessment parameters listed under "Defining Characteristics." Additionally, a serum lactate level > 3 mosm is felt to represent cellular perfusion failure at its earliest stage.
2. Secure airway and administer oxygen.
3. Position patient supine with legs elevated *to increase preload and therefore cardiac output in late-stage shock.*
4. Administer intravenous solutions as prescribed using the fluid challenge technique: infuse precise amounts of fluid (usually 5 to 20 ml/min) over 10-minute periods and monitor cardiac loading pressures serially to determine successful challenging. If the PAWP or PADP elevates more than 7 mm Hg above beginning levels, the infusion should be stopped. If the PAWP or PADP rises only to 3 mm Hg above baseline, or falls, another fluid challenge should be given.
5. Assess for signs and symptoms of fluid overload once fluid replacement has begun. These may include elevations above normal of PAP or CVP levels, pulmonary crackles, or dyspnea.
6. With physician collaboration, administer intravenous antimicrobials and closely monitor their effectiveness and specific side effects. Carefully assess patient for hypersensitivity reaction to antimicrobials.
6. With physician collaboration, administer vasopressor agents and positive inotropic drugs *to maintain perfusion and cardiac output.*
7. With physician collaboration, administer steroids.

Decreased Cardiac Output related to vasodilation and bradycardia secondary to sympathetic blockade of neurogenic (spinal) shock following spinal cord injury above T-6 level

DEFINING CHARACTERISTICS

- Postural hypotension, such as turning from supine to prone
- SBP < 90 mm Hg or below patient's norm
- Decreased PAP, PAD, and PCWP
- Decreased cardiac index
- Decreased SVR
- Bradycardia
- Cardiac dysrhythmias
- Decreased urinary output
- Hypothermia as a result of inability to retain body heat (See section on Neurological Alterations for the assessment and treatment of other neurological manifestations of spinal shock.)

OUTCOME CRITERIA

- SBP is > 90 mm Hg or within patient's norm.
- Fainting/dizziness with position change is absent.
- <10 mm Hg DBP drop with position change.
- HR is 60-100 beats/min.
- <20 beats/min HR increase with position change.
- PAP is 4 to 6 mm Hg.
- PCWP is 4 to 12 mm Hg.
- PAD is 8 to 14 mm Hg.
- SVR is 950 to 1300 dynes/sec/cm.
- Cardiac index is 2.5 to 4.0.
- Urinary output is > 30 ml/hr.
- Normothermia is present.

NURSING INTERVENTIONS *AND RATIONALE*

1. Continue to monitor the assessment parameters listed under "Defining Characteristics."
2. Implement measures *to prevent episodes of postural hypotension.*
   - Change patient's position slowly.
   - Apply antiembolic stockings *to promote venous return.*
   - Perform range of motion exercises every 2 hours *to prevent venous pooling.*
   - Collaborate with physical therapy regarding use of a tilt table *to progress patient from supine to upright position.*
3. Administer crystalloid intravenous fluids using fluid challenge technique: infuse precise amounts of fluid (usually 5 to 20 ml/min) over 10-minute periods; monitor cardiac loading pressures serially to determine successful challenging.
4. Anticipate the adminstration of colloids.
5. Anticipate administration of vasopressors if fluid challenges ineffective.
6. Monitor cardiac rhythm. Be especially vigilant during vagal stimulating procedures such as suctioning *because serious bradycardia can result.*
7. Administer atropine per critical care emergency standing orders for symptomatic bradycardia.
8. Maintain normothermia by increasing temperature in patient's room and applying blankets. Avoid use of electronic warming devices *because of decreased peripheral blood flow and sensation.*

THEORETICAL CONCEPTS OF ALTERED TISSUE PERFUSION

The function of cells throughout the body depends on an adequate supply of oxygen and nutrients and the removal of waste products. Therefore tissue perfusion is the ultimate goal of circulation. Perfusion is determined by the body's metabolic needs, primarily the need to provide adequate oxygen delivery to all cells. Flow to any organ depends on enough pressure within the system to overcome the vascular resistance of the organ. Blood flows from areas of higher pressure to areas of lower pressure; this pressure gradient must be maintained for flow to progress from one area to another. In the body blood flows from the higher pressure arterial system (average pressure 100 mm Hg) to the low pressure venous system (RA pressure 0 mm Hg.). Thus blood flows as the pressure progressively declines.[19]

The arterial blood pressure is the major determinant of perfusion to an organ. Conditions that would alter perfusion to tissues are: (1) closure or occlusion of a vessel that impedes or prevents delivery of blood, (2) inadequate car-diac output, (3) constriction of a vessel or high systemic vascular resistance preventing delivery of blood, and (4) decreased systemic vascular resistance resulting in lowered arterial pressure inadequate for perfusion.[1]

Flow to any organ depends on the arterial blood pressure and the vascular resistance of that organ. Vascular resistance is predominantly related to the diameter of the blood vessels. Several mechanisms, mainly neural, humoral, and local regulation, have the ability to change vascular resistance. Study of these mechanisms will help in understanding circulatory control.

Control Mechanisms

Neural control

Autonomic regulation. The sympathetic nervous system, via the transmitter norepinephrine, has an adrenergic effect on the heart and blood vessels that results in an increase in heart rate, contractility, and constriction of blood vessels. This effect is mediated through alpha and beta receptors.

Alpha receptors are primarily located in blood vessels

where their stimulation results in vasoconstriction.

Beta receptors are located in blood vessels and in the myocardium. Beta-1 receptors, located in the myocardium, stimulate the heart to increase its rate and contractility. Beta-2 receptors, located in the peripheral blood vessels, cause vasodilation when stimulated. Catecholamines can activate both alpha and beta receptors. The effect is dependent on the dose and the target organ.[1]

The parasympathetic nervous system has a cholinergic effect. Acetylcholine vasodilates blood vessels, allowing more blood to pool in the periphery and less to return to the heart.

Effect of medications. Some medications (for example, vasopressors) act by mimicking the sympathetic nervous system. When these drugs are given to combat hypotension, blood pressure is maintained by constriction of peripheral blood vessels. Subsequently, blood is shunted from the extremities to vital areas such as the brain, heart, and kidneys. If vasopressor doses are high enough, perfusion to the extremities will be diminished, resulting in pale or cyanotic digits.

Pressor and chemoreceptors. The vasomotor center is located in the lower third of the pons and the upper medulla. The vasomotor center responds to signals sent by: (1) afferent neurons of baroreceptors located in the heart, lungs, and arteries, (2) chemoreceptors located in the carotid body, aortic arch, and skeletal muscle, and (3) thermoreceptors. Baroreceptors located in the aortic arch, carotid sinus, atria, vena cava, and pulmonary arteries respond to changes in mean arterial pressure. When baroreceptors, which are influenced by stretch, sense an elevated mean arterial pressure, messages are sent to the vasomotor center, which inhibits sympathetic stimulation. There is a decrease in sympathetic vasoconstrictor tone and in sympathetic tone to the heart, and this results in a tendency for the blood pressure to fall or return toward normal.

A drop of pressure over a baroreceptor causes the opposite effect and leads to an increase in sympathetic activity. This is a rapid response system occurring within seconds.

Chemoreceptors are stimulated by reduction in arterial oxygen concentration, increases in carbon dioxide concentration, and elevation in hydrogen ion concentration. The principle role of chemoreceptors is to increase ventilation; however, they also respond to pressure changes, possibly because decreased tissue oxygenation occurs with decreased perfusion pressure. Stimulation results in increased vascular resistance in skeletal muscle. Chemoreceptors also respond promptly but less effectively than baroreceptors.

Humoral control. Humoral regulation means regulation by substances in body fluids such as hormones and ions. An example of humoral control can be seen when atrial pressure falls. A decrease in atrial pressure causes the kidney to release renin. Release of renin leads to formation of angiotensin 1. Angiotensin 1 is then converted in the pulmonary circulation to angiotensin 2, a potent vasoconstrictor. In addition, angiotensin 2 stimulates release of aldosterone from the adrenal cortex, which results in sodium and water retention and increases fluid volume. Response time for this system is 20 to 30 minutes.[30]

Control of intravascular volume. Urinary output of water and electrolytes is related to arterial pressure. With elevated pressure urine output increases, and with decreased pressure urine output drops. Intravascular volume is determined by intake, sodium, insensible water loss, and urinary output. A decreased intravascular volume, such as might occur with dehydration, reduces renal output of sodium and water. If the fluid is replaced and pressure normalizes, the kidney will again maintain an output related to intake (in the normal kidney). This system requires a long time to normalize pressure (days to weeks) without assistance of other control mechanisms.[30]

Local control. Local factors that regulate vascular resistance and therefore perfusion to specific organs in response to increased demand for oxygen or nutrients are also important. The muscle is an example of local control. Blood flow to the muscle can be greatly increased during exercise to meet the increased need for oxygen. Neural and humoral factors play a larger part in regulating blood flow at rest and exert almost no effect during maximal exercise.

Some organs show no relationship between metabolic activity and blood flow. The kidney is an example. Flow to the kidney is much greater than that demanded for delivery of nutrients. The kidney filters a large proportion of the cardiac output on a continuous basis, and its vascular resistance is low.[30]

Occlusion of a Vessel

Occlusion of a vessel can occur slowly, as with atherosclerosis, or rapidly, as the result of an embolus. Slow occlusion allows the development of collateral circulation and other compensatory measures, whereas massive acute insult can result in shock or sudden death. The results of thrombosis are most evident when an artery is involved. If an artery is occluded, tissues served by that artery will lose their blood supply. Venous thrombosis generally has less-serious consequences, unless the vein thrombosed is a major one and local swelling results. Occlusion of smaller veins causes diversion of the blood supply into adjacent veins for transport back to the heart. The most serious consequence of venous thrombi occurs when pieces break off and travel to other areas. When this occurs, the pieces travel through the venous system to the right side of the heart and then to the pulmonary artery and smaller vessels. Most venous emboli terminate as pulmonary emboli.

Emboli that lodge in the arterial system usually originate in the left side of the heart or the large arteries. Travel to the brain results in a cerebral embolus; travel to the renal artery results in possible failure of one kidney.

Pulmonary thromboembolism is fairly common. Many substances can impact in pulmonary arteries and occlude them: blood clots, air, amniotic fluid, fat (from fractured long bones), tumor cells, ova of parasites, and endocarditic vegetations from the right side of the heart.[14]

In nearly all cases the embolus originates as deep vein thrombosis (DVT) in the proximal deep venous system in the lower legs. A large number of disorders predispose to thromboembolism. Among those at risk are patients who have a history of venous thrombosis, thrombocytopenia, a recent surgical procedure (particularly orthopedic), trauma to the lower extremities, congestive heart failure, and a malignancy and those who are on bed rest and contraceptive agents and are obese or elderly (atherosclerosis).[27]

Potential for Altered Peripheral Tissue Perfusion

RISK FACTORS
- Vasopressor therapy

DEFINING CHARACTERISTICS
- Pale or cyanotic digits
- Ischemic pain
- Delayed capillary refill
- Weak peripheral pulses

OUTCOME CRITERIA
- Digits are free from pallor or cyanosis.
- Ischemic pain is absent.
- Capillary refill is immediate.
- Peripheral pulses are full and equal.

NURSING INTERVENTIONS *AND RATIONALE*

1. Continue to monitor the assessment parameters listed under "Defining Characteristics."
2. Careful evaluation of the adequacy of peripheral perfusion is essential in patients receiving infusions of the following vasopressor drugs. Additionally, *extravasation of these agents into tissues results in localized ischemic necrosis and therefore are infused through central lines when possible.* Dopamine infusions: at dosages > 10 mcg/kg/min, alpha adrenergic receptors are stimulated *producing moderate peripheral vasoconstriction;* at dosages > 20 µg/kg/min intense peripheral vasoconstriction results, *producing serious perfusion alterations.* Levarterenol bitartrate infusions: at all dosages alpha adrenergic receptors are stimulated *producing the potential for perfusion alterations.*
3. Avoid high-dose vasopressor therapy. Titrate vasopressor drips to achieve and maintain SBP of 90 or MAP above 70. Further augmentation of SBP or MAP should be accomplished by means of other modalities.
4. Immediate physician notification is indicated at the earliest sign of peripheral perfusion alterations.

Potential for Altered Peripheral Tissue Perfusion

RISK FACTORS
- Orthopedic injury or manipulation of an extremity
- Orthopedic devices applied to an extremity

DEFINING CHARACTERISTICS
- Weak and/or unequal peripheral pulses
- Delayed capillary refill
- Ischemic pain distal to injury/manipulation/device
- Cool skin distal to injury/manipulation/device
- Paresthesias

OUTCOME CRITERIA
- Peripheral pulses are full and equal bilaterally.
- Capillary refill is equal bilaterally.
- There is no ischemic pain distal to injury/manipulation/device.
- There is equal skin temperature distal to injury/manipulation/device.
- Paresthesias are absent.

NURSING INTERVENTIONS *AND RATIONALE*

1. Continue to monitor the assessment parameters listed under "Defining Characteristics."
2. Elevate extremity above heart level *to promote venous and lymphatic drainage, thereby reducing interstitial swelling.*
3. Apply ice over or beside area of injury or manipulation for the first 24 hours. Follow a schedule of ice on 20 minutes, off 20 minutes, repeat. *This optimizes the therapeutic effect of ice in prevention and/or reducing swelling.*
4. Maintain patency of wound drainage device *to prevent excessive interstitial swelling or blood accumulation.*
5. Assess dressings for fit and loosen if constrictive to superficial blood vessels.

THEORETICAL CONCEPTS OF ACTIVITY INTOLERANCE

After varying lengths of bed rest, patients are often unable to tolerate activity without displaying symptoms of hypotension, tachycardia, and dyspnea (see box below). Hundreds of research studies have been conducted to determine the reason for this activity intolerance.

When the patient is in the supine position, more than 50% of the total blood volume is contained in the systemic veins, about 30% in the intrathroacic vessel compartments, and less than 15% to 20% in the systemic arteries. During changes in posture from standing to supine to head-down tilt, great quantities of blood shift between extreme ends, while the middle or abdominal region remains relatively unaffected.[8] When the patient assumes an upright position, approximately 500 ml of blood is displaced into dependent parts of the body, primarily to the leg veins. Most of this shifting blood volume is derived from the intrathoracic vascular compartment. This shift in blood from the intrathoracic vessels to the dependent parts of the body results in a reduction of preload, ventricular end diastolic volume, and stroke volume (to about 50% to 60% of normal). Because of the fall in CO, compensatory mechanisms are activated primarily via baroreceptors, which increase heart rate and maintain blood pressure.

Effects of bed rest were found to be decreased cardiac output,[22,29] increased heart rate,[22,29] decreased total blood volume,[22] decreased red cell mass,[22] decreased total body water,[9,22] decreased intracellular fluid volume,[9,22] decreased plasma volume,[6,22,29] decreased stroke volume,[6,22,29] decreased left ventricular end diastolic volume,[6,11] and decreased maximal oxygen uptake.[6,11,22,29]

During research studies, maximal oxygen uptake was considered an important parameter to monitor during bed rest and activity. This is a measure of the ability of the respiratory and circulatory systems to deliver oxygen to the tissues. It represents the maximal rate at which oxygen can be delivered to the tissues and is the equivalent of the aerobic work power of the body.[22]

Saltin and others[22] studied the effects of 20 days of bed rest on six healthy young men. The most striking results were found to be the greatly decreased ability of the circulatory system to adapt to exercise after bed rest. Compared with levels before bed rest, maximal cardiac output fell by 26%, heart rate increased, and stroke volume decreased 30%. Maximal oxygen uptake ($\dot{V}_{O_2}$ max) decreased 28%.

Stremel and others[29] studied bed rest deconditioning in seven healthy men (19 to 22 years) following three 14-day periods of controlled activity in the supine position. The three exercise regimens consisted of: (1) 14 days of two 30 minute periods daily of intermittent static exercise at 21% maximal leg extension force; (2) 14 days of two 30 minute periods of dynamic bicycle ergometer exercise daily at 68% of $\dot{V}_{O_2}$ max; and (3) 14 days of no exercise.

They found maximal oxygen uptake decreased under all exercise conditions, 12.3% with no exercise, 9.2% with dynamic exercise, but only 4.8% with static exercise. Maximal heart rate increased 3.3% to 4.9% under the three exercise conditions, while plasma volume decreased 15.1% with no exercise, 10.1% with static exercise, and 7.8% with dynamic exercise.

In healthy individuals, the effect of exercise and training is to increase the ability of the heart to supply the muscles with oxygen and to increase the muscle's ability to utilize oxygen. Physical training gradually increases $\dot{V}_{O_2}$ max. Athletes have a lower resting heart rate, greater stroke volume, and lower peripheral resistance than they had before training or after deconditioning (sedentary lifestyle or bed rest).[4] In other words, bed rest results in the opposite effect of physical conditioning. It decreases the ability of the body to maximally deliver and utilize oxygen.

Convertino and others[6] studied the effects of 10 days of bed rest deconditioning in 12 healthy men aged 50 ± 4 years. The men underwent supine and upright graded maximal exercise testing before and after bed rest. The researchers concluded the lack of orthostatic stress is the most important factor limiting exercise tolerance after bed rest in normal middle-aged men.

Humans spend two thirds of the time in an upright position; standing and weight bearing is known as orthostatic stress. Orthostatic stress results in pressure on skeletal long bones and muscles and prevents loss of calcium and muscle tone. It provides for functioning of the venopressor mechanism (a muscle contraction that puts pressure on veins and assists with return of blood to the heart). Without orthostatic stress the autonomic nervous system loses its ability to maintain blood pressure in the standing position as a result of loss of the vasopressor mechanism. Without this, blood tends to pool in the lower parts of the body, thereby decreasing venous return to the heart.

Recent studies associated with the U.S. space program have shown that weightlessness, bed rest, and a head-down tilt position produce similar consequences. The head-down tilt position has been used to study the effects of bed rest and weightlessness, because it produces effects in a shorter period of time.[32]

Hargens and others[9] studied fluid shifts and muscle function during acute simulated weightlessness by using the head down tilt position. Studies of both simulated and actual weightlessness showed a significant fluid shift from the legs

---

INDICATIONS OF ACTIVITY INTOLERANCE

Diaphoresis

Tachycardia of 120 beats/min or an increase of 15 beats/min over resting heart rate in patients receiving beta-blocking drugs

Dizziness

Fatigue

Chest pain

Dysrhythmias

Postural hypotension (an SBP drop greater than 20 mm Hg and/or a heart rate increase of greater than 20 mm Hg on standing)

Syncope

to the upper body, ranging between 10% to 19% of initial leg volume. The fluid shifted out of lower limb tissues into the bloodstream. As a result of the increased blood volume, urine output increased, leading to a dehydrating effect on leg muscles and possible effects on muscle function.[9]

Convertino and others[5] used a reverse gradient garment (RGG) to deliberately induce venous pooling in the legs of bed-rested subjects to determine whether such venous distention would reverse the reduction in maximal oxygen uptake usually observed after bed rest. Compared with pre-bed rest values $\dot{V}O_2$ maximum was reduced by 14%, heart rate maximum was increased by 4.2%, and endurance time for the exercise test was decreased by 9.2% in the control group. In the RGG group $\dot{V}O_2$ maximum, heart rate maximum, and endurance time were essentially unchanged after bed rest. The plasma volume in the control group decreased by 16.7% compared with a statistically insignificant 10.3% in the RGG group. The researchers found that data supported the hypothesis that lack of venous pooling (such as normally occurs when we stand many times a day) and associated fluid shifts contribute to the decrease in $\dot{V}O_2$ maximum after bed rest deconditioning.

Hung and others[11] studied the mechanisms responsible for the decrease in exercise capability after bed rest in 12 apparently healthy men 50 ± 4 years. The men underwent gated pool scanning during supine and upright multistage bicycle ergometry before and after 10 days of bed rest. The researchers found that after bed rest increased left ventricular ejection fraction and heart rate largely compensated for decreased cardiac volume during exercise while the subject was lying down; however, during upright exercise, these mechanisms were unable to maintain pre-bed rest oxygen transport capacity. Their results indicated that fluid shifts from the thorax to the legs, leading to decreased blood return to the heart when an individual assumes a standing position after bed rest, was the major cause of reduced exercise tolerance after 10 days of bed rest in normal middle-aged men.

The studies reviewed have shown that body fluid shifts during bed rest, the lack of orthostatic stress, and a redistribution of 300 to 800 ml of blood to the legs on standing lead to the activity intolerance experienced after bed rest of 1 week or more.[8,11,22] The subsequent decreased preload, increased ejection fraction, and heart rate lead to an increased myocardial oxygen demand that can be hazardous to a patient with coronary artery disease or a myocardial infarction.

Any condition that decreases preload, such as the administration of medication (morphine, nitrates, antihypertensives), dehydradation, hemorrhage, or shock can produce the same effects as prolonged bed rest. Decreased preload leads to decreased cardiac output, which impairs oxygen delivery. If tissues do not receive an adequate oxygen supply, lactic acid accumulates and ischemic pain occurs, further decreasing activity tolerance.

Nursing Care

Nursing measures to counteract the fluid shifts that occur during bed rest consist of getting the patient out of bed as soon as he or she is physiologically able and encouraging low-level activity, such as sitting in a chair two or three times a day, to help avoid the hypovolemia experienced with prolonged bed rest.

The plasma volume contracts more than the red cell mass and lays the groundwork for thromboembolism. The risk is further increased secondary to loss of the leg muscle pump at bed rest.[31]

Other problems encountered are negative nitrogen, calcium, and potassium balance, depression, and anxiety, all of which contribute to activity intolerance.

If bed rest is required, a sitting position, preferably with the legs down, as in a chair-bed, would be useful. If the medical condition permits, the patient, while sitting, can do self-care activities such as washing, grooming, active or passive range-of-motion exercises, and ankle plantar flexion and dorsiflexion. Once the patient is allowed up, his or her response to standing and/or activity should be monitored. Diaphoresis, tachycardia of 120 beats/min or greater, an increase of greater than 15 beats/min over resting heart rate in patients receiving beta blocking drugs, dizziness, fatigue, chest pain, dysrhythmias, or hypotension may mean the patient needs to sit and rest or temporarily return to bed.[16,31] In this case the patient should change from a supine to an upright position slowly, perhaps sitting on the edge of the bed 5 to 10 minutes before standing.[31,32]

One should think carefully about the need for continued bed rest, especially in view of the serious side effects of bed rest deconditioning (see the box below). The detrimental effects of bed rest deconditioning can be prevented merely by getting patients up before meals. Health care can be improved and costs reduced by judicious use of increased activity in those patients assessed to be ready.

EFFECTS OF BED REST DECONDITIONING

Decreased cardiac output
Increased heart rate
Decreased stroke volume
Decreased left ventricular end diastolic volume
Decreased maximal oxygen uptake
Decreased total blood volume
Decreased red cell mass
Decreased total body water
Decreased intracellular fluid volume
Decreased plasma volume

Activity Intolerance related to postural hypotension secondary to prolonged immobility, narcotics, vasodilator therapy

DEFINING CHARACTERISTICS

- SBP drop > 20, heart rate increase > 20 on postural change
- Vertigo on postural change
- Syncope on postural change

OUTCOME CRITERIA

- SBP drop is < 10, heart rate increase is < 10 on postural change.
- Vertigo or syncope is absent on postural change.

NURSING INTERVENTIONS *AND RATIONALE*

1. Continue to monitor the assessment parameters listed under "Defining Characteristics."
2. *To increase muscular and vascular tone,* instruct and assist in the following bed exercises: straight leg raises, dorsiflexion/plantar flexion, and quadriceps setting and gluteal setting exercises.
3. Determine that the patient is hydrated to 24 hour fluid requirements per BSA *to increase preload and thus stroke volume and cardiac output.* Hydrate accordingly if not contraindicated by cardiac or renal disorders.
4. Assist with postural changes accomplished in increments:
   - Head of bed to 45 degrees and hold until symptom free
   - Head of bed to 90 degrees and hold until symptom free
   - Dangle until symptom free
   - Stand until symptom free and ambulate
5. As soon as it is medically safe, assist patient to sit at bedside for meals.
6. When treating pain with narcotic analgesics, plan ambulation to occur well before peak action of the drug.

Activity Intolerance related to knowledge deficit of energy-saving techniques

DEFINING CHARACTERISTICS

- Dyspnea on exertion
- Subjective fatigue on activity
- Heart rate elevations 30 beats above baseline on activity; heart rate 15 beats above baseline on activity for patients on beta blockers or calcium channel blockers

OUTCOME CRITERIA

- The patient has subjective tolerance of activity.
- Heart rate elevations are < 20 beats above baseline on activity and are < 10 beats above baseline on activity for patients on beta blockers or calcium channel blockers.

NURSING INTERVENTIONS *AND RATIONALE*

1. Continue to monitor the assessment parameters listed under "Defining Characteristics."
2. Teach and supervise energy-saving techniques based on the principle of performing work on exhalation, that is, standing up from a bed or chair, repositioning self in bed with or without help, reaching, washing face, brushing hair or teeth.
3. To the extent possible, have the patient perform work while seated.
4. Teach and supervise muscle-toning exercises, *observing that a toned muscle uses less oxygen,* such as arm bends with elbows down, elbow bends with arms up, straight arm raises inward and outward, plantar flexion and dorsiflexion of the feet, straight leg raises.

Activity Intolerance related to decreased cardiac output and/or myocardial tissue perfusion alterations

DEFINING CHARACTERISTICS

- Heart rate elevations 30 beats above baseline upon activity; heart rate elevations 15 beats above baseline upon activity for patients on beta blockers or calcium channel blockers
- Heart rate elevations above baseline 5 minutes after activity
- Ischemic pain on activity
- Electrocardiographic changes on activity
- Subjective fatigue on activity

OUTCOME CRITERIA

- Heart rate elevations are < 20 beats above baseline on activity and are < 10 beats above baseline on activity for patients on beta blockers or calcium channel blockers.
- Heart rate returns to baseline 5 minutes after activity.
- Ischemic pain is absent on activity.
- The patient has subjective tolerance to activity.

NURSING INTERVENTIONS *AND RATIONALE*

1. Continue to monitor the assessment parameters listed under "Defining Characteristics."
2. Encourage active or passive range-of-motion exercises while the patient is in bed *to keep joints flexible and muscles stretched.* Teach patient to refrain from holding breath while performing exercises, *avoiding Valsalva maneuver.*
3. Encourage performance of muscle-toning exercises at least 3 times daily, *because a toned muscle uses less oxygen when performing work than an untoned muscle.*
4. Progressive ambulation.
5. Teach patient pulse taking *to determine activity tolerance:* take pulse for full minute before exercise, then for 10 seconds and multiply by 6 at exercise peak.

THEORETICAL CONCEPTS OF POTENTIAL FOR INFECTION

Arterial catheters, pulmonary artery catheters, and central venous pressure lines, increasingly used as invasive patient care monitoring modalities, predispose a patient to the possibility of nosocomial infection. The nurse working with this equipment must be aware of the risk of infection and use utmost caution when involved with dressing changes, preparation of equipment, manipulation of any part of the system (such as zeroing the transducer), withdrawing blood, or injecting solutions or the catheter itself.[13]

Categories of infections related to intravascular monitoring include the following[12]:
1. Significant versus insignificant catheter colonization without obvious infection
2. Local cutaneous infection
3. Local vascular infection
4. Bacteremia
5. Complicated bacteremia (such as endocarditis)

Infection may occur as a result of contaminated infusion solutions, poor technique during insertion, equipment contamination during manufacture, poor technique during assembly, or manipulation of lines when withdrawing blood, injecting solutions, or during dressing changes. An increased rate of infection is reported associated with cutdown versus percutaneous insertion.[2,13]

Studies showed line related sepsis occurring in 7% to 18% of lines inserted.[2,15,17,27] In a 3-month study of 51 patients (54 arterial lines and 37 pulmonary artery lines) it was found that 10% of the catheters were colonized at the time of removal, and of these 10%, 4% to 44% were as-

sociated with bacteremia.[27] An 8-month study of 172 arterial lines, 82 central venous catheters, and 37 pulmonary artery lines showed 92% noninfected and 8% infected.[17]

Some studies demonstrate increased incidence of infection with catheters left in place more than 72 hours[17,18] whereas others found no correlation to duration of insertion[1,27] stating that technique of insertion and maintenance were more important.[27]

Band and Maki[3] conducted a 2-year study of 130 arterial catheters from 95 patients at high risk of nosocomial infection. Twenty-three (18%) produced local infection and five (4%) septicemia. Sixteen of the 23 local infections and all septicemias occurred with catheter placement exceeding 4 days. They recommended catheter sites be changed after 96 hours (4 days).

Three-way stopcocks within the infusion system are frequently found to be contaminated.[12] Microorganisms may come from the hands of staff members, syringes used to flush or draw specimens, blood left in the port after use, or failure to treat the port with asceptic technique by maintaining a closed system and leaving ports capped between use.

Singh and others[27] found that preexistent sepsis, such as urinary tract infections, pneumonia, or peritonitis, did not increase the probability of catheter colonization; however, Band and Maki[3] stated that inflammation of the insertion site did.

In the studies reviewed, predominant organisms reported in catheter-related infections were *Staphylococcus epidermidis* and *Staphylococcus aureus*.[2,15,17,18] These organisms could have been part of the patient's normal cutaneous flora or transmitted to the patient by health care personnel via hair, nose, or, more likely, hands. Many other organisms are also associated with line-related infections; *Candida albicans, Escherichia coli, Klebsiella, Enterococcus, Enterobacter, Pseudomonas, Aeruginosa pneumoniae,* and *Candida sp.* are among those more frequently mentioned.[3,18]

Systemic antimicrobial therapy given to 80% of the entire group and four of the five with septicemia did not protect against catheter-related infection.[3] It should not be assumed that simultaneous antibiotic administration prevents a line-related infection.

For techniques to prevent line-related infections, see the Care Plan box below.

To protect health care workers as well as patients, many institutions are currently instituting a system known as "universal blood and body fluid precautions." This method advocates routine use of gloves for all blood drawing or handling, gowns, masks, and goggles, when appropriate, to prevent blood or body fluid exposure to skin or mucous membranes.

Potential for Infection

RISK FACTOR

- Invasive monitoring devices

DEFINING CHARACTERISTICS

- Fever of undetermined origin
- Tachycardia
- Elevated white blood cells
- Reddened, inflamed catheter insertion sites
- Drainage from catheter insertion sites

OUTCOME CRITERIA

- Patient is afebrile.
- HR is within range of baseline.
- Catheter insertion sites are clear and dry.

NURSING INTERVENTIONS *AND RATIONALE*

NOTE: *The rationale for each of the following interventions is the avoidance of contamination and colonization of invasive lines and is based on national standards and supported with research.*

1. Continue to monitor the assessment parameters listed under "Defining Characteristics."
2. Practice handwashing consisting of 15 seconds using mechanical friction and soap and water before drawing blood or any line manipulation in which the closed system is interrupted.
3. Secure catheters to prevent piston movement (in and out).
4. Maintain an occlusive, sterile dressing. Gauze dressings over arterial lines are recommended.
5. Eliminate all nonessential stopcocks. When stop-

cocks are necessary, they should have as few ports as possible. Stopcocks should be replaced every 24 hours or when soiled, and they should be covered at all times.

6. A new anatomical site should be selected for each catheter inserted.
7. To the extent possible, limit blood drawing by obtaining all specimens at the same time.
8. Use uniform, prepackaged, sterile transducer/pressure monitoring and flush assembly.
9. Maintain a strict protocol for skin preparation. Clean the skin with iodofor after degreasing and defatting with acetone. Wear gloves, mask, and cap and use sterile drapes. A sterile gown should be worn when inserting central lines.
10. Use sterile normal saline as the flush solution.
11. Before obtaining a sample of blood, the stopcock port must be cleansed thoroughly with 70% alcohol with a sterile towel placed under the port being entered.
12. Transparent, occlusive dressings should be changed every 72 hours or when integrity is disrupted. Gauze dressings should be changed every 48 hours or sooner if soiled, saturated, or disrupted.
13. Catheters inserted in an emergency, without proper asepsis, should be removed and, if necessary, replaced under aseptic conditions.
14. At any sign of infection, (localized pain, inflammation, sepsis, fever of undetermined origin) catheters should be removed and cultured.

REFERENCES

1. Abbound F: Pathophysiology of hypotension and shock. In Hurst W, editor: The heart, arteries and veins, ed 6, New York, 1986, McGraw-Hill Book Co.
2. Abbott N and others: Infection related to physiologic monitoring: venous and arterial catheters, Heart Lung 12(1):28, 1983.
3. Band J and Maki D: Infections caused by arterial catheters used for hemodynamic monitoring, Am J Nurs 11(67):735, 1979.
4. Berne R and Levy M: Cardiovascular physiology, ed 5, St Louis, 1986, The CV Mosby Co.
5. Convertino YA and others: Induced venous pooling and cardiorespiratory responses to exercise after bed rest, J Appl Physiol 52:1343, 1982.
6. Convertino Y and others: Cardiovascular responses to exercise in middle-aged men after 10 days of bed rest, Circulation 65(1):134, 1982.
7. Dalen J and Albert J: Pulmonary embolism. In Hurst W, editor: The heart, arteries and veins, ed 6, New York, 1986, McGraw-Hill Book Co.
8. Gauer OH and Thron HL: Postural changes in the circulation. In Hamilton WF and Dow P, editors: Handbook of physiology. Section 2: Circulation, Washington, 1965, American Physiological Society.
9. Hargens AR and others: Fluid shifts and muscle function in humans during acute simulated weightlessness, J Appl Physiol 54(4):1003, 1983.
10. Hudson-Civetta J and Banner T: Intravascular catheters: current guidelines for care and maintenance, Heart Lung 12(5):466, 1983.
11. Hung J and others: Mechanisms for decreased exercise capacity after bed rest in normal middle-aged men, Am J Cardiol 51:344, 1983.
12. Kaye W: Catheter and infusion related sepsis: the nature of the problem, Heart Lung 1(3):221, 1982.
13. Keeler C and others: A review of infection control practices related to intravascular pressure monitoring devices, Heart Lung 16(2):201, 1987.
14. Kluida H: Pulmonary hypertension: mechanism and recognition. In Hurst W, editor: The heart, arteries and veins, ed 6, New York, 1986, McGraw-Hill Book Co.
15. Miller J and others: Comparison of the sterility of long-term central venous catheterization using single lumen, triple lumen, and pulmonary artery catheters, Crit Care Med 12(8):634, 1984.
16. O'Reilly MY and Kilshaw M: Recent advances in the management of acute uncomplicated myocardial infarction. II. The post-acute phase, J Irish Coll Phys Surg 4(2):54, 1974.
17. Pinilla J and others: Study of the incidence of intravascular catheter infection and associated septicemia in critically ill patients, Crit Care Med 11(1):21, 1983.
18. Ponce De Leon S and others: Polymicrobial bloodstream infections related to prolonged vascular catheterization, Crit Care Med 12(1):856, 1984.
19. Price S and Wilson L: Pathophysiology, clinical concepts of disease processes, ed 3, New York, 1986, McGraw-Hill Book Co.
20. Rice Y: Shock management. Part II. Pharmacologic intervention, Crit Care Nurse 5(1):42, 1985.
21. Roberts S: Pulmonary tissue perfusion altered: embolic, Heart Lung 16(2):128, 1987.
22. Saltin B and others: Response to exercise after bed rest and after training, Circulation 38(5), Supplement 7:1, 1968.
23. Schlant R and Sonnenbleck E: Normal physiology of the cardiovascular system. In Hurst W, editor: The heart, arteries and veins, ed 6, New York, 1986, McGraw-Hill Book Co.
24. Sedlock S: Cardiac output: physiologic variables and therapeutic interventions, Crit Care Nurs 1(2):14, 1981.
25. Shabetai R: Diseases of the pericardium. In Hurst W, editor: The heart, arteries, and veins, ed 6, New York, 1986, McGraw-Hill Book Co.
26. Shepard N, Vaughn P, and Rice Y: A guide to arrhythmia interpretation, Crit Care Nurs 2(5):59, 1982.
27. Singh S and others: Catheter colonization and bacteremia with pulmonary and arterial catheters, Crit Care Med 10(11): 736, 1982.
28. Smith T: Heart failure. In Wyngaarden J and Smith L, editors: Cecil testbook of medicine, ed 18, Philadelphia, 1988 WB Saunders Co.
29. Stremel RW and others: Cardiorespiratory deconditioning with static dynamic leg exercise during bed rest, J Appl Physiol 41(6):905, 1976.
30. Wallace A and Waugh R: Pathophysiology of cardiovascular disease. In Smith L and Thier S, editors: Pathophysiology: the biological principles of disease, ed 2, Philadelphia, 1985, WB Saunders Co.
31. Wegner N: Early ambulation physical activity: myocardial infarction and coronary artery bypass surgery, Heart Lung 13(1):14, 1984.
32. Winslow EH: Cardiovascular consequences of bed rest, Heart Lung 14(3):236, 1985.

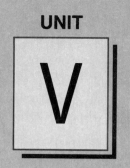

PULMONARY ALTERATIONS

Pulmonary Anatomy and Physiology

- *List important functions of pulmonary surfactant and the clinical effects of a decrease in its amount.*
- *Explain why the lungs stay inflated and relate this explanation to pneumothorax.*
- *Explain oxygen transport in the bloodstream.*
- *Explain what "work of breathing" means and relate how increased work of breathing uses excess energy.*
- *Discuss clinical implications of excessive methemoglobin, carboxyhemoglobin, and deoxygenated hemoglobin.*

The primary function of the pulmonary system is gas exchange, that is, the movement of oxygen from the atmosphere into the bloodstream and the movement of carbon dioxide from the bloodstream into the atmosphere. Since the anatomical structures that constitute the pulmonary system are intimately related to function and since structural abnormalities can readily translate into pulmonary disorders, an applicable knowledge of anatomy and physiology is imperative in pulmonary care. Where possible in this chapter, care has been taken to relate nursing actions and pathophysiology to normal anatomy and physiology.

Because the focus of this book is critical care nursing and because upper airway pathology is infrequently seen in critical care, the anatomy and physiology of the airway structures above the larynx are not reviewed in this chapter.

STRUCTURES OF THE THORAX AND THE LUNGS
Thorax and Ribs

The thorax is cone shaped, and although it must be somewhat rigid to protect the underlying structures, it must also be flexible to accommodate inhalation. The thorax consists of 12 thoracic vertebrae, each with a respective pair of ribs. Each rib is attached posteriorly to its own vertebrae, but the anterior attachment varies (Fig. 17-1). The first seven pairs of ribs are attached directly to the sternum. The eighth,

ninth, and tenth pairs are attached by cartilage to the rib above. The eleventh and twelfth ribs have no anterior attachment and for this reason are sometimes referred to as "floating ribs."

The second rib is attached to the sternum at the angle of Louis, which is the raised ridge that can be felt just below the suprasternal notch. Location of the second rib is essential in cardiac assessment because the second intercostal space, just below the rib, is an area of cardiac valve auscultation. Specifically, the second intercostal space on the right of the sternum is the point for aortic valve auscultation, whereas the second intercostal space to the left of the sternum is the point for pulmonic valve auscultation. These and other cardiac valve auscultation areas can be found on the chest by counting intercostal spaces, beginning with the second and locating the third, fourth, and fifth spaces (Chapter 12 provides details about cardiac assessment).

Lung Divisions

The lungs are cone shaped; the superior portion is termed the apex and the inferior portion, the base. Because the apex of each lung rises a few centimeters above the clavicle (see Fig. 17-1), the apical portion of a lung can be involved in a pneumothorax during insertion of a subclavian intravenous line. Each lung is firmly attached to the thoracic cavity at the hilum and at the pulmonary ligament.

The lungs are divided into lobes and segments. Lobes are separated by pleural membrane–covered fissures. The right lung, which is larger and heavier than the left, is divided into upper, middle, and lower lobes, whereas the left lung has only an upper and a lower lobe. A portion of the left lung, the lingula, corresponds anatomically with the right middle lobe.

The horizontal fissure divides the right upper lobe from the right middle lobe. The oblique fissure divides the right upper and middle lobes from the lower lobe and the left upper lobe from the lower lobe. The lobes are divided into 18 segments, each of which has its own bronchus branching immediately off of a lobar bronchus. Ten segments are in the right lung and eight in the left lung.

The area between the two lungs, the *mediastinum*, con-

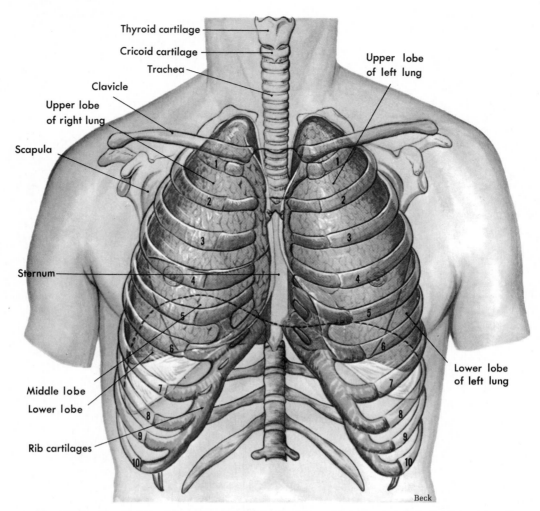

Fig. 17-1 Ventilatory structures of the chest wall and lungs, showing ribs (numbered) and lobes of the lungs. Each intercostal space takes the number of the rib above it. Dotted line indicates the location of the diaphragm at inhalation and exhalation. Note the apex of each lung rises above the clavicle. (From Anthony CP and Thibodeau GA: Textbook of anatomy and physiology, ed 12, St Louis, 1987, Times Mirror/Mosby College Publishing.)

tains the heart, great vessels, lymphatics, and esophagus. A portion of the mediastinal area contains the *hilum,* also known as the root of the lungs, in which the visceral and parietal pleura form a sheath around the mainstem bronchi, the major blood vessels, and the nerves that enter and exit the lungs. Hilar masses and hilar lymphadenopathy that are seen on a chest radiograph are located in this area.

THE CONDUCTING AIRWAYS

The conducting airways are the passageways to the respiratory regions of the lung. No gas exchange occurs within the conducting airways, which include all of the area beginning with the nose and mouth and ending at the terminal bronchioles.

Trachea

The trachea is a hollow tube approximately 11 cm (4.5 inches) in length and 2.5 cm (1 inch) in diameter. Fig. 17-2 illustrates that the trachea begins at the cricoid cartilage and ends at the bifurcation (the major carina) from which the two mainstem bronchi arise. The carina is approximately at the level of the aortic arch,[19] the fifth thoracic vertebrae,[19] or just below the level of the angle of Louis.[18] The trachea consists of smooth muscle supported anteriorly by 16 to 20 C-shaped cartilaginous rings, which prevent tracheal collapse during bronchoconstriction of its smooth muscle fibers and during strong coughing. The posterior wall of the trachea lies contiguous with the anterior wall of the esophagus. Having no cartilaginous support, this wall is composed only of muscle tissue, which is separated from the anterior esophageal wall by loose connective tissue (see insert, Fig. 17-2). For this reason, tracheal damage and tracheoesophageal fistulas, resulting from cuffed airway tubes (both endotracheal and tracheostomy) develop first in the posterior tracheal wall. A tracheostomy is usually performed at the second or third tracheal ring because this region contains less vasculature.

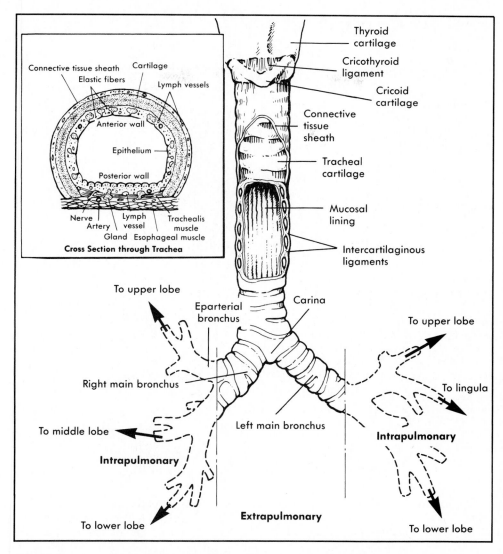

Fig. 17-2 Anterior view of the trachea and primary bronchi and a cross section through a part of the trachea, including a C-shaped cartilagenous element. (From Martin DE: Respiratory anatomy and physiology, St Louis, 1988, The CV Mosby Co.)

Bronchial Tree

As shown in Fig. 17-2, the two mainstem bronchi are structurally different. The left bronchus is slightly narrower than the right, and because of its position above the heart, the left bronchus angles directly toward the left lung at approximately 45 to 55 degrees from the midline. This sharp inclination causes less likelihood of aspiration into the left bronchus. The right bronchus is wider and angles at 20 to 30 degrees from midline. Because of this angulation and the forces of gravity, the most common site of aspiration of foreign objects is through the right mainstem bronchus into the lower lobe of the right lung.

Every branching of the tracheobronchial tree produces a new *generation* of tubes as is indicated in Table 17-1. The mainstem bronchi are the first generation; the next branch, the five lobar bronchi, is the second generation. The third generation includes the 18 segmental bronchi.

The fourth through approximately the ninth generations are referred to as the small bronchi, beginning with the subsegmental bronchi. In these bronchi, diameters decrease; however, since the number of bronchi increases with each generation, the total cross-sectional area increases with each generation. Table 17-1 shows the number of airways increasing from 20 per generation at the fourth generation to approximately 1020 per generation at the tenth generation. The eleventh generation has approximately seven times the cross-sectional area of the lobar bronchi.[31] This great increase in the cross-sectional area of the lung is extremely significant in that it allows easy ventilation in spite of the small airway lumens through which air is passing.

The final subdivision of the conducting airways is the *bronchioles,* which are tubes less than 1 mm in diameter

Table 17-1 Subdivisions of the respiratory tree*

Generation	Name	Diameter (cm)	Length (cm)	Number per generation	Histological notes
0	Trachea	1.8	12	1	Wealth of goblet cells
1	Primary bronchi	1.2	4.8	2	Right larger than left
2	Lobar bronchi	0.8	0.9	5	3 right, 2 left
3	Segmental bronchi	0.6	0.8	18	10 right; 8 left
4	Subsegmental bronchi	0.5	1.3	20	
5 ↓	Small bronchi	0.4	1.1	40	Still have cartilage; many cell types as well as respiratory
10		0.1	0.5	1,020	epithelium
11 ↓	Bronchioles—primary and secondary	0.1	0.4	2,050	No cartilage; smooth muscle, cilia, goblet cells present
13		0.1	0.3	8,190	
14 ↓	Terminal bronchioles	0.1	0.2	16,380	No goblet cells; smooth muscle, cilia, and cuboidal cells
15		0.1	0.2	32,770	
16 ↓	Respiratory bronchioles	0.1	0.2	65,540	No smooth muscle; cilia, cuboidal cells; cilia disappear
18		0.1	0.1	262,140	
19 ↓	Alveolar ducts	0.05	0.1	524,290	No cilia; cuboidal cells
23		0.04	0.05	8,390,000	
24	Alveoli*	244	238	300,000,000	

From Martin DE: Respiratory anatomy and physiology, St Louis, 1988, The CV Mosby Co; modified from Weibel ER: Morphometry of the human lung, Berlin, 1973, Springer Verlag.
*Alveolar dimensions given in micrometers.

that are distinguished by having a lack of connective tissue and cartilage within their walls. Their walls do, however, contain smooth muscle. When smooth-muscle constriction occurs, these airways may close completely from lack of structural support. Some of the wheezing and dyspnea associated with asthma can be traced to bronchoconstriction of the bronchioles. The *terminal bronchioles* form the last branch of the conducting airways, after which the gas exchange areas of the lung begin. As Table 17-1 shows, there are more than 32,000 terminal bronchioles.

Functions of the Conducting Airways

The major functions of the conducting airways are (1) to condition the inhaled air, (2) to act as a protective mechanism that prevents the entrance of foreign matter into the gas exchange areas, and (3) to serve as a passageway for air entering the gas exchange regions of the lungs.

Conditioned air has been warmed, humidified, and cleaned of some irritants. Warming and humidifying, which are essential to achieve a nonirritant effect on the lower airways, occur mainly within the nose through a dense vascular network that lines the nasal passages. Many irritants are filtered by coarse hairs, which line the nasal passages.

Within the airways, the main defense system is the mucociliary escalator, or mucous blanket, a combination of mucus and cilia. The mucus, which floats atop the cilia (Fig. 17-3), traps foreign particles, whereas ciliary move-

ment propels the entire mucous blanket and, with it, any trapped particles upward toward the pharynx at an average speed of 1 to 2 cm/minute.[9,31] The submucous glands of the airways produce approximately 100 ml of mucus per day. So efficient is the mucociliary escalator that almost no particles larger than the size of a red blood cell (4 to 6 μm) reach the alveoli.

In addition to removing foreign particles from the air, the conducting airways protect the lungs by other means. A *cough* is a protective mechanism that removes foreign matter that has reached the carina, the mainstem bronchi, or farther into the tracheobronchial tree. The carina is a particularly sensitive area as is often demonstrated clinically when a suction catheter is advanced into the trachea. During the advancement when the patient begins coughing, often violently, the catheter has reached the carina.

The *epiglottis* protects the lower airways by closing the opening to the trachea during swallowing so that food passes into the esophagus. The epiglottis is a thin, leaf-shaped elastic cartilage located directly posterior to the root of the tongue and is attached to the thyroid cartilage. It opens widely during inhalation, permitting air to pass through the trachea and into the lower airways. Because the epiglottis covers the trachea during swallowing, stomach tubes are best advanced during swallowing. On the other hand, because the epiglottis is open during inhalation, suction catheters are best advanced during inhalation.

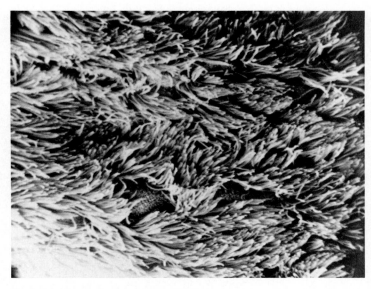

Fig. 17-3 Scanning electron micrograph of the luminal surface and cilia of a bronchiole from a normal adult male. (×2000.) (From Murray JF: The normal lung, ed 2, Philadelphia, 1986, WB Saunders Co, originally from Ebert RV and Terracio MJ: Am Rev Resp Dis 111:130, 1975.)

RESPIRATORY AIRWAYS

The respiratory airways of the lungs are the gas exchange regions and include the respiratory bronchioles, alveolar ducts, and alveolar sacs. Gas exchange at this level is referred to as external respiration, whereas the gas exchange that occurs at the cellular level is termed internal respiration. This discussion concentrates on external respiration.

Respiratory Bronchioles

Each terminal bronchiole gives rise to an average of three respiratory bronchioles, each of which gives rise to several alveolar ducts (Fig. 17-4). The respiratory bronchioles themselves do not permit gas exchange except where alveoli branch off their walls.

Alveoli

Within the two lungs are approximately 300 million alveoli composed of several types of cells, including type I alveolar epithelial cells and type II alveolar epithelial cells.

Type I alveolar epithelial cells. Type I alveolar epithelial cells (Fig. 17-5) compose approximately 90% of the total alveolar surface within the lungs.[19] They are the chief structural cells of the alveolar wall and play the major role in maintenance of the gas-blood barrier and in gas exchange. Type I cells are extremely susceptible to injury and become inflamed when exposed to inhaled toxins. Whether type I cells can regenerate is in question; however, research suggests that type II cells can regenerate and change to type I cells.[19]

Within the walls of the type I cells are the pores of Kohn (Fig. 17-6) which are thought to allow collateral movement

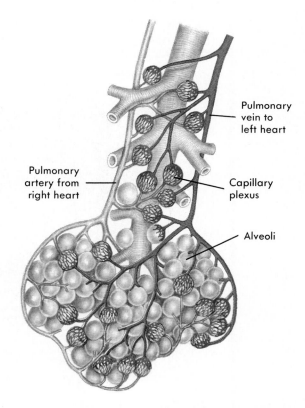

Fig. 17-4 Terminal ventilation and perfusion units of the lung. Pulmonary arterial blood is venous *(dark grey)* and pulmonary venous blood is oxygenated (red). (From Thompson JM and others: Mosby's manual of clinical nursing, ed 2, St Louis, 1989, The CV Mosby Co.)

Labels on Fig. 17-4: Pulmonary vein to left heart; Pulmonary artery from right heart; Capillary plexus; Alveoli

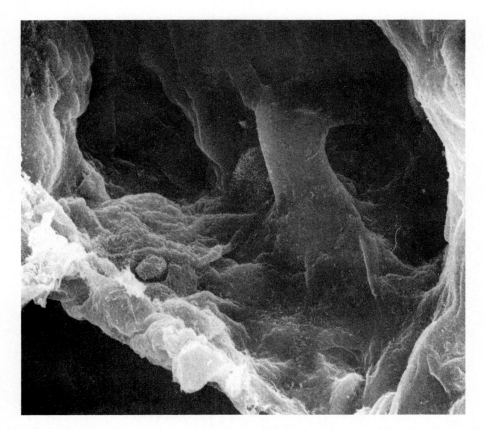

Fig. 17-5   Detail of an alveolar surface comprised chiefly of type I alveolar epithelial cells. (Picture width—1 cm equals 3.46 μm.) (From Martin DE: Respiratory anatomy and physiology, St Louis, 1988, The CV Mosby Co.)

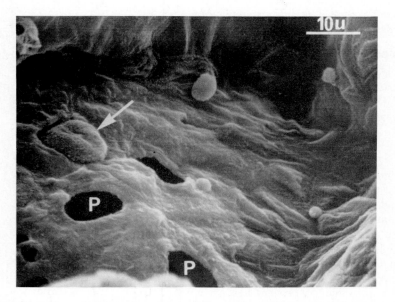

Fig. 17-6   Scanning electron micrograph of the surface of a human alveolus, showing pores of Kohn *(P)* and a macrophage *(arrow).* (×1500.) (From Murray JF: The normal lung, ed 2, Philadelphia, 1986, WB Saunders Co; courtesy Dr. NS Wang.)

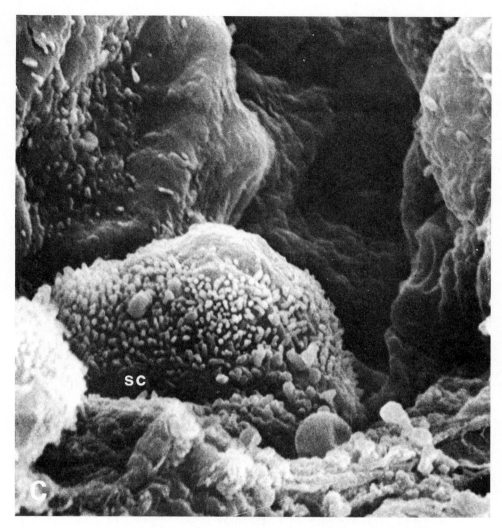

Fig. 17-7 Type II alveolar epithelial cell. Note the presence of brush microvilli on all except the bald top of the round luminal surface. Type II cells produce surfactant. (Picture width—1 cm equals 0.85 μm.) (From Martin DE: Respiratory anatomy and physiology, St Louis, 1988, The CV Mosby Co.)

of air between alveoli,[19] although recently this long-held belief has been questioned.[23] The canals of Lambert are collateral air pathways that exist between type I cells and respiratory and terminal bronchioles. When a respiratory bronchiole is blocked or collapsed, gas may still be able to pass into alveoli distal to the block through the canals of Lambert. Thus collateral air passages are of significant benefit in any lung pathology that results in obstruction of airflow into a portion of the lungs. In contrast, however, these pores and canals also allow the efficient movement of microorganisms through lung tissue.

Type II alveolar epithelial cells. Type II alveolar epithelial cells occur in much greater numbers than type I cells, but because of their minute size, they comprise a smaller portion of the total alveolar wall. After injury to the alveolar wall, type II cells rapidly divide to line the surface; later, they transform into type I cells. By far, however, the most important function of the type II cells is their ability to produce, store, and secrete pulmonary surfactant (Fig. 17-7).

Surfactant. Surfactant is a phospholipid composed of fatty acids bound to lecithin. Like other surfactants such as detergents and soaps, pulmonary surfactant functions to lower surface tension. Whereas with detergents and soaps this decrease in surface tension cleans clothes, within the lungs it stabilizes the alveoli, increases lung compliance, and eases the work of breathing. When pulmonary disease disrupts the normal synthesis and storage of surfactant, the lungs become less compliant, and the work of breathing increases. Severe loss of surfactant results in alveolar instability, collapse (atelectasis), and impairment of diffusion. The classic example of this pathology occurs in adult respiratory distress syndrome (ARDS) in which the increased permeability of the alveolar-capillary bed allows vascular fluid to move into the alveoli, interfering with the production of surfactant. The refractory hypoxemia, tissue hypoxia, and mortality from ARDS result from altered alveolar-capillary permeability, disruption of surfactant production, alveolar instability, and atelectasis.

Sighing is thought to contribute to the spread of surfactant throughout the lungs because the large volume of air generated by the sigh opens otherwise partially closed alveoli and spreads surfactant over their walls.[16] This theory is supported by studies that have shown that continuous ventilation with the same volume of air, as in controlled mechanical ventilation, can result in decreasing lung compliance, meaning that the lungs become "stiffer" and more difficult to inflate.[1,8]

Surfactant has a half-life of only 14 hours; this short time period accounts for the high metabolic activity of the type II cells. Because of its function in lipid metabolism, thyroxine is thought to play a role in surfactant production. Studies in animals and humans have shown an increased production and storage of surfactant when thyroxine has been administered. Acetylcholine, prostaglandins, and estradiol are also known to increase surfactant synthesis.[23]

Alveolar macrophages. Alveolar macrophages (Fig. 17-8) are monocytes that originate in the bone marrow; when traveling through the pulmonary capillary circulation, they move out of the capillaries into the interstitial space and the alveoli. Once in the alveoli, these monocytes transform into macrophages and assume a phagocytic role. In that capacity, they move from alveoli to alveoli through the pores of Kohn (Fig. 17-6), functioning to keep the alveoli clean and sterile through phagocytosis and through microbial killing activity, which includes the secretion of hydrogen peroxide, lysozyme, and other substances that kill microorganisms.

An increase or decrease in the number of alveolar macrophages is thought directly related to an individual's resistance to lung infection. Depression of macrophage activity can occur with the presence of cigarette smoke, hypoxia, hyperoxia, metabolic acidosis, uremia, ozone, nitrogen dioxide, ethanol ingestion, and corticosteroid ingestion and after viral infections.[19,24]

Alveolar Capillary Membrane

The vessels of the alveolar-capillary membrane form a network around each alveolus that is so dense it forms an almost continuous sheet of blood covering the alveoli. The interior diameter of each capillary segment is approximately 10 μm, just large enough to allow red blood cells to squeeze by in single file so that their cell membranes touch the capillary walls, as illustrated in Fig. 17-9. In this way, oxygen and carbon dioxide need not pass through significant amounts of plasma when diffusing into and out of the alveoli, making a highly efficient vehicle for gas exchange.[9]

Each red blood cell spends approximately three fourths of a second in the alveolar-capillary network and is exposed to the alveolar gas of two or three alveoli.[44] In that short time hemoglobin is brought from its normal venous blood saturation level of 75% to its arterial blood level of >96%. However, hemoglobin levels have been shown to reach normal within only a 0.25 second exposure to alveolar gas; thus under conditions such as in tachycardia in which the red blood cells spend less time within the pulmonary capillary network, normal oxygenation will still occur.[44]

The alveolar-capillary membrane is composed of several layers of cells: the alveolar epithelium, the alveolar base-

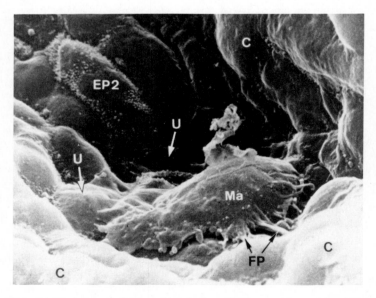

Fig. 17-8 Scanning electron micrograph of a healthy human lung, showing an alveolar macrophage *(Ma)* attached to the epithelium partly by filopodia *(FP)* and forming an undulating membrane *(U)* in the direction of forward movement to the left. Several capillaries *(C)* are evident, and a type II alveolar epithelial cell *(EP2)* can be seen in the background. (Original magnification ×3700.) (From Murray JF: The normal lung, ed 2, Philadelphia, 1986, WB Saunders Co; originally from Gehr P and others: Respir Physiol 32(2):130, 1978.)

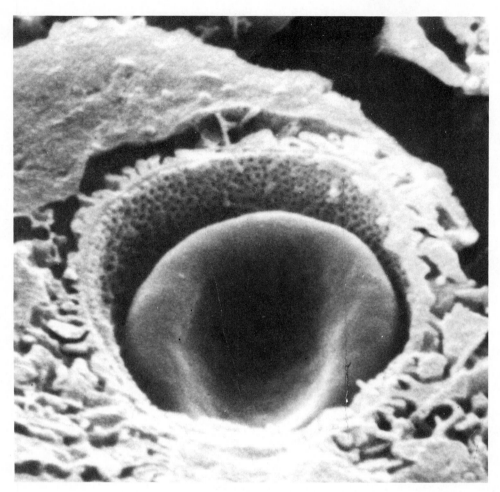

Fig. 17-9 Scanning electron micrograph of a red blood cell in a capillary. Note that the diameters of both are similar. In many instances the red blood cells course through even smaller capillaries, often through capillaries that are one half the diameter of the red blood cell. This is possible because the cells are pliable, mainly as a result of their biconcave disk shape.[19] (From Martin DE: Respiratory anatomy and physiology, St Louis, 1988, The CV Mosby Co.)

ment membrane, the interstitial space, the capillary basement membrane, and the capillary endothelium. Oxygen and carbon dioxide traverse easily across these layers, which present no barrier to diffusion because the membrane is less than 0.5 μg thick. However, there are pulmonary disorders such as cardiogenic pulmonary edema and ARDS which increase the thickness of the membrane enough that a barrier to diffusion results.

PULMONARY BLOOD AND LYMPH SUPPLY

Two vascular systems and one lymphatic system make up the pulmonary blood and lymph supply. The *pulmonary circulation* arises from the right side of the heart with the pulmonary artery and is the gas exchange network that surrounds the alveoli and empties into the left side of the heart. The *bronchial circulation* is the vascular system that perfuses the tracheobronchial tree.

Pulmonary Circulation

The pulmonary circulatory system begins at the pulmonary artery, which receives venous blood from the right ventricle. The pulmonary artery then divides into mainstem left and right branches and continues to branch until it forms the capillaries that surround the alveoli (see Fig. 17-4). Once blood is oxygenated, it returns to the left side of the heart through the pulmonary veins.

The pulmonary circulation is, by far, the largest vascular bed within the body and is the only one that receives the entire cardiac output.

Just as the systemic circulation has a systolic and a diastolic blood pressure, so does the pulmonary circulation. However, because of the relative lack of smooth muscle within the vessels of the pulmonary circulation, the pressures are vastly lower than within the systemic circulation.[7] Placement of a pulmonary artery catheter, a common practice in critical care, allows direct measurement of the blood pressure within the pulmonary system. Pulmonary artery systolic (PAS) pressure averages 25 mm Hg, pulmonary artery diastolic (PAD) pressure averages 10 mm Hg, and pulmonary artery mean (PAM) pressure is 15 mm Hg, considerably lower than the systemic systolic pressure of 120 mm Hg, diastolic of 70 mm Hg, and mean of 80 mm Hg. Because of the low pulmonary artery pressures, right-ventricular wall thickness needs to be only approximately one third of left-ventricular wall thickness. However, just as hypertension can occur within the systemic circulation, it can also occur within the pulmonary circulation.

Pulmonary hypertension. Pulmonary hypertension is defined as increased pressure (PAS greater than 30 mm Hg and PAM greater than 18 mm Hg) within the pulmonary arterial system. Pulmonary hypertension can develop as a result of both cardiac and pulmonary pathologies. Cardiac pathologies include mitral stenosis, left-ventricular failure, and congenital heart disease. Cardiac-generated pulmonary hypertension is sometimes called "passive pulmonary hypertension" because the rise in pressure is caused, not by disease of the pulmonary vascular bed, but by a rising left atrial pressure.

The most common cause of pulmonary hypertension, however, is pathology of the lungs such as pulmonary embolism, and obliteration of the vascular bed associated with emphysema or hypoxic vasoconstriction (see the box at right).

The pulmonary hypertension resulting from hypoxic vasoconstriction, although caused, in part, by vasospasm, is largely a result of alterations in the structure of the blood vessels of the pulmonary circulation, which results in an increase in the medial thickness and a reduction in the size of the vascular lumen.[38] Pulmonary hypertension increases the afterload of the right ventricle and, when chronic, can result in right-ventricular hypertrophy.

Pulmonary hypertension resulting from a pulmonary embolism can have serious consequences if the embolism is large. Significant pulmonary hypertension occurs when the pulmonary tree is 30% to 50% occluded; severe hypertension results with greater than 60% occlusion. Chronic thromboembolic pulmonary hypertension can produce pulmonary artery mean pressure greater than 60 mm Hg and a pulmonary vascular resistance greater than 900 dynes/sec/cm^{-5} (normal is 100 to 250 dynes/sec/cm^{-5}).[22]

Bronchial Circulation

The bronchial circulation, also known as the "systemic" blood supply to the lungs,[4] is a system that perfuses the tracheobronchial tree, visceral pleura, interstitial and connective tissue, some arteries and veins, lymph nodes, and the nerves within the thoracic cavity. The bronchial arteries that perfuse structures in the left side of the thorax branch off the aorta, whereas those that perfuse the right side's structures branch from the intercostal, subclavian, or internal mammary artery. After perfusing the specific lung structures, most of the venous blood returns to the right side of the heart; however, some venous blood from the bronchial circulation returns directly into the pulmonary veins and the left atrium.[4] The left atrium contains pure oxygenated blood with a hemoglobin saturation at 100% (assuming healthy

---

PATHOPHYSIOLOGY OF HYPOXIC VASO-CONSTRICTION

Hypoxic vasoconstriction refers to vasoconstriction of any portion of the pulmonary-capillary bed that perfuses unventilated or underventilated alveoli. Although most blood vessels in the body dilate in response to hypoxia to deliver more blood flow to the hypoxic tissue, the pulmonary vessels do the opposite and constrict in response to hypoxia. Hypoxic vasoconstriction occurs in lung regions where the partial pressure of oxygen in alveolar gas (Pao$_2$) falls below 60 mm Hg. Research indicates that the lower the Pao$_2$, the greater will be the hypoxic vasoconstriction.[38] The mediator of this response is as of yet unknown, but the vasoconstriction has the effect of directing blood flow away from the hypoxic alveoli to alveoli in which the Pao$_2$ is or might be normal.

The drop in Pao$_2$ can result from various conditions associated with chronic pulmonary disease such as bronchoconstriction and chronic blockage of airways by mucus or from breathing low concentrations of oxygen such as happens to individuals living at a high altitude. Indeed, high altitude dwellers do experience the same vascular changes in their pulmonary arterioles as do individuals who develop hypoxic vasoconstriction as a result of chronic pulmonary disease.

Hypoxic vasoconstriction is not necessarily bad. When it occurs regionally within the lung such as in atelectatic areas, it protects against severe hypoxemia by limiting shunt.[41] However, when hypoxic vasoconstriction becomes generalized throughout the lung, pulmonary hypertension will result.

Prolonged hypoxic vasoconstriction such as commonly occurs in patients with chronic bronchitis can lead to pulmonary hypertension and cor pulmonale. Pulmonary hypertension develops when the hypoxic vasoconstriction is diffuse and affects a significant amount of the pulmonary vascular bed.

---

lungs). The mixing of venous blood from the bronchial circulation with the oxygenated blood in the left atrium decreases the saturation of left atrial blood to 96% to 99%. For this reason, while an individual is breathing room air, the oxygen saturation of arterial blood will be less than 100%. The dumping of venous blood into the left atrium is called the *physiological shunt,* a term that expresses two thoughts; physiological means that this is a normal part of physiology, not a pathological event, and shunt refers to the mixing of venous blood with arterial blood. Another system responsible for the addition of venous blood to the left atrium, thus contributing to the normal physiological shunt, is the thebesian system, which perfuses the coronary arteries. These two systems constitute the normal physiological shunt, which comprises approximately 3% to 5% of the total cardiac output.

Lymphatic Circulation

The lungs are more richly supplied with lymphatic tissue than any other organ perhaps because of the lungs' constant exposure to the foreign, external environment.[23] The lymphatic vessels parallel much of the pulmonary vasculature and the tracheobronchial tree to the level of the terminal and respiratory bronchioles. Lymphatic vessels are also located within the connective tissue of lung parenchyma and within the pleural membranes. These vessels eventually drain into the primary lymph nodes located at the hilum of the lungs. Lymph tissue and vessels are probably responsible for both antibody and cell-mediated immune responses within the lung and for removing fluid from the lungs.

PLEURAL MEMBRANES

The pleural membranes consist of two serous membranes—the parietal and visceral pleurae. The parietal pleura is attached to the thoracic wall; the visceral pleura is attached to the lungs and covers them completely. Both surfaces have a blood and lymphatic supply through which they secrete and absorb fluid. In healthy individuals, there is a continuous filtration of fluid from the capillaries of the parietal pleura into the capillaries of the visceral pleura. Figure 17-10 illustrates this filtration. However, since pleural fluid is constantly being secreted and absorbed, at any one time there are only 3 to 5 ml within the pleural space, and excess fluid is removed by the lymphatic system.[29] Approximately 1 to 2 L of fluid moves across the pleural space each day.[6] Pleural fluid allows the visceral and parietal pleural membranes to glide against each other during inhalation and exhalation. Patients who have experienced a loss of pleural fluid or inflammation of the pleural space (pleuritis) often report severe, painful breathing.

Pleural Space

There are two main issues of importance regarding the pleural space. First, the pleural space has a pressure within

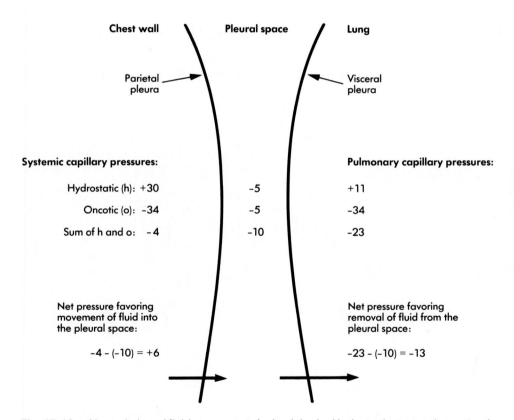

Fig. 17-10 Normal pleural fluid movement. A physiological balance between the systemic and pulmonary capillaries provides continuous movement of fluid from parietal pleural capillaries into the pleural space and then into the visceral pleural capillaries. All pressures are in cm H_2O. Pressures that tend to force fluid out of the capillaries are shown with a plus *(+)* sign; pressures that tend to hold fluid in the capillaries or pleural space are shown with a *(−)* sign. There is a net +6 cm H_2O pressure favoring fluid movement into the pleural space and a net −13 cm H_2O pressure favoring removal of fluid from the pleural space. In this diagram the two pleural membranes are shown apart, but in healthy persons, the membranes touch, separated only by a thin (and radiologically invisible) film of pleural fluid. (From Martin L: Pulmonary physiology in clinical practice: the essentials for patient care and evaluation, St Louis, 1987, The CV Mosby Co.)

it called *intrapleural pressure,* which differs in value from intraalveolar and atmospheric pressures. Second, the pleural space has the capacity to hold much more fluid than its normal volume of a few milliliters.

Intrapleural Pressure

Normally, intrapleural pressure is less than intra-pulmonary pressure* and less than atmospheric pressure. Atmospheric pressure, in pulmonary physiology, is assigned a value of zero; any pressure less than atmospheric pressure is negative, and any pressure greater than atmospheric pressure is positive.[20] Zero is used in reference to atmospheric pressure to simplify terminology. Atmospheric pressure at sea level is approximately 760 mm Hg; intrapleural pressure and intrapulmonary pressure vary from slightly above to slightly below 760 mm Hg.

Since under normal conditions intrapleural pressure is less than atmospheric pressure, it is recorded as a negative number, with a normal range of -4 cm H_2O to -10 cm H_2O during exhalation and inhalation, respectively. Fig. 17-11 illustrates these pressures. A deep inhalation can generate intrapleural pressures of -12 to -18 cm H_2O.

This negative intrapleural pressure results because forces within the chest wall exert pressure to pull the parietal pleura

*Intrapulmonary pressure is also known as intraalveolar pressure and reflects pressure inside the lungs.

(attached to the chest wall) outward and away from the visceral pleura (attached to the lungs) while the elastic fibers within the lungs exert pressure to pull the visceral pleura inward away from the parietal pleura. The constant "pull" of the two pleural membranes in opposite directions from each other causes the pressure within the space to be subatmospheric.

This subatmospheric pressure functions in a very important manner—it keeps the lungs inflated (see the box on p. 361). If atmospheric pressure enters the pleural space, all or part of a lung will collapse, producing a pneumothorax (frequently, a pneumothorax affects only a portion of one lung).

Intrapleural Fluid Volume

The pleural space is considered a "potential" space because, although it normally contains only a few milliliters of fluid, it has the capacity to hold much more. Pathologies such as congestive heart failure, cancer, pancreatic disease, or liver disease can result in an accumulation of fluid within this space[29]; the term for excess pleural fluid is *pleural effusion.* Bacterial and viral pneumonias can cause inflammation of the pleural membranes and altered pleural membrane permeability, which may allow protein to move into the pleural space. Water will follow the protein resulting in a pleural effusion.

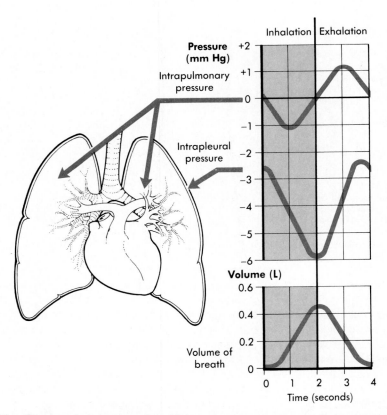

Fig. 17-11 Changes in intrapleural and intrapulmonary pressures during inhalation and exhalation. Just before inhalation, the intrapulmonary pressure falls, and intrapleural pressure becomes more negative. Just before exhalation, the intrapleural pressure rises, and intrapleural pressure becomes less negative.

WHY THE LUNGS STAY INFLATED

The lungs stay inflated because the pressure surrounding them (intrapleural) is always less than the pressure within them (intrapulmonary).

WHY IS THE INTRAPLEURAL PRESSURE LESS THAN THE INTRAPULMONARY PRESSURE?

The intrapleural pressure is always (1) less than intrapulmonary pressure, (2) less than atmospheric pressure, and (3) considered negative because of the "pull" of the two pleural membranes in opposite directions. The parietal pleura is pulled outward by forces within the chest wall while the visceral pleural is pulled inward by the force of the elastic fibers within the lungs.

WHY DO THE TWO PLEURAL MEMBRANES "PULL" IN OPPOSITE DIRECTION?

The parietal pleura, attached to the chest, is pulled outward because the elastic fibers within the intercostal muscles exert outward pressure on the ribs. These fibers are in a relaxed state when the rib cage is fully expanded such as during a deep inhalation.[6] The visceral pleural, attached to the lungs, is pulled inward because the elastic fibers within the lungs, responsible for elastic recoil, exert pressure to make the lungs smaller. Elastic fibers in the lungs are only in a relaxed position when the lung is at its smallest configuration such as occurs with a pneumothorax. Hence, because of the opposite pull of the chest wall and the lung and because the pleural membranes are attached to these structures, there is a constant pull of the two membranes in opposite directions. The subatmospheric pressure, which results within the pleural space, plus the greater than atmospheric intrapulmonary pressure within the lungs allow the lungs to remain inflated. Anything that causes the pressure within the pleural space to rise to atmospheric pressure or above will cause the lung(s) to collapse—a pneumothorax.

MUSCLES OF VENTILATION

The muscles of ventilation (Fig. 17-12) are governed by the regulatory activity of the medulla oblongata, which sends messages to the muscles to stimulate contraction and relaxation. This muscular activity controls inhalation and exhalation. Muscles that increase the size of the chest are called muscles of inhalation; those which decrease the size of the chest are called muscles of exhalation.

Muscles of Inhalation

The *diaphragm* is a dome-shaped fibromuscular septum that separates the thoracic and abdominal cavities and is connected to the sternum, ribs, and vertebrae. During normal, quiet breathing the diaphragm does approximately 80% of the work of breathing. When the diaphragm contracts, it pushes down on the viscera and displaces the abdomen outward. Diaphragmatic contraction also lifts and expands the rib cage to some extent.

The action of the diaphragm is governed by the medulla oblongata, which sends its impulses through the phrenic nerve. The phrenic nerve arises from the cervical plexus through the fourth cervical nerve, with secondary contributions by the third and fifth cervical nerves. For this reason and because the diaphragm does most of the work of inhalation, trauma involving C_3, C_4, and C_5 levels causes ventilatory dysfunction.

Other muscles of inhalation include the *external intercostal* muscles, which elevate the ribs, expanding the chest cage outward. The *scalene, anterior serrati,* and *sternocleidomastoid* muscles elevate the first two ribs and sternum.

Muscles of Exhalation

Exhalation in the healthy lung is a passive event requiring very little energy in comparison to that needed for inhalation. Exhalation occurs when the diaphragm relaxes and moves back up toward the lungs. The intrinsic elastic recoil of the lungs assists with exhalation.

Since exhalation is a passive act, there are no true muscles of exhalation other than the *internal intercostal* muscles, which assist the inward movement of the ribs. However, during exercise exhalation becomes a more active event, requiring some participation of the accessory muscles of ventilation. Several muscles of the abdomen have long been thought to contribute to active exhalation.

Accessory Muscles of Ventilation

The accessory muscles of ventilation are usually considered those muscles that enhance chest expansion during exercise but are not active during normal, quiet breathing. The accessory muscles include the *scalene, sternocleidomastoid,* and other chest and back muscles such as the *trapezius* and *pectoralis major.* Use of the accessory muscles at rest, which is common in patients with chronic pulmonary disease, is hard work since accessory muscle use requires great amounts of energy and oxygen. The accessory muscles sometimes are referred to as "oxygen robbers" because of the excessive amount of oxygen their use requires, depleting the amount available to other parts of the body.

Work of Breathing

The work of normal breathing occurs during inhalation and results from the muscular work needed to overcome lung recoil, chest wall recoil, and airway resistance during inhalation.[41] However, even exhalation can be a strain when lung recoil, chest wall recoil, and/or airway resistance is abnormal such as can occur in patients with emphysema, chronic bronchitis, asthma, pulmonary edema, and other pulmonary disorders.

During normal, quiet ventilation only 2% to 3% of the total energy expended by the body is required by the pulmonary system. During heavy exercise the amount of energy required by the pulmonary system will increase but only to 4% or 5% of the total body energy expended,[9] illustrating efficient energy use by a system that, when healthy, is well suited to its function.

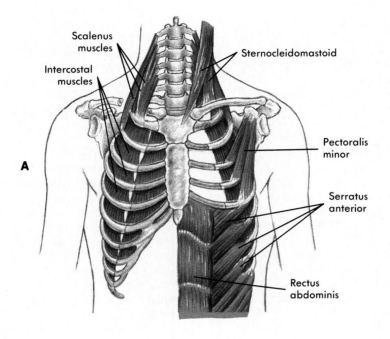

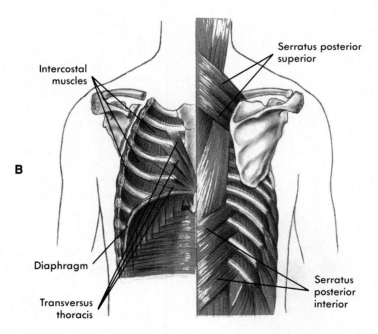

Fig. 17-12   Muscles of ventilation **A,** Anterior view. **B,** Posterior view.

Pathology of the pulmonary system, however, drastically changes the energy requirement for ventilation. Pulmonary diseases that decrease lung compliance (atelectasis, pulmonary edema), decrease chest wall compliance (kyphoscoliosis), increase airway resistance (bronchitis, chronic obstructive pulmonary disease [COPD]), or decrease lung recoil (emphysema) can increase the work of breathing so much that one third or more of the total body energy is used for ventilation.[9] Understanding this concept is vital since the increased work of breathing alone requires great energy, which, coupled with an acute illness, may postpone a critically ill patient's recovery (see the section in Chapter 22 on ineffective breathing patterns for more information about how increased work of breathing can alter breathing patterns).

VENTILATION

Ventilation is defined as the movement of air into and out of the lungs and is distinct from respiration, which refers to gas exchange, not movement of air. The difference between ventilation and respiration may be clarified when considering a mechanical ventilator (in previous years, sometimes incorrectly called a respirator). The mechanical ventilator is a machine designed to perform one lifesaving function—to move oxygen into a patient's lungs. The machine cannot make the oxygen diffuse into the pulmonary capillary; it can only act as a bellows to move gas into the lung. Patients succumb to serious pulmonary infections and diseases (adult respiratory distress syndrome [ARDS], for example) when on mechanical ventilation because, even though the machine can deliver 100% oxygen to the patient's lungs, it cannot effectively assist in the diffusion of that oxygen across the alveolar-capillary membrane. The closest science has come to designing a true respirator is the heart-lung machine used during cardiac surgery.

Inhalation

Air moves into and out of the lungs because of changes in the pressure inside the lungs (intrapulmonary pressure) compared to atmospheric pressure. When intrapulmonary pressure is less than atmospheric pressure, air, following normal gas laws, will move from the area of higher pressure to the area of lower pressure. Thus when the intrapulmonary pressure falls below atmospheric pressure, air will flow into the lungs. The question then arises, why does the intrapulmonary pressure fall below atmospheric pressure?

Intrapulmonary pressure falls below atmospheric pressure when the muscles of inhalation cause the chest and lungs to expand. As this expansion occurs, the volume of gas within the lungs moves into a larger space. Applying normal gas laws, *when a fixed volume moves into a larger space, the pressure within the space will fall*. Hence, at the command of the medulla oblongata, the muscles of ventilation contract, the thorax and lungs expand, and the intrapulmonary pressure falls. When it falls below atmospheric pressure, air from the atmosphere will enter as an inhalation.

Exhalation

Air moves out of the lungs because of the same principles that caused it to enter. When the intrapulmonary pressure

is greater than the atmospheric pressure, air will move from the lungs into the atmosphere. Intrapulmonary pressure rises above atmospheric pressure when, just after inhalation, the muscles of ventilation relax, causing the thorax and ribs to lower and the lung to be compressed. This compression forces the gas within the lungs into a smaller area. Once more, applying normal gas laws, *when a fixed volume of gas is compressed into a smaller area, the pressure within the area will rise*. As the lungs are compressed, intrapulmonary pressure rises. When it rises above atmospheric pressure, exhalation occurs.

How Lung Disease Can Alter Ventilation

Normal *muscular action of the diaphragm, flexibility of the rib cage, elasticity of the lungs, and airway diameter* are instrumental in allowing easy inhalation and exhalation. Anything that interferes with these actions will impair normal ventilation.

Many authorities categorize pulmonary diseases into *obstructive* or *restrictive* diseases. In some part, these terms refer to failure of the diaphragm, the rib cage, the lungs, and/or the airways to allow normal ventilation. Restrictive diseases "restrict" lung or chest wall movement and include, among others, diffuse interstitial lung fibrosis, atelectasis, kyphoscoliosis, and severe chest wall pain. These conditions can be either acute or chronic, and because they restrict lung and/or chest wall expansion, patients will have smaller tidal volumes but an increased ventilatory rate to maintain minute ventilation. Obstructive diseases result in obstruction to normal airflow. The classic examples are emphysema, in which airflow is decreased because of a decrease in lung recoil, and asthma, in which airflow is decreased because of diffuse airway narrowing.

Emphysema results in lungs that inflate easily but, lacking the normal elastic recoil, do not compress to assist with exhalation. Patients with emphysema may have little difficulty inhaling but struggle to exhale.

Normal ventilation depends on many factors, the most important of which are flexibility of the rib cage and elasticity of the lungs, as well as normal action of the muscles of ventilation and normal airway diameter. When patients are critically ill with a disease that alters the function of any of these factors, assessment of the efficiency or inefficiency of ventilation is mandatory.

Pulmonary Volumes and Capacities

Pulmonary volumes and capacities refer to the various parts of the total lung capacity. These volumes and capacities are a part of the pulmonary function tests that assist in the diagnosis of pulmonary disease.

The following discussion concerns only those tests that are of value in critical care and with which the critical care nurse should be familiar to assist in providing efficient patient care. Table 17-2 provides a review of these tests.

Volumes and capacities vary with a person's age, sex, and size. A 25-year-old man has a total lung capacity of approximately 6000 cc, a vital capacity of 4800 cc, and a residual volume of 1200 cc, whereas a 25-year-old woman has a total lung capacity of 4200 cc, a vital capacity of 3200 cc, and a residual volume of 1000 cc.[41]

Table 17-2 Pulmonary volumes and capacities relevant to critical care

Volume capacity	Definition	Relevance
Tidal volume (VT)	Volume of air exhaled after normal inhalation; estimated at 500 cc or 6 to 8 cc/kg, while off ventilator, or 10 to 15 cc/kg while on ventilator	Used to assess weaning from mechanical ventilation Must be significantly greater than dead space
Minute ventilation (V̇E)	Volume of air inhaled per minute—VT × RR* Normal, 4 to 8 L/min (adult)	Must be high enough to prevent accumulation of carbon dioxide (PaCO₂) Used to assess weaning from mechanical ventilation
Minute alveolar ventilation (V̇A)	Volume of air reaching alveoli per minute—(VT − VD)† × RR	Same as V̇E Not routinely measured
Vital capacity (VC)	Volume of air exhaled after the deepest inhalation Normal, 3 to 5 L	Essential to weaning Usually must be >1 L or 10 to 15 cc/kg for successful weaning from mechanical ventilation
Functional residual capacity (FRC)	Volume of air in lung after normal exhalation Normal, 2500 cc	Keeps the lung minimally inflated, decreasing the work of breathing Provides gas exchange between breaths

*RR, Respiratory rate.
†VD, Volume of dead space.

Tidal volume (VT) represents the volume of air that is exhaled after a normal inhalation. During normal, quiet breathing in a healthy individual, VT ranges from 450 to 600 cc, with an average of 500 cc per breath[35]; however, VT varies with a person's age, size, and state of health. Another method of predicting VT is to use the following amounts: (1) 6 to 8 cc/kg for patients not on a ventilator and (2) 10 to 15 cc/kg for patients on a ventilator. As is apparent using the second formula, patients on mechanical ventilation have high VTs.

When the VT is multiplied by the respiratory rate (RR), the patient's *minute ventilation (V̇E)* is calculated. The assessment of V̇E is as important to evaluating the pulmonary system as is the assessment of cardiac output to evaluating the cardiac system. V̇E represents the volume of air needed each minute for the body to maintain normal metabolism. Because a normal V̇E is essential, the body will compensate by various means to maintain the V̇E. Generally, compensation becomes necessary when a patient's VT falls and, to keep V̇E within normal limits, the ventilatory rate rises. A rise in the ventilatory rate can compensate only so far because as the rate rises, the work of breathing increases. VT and ventilatory rate should be considered when checking the V̇E. Even in situations in which the V̇E is not calculated, the VT and respiratory rate should be checked to assess whether each is *effective* for maintaining metabolism and that each *can be maintained* by the patient.

V̇E is not an accurate assessment of the amount of air reaching the alveolar portion of the lungs because, by using the full VT in the formula (VT × RR), the amount of air ventilating the conducting airways in which no gas exchange takes place is included. To assess the amount of air reaching the alveolar portion of the lungs, the volume of gas ventilating the conducting airways must be subtracted to yield

the *minute alveolar ventilation (V̇A)*. Since the volume of air filling the conducting airways can be estimated at 150 ml, the formula for calculating the V̇A is simply (VT − 150 ml) × RR = V̇A.

Air remaining within the conducting airways that does not reach the alveoli is termed air occupying *dead space*. There are three types of dead space—anatomic, alveolar, and physiologic (see the following box). Any clinician planning to work in critical care should be familiar with these concepts because they are requisite to the understanding of

---

TYPES OF DEAD SPACE

ANATOMIC DEAD SPACE

The volume of the conducting airways
Usually estimated at 150 cc
Formula: 1cc/lb ideal body weight or 2 cc/kg ideal body weight

ALVEOLAR DEAD SPACE

Any area within the gas exchange region of the lungs in which ventilation occurs without perfusion
Not found in the normal lung

PHYSIOLOGIC DEAD SPACE

The combination of both the anatomical and the alveolar dead space

mechanical ventilation, of ventilation-perfusion inequalities, and of some pulmonary disorders and treatment modalities.

Anatomic dead space is defined as the area from mouth and nose to terminal bronchioles and is usually estimated at approximately 150 cc. A more specific method of assessing the volume of anatomic dead space uses the following formula: 1 cc of dead space per pound or 2 cc of dead space per kilogram of *ideal* body weight. Anatomic dead space is so termed because it is a component of normal pulmonary anatomy and, under normal conditions, is the only lung area in which dead space exists.

At times, however, pathology within the pulmonary system leads to dead space in areas other than the conducting airways. *Alveolar dead space* is pathological and occurs when a gas exchange area is no longer normally perfused. One pathology that produces alveolar dead space is pulmonary embolism. In this circumstance, the embolism decreases blood flow to the lung area distal to it, but the area may still receive ventilation. The result is an area of ventilation with no perfusion, that is, dead space. Normally, there is no measurable alveolar dead space within the lung. Other pathologies that can lead to alveolar dead space include hypotension from decreased cardiac ouput or hemorrhage. In this case, a redistribution of blood flow and volume favors the dependent parts of the lungs, causing decreased perfusion in many well-ventilated alveoli in the upper lung areas. Positive pressure mechanical ventilation may cause alveolar dead space because the positive pressure can restrict blood flow through some pulmonary capillaries.[20]

Physiologic dead space refers to the combination of anatomic and alveolar dead space. Since there is normally no alveolar dead space, physiologic dead space should equal anatomical dead space in healthy lungs.

Vital capacity (VC) is the volume of gas that can be expelled from the lungs after a maximal inhalation. In healthy lungs VC represents approximately 80% of total lung capacity. Normal values can vary significantly, depending on age, sex, and position of the patient's body at the time of testing.[35] VC is used as a weaning and an extubation parameter because it is a measure of the strength of the ventilatory muscles and thus yields some information about the patient's ability to sustain his ventilations after mechanical ventilation. Generally, a VC of 10 to 15 ml/kg of body weight is necessary for successful weaning.[10,16]

The *residual volume (RV)* is the volume of air left in the lung after the most forceful exhalation and represents a volume that can never be fully expelled.

Similar in definition to RV is *expiratory reserve volume (ERV),* which is defined as the amount of air that can be further exhaled after a normal exhalation. The ERV does not include the RV (the volume that cannot be exhaled). In the healthy lung there is always a volume of air that can be exhaled further after a normal, quiet exhalation. It represents approximately 1000 cc. Together, these two volumes, the RV and the ERV, reflect the volume of air that remains within the lung after a normal exhalation. Neither is generally measured at the bedside but requires specialized equipment found in the pulmonary function laboratory.

When added together, the RV and the ERV compose the *functional residual capacity (FRC).*

The FRC is the amount of air left in the lung after exhalation. One may wonder why have any air left in the lung after exhalation? One reason is that it is easier to inflate the lungs again if they are already partially inflated (in the same way that it is easier to blow up a partially inflated balloon than a completely deflated one). Thus the work of inhalation is decreased if some air remains within the lungs after exhalation.

In addition to assisting inhalation, the FRC fills the lungs with air that can be used for gas exchange between breaths. With every heartbeat, new blood is moved into the pulmonary capillaries for gas exchange. If there were no air within the lungs between inhalations, there would be no mechanism for gas exchange between inhalations; thus the FRC increases the efficiency of oxygenation.

RESPIRATION

Respiration refers to the movement of oxygen and carbon dioxide. These gases diffuse across the alveolar-capillary membrane, an event referred to as external respiration, and they diffuse into and out of the cells, an event referred to as internal respiration. This section focuses only on the movement of these gases across the alveolar-capillary membrane. See the next section, "Gas Transport," for a discussion of diffusion at the cellular level.

All gases of concern in respiratory physiology are simple molecules free to move among each other in the atmosphere, where they remain in the gaseous state, and in tissue fluids such as blood, where they remain in either a gaseous or a liquid state. These gases are often called volatile because of their unique ability to move from a liquid to a gaseous state and vice versa. An example can be seen with the change in oxygen as it moves from its gaseous state in the alveoli into its liquid state in the pulmonary capillaries. Gases other than oxygen and carbon dioxide are volatile and are of some importance when studying pulmonary physiology and pulmonary disease. Carbon monoxide and nitrogen are two such gases, although carbon monoxide is not plentiful in the atmosphere and nitrogen will only diffuse across the alveolar-capillary membrane under greater than atmospheric pressure such as occurs during scuba diving.

Diffusion

Oxygen and carbon dioxide move throughout the body by diffusion. Diffusion moves molecules from an area of high concentration to an area of low concentration and functions only when there is a source of energy or "drive." Within the lungs this energy is generated because of the difference in the pressure that is exerted by the concentration of each gas within the pulmonary capillaries and within the alveoli. Oxygen is in high concentration and thus exerts a high pressure within the alveoli as compared to the pressure it exerts within the pulmonary capillary. Therefore oxygen moves by diffusion from the alveoli into the pulmonary capillaries. On the other hand, carbon dioxide is in higher concentration within the pulmonary capillary than within the alveoli; carbon dioxide, therefore, diffuses out of the

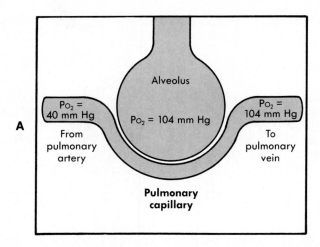

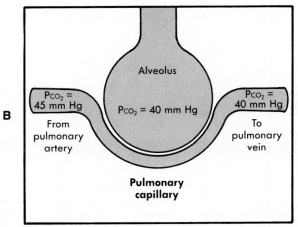

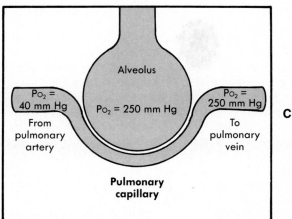

Fig. 17-13 **A,** Diffusion of oxygen from the alveolus into pulmonary capillary blood. The alveolar partial pressure of oxygen (P_{AO_2}) of 104 mmHg assumes room air has been breathed at sea level by a healthy subject. **B,** Diffusion of carbon dioxide from the pulmonary capillary blood into the alveolus. **C,** Diffusion of oxygen from the alveolus into pulmonary capillary blood. The P_{AO_2} is elevated because supplemental oxygen is being administered.

capillaries into the alveoli where it is exhaled. Fig. 17-13, *A* and *B* illustrates these two concepts.

There are several factors that affect diffusion and which, under certain circumstances, critical care nurses have the ability to control and thus must understand.

How oxygen therapy alters diffusion. To understand how oxygen therapy affects diffusion, one must be familiar with basic concepts of gas movement. One essential concept is that the greater the difference in pressure across the alveolar-capillary membrane, the greater will be diffusion. It follows, then, that a higher concentration of oxygen within the atmosphere will result in more oxygen available to the alveoli and a greater amount of oxygen transferred by diffusion. (This concept assumes the individual has healthy lungs and a normal ventilatory pattern.)

The pressure oxygen exerts within the alveoli is referred to as P_{AO_2} (P, pressure; A, alveoli; O_2, oxygen). Breathing room air at sea level will yield a P_{AO_2} of approximately 104 mm Hg. Diffusion takes place across the alveolus because the P_{AO_2} is so much higher than the pressure of oxygen in

the pulmonary capillaries, which is normally only approximately 40 mm Hg. Thus there exists a large difference in the pressures, and this creates the drive for diffusion.

This drive could be made even stronger by increasing the P_{AO_2}. How can this be done? It is accomplished everyday in hospitals through the administration of supplemental oxygen. Fig. 17-13, *C*, shows the change in P_{AO_2} associated with oxygen adminstration. In the healthy lung when the P_{AO_2} is increased, the additional oxygen will diffuse into the capillary in which it is reflected as a rise in the partial pressure of oxygen within the arterial blood (P_{aO_2}).

How altitude alters diffusion. As long as one stays at sea level, the P_{AO_2} will remain at approximately 104 mm Hg. However, the farther above sea level one climbs, the lower will be the barometric pressure and the lower will be the P_{AO_2}. Table 17-3 shows how various altitudes will lower the P_{AO_2}. Of particular interest to the nursing community is the change in P_{AO_2} that occurs when flying in the passenger cabin of a commercial airliner. Because airline cabins are pressurized only to approximately 6000 to 8000 feet (not

Table 17-3   Inspired and alveolar oxygen pressure at various altitudes*

Location	Altitude (feet)	PB (mm Hg)	PIO$_2$ (mm Hg)	PAO$_2$† (mm Hg)
Miami	0	760	160	102
Denver	5,280	629	132	74
Airplane—passenger cabin	6,000	608	128	70
Mexico City	7,347	578	121	64
Leadville, Colorado	10,200	517	109	51
Top of Mt. Everest‡	29,028	253	53	−5
Air outside plane while cruising	35,000	160	34	−24

From Martin L: Pulmonary physiology in clinical practice: the essentials for patient care and evaluation, St Louis, 1987, The CV Mosby Co.
*At all altitudes, FIO$_2$, 0.21; PB, barometric pressure; PIO$_2$, partial pressure of oxygen in atmosphere (dry air); PAO$_2$, alveolar PO$_2$.
†PAO$_2$ is calculated using the formula PAO$_2$ = FIO$_2$(PB − 47) − 1.2(PCO$_2$), where PCO$_2$ = 40 mm Hg. Normally there is compensatory hyperventilation with increasing altitude so that the actual PAO$_2$ will be higher than is shown, depending on the degree of hyperventilation.
‡Calculations for Mt. Everest are based on data from West JB and others: J Appl Physiol 55:678, 1983. On the top of Mt Everest alveolar PCO$_2$ was measured at 7.5 mm Hg, and PAO$_2$ measured as 35 mm Hg; the calculated PAO$_2$ without supplemental oxygen is 28 mm Hg.

to sea level), the barometric pressure within the atmosphere of the cabin is equivalent to that at 6000 to 8000 feet above sea level.[1,11,20] Hence, the PAO$_2$ is less, there is a decreased drive for diffusion across the alveolar-capillary membrane, and the PaO$_2$ falls. For this reason, some patients cannot fly without supplemental oxygen use and cannot live at extreme altitudes. High altitude dwellers compensate for the lowered PAO$_2$ through means such as polycythemia.

How loss or gain of lung tissue alters diffusion. The total lung area available for diffusion averages greater than 70 m². This means that if the respiratory portions of the lungs were laid on a floor, they would cover an area at least 30 × 25 feet in size.[9] Anything that decreases or increases that surface area will alter the total amount of gas that can be diffused.

Lobectomy or pneumonectomy results in loss of the diffusion membrane, although arterial blood gas values are often normal after either procedure, particularly when the patient is resting. When enough of the respiratory portion of lung area is lost; however, blood gas values will show abnormalities.

The area for diffusion is increased naturally every time a person sighs because the sigh opens partially inflated alveoli, therefore increasing the area available for diffusion. For a long time *artificially* increasing the area for diffusion was not a reality. Now, however, this can be accomplished artificially through the use of positive end-expiratory pressure (PEEP) on mechanically ventilated patients. PEEP exerts a pressure within the lungs that holds alveoli open somewhat wider than they would be without its use and, as does the sigh, opens partially inflated alveoli. PEEP results in an increase in the FRC and the available alveolar surface area, thereby improving ventilation-perfusion relationships and the PaO$_2$.[8,27]

GAS TRANSPORT

Gas transport refers to the movement of oxygen and carbon dioxide to and from the tissue cells. The transportation vehicle is the bloodstream, which is moved by the pumping action of the heart. At the tissue level, both oxygen and carbon dioxide move into and out of the cell by diffusion. Fig. 17-14 illustrates the movement of oxygen and carbon dioxide.

How Changes in PaO$_2$ Alter Tissue Oxygenation

Fig. 17-14, *A*, illustrates the pressure difference between the arterial partial pressure of oxygen (PaO$_2$) and the oxygen level of a tissue cell. (Intracellular oxygen levels vary widely from tissue to tissue, sometimes being much lower than the 40 mm Hg used for Fig. 17-14, *A*.) Oxygen diffuses because of the pressure gradient that exists between oxygen in the blood and oxygen in the cell. Suppose, because of pulmonary disease, the PaO$_2$ has fallen from 95 to 55 mm Hg. This would cause the pressure gradient to be less, although diffusion would still occur. Now suppose the pulmonary disease worsens, causing the PaO$_2$ to fall further, severely compromising the pressure gradient. Tissue hypoxia would result when the PaO$_2$ falls to the point at which a functional diffusion gradient no longer exists.

What happens when the PaO$_2$ is elevated above normal by the application of supplemental oxygen? The addition of supplemental oxygen may raise the PaO$_2$ to a level at which a more functional gradient exists. Considering Fig. 17-14, *A*, once more, it is easy to see that elevation of PaO$_2$ will increase the gradient between oxygen in the arterial blood and oxygen in the tissue cell, thus improving diffusion.

Oxygen Transport Within the Blood

Oxygen is transported to the tissue cells by the blood in two ways. It is either *dissolved in plasma (PaO$_2$)* or *bound to hemoglobin molecules (SaO$_2$)*. Most of the oxygen is transported by hemoglobin, with the portion of oxygen dissolved in plasma equal to approximately 3% of the total oxygen within the blood. However, whereas only a small portion of the total amount of oxygen carried by the blood is dissolved in plasma, it is this dissolved portion that is significant to cellular oxygenation. The pressure exerted by the oxygen dissolved in plasma is important because this oxygen diffuses across the capillary membrane into the cells first and serves as the vehicle for the unloading of the oxygen from the hemoglobin molecule. As molecules of dissolved

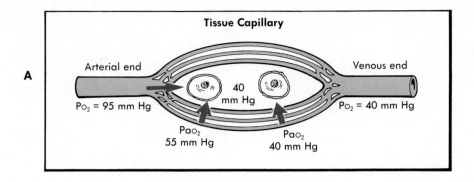

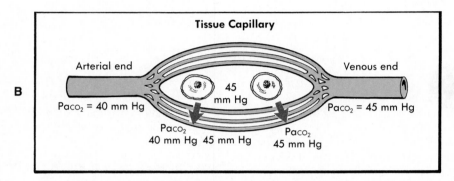

Fig. 17-14 **A,** Diffusion of oxygen from a tissue capillary into a tissue cell. **B,** Diffusion of carbon dioxide from a tissue cell into a tissue capillary.

oxygen leave the plasma and diffuse into the cells, the molecules of oxygen move off the hemoglobin, dissolve into the plasma, and, in turn, diffuse into the cells. For this procedure to begin, the PaO_2 must be greater than the oxygen level within the cell.

Oxyhemoglobin dissociation curve. The relationship between dissolved oxygen and hemoglobin-bound oxygen is illustrated graphically as the oxyhemoglobin dissociation curve (Fig. 17-15). The sigmoid shape of the oxyhemoglobin dissociation curve illustrates several essential points about the relationship between the two ways oxygen is carried. The *steep lower portion* of the curve, at PaO_2 levels of 10 to 50 mm Hg, shows that the peripheral tissues can withdraw large amounts of oxygen from the hemoglobin molecule with only a small change in PaO_2, thus preserving the gradient for the continued unloading of hemoglobin.

The area at PaO_2 levels of 60 to 100 mm Hg is called the *flat upper portion* of the curve. This portion shows that the saturation of hemoglobin remains high even as the PaO_2 declines. For example, in a healthy person, a PaO_2 of 60 mm Hg yields a saturation of 89%, whereas a PaO_2 of 100 mm Hg yields a saturation of 98%. The great drop in PaO_2 (from 100 to 60 mm Hg) causes only a small drop in oxygen saturation (from 98% to 89%). For this reason, many patients with chronic lung disease manage quite well with a PaO_2 as low as 55 or 60 mm Hg since that level (1) provides sufficient loading of hemoglobin with oxygen and (2) provides a PaO_2 gradient sufficient for the unloading of hemoglobin.

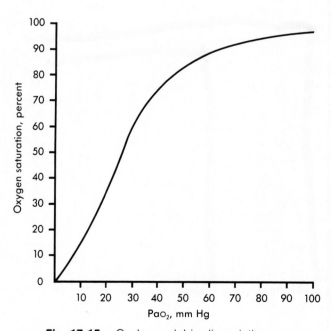

Fig. 17-15 Oxyhemoglobin dissociation curve.

Table 17-4 Predictable relationship of Pa_{O_2} and Sa_{O_2} on the normal oxyhemoglobin dissociation curve

Pa_{O_2} (mm Hg)	Sa_{O_2} (%)
100	98
90	97
80	95
70	93
60	89
50	84
40	75
30	57
20	35
10	14

The ability of human beings to live comfortably at high altitudes is based on the unique relationship between dissolved oxygen and hemoglobin-bound oxygen, illustrated by assessing the flat upper portion of the curve. At high altitudes, because of the decreased barometric pressure, the Pa_{O_2} will fall. There exists a wide range in which the Pa_{O_2} can fall, yet loading of the hemoglobin molecule remains quite sufficient.

Shifting of the oxyhemoglobin dissociation curve. Under normal circumstances, hemoglobin has a steady and predictable affinity for oxygen. The combination of oxygen and hemoglobin based on this affinity is responsible for the position of the oxyhemoglobin dissociation curve wherein a given Pa_{O_2} will yield a predictable oxygen saturation. Table 17-4 illustrates this predictable relationship between the Pa_{O_2} and the Sa_{O_2}.

Occasionally, particularly in critically ill individuals, events will occur that alter the affinity hemoglobin has for oxygen. Anytime this affinity is altered, the position of the oxyhemoglobin dissociation curve will shift (Fig. 17-16). Shifts in the position of the curve mean there is a change in the way oxygen is taken up by the hemoglobin molecule at the alveolar level, as well as a change in the way oxygen is delivered at the tissue level.

Clinical implications of a shifted curve. When the curve is shifted to the right (Fig. 17-16, *curve C*), there is a lower oxygen saturation for any given Pa_{O_2}; in other words, hemoglobin has less affinity for oxygen. Although the saturation is lower than expected, a right shift enhances oxygen delivery at the tissue level because hemoglobin unloads more readily. Factors that cause this change in oxygen-hemoglobin affinity and thus shift the curve include fever, increased Pa_{CO_2}, acidosis, and an increase in 2,3-diphosphoglycerate (2,3-DPG) (see the box on p. 371).

When the curve is shifted to the left (Fig. 17-13, *curve A*), quite the reverse occurs; there is a higher arterial saturation for any give Pa_{O_2} because hemoglobin has an increased affinity for oxygen. Although the saturation is higher, oxygen delivery to the tissues is impaired because

hemoglobin does not unload as easily. Factors that contribute to the effect include hypothermia, alkalemia, decreased Pa_{CO_2}, and decreased 2,3-DPG.

To assess whether the curve is shifted to the left or to the right, the Pa_{O_2} at the 50% saturation level (P_{50}) must be assessed. Fig. 17-16 shows that when the curve is in its normal position, a P_{50} is associated with a Pa_{O_2} of 26.6 mm Hg. If, when looking at the P_{50}, the Pa_{O_2} is higher, the curve is shifted to the right (Fig. 17-16, *curve C*). On the other hand, if, when looking at the P_{50}, the Pa_{O_2} is less than 26.6 mm Hg, the curve is shifted to the left (Fig. 17-16, *curve A*).

When working in a clinical situation in which a P_{50} is not available, one need only remember the above clinical situations that are responsible for left and for right shift of the curve.

Abnormalities of hemoglobin structure. Hemoglobin carries approximately 97% of the total amount of oxygen held within the bloodstream. This great carrying capacity is dependent on hemoglobin's being normal in amount and molecular structure. Normal adult hemoglobin is labeled hemoglobin A (Hb A). Abnormal hemoglobins do exist, and situations occur in which normal hemoglobin becomes abnormal. Most hemoglobin abnormalities affect the oxygen-carrying capability of this molecule. Methemoglobin and carboxyhemoglobin are abnormalities of hemoglobin that are sometimes present in the critically ill patient.

Methemoglobin. Certain drugs (Table 17-5), particularly nitrates and sulfonamides, will change normal hemoglobin into methemoglobin (metHb). Methemoglobin occurs when the iron atoms within the Hb A molecule are oxidized from the ferrous state to the ferric state. Methemoglobin does not carry oxygen, and, in high enough levels, will cause tissue hypoxia. It will also cause cyanosis because metHb darkens the color of the oxidized hemoglobin. Normally, approximately 1.5% of hemoglobin is in this oxidized state; an amount greater than 1.5% defines a state of methemoglobinemia.[20] Mild methemoglobinemia (metHb <30%) is treated with supplemental oxygen and removal of the offending drug. More severe cases can be treated with methylene blue, which acts as a reducing agent that converts the ferric state back to the ferrous state and returns the metHb to Hb A.

Carboxyhemoglobin. Carboxyhemoglobin (HbCO) occurs when carbon monoxide (CO) combines with Hb A. HbCO exposure can be lethal because the carbon monoxide molecule uses the same binding site on the Hb molecule that oxygen uses. However, carbon monoxide's affinity for Hb is approximately 220 times that of oxygen; thus, when in competition with oxygen for the Hb binding site, carbon monoxide will always bind before oxygen can. Unfortunately, the body cannot use carbon monoxide for metabolism; hence, when enough Hb becomes bound with carbon monoxide and not oxygen, tissue hypoxia will result. Normal HbCO levels are less than 2%, but levels of only 10% can lead to symptoms, whereas levels of 20% or more are indicative of cellular hypoxia. Table 17-6 shows the clinical effects of carbon monoxide poisoning.

Exposure to heavy automobile traffic or to cigarette smoke can raise HbCO from its normal level up to 10%. Patients

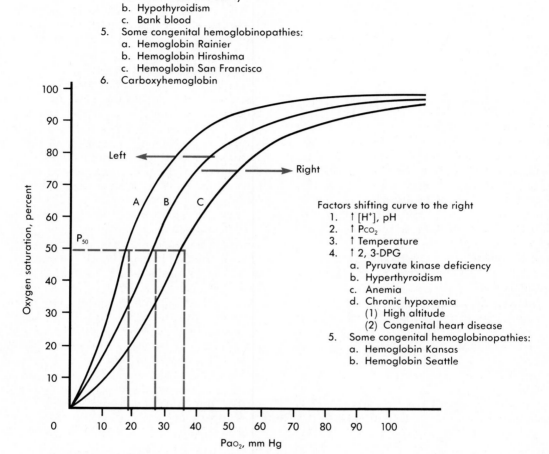

Factors shifting curve to the left
1. ↓ [H⁺], pH
2. ↓ Pco₂
3. ↓ Temperature
4. ↓ 2, 3-DPG
   a. Hexokinase deficiency
   b. Hypothyroidism
   c. Bank blood
5. Some congenital hemoglobinopathies:
   a. Hemoglobin Rainier
   b. Hemoglobin Hiroshima
   c. Hemoglobin San Francisco
6. Carboxyhemoglobin

Factors shifting curve to the right
1. ↑ [H⁺], pH
2. ↑ Pco₂
3. ↑ Temperature
4. ↑ 2, 3-DPG
   a. Pyruvate kinase deficiency
   b. Hyperthyroidism
   c. Anemia
   d. Chronic hypoxemia
      (1) High altitude
      (2) Congenital heart disease
5. Some congenital hemoglobinopathies:
   a. Hemoglobin Kansas
   b. Hemoglobin Seattle

Fig. 17-16 Curve B is the standard oxyhemoglobin dissociation curve. Curve A shows the curve shifted to the left because of hemoglobin's increased affinity for oxygen. Curve C shows the curve shifted to the right because of hemoglobin's decreased affinity for oxygen. Factors responsible for shifting the curve are listed adjacent to curves A and C. (From Kinney MR and others: AACN's clinical reference for critical care nursing, St Louis, 1988, The CV Mosby Co.)

WHAT IS 2,3-DPG?

2,3-Diphosphoglycerate (2,3-DPG), an organic phosphate found primarily in red blood cells, has the ability to alter the affinity of hemoglobin for oxygen. When the level of 2,3-DPG increases within the red blood cells, hemoglobin's affinity for oxygen is decreased (a shift in the oxyhemoglobin curve to the right), thus making more oxygen available to the tissues. Increased synthesis of 2,3-DPG apparently is an important component of the adaptive responses in healthy persons to an acute need for more tissue oxygen. Tissue hypoxia acts as the stimulus for production of 2,3-DPG, and increased amounts have been found in patients with anemia, right-to-left shunts, and congestive heart failure and in persons residing at high altitudes.[23]

A decrease in the amount of 2,3-DPG is detrimental to tissue oxygenation because this decrease causes hemoglobin's affinity for oxygen to increase (a shift in the oxyhemoglobin curve to the left). Situations resulting in decreased 2,3-DPG levels include hypophosphatemia, septic shock, and the use of banked blood. Blood preserved with acid citrate dextrose loses most of its red cell 2,3-DPG within several days. Blood preserved with citrate phosphate dextrose maintains its 2,3-DPG levels for several weeks. Transfusion of blood with low 2,3-DPG will not be beneficial for tissue oxygenation until the 2,3-DPG level is restored, which may take 18 to 24 hours.[1]

Table 17-5 Some drugs implicated in causing methemoglobinemia

Generic name	Use
Dapsone	Skin protectant
Benzocaine	Local anesthetic
Metoclopramide	Gastric stasis
Nitroglycerin	Angina
Phenazopyridine	Urinary tract analgesic
Prilocaine	Local anesthetic
Primaquine	Malaria prophylaxis and treatment
Trimethoprim	Urinary antibacterial
Amyl nitrite	Rarely used clinically; often used by drug abusers

From Martin L: Pulmonary physiology in clinical practice: the essentials for patient care and evaluation, St Louis, 1987, The CV Mosby Co.

Table 17-6 Correlation of symptoms and signs with carbon monoxide level

Percent of carbon monoxide in inspired air	Percent of HbCO in blood	Signs and symptoms
0.007	10	Common in cigarette smokers; dyspnea during vigorous exertion; occasional tightness in forehead; dilation of cutaneous blood vessels
0.012	20	Dyspnea during moderate exertion; occasional throbbing headache in temples
0.022	30	Severe headache; irritability; easy fatigability; disturbed judgment; possible dizziness and possible dimness of vision
0.035-0.052	40-50	Headache; confusion; fainting on exertion
0.080-0.122	60-70	Unconsciousness; intermittent convulsions; respiratory failure; death if exposure prolonged
0.195	80	Fatal

From Martin L: Pulmonary physiology in clinical practice: the essentials for patient care and evaluation, St Louis, 1987, The CV Mosby Co; modified from Winter PM and Miller JN: JAMA 236:1503, 1976, Copyright 1976, American Medical Association.

with preexisting chronic hypoxemia have decreased exercise tolerance at levels of 4% or more HbCO.[20] At levels of 5% to 8% HbCO, healthy coronary arteries will dilate to bring more blood to the myocardium to compensate for the decreased oxygen content. In persons with fixed coronary artery obstruction, dilation may not be possible, leading to compromise of cardiac oxygenation. There is also evidence that HbCO leads to a decrease in the threshold for ventricular fibrillation, possibly relating to the sudden death of smokers with coronary disease.[20]

Treatment of HbCO includes removing the source of the carbon monoxide poisoning and administering oxygen. The half-life of HbCO when an individual is breathing room air is approximately 4 to 6 hours. With administration of 100% oxygen, the half-life can be shortened to 1 hour.[16] Patients with severe poisoning may require endotracheal intubation followed by administration of 100% oxygen. Hyperbaric oxygen therapy, although not always available or practical, is highly effective. Hyperbaric therapy can dissolve enough oxygen in plasma (6 ml/100 ml plasma when breathing 100% oxygen at 3 atm) to sustain life, even if HbCO is 100%.[20]

Abnormalities of hemoglobin quantity. "Deoxygenated hemoglobin" (previously known as reduced hemoglobin) refers to the amount of hemoglobin not saturated with oxygen and means that the oxygen binding site is empty. Therefore some portion of the hemoglobin content is desaturated.

Deoxygenated hemoglobin results for various reasons, including low quantity of oxygen in the atmosphere, hypoventilation, and acute or chronic pulmonary disease. When 5 g or more of hemoglobin per 100 ml of blood are desaturated, cyanosis will be present because the color of desaturated blood is darker than the color of saturated blood. Venous blood is desaturated, hence its dark color when compared to arterial blood.

Carbon Dioxide Transport Within the Blood

Carbon dioxide (CO_2), one of the end products of aerobic cellular metabolism, is produced continuously within the cells. On its way from the cells to the lungs, carbon dioxide is transported within the plasma and the erythrocytes. Plasma carbon dioxide is transported (1) physically dissolved as the Pa_{CO_2}, (2) bound to plasma proteins to form carbamino compounds, or (3) combined with water to form carbonic acid, some of which dissociates into hydrogen ions and bicarbonate. Most of the carbon dioxide, however, diffuses into the red blood cells and is carried and (1) dissolved, (2) combined with water to form carbonic acid, then hydrogen ions and bicarbonate, and (3) combined with hemoglobin.

In the lungs, these methods of carbon dioxide carriage are reversed as the carbon dioxide leaves the plasma and erythrocytes for exhalation.[23]

REGULATION OF VENTILATION

Regulation of ventilation by the brain is complex and not completely understood. The simple overview presented here provides a basic understanding of the control of ventilation.

Ventilation is regulated by a triad comprising a *controller* (located within the central nervous system), a group of *effectors*, which are the muscles of ventilation, and a group of central (located in the brainstem and medulla oblongata) and peripheral *chemoreceptors* (located within the aortic arch and the carotid arteries).

The Controller

The central nervous system houses what is known as the controller of ventilation. Actually, the controller is not located in one specific area; rather, it is in several areas that work in conjunction to provide coordinated ventilation. The brainstem regulates automatic ventilation, the cerebral cortex allows voluntary ventilation, and neurons housed in the spinal cord process information from the brain and from the peripheral receptors, allowing them to send final information to the muscles of ventilation (Fig. 17-17).

In the brainstem, both the medulla oblongata and the pons function during ventilation. The reticular formation of the medulla houses cells that regulate both inhalation and exhalation. One popular, although not universally accepted theory, concludes that some of the cells located in the dorsal region of the medulla automatically fire, triggering inhalation in much the same way as the sinoatrial node fires to trigger depolarization of the heart.[44] Other cells located in the ventral medullar area are believed to function during exercise when exhalation is less passive and more active.

Neurons with ventilatory activity have also been identified in the pons. Pontine neurons exhibit both inhalatory and exhalatory activity, and they may serve to smooth the transition from one phase of ventilation to the next. Two ventilatory centers within the pons are the apneustic center and the pneumotaxic center, which function together to "fine tune" inhalation and exhalation.

The cerebral cortex functions by allowing voluntary ventilation to override the automatic controls of the medulla and pons. Voluntary ventilatory control is most important during behavioral states such as crying, laughing, singing, and talking. During these states, voluntary control may override the automatic control, which responds chiefly to chemical stimuli and to changes in lung inflation.[23]

Effectors

The effectors of ventilation are the muscles of ventilation (see section entitled "Muscles of Ventilation"). When considering their function in the control of ventilation, however, the most important issue is that they function in a coordinated fashion. The central nervous system regulates this function.

Sensors

The sensors are composed of central and peripheral chemoreceptors, lung receptors, and other receptors.

Chemoreceptors respond to a change in the chemical composition of the blood or other fluid around them.[44]

Central chemoreceptors. The central chemoreceptors are located near the ventral surface of the medulla oblongata. Animal experiments have shown that local application of hydrogen ions or dissolved carbon dioxide to this area will stimulate ventilation within a few seconds.[33] These chemoreceptors are surrounded by the brain's extracellular

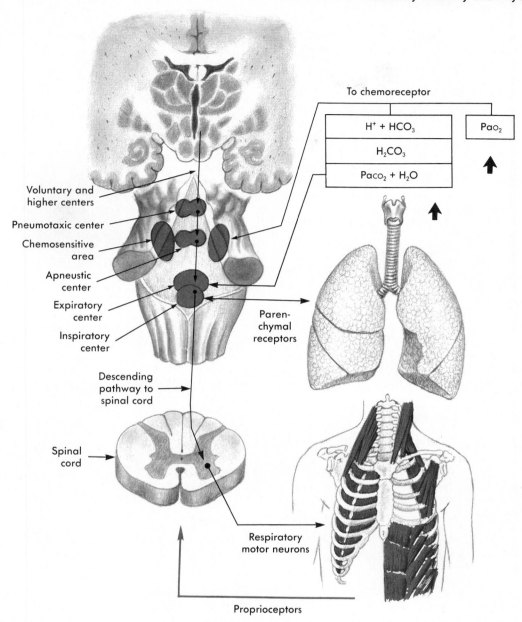

To chemoreceptor

| $H^+ + HCO_3$ |
| H_2CO_3 |
| $Pa_{CO_2} + H_2O$ |

Pa_{O_2}

Voluntary and
higher centers

Pneumotaxic center

Chemosensitive
area

Apneustic
center

Expiratory
center

Inspiratory
center

Paren-
chymal
receptors

Descending
pathway to
spinal cord

Spinal
cord

Respiratory
motor neurons

Proprioceptors

Fig. 17-17 Respiratory control system. (From Thompson JM: Clinical nursing, St Louis, 1986, The CV Mosby Co.)

fluid, and they respond to changes in the hydrogen ion concentration of that fluid. Ventilation is increased when the hydrogen ion concentration increases and is decreased when the hydrogen ion concentration falls. A rise in the plasma Pa_{CO_2} causes movement of carbon dioxide into the cerebral spinal fluid, stimulating the movement of hydrogen ions into the brain's extracellular fluid. These hydrogen ions then stimulate the chemoreceptors, and ventilation is increased. Consequently, the increased ventilation causes exhalation of the excess carbon dioxide, the Pa_{CO_2} falls, and ventilation returns to normal.

Peripheral chemoreceptors. The peripheral chemoreceptors are located above and below the aortic arch and at the bifurcation of the common carotid arteries. The most important action of the carotid chemoreceptors is their re-

sponse to changes in the Pa_{O_2}. The peripheral chemoreceptors are believed the only receptors that increase ventilation in response to arterial hypoxemia. Thus immediate hyperventilation, one of the principle compensatory mechanisms in response to hypoxemia, is governed by these chemoreceptors. It seems evident that the carotid bodies are responsible for this effect because it has been shown that patients have lost the ventilatory response to hypoxemia subsequent to bilateral carotid body resection or denervation.[23,44]

The peripheral chemoreceptors also act to increase ventilation when Pa_{CO_2} is elevated. The response to pH apparently is found only in the carotid bodies, which respond to a fall in pH by increasing ventilation.

Lung receptors. Irritant receptors lie between airway epithelial cells and function to stimulate bronchoconstriction and hyperpnea in response to inhaled irritants. "J" receptors lie in the alveolar walls close to the capillaries. Evidence indicates that the J receptors stimulate ventilation in response to engorgement of the pulmonary capillaries and to increases in the interstitial fluid volume of the alveolar wall.

REFERENCES

1. Burton GG and Hodgkin JE: Respiratory care: a guide to clinical practice, Philadelphia, 1984, JB Lippincott Co.
2. Chatburn RL: Dynamic respiratory mechanics, Respir Care 31(8): 703, 1986.
3. Dantzker DR and Tobin MJ: Monitoring respiratory muscle function, Respir Care 30(6):422, 1985.
4. Deffebach ME and others: The bronchial circulation: small but a vital attribute of the lung, Am Rev Respir Dis 135(2):463, 1987.
5. De Troyer A and Estenne M: Functional anatomy of respiratory muscles, Clin Chest Med 9(2):175, 1988.
6. Fishman AP: Pulmonary diseases and disorders, ed 2, New York, 1988, McGraw-Hill Book Co.
7. Gil J: The normal lung circulation: state of the art, Chest 93 (suppl 3):80S, 1988.
8. Grum CM and Chauncey JB: Conventional mechanical ventilation, Clin Chest Med 9(1):37, 1988.
9. Guyton AG: Textbook of medical physiology, ed 7, Philadelphia, 1986, WB Saunders Co.
10. Hess D: Perspectives on weaning from mechanical ventilation—with a note on extubation, Respir Care 32(3):167, 1987.
11. Hodgkin JE and Petty TL: Chronic obstructive pulmonary disease: current concepts, Philadelphia, 1987, WB Saunders Co.
12. Hogg JC: Primary pulmonary hypertension, Chest 93(suppl 3):172S, 1988.
13. Hurewitz AN and Bergofsky EH: Pathogenic mechanisms in chronic pulmonary hypertension, Heart Lung 15(4):327, 1986.
14. Kline JL and others: The use of calculated relative inspiratory effort as a predictor of outcome in mechanical ventilation weaning trials, Respir Care 32(10):870, 1987.
15. Luce JM, Tyler ML, and Pierson DJ: Intensive respiratory care, Philadelphia, 1984, WB Saunders Co.
16. MacDonnell KF, Fahey PJ, and Segal MS: Respiratory intensive care, Boston, 1987, Little Brown and Co, Inc.
17. MacIntrye NR: Weaning from mechanical ventilatory support: volume assisting intermittent breaths versus pressure-assisting every breath, Respir Care 33(2):121, 1988.
18. Malasanos L and others: Health assessment, St Louis, 1986, The CV Mosby Co.
19. Martin DE: Respiratory anatomy and physiology, St Louis, 1988, The CV Mosby Co.
20. Martin L: Pulmonary physiology in clinical practice: the essentials for patient care and evaluation, St Louis, 1987, The CV Mosby Co.
21. Miyagawa CI: Sedation of the mechanically ventilated patient, Respir Care 32(9):792, 1987.
22. Moser KM, Daily PO, and Peterson K: Chronic thromboembolic disease—results of pulmonary thromboendarectomy in 42 patients, Ann Intern Med 107(4):560, 1987.
23. Murray JF: The normal lung: a basis for diagnosis and treatment of pulmonary disease, ed 2, Philadelphia, 1986, WB Saunders Co.
24. Murray JF and Nadel JA: Textbook of respiratory medicine, Philadelphia, 1988, WB Saunders Co.
25. Parrillo JP: Current therapy in critical care medicine, Toronto, 1987, Brian C Decker, Publisher.
26. Peil ML and Rubin LJ: Therapy of secondary pulmonary hypertension, Heart Lung 15(5):450, 1986.
27. Petty TL: The use, abuse and mistique of positive end expiratory pressure, Am Rev Respir Dis 138(2):475, 1988.
28. Rochester DF: Respiratory muscle function in health, Heart Lung 13(4):349, 1984.
29. Sahn S: The pleura, Am Rev Respir Dis 138(1):184, 1988.
30. Shapiro BA, Harrison RA, and Walton JR: Clinical application of blood gases, ed 3, Chiciago, 1982, Year Book Medical Publishers, Inc.
31. Shapiro BA, and others: Clinical application of respiratory care, ed 3, Chicago, 1985, Year Book Medical Publishers, Inc.
32. Sharp JT: The respiratory muscles in chronic obstructive pulmonary disease, Am Rev Respir Dis 134(4):1089, 1986.
33. Sieck GC: Diaphragm muscle: structural and functional organization, Clin Chest Med 9(2):195, 1988.
34. Sleigh MA, Blake JR, and Liron N: The propulsion of mucus by cilia, Am Rev Respir Dis 137(3):726, 1988.
35. Spearman CB and Sheldon RL: Egan's fundamentals of respiratory therapy, ed 4, St Louis, 1982, The CV Mosby Co.
36. Sporn HS and Morganroth ML: Discontinuation of mechanical ventilation, Clin Chest Med 9(1):113, 1988.
37. Staub NC: Pulmonary intravascular macrophages, Chest 93(suppl 3):84S, 1988.
38. Thompson BT and Hales CA: Hypoxic pulmonary hypertension: acute and chronic, Heart Lung 15(5):457, 1986.
39. Tisi GM: Clinical pulmonary physiology. In Moser KM and Spragg RG: Respiratory emergencies, St Louis, 1982, The CV Mosby Co.
40. Tobin MJ: Respiratory muscles in disease, Clin Chest Med 9(2):263, 1988.
41. Traver GA: Personal communication, October, 1988.
42. Traver GA: Respiratory nursing: the science and the art, New York, 1982, John Wiley & Sons, Inc.
43. Wagenvoort CA: Lung biopsy findings in secondary pulmonary hypertension, Heart Lung 15(5):429, 1986.
44. West JB: Respiratory physiology: the essentials, ed 3, Baltimore, 1985, Williams & Wilkins.
45. Wollschlager CM and Khan FA: Secondary pulmonary hypertension: clinical features, Heart Lung, 15(4):429, 1986.
46. Wright JR and Clements JA: Metabolism and turnover of lung surfactant, Am Rev Respir Dis 136(2):426, 1987.

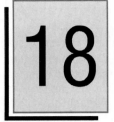

CHAPTER

18

Pulmonary Clinical Assessment

CHAPTER OBJECTIVES

- *Discuss the rationale involved in developing a consistent, sequential format for performing a pulmonary nursing assessment.*
- *Perform a thorough nursing assessment of the pulmonary system on a critically ill patient, interpret the results, and plan nursing interventions that will treat abnormal findings when possible.*
- *Identify and state where normal lung sounds are auscultated on the thorax.*
- *Name the three types of adventitious lung sounds.*
- *Describe the assessment findings most commonly associated with the following pulmonary disorders: asthma, atelectasis, chronic bronchitis, emphysema, pneumonia,. pleural effusion, and pneumothorax.*

As with assessment of any body system, examination of the patient's respiratory status must be a systematic process of garnering clues leading to a diagnosis. This process can be of brief duration (for example, determining breathlessness) or can involve a detailed history and examination, depending on the nature and immediacy of the patient's situation. Whatever the setting, the nurse should develop and practice a sequential pattern of assessment to avoid omitting portions of the examination.[1,6] Since the thorax is arranged symmetrically, it is necessary to compare areas of the left thorax to areas of the right thorax in an effort to observe significant differences. For example, the left apex of the lung should be compared with the right apex of the lung, as opposed to the lower lung field on the same or opposite side.

Proper assessment includes an investigation into the chronology of symptoms (history), physical signs (physical examination), and findings (laboratory diagnostic tests). Evaluation of data uncovered using these three components will generally yield a reliable determination of the patient's condition.

HISTORY

The history of the illness is considered extremely important in determining the patient's condition. Throughout the interview, the patient's chief complaint is evaluated in an attempt to reveal the underlying cause(s). The nurse seeks to expose key signs and symptoms that can determine causation and lead to proper intervention. Table 18-1 reviews the key symptoms associated with respiratory disease. Although the elucidation of key symptoms is important, attention must also be given to assessing the chronology of events. For example, cough associated with fever, chills, and pleural chest pain of acute onset is a classic description of pneumonia.[3,5]

During the discussion of symptoms, it is important to note the absence of a symptom from a usual cluster or grouping. For example, cough is generally associated with pulmonary infection; absence of any cough would be noted as a significant negative in symptoms of this disorder and could help refine the list of possible causes.

Symptoms

Shortness of breath. Shortness of breath is probably one of the most frequent complaints that prompts patients to seek assistance. It is a common symptom of respiratory and cardiac disease. Careful questioning should be used to clarify the patient's meaning of the terms "shortness of breath," "breathlessness," and "loss of wind." Some patients refer to the tightness and pressure that can accompany myocardial infarction as loss of breath; this difference must be explored. Since breathlessness is a subjective complaint, it is difficult to assess its severity. Often a patient's complaints of dyspnea do not correlate with the findings of pulmonary function tests, arterial blood gas values, or other available objective measurements. One method that seems to provide quantitative data is having the patient rate dyspnea using the Visual Analog Scale (VAS) or the Modified Borg Scale.[2,8,11,16]

The VAS consists of a horizontal line with "not at all breathless" to "very breathless" at either end of the continuum.[16] The patient is asked to locate his or her sensation of breathlessness on this line. Changes in severity or im-

Table 18-1 Key symptoms in respiratory disease

Symptoms	Possible causes
Dyspnea/shortness of breath, breathlessness, inability to catch breath, smothering tightness in chest, dyspnea on exertion, orthopnea	Airway obstruction; e.g., foreign body, bronchitis, mucus, asthma, chronic obstructive pulmonary disease (COPD), atelectasis, tumors, pneumothorax
	Altered mechanics of breathing; e.g., congestive heart failure (CHF), pulmonary embolism, pulmonary contusion, acute blood loss, anemia, splinting, chest wall deformity
	Hyperventilation syndrome
Chest pain accentuated by breathing, coughing, sneezing, laughing; usually sharp, knifelike burning quality to pain	Inflammation or trauma of ribs, muscles, nerves, and pleurae; pleurisy, rib fracture, costochondritis, intercostal myositis
Cough with or without sputum production	Exacerbation of COPD, pneumonia, interstitial lung disease, aspiration lung disorders, CHF, pulmonary embolism, noncardiogenic pulmonary edema, chronic irritation of respiratory mucosa

provement can then be plotted along the continuum during the course of therapy. The Modified Borg Scale has a vertical continuum on which the patient is asked to quantify dyspnea[11] (see the box at right).

Dyspnea can be caused by one or all of the following: (1) hypercapnia or hypoxemia, (2) discrepancy in work demanded and work achieved, and (3) reflexes originating in airways and parenchyma.[11] Dyspnea may be acute or chronic in onset, or it may be associated with activity and position. Orthopnea is the term used to describe dyspnea that is only relieved by assuming an upright position. Functional dyspnea is used to describe dyspnea at rest that is not present during exercise. This phenomenon is not associated with pathological changes but is of a psychological nature.[8]

Cough. Cough is a frequent complaint, although it is nonspecific as an indicator of pulmonary disease. Like other nonspecific complaints, cough requires careful investigation by the interviewer. One should inquire about the onset, frequency, precipitating events, and whether the cough is productive. If the cough is productive, visualization of sputum is desirable, and the patient should be asked to quantify sputum production. The investigator should also inquire about the presence or absence of hemoptysis. Table 18-2 lists abnormal sputum characteristics and their likely causes.

Chest pain. Chest pain is one of the most frequently seen initial symptoms. When not associated with trauma, chest pain may be accompanied by a heightened emotional state because of the association of chest pain with heart attack. Since there may not be physical signs associated with pain, careful questioning about the pain is essential.[8,10]

Using the PQRST mnemonic can assist the practitioner in compiling a complete description of the pain complaint, allowing significant reduction in possible causes. *P* stands for provocative-palliative factors of pain; *Q* refers to quality of pain; *R* relates to region of pain and radiation to other areas; *S* refers to a description of the severity of pain; and *T* refers to the temporal characteristics of pain[4] (see the box on p. 377).

Along with the current history, the nurse should know

MODIFIED BORG SCALE

Circle the number that best matches your shortness of breath

0	None at all
0.5	Very, very slight (just noticeable)
1	Very slight
2	Slight
3	Moderate
4	Somewhat severe
5	Severe
6	
7	Very severe
8	
9	Very, very severe (almost maximal)
10	Maximal

Dyspnea Visual Analogue Scale

Mark the line at the point that best describes your breathing.

No difficulty breathing　　　　Extreme difficulty breathing

From Lush M and others: Heart Lung 17(5):528, 1988.

---

the patient's past medical nursing history. Awareness of other disease conditions has significant bearing on planning patient care, because morbidity and mortality are affected by associated disease states.

PHYSICAL EXAMINATION

Once the history has been obtained, the nurse should begin the physical examination (the search for key signs), which will move her or him further toward a diagnosis.

Table 18-2 Sputum characteristics seen in various respiratory disorders

Appearance	Likely cause
Bloody gelatinous sputum (current-jelly sputum)	*Klebsiella pneumoniae*
Rusty sputum (prune-juice sputum)	Pneumococcal pneumonias
Thick, greenish sputum with blood streaking it	*Klebsiella pneumoniae*
Stringy mucoid sputum	Asthmatic attack
Frothy sputum	Pulmonary edema
Purulent sputum of yellow, green, gray nature	Pneumonias

Inspection

Surveying the general appearances of the patient should be the initial component of inspecting any body system. How does the person appear as a whole? Does he or she appear ill? What are his or her skin color, body configuration, muscle tone, motor activity, nutritional state, behavior, speech, and/or outstanding anatomical changes or malfunctions? Inspection is the most difficult physical examination technique to master, possibly because of the difficulty in systemizing it, the impatience to begin the hands-on examination, or the fact that recognition of signs is dependent on the knowledge of the observer. We see what we know. Therefore inspection is often too superficial to reveal signs that are pertinent clues in the diagnostic process. Much can be gleaned about the respiratory status during the inspection, and the nurse should focus on (1) general signs of respiratory disease, (2) chest wall movement and deformity, (3) ventilatory pattern, and (4) discharges of sputum, pus, or hemoptysis.

General signs associated with respiratory problems are numerous. Clubbing of the fingers may be a sign of respiratory or other disease processes. Clubbing includes loss of angulation at the nail plate, change in the curvature of the nail, and floating of the nail root (Fig. 18-1).[4,12]

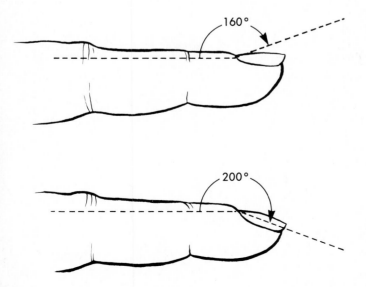

DESCRIBING PAIN USING THE PQRST APPROACH

PROVOCATIVE-PALLIATIVE

Document factors that aggravate or alleviate pain. Distinguish if pain is increased or unchanged during ventilation. Pain associated with movement can often be localized to displaced tissues. Assess whether pain is affected by position or inactivity.

QUALITY

Pain is usually described as (1) burning, (2) pricking or sharp, and (3) deep or aching. Superficial pain is often associated with burning, pricking, and sharp characteristics and is localized. Throbbing or cramping may be described. Deep pain is usually longer in duration and is associated with pressure and aching.

REGION-RADIATION

Ask the patient to indicate the area of pain; with superficial pain, the patient can often identify the exact spot. Any radiation of pain should be determined. Radiation is usually associated with deep, visceral pain.

SEVERITY

Pain's severity defies precise measurement; use a pain-rating scale for quantification of patient's pain (0 equals pain free, 10 equals worst pain imaginable). Studies show pain rated <7 on a 0 to 10 scale usually responds to nonnarcotic drugs and/or nursing measures that increase naturally occurring endorphins. Pain rated as >7 on a 0 to 10 scale usually requires narcotic drug intervention and cannot be relieved by nursing measures alone. Intense pain is usually associated with other signs such as tachycardia, diaphoresis, facial grimacing, posturing, splinting, and/or nausea and vomiting.[7,9,10,13,14]

TEMPORAL

These characteristics of pain give information about onset and duration of pain. Assess whether pain is acute or chronic, periodic in occurrence, and brief or extended in duration.

Fig. 18-1 Clubbing of the fingers. Top view is normal; bottom view shows loss of normal nail bed angulation. (From Andreoli KG and others: Comprehensive cardiac care, ed 6, St Louis, 1987, The CV Mosby Co.)

Central cyanosis may be associated with hypoxic pulmonary disease and is seen as a blue color of the skin and mucous membranes. Cyanosis occurs when large amounts of unsaturated hemoglobin are present in the capillaries (>5 g/dl blood).[4,9] Inspection of lips, ears, and molar regions helps to differentiate central from local peripheral cyanosis.[9] Other general findings may include various lesions such as petechiae, Osler nodes, and erythema multiforme, which can be associated with staphylococcal pneumonias.[3] Osler nodes are tender reddish bumps on the hands that develop as embolic lesions of the bacteria, and erythema multiforme is an associated skin lesion characterized by redness.

Chest wall movement and symmetry should be carefully observed. Whenever possible, observation of the thorax and chest wall movement should be accomplished with the patient in a sitting position. Since sitting is not feasible for many critically ill patients, the nurse must adjust for the variation of chest wall movements created by the patient's position. The shape of the chest should be assessed for structural deformities such as kyphosis, scoliosis, or pectus excavatum. Any scars should be noted, as should all surgical incisions. The presence of other iatrogenic features such as chest tubes, central venous lines, artificial airways, and/or nasogastric tubes must be noted since they may affect assessment findings.

Breathing should be observed for the effort it necessitates. Normal, quiet breathing is relatively effortless, whereas difficult breathing can range from mild to extreme dyspnea. Extreme dyspnea is exemplified by the breathing of a patient suffering an exacerbation of chronic obstructive pulmonary disease (COPD) who sits in high-Fowler's position and leans forward, using neck and chest accessory muscles to inhale and pursed-lip breathing to exhale. Gasps for air may make the distress readily apparent. Lesser degrees of dyspnea are reflected by the same factors—patient position, active effort to breathe, use of the accessory muscles of ventilation, presence of intercostal retraction, unequal movement of chest and thoracic wall, flaring of nares, or pausing midsentence to take a breath.

Inspection would not be complete without determining the patient's breathing pattern, since several types of irregular breathing patterns may occur in certain disease states. Table 18-3 outlines irregular breathing patterns. The depth of inhalation should also be grossly determined during observation of the respiratory cycle. Kussmaul respiration (air hunger) is a deep, regular, sighing breathing that may be associated with a slow or fast rate. It occurs in response to metabolic acidosis, peritonitis, severe hemorrhage, and pneumonia.[9] Noting noisy breathing, especially stridulous breathing, which is the high-pitched whistling or crowing sound associated with glottic narrowing, gives additional clues. Stridulous breathing may presage complete airway obstruction and requires immediate intervention.

Palpation

Palpation of the chest wall should reveal areas of tenderness and lumps or bony deformities. Tracheal position should be assessed by placing the fingers on the middle of the top of the manubrium and moving upward. The trachea should be located in the midline. Deviations to either side may indicate a pneumothorax, a large pleural effusion, or severe atelectasis.

Vibratory palpation (tactile fremitus) involves using the examiner's hands to evaluate air vibration. As the patient speaks, the palmar surface of each hand is held firmly against the patient's chest to assess the chest wall vibrations that occur during speech (Fig. 18-2). Alterations within the lung or pleura change the ease with which vibrations are transmitted to the chest wall. Pleural effusions decrease the vibrations, whereas consolidation of lung tissue increases the vibrations (Table 18-4).

Respiratory excursion is measured by placing the hands on either side of the posterior thorax while the patient breathes. Excursion should be evaluated in the upper, middle, and lower posterior thorax. Evaluation of posterior excursion is facilitated by placing the thumbs together on the spinal column with fingers reaching around each side of the chest wall (Fig. 18-3). Noting movement of thumbs away from each other allows estimation of respiratory excursion

Table 18-3 Irregular breathing patterns

Pattern	Defining characteristics	Possible causes
Cheyne-Stokes respiration	A pattern of breathing characterized by shallow ventilations, which increase in depth, reach a peak, and decline. A period of apnea occurs as the ventilations decline, after which the pattern is repeated.	Normal variation in children and in elderly people; left cardiac failure, aortic valvular problems, low diastolic pressure, increased cerebral pressure, brain injury, morphine and its derivatives, barbiturates
Biot's breathing	Uncommon variant of Cheyne-stokes respiration. Periods of apnea irregularly interrupt breaths of equal depth.	Meningitis
Painful breathing	Normal breathing interrupted by pain and splinting.	Pleurisy, inflamed and traumatized muscle, fractured ribs or cartilages, subphrenic inflammation
Sighing respirations	Normal rhythm periodically interrupted by deep sighing.	Psychoneurosis, physiological sighing

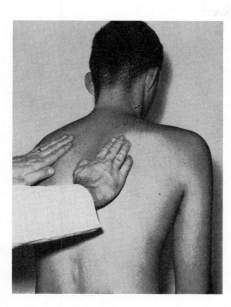

Fig. 18-2 Palpation of fremitus, showing simultaneous application of the fingertips of both hands to compare sides. (From Malasanos L and others: Health assessment, ed 4, St Louis, 1989, The CV Mosby Co.)

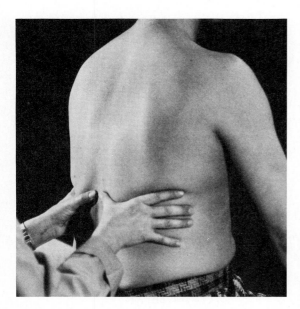

Fig. 18-3 Assessment of thoracic excursion. (From Malasanos L and others: Health assessment, ed 4, St Louis, 1989, The CV Mosby Co.)

Table 18-4 Characteristics of normal and abnormal tactile fremitus

Type	Discussion of characteristics
Normal fremitus	Varies greatly from person to person and is dependent on the intensity and pitch of the voice, the position and distance of the bronchi in relation to the chest wall, and the thickness of the chest wall. Fremitus is most intense in the second intercostal spaces at the sternal border near the area of bronchial bifurcation.
Increased fremitus	May occur in pneumonia, compressed lung, lung tumor, or pulmonary fibrosis (a solid medium of uniform structure conducts vibrations with greater intensity than a porous medium).
Decreased or absent fremitus	Occurs when there is a diminished production of sounds, a diminished transmission of sounds, or the addition of a medium through which sounds must pass before reaching the thoracic wall as, for example, in pleural effusion, pleural thickening, pheumothorax, bronchial obstruction, or emphysema.
Pleural friction rub	Vibration produced by inflamed pleural surfaces rubbing together. It is felt as a grating, is synchronous with respiratory movements, and is more commonly felt on inspiration.
Rhonchal fremitus	Coarse vibrations produced by the passage of air through thick exudates in the large air passages. These can be cleared or altered by coughing.

From Malasanos L and others: Health assessment, ed 4, St Louis, 1989, The CV Mosby Co.

and determination of symmetry. Asymmetrical movement of the chest can occur in pneumothorax, pneumonia, splinting, or other disorders that interfere with lung inflation.

Percussion

The density of organs and tissues is evaluated by percussion. When struck, different tissues emit characteristic sounds described as resonant, tympanic, dull, or flat, depending on the pitch and timbre. These sounds defy verbal description and are best distinguished by the examiner through practice. The sound emitted by air-filled lung is referred to as resonance, percussion of the stomach yields tympany, the heart sounds dull, and muscle sounds flat when percussed (Fig. 18-4). The sound emitted when percussing over a pneumothorax is termed hyperresonance. In the acute care setting, percussion of lung fields is infrequently used after the initial baseline assessment has been completed. During percussion, as with other maneuvers, like areas of the lungs should be compared; that is, percussion of the posterior left apex should be compared with the posterior right apex, using a back-and-forth movement. Both anterior and posterior chest fields should be percussed.

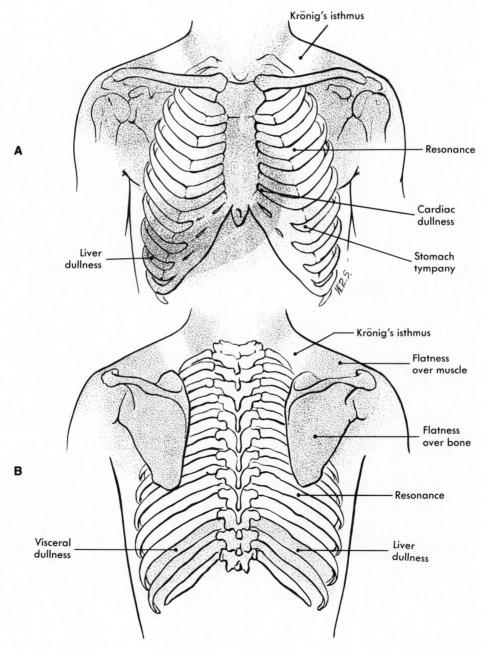

Fig. 18-4   Percussion sounds of the anterior, **A**, and posterior, **B**, thorax. (From Malasanos L and others: Health assessment, ed 4, St Louis, 1989, The CV Mosby Co.)

Table 18-5 Characterisitcs of normal breath sounds

Sound	Characteristics	Findings
Vesicular	Heard over most of lung field; low pitch; soft and short exhalation and long inhalation	
Bronchovesicular	Heard over main bronchus area and over upper right posterior lung field; medium pitch; exhalation equals inhalation	
Bronchial	Heard only over trachea; high pitch; loud and long exhalation	

Modified from Thompson JM and others: Mosby's manual of clinical nursing, ed 2, St Louis, 1989, The CV Mosby Co.

Auscultation

Listening over the lung fields with a stethoscope permits the nurse to evaluate air movement and the presence of adventitious sounds. Air movement creates turbulence as it flows through the branching network of airways. Because of the variation in airway size encountered, *normal breath sounds* change as airway size changes. Air movement heard over large airways such as the trachea or mainstem bronchi is referred to as bronchial breath sounds. Other breath sounds include vesicular and bronchovesicular sounds. Table 18-5 reviews the characteristics of these normal breath sounds.

Besides listening to breath sounds, the nurse should assess voice sounds. Voice sounds are particularly useful in detecting consolidation. The two types of voice sounds assessed are whispered pectoriloquy and bronchophony. In healthy lungs, whispered and spoken words will not be clearly heard during auscultation. An increase in the loudness and distinctiveness of whispered or spoken words indicates pathology (Table 18-6).

Egophony is a form of bronchophony. It is also referred to as an "e" to "a" change.[4] If the lung is compressed such as with a pleural effusion, the letter "e" will be heard as "a" when spoken by the patient.

Although a multitude of names exist for extra or adventitious sounds heard in the lung, the Joint Committee on Pulmonary Nomenclature has recommended use of the terms "crackles and wheezes."[6]

Crackles is used to describe the sounds previously called *rales*. Once thought caused by air passing through fluid-filled airways, acoustical studies show that these sounds are caused by pressure variations in the airways and reflect the opening of collapsed alveoli in the lung. *Wheezes* are associated with bronchial wall oscillations and the airways'

Table 18-6 Voice sounds, normal and abnormal results

Voice sounds	Results
Bronchophony: using diaphragm of stethoscope, listen to posterior chest as patient says "ninety-nine"	Normal response: muffled "nin-nin" sound heard Abnormal response: clear, loud "ninety-nine" response heard because the lung tissue is consolidated
Whispered pectoriloquy: listen to posterior chest as patient whispers "one, two, three" or "ninety-nine"	Normal response: muffled sounds heard Abnormal response: clear "one, two, three" or "ninety-nine" heard because of lung consolidation
Egophony: listen to posterior chest as the patient says "e-e-e"	Normal response: muffled "e-e-e" sound heard Abnormal response: sound of e changes to an "a-a-a" sound, referred to as e to a change, because of consolidation

From Thompson JM and others: Mosby's manual of clinical nursing, ed 2, St Louis, 1989, The CV Mosby Co.

Table 18–7 Causes and characteristics of adventitious sounds

Sound	Causes	Characteristics
Crackles	Pressure variations in airways	Discontinuous and categorized as early or late inspiratory
Early inspiratory crackles	Same	Low pitched and few in number; vary in loudness and not abolished by cough or deep breathing; frequently audible at mouth, as well as over lung fields
Late inspiratory crackles	Same	Numerous, gravity dependent, and affected by position changes; may be abolished or decreased by deep breathing or coughing; heard only over lung fields
Wheezes	Bronchial wall oscillations and opening and closing of airways	Continuous sounds heard during inhalation and/or exhalation; musical or snoring in character
Friction rubs	Rubbing together of inflamed and roughened pleural surfaces	Creaking or grating quality during inhalation and exhalation; heard best in lower anteriorlateral chest (area of greatest thoracic expansion); not affected by coughing; disappears when patient pauses in breathing

opening and closing. Table 18-7 outlines adventitious sounds.

Other adventitious sounds that can be heard are pleural friction rub and mediastinal emphysema (Hammans' sign).[5] Pleural friction rub is a grating, rough sound caused by inflammation within the pleura. The sound corresponds to ventilation and disappears with breath holding[2,12,17]; thus it can be differentiated from pericardial friction rub, which does not vary with ventilation. Mediastinal emphysema is caused by air in the mediastinum and sounds like high-pitched crunching and crackling heard around the mediastinum.[4] Table 18-8 reviews the pulmonary assessment findings from many disorders that occur in the critically ill patient.

When listening for adventitious sounds, it is necessary to eliminate any outside source of sounds (for example, the sound of the bubbling of water from ventilator tubing, which can be transmitted to a patient's chest during auscultation) that could be transmitted to the lung. Before auscultation, listening to the environmental sounds created by equipment supporting the patient can help the nurse identify potential sources of random sounds that could be confused during the auscultory process.

Table 18-8 Assessment findings frequently associated with common lung conditions

Condition*	Breath sound†	Description	Inspection	Palpation	Percussion	Auscultation
Healthy lung		Tracheobronchial tree and alveoli are clear; pleurae are thin and close together; chest wall is mobile.	Symmetrical rib and diaphragmatic movement—absence of accessory muscle activity Regular respiratory rhythm	Trachea—midline Expansion—equal bilaterally Tactile fremitus—present Diaphragmatic excursion—3 to 5 cm	Resonant	Breath sounds—vesicular over periphery areas Voice sounds—normal Adventitious sounds—none except for a few transient crackles at the bases that clear with deep breathing
Asthma	Normal bronchial lumen Bronchospasm	Asthma is characterized by intermittent episodes of airway obstruction caused by bronchospasm, excessive bronchial secretion, or edema of bronchial mucosa.	Central cyanosis Tachypnea with audible wheezing Use of accessory muscles of ventilation	Tactile fremitus—decreased	Hyperresonant	Breath sounds—distant, decreased Voice sounds—decreased Adventitious sounds—wheezes

Continued.

Modified from Malasanos L and others: Health assessment, ed 4, St Louis, 1989, The CV Mosby Co.
*Although some disease conditions are bilateral, one diseased lung and one healthy lung are illustrated for each condition to provide contrast. pathological condition is illustrated on the left side, and the normal lung is on the right side.
† ⊙∴ Denotes auscultation of crackles; ∿∿, denotes auscultation of wheezes.

Table 18-8 Assessment findings frequently associated with common lung conditions—cont'd

Condition*	Breath sound†	Description	Inspection	Palpation	Percussion	Auscultation
Atelectasis Collapsed portion of lung		Atelectasis is the collapse of alveolar lung tissue, and findings reflect the presence of a small, airless lung; this condition is caused by complete obstruction of a draining bronchus by a tumor, thick secretions, or an aspirated foreign body, by persistent hypoventilation, and by lack of sighing.	Decreased chest motion on affected side Affected side retracted, with ribs appearing close together Cough may or may not be present Intercostal retraction on affected side during inhalation and bulging during exhalation	Trachea—shifted to affected side Expansion—decreased on affected side Tactile fremitus—decreased or absent over atelectasis	Dull to flat over affected area	Breath sounds—decreased or absent over affected area; high-pitched bronchial sounds when partial obstruction present Adventitious sounds—high pitched; possible crackles during terminal portion of inspiration
Bronchiectasis Dilated bronchi		Bronchiectasis is abnormal dilation of the bronchi or bronchioles or both. It results in copious amounts of thick mucus.	If mild, normal respirations; if severe, tachypnea Less expansion on affected side Cough with purulent sputum	Expansion—decreased on affected side Tactile fremitus—increased	Resonant or dull	Breath sounds—usually vesicular Voice sounds—usually normal Adventitious sounds—crackles

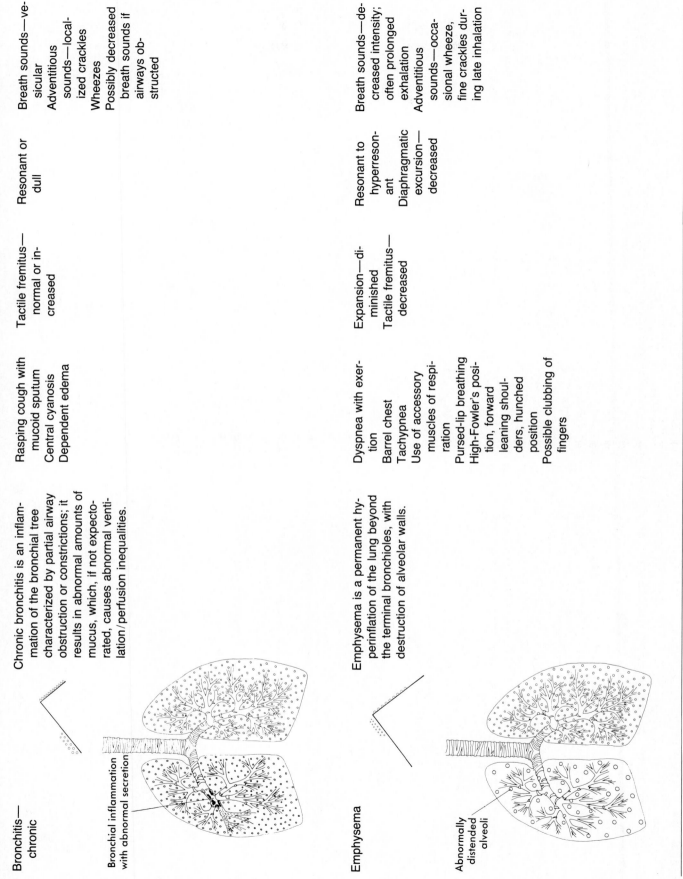

Bronchitis—chronic

Chronic bronchitis is an inflammation of the bronchial tree characterized by partial airway obstruction or constrictions; it results in abnormal amounts of mucus, which, if not expectorated, causes abnormal ventilation/perfusion inequalities.

Bronchial inflammation with abnormal secretion

Rasping cough with mucoid sputum
Central cyanosis
Dependent edema

Tactile fremitus—normal or increased

Resonant or dull

Breath sounds—vesicular
Adventitious sounds—localized crackles
Wheezes
Possibly decreased breath sounds if airways obstructed

Emphysema

Emphysema is a permanent hyperinflation of the lung beyond the terminal bronchioles, with destruction of alveolar walls.

Abnormally distended alveoli

Dyspnea with exertion
Barrel chest
Tachypnea
Use of accessory muscles of respiration
Pursed-lip breathing
High-Fowler's position, forward leaning shoulders, hunched position
Possible clubbing of fingers

Expansion—diminished
Tactile fremitus—decreased

Resonant to hyperresonant
Diaphragmatic excursion—decreased

Breath sounds—decreased intensity; often prolonged exhalation
Adventitious sounds—occasional wheeze, fine crackles during late inhalation

Continued.

Table 18-8 Assessment findings frequently associated with common lung conditions—cont'd

Condition*	Breath sound†	Description	Inspection	Palpation	Percussion	Auscultation
Pleural effusion and thickening	Fluid in the pleural space	Pleural effusion is a collection of fluid in the pleural space; if pleural effusion is prolonged, fibrous tissue may also accumulate in the pleural space. The clinical picture depends on the amount of fluid or fibrosis present and the rapidity of development; fluid tends to gravitate to the most dependent areas of the thorax, and the adjacent lung is compressed.	Tachypnea Decreased chest expansion on the affected side (expansion may be normal when effusion is small)	Trachea—no deviation in small effusions; deviation toward normal side with large effusion Expansion—decreased on affected side with large effusions Tactile fremitus—decreased or absent	Dull to flat over effusion area	Breath sounds—decreased or absent over area involved in the effusion Adventitious sounds—sometimes pleural friction rub; possible crackles in thoracic area overlying effusion/normal lung interface
Pneumonia with consolidation	Consolidation	Pneumonia with consolidation occurs when alveolar air is replaced by fluid or tissue; physical findings depend on the amount of parenchymal tissue involved.	Tachypnea Guarding and less motion on the affected side or on both sides when bilateral pneumonia present Cough Possible sputum production	Expansion—limited on the affected side or bilaterally Tactile fremitus—usually increased but may be decreased if a bronchus leading to the affected area is plugged Trachea—no deviation or deviation to unaffected side in unilateral pneumonias	Dull to flat	Breath sounds—increased in intensity; bronchovesicular or bronchial breath sounds over affected area Voice sounds—increased bronchophony, egophony, whisper pectoriloquy Adventitious sounds—crackles when consolidation is small Changes may be minimal or absent

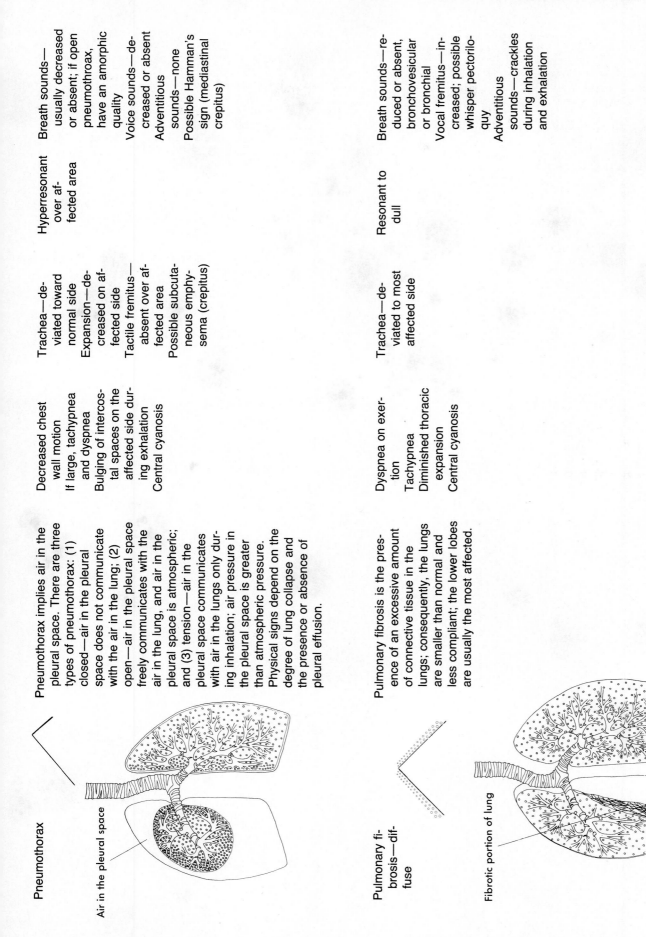

Pneumothorax

Air in the pleural space

Pneumothorax implies air in the pleural space. There are three types of pneumothorax: (1) closed—air in the pleural space does not communicate with the air in the lung; (2) open—air in the pleural space freely communicates with the air in the lung, and air in the pleural space is atmospheric; and (3) tension—air in the pleural space communicates with air in the lungs only during inhalation; air pressure in the pleural space is greater than atmospheric pressure. Physical signs depend on the degree of lung collapse and the presence or absence of pleural effusion.

Decreased chest wall motion
If large, tachypnea and dyspnea
Bulging of intercostal spaces on the affected side during exhalation
Central cyanosis

Trachea—deviated toward normal side
Expansion—decreased on affected side
Tactile fremitus—absent over affected area
Possible subcutaneous emphysema (crepitus)

Hyperresonant over affected area

Breath sounds—usually decreased or absent; if open pneumothorax, have an amorphic quality
Voice sounds—decreased or absent
Adventitious sounds—none
Possible Hamman's sign (mediastinal crepitus)

Pulmonary fibrosis—diffuse

Fibrotic portion of lung

Pulmonary fibrosis is the presence of an excessive amount of connective tissue in the lungs; consequently, the lungs are smaller than normal and less compliant; the lower lobes are usually most affected.

Dyspnea on exertion
Tachypnea
Diminished thoracic expansion
Central cyanosis

Trachea—deviated to most affected side

Resonant to dull

Breath sounds—reduced or absent, bronchovesicular or bronchial
Vocal fremitus—increased; possible whisper pectoriloquy
Adventitious sounds—crackles during inhalation and exhalation

REFERENCES

1. Blackburn N and Cebenka D: Honing your respiratory assessment technique, RN 5:28, 1980.
2. Burdon J and others: The perception of breathlessness in asthma, Am Rev Respir Dis 126:825, 1982.
3. Chase RA and Gordon J: Overwhelming pneumonia, MCN 70(4):945, 1986.
4. DeGowan E and DeGowan R: Bedside diagnostic examination, London, 1976, MacMillan, Inc.
5. Griffith D and Wallace R: Bacterial pneumonia in the adult: diagnoses and therapy, Hosp Med 24:188, 1988.
6. Harper R: A guide to respiratory care, Philadelphia, 1981, JB Lippincott Co.
7. Jacox A: Assessing pain, Am J Nurs 79(5):895, 1979.
8. Jansen-Bjerklie S, Camierei V, and Hudes M: The sensation of pulmonary dyspnea, Nurs Res 35(3):25, 1986.
9. Lane G, Cronin K, and Peirce A: Flow charts: clinical decision-making in nursing, Philadelphia, 1983, JB Lippincott Co.
10. Linn A: Evaluating pain: the most subjective symptom, Aches Pain 2(6):24, 1981.
11. Lush M and others: Dyspnea in the ventilator-assisted patient, Heart Lung 17(5):528, 1988.
12. Malasanos L and others: Health assessment, ed 4, St Louis, 1989, The CV Mosby Co.
13. McCaffery M: Relieve your patient's pain fast and effectively with oral analgesics, Nursing 80 10(11):58, 1980.
14. McCaffery M: Relieving pain with non-invasive techniques, Nursing 80 10(12):54, 1980.
15. McCaffery M: Understanding your patient's pain, Nursing 80 10(9):26, 1980.
16. Stark R and Chatterjee M: A new exercise test for clinical dyspnea, Pract Cardiol 9(6):86, 1983.
17. Traver GA: Assessment of thorax and lungs, Am J Nurs 3:466, 1973.
18. Washington JA II: Maximizing diagnostic yield from sputum examination, J Resp Dis p. 81, July, 1981.
19. West BA: Understanding endorphins: our natural pain relief system, Nursing 81 11(2):50, 1981.

Pulmonary Laboratory Assessment and Diagnostic Procedures

CHAPTER OBJECTIVES

- *Identify abnormal arterial blood gas levels and initiate nursing interventions that will assist in correcting the abnormalities.*
- *Identify the parameters that must be evaluated to assess total oxygenation of arterial blood.*
- *List the indications and nursing care for patients undergoing a bronchoscopy or thoracentesis.*
- *Discuss the importance of pulmonary function tests in diagnosing pulmonary disorders.*
- *List essential nursing care of a patient with excessively low Pao_2 or high $Paco_2$ values.*

LABORATORY ASSESSMENT
Arterial Blood Gas Analysis

Interpretation of arterial blood gas levels can be difficult, especially if one is under pressure to do it quickly and accurately as is so often the case in critical care. One way that the nurse can help to ensure accuracy when analyzing arterial blood gas levels is by following the same steps of interpretation each time.

A specific method to be used each time blood gas values must be interpreted is presented here. Understanding this method and the normal blood gas values will greatly assist in successful interpretation.

Step 1: Look at the Pao_2 and answer the question, "Does the Pao_2 show hypoxemia?" The Pao_2 is a measure of the partial pressure of oxygen dissolved in arterial blood plasma, with *P* standing for "partial pressure" and *a* standing for "arterial." Sometimes Pao_2 is shortened to Po_2. It is reported in millimeters of mercury (mm Hg).

The normal range for Pao_2 on room air breathed at sea level is 80 to 100 mm Hg. However, the normal range is age-dependent in two groups: persons aged 60 years and older and infants. The normal level for infants breathing room air is 40 to 70 mm Hg.[32] The normal level for persons

60 years of age and older decreases with age as changes occur in the ventilation-perfusion ratio in the aging lung.[6] The correct Pao_2 for older persons can be ascertained by subtracting 1 mm Hg for every year that a person is over 60 years of age from 80 mm Hg (the lowest normal value). Using this formula, it will be found that a 65-year-old individual can have a Pao_2 as low as 75 mm Hg and still be within the normal range. (Formula: 5 years over 60 years of age; 80 mm Hg − 5 mm Hg = 75 mm Hg.) In the same way, an acceptable range for an 80-year-old person would begin at 60 mm Hg. (Formula: 20 years over the age of 60; 80 mm Hg − 20 mm Hg = 60 mm Hg.) At any age, a Pao_2 less than 40 mm Hg represents a life-threatening situation that requires immediate action. If the Pao_2 is less than the predicted lowest value, it shows *hypoxemia,* which means that a lower than normal amount of oxygen is dissolved in plasma. That is why the question "Does the Pao_2 show hypoxemia?" is asked.

There are several reasons supporting analysis of the Pao_2 level before those of other blood gas components. First, the Pao_2 may be the most crucial finding. As is pointed out in Chapter 17, a Pao_2 of less than 40 mm Hg severely compromises tissue oxygenation and calls for the immediate administration of supplemental oxygen and/or mechanical ventilation. Another reason the Pao_2 should be examined first is that the test results for the Pao_2 level can be quickly analyzed; if it is above the lowest value for the patient's age, it is normal. When the Pao_2 level is normal, it can be put aside so that the values for the acid-base components of arterial blood gases can be assessed.

All of the other components of normal arterial blood gases (pH, $Paco_2$ and HCO_3) are acid-base components and should be analyzed sequentially. Unless the Pao_2 falls low enough to trigger tissue hypoxia and lactic acid production, it does not contribute to acid-base production.

Step 2: Look at the pH level and answer the question, "Is the pH on the acid or alkaline side of 7.40?" The pH is the hydrogen ion concentration of plasma. The normal range is 7.35 to 7.45 with the mean being 7.40. If the pH is less than 7.40, it is on the acid side of the mean. Less than 7.35 is called *acidemia,* and the overall condition is called *acidosis.*

If the pH is greater than 7.40, it is on the alkaline side of the mean. Greater than 7.45 is called *alkalemia,* and the overall condition is called *alkalosis.* Calculation of the pH is accomplished by using the partial pressure of carbon dioxide ($PaCO_2$) and the plasma bicarbonate level (HCO_3). The formula used is the Henderson-Hasselbalch equation (see the box below).

Step 3: Look at the $PaCO_2$ and answer the question, "Does the $PaCO_2$ show respiratory acidosis, alkalosis, or normalcy?" The $PaCO_2$ is a measure of the partial pressure of carbon dioxide dissolved in arterial blood plasma, and it is reported in mm Hg. It is the acid-base component that reflects the effectiveness of ventilation in relation to the metabolic rate. In other words, the $PaCO_2$ value indicates whether the patient can ventilate well enough to rid his or her body of the carbon dioxide produced as a consequence of metabolism. When the patient cannot ventilate well enough, the $PaCO_2$ will rise.

A buildup of carbon dioxide in the body is a serious health matter; thus the importance of accurate assessment of the $PaCO_2$ level cannot be overemphasized. The normal range for the $PaCO_2$ is 35 to 45 mm Hg. This range does not change as a person ages. A $PaCO_2$ greater than 45 mm Hg defines *respiratory acidosis,* which results from alveolar hypoventilation or ventilation-perfusion inequality. Another way of stating this is to say that respiratory acidosis occurs because the patient's ventilation is not effective in removing the carbon dioxide produced by metabolism.

```
        ┌─────────────────────────────────────┐
        │  THE HENDERSON-HASSELBALCH          │
        │  EQUATION FOR BLOOD pH              │
        └─────────────────────────────────────┘
```

THE HENDERSON-HASSELBALCH EQUATION FOR BLOOD pH

The blood pH depends on the ratio of bicarbonate to dissolved carbon dioxide. As long as the ratio is 20:1, the pH will be 7.4.

$$pH = pK^* + \log \frac{base}{acid}$$

$$pH = pK + \log \frac{HCO_3^-}{CO_2}$$

$$pH = 6.1 + \log \frac{24\ mEq/L}{40 \times .03\ mEq/L}$$

$$pH = 6.1 + \log 20$$

$$pH = 6.1 + 1.3$$

$$pH = 7.4$$

---

*pK is the pH at which the substance is half dissociated and half undissociated—value here is 6.1; HCO_3 normal is 24 mEq/L; CO_2 normal for arterial blood is 40 mm Hg and must be converted to mEq/L to be used in this equation. Therefore the 40 mm Hg is multipled by .03 to convert to mEq/L.

Ventilatory failure is diagnosed whenever the $PaCO_2$ level rises above 50 mm Hg. Acute ventilatory failure occurs when the $PaCO_2$ level is above 50 mm Hg with a pH below normal, usually less than 7.30.[6,32] It is referred to as acute because the pH is abnormal, thereby not allowing enough time for the body to compensate by returning the pH to normal. The student of respiratory nursing should remember ventilatory failure occurs because the patient is not breathing or *ventilating* effectively. It will be of little or no help to administer oxygen without also improving ventilation. These patients need assistance to *ventilate,* not necessarily to *oxygenate.*

Interventions that will assist the patient in ventilation include elevating patent's chest to ease diaphragmatic descent; teaching the patient deep-breathing exercises; encouraging the patient to expectorate mucus, or if this is not possible, suctioning the mucus; and when vital capacity and tidal volume fall severely low while $PaCO_2$ continues to climb, providing mechanical ventilation.

A $PaCO_2$ value that is less than 35 mm Hg defines *respiratory alkalosis,* which is caused by alveolar hyperventilation. Hyperventilation can result from pain, fever, chills, anxiety, overvigorous mechanical ventilation, sepsis, or as a compensatory mechanism to metabolic acidosis.

Although respiratory alkalosis does not produce the life-threatening situation of respiratory acidosis, it must not be overlooked because the alkalemia can result in cardiac, cerebral, and neuromuscular irritability.[20] Interventions are usually aimed at correcting the underlying cause of the alkalemia.

Step 4: Look at the HCO_3^- level and answer the question, "Does the HCO_3 show metabolic acidosis, alkalosis, or normalcy?" The bicarbonate (HCO_3) is the "base" component of acid-base blood gas analysis and reflects kidney function. The bicarbonate is reduced or increased in the plasma by renal mechanisms. The normal range is 22 to 26 mEq/L. A bicarbonate level of less than 22 mEq/L defines *metabolic acidosis,* which can result from ketoacidosis, lactic acidosis, renal failure, or diarrhea. A bicarbonate level that is greater than 26 mEq/L defines *metabolic alkalosis,* which can result from fluid loss from the upper GI tract (vomiting or nasogastric suction), diuretic therapy, severe hypokalemia, alkali administration, or corticosteroid therapy.

Step 5: Look back at the pH level and answer the question, "Does the pH show a compensated or an uncompensated condition?" If the pH level is abnormal, that is, less than 7.35 or greater than 7.45, the $PaCO_2$, the HCO_3, or both will also be abnormal. This is an uncompensated condition, because there has not been enough time for the body to return the pH to its normal range. Two examples of uncompensated arterial blood gases follow:

1. PaO_2: 90 mm Hg
   pH: 7.25
   PCO_2: 50 mm Hg
   HCO_3: 22 mEq/L
   This is diagnosed as *uncompensated respiratory acidosis.*

2. PaO_2: 90 mm Hg
   pH: 7.25

Pco_2: 40 mm Hg
HCO_3: 17 mEq/L

This is diagnosed as *uncompensated metabolic acidosis*.

If the pH is within normal limits and both the $Paco_2$ and the HCO_3 are abnormal, the condition is *compensated* because there has been enough time for the body to restore the pH to within its normal range. Two examples of compensated arterial blood gases follow:

1. Pao_2; 90 mm Hg
   pH: 7.37
   Pco_2: 60 mm Hg
   HCO_3: 38 mEq/L

   This is diagnosed as *compensated respiratory acidosis with metabolic alkalosis*. The acidosis is considered the main disorder and the alkalosis the compensating disorder, because the pH is on the acid side of 7.40.

2. Pao_2: 90 mm Hg
   pH: 7.42
   Pco_2: 48 mm Hg
   HCO_3: 35 mEq/L

   This is diagnosed as *compensated metabolic alkalosis with respiratory acidosis*. The alkalosis is considered the main disorder and the acidosis the compensating disorder, because the pH is on the alkaline side of 7.40.

This method of blood gas interpretation is reviewed in the box below.

STEPS FOR INTERPRETATION OF BLOOD GAS LEVELS

STEP 1

Look at the Pao_2 level and answer the question, *"Does the Pao_2 level show hypoxemia?"*

STEP 2

Look at the pH level and answer the question, *"Is the pH level on the acid or alkaline side of 7.40?"*

STEP 3

Look at the $Paco_2$ level and answer the question, *"Does the $Paco_2$ level show respiratory acidosis, alkalosis, or normalcy?"*

STEP 4

Look at the Hco_3 level and answer the question, *"Does the Hco_3 show metabolic acidosis, alkalosis, or normalcy?"*

STEP 5

Look back at the pH level and answer the question, *"Does the pH show a compensated or an uncompensated condition?"*

Other Considerations When Interpreting Arterial Blood Gases

Oxygen saturation (Sao_2). Oxygen saturation is a measure of the amount of oxygen bound to hemoglobin compared to hemoglobin's maximum capability for binding oxygen.[4] It is reported as a percentage or as a decimal with the normal being greater than 96% (.96) on room air. The Sao_2 level cannot reach 100% (on room air) because of the normal physiological shunting of venous blood into the arterial system via the bronchial, thebesian, and other minor systems within the lungs and heart. (See "Bronchial Circulation" in Chapter 17.) However, when supplemental oxygen is administered, the Sao_2 level may approach 100% so closely that it is reported as 100%.

Proper evaluation of the Sao_2 level is vital. For example, an Sao_2 of 97% means that 97% of the available hemoglobin is bound with oxygen. The word *available* is essential to evaluating the Sao_2 level, because the hemoglobin level is not always within normal limits and oxygen can only bind with what is available. A 97% saturation level associated with 10 grams of hemoglobin does not deliver as much oxygen to the tissues as does a 97% saturation associated with 15 grams of hemoglobin. Thus assessing only the Sao_2 level and finding it within normal limits should not lead one to believe that the patient's oxygenation status is normal. The hemoglobin level must also be evaluated before a decision on oxygenation status can be made.

Oxygen content. Oxygen content (Cao_2 or O_2Ct) is a measure of the total amount of oxygen carried in the blood including the amount dissolved in plasma, measured by the Pao_2, and the amount bound to the hemoglobin molecule, measured by the Sao_2. Cao_2 is reported in milliliters (ml) of oxygen carried per 100 ml of blood. The normal value is 18 to 20 ml of oxygen carried per 100 ml of blood; this can also be stated as 18 to 20 vol%.

To calculate the oxygen content, the Pao_2, the Sao_2, and the hemoglobin level are used; therefore a change in any of these factors will change the Cao_2. For instance, a low hemoglobin concentration will yield a low Cao_2. The formula for calculating the Cao_2 can be found in Appendix C.

The value of assessing the Cao_2 is best illustrated by the example in Table 19-1. Here, the arterial blood gas parameters that are most commonly used to evaluate oxygenation status (Pao_2 and Sao_2) are both normal. Assessing only the Pao_2 and the Sao_2 would lead to the false belief that, in Patient B, oxygenation status is normal. However, it can be seen by looking at the hemoglobin and the Cao_2 that the oxygenation of Patient B's blood is far from normal.

Table 19-1 illustrates two essential facts of oxygenation assessment: (1) checking the Pao_2 and the Sao_2 are not

Table 19-1 Assessing oxygenation status

Patient	Pao_2 level (mm Hg)	Sao_2 level (%)	Hb level (gm%)	Cao_2 level (vol%)
A	100	97	15	19.8
B	100	97	10	13.3

Table 19-2 The expected Pao_2 versus the actual Pao_2

Patient*	Flo_2 level (%)	Expected Pao_2 level (mm Hg)	Actual Pao_2 level (mm Hg)
A	30	150	160
B	50	250	85
C	50	250	60

*Patients are all under 60 years of age.

Table 19-3 Guidelines for estimating Flo_2 with low-flow oxygen devices

100% O_2 flow rate (L)	Flo_2 (%)
NASAL CANNULA OR CATHETER	
1	24
2	28
3	32
4	36
5	40
6	44
OXYGEN MASK	
5-6	40
6-7	50
7-8	60
MASK WITH RESERVOIR BAG	
6	60
7	70
8	80
9	90
10	99 +

Note: Normal ventilatory pattern assumed.
From Shapiro BA, Harrison, RA, and Walton JR: Clinical application of blood gases, Chicago, 1989, Year Book Medical Publishers, Inc. Reproduced with permission.

enough and (2) a patient may not be *hypoxemic* but may be *hypoxic*. Hypoxemia versus hypoxia is discussed in more detail in Chapter 20.

Expected Pao_2. When a patient is put on supplemental oxygen, his or her Pao_2 level is expected to rise. Knowing the level to which the Pao_2 *should* rise in normal subjects on a given FIO_2 and comparing that to the level in which the Pao_2 actually *does* rise in patients with pulmonary disease has value, because it illustrates how well the lung is functioning.

Calculating the expected Pao_2 is accomplished by multiplying the FIO_2 value by 5.[32] Thus the expected Pao_2 on an FIO_2 of 30% should be at least 150 mm Hg (30 × 5), whereas the expected Pao_2 on an FIO_2 of 50% should be 250 mm Hg (50 × 5). These expected Pao_2 values represent the oxygen level achievable with healthy lungs. Pulmonary disease can radically decrease the expected Pao_2 level. Table 19-2 illustrates three examples of what can occur when the expected Pao_2 level does not reach normal.

Patient A shows a normal expected Pao_2 level; thus it is assumed that his or her lungs are performing normally. The fact that the expected Pao_2 level is reached means he or she may not require supplemental oxygen. Patient B does not reach the expected Pao_2 level, but at least he or she is not hypoxemic; supplemental oxygen, administered at an FIO_2 of .50, allows the Pao_2 level to be above 80 mm Hg. However, because the expected Pao_2 level is not achieved, an assumption should be made that removal of oxygen will result in hypoxemia.[32] Therefore in situations like this, nursing care must include education of the patient, his or her family, and all caregivers about the importance of the oxygen remaining in place. Patient C does not reach the expected Pao_2 level, and he or she is hypoxemic; he or she needs more help. This may include emphasis on coughing or suctioning of mucus to remove a possible source of ventilation-perfusion inequality, repositioning to allow for better lung inflation and for better matching of ventilation with perfusion, and increasing the FIO_2 or applying positive end-expiratory pressure (PEEP) if the patient is mechanically ventilated.

It is impossible to apply the "FIO_2 value × 5" rule to achieve the expected Pao_2 value when the patient is on a system that delivers oxygen by liters per minute. For these situations, Table 19-3 shows the FIO_2 levels that correspond to various oxygen delivery systems.

Body temperature. The discussion of how body temperature affects arterial blood gas levels assumes the reader is familiar with the content in Chapter 17 covering "Oxygen Transport Within The Blood." A review of that content is suggested if necessary.

Body temperature will alter the normal affinity that exists between oxygen and hemoglobin. For this reason, either the patient's temperature must be taken when the arterial blood gases are drawn, or the computer that measures and records the blood gas levels must also measure the blood temperature.

Fever will decrease the normal affinity that exists between oxygen and hemoglobin, which results in a decrease in oxyhemoglobin but an increase in the oxygen dissolved in plasma. In the presence of fever, less oxygen will bind to hemoglobin, but because of its lessened affinity for hemoglobin, the oxygen will unload more readily at the tissue level. This physiology is illustrated by a rightward shift in the oxyhemoglobin dissociation curve. Clinically, any factor (such as fever or acidosis) responsible for a rightward shift of the curve improves tissue oxygenation (within limits).

Hypothermia will increase the normal affinity that exists between oxygen and hemoglobin, resulting in more oxyhemoglobin and a lower Pao_2 for any given saturation. Oxygen will less readily unload at the tissue level. This physiology is illustrated by a leftward shift of the oxyhemoglobin dissociation curve.

A general rule is that fever helps the unloading of oxygen at the tissue level (within limits), whereas hypothermia interferes with the unloading of hemoglobin.

Base excess and base deficit. Base excess or base deficit reflects the nonrespiratory contribution to acid-base balance and are reported in milliequivalents per liter above or below the normal range of -2 mEq/L to $+2$ mEq/L. A negative base level is reported as a *base deficit*, which correlates with metabolic acidosis, whereas a positive base level is reported as a *base excess*, which correlates with metabolic alkalosis.

Alveolar–arterial oxygen tension difference. The alveolar–arterial oxygen tension difference [(A-a)DO$_2$] is also written as P(A-a)O$_2$ and referred to as the A-a gradient. It measures the difference between the oxygen tension within the alveoli (A) and the artery (a) and provides information on the efficiency of the transfer of oxygen into the blood at the alveolar-capillary level. Serial determinations of the A-a gradient provide clinically useful data on lung function and are useful guides to therapy.[25]

The normal gradient for persons under 61 years of age is 10 mm Hg (measured while breathing room air). However, the normal gradient elevates in at least two instances not related to acute lung pathology. First, age elevates the gradient, because the lungs develop ventilation-perfusion (V/Q) inequalities as a normal part of aging, thereby resulting in less efficient oxygen exchange; in one study, persons aged 61 to 75 years had an average A-a gradient of 16 mm Hg.[24] Second, the use of supplemental oxygen will elevate the gradient at least up to an FIO$_2$ of 60%.[21] Fig. 19-1 illustrates the change in the A-a gradient in response to increase in FIO$_2$. Changes in PaCO$_2$ will not affect the A-a gradient.

Recently, the clinical usefulness of the A-a gradient has been questioned, particularly because of its variability when calculated on levels of oxygen above room air[31] and because of the need to calculate the PAO$_2$.[15] See Appendix C for the PAO$_2$ formula. An elevated A-a gradient can result from V/Q inequalities, from shunt abnormality (Qs/Qt), or from diffusion limitations; changes with hypoxemia are shown in Table 19-4.

The arterial/alveolar oxygen tension ratio. The relationship between the PaO$_2$ and the PAO$_2$ can also be expressed as a ratio, PaO$_2$/PAO$_2$. Like the A-a gradient, the arterial/alveolar oxygen tension ratio (PaO$_2$/PAO$_2$) also requires the calculation of the alveolar PO$_2$. Unlike the A-a gradient, the PaO$_2$/PAO$_2$ remains relatively stable when the FIO$_2$ changes as long as the underlying lung condition is stable.[15] (See Fig. 19-1.)

The normal PaO$_2$/PAO$_2$ ratio is 0.75 to 0.90 for any FiO$_2$. A ratio of less than 0.75 indicates V/Q inequality, shunt, or diffusion limitation. Table 19-4 shows the change in the PaO$_2$/PAO$_2$ seen in a hypoxemic patient.

The PaO$_2$/FiO$_2$ Ratio. The oxygen ratio, PaO$_2$/FiO$_2$, is easier to calculate than the A-a gradient or the PaO$_2$/PAO$_2$, because it does not require use of the alveolar gas equation in its calculation. However, it has the disadvantage of being affected by changes in the PaCO$_2$, and there is much controversy over its usefulness as a predictor of pulmonary dysfunction.[21,22] Specifically, some studies have shown it to be an insensitive indicator of changes in shunt.[15,33] Changes in the PaO$_2$/FiO$_2$ ratio seen in the hypoxemic patient are illustrated in Table 19-4.

Arterial-mixed venous oxygen content difference. When both arterial blood samples and pulmonary arterial blood samples are available, the arterial-mixed venous oxygen content difference (A-VDO$_2$) can be calculated. The A-VDO$_2$ represents an assessment of the cardiac output in relation to metabolic needs and is useful in determining oxygen extraction and whether cardiac output is sufficient enough to meet the body's metabolic needs.

In healthy persons, the A-VDO$_2$ is 5.0 vol% with the normal range being 4.5 to 6.0 vol%.[33] Critically ill patients with adequate cardiovascular function can maintain an A-VDO$_2$ of 2.5-4.5 vol%, whereas critically ill patients with inadequate cardiovascular reserves may show an A-VDO$_2$ greater than 6.0 vol%.

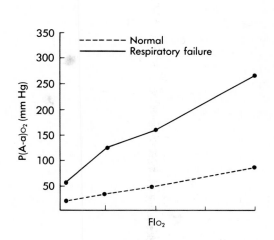

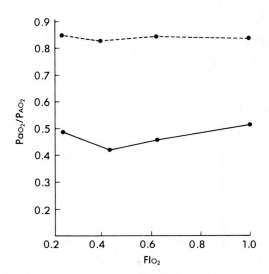

Fig. 19-1 Changes in P(A-a)O$_2$ and PaO$_2$/PAO$_2$ with increasing FIO$_2$ in a healthy subject and in a patient with respiratory failure. With increasing FIO$_2$, PaO$_2$/PAO$_2$ varies much less than does P(A-a)O$_2$. (From Martin L: Pulmonary physiology in clinical practice: the essentials for patient care and evaluation, St Louis, 1987, The CV Mosby Co.

Table 19-4 The effects of increasing FIO_2 on PaO_2, PAO_2, $P(A-a)O_2$, PaO_2/PAO_2, and PaO_2/FIO_2 in a normal subject and a hypoxemic (right to left shunt) patient

FIO_2	PaO_2 (mm Hg)	PAO_2 (mm Hg)	$P(A-a)O_2$ (mm Hg)	PaO_2/PAO_2	PaO_2/FIO_2
NORMAL SUBJECT					
0.21	90	97	7	0.93	429
0.50	280	300	20	0.93	560
1.0	560	610	50	0.92	560
HYPOXEMIC PATIENT					
0.21	40	97	57	0.41	190
0.50	80	300	220	0.27	160
1.0	150	610	460	0.25	150

From Murray JF and Nadel JA: Textbook of respiratory medicine, Philadelphia, 1988, WB Saunders Co.

Blood Studies

Blood studies usually involve obtaining the patient's complete blood cell count (CBC), electrolytes, and general chemistry profile. Other studies are added depending on the patient's history and physical condition. Isoenzymes of creatine phosphokinase (CPK) are appropriate in chest injury when myocardial damage is questioned.

The CBC and white blood cell count (WBC) differential are general screening tests. Increased WBCs with a shift to the left (high numbers of immature neutrophils) suggest bacterial as opposed to viral infections[9,11,23,29] and, therefore, assist in delineating treatment of pneumonia, especially in situations where sputum analysis, for one reason or another, has not been achieved. Elevated eosinophils (more than 500/mm³) accompany asthma and certain allergic lung conditions. Lung disease is often associated with polycythemia because of chronic tissue hypoxia.[8] Polycythemia will develop even if tissue hypoxia is only present during part of the 24-hour period, such as at night when decreased ventilation and oxygen intake cause oxygen desaturation of the hemoglobin molecule.[23] The presence of anemia may explain tachypnea and persistent tissue hypoxia despite normal PO_2 and O_2 saturations.

Evaluation of electrolytes can yield important information about the patient's overall condition, and the effects of therapy or the need for therapy. Sodium levels can shed light on the fluid status of the patient, which becomes crucial in the patient critically ill with pulmonary disease. Evaluation of sodium levels in urine and blood may identify the syndrome of inappropriate secretion of antidiuretic hormone (SIADH), which can occur in ventilator-supported patients or patients receiving frequent intermittent positive-pressure breathing (IPPB) treatments.[17]

Maintaining a normal potassium level is important in treating acid-base abnormalities. The body cannot fully correct an alkalosis that occurs along with hypokalemia, because potassium is the exchange ion in the kidney that allows for retention of hydrogen ion (H^+) and thus lowers pH.[13] The opposite is true in acidosis associated with hyperkalemia.

Recently the role of phosphate in adequate diaphragmatic contractility has surfaced. Phosphate levels should be evaluated in patients with acute respiratory failure to determine if hypophosphatemia is contributing to poor venitilatory dynamics.[2]

An analysis of serum enzymes may be helpful in identifying patients who may have experienced pulmonary infarction. Because enzymes are present in many body tissues, more definite radiological tests are usually performed to confirm pulmonary injury.

Sputum Studies

Sputum should always be carefully evaluated. The most difficult aspect of sputum examination is proper collection of the specimen. When the patient has difficulty producing sputum, inducing sputum with heated, nebulized saline may help to loosen secretions for expectoration. Chest physiotherapy combined with nebulization will improve the success rate. Collection of a sputum specimen is best done in the morning, because secretions have a greater volume caused by nighttime pooling.[8,25,36] The presence of an effective, forceful cough is helpful; however, many critically ill patients are unable to cough effectively and thus sputum collection by other means, such as transtracheal aspiration, is required.

Transtracheal aspiration. Transtracheal aspiration (TTA) in nonintubated patients is preferred over nasotracheal or bronchial washings.[9] In this technique, a catheter is introduced by cricoid stick into the trachea. This eliminates contamination of sputum by resident flora of mouth and pharynx. The TTA maneuver should be performed by an experienced physician, because major complications can occur.[11,29] Massive intraairway hemorrhage is possible, dysrhythmias can occur, and subcutaneous emphysema can develop.

Endotracheal/tracheal specimen collection. Many critically ill patients will have endotracheal or tracheal tubes already in place. Collecting sputum specimens from these patients requires special attention to technique (see the box "Procedure for Collection of Tracheal or Endotracheal

---

PROCEDURE FOR COLLECTION OF TRACHEAL OR ENDOTRACHEAL SPECIMEN

1. Clear the endotracheal or tracheostomy tube of all local secretions, avoiding deep airway penetration.
2. Attach a sputum trap to a sterile suction catheter and advance the catheter into the trachea while trying to avoid contact with the endotracheal tube or tracheostomy tube.
3. After catheter is fully advanced, apply suction until secretions return to the sputum trap. When enough secretions are collected, discontinue suctioning and remove catheter.

4. Do not apply suction while the catheter is being withdrawn, because this can contaminate the sample with sputum from the upper airway. Do not flush with sterile water since this dilutes the sample.
5. If the catheter becomes plugged with secretions, place it in a sterile container and send it to the laboratory. The specimen should be transported immediately or refrigerated if a delay is necessary.

Specimen[1]). Deep specimens should be obtained to avoid resident upper airway flora that may have migrated down the tube. This colonization of the lower airways with upper airway flora can occur within 24 hours of intubation of tracheostomy.[23,39]

Other methods of specimen collection. Proper specimen retrieval may require more invasive measures, such as the use of a fiberoptic bronchoscopy in association with a sheath-protected catheter specimen, a transbronchial biopsy and bronchoalveolar lavage, a transthoracic needle aspiration of lung, or an open lung biopsy.

The fiberoptic bronchoscopy is the most frequent invasive procedure used in the diagnosis of pulmonary infections. It is versatile with respect to options (that is, it can be used for simple specimen collection, biopsy, lavage, or all three) and has few side-effects. Bleeding occurs in up to 7% of patients, and hypoxemia can be associated with the procedure.[12,34]

Although transthoracic needle aspiration can be selectively guided by fluoroscopy, complications are frequent and significant. Hemoptysis occurs in 3% to 10% of patients, and pneumothorax occurs in 20% to 30%.[3,34]

Open biopsy offers the best opportunity for the investigation of pulmonary infection. Theoretically, by locating the proper area for specimen collection and biopsy, ineffective results should be eliminated. However, one study showed that only 70% of the cases of open biopsy yielded identification of the causative organism.[12] The mortality rate is around 5%, which poses a major disadvantage to this approach. Critically ill patients may not be able to tolerate such a procedure, and all other methods of diagnosis are generally employed first.

Once a sputum specimen is obtained, a Gram's stain followed by a culture and sensitivity (C&S) should be performed. A Gram's stain allows for cellular quantification and evaluation of the value of the specimen.

DIAGNOSTIC PROCEDURES
Bronchoscopy

Indications. Bronchoscopy is a relatively safe procedure that is most often used as a diagnostic tool (see the box

---

INDICATIONS FOR BRONCHOSCOPY

Persistent, unexplained cough
Hemoptysis of unknown origin
Aspiration of gastric contents, foreign body, mucus
Bronchial obstruction
Pleural effusion of unknown origin
Suspected pulmonary tumor
Tissue biopsy
Retrieval of cellular elements and secretions for culture and cytology
Bronchial lavage
Staging of lung tumors
Evaluation of inhalation injury
Suspected lung cancer
Interstitial or alveolar infiltrates of unknown origin
Lung infections
Atelectasis
Guide patient intubation in neck injury

"Indications for Bronchoscopy"). Therapeutic uses include the removal of foreign bodies, removal of obstructing secretions, and resection of small, benign growths from the airway.

Procedure. Bronchoscopy can be performed with a rigid or flexible scope. Table 19-5 outlines the indications and disadvantages of both apparatuses. Some operators use one type of scope to supplement the capabilities of the other type, although the flexible fiberoptic scope has become the instrument of choice in most situations.

Before the bronchoscopy, a complete patient history and examination, including a chest x-ray examination, should be performed.[3,35] Preoperative evaluation of the patient should also include clotting studies (PT, PTT, and platelet count) and evaluation of the arterial blood gas levels. When the platelet count is less than 50,000, platelet transfusions before and during the procedure should be given.[10] Hyp-

Table 19-5 Comparison of rigid and flexible bronchoscope

Indications	Disadvantages
RIGID BRONCHOSCOPE	
Evaluate large lung hemorrhage (>200 cc)	Limited visualization of distal airways
Removal of foreign body	Cannot be used with mechanically ventilated patients
Surgical excision of tracheal or main bronchial lesions	Limited in patients with cervical problems
Biopsy of vascular tumor	Less patient comfort, especially with local anesthesia
FLEXIBLE BRONCHOSCOPE	
Applied in full variety of diagnostic and therapeutic situations	View may be inferior in quality and easily obscured
	May be difficult to control massive hemorrhage
	May necessitate several withdrawals and reinsertions during procedure
	Size can limit removal of foreign bodies and secretions

oxemic patients (less than 70 mm Hg PaO$_2$) need supplemental oxygen during the procedure. The patient should have nothing by mouth for 4 to 6 hours before the bronchoscopy to reduce the risk of aspiration.[17]

Although topical anesthesia can be used alone, it is generally supplemented by systemic anesthesia or analgesia. Diazepam (Valium) and midazolam HCl (Versed) are two agents frequently administered intravenously during the procedure. Preoperative medications for a diagnostic bronchoscopy may include atropine and intramuscular codeine. The atropine lessens the vasovagal response and reduces the secretions, whereas codeine decreases the cough reflex. When a bronchoscopy is performed therapeutically to remove secretions, medications other than analgesics are avoided because intratracheal topical anesthesia tends to decrease cough and impair secretion clearance.

The bronchoscopy should not be performed within a few days of other operative procedures because of increased secretions that result from local irritation. By the same token, after a bronchoscopy, patients often experience an increased cough and throat discomfort. A small amount of blood may be present in the sputum and a slight fever, should it occur, is usually self-limiting.

Nursing care. The nursing care of patients undergoing theapeutic or diagnostic bronchoscopy involves (1) preparation of the patient psychologically and physically for the procedure and (2) monitoring the patient's responses to the procedure and assessing the patient after the bronchoscopy.

Many of the bronchoscopies performed on the critically ill patient are carried out to remove secretions interfering with proper aeration. Anxiety is often present because of the concomitant tissue hypoxia, the artificial airway, and possible ventilator support. The patient may fear the insertion of the bronchoscope because he or she assumes that it will interfere with breathing and therefore lead to suffocation. The nurse must reassure the patient that proper ventilation will occur.

The nonintubated patient undergoing a bronchoscopy should receive nothing by mouth both before the procedure and until the gag reflex returns afterwards. Periodical assessment of the gag reflex should be performed.

During the procedure, the nurse should monitor the patient's vital signs and oxygenation and inform the physician of changes. If specimen retrieval is performed during the bronchoscopy, the nurse may need to assist in preparing the specimen for transport to the laboratory.

Following the procedure, the patient must be observed for the development of complications, degree of oxygenation, and return of the cough and gag reflexes.

When a tissue biopsy is performed, some hemoptysis may occur immediately after the bronchoscopy. Frank bleeding is not usual and may mean hemorrhage is occurring.

In the nonintubated patient, equipment for emergency airway management should be available to treat tracheal edema, which may result from the procedure. The patient may complain of a sore throat and hoarseness, but these side effects are generally self-limiting.

Thoracentesis

Indications. Thoracentesis is a simple, usually uncomplicated procedure for the removal of fluid from the pleural space. It is most frequently used as a diagnostic measure, although in rare circumstances it may be performed therapeutically as in the case of pleural effusion drainage.

Most pleural effusions are self-limiting, and unless the cause is unknown or therapy for the patient may be altered by the results, thoracentesis is unwarranted. When a pleural effusion persists despite treatment of the primary cause, thoracentesis should be considered. Table 19-6 outlines causes of pleural effusions and appropriate diagnostic testing.

Procedure. The patient should be in a sitting position with legs over the side of the bed and hands and arms supported on a padded overbed table. If the patient's condition precludes sitting, the side-lying position with back flush with the edge of the bed can be used. The patient should be cautioned not to move or cough during the procedure.

During the thoracentesis, the site of the needle insertion is usually determined by previous chest x-ray examination results, CT scan, or chest percussion. A local anesthetic is used to minimize patient discomfort during insertion of the

Table 19-6 Diseases involving the pleura and confirming diagnostic tests

Pleural process	Clinical setting	Useful tests	Diagnostic criteria
Transudative	Congestive heart failure, nephrotic syndrome, hypoalbuminemia	Serum and pleural fluid, protein, LDH	Any one of these criteria make it an exudate: PF protein/plasma > 0.5 PF LDH/serum LDH > 0.6 PF LDH > 200
Infective	Aerobic, anaerobic bacteria	Gross appearance, smell, Gram's stain, aerobic and anaerobic cultures, glucose, pH, LDH	Empyema is considered when the fluid is purulent, organisms can be demonstrated in Gram's stain or culture. Foul smell is seen with anaerobic infection. pH of pleural fluid is to be obtained only with clear fluids. Complicated parapneumonic effusions are clear fluids with no demonstrable organisms but have pH <7.00 and LDH > 1000.
	Viral, mycoplasmal		Virus and *Mycoplasma* are considered causes by association and exclusion.
	Parasitic		Parasite to be considered in patients coming from endemic areas.
Granulomatous	Tuberculosis (TB)	Pleural fluid, pleural tissue for smears and cultures of AFB and fungus, PPD results	Pleural granuloma with stainable AFB or positive culture is diagnostic of tuberculosis.
	Fungi		Pleural granuloma with fungus on stain or culture is diagnostic of fungal infection.
	Sarcoidosis		Pleural granuloma with negative cultures for AFB and fungi and negative PPD are suggestive of sarcoidosis in the appropriate clinical setting.
Malignant	Metastatic lymphoma, leukemia, mesothelioma	Pleural fluid cytology, pleural biopsy	Class V cytology or pleural tissue showing malignancy. Mesothelioma is rarely diagnosed by cytology and pleural biopsy. Hyaluronic acid levels are high but not specific.
Chylothorax	Tear of thoracic duct (trauma, lymphoma, cancer, mediastinal surgery)	Gross appearance, smell, centrifugation, lipoprotein electrophoresis, triglyceride, cholesterol, fat globules, cholesterol crystals	Chylothorax is milky, no odor, clears with ether; supernatant is cloudy; triglycerides are elevated with chylomicrons.
Hemothorax	Trauma, dissecting aneurysm	CBC, Hct	Hct is the best way to distinguish hemothorax from serosanguineous effusion. In hemothorax the Hct is usually >10.
Reactive	Abdominal surgery, pneumonia, pulmonary embolism		Effusion is nonspecific. Diagnosis is by exclusion, association, and evolution.
Miscellaneous	Pancreatitis	Serum and pleural fluid amylase	PF amylase is higher than serum and is of pancreatic type.
	Asbestosis		Eosinophilic; otherwise nonspecific. Diagnosis is by exclusion, association, and evolution.
	Radiation		Nonspecific. Diagnosis by history and exclusion.

LDH, lactic dehydrogenase; AFB, acid-fast bacilli; PPD, purified protein derivative; PF, pleural fluid; ANA, antinuclear antibody; CBC, complete blood count; Hct, hematocrit; SLE, systemic lupus erythematosus.
Adapted from McDonnell KF, Fahey PJ, and Segal MS: Respiratory intensive care, Boston, 1987, Little, Brown & Co.

thoracentesis needle. Most institutions now have disposable thoracentesis trays, which contain all the equipment required for the procedure.

Relative contraindications. No absolute contraindications to thoracentesis exist, although there are risks that generally contraindicate the procedure in all but emergency situations. Factors that heighten the risk of thoracentesis include unstable hemodynamics, coagulation defects, mechanically ventilated patients, the presence of an intraaortic balloon pump,[30] or patients who are uncooperative. In most clinical situations, diagnostic thoracentesis can be delayed until these risk factors are eliminated.

Complications. Complications associated with thoracentesis include pain, pneumothorax, and reexpansion pulmonary edema. The risk of pain or pneumothorax is significantly reduced when the thoracentesis is performed by an experienced clinician. Reexpansion pulmonary edema can occur when a large amount of effusion fluid is removed from the pleural space.[21,28,30] Removal of the fluid increases the negative intrapleural pressure which, when the lung does not reexpand to fill the space, can lead to edema. The patient can experience severe coughing and shortness of breath. The onset of these symptoms is an indication to discontinue the thoracentesis. If the physician is measuring the negative pressure during the thoracentesis, withdrawal of fluid should stop when pressure exceeds -20 cm of water pressure.[23]

The removal of a large amount of fluid has been associated with higher morbidity and decreased arterial oxygenation in association with reexpansion pulmonary edema.[16] There is little evidence of improvement in a patient's condition with removal of large effusions and subjective reports of dyspnea relief have varied.[30]

Nursing care. Nursing care of patients undergoing thoracentesis is directed at (1) preparing the patient both psychologically and physically, and (2) monitoring the patient's condition during and following the procedure. In critical care patients, performing a thoracentesis may be more problematic because of the patient's being confused and less alert or resulting from an unstable hemodynamic state or positioning limitations imposed by the patient's condition. The nurse must adjust her or his plans and responses based on the presence of complicating patient situations.

A thorough explanation should be given to patients about what will be done to them and expected from them during the thoracentesis procedure. Patient cooperation and understanding increases the safety and ease of the procedure. Supplemental oxygen should be provided, and proper positioning of the patient accomplished. Baseline vital signs should be taken, and provisions made for ongoing monitoring of these parameters.

When possible, oxygenation should be monitored by oximetry or other instantaneous measuring devices. Removal of a large pleural effusion is often accompanied by a reduction in the PaO_2, which can continue up to 24 hours after the procedure. Administering supplemental oxygen can lessen the hypoxemia. The removal of effusion fluid can also result in reexpansion pulmonary edema, which can be evidenced by increasing dyspnea and coughing and decreasing oxygen saturation.[30]

After the thoracentesis, a chest x-ray examination should be performed to rule out accidental pneumothorax, which is a potential complication.[28] The patient's vital signs should be checked every 15 minutes until stable, and the nurse should periodically assess lung sounds and oxygen saturation. The patient should be encouraged to lie with the uninvolved lung facing down, because research shows this position to improve oxygenation. Bleeding is a possibility, and the nurse should evaluate the patient for any signs and symptoms of hemorrhage.

Pulmonary Function Tests

Pulmonary function tests are designed to quantify respiratory function. They are utilized in five primary ways (see the box "Uses of Pulmonary Function Tests"). Tests of lung function can be divided into assessment of mechanical functioning, distribution of ventilation and blood flow, and arterial blood gases. Variations in the normal pulmonary function occur with age, gender, and body size.

The thorax functions as a bellows, bringing air to and from the lungs. Measurements can be taken to evaluate the static and dynamic properties of the lung-thorax system. Static properties of the lung refer to the elasticity of thorax and lung tissue. During inhalation, the ventilatory muscles contract and lung tissue is expanded or stretched. When the muscles relax, the stretching force is released and the elastic lung tissue recoils to its original shape and size. Measurement of lung volumes and capacities reflect static pulmonary parameters. Lung volumes and capacities measure the amount of air that the resting patient can inhale and exhale. The procedures for this require patient understanding and cooperation so that an accurate reflection of lung function can be obtained. Pulmonary volumes can be measured by gas dilution techniques, body plethysmography, or spirometry. (see the box "Lung Volumes and Capacities;" Fig. 19-2 is a schematic representation of these same lung capacities and volumes).

Gas dilution techniques. Gas dilution techniques are used to measure the residual volume and the functional residual capacity. Determining functional residual capacity (FRC) involves the use of a gas that is relatively insoluble in the blood. The gases predominantly used are helium and nitrogen. When helium is used, the patient breathes from a spirometer that contains a mixture of air and helium. When the amount of helium in the spirometer stabilizes during inhalation and exhalation, the concentration in the spirom-

---

USES OF PULMONARY FUNCTION TESTS

- Initial evaluation of patients with a complaint of breathlessness
- Initial evaluation of patients with known respiratory disease
- Document course of patients with respiratory disease
- Preoperative evaluation of patients with respiratory complication
- Screening for subclinical disease

LUNG VOLUMES AND CAPACITIES

Tidal Volume (V$_T$): The volume of air exhaled after a normal resting inhalation. V$_T$ × respiratory rate = minute ventilation.

Inspiratory Reserve Volume (IRV): The amount of additional air that can be taken in after a normal inhalation.

Inspiratory Capacity (IC): The maximal amount of air that can be inhaled after a normal exhalation.

Expiratory Reserve Volume (ERV): The additional amount of air that can be exhaled after a normal resting exhalation.

Vital Capacity (VC): The maximal amount of air that can be exhaled after a maximal inhalation.

Residual Volume (RV): The amount of air left in the lung after maximal exhalation.

Functional Residual Capacity (FRC): The amount of air left in the lung after a normal exhalation. The total of the ERV and RV.

Total Lung Capacity (TLC): The maximal volume of air in the lung following a maximal inspiration. The total of all lung volumes.

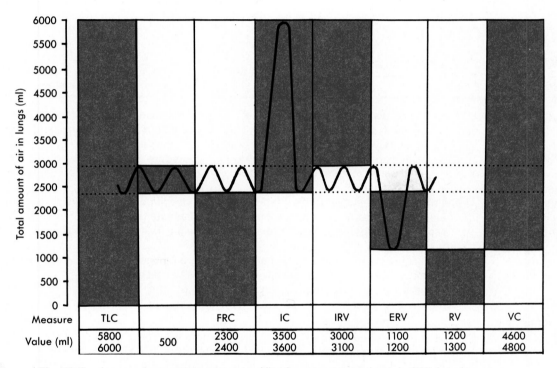

Measure	TLC		FRC	IC	IRV	ERV	RV	VC
Value (ml)	5800 6000	500	2300 2400	3500 3600	3000 3100	1100 1200	1200 1300	4600 4800

Fig. 19-2 Lung volume measurements. All values are approximately 25% less in women. TLC, total lung capacity; V$_T$, tidal volume; FRC, functional residual capacity; IC, inspiratory capacity; IRV, inspiratory reserve volume; ERV, expiratory reserve volume; RV, residual volume; VC, vital capacity.

eter and the patient's lungs has equalized. The helium remaining in the spirometer is then used to calculate the patient's FRC. The residual volume (RV) is determined by subtracting the expiratory reserve volume (ERV) from the FRC. This is often expressed as a ratio of the total lung capacity (TLC) as RV/TLC. The functions of both the RV and FRC are discussed in Chapter 17, p. 365.

When nitrogen is used, the patient inhales 100% oxygen. The exhaled gas is collected, and the percent of nitrogen present is constantly measured. As 100% oxygen is breathed, nitrogen is "washed out" of the lungs (over approximately a 7-minute period).[17] The amount of nitrogen exhaled is measured, and the FRC calculated.

Body Plethysmography. Body plethysmography involves an airtight box or compartment in which the patient sits. The patient breathes air through a tube or mouthpiece that is connected to an outside air source. At the end of exhalation, the tube is briefly occluded and the patient is instructed to pant into the mouthpiece. Changes in the patient's lung pressures and the pressure within the box are recorded during this maneuver. Using the pressure measurement, the therapist can calculate the patient's TLC and derive the FRC from that.[1] When patients have lung disease that results in air trapping, body plethysmography provides a more reliable measurement of lung volumes than gas dilution techniques.

Spirometry. Spirometry, the simplest measuring technique, can be performed at the bedside as well as in the pulmonary laboratory. It is most frequently used to measure tidal volume, vital capacity, and minute ventilation. Spirometry cannot measure residual volume or functional residual capacity. If these parameters are essential, the gas dilution technique or body plethysmography must be used.

Dynamic pulmonary function tests are designed to evaluate the function of the respiratory muscles, the thorax, and the lungs.[38] Ventilation is accomplished by overcoming inertia and resistance to air flow. Timed breathing studies reflect the ease of ventilation and include forced vital capacity, forced expiratory flow at midpoint of vital capacity, forced expiratory flow at 1 and 3 seconds, and maximal voluntary ventilation. Table 19-7 defines these tests. Flow volume loops are a more recent method used to study the dynamics of ventilation.[1,38]

Flow volume loops. Flow volume loops are a continuous recording of air flow rate and lung volume during forced vital capacity maneuvers (Fig. 19-3). Inspiratory and expiratory curves make up the graph and form a loop configuration. Flow volume loops are replacing timed vital capacity measurements in the pulmonary specialist's array of diagnostic tests. The portion of the graph that comprises the expiratory flow volume curve (upper half) is more helpful in distinguishing between restrictive and obstructive disorders, whereas the inspiratory portion (lower half) assists in differentiating extrathoracic from intrathoracic airway obstructions.

Chronic obstructive pulmonary disease (COPD) alters the characteristic of the expiratory curve with the peak flow rate that occurs earlier than usual and an overall reduced rate of flow throughout exhalation (see Curve 2, Fig. 19-3).[38] These alterations result from pressure changes and early airway closure.

Table 19-7 Dynamic pulmonary function tests

Test	Description	Abnormal value
Forced vital capacity (FVC)	The maximal amount of gas a patient can exhale into a spirometer as forcefully and as quickly as possible	Flow reduced with obstructive pulmonary disease because of early airway closure caused by forced exhalation
Forced expiratory flow in 1 and 3 seconds (FEV$_1$ and FEV$_3$)	The maximal amount of gas a patient can exhale into a spirometer during 1 and 3 seconds of a forced exhalation	Flow reduced in obstructive disease because of early airway closure caused by forced exhalation
Forced expiratory flow at midpoint of vital capacity (FEF 25%-75%)	The measure of the average flow rate during the middle 50% of exhalation; also a good measure of small or distal airway function	Reduced in obstructive airway disease and is considered a good indicator of early changes indicating obstructive lung disease
Maximal voluntary ventilation (MVV)	The maximal amount of gas that a patient can move in 1 minute. Test usually occurs in a 10-15 second period, with L/min value calculated	Value reduced in moderate to severe obstructive airway disease

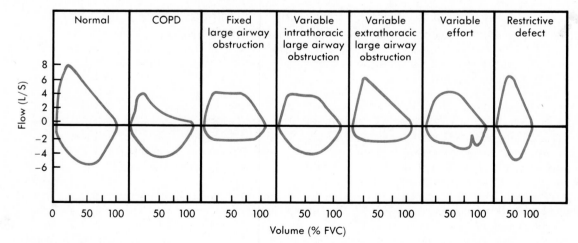

Fig. 19-3 Characteristic flow volume loops from various pulmonary dysfunctions. The total lung capacity (TLC) is to the left of each panel. (From Burton GG and Hodgkin JE: Respiratory care: a guide to clinical practice, Philadelphia, 1984, JB Lippincott Co. Courtesy of Lauer J: Computer methods in spirometry: diagnosis and flow-volume curve analysis, unpublished thesis, Loma Linda University Graduate School, Loma Linda, Calif, 1973.)

Table 19-8 Pulmonary function findings in lung disorders

Test	Predominantly reversible air flow obstruction (asthma)	Predominantly irreversible air flow obstruction	Interstitial lung disease (restrictive disease)	Emphysema (obstructive disease)
FEV₁	↓ ↓	↓ ↓	↓	↓ ↓
FVC	↓	↓	↓ ↓	↓
FEV₁/FVC%	↓	↓	N or ↑	↓
TLC	N or ↑	N or ↑	↓	↑ ↑
RV	↑	↑	↓	↑ ↑
DL₍CO₎	N or ↑	↓	N or ↓	↓ ↓

↑, increased; ↑ ↑, greatly increased; ↓, decreased; ↓ ↓, greatly decreased; N, normal; FEV₁, forced expiratory volume in 1 second; FVC, forced vital capacity; RV, residual volume; TLC, total lung capacity; D₍LCO₎, the diffusing capacity of carbon monoxide.

In restrictive disorders, lung volumes are reduced because of a loss of lung parenchyma and/or respiratory muscle weakness. Rate of air flow is generally normal or increased. As a result, the flow volume loop will be narrow and tall reflecting the smaller volume, but normal flow, rates (see Curve 7, Fig. 19-3).

The easy visualization of lung mechanics shown by flow volume curves makes them particularly valuable in monitoring the clinical status of patients with varying conditions. Since the loop reflects both volume and flow, the efficacy of various therapeutic modalities can be concretely evaluated.

Lung Disorders and Pulmonary Function Tests

The static and dynamic measurements allow separation of lung disorders into the two categories: restrictive and obstructive. *Restrictive disorders* can be intrinsic (within the lungs) or extrinsic (outside the lungs). An example of an intrinsic disorder is pulmonary fibrosis or interstitial lung disease, whereas kyphoscoliosis is an example of extrinsic disorder. Regardless of the cause, restrictive disorders limit lung expansion and therefore reflect diminished volumes and capacities. Restrictive disorders may have little or no effect on air flow in and out of the lungs; therefore timed studies may be normal[1,6,21] (see Table 19-8).

Obstructive disorders affect air flow; consequently, timed ventilatory values will be decreased in relationship to normal values. Volume and capacity measurements in individuals with obstructive disorders may be normal or increased[1] (see Table 19-8). As air flow out of the lung is impeded, air trapping occurs and lung overinflation results. This process tends to progress as the disease worsens (see the box "Pulmonary Function Patterns in Disease States," which presents the usual pattern of results from pulmonary function studies seen in restrictive and obstructive disorders). In obstructive disorders, the vital capacity reduction results from air trapping and increased residual lung volume which compromises the vital capacity.[1,38]

Because critically ill patients may not be able to actively cooperate in pulmonary function studies, complete batteries are infrequently performed and results must be considered in relation to the total picture. The constraints involved with mechanical ventilation or artificial airways preclude accurate pulmonary function studies. Nevertheless, some parameters that provide information about the static and dynamic properties of the lung can be gathered.

PULMONARY FUNCTION PATTERNS IN DISEASE STATES

RESTRICTIVE PATTERN IN PULMONARY FUNCTION TESTS

Decreased vital capacity <80% predicted
Normal FEV₁
Normal maximal voluntary ventilation
Decreased total lung capacity

OBSTRUCTIVE PATTERN IN PULMONARY FUNCTION TESTS

Normal or decreased vital capacity
Decreased FEV₁
Decreased maximal voluntary ventilation
Increased residual volume
Increased airway resistance

If the patient is being mechanically ventilated, the results of some of these pulmonary function tests may be readily available for interpretation. When using this data to assess a patient's status, evaluation of the trend is more important than evaluation of an isolated finding.

In patients on IMV/SIMV ventilation, parameters that can reflect changes in the patient's condition include increasing respiratory rate, decreasing tidal volume, and increased resistance as seen by changes in pressure needed to ventilate. This can reflect airway obstruction, the need for secretion clearance, and respiratory muscle fatigue.

Ventilation-Perfusion Scanning

Indications. The major goal of the lungs is to provide adequate gas exchange between people and their environment. Intimate contact between the alveolar-capillary membrane is provided by millions of alveoli with billions of capillaries draped around them in a sheetlike fashion. With ideal matching of ventilation (air) and perfusion (blood), each alveolar-capillary unit would receive an equal amount of air and an equal amount of blood simultaneously. This would result in a ventilation-perfusion (V/Q) ratio of 1.0.[7,14] The ideal, however, never exists even in normal lungs, because of physiological and anatomic shunting of blood. In normal subjects, mismatching of V/Q relationships is not detrimental, but illnesses or diseases that substantially alter V/Q ratios can result in serious impairment of gas exchange. Ventilation-perfusion scanning is indicated where a serious alteration of the normal V/Q relationship is suspected.

Ventilation-perfusion studies are most frequently ordered to diagnose pulmonary emboli. When pulmonary emboli are suspected, V/Q scanning approaches 92% accuracy in determining this diagnosis. When the perfusion portion alone is performed, the sensitivity of detecting pulmonary emboli is reduced to 75% for true positives and 64% for true negatives.[14] Comparing the perfusion scan with the results of a regular chest x-ray examination may improve these percentages somewhat. As results are less than 100% accurate in predicting pulmonary emboli, most V/Q scans will be interpreted by the nuclear radiologist in one of four ways[14]:

1. Normal. This interpretation can be used when the perfusion scan is normal and the probability of pulmonary embolism approaches zero.
2. Low probability. This interpretation can be used when there are small V/Q mismatches, when there are focal V/Q matches with no corresponding radiographic abnormalities, or when the perfusion defects are considerably smaller than the radiographic abnormalities.
3. Intermediate probability. This interpretation can be used when there are severe diffuse air flow obstructions, perfusion defects corresponding in size and position to radiographic abnormalities, and a single moderate V/Q mismatch without a corresponding radiographic abnormality.
4. High probability. This interpretation can be used when the perfusion defects are substantially larger than the radiographic abnormalities or when there is one or more large or two or more moderate V/Q mismatches with no corresponding radiographic abnormalities.

Frequently, in suspected pulmonary embolism, anticoagulation (unless contradicted) is initiated before the V/Q study. Once the study is completed, the results can be used to further guide therapy along the following rationale[14]:

1. If the perfusion scan is normal, anticoagulation can be stopped.
2. If the V/Q study shows a high probability for pulmonary embolism, anticoagulation should be continued.
3. If the V/Q study shows a low probability for pulmonary embolism, anticoagulation can be discontinued.
4. If no definite conclusions can be drawn from the V/Q study and if the probability for pulmonary embolism falls in the intermediate range, pulmonary angiography should be considered.[16]

Other uses of V/Q studies are included in the box "Diagnostic Uses of Ventilation-Perfusion Scanning."

Procedure. V/Q scans are one method to evaluate the relationship of air distribution and blood flow in lungs. The V/Q scan involves the use of radioisotopes, most commonly xenon or technetium, which are administered by inhalation and intravenous techniques.

Scintillation cameras record the gamma radiation images produced by the isotope as it is breathed or perfused into the lung. When an obstruction of the isotope's flow into an area of the lung occurs, the diminished radioactivity will be reflected in the camera image of that zone. Newer portable cameras have been developed that allow bedside V/Q studies to be performed on critically ill patients who are too unstable to be moved to the nuclear medicine departments.

Perfusion scans are usually obtained by injecting a radioactive nucleotide, often technetium (^{99m}Tc) intravenously. These particles are 50 to 1,000 times larger than other radioactive colloids and are trapped in the vascular bed as they pass through the lungs. A scintiograph camera measures the concentrations and reflects it on a cathode tube. Areas of the lung receiving more perfusion will show a more dense collection than will a less perfused lung tissue. Pulmonary emboli alter the normal perfusion pattern, hence the resulting concentration of radioactivity.

Ventilation scans may be achieved by having the patient inhale a radioactive gas. The distribution of gas in the lungs is then documented both by the concentration of radioactivity displayed on the scanner and by the time that it takes to clear the gas from the lungs. Ventilation disturbances occur in bronchitis, pneumonia, and obstructive processes.

DIAGNOSTIC USES OF VENTILATION-PERFUSION SCANNING

Perfusion abnormalities

Vasculitis
Arteriovenous fistula
Pulmonary hypertension
Tumors of hilum
Bullous emphysema
Diffuse interstitial fibrosis
Pulmonary infarction
Conditions creating regional lung hypoxia

Evaluation of function before lung resection surgery

Ventilation abnormalities

Chronic obstructive pulmonary disease
Bronchiectasis
Cystic fibrosis
Airway obstruction
Pneumonia
Pulmonary infarction
Severe pulmonary edema

REFERENCES

1. Altose M: The physiologic basis of pulmonary function testing, Clin Sump 31(2):3, 1979.
2. Aubier M and others: Effect of hypophosphatemia on diaphragmatic contractility in patients with acute respiratory failure, N Engl J Med 4:313, 1985.
3. Baum G and Wolinsky E: Textbook of pulmonary disease, ed 3, Boston, 1983, Little, Brown & Co, Inc.
4. Burton GG and Hodgkin JE: Respiratory care: guide to clinical practice, Philadelphia, 1984, JB Lippincott Co.
5. East T, Pace N, and Westenkow D: Lateral position with differential lung ventilation and unilateral PEEP following unilateral lung acid aspiration in the dog, Acta Anaesthesiol Scand 28:529, 1984.
6. Fishman AP: Pulmonary diseases disorders, ed 2, New York, 1988, McGraw-Hill Inc.
7. Freeman L and Johnson P: Clinical radionuclide imaging, vols 1 and 2, ed 3, Orlando, Fla, 1984, Grune & Stratton, Inc.
8. Fromm G: Using basic laboratory data to evaluate patients with acute respiratory failure, CCQ 1(4):43, 1979.
9. Gantz NM: Respiratory infections in the elderly, Geriatr Med Today 12:13, Dec 1967.
10. Glenn W and others: Thoracic and cardiovascular surgery, ed 4, Norwalk, Conn, 1983, Appleton-Century-Crofts.
11. Griffith D and Wallace R: Bacterial pneumonia in the adult: diagnosis and therapy, Hosp Med 24:188, Jan 1988.
12. Guenter C and Welch M: Pulmonary medicine, ed 2, Philadelphia, 1982, JB Lippincott Co.
13. Guyton A: Textbook of medical physiology, Philadelphia, 1981, WB Saunders Co.
14. Harbert J and DaRocha AF: Textbook of nuclear medicine, ed 2, Philadelphia, 1984, Lea & Febiger.
15. Hess D and Maxwell C: Which is the best index of oxygenation—$P(A-a)O_2$, PaO_2/PAO_2 or PaO_2/FiO_2, Respir Care 30(11): 961, 1985.
16. Iberti T and Gentili D: Pleural effusions, emergency decision (pamphlet) 2(8):, Sept 1986.
17. Kaye W: Invasive therapeutic techniques, Heart Lung 12(3):122, 1983.
18. Lane G and Pierce A: When persistence pays off, Nursing 82, 12:44, Jan 1982.
19. Light RW and others: Pleural effusions: the diagnostic separation of transudates and exudates, Ann Intern Med 77:506, 1972.
20. Luce JM, Tyler ML, and Pierson DJ: Intensive respiratory care, Philadelphia, 1984, WB Saunders Co.
21. Martin L: Pulmonary physiology in clinical practice: the essentials for patient care and evaluation, St Louis, 1987, The CV Mosby Co.
22. Maxwell C, Hess D, and Shefet D: Use of the arterial/alveolar oxygen tension ratio to predict the inspired oxygen concentration needed for a desired arterial oxygen tension, Respir Care 29(11):1135, 1984.
23. McDonnell K, Fahey P, and Segal M: Respiratory intensive care, New York, 1987, Little, Brown & Co.
24. Murray JF: The normal lung, Philadelphia, 1986, WB Saunders Co.
25. Murray JF and Nadel JA: Textbook of respiratory medicine, Philadelphia, 1988, WB Saunders Co.
26. Nadel JA: Pulmonary function testing, Basics of RD 1(4):5, 1975.
27. Peris LV and others: Clinical use of the arterial/alveolar oxygen tension ratio, Crit Care Med 11:(11), 888, 1983.
28. Prosperi A, Mitchell T, and Govi J: Thoracentesis for pleural effusions, Fam Prac Recertification 8(5):29, 1986.
29. Raju L and Kahn F: Pneumonia in the elderly: review, Geriatrics 43(10):51, 1988.
30. Sahn S: Pleural effusion: diagnosis and management, Hosp Med 24(8):77, 1988.
31. Shapiro BA: Respiratory critical care: state of the art—controversies—new horizons, vol 8, Chicago, 1988, Respiratory Care Seminars, Inc.
32. Shapiro BA, Harrison RA, and Walton JR: Clinical application of blood gases, Chicago, 1982, Yearbook Medical Publishers, Inc.
33. Shapiro BA, and others: Clinical application of respiratory care, Chicago, 1985, Yearbook Medical Publisehrs, Inc.
34. Sheldon RL: Flexible fiberoptic bronchoscopy, Prim Care 12(2):299, 1985.
35. Stradling P: Diagnostic bronchoscopy: an introduction, ed 3, New York, 1976, Churchill Livingstone, Inc.
36. Washington JA: Maximizing diagnostic yield from sputum examination, J Resp Dis 7:81, 1981.
37. Wegmann JA and Forshee T: Malignant pleural effusions: pertinent issues, Heart Lung 12(5):533, 1983.
38. Williams D and Cugell D: Pulmonary function tests: indications and interpretation, Hosp Med 24(5):23, 1988.
39. Wu, WH and Huang S: Tracheal intubation, Consultant 26:34, 1986.

CHAPTER

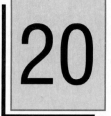

20

Pulmonary Disorders

CHAPTER OBJECTIVES

- Differentiate between hypoxemia and tissue hypoxia according to cause, symptoms, and treatment.
- Discuss important aspects of nursing care for the patient with a restrictive pulmonary disorder.
- Discuss important aspects of the nursing care that will prevent and/or treat atelectasis.
- Identify and describe the two major problems faced by patients with obstructive pulmonary disorders.
- Briefly describe important aspects of the care of patients with pneumonia, aspiration lung disorder, respiratory failure, and adult respiratory distress syndrome.

HYPOXEMIA

Hypoxemia is a word used to define a lower than normal amount of oxygen dissolved in plasma (see the box at right.) Thus, when the PaO_2 is less than predicted for the patient's age, hypoxemia is diagnosed. The etiological categories of hypoxemia to be discussed are listed in Table 20-1 and include alveolar hypoventilation, pulmonary shunting, and ventilation-perfusion (V/Q) inequalities. Most authorities now agree that diffusion impairment is not an etiological category of hypoxemia. Conditions once listed as causes of the hypoxemia related to diffusion impairment have been shown to mediate hypoxemia by one of the other three routes. Diffusion impairment is much more likely to result in hypoxemia during exercise or at high altitude, particularly in patients with chronic pulmonary disease.[67] Exercise-induced desaturation of hemoglobin and hypoxemia can occur because of disease that either increases the diffusion pathway across the alveolar-capillary membrane (adult respiratory distress syndrome) or because of a decrease in the volume of the pulmonary-capillary bed (emphysema).

Cause

Alveolar hypoventilation. Alveolar hypoventilation occurs when the amount of oxygen being brought into the

---

RELATED DEFINITIONS
Hypoxemia
A PaO_2 less than predicted for the patient's age.
Arterial hypoxia
A decreased amount of oxygen in the plasma; the same as hypoxemia; this term may have been responsible for the incorrect assumption that hypoxemia and hypoxia are one and the same.
Tissue hypoxia
A lower than normal amount of oxygen delivered to the tissues.

Table 20-1 Causes of hypoxemia

Etiological category	Medical disorder
Alveolar hypoventilation	CNS depression, disease of the medulla and spinal cord, Guillain-Barré syndrome, myasthenia gravis, muscular dystrophy, restriction to chest wall expansion, obesity
Shunt	Pulmonary edema, pneumonia, adult respiratory distress syndrome, atelectasis
V/Q inequality	Asthma, chronic bronchitis, chronic obstructive pulmonary disease, pneumonia, atelectasis

Table 20-2 Causes of alveolar hypoventilation

Disorder	Cause
Depressed respiratory center activity	Drugs, neurological disease
Reduced chest expansion	Pain, surgical incision, fatigue, chest wall deformity, poor patient positioning, or failure to frequently reposition patient
Restriction to lung expansion	Pulmonary fibrosis, pneumothorax, pleural effusion

---

Nursing Diagnosis and Management
Hypoxemia

- Impaired Gas Exchange related to alveolar hypoventilation secondary to (specify), p. 488
- Impaired Gas Exchange related to ventilation-perfusion inequality secondary to (specify), p. 487

---

alveoli is insufficient to meet metabolic needs. The hypoxemia caused by alveolar hypoventilation is often associated with an elevated $PaCO_2$[107] and commonly results from disorders outside the lungs. Table 20-2 is a review of some of these disorders. This type of hypoxemia is usually corrected by administration of supplemental oxygen and, in some cases, depending on the cause, assistance with ventilation.

Shunt. Shunt occurs when blood reaches the arterial system without passing through ventilated regions of the lungs. Shunts can occur as a result of congenital heart defects or pulmonary arteriovenous fistulas. A shunt can also occur because a portion of a lung is not ventilated as the result of either alveolar collapse (example, atelectasis), alveolar consolidation (example, pneumonia), or excessive mucus accumulation (example, chronic bronchitis).

When a patient with a shunt is given 100% oxygen to breathe, the PaO_2 will fail to rise to the level seen in normal subjects or to the expected PaO_2. Indeed, with pure shunt and no accompanying ventilation-perfusion inequality, the PaO_2 will not rise at all upon the administration of oxygen. This happens because when a shunt occurs there is no ventilation to the affected area of the lung and no inspired air reaches that region; therefore no amount of supplemental oxygen will reach the affected region. Only shunts behave in this way. The hypoxemia mediated by alveolar hypoventilation and ventilation-perfusion inequality will show some or complete correction with administration of 100% oxygen.[108]

The shunt can be calculated with the resulting figure showing the percentage of total blood flow that is not exposed to ventilated alveoli. The calculation is:

$$\frac{Qs}{Qt} = \frac{Cco_2 - CaO_2}{Cco_2 - CvO_2}$$

Total blood flow is designated Qt; shunt flow is Qs. The oxygen content in the pulmonary capillary (c) is derived by assuming that the capillary PO_2 is equal to the alveolar PO_2. Normally, only 2% to 5% of the cardiac output should be made up of shunted blood. In severe cases of oxygen failure, as much as 40% of the cardiac output may be shunted.[63] In most cases, the higher the Qs/Qt, the more ominous is the pulmonary pathology.

Ventilation-perfusion inequalities. Ventilation-perfusion (V/Q) inequality occurs when ventilation and blood flow are mismatched in various regions of the lung. In the normal lung, there is always some ventilation-perfusion inequality, since not all alveoli are completely ventilated and completely perfused. The ventilation-perfusion inequality referred to in this discussion and in pulmonary pathology means that there is an *abnormal and excessive* amount of ventilation and perfusion inequality. While with shunt blood passes through alveoli that are *unventilated,* in many causes of V/Q inequality, blood passes through alveoli that are *underventilated.* In other words, although some air passes into these alveoli, it is not the normal amount. Because of this, supplemental oxygen is usually helpful in correcting the hypoxemia resulting from V/Q inequality. V/Q inequality is the most common cause of hypoxemia and is responsible for most, if not all, of the hypoxemia of chronic obstructive pulmonary disease (COPD), interstitial lung disease, and pulmonary embolism.[108]

Symptoms

Until hypoxemia proceeds to tissue hypoxia (in most cases a PaO_2 of <50 mm Hg), there are no symptoms other than the low PaO_2. Any clinician new to pulmonary care is advised to become familiar with the causes of hypoxemia in order to anticipate hypoxemia. Many times, the progression from hypoxemia to tissue hypoxia is rapid.

Treatment

Treatment of hypoxemia depends on its severity. Mild hypoxemia may not require oxygen therapy, whereas severe hypoxemia will always necessitate some period of oxygenation. Further, severe hypoxemia as a result of massive ventilation-perfusion inequality or pulmonary shunt may not respond to oxygen alone and may require mechanical ventilation with positive end expiratory pressure (PEEP). The box on p. 406 presents essential information for the evaluation of hypoxemia. In all cases of hypoxemia, the cause must be sought and treatment instituted against it, since hypoxemia is a *symptom* of a disorder, not a cause of a disorder.

TISSUE HYPOXIA

Tissue hypoxia denotes a lower than normal amount of oxygen being delivered to the tissue cells. (See the box on p. 404). Causes of tissue hypoxia include: (1) hypoxemia, (2) abnormal hemoglobin, (3) low cardiac output, (4) increased oxygen requirements, and (5) toxic substance preventing normal O_2 utilization.

EVALUATION OF HYPOXEMIA

DEFINING HYPOXEMIA

Patient under 60 years old breathing room air
Mild hypoxemia	PaO_2 < 80 mm Hg
Moderate hypoxemia	PaO_2 < 60 mm Hg
Severe hypoxemia	PaO_2 < 40 mm Hg

For each year patient over 60 years, subtract 1 mm Hg to determine lower limits of normal for patient's age

DETERMINING HYPOXEMIA

Look at the PaO_2 to answer the queston, "Does the PaO_2 show hypoxemia?" Less than predicted for age means hypoxemia

EVALUATING OXYGEN THERAPY TO CORRECT HYPOXEMIA

Corrected hypoxemia	PaO_2 ≥ predicted for patient's age
Uncorrected hypoxemia	PaO_2 < predicted for patient's age
Overcorrected hypoxemia	PaO_2 > 100 mm Hg

Modifed from Shapiro BA, Harrison RA, and Walton JR: Clinical application of blood gases, ed 4, Chicago, 1989, Year Book Medical Publishers.

Nursing Diagnosis and Management
Tissue hypoxia

- Potential Altered Peripheral Tissue Perfusion related to compromised arterial flow, p. 341

- Potential Altered Peripheral Tissue Perfusion risk factor: vasopressor therapy, p. 341

- Potential Altered Peripheral Tissue Perfusion risk factor: orthopedic injury or manipulation of an extremity, p. 341

- Potential Impaired Skin Integrity risk factor: altered circulation, p. 725

- Activity Intolerance related to decreased cardiac output and/or myocardial tissue perfusion alterations, p. 345

Causes

Hypoxemia. A PaO_2 of less than 50 mm Hg can produce tissue hypoxia. Some patients with chronic pulmonary disease and persons who reside at high altitudes maintain a PaO_2 as low as 55 mm Hg without tissue hypoxia because of compensatory mechanisms, such as increased cardiac output and polycythemia. In these cases, the elevated cardiac output and red blood cell count allow for a greater oxygen-carrying capacity of the blood. In most cases, however, severe acute hypoxemia will result in tissue hypoxia.

Abnormal hemoglobin. The effect that abnormal hemoglobin has on its oxygen-carrying capacity was discussed thoroughly in Chapter 17. It is recommended at this time that those sections (pp. 369 to 372) be reread. As a quick review, methemoglobin, carboxyhemoglobin, and deoxygenated hemoglobin each prevent normal oxygen delivery to the tissues that does not result in hypoxemia but may result in tissue hypoxia. It is the classic example of tissue hypoxia occurring without concomitant hypoxemia.

The occurrence of tissue hypoxia without hypoxemia can be a confusing issue to students of pulmonary care; however, it may be clarified if the student remembers that hypoxemia is defined as a lower than predicted amount of oxygen *dissolved in plasma, measured as the PaO_2*. Abnormal hemoglobins may not affect the amount of oxygen dissolved in plasma; thus the PaO_2 can be normal in the event of a great volume of abnormal hemoglobin. The patient will not be diagnosed as being hypoxemic but may very well be hypoxic at the tissue level because the hemoglobin level is either too low or will not properly carry oxygen.

Correction of tissue hypoxia related to abnormal hemoglobin must be directed at returning the hemoglobin to a normal structure at normal levels. Supplemental oxygen can be administered to raise the PaO_2 in hopes of providing some added oxygen to the tissues. Oxygen therapy is particularly helpful in correcting the hypoxia resulting from carboxyhemoglobin.

Low cardiac output. A low cardiac output can result in tissue hypoxia because of failure of the heart to perfuse enough blood through the systemic circulation to meet the body's metabolic needs. This can follow myocardial infarction(s), cardiac dysrhythmias, heart failure, hypovolemic shock, cardiogenic shock, and other acute and chronic diseases of the cardiovascular system. Interventions to correct tissue hypoxia resulting from low cardiac output should be directed toward that system, assuming oxygenation via the pulmonary system is normal.

Increased oxygen requirements. Increased oxygen requirements occur in obese persons, patients with fever, and particularly in burn patients. The change in oxygen requirements of the burn patient is covered in Chapter 43.

Toxic substance tissue hypoxia. This form of hypoxia is rare. An example potentially seen in critical care is the toxicity that occurs with cyanide poisoning. Cyanide prevents the use of oxygen by the cellular enzyme cytochrome oxidase. Dissolved oxygen (PaO_2) is unaffected; hence this is another example of tissue hypoxia occurring without hypoxemia. Patients with cyanide poisoning will not respond to oxygen therapy but must be given the antidote containing sodium nitrite, which combines with the cyanide, thus freeing cytochrome oxidase. Administration of sodium thiosulfate further degrades the cyanide. A byproduct of this antidote is methemoglobin, which can then be reduced by administration of methylene blue.[58]

Symptoms

Symptoms of tissue hypoxia are best organized into systems, as presented in Table 20-3. Tachycardia and tachypnea

Table 20-3   Symptoms of tissue hypoxia

System	Symptoms
Cardiovascular	Tachycardia, hypertension, dysrhythmias, polycythemia
Respiratory	Tachypnea, dyspnea, cyanosis, hypoxemia
Renal	Low urine output
Neurological	Headache, anxiety, agitation, confusion, weakness, double vision, impaired judgment, weakness, drowsiness, coma

are normal body compensatory mechanisms triggered to correct the hypoxia. Other symptoms such as dysrhythmias, confusion, double vision, and drowsiness are manifestations of hypoxia of specific body cells.

Treatment

The specific treatment of each cause of hypoxia was discussed in the previous sections. In general, tissue hypoxia is treated by identifying and treating the cause, such as abnormal hemoglobin, hypoxemia, or low cardiac output. Regardless of the cause, the tissue oxygen delivery must be brought back to normal by the administration of supplemental oxygen and, when the patient is not effectively ventilating, by mechanical ventilation. If the presence of mucus is suspected, it must be cleared via effective cough, suctioning, intermittent positive pressure breathing, chest physiotherapy, or, as a last resort, bronchoscopy.

OBSTRUCTIVE AND RESTRICTIVE LUNG DISORDERS

Pulmonary diseases are often categorized by the manner in which they alter a patient's breathing pattern. Two patterns predominate: diseases that result in obstruction of ventilation and those that result in restriction of ventilation. The following discussion will explain how these disorders affect the lower airways, resulting in the diseases often seen in critical care.

Obstruction of Ventilation

Obstruction of ventilation means that airflow during exhalation, particularly during forced exhalation, is abnormally slow. This is usually a result of airway narrowing and/or airway collapse. Some of the diseases that are associated with this pattern of ventilation and are often seen in the critical care unit include asthma, chronic bronchitis, emphysema, and chronic obstructive pulmonary disease (COPD). Cystic fibrosis and bronchiectasis are also obstructive diseases but are not commonly seen in adult critical care.

For the most part, diseases that have an obstructive component are chronic in nature, such as bronchial asthma, chronic bronchitis, bronchiectasis, and emphysema. Acute bronchitis is an exception.

Airway narrowing or airway collapse can result from several factors. One factor is mucus within the airways, which, if it is in a large volume such as occurs in chronic bronchitis or bronchiectasis and is not expectorated, will result in obstruction to normal airflow.

Another factor involved in airway narrowing is edema of the lung tissue surrounding the bronchioles, which can compress these airways. This can occur in left-sided heart failure and pulmonary edema.

Finally, when the obstruction is caused by airway collapse, it is most often associated with emphysema, because this disease process weakens the respiratory bronchioles so that they remain open during inhalation but collapse as a result of the forces produced during exhalation.

Obstruction of ventilation is diagnosed when pulmonary function tests such as the forced vital capacity (FVC) and the forced expiratory volume measured over one second (FEV_1) show excessively prolonged exhalation.

Two main problems associated with airway obstruction are: difficulty breathing and excessive mucus production with or without cough. These are problems related to the pathophysiological process of obstructive airway disease and are treated by medical interventions such as bronchodilators, expectorants, or mechanical ventilation. However, both difficulty breathing and excessive mucus production lead to other patient problems that need to be resolved and that, in many situations, are evaluated for and resolvable by nursing care.

Difficulty breathing. How does obstruction of ventilation affect a patient's breathing? This question can be answered if the reader will perform the short experiment outlined in the box on p. 408 (bottom).

Patients with chronic airway obstruction live with this breathing difficulty constantly, and it impairs not only their physical wellness but also their emotional and social wellness. They alter their lifestyles to fit their breathing patterns, often decreasing or stopping activities they enjoy but can no longer tolerate. While a chest infection may not present a serious problem to a healthy person, it can and often does mean hospitalization to someone with obstructive lung dysfunction.

Excessive mucus with or without cough. In addition to difficulty breathing as a result of airway narrowing, many patients with obstructive lung disease have chronic, excessive mucus production, which further complicates breathing and can lead to chronic cough. Cough is reported by patients with chronic bronchitis as their single most debilitating health problem.[108]

Regarding mucus production, two important issues should be identified. The first is that some obstructive dysfunctions are *not* accompanied by mucus production. Emphysema in its pure form, without accompanying bronchitis or an acute chest infection, is an obstructive disease that is not complicated by mucus production. Second, when a patient develops an acute chest infection superimposed on chronic obstructive lung disease, the amount of mucus normally produced will increase.

It is impossible to discuss mucus production without including cough. Patients with excessive production of mucus should be encouraged to cough, because it is a lack of an

Nursing Diagnosis and Management
Obstructive lung dysfunction

- Ineffective Airway Clearance related to excessive secretions, p. 475

- Ineffective Airway Clearance related to knowledge deficit of controlled cough and hydration techniques, p. 476

- Ineffective Breathing Pattern related to chronic airflow limitations, p. 481

- Impaired Gas Exchange related to ventilation-perfusion inequality secondary to chronic obstructive lung dysfunction, p. 487

- Impaired Gas Exchange related to alveolar hypoventilation secondary to (specify), p. 488

- Activity Intolerance related to knowledge deficit of energy-saving techniques, p. 344

- Altered Nutrition: Less Than Body Protein-Calorie Requirements related to lack of exogenous nutrients and increased metabolic demand, p. 713. (See also discussion of metabolic results from carbohydrate overfeeding, Chapter 10.)

- Potential for Infection risk factors: protein-calorie malnourishment, steroid therapy, pp. 346 and 720

- Sleep Pattern Disturbance related to fragmented sleep, p. 88

- Sensory-Perceptual Alterations related to sensory overload, sensory deprivation, sleep pattern disturbance, p. 601

- Potential Impaired Skin Integrity risk factors: reduced mobility, protein-calorie malnourishment, steroid therapy, p. 725

- Sexual Dysfunction related to activity intolerance secondary to chronic lung disease, p. 867

- Altered Health Maintenance related to lack of perceived threat to health, p. 67

- Noncompliance: Energy-Saving Techniques, Breathing Techniques (Diaphragmatic, Pursed Lip), Hydration, Avoidance of Environmental Pollutants (Smoking), Medication Regimen, Muscle Toning Exercises related to lack of resources, p. 68

- Body Image Disturbance related to actual change in body structure, function, and appearance, p. 833.

- Self-Esteem Disturbance related to feelings of guilt over physical deterioration, p. 835

- Altered Role Performance related to physical incapacity to resume usual or valued role, p. 835

- Powerlessness related to health care environment or illness-related regimen, p. 837

- Hopelessness related to perceptions of deteriorating physical condition, p. 839

- Anxiety related to threat to biological, psychological, and/or social integrity, p. 852

SIMULATING DIFFICULTY BREATHING

Imagine yourself in the position of the patient with difficulty breathing caused by an obstructive airway disease. To help with this, place a straw in your mouth and breathe through it with your nose pinched shut. Make a tight seal so that you cannot draw in air around the straw. You have just simulated airway narrowing; hence obstructon of ventilation. You are probably noticing that breathing is more difficult through the straw. Perhaps you are breathing much harder than normal because the work of drawing air in and pushing it through the small lumen of the straw is much more difficult than it is to draw it through your mouth and nose. The work of breathing has increased; it can be tiring. Wouldn't it be nice to have a straw with a bigger lumen? It would make breathing easier and would be like taking a bronchodilator.

effective cough combined with excessive mucus production that results in ventilatory and respiratory failure. Therefore the teaching and assessment of effective cough are imperative, since the only other means to remove mucus is by nasopharyngeal suctioning or bronchoscopy. Chapter 22 contains information on effective coughing and the nursing care plans "Ineffective Airway Clearance related to excessive secretions" and "Ineffective Airway Clearance related to knowledge deficit of controlled cough and hydration techniques," in which many nursing interventions are listed that are extremely effective in assisting with cough.

Restriction of Ventilation

Restriction of ventilation means that the expansion of the lung is limited (restricted). To the patient, it means that he or she is unable to take a full, deep breath. This abnormal pattern of ventilation can be either acute or chronic and is caused by pathological conditions that fit into one of four groups: (1) lung parenchymal dysfunctions, (2) pleural membrane dysfunctions, (3) chest wall dysfunctions, and (4) neuromuscular impairment. Table 20-4 lists causes that

Table 20-4 Restrictive lung dysfunction

Group classification	Diseases
Lung parenchymal dysfunction	Sarcoidosis, atelectasis, diffuse interstitial fibrosis
Pleural membrane dysfunction	Pneumothorax, pleural effusion, pleuritis
Chest wall dysfunctions	Kyphoscoliosis, rib fractures/trauma, tight chest strapping, chest or upper abdominal incision, abdominal distention obesity
Neuromuscular disorders	Polio, Guillain-Barré syndrome, muscular dystrophy, myasthenia gravis, amotrophic lateral sclerosis

fall into each of the four groups of restrictive dysfunction. It should be noted that a number of the acute pathological conditions such as atelectasis, pneumothorax, and pleural effusion often occur in patients who do not have primary pulmonary disease.

Even though the causes in Table 20-4 have differences such as pathophysiology and chronicity, they each have one commonality. Each restricts lung expansion resulting in the predictable ventilatory pattern of restrictive lung dysfunction—that of a smaller, fixed tidal volume (Vt) associated with a more rapid ventilatory rate as a compensatory mechanism to maintain minute ventilation ($\dot{V}E$). Persons with restrictive pulmonary disease, whether acute or chronic, will demonstrate this pattern of breathing regardless of the disease responsible for pulmonary restriction. The severity of the disease plus the patient's relative health will both affect the degree to which the restriction to ventilation is manifested.

What are the consequences of this altered ventilatory pattern? One consequence may be activity limitations. The patient with restrictive disease cannot effectively increase tidal volume during stress, such as when moving about in bed, ambulating, or coughing. As the patient's metabolic rate increases in these situations a greater minute ventilation becomes necessary. With a relatively fixed tidal volume, minute ventilation can increase only through an increased ventilatory rate. However, the patient with a restrictive ventilatory pattern may already be breathing more rapidly than most persons—thus a further increase in ventilatory rate can be difficult, if not exhausting. Any exertion on the part of the patient requires a precise nursing assessment, evaluating the patient's ability to tolerate the exertion.

Another consequence of restrictive disease is an increase in the work of breathing. This occurs because many of the diseases that result in the restrictive breathing pattern also reduce lung compliance and impede lung inflation. Some of these diseases include diffuse interstitial lung fibrosis, atelectasis, pleural effusion, sarcoidosis, and pneumothorax. The increased work of breathing and the altered ventilatory pattern (low Vt–high rate) can seriously interfere

with recovery of the critically ill patient.

Nursing care. The most important consideration when caring for a patient with a restrictive pulmonary dysfunction is evaluation of the activity level the patient can tolerate. Nursing care should be planned so that the patient's activity level does not put excessive stress on his or her breathing pattern. Assessment of a tolerable activity level is very individual. One patient may become exhausted after turning in bed or having had a portable chest x-ray taken, whereas another patient may easily tolerate sitting at the bedside. When the resting ventilatory rate is significantly elevated, for example, as high as 28 per minute or more, the patient can be so exhausted maintaining this rate that further activity is not possible. At other times, however, with other patients, a rate of 28 per minute may be tolerable even if the activity level is increased. In any situation in which there is an elevated ventilatory rate, the assessment of a patient's tolerance of activity must be made, and generous rest periods should be spaced between activities.

It is most important that critical care nurses understand that restrictive dysfunctions do not necessarily need to involve the pulmonary system and that they are, many times, acute rather than chronic. A review of Table 20-4 reveals that upper abdominal surgery, abdominal distention, tight abdominal strapping, and obesity can alter lung inflation without direct involvement of the pulmonary system. These conditions impede diaphragmatic descent and intercostal muscle action, impairing both inhalation and exhalation. Pulmonary conditions that might not be considered serious, such as kyphoscoliosis and rib fractures, can actually present a severe pulmonary restriction when coupled with other problems for which the patient may have been admitted to the critical care unit.

Impaired inhalation, in particular, is a serious problem because it is a risk factor for development of atelectasis. Abdominal distention and tight strapping of the abdomen, most often seen by the use of an abdominal binder, hinder diaphragmatic descent and the normal outward abdominal movement occurring during inhalation; hence, patients tend toward a shallow, monotonous breathing pattern. This situation can be made worse if the abdominal binder works its way to the upper abdomen or lower chest, as sometimes is the case with bedridden patients. Because the potential pulmonary problems (atelectasis, pneumonia) outweigh the need for the binder, many surgeons no longer order them. However, in those situations in which one is used, it must be repositioned whenever it is found to have slipped up toward the chest or rib cage, and nursing care should include the interventions listed in the next section that can assist in preventing atelectasis.

Kyphoscoliosis can impair intercostal rib action, thus chest and lung expansion. This chest deformity compresses the underlying lung tissue so that it may not be ventilated well enough to contribute to gas exchange. When a patient with kyphoscoliosis is admitted to the critical care unit, the chest deformity itself can be a serious enough ventilatory limitation to put him at risk for development of atelectasis or pneumonia, particularly because both bed rest and acute critical illness will put additional stress or limitation on the ventilatory pattern. Vigilance is necessary in the assessment

---

Nursing Diagnosis and Management
Restrictive lung dysfunction

- Ineffective Breathing Pattern related to modifiable chest wall restrictions secondary to pneumothorax or pleural effusion, p. 481

- Ineffective Breathing Pattern related to unmodifiable chest wall restrictions secondary to kyphoscoliosis or obesity, p. 484

- Activity Intolerance related to knowledge deficit of energy-saving techniques, p. 344

- Body Image Disturbance related to actual change in body structure, function, and appearance, p. 833

- Powerlessness related to physical deterioration despite compliance, p. 838

- Sexual Dysfunction related to activity intolerance secondary to chronic lung disease, p. 867

---

of breath sounds, ventilatory rate, blood gases, and changes in activity tolerance, as well as in the application of the nursing interventions that prevent atelectasis.

Rib fractures can present the same risk as kyphoscoliosis. In this case however, pain medication may be ordered and should be provided at a level that will allow full lung inhalation without the dosage being so high as to unnecessarily prolong sleep or naps when ventilations decrease in rate and depth.

Probably the most frequently seen restrictive dysfunction resulting from hospitalization is atelectasis. Because of this and because it is so responsive to nursing interventions, it will be discussed next, under its own heading. Restrictive dysfunctions that are not frequently seen in critical care, such as those related to neuromuscular disorders and some that fall under lung parenchymal dysfunction (sarcoidosis, DIF), will not be discussed in this text. The reader is referred to a medical-surgical nursing text or a pulmonary text for these discussions. Further though, the reader is reminded that *any* disease or dysfunction that presents a restriction to ventilation should be treated with the previous nursing care section in mind.

ATELECTASIS
Description

Pulmonary atelectasis is collapse of lung tissue. This should not be confused with pneumothorax. While there is alveolar collapse in both conditions, the cause of the collapse is very different. Atelectasis occurs because alveoli become underinflated or uninflated. Pneumothorax occurs because air enters the pleural space. In most cases, pneumothorax is not preventable. Atelectasis, however, in most cases is preventable by appropriate nursing interventions, as will be elucidated in the following discussion.

Many different terms have been used to describe atelectasis, and because of this some confusion has resulted. Atelectasis has been described according to its mechanism of occurrence, clinical setting, duration, and radiological appearance. Table 20-5 lists some of these descriptions. Regardless of the number of terms or methods one can find in the literature that have been used to describe atelectasis, they each refer to the one entity—collapse of alveoli.

Cause and Pathophysiology

Atelectasis can be the result of a variety of abnormalities including: localized airway obstruction, a ventilatory pattern of shallow monotonous breathing, patient positioning that impairs adequate lung expansion, a change in the distending forces within the lung, negative airway pressure, and a deficiency of surfactant.

Localized airway obstruction. Local airway obstruction has long been considered a pathogenesis of atelectasis, with the offending agent believed to be an abnormal accumulation of mucus in the airways. Atelectasis then develops because the mucus completely or partially blocks the entry of fresh

Table 20-5 Various means of classifying atelectasis

Means	Classification
Etiology	Absorption
	Adhesive
	Compressive
	Congestive
	Contraction
	Functional
	Obstructive
	Reinflation
Radiological appearance	Massive (whole lung)
	Multilobar
	Lobar
	Segmental
	Subsegmental
	Discoid (platelike, linear, Fleischner's lines)
	Micro (invisible on radiograph)
	Miliary
	Round (rounded peripheral lung mass)
	Presence/absence of air bronchogram sign
	Hilar
Duration	Acute
	Chronic
	Migratory
	Recurrent
	Refractory
Clinical setting	Postoperative
	Postanesthetic
	Postextubation

Modified from Johnson NT and Pierson DJ: Respir Care 31(11):1108, 1986.

air into the distal areas. Lack of new ventilation to these areas promotes the absorption of what air is available until collapse results. This is sometimes termed, absorption atelectasis, which is further discussed in the box on p. 413. The development of atelectasis through this process is somewhat attenuated by the Pores of Kohn and the Canals of Lambert that can provide collateral air circulation to blocked airways. However, the mucus accumulation can be diffuse enough to block even these collateral pathways. Diseases associated with the development of atelectasis through this means are those notable for producing mucus, such as cystic fibrosis, chronic bronchitis, COPD, and bronchectasis. Further, any acute pulmonary disease, such as a pneumonia, superimposed on these chronic diseases further increases mucus and heightens the risk for development of atelectasis.

Shallow, monotonous breathing pattern. A shallow, monotonous breathing pattern has also long been considered a cause of atelectasis. Changes in ventilation that result from this breathing pattern include decreased lung volume, decreased compliance ("stiff" lungs), and pulmonary shunting.[9] The breathing pattern is found most commonly in patients who have had upper abdominal surgery, but it occurs to some extent following all surgeries and appears to result because the recumbent position in which most patients are placed during surgery reduces lung inflation. The functional residual capacity (FRC) declines as much as 30% with a position change from upright to supine, thus the lung is less well inflated when the patient is placed in the supine position.[9] Position is not the only surgical factor that can increase the risk for atelectasis caused by shallow, monotonous breathing; general anesthesia is known to alter normal lung mechanics and promote development of atelectasis. General anesthesia reduces lung and chest wall compliance[59] and impairs normal diaphragmatic action to the extent that FRC, and therefore lung inflation, is reduced.[27] Recently, it has been reported that general anesthesia alone, regardless of the surgery, can result in 24 hours of impaired diaphragmatic activity.[103] However, the likelihood of pulmonary complications resulting from anesthesia and surgery is more a function of the type and duration of the surgery[59] and of the postoperative care.

Surgery of the upper abdomen and thorax heightens the risk of atelectasis because total lung capacity, FRC, and vital capacity can be decreased for as long as 5 to 7 days.[96] The incidence of clinically important atelectasis increases as the incision approaches the diaphragm.[3]

The potential for the development of atelectasis after surgery is compounded by the tendency of patients to breathe lower tidal volumes at higher respiratory rates because this is the easiest, most pain-free pattern. Additionally, both pain and the analgesics used for pain relief disrupt the normal sighing pattern thought to open underventilated alveoli and enhance the spread of surfactant.

The shallow, monotonous breathing pattern is also found in patients who have not had surgery but whose illnesses require bed rest or prevent normal lung expansion such as will occur with chest or abdominal wall trauma. Additionally, any trauma or disease that might interfere with the normal functioning of the respiratory control centers of the central nervous system should be viewed as presenting a risk for the development of atelectasis.

Improper patient positioning. To the extent that position impairs normal lung inflation, atelectasis can develop as a result of improper patient positioning. In particular, any position that interferes with diaphragmatic descent or chest wall expansion can restrict lung inflation to the degree that atelectasis becomes a risk. Because of this, clinical assessment of the pulmonary system must include the evaluation of the effectiveness of ventilation in patients who cannot readily change position or who are reluctant to change position as a result of pain or decreased movement capability. Lung inflation is best achieved with the chest at least semi-upright, such as in semi-Fowler's position with the thorax elevated from waist level and in an even right to left position.

Decreased distending forces. The lung remains inflated as a result of the normal distending pressures that exist because of the opposing forces exerted by the natural recoil of the lung and by negative intrapleural pressure. (See Chapter 17 for a review of intrapleural pressure.) When a pulmonary dysfunction occurs that interferes with the action of these two forces, normal lung inflation is interrupted, and the risk of developing atelectasis is increased. The loss of the normal inflation forces alone does not necessarily result in atelectasis. However, the patient is put in a position of increased risk. The clinician should be aware of the disorders that alter normal lung inflation forces so that interventions can be initiated to prevent the development of atelectasis when appropriate. These disorders include pneumothorax, pleural effusion, chest wall/rib disorders, impairment of normal diaphragmatic functioning, and bullae formation resulting from emphysema.

Assessment

Symptoms resulting from atelectasis develop in proportion to the underlying respiratory impairment, the extent of the atelectasis, and the abruptness of onset. Atelectasis that develops slowly in a segment or lobe of an otherwise well-compensated patient generally causes few symptoms.[62] However, a patient who develops atelectasis and who may have an ongoing acute or chronic disease may exhibit severe symptoms.

Physical signs of atelectasis vary depending on how large an area is affected and on the patency of the airways that lead into the atelectatic area. Crackles, bronchial breath sounds, and egophony may be present if the airways are open, whereas decreased breath sounds will be found when the airways are occluded.[62] Crackles can be auscultated on the periphery of the atelectatic area, while decreased to absent breath sounds may be heard directly over the area. Large amounts of atelectatic lung tissue can produce a tracheal deviation toward the affected side, a dull percussion finding instead of the normal resonance, and decreased chest excursion on the affected side.

Arterial blood gas levels may or may not be altered by atelectasis. When they are altered, the PaO_2 usually shows hypoxemia. This results because blood passing through the atelectatic area does not come into contact with oxygen and proceeds to the left side of the heart in its venous concentration. There it mixes with normally oxygenated blood that has come from ventilated (nonatelectatic) lung areas. The resultant mixture shows a reduction in both PaO_2 and SaO_2 and is a consequence of what is known as right-to-left pulmonary shunting. Hypoxemia is relatively uncommon when all cases of atelectasis are considered, and it occurs most often in acute atelectasis when one or more lobes are involved.[49]

Fever may be present but has not been shown to be a reliable indicator of atelectasis.[49,80] Nevertheless, a fever occurring in conjunction with the risk factors outlined under the section describing cause and pathophysiology should be investigated as a sign of potential atelectasis. Fever that does accompany atelectasis is most likely related to lung infection distal to the obstructed airway.[49]

Atelectasis is most often first noticed on chest radiograph by abnormalities such as displacement of lobar fissures[62] (which occurs as a result of loss of lung volume), opacity of an area, obliteration of known borders such as one of the cardiac borders,[49] or elevation of the diaphragm on the affected side. It remains one of the many dysfunctions in which the diagnosis is best confirmed by chest x-ray examination.

Prevention

Prevention is not a usual heading under the discussion of diseases/disorders found in most critical care texts; however, atelectasis is one of the few dysfunctions in the hospitalized patient that can be prevented so easily that this discussion seems vital and will thus be included here. Very simply, atelectasis can, in many instances, be prevented with delivery of inspiratory volumes that will adequately ventilate the lung on a regular basis, such as several times every hour. Adequate ventilation can be assumed if auscultation of the lung during ventilation reveals breath sounds throughout all lung fields (discounting any previous pathology), especially at the lung bases.

There are many methods that can be used to achieve adequate ventilation, including incentive spirometry, intermittent positive pressure breathing (IPPB), mechanical ventilation, and repeated coaching by a nurse or respiratory therapist. Regardless of the method used, adequate lung ventilation must result or the efforts will be ineffective. The principle on which all prevention and treatment of atelectasis is based is that of providing regular, adequate inflation of the lung.

At this point, the reader should be assisted to understand those interventions that have not been shown to be effective in preventing atelectasis, so that ineffective interventions can be avoided in practice. It is impossible for alveoli to inflate during exhalation; therefore forced coughing (in the absence of secretions), tracheal irritation that induces coughing, and blowing into devices have not been shown to be effective in preventing or treating atelectasis. According to Bartlett[9]: "While it may be common practice to encourage patients to cough, it is uncomfortable and has no rational basis." Unless a patient has mucus in the airways (evaluated on chest auscultation) or is spontaneously coughing, he or she should not be encouraged to do so regardless of the much taught postoperative nursing care routine of cough-turn–deep breathe (CTDB). The only benefit that can be attributed to expiratory maneuvers may be the inhalation that occurs before coughing or use of the exhaling device.[9]

Nursing Care to Help Prevent Atelectasis

Nursing interventions can be extremely instrumental in preventing atelectasis, and their focal points should be teaching the patient proper ventilatory techniques and confirming maximum lung ventilation.

Maximal deep inhalations held for approximately 3 seconds or longer (without the patient inadvertently initiating the Valsalva maneuver, prevented by keeping an open glottis) should be incorporated into the care plans for any patient at risk for developing atelectasis. Both the duration and the depth of inflation, which should be at least twice the tidal volume, are important in preventing as well as treating alveolar collapse.[62] The chest should be auscultated during inflation to ensure that all dependent parts of the lung are well ventilated and to help the patient understand the depth of breath necessary for optimum effect. In this way, when a nurse is not present for chest auscultation, the patient will know what depth yields adequate ventilation. Incentive spirometry is not necessary to prevent atelectasis, if the patient can be relied on to follow through with his or her own sustained maximal ventilations.

When an incentive spirometer is ordered, correct use is mandatory; this includes at least ten deep, effective breaths be taken per hour. Ten breaths has been recommended, because research has shown it to be the average number of deep breaths (sighs) taken per hour by normal, healthy persons.[62] An hourly regimen of deep breathing is recommended because studies have indicated that some alveoli remain open for only 1 hour after the onset of hypoventilation; thus hourly hyperventilation is mandatory.[89] Close supervision of patient compliance with the prescribed regimen is recommended, as is the auscultation for breath sounds during the patient's maximum inhalations.

Many patients are reluctant to use the incentive spirometer or perform deep breathing because of associated discomfort or pain. Care must be taken to assess the level of analgesic necessary to relieve pain yet allow maximal lung inflation without oversedation so that the breathing pattern reverts to one of shallow, monotonous ventilations.

Frequent repositioning (a minimum of every 2 hours while the patient is awake) is essential because it most often results in a change in ventilatory pattern to that of deeper, more frequent ventilations. Although patients in the critical care unit are not often ambulated, those in the step-down units are, and early ambulation is essential in restoring lung function, providing several points are kept in mind.

When sitting at the bedside or ambulating, patients must be encouraged to keep the thorax in straight alignment while they breathe deeply. This position best accommodates diaphragmatic descent and intercostal muscle action, thus the breathing benefits. Also, the sitting or standing position provides enhanced ventilation to areas of the lung that are dependent in the supine position, thus accommodating maximal inflation and, in some instances, gas exchange.[70]

Adequate fluid intake is essential, in particular if the nursing assessment of a patient reveals him or her to be at increased risk for mucus production such as those patients with previous mucus history and those with an underlying mucus-producing disease, such as chronic bronchitis, pneumonia, or bronchiectasis. Collaboration with the physician and/or a nutritionist may be necessary to establish a fluid intake that will allow mobilization of secretions without causing fluid volume overload. Many patients with mucus history maintain the fluid intake at one and one half or more quarts of decaffeinated beverage per day. For patients who are not on oral intake, 24-hour intake by other means must be given at a level that allows mobilization of secretions. Whenever tenacious mucus is suctioned or expectorated, inadequate fluid intake should be suspected. Additionally, those patients with an artificial airway require humidification to that airway so that pulmonary secretions remain mobile. Collaboration with a respiratory therapist may be necessary if insufficient humidification is suspected.

Patient teaching cannot be overlooked in the prevention of atelectasis. All of the above interventions require patient cooperation and thus should be incorporated into a patient teaching plan. Preoperative teaching is most effective and should include as many of the above nursing interventions as time will allow, including practice with an incentive spirometer if postoperative orders will include its use.

Treatment

Once atelectasis has been diagnosed, treatment should ensue with vigor as any amount of alveolar collapse increases the work of breathing by decreasing lung compliance. This means patients must work harder to achieve lung inflation, and, if they are too weak to do so alone, they will require assistance or the atelectasis will worsen. Medical interventions include use of incentive spirometry, IPPB, mechanical ventilation if respiratory failure occurs, chest physiotherapy (CPT), administration of bronchodilators and/or mucolytics, oxygen for hypoxemia, and antibiotics when pneumonia is suspected. Atelectasis is often associated with pneumonia because it reduces both blood and lymph flow in the atelectatic area, thus hindering two major defense systems for preventing infection.[89]

Use of incentive spirometry was discussed in the section on prevention of atelectasis. The same recommendations for use apply when it is prescribed as a treatment for atelectasis.

IPPB is used more often as a treatment for atelectasis than it is as a prevention. It must be used correctly to be effective. This means that during the inhalation period of IPPB, air flow should be auscultated throughout all lung fields to ascertain the adequacy of ventilation. One of the major limitations of IPPB use occurs because patients are not supervised during the treatment. Many patients, as a result of the discomfort associated with chest inflation, stop air flow out of the machine before full lung inflation is achieved, thus negating the effectiveness of the treatment. IPPB treatments require supervision by a nurse or therapist who can instruct the patient about the depth of breath necessary to achieve maximal effect. Mechanical ventilation is used when atelectasis is associated with ventilatory failure.

CPT, the percussion and clapping of the thorax, involves positioning the atelectatic lung areas for favorable drainage followed by low-frequency (clapping) or high-frequency (vibration) percussion against the chest wall to jar secretions loose.[49] CPT is often used in conjunction with bronchodilator and mucolytic therapy.

Hypoxemia associated with atelectasis requires oxygen

ABSORPTION ATELECTASIS

According to Shapiro[90]: "Absorption atelectasis is the most common type of acute lung collapse and is usually caused by retained secretions." Secretions that obstruct bronchi or bronchioles prevent air from entering the alveoli distal to the obstruction. This lack of fresh air with which to inflate the alveoli after each exhalation results in deflation of the alveoli and atelectasis. Collapse is not complete however, because alveoli will remain inflated with nitrogen from the atmosphere, since nitrogen does not diffuse into the pulmonary capillary.

Absorption atelectasis can also result from the administraton of an oxygen concentration that is both too high and administered over too long a period of time. Normally, alveoli are held open because they are filled by atmospheric gas largely composed of nitrogen that remains within the alveoli after all of the oxygen has diffused into the pulmonary capillary. When a concentration of oxygen above the normal atmospheric level of 21% is administered, some of the nitrogen is "washed out" or replaced by oxygen. The higher the concentration of oxygen, the greater the amount of nitrogen washed out. When nitrogen is replaced by oxygen, alveoli do not remain well inflated, since all of the oxygen diffuses into the pulmonary capillary leaving alveoli empty. Thus the higher the concentration of oxygen administered, the less well inflated will be the alveoli. This is referred to as "nitrogen wash out absorption atelectasis." Because of this pathology, it is not recommended that oxygen be administered at an FIo_2 above 40% to 50%.

---

therapy and vigorous means of lung inflation. However, the fraction of inspired oxygen concentration (FIO_2) chosen should be high enough only to return the patient's PaO_2 to within normal limits for his or her age, as excessive amounts of oxygen are unnecessary and can be detrimental to surfactant production (see the box above). Some authorities suggest that the FIO_2 be kept at a level that maintains the PaO_2 at 60 to 80 mm Hg, as that level will prevent tissue hypoxia at the lowest FIO_2.[69] Others feel the PaO_2 should be restored back to its nonhypoxemia level.

Nursing Care of a Patient with Atelectasis

Nursing care can and should encompass any of the interventions listed under the section on nursing care to help prevent atelectasis. Preventive interventions should also be used for treatment interventions as they achieve the same result—maximal lung inflation. However, once atelectasis has developed, more vigilance is needed on the part of patient, nurse, and respiratory therapist in performing the interventions. Because atelectasis, depending on its extent, can increase the work of breathing, significant encouragement may be necessary when the patient is performing max-

---

Nursing Diagnosis and Management
Atelectasis

- Ineffective Breathing Pattern related to abdominal or thoracic pain, p. 483

- Ineffective Breathing Pattern related to modifiable chest wall restrictions secondary to pneumothorax or pleural effusion, p. 481

- Ineffective Airway Clearance related to excessive secretions, p. 475

- Impaired Gas Exchange related to alveolar hypoventilation secondary to (specify), p. 488

- Impaired Gas Exchange related to ventilation-perfusion inequality secondary to (specify), p. 487

---

imal lung inflations. Also, the assessment of the length of time a patient is able to spend on lung inflation corresponding with the length of rest necessary to recover will assist in the development of a daily care plan that best accommodates patient care.

Once this dysfunction has been diagnosed, careful assessment of lung sounds, breathing pattern, presence of fever, and patient ability to withstand the current nursing and medical interventions is necessary to establish whether the atelectasis is being resolved or is progressing.

PNEUMONIA
Description

Once the leading cause of human death, pneumonia continues to be a major health problem. Despite antibiotics, it is still the most frequent cause of infectious mortality and remains the fifth leading cause of death in the United States.[23,33,111,38] Nosocomial pneumonias account for 15% of hospital-acquired infections, with the majority of cases occurring in critical care units or similar areas.[23,33,111] The morbidity and mortality associated with such cases is 20% to 50%.[23,33,111]

Cause

Pneumonia is caused when virulent organisms are able to multiply in the lower respiratory system. Host defenses are multiple and bacteria must overcome these defenses to colonize the lower respiratory tract. The protective mechanisms that maintain sterility below the glottis include aerodynamic energy, mucociliary action, antibody secretion, phagocytic activity, and the lymphatic response.[10,41]

Pneumonias experienced in the critical care unit population can be community acquired or nosocomial infections, that is, those acquired in the hospital. The most frequently seen community-acquired pneumonia is pneumococcal.[38,64]

Although pneumococcal pneumonia continues to be seen in patients, the spectrum of bacterial pneumonias encountered is changing. Pathogens such as *Legionella pneumophilia* and *Branhamella catarrhalis* have been identified as pneumonia agents in some populations. *Staphylococcus, Haemophilus influenzae,* and *Klebsiella* are less common community-acquired pneumonias but are severe in nature.

Nosocomial infections are generally gram-negative enteric bacteria. *Klebsiella, Enterobacter, Escherichia coli, Proteus, Pseudomonas,* and *Serratia* are those most frequently encountered. Often, institutions have their own resident flora that predominate in nosocomial infections. Table 20-6 outlines some pneumonias encountered by the practitioner in the critical care patient population.

Pathophysiology

Development of acute pneumonia implies (1) a defect in host defenses, (2) a particularly virulent organism, or (3) an overwhelming inoculation event. Bacterial invasion of the lower respiratory tract can occur by inhalation, aspiration, migration from adjacent sites, or, less commonly, hematogenous seeding.[19,111] The most common method appears to be that of microaspiration of bacteria colonized in the upper airway.[36]

The oropharynx has a stable population of resident flora that may be of an anaerobic or aerobic nature. When stress occurs, such as with illness, surgery, or viral infection, pathogenic organisms replace normal resident flora.[66] Prior antibiotic therapy affects the resident flora population, making replacement by pathological organisms more likely.[64] The pathogens are then poised for invasion into the sterile lower respiratory tract. It has been demonstrated that 80% to 90% of critical care patients have gram-negative bacteria present in the oropharynx, and the prevalence increases with intensity of medical care.[48] Disruption of the mechanical defenses of cough and ciliary motility leads to colonization of the lungs and subsequent infection. (See Table 20-7 for a summary of altered host defenses.)

Infection results in pulmonary inflammation with or without significant exudates. Ventilation-perfusion inequality and hypoxemia occur as lung consolidation progresses. Untreated pneumonia can result in respiratory failure and septicemia. Mortality increases with associated disease states, such as diabetes, malnutrition, immunosuppression or chronic obstructive lung disorders, and patient age.

Assessment and Diagnosis

Dyspnea is the primary symptom experienced in diffuse pneumonia. Coughing and wheezing with sputum production may be present. Often the patient complains of fever or chills, although this may be less frequent in the elderly and immunosuppressed population.[36] Pleuritic pain may be a prominent feature. Generally, the onset will be acute with the patient feeling quite unwell in a brief period of time. However, in the hospitalized patient the onset can also be insidious.

In critically ill patients, many of whom have multiple-system problems and various invasive monitoring devices in place, the cause of an infection that presents an indolent course can be easily obscured.

Table 20-6 Characteristics of common pneumonias

Parameter	*Pseudomonas aeruginosa*	Staphylococcal pneumonia	Streptococcal pneumonia	*Hemophilus influenzae*	Mycoplasmal pneumonia
Seasonal predominance	None—a nosocomial infection	None	Winter	Winter	None
Patient types	Critically ill patients and elderly debilitated patients	Chronically ill patients and children under 2 years	Middle-aged to elderly, young adults can be infected	Middle-aged and elderly	Adolescents and young adults (teens to 20 years), rarely in people over 40 years
Associated conditions	Associated with burns, chronic bronchitis and COPD, neutropenia, congestive heart failure, respiration inhalation equipment, aspiration lung disorder, cystic fibrosis, and tracheal intubation	Viral influenza, recent surgery, infected wounds, COPD, TB, lung cancer, intravenous drug users, recent hospitalization, nursing home residents	Viral influenza and epidemics, alcoholism, immune diseases, bone marrow depression, splenectomy, diabetes, AIDS	Associated with chronic bronchitis, alcoholism, viral infections, COPD, AIDS	Community or family epidemics over several months
Classic signs and symptoms	Fever, especially in morning, chills, severe dyspnea, copious purulent sputum	Sudden or insidious onset, sustained fever and pleuritic chest pain, productive cough, shaking chills, dyspnea, cyanosis, tachypnea, pleural effusion, rapid development of respiratory failure	Abrupt onset, fever, cough, chest pain, afternoon-evening temperature, diaphoresis, rusty sputum, chills, myalgias; consolidation with egophony, bronchophony, bronchial breathing; chest dull to percussion, crackles, wheezes auscultated	Cough, sputum production, fever, chills, dyspnea, pleuritic chest pain, increasing respiratory insufficiency	Gradual onset with sore throat, pounding headache, myalgias; dry persistent hacking cough, fatigue, low-grade fever, scant sputum/or none; crackles appear later in disease, dull to percussion, wheezes, pleural friction, rub; acute 80% cough, temperature $> 101°$, erythema multiforme, bullous myringitis
X-ray findings	Diffuse bronchopneumonia, typically bilateral, nodular infiltrates, small pleural effusions	Consolidation in segments or lobes; patchy bilateral infiltrates, pleural fluid common; when hematogenous route, large confluent, bilateral infiltrates seen	Dense homogenous shadows involving all of one or more lobes	Variable ranges from patchy infiltrates to dense consolidation effusion common	Patchy perihilar, lobar, or diffuse infiltrates; 50% infiltrates multilobar; significant effusion rare, if present, reconsider diagnosis

Modified from Johnson MA: Fam Pract Recert 8(8):49,1986.
PMNs, polymorphonuclear leukocytes.

Continued.

Table 20-6 Characteristics of common pneumonias—cont'd

Parameter	*Pseudomonas aeruginosa*	Staphylococcal pneumonia	Streptococcal pneumonia	*Hemophilus influenzae*	Mycoplasmal pneumonia
Sputum gram stain	PMNs gram-negative rods, appear as single, pairs, or chains	PMNs, round cocci in clusters	Gram-negative diplococci pneumococcal antigen present or in plasma/sputum; PMNs	PMNs, small, gram-negative coccobacilli	Sometimes PMNs, mononuclear cells, no organisms
Diagnostic tests	Sputum culture, blood culture	Sputum and blood cultures	Sputum and blood cultures	Sputum culture, blood culture	Cold agglutinin testing 1-4 weeks after infection serology, antibody-specific titer
Therapy	Gentamicin, tebramycin, amikacin	Oxacillin, penicillinase-resistant semisynthetic penicillin, cephalosporin, clindamycin, tobramycin, gentamycin as last resort	Penicillin, if resistant to erythromycin, vancomycin; if allergy to penicillin, then tetracyclines, lincomycin, cephalosporins, chloramphenical	Second-generation cephalosporins, then ampicillin, if sensitive; trimethoprimsulfamethoxazole; after hospital discharge, ampicillin or cefaclor, chloramphenical	Erythromycin, tetracycline
Preventive measures	Proper sterilization and use of disposable respiratory therapy devices, suction apparatus, proper hand washing		Polyvalent pneumococcal vaccine for high risk people	Vaccine for encapsulated hemophilus influenza type B; usual infection in critical care unit involves encapsulated forms	Erythromycin for high-risk contacts in family setting, tetracyclines

Table 20-7 Altered host defenses

Condition	Cause
Depressed epiglottal and cough reflex	Unconsciousness, neurological disease, endotracheal or tracheal tubes, anesthesia, aging
Decreased cilia activity	Smoke inhalation–smoking history, oxygen toxicity, hypoventilation, intubation, viral infections, aging, COPD
Increased secretion	COPD, viral infections, bronchiectasis, general anesthesia, endotracheal intubation, smoking
Atelectasis	Trauma, foreign body obstruction, tumor, splinting, shallow ventilations, general anesthesia
Decreased lymphatic flow	CHF, tumor
Fluid in alveoli	CHF, aspiration, trauma
Abnormal phagocytosis and humoral activity	Neutropenia, immunocompetent disorders such as AIDS, patients receiving chemotherapy
Impaired alveolar macrophages	Hypoxemia, metabolic acidosis, cigarette smoking history, hypoxia, alcohol use, viral infections, aging

CHF, congestive heart failure.

Examination reveals hyperpnea or tachypnea, possibly associated with crackles and wheezes over the area of involvement. Chest x-ray evaluation may show infiltrates, depending on the length of illness and absence of other lung problems. An elevated leukocyte count with a shift to the left is seen in bacterial pneumonias. A normal or decreased white blood cell count in the presence of pneumonia suggests an overwhelming infection and a poor prognosis. Sputum cultures and blood cultures should be obtained to completely assess the patient's condition. Sputum collection technique is important to the success of adequate specimen retrieval. Because of the difficulty involved with sputum collection and culture, the causative agent may not be identified. Gram stain is very useful, since the results are immediately available and can indicate the probable bacteria.

Invasive tests such as a thoracentesis for pleural fluids, transtracheal aspiration, bronchoscopy, and open biopsy are further diagnostic measures that can be used in cases in which attempts to identify the pathogen have been otherwise ineffective.

Treatment

Treatment of pneumonia should include specific antibiotic therapy, support of respiratory function, support of nutrition, treatment of associated medical problems and complications, and proper fluid and electrolyte management. Special attention should be aimed at preventing the spread of infection, along with prompt recognition and treatment.

Although bacteria-specific therapy is the goal, this may not always be possible because of difficulties in identifying

the organism and the seriousness of the patient's condition. The time involved obtaining bacterial specimens should be balanced against the need to begin some treatment based on patient condition. Empirical therapy has become a generally acceptable approach.[33,38,46,47]

In this approach, choice of antibiotic treatment is based on the most likely etiological organism while avoiding drug toxicity or super infection. If available, Gram stain results should be used to guide choices of antibiotics. Antibiotics should be chosen that offer broad coverage against gramnegative and gram-positive organisms. Factors such as atypical features, COPD with high risk of *Haemophilus* infection, and other exposure risks should be considered when selecting the antibiotic. Efforts to isolate the particular organism should continue. Failure of the patient to improve or further worsening indicates the need to reevaluate therapy. A persistent fever in a patient who otherwise seems to be improving may represent drug fever and should be considered if other sources of infection have been excluded. The antibiotic therapy used should be refined as data completion occurs. This helps reduce the unnecessary risks of toxicity or development of multiresistant bacteria. Care should always be given to antibiotic choice when renal, hepatic, or hematopoietic impairment exists.

Table 20-8 Comparative antibiotic costs, Cheshire Medical Center, 1988

Antibiotic	Typical daily adult dose	Cost to pharmacy per day of therapy
Gentamicin	300 mg	1.00
Amikacin	1000 mg	57.60
Streptomycin	1.0 g	1.78
Oral metronidazole	1.0 g	0.32
Oral vancomycin	2.0 g	48.00
Clindamycin	2.4 g	35.16
Metronidazole (IV)	1.5 g	3.18
Chloramphenicol	2.0 g	5.20
Cefotan	4.0 g	35.26
Ampicillin	6.0 g	4.20
Penicillin G	1.0 million U	0.51
	20.0 million U	3.84
Methicillin NA	6.0 g	11.00
Oxacillin	6.0 g	7.44
Rifampin	600 mg	2.40
Piperacillin	18 g	56.70
Cefazolin (Kefzol)	3.0 g	12.00
Cephalothin (Keflin)	6.0 g	8.28
Ceftriaxone (Rocephin)	2.0 g	47.40
Cefoperazone (Cefobid)	6.0 g	60.75
Vancomycin (IV)	2.0 g	52.10
Trimethoprim/sulfamethoxazole (Bactrim/Septra)	6 vials	15.18
Doxycycline	200 mg	1.20
Erythromycin	4.0 g	10.32

Costs are for antibiotics only and do not include costs of intravenous fluid, the intravenous line, and preparation.

Selection of the antibiotic should reflect clinical efficacy, microbiological activity, antibiotic penetration, metabolism, and side effects. With increasing awareness of the need to control cost of medical care, expense of an antibiotic can become a factor in selection (see Table 20-8). Recent literature has focused on the ability of antibiotics to penetrate the blood bronchus barrier as a criterion for successful treatment of pneumonia in some populations. Generally, this becomes a concern in people with chronically damaged or hypersecreting bronchial systems who may be significant in number in critical care settings. Some of the new cephalosporins show better penetration in research studies.[56]

Another common antibiotic group, aminoglycosides, are frequently used in gram-negative bacillary pneumonia. Because of the narrow therapeutic range and low penetration, addition of a beta-lactamase antibiotic is recommended. Aminoglycosides have been instilled directly into the respiratory tract by endotracheal or tracheal routes. No clear consensus on the usefulness of such an approach has been reached.[20] This technique has resulted in increased resistance of pathogens when used as a prophylactic therapy.[20] Passive immunity by administration of antibodies collected from immune species has been explored in gram-negative bacilli, but this methodology remains experimental.[64] Table 20-9 summarizes current antibiotic choices according to infecting organism.

Stopping antibiotic therapy is generally indicated when the patient has been afebrile for several days with a previously abnormal (elevated or depressed) white blood cell count close to or at normal levels. Reexamination of the sputum should demonstrate freedom from bacteria. X-ray infiltrates can persist for extended periods after the pneumonia has resolved and should not be considered a reason to continue drug therapy.[55,64]

Patients in critical care units, being sicker and with multiple problems, may require a longer course of antibiotic therapy. Gram-negative pneumonias, *Legionella*, and staphylococcal pneumonia may require treatment for up to 3 weeks.[64]

Despite medical progress, pneumonia remains a constant threat to the critical care patient population. Prevention is the best approach, and efforts to develop vaccines for use in the high-risk patient population continue. Some vaccines being developed include vaccines for *Staphylococcus aureus*, *Mycoplasma pneumoniae*, *Pseudomonas aeruginosa*, and *Branhamella catarrhalis*. Pneumococcal polysaccharide vaccine is available for the patient recovering from pneumococcal pneumonia.

Table 20-9 Antibiotic choices for pneumonias when infecting organism is known or highly suspected

Organism	First choice	Second choice
Streptococcus pneumoniae	Penicillin G, 2 million U, every 2-4 hr	Erythromycin, 1 g every 6 hr
Mycoplasma pneumoniae	Erythromycin, 1 g every 6 hr	Doxycycline 100 mg every 12 hr
Legionella sp.	Erythromycin, 1 g every 6 hr ± rifampin, 600 mg/day	Rifampin 600 mg/day
Staphylococcus aureus, methicillin sensitive	Oxacillin, 3 g every 6 hr	Vancomycin, 1 g every 12 hr
Staphylococcus aureus, methicillin resistant	Vancomycin, 1 g every 12 hr	Trimethoprim-sulfamethoxazole 4 mg/kg every 6 hr
Haemophilus influenzae	Ampicillin, 2 g every 6 hr	Trimethoprim-sulfamethoxazole 4 mg/kg every 6 hr
Klebsiella sp.	Cefazolin, 2 g every 8 hr plus gentamicin, 1.7 mg/kg every 8 hr	Ceftizoxime, 1 g every 8 hr plus amikacin 5 mg/kg every 8 hr
Pseudomonas aeruginosa	Ticarcillin, 3 g every 4 hr plus gentamicin, 1.7 mg/kg every 8 hr	Piperacillin, 3 g every 4 hr plus tobramycin 1.7 mg/kg every 8 hr
Branhamella catarrhalis	Trimethoprim-sulfamethoxazole, 4 mg/kg every 6 hr	Erythromycin, 1 g every 6 hr
Group B streptococcus	Penicillin G, 2 million U every 2-4 hr	Erythromycin, 1 g every 6 hr
Chlamydia psittaci (psittacosis)	Doxycycline, 100 mg every 12 hr	Chloramphenicol, 1 g every 6 hr
Francisetta tularensis (tularemia)	Gentamicin, 1.7 mg/kg every 8 hr	Doxycycline, 100 mg every 12 hr
Coriella burnetti (Q fever)	Doxycycline, 100 mg every 12 hr	Chloramphenicol, 1 g every 6 hr
Yersinia pestis (plague)	Streptomycin, 500 mg every 12 hr, IM only	Doxycycline, 100 mg every 12 hr
Bacillus anthracis (anthrax)	Penicillin G, 2 million U every 2-4 hr	Doxycycline, 100 mg every 12 hr
Bacteroides fragilis (aspiration)	Penicillin G, 2 million U every 2-4 hr	Metronidazole 15 mg/kg (1 dose), then 7.5 mg/kg every 6 hr

From McDonnell K, Fahey P, and Segal M: *Respiratory intensive care*, Boston, 1987, Little, Brown & Co.

Nursing Care

Nursing care of patients with pneumonia requires a multifaceted approach: (1) safe and timely administration of antibiotic therapy, (2) monitoring and support of the patient's ventilatory efforts, and (3) prevention of further contamination by other organisms from infected patients to other critically ill patients.

The nurse has a major role in assisting with antibiotic therapy, as planned and prescribed by the physician. Often, if not always, the nurse is responsible for collecting the sputum specimens on which therapy will be based. The nurse also monitors the patient's response to antibiotic therapy by continually evaluating the patient's status. Changes in vital signs, sputum production, and sputum characteristics will generally be noticed initially by the nurse through routine patient monitoring. In most instances the nurse manages the intravenous access by which the antibiotic is administered.

Throughout the course of the pneumonia, the critical care nurse monitors and supports the patient's ventilatory function. Lung sounds are assessed at least every 4 hours, along with other vital signs (temperature, pulse, respiratory rate, and blood pressure). Efforts to support airway clearance and adequate ventilation are directed by nursing. This will include various measures of pulmonary toilet, depending on the patient's individual condition and proper patient positioning to facilitate lung expansion. Recent research shows coached deep breathing with coughing to be more effective in raising sputum in acute pneumonias than does postural drainage and vibration techniques.[50] See Chapters 21 and 22 for a complete presentation of airway management and patient positioning.

Frequent changes of the patient's position should be implemented to maximize ventilation and perfusion in different areas of the lungs. When unilateral pneumonia exists, positioning the patient on the unaffected side (with the good lung down) can improve ventilation-perfusion matching.

Prevention should also be directed at eradicating pathogens from the environment and interrupting the spread of organisms from person to person. Significant progress has been made in removing contaminants from the patient environment through proper disinfection of respiratory equipment and increased use of disposable supplies. Other possible environmental sources of pathogens include suctioning equipment and indwelling lines. Proper aseptic care must be directed at the management of these invasive tools. Proper hand-washing technique is the single most important measure available to prevent spread of bacteria from person to person.[48]

ASPIRATION LUNG DISORDER
Description

Aspiration pneumonia, a special type of pneumonia that may be seen in critical care units, is a major cause of morbidity and mortality. Aspiration has been recorded in as many as 38% of critically ill, intubated patients receiving feeding through small-bore nasogastric tubes, despite maintenance of the integrity of cuffed tracheal tubes.[20,65] Many of the risk factors leading to aspiration are present in critical care patients (see the box below).

Cause

The presence of abnormal substances in the airways and alveoli as a result of aspiration is misleadingly called aspiration pneumonia. The title is misleading because the aspiration of toxic substances into the lung may or may not involve bacterial infection. Aspiration lung disorder would be a more meaningful title, because injury to the lung can

---

Nursing Diagnosis and Management
Pneumonia

▪ Impaired Gas Exchange related to ventilation-perfusion inequality secondary to alveolar infiltrates, p. 487
▪ Impaired Gas Exchange related to ventilation-perfusion inequality secondary to (specify), p. 487
▪ Impaired Gas Exchange related to alveolar hypoventilation secondary to (specify), p. 488
▪ Ineffective Airway Clearance related to excessive secretions, p. 475
▪ Acute Pain related to transmission and perception of noxious stimuli secondary to pneumonia, p. 594
▪ Altered Nutrition: Less Than Body Protein-Calorie Requirements related to lack of exogenous nutrients and increased metabolic demand, p. 713. (See also discussion of metabolic results from carbohydrate overfeeding, Chapter 10.)
▪ Powerlessness related to health care environment or illness-related regimen, p. 837
▪ Anxiety related to threat to biological, psychological, and/or social integrity, p. 852

RISK FACTORS ASSOCIATED WITH ASPIRATION

Impaired consciousness
Compromised glottal closure
Compromised cough reflex
Ileus or gastric dilation
Nasogastric feeding tubes (large or small bore)
Artificial airways
Disorders affecting pharyngeal and/or esophageal motility
Tracheoesophageal fistulas
General anesthesia
Cardiopulmonary resuscitation
Improper patient positioning during tube feeding
Esophageal strictures

Table 20-10 Clinical entities associated with aspiration lung disorder

Inoculum	Pulmonary sequelae	Clinical features	Therapy
Acid	Chemical pneumonitis, late bacterial infection possible	Acute dyspnea, tachypnea, tachycardia; hypoxemia, bronchospasm, fever; sputum: pink, frothy; x-ray film: infiltrates in one or both lower lobes	Correct hypoxemia, intravenous fluids, monitor blood gases, antibiotics for associated bacterial infections
Oropharyngeal bacteria	Bacterial infection, lung abscess, empyema	Usually insidious onset, cough, fever, purulent sputum, leukocytosis; x-ray film: infiltrate involving dependent pulmonary segment or lobe ± cavitation	Antibiotics
Inert fluids (water, blood, barium)	Mechanical obstruction, reflex airway closure	Acute dyspnea, cyanosis ± apnea, pulmonary edema, hypoxemia	Tracheal suction during or immediately following aspiration event, correct hypoxemia
Particulate matter, foreign bodies	Mechanical obstruction	Dependent on level of obstruction: range from acute apnea and rapid death to irritating chronic cough ± recurrent infections	Extraction of large particulate matter via bronchoscopy, antibiotics for infections

Modified from Baum G, and Wolinsky E, Textbook of pulmonary disease, ed. 3, Boston, 1983, Little Brown & Company.

result from chemical, mechanical, and/or bacterial characteristics of the aspirate. Each gives rise to a specific clinical entity (see Table 20-10).

Pathophysiology

Characteristics of the aspirated material are crucial to the ultimate effects on lung tissue. Generally, an aspirate with a low pH spreading throughout the lung fields may quickly result in adult respiratory distress syndrome. As seen in animal studies, the "critical pH" of less than 2.5 is thought to cause severe chemical lung injury.[20,41] The coupling of a low pH and virulent pathogens may quickly overwhelm normal defenses of the lung. Aspiration of material from the oropharynx carries resident flora to the sterile lower respiratory tract. Elderly and hospitalized patients show a prevalence of gram-negative bacteria in the oropharynx, which increases the likelihood of gram-negative pneumonias associated with aspiration.[12,20,31,41,94]

The outcome of an aspiration event depends on the amount and type of aspirate, the distribution of aspirate in the lungs, and the patient's overall condition and defense mechanisms. Recognition of the aspiration event also plays a role in outcome. Aspiration of significant amounts can be readily noticed with respiratory distress, dyspnea, wheezing, and coughing. However, aspiration of smaller amounts (silent aspiration) can occur without recognition, especially in patients with altered levels of consciousness.

Aspiration of gastric juices that have a pH of less than 2.5 results in a chemical burn to the lung. If significant amounts of acid are aspirated, extensive atelectasis can occur. Bronchospasm occurs later and is followed by epithelial injury and disruption of the alveolar membrane. Changes in the alveolar membrane result in fluids and cellular elements leaking into the interstitial space and to the alveoli. The fluid decreases surfactant production, which results in atelectasis. Hyaline membrane formation has been demonstrated in animal studies. These sequelae lead to decreased lung compliance ("stiff lung"), alveolar-arterial oxygen difference (A-aDo$_2$), hypoxemia, and loss of intravascular volume from the fluid shift.[24,64]

Aspiration of particulate matter may have an immediate life-threatening result if large particles mechanically block the major airways. In less dramatic situations, small particles cause small segmental atelectasis by occluding bronchioles. The presence of foreign matter causes an inflammatory response in the lung, though not the dramatic fluid shift seen in acid aspiration.

Bacterial inoculation by aspiration usually follows an indolent course. Bacteria invade the lung, resulting in a clinical picture that can range from patchy bronchopneumonia to empyema and purulent lung abscesses. Anaerobic organisms predominate in community aspirations, whereas gram-negative aerobic organisms are seen in the majority of aspirations occurring in hospitalized patients.[109]

Assessment and Diagnosis

When aspiration of a significant volume or repeated aspiration of smaller volumes occurs, the patient will develop increasing dyspnea, fever, tachypnea, and cyanosis.[20] If the cough reflex is intact, increased coughing occurs. Intubated patients may require more frequent suctioning, and aspirated material may be present in secretions. Auscultation of the lung fields demonstrates decreased breath sounds in the affected area with associated wheezes.

Arterial blood gases reflect hypoxemia and a widened A-a Do$_2$, while an increased FIo$_2$ is needed to maintain satisfactory oxygenation.[20] Intubation followed by mechanical ventilation may be required. The system pressures required to deliver the prescribed volume in ventilated patients will increase as compliance within the lungs decreases. If bacterial infection becomes established, the white blood cell count may become elevated. A normal or decreased white blood cell count in the setting of infection suggests overwhelming host invasion and a poor prognosis.

Chest x-ray changes appear 12 to 24 hours after the initial aspiration. The validity of the chest x-ray in diagnosing aspiration lung disorder is related to the prior status of the patient. Patients with underlying lung involvement, as commonly seen in critical care units, may already have significant pulmonary infiltrates present on chest x-ray evaluation, clouding the interpretation. In massive aspiration, diffuse bilateral infiltrates suggest pulmonary edema is present, whereas lesser aspirations show atelectasis in the early period.[20] Later chest films show large, fluffy infiltrates.

Because of the acute vertical descent of the right mainstem bronchus, the right lung is more often the site of involvement in aspirations. The lower right and left lobes and the right middle lobe are common sites of aspiration[20] involvement with occurrences being 60%, 42%, and 32%, respectively.[41] The patient position at the time of aspiration affects the distribution pattern of the aspirate in the lungs. Patients at risk for aspiration are best kept in a head-down position, or at least supine and lateral.

Since most aspiration events are unwitnessed, a high degree of suspicion coupled with an ability to recognize the at-risk patient is paramount to diagnosing aspiration lung disorder. Purposeful data collection is followed to delineate the presence or absence of aspiration lung disorder. Radiographic and bacteriological studies should be undertaken.

Recognizing aspiration lung disorder requires understanding of the clinical spectrum of events, recognition of the factors that predispose to aspiration, chest x-ray and laboratory data, and the identification of pathogens from the aspirated material or uncontaminated sputum specimens. Diagnosis of aspiration-acquired pneumonia is confirmed by the identification of bacterial organisms. Transtracheal or bronchoscopic sputum specimens are most reliable when appropriately collected, since they avoid contamination of the specimen by oropharyngeal contact (see Chapter 19).

Treatment

Management includes emergency treatment and follow-up treatment. When aspiration is witnessed, emergency treatment should be instituted to secure the airway and minimize pulmonary damage. The patient should be placed in slight (6 to 8 inches head-down) Trendelburg's position and turned to right lateral decubitus position to aid drainage and avoid involvement of other lung areas.[20,64] Oropharyngeal suctioning should immediately follow. Direct visualization by bronchoscopy is indicated when large particulate aspirate blocks airways. Bronchial and pulmonary lavage is not recommended, because studies have demonstrated that this practice disseminates aspirate in lungs and increases damage.[20,64]

Following airway clearance, attention should be given to hemodynamic support, arterial blood gas monitoring, and respiratory support. Hemodynamic changes result from fluid shifts occurring in massive aspirations causing noncardiogenic pulmonary edema. Transudation of large amounts of cellular and colloidal fluids causes a disarray of pulmonary defenses and cellular injury. Monitoring intravascular volume is essential, and judicious amounts of replacement fluids should be instituted to maintain adequate urinary output and vital signs.

Arterial blood gas analysis should be obtained immediately and sequentially throughout the patient course to direct oxygen therapy. Inability to correct hypoxemia, despite supplemental oxygen, is an indication that aggressive treatment is needed. Positive end expiratory pressure (PEEP) ventilation may help maintain acceptable oxygenation with lower concentrations of inspired oxygen. However, at the same time that PEEP provides for a lower FIO_2, it can also decrease cardiac output, thus lowering tissue oxygenation; therefore the lowest level of PEEP needed for satisfactory oxygenation should be used.[15]

Other medical intervention involves drug therapy. Bronchodilators may be useful in situations associated with bronchospasm. Benefits of steroidal drugs remain unclear; they are frequently used in aspiration, even though current studies do not support the use of steroids.[24,26,105,106] Osmotic agents such as albumin should not be utilized as the albumin extravasates into the lung, further decreasing gas exchange at the alveolus.[20,64,75] Antibiotics should be instituted according to positive Gram's stain or culture results. When anaerobic contamination is present, Levinson[56] noted a greater response to clindamycin than to penicillin. In hospital-acquired aspiration pneumonia, a broad-spectrum antibiotic such as a cephalosporin has been shown to improve patient outcome. When *Pseudomonas* is present, an aminoglycoside or betalactamase penicillin should be administered.[20]

Recent studies regarding the efficiency of administering prophylactic H^2 blockers to lessen gastric acidity in preoperative patients have been performed.[20] Results have shown that lessening of the acid level of gastric secretions minimizes lung injury when aspiration occurs.[13] Alteration of gastric pH in other at-risk patients may be warranted. The use of oral antacids has been efficacious in increasing the gastric pH of gastric secretions, but nonparticulate antacids such as sodium citrate appear to be preferred in high-risk patients, such as patients in the critical care unit. Metoclopramide hydrochloride, a dopamine antagonist, has been shown to decrease gastric volume and increase upper gastrointestinal motility and gastric sphincter tone.[64] It may therefore be advantageous when given preoperatively.

Nursing Care

During the course of caring for the critically ill patient, the nurse must implement measures for preventing aspiration lung disorder. If the aspiration event occurred before the patient's admission to the critical care unit, the nurse must direct interventions toward (1) maintaining the airway and supporting respiratory function, (2) early recognition and treatment of complications of aspiration lung disorder, and (3) preventing further aspiration events. Chapter 22 includes a detailed discussion of nursing approach to problems associated with airway clearance air and gas transport.

In at-risk patients, nursing interventions should be directed at preventing aspiration. Decisions regarding patient positioning should reflect consideration of the potential for aspiration. Unless contraindicated, the unconscious patient should be placed on the side in a slight Trendelburg's position to promote drainage and discourage aspiration. Place-

---

Nursing Diagnosis and Management
Aspiration lung disorder

- Impaired Gas Exchange related to ventilation-perfusion inequality secondary to aspiration, p. 487
- Potential for Aspiration risk factors: reduced level of consciousness, depressed cough and gag reflexes, presence of tracheostomy or endotracheal tube, gastrointestinal tube, enteral tube feedings, decreased gastrointestinal motility, impaired swallowing, facial/oral/neck surgery or trauma, situations hindering evaluation of upper body, p. 489
- Sensory-Perceptual Alterations related to sensory overload, sensory deprivation, sleep pattern disturbance, p. 601
- Anxiety related to threat to biological, psychological, and social integrity, p. 852

---

ment of nasogastric (NG) tubes for gastric decompression requires careful consideration, as NG tubes paradoxically increase the risk of aspiration and have been frequently shown to empty the stomach incompletely.[64] Patients receiving continuous or intermittent tube feeding should be maintained in at least a 30-degree head elevation. If a recumbent or head down position is necessary, feedings should be interrupted every 30 minutes to 1 hour before assuming a flat position. When head elevation is contraindicated, the right lateral decubitus position is preferred, because it aids passage of gastric contents through the pylorus.[65] Also, in this situation the choice of the type of feeding tube takes on added importance. Most sources recommend intestinal feedings via a small-bore weighted tube to reduce the risk of aspiration.[20,64]

Tube feeding into the stomach should be avoided in all unconscious patients or patients with an absent or compromised cough reflex. These patients should receive feeding into the intestine by means of a small-bore weighted tube, since these tubes are associated with a lower incidence of aspiration than the larger bore tubes. Frequent checking of tube location, as well as checking for gastric retention of the feeding, is necessary to prevent aspiration. The standard technique used to check retention may be difficult in small-bore, pliable catheters, because drawing back can collapse the lumen. Therefore abdominal girths should be monitored on a serial basis. An increase in abdominal measurements of 8 to 10 cm above the baseline should be interpreted as a significant sign of gastric retention, and feedings should temporarily be postponed.[52,65] When the residual can be checked by aspiration, amounts greater than 150 ml of a bolus feeding or greater than 10% to 20% of the hourly flow rate in continuous feeding indicate that feeding should be withheld until emptying occurs.[40] Consistent elevation in residual amounts indicates that the feeding should be discontinued until the cause of the elevated residual can be determined and eliminated.

Gastrointestinal motility should be assessed regularly by auscultation of bowel sounds. Absence of bowel sounds (5 minutes without sounds), presence of persistent distention, or nausea and vomiting indicate that feedings should be discontinued.[52]

Monitoring nasogastric tube placement regularly is a necessary nursing task. Placement of any tube should be initially verified by x-ray examination or whenever the possibility of dislodgement is suspected. There have been several reports about small-bore tubes being inadvertently placed or dislodged into the respiratory tract.[65]

Glucose oxidase reagent strips can be used to check for glucose in tracheobronchial secretions of tube-fed patients, since normal sputum is free from detectable glucose. Small amounts of blood in the secretions can create a false-positive test, and this should be considered when oxidase strips are used.

Frequent suctioning of the oropharynx should be performed in patients with artificial airways. This prevents pooling of secretions on the cuff and subsequent aspiration to the lower respiratory tract. Aspiration past a properly inflated, functioning cuffed tube has been seen in 58% to 87% of patients.[12,94]

RESPIRATORY FAILURE
Description

Respiratory failure is commonly seen in critical care patients as a primary disorder or as a complication of other system failures or traumatic injuries. Respiratory failure is generally accepted as being present when the PaO_2 is <50 mm Hg, and/or the $PaCO_2$ is >50 mm Hg at an FIO_2 of 21%.[8,13,61] When hypoxemia without associated hypercapnia is present (type I), respiratory failure is said to exist. Type II respiratory failure exists when the patient is both hypoxemic and hypercapnic. Clearly, as seen in Table 20-11 and as experienced clinically, some conditions deteriorate from type I to type II respiratory failure in the course of the disease or when intervention is delayed or unsuccessful.

Cause

As Table 20-11 indicates, many causative agents or conditions can lead to respiratory failure. When disease and disability result in an insufficient exchange of air and gas in relation to the amount needed to maintain metabolism, respiratory failure exists.[25,82]

Pathophysiology

Respiratory failure can be acute or chronic, depending on the speed of onset and duration of the illness. It can result from changes in the functioning of the components of the respiratory system such as the airways, the alveoli, or the alveolar-capillary membrane. Changes in how these components function in relation to the whole can result in hypoventilation, impeded diffusion, ventilation-perfusion mismatch, and increased pulmonary shunting. Combinations of these abnormalities are frequently seen in patients with respiratory failure. Type I hypoxemic respiratory failure results from V/Q mismatch, shunt, or diffusion abnormalities.[57] Type II respiratory failure results from the same

Table 20-11 Causes of respiratory failure

Type I (hypoxemia without hypercapnia)	Type II (ventilatory failure, hypoxemia with hypercapnia)
Chronic bronchitis and emphysema	Chronic bronchitis and emphysema
Pneumonia	Bronchial asthma
Pulmonary edema	Crushed chest injury
Pulmonary fibrosis	Drug overdose (narcotic, sedative, and so on)
Bronchial asthma	Central alveolar hypoventilation syndrome
Atelectasis	Obstructive sleep apnea syndrome
Aspiration (acid-bile)	Myasthenia gravis
Adult respiratory distress syndrome (ARDS)	Tetanus
Bronchiectasis	Polyneuropathies, myopathies
Smoke inhalation	Cervical cord injuries
Pulmonary embolism	Head injuries
Cardiogenic shock	Poliomyelitis
Cyanotic congenital heart disease	Hypothermia
Pulmonary arteriovenous fistulas	Hypertrophy of the tonsils and adenoids
Kyphoscoliosis	Near-drowning
Massive obesity	Curariform drugs
Postoperative	Barbiturate poisoning
Crushed chest injury	
Fat embolism	

From MacNee W: J Roy Soc Med 78:61, 1985.

conditions that cause type I failure and includes hypoventilation. Treatments directed at improving dynamics or breathing are necessary to correct the hypercapnia, hypoxemia, and subsequent acidosis.[57]

Assessment and Diagnosis

Diagnosing and following the course of respiratory failure is best accomplished by blood gas analysis. Clinical symptoms displayed by the patients are not reliable in predicting the degree of hypoxemia or hypercapnia. Blood gas analysis confirms the level of $PaCO_2$, PaO_2, and blood pH.

Treatment

In type I failure, aggressive treatment of hypoxemia using a high FIO_2 is necessary, as severe hypoxemia ($PaO_2 < 40$ mm Hg) is rapidly fatal.[57,82] Although the absolute level of hypoxemia varies in each individual, circumstances as a result of age, and the underlying disease, most treatment approaches aim to keep the oxygen saturation at 90% or above. Correcting hypoxemia by increasing the FIO_2 is effective in treating V/Q inequalities and diffusion impairments. When shunt exists (blood flowing through a nonventilated alveoli), increasing the FIO_2 of inspired air alone is ineffective.[82] In these situations, alveolar ventilation, hence PaO_2 may be increased by constant positive airway pressure (CPAP) or PEEP in addition to mechanical ventilation.

In type I patients, the mixed venous PO_2 (PvO_2) is an assessment parameter that reflects tissue oxygenation and cardiac output more accurately than arterial blood gas analysis.[29] Mixed venous O_2 monitoring requires a pulmonary artery catheter, and the recent development of a catheter with fiberoptic bundles has allowed for constant monitoring of the PvO_2 as opposed to intermittent sampling. Along with the importance of providing adequate oxygen, prolonged administration of a high FIO_2 should be avoided, because this results in oxygen toxicity and aggravates low V/Q ratios. When faced with a $PaO_2 < 50$ mm Hg, despite an FIO_2 of 50%, significant intrapulmonary shunt exists.[61] ARDS is a common example of this respiratory failure. Patients with ARDS generally require mechanical ventilation with PEEP, yet still experience high mortality.

Ventilatory support in type I respiratory failure should be considered when (1) inadequate oxygenation continues despite FIO_2 increases, (2) retention of CO_2 occurs leading to increased $PaCO_2$, mental depression, or increased fatigue, and (3) secretion control becomes difficult.[8,61]

Type II respiratory failure, associated with hypoventilation, requires methodology aimed at improving respiratory dynamics. Intervention may require lowering the FIO_2 in patients who chronically retain carbon dioxide and thus are dependent on the hypoxic respiratory drive. Other interventions in type II respiratory failure include narcoleptic drugs, reversal of drug overdose, or mechanical ventilation if the respiratory failure results from neurological or muscle disorders of ventilatory muscle fatigue.

One of the most frequent situations leading to type II respiratory failure is acute exacerbation of chronic obstructive pulmonary disease as a result of a new pulmonary infectious process.[61] Acute deterioration in a chronic setting can be detected by the presence of acidosis in a previously compensated patient. Therapy is aimed at treating the pulmonary infection, relieving the hypoxemia, stimulating the respiratory drive, and, if necessary, providing mechanically assisted ventilation. Each approach must be evaluated on the basis of the individual patient situation.

Treating hypoxemia is a primary aim, because hypoxemia gives rise to systemic complications and, if untreated, will result in death. In most situations, conservative treatment of hypoxemia has proved more satisfactory than aggressive therapy involving intubation and assisted ventilation.[61] Low levels of FIO_2 are warranted to avoid depressing any hypoxic respiratory drive that might exist in patients with chronic CO_2 retention.

The process of ventilation is driven by many forces. One of the predominant chemical factors stimulating ventilation is the level of hydrogen ions (H^+) circulating in the medulla and the brain. In normal states, small increases in hydrogen ion concentration result in increasing the ventilatory drive (rate and depth of inspiration), which in turn increases the removal of CO_2 (an H^+ precursor) from the lungs. However, if the CO (and subsequently the H^+ level) climbs slowly over time (as in COPD), the chemoreceptors in the medulla become less and less responsive to hydrogen ion concentration. When this occurs, low tissue oxygen levels (hypoxemia) stimulate ventilation.[82] Giving the patient too much supplemental FIO_2 can abolish the hypoxic drive and result in apnea. Generally, oxygen should be titrated to produce a PaO_2 of 50 to 60 mm Hg.[8,57]

Small increases in FIO_2 will often produce significant rises in oxygen saturation, because the patient's hemoglobin is partially unsaturated. According to the oxyhemoglobin dissociation curve, a $PaO_2 < 50$ mm Hg will result in less than 85% of hemoglobin being saturated with oxygen (normal saturation 96% to 100%). Therefore giving the patient just enough supplemental FIO_2 to raise the PaO_2 into the 50 to 60 mm Hg range can improve the oxygen-carrying capacity of the blood significantly. Methods frequently chosen to deliver lower oxygen concentrations include Venturi masks or nasal prongs at 1 to 3 L/min. Patient compliance with oxygen therapy is often better with nasal prong use than with face mask use because of perceived comfort by the patient. When the face mask is used to treat hypoxemia, the patient will often complain that the mask compromises breathing, talking, and eating and may even remove the mask. Nasal prongs allow patients to be active while continuing to receive oxygen, therefore providing a more consistent level of oxygenation.

Even careful administration of oxygen has the potential for decreasing the hypoxic drive to ventilate in patients who chronically retain carbon dioxide. As previously mentioned, clinical signs of hypercapnia and hypoxia are not reliable in reflecting the degree of abnormality. Arterial blood gases should be utilized. Frequency of sampling warrants arterial catheterization that will also allow for continuous monitoring of the blood pressure. Warren and others[105] suggested treatment with oxygen in this group of patients should be aimed at keeping the PaO_2 at 50 mm Hg and a pH of >7.26. In their opinion, arterial $PaCO_2$ level is unimportant if the pH remains in a satisfactory range.

Air flow problems may result from airway narrowing, secretions, or muscle fatigue. Bronchodilation can improve air flow in patients and lessen hypoxemia. Although theophylline preparations are commonly chosen, beta blockers have proved effective, especially when delivered by nebulized inhalation. Two drugs that may be used are ipratropium bromide and salbutamol.[61] Nebulizing the drugs in saline is recommended to decrease the bronchoconstriction that can be associated with distilled water. Oxygen should be the gas used for nebulization as opposed to air, because this will help alleviate the hypoxemia.[61]

The use of steroids or respiratory stimulants in the treatment of respiratory failure as a result of COPD remains controversial. In respiratory failure associated with ARDS or aspiration lung disorder, steroids have clearly been shown to be unwarranted, because steroids reduce the lung's ability to clear bacteria.[24,64] When respiratory failure occurs in patients with COPD because of acute infections, the beneficial results from the use of steroids seems doubtful.

When the patient has CO_2 narcosis from respiratory depression as a result of drugs or oxygen, doxapram is helpful. Doxapram has been administered in a continuous drip in an attempt to increase patients' levels of alertness and improve their ability to participate in bronchial hygiene activities.[61] Respiratory stimulants such as nikethamide offered no improvement in the course of respiratory failure. Almitrine is a newer respiratory stimulant that may have advantages not seen in other drugs. Specifically, almitrine stimulates the carotid and aortic bodies to increase ventilation. Studies in France show improvement in PaO_2 and decrease in the $PaCO_2$ when almitrine was given in a continuous intravenous drip.[57] (Oral forms of the drug are also available.)

When conservative measures fail to reverse the elevated $PaCO_2$ and improve oxygenation, mechanical ventilation may be necessary. Complications of mechanical ventilation such as barotrauma can occur and difficulty in weaning the patient from a mechanical ventilator is a real possibility. Mechanical ventilation in COPD patients should be brief and instituted for short-term problems that can be aggressively reversed. Since conservative management (without mechanical ventilation) in COPD patients is as successful as the use of mechanical ventilation and carries fewer risks of complications, it should be tried first.

Nursing Care

Respiratory failure can result from a myriad of precipitating events with varying treatment approaches. Nursing care will be directed by the specific cause of the respiratory failure, although some common interventions are utilized. The nurse has a significant role in (1) monitoring the patient's course, (2) supporting and improving the ventilatory dynamics, (3) maintaining a patent airway and aiding secretion clearance, and (4) proper administration of drugs, including oxygen.

Monitoring the course of an illness is a major nursing responsibility. Since the nurse provides care on a continuous basis, changes in the patient's status are initially recognized and evaluated by the nurse caregiver. Baseline and ongoing respiratory assessment should include airway patency, respiratory rate and depth, pattern of respirations, presence of or changes in adventitious lung sounds, arterial blood gas analysis, and secretion production and clearance.

The reader is referred to Chapter 18 for a complete discussion of respiratory assessment. Establishing the baseline state of the patient's monitoring parameters is important, since it is the reference point from which progress or deterioration is judged. Next, the nurse should establish the levels of change necessary to trigger alterations in intervention. For example, if arterial blood gases are being periodically assessed, what goal is desired? Once this is established, the intervention techniques can be preplanned. In this situation, the nurse knows in advance what to do for specific blood gas results without having to recontact the physician. When clear plans are articulated in advance, unnecessary loss of time and effort is eliminated.

Chapter 22 includes a detailed discussion of interventions and nursing management of patients with ineffective airway clearance, ineffective breathing patterns, and/or air and gas exchange problems.

ADULT RESPIRATORY DISTRESS SYNDROME (ARDS)
Description

Adult respiratory distress syndrome (ARDS) is a well-recognized syndrome erupting as the final common pathway

Nursing Diagnosis and Management
Respiratory failure

- Impaired Gas Exchange related to alveolar hypoventilation secondary to (specify), p. 488

- Impaired Gas Exchange related to ventilation-perfusion inequality secondary to (specify), p. 487

- Ineffective Breathing Pattern related to chronic airflow limitations, p. 481

- Ineffective Breathing Pattern related to respiratory muscle deconditioning secondary to mechanical ventilation, p. 482

- Ineffective Airway Clearance related to excessive secretions, p. 475

- Ineffective Airway Clearance related to impaired cough secondary to loss of glottic closure with cuffed endotracheal/tracheostomy tube, p. 476

- Potential for Aspiration risk factors: reduced level of consciousness, depressed cough, and gag reflexes, presence of tracheostomy or endotracheal tube, p. 489

- Decreased Cardiac Output related to decreased preload secondary to mechanical ventilation with or without PEEP, p. 335

- Altered Nutrition: Less Than Body Protein-Calorie Requirements related to lack of exogenous nutrients and increased metabolic demand, p. 713. (See also discussion of metabolic results from carbohydrate overfeeding, Chapter 10.)

- Potential for Infection risk factor: invasive monitoring devices, p. 346

- Sensory-Perceptual Alterations related to sensory overload, sensory deprivation, sleep pattern disturbance, p. 601

- Sleep Pattern Disturbance related to circadian desynchronization, p. 89

- Potential for Impaired Skin Integrity risk factors: immobility, nutritional deficit, steroid therapy, enteral tube feedings, stool incontinence, p. 725

- Body Image Disturbance related to actual change in body structure, function, and appearance, p. 833

- Body Image Disturbance related to functional dependence on life-sustaining technology, p. 834

- Powerlessness related to health care environment or illness-related regimen, p. 837

- Ineffective Individual Coping related to situational crisis and personal vulnerability, p. 850

---

of various insults that cause damage to the alveolar-capillary interface. Despite the advancement in techniques available to monitor and support critically ill patients, the outcome for patients with ARDS has improved little. Mortality rates remain at 50% to 60%.[11,15,64] A National Institutes of Health (NIH) study reports that mortality rates increase significantly when organ failure is present: one organ (lung only), 40%; two organs, 54%; four organs, 84%; and with five organs failing, 100%.[15] No clear understanding of the pathology or the approach to treatment exists, making ARDS a challenging and frustrating phenomenon.

In 1967 Ashbaugh and others[5] described the criteria for diagnosing ARDS. They identified a syndrome preceded by a catastrophic event, such as multiple trauma, followed by increased intrapulmonary shunting, increased dead space, and loss of pulmonary compliance with resulting hypoxemia despite increasing levels of FIO_2. Changes revealed by chest x-ray evaluation, with the appearance of diffuse bilateral infiltrates, confirmed the diagnosis. Studies continue to be done to clarify the etiological factors related to ARDS and to find treatment modalities that will lower the mortality.

Etiology

Many factors have been implicated as causative agents of ARDS, but the mechanisms of pulmonary injury are unclear in many cases. The box on p. 426 lists situations frequently leading to adult respiratory distress syndrome. Of those implicated, patients with direct lung injury and/or systemic sepsis are at highest risk of developing ARDS.[11] Fein and others[30] demonstrated in a retrospective study that 18% of all patients admitted to the hospital with sepsis developed ARDS. When sepsis is associated with trauma, the incidence of ARDS is probably higher. Patients with indirect lung injury should be carefully monitored for early signs of respiratory insufficiency, which may signal the development of ARDS.

Pathophysiology

Research on the biochemical processes involved in the pathological states related to ARDS has resulted in diverse theories. No single element or common mechanism has yet been identified. Some areas being studied include arachidonic acid, the complement system, free radicals, and platelet and neutrophil activity.[8,11,16,64] These factors are briefly outlined in Table 20-12.

After the injury event, the earliest alterations are interstitial lung edema, defects of the alveolar epithelium, and microthrombosis.[18] Changes in the alveolar-capillary endothelium allow for larger than normal amounts of fluid and protein to leak into the pulmonary interstitium and even-

CONDITIONS LEADING TO ARDS

DIRECT PULMONARY INJURY

Aspiration of gastric contents or other toxic substances
Near-drowning
Inhalation of toxic substances
Diffuse viral pneumonia
Diffuse mycoplasmal pneumonia
Diffuse rickettsial pneumonia
Pulmonary contusion secondary trauma
Drugs: heroin, panaquat, salicylates
Embolism: fat, air, amniotic fluid

INDIRECT PULMONARY INJURY

Sepsis—especially gram-negative
Severe pancreatitis
Multiple emergency blood transfusions
Multiple trauma
Disseminated intravascular coagulation (DIC)
Shock from any cause
Neurogenic states: head trauma, increased intracranial
    pressure
Nonpulmonary systemic diseases
Postcardiopulmonary bypass
Anaphylaxis

Modified from Bernard G and Brigham K: Ann Rev Med 36:195, 1985.

Table 20-12 Substances implicated in lung injury associated with ARDS

Substance	Source	Actions	Pathological results
Complement fragments	From activation of the complement system that is involved in the antigen-antibody reactions and cell lysis reactions	Activate or attract inflammatory cells; cause clumping and lysis of cells, releasing lysosomes; activate neutrophils	Increase permeability of vascular tissue; free oxygen radicals causing tissue damage
Free radicals (atom or molecules with an impaired electron) such as superoxide free radicals	Formed by oxidative processes in body (usually rapidly neutralized by superoxide disputase and other antioxidants)	Attack lipids of cell membrane, changing membrane permeability	Leakage of protein fluid into interstitium of lung and flooding of alveoli
Arachidonic acid	Unsaturated fatty acid precursor of certain prostaglandins	Form prostaglandins that stimulate platelet aggregation, vasoactive actions of prostaglandin, regulate blood flow and fluid leak in inflamed tissues	Thrombosis of small arterioles; pulmonary vasoconstriction; change in vascular permeability
Neutrophils	Type of polymorphonuclear granulocyte circulating in blood and in bone marrow	Attach to damaged endothelium; release enzymes that affect vascular membrane permeability and increase chemotaxis through release of leukotrines; contain oxidase enzymes that give rise to free radicals	Increase permeability of vascular membranes leading to fluid leakage; phosphatases present in neutrophils interact with arachidonic acid to perpetuate prostaglandin activity
Platelets	Blood cellular element	Stimulate clotting process as activated platelets release thromboxane A—a vasoconstrictor	Increase pulmonary artery pressures—lung congestion; microthrombosis of small pulmonary vessels

Table 20-13 Clinical presentation of adult respiratory distress syndrome

Clinical features	X-ray findings	Pulmonary function
Tachypnea and dyspnea	Diffuse or localized condensation images, interstitial pattern with increased vascular shadows	Reduced Pa_{O_2} Reduced Pa_{CO_2}
Progressive dyspnea, irritability, cyanosis, confusion, hypoxemia (partially reversible with FI_{O_2})	Alveolar edema pattern, normal vascular shadows, normal heart size	Reduced Pa_{O_2} Reduced Pa_{CO_2} Reduced compliance Reduced functional residual capacity
Severe hypoxemia despite FI_{O_2} of 1.0	Alveolar edema pattern with progression to massive fibrosis in some cases	Increased A-a_{O_2} Reduced functional residual capacity Reduced compliance Reduced Pa_{O_2} Increased Pa_{CO_2}

From Cadierno-Carpintero M and others: Cardiovasc Rev Rep 8(3):35, 1987.
FI_{O_2}, concentration of inspired oxygen; Pa_{O_2}, arterial oxygen pressure; Pa_{CO_2}, arterial carbon dioxide pressure; A-a_{O_2}, alveolar-arterial oxygen gradient.

tually into the alveoli causing noncardiogenic (increased permeability versus increased pressure) pulmonary edema. The process of pulmonary noncardiogenic edema is a progressive one with fluid and proteins first accumulating in the interstitium, which in itself does not interfere with gas exchange.[8,16] However, as the interstitial fluid overwhelms the local controlling factors (oncotic pressure, capillary hydrostatic pressure, lymphatic drainage), the increased hydrostatic pressure compresses and eventually collapses the terminal bronchioles. At this point, diminished gas exchange occurs and hypoxemia is seen. Eventually, fluid and protein enter the alveoli, decrease the activity of surfacant, and promote alveolar collapse. Pulmonary shunting increases, and the hypoxemia worsens. In severe ARDS, shunting can involve 50% of blood flow through the lungs that is reflected in arterial blood gas results showing acidosis, hypercapnia, and hypoxemia despite supplemental FI_{O_2}. As fluid continues to flood the pulmonary interstitium and alveolar spaces, lung compliance and functional residual capacity decrease, while the work of breathing, oxygen consumption, and dead space area increase.[7,11] Eventually, the protein that has leaked out of the vascular space into the interstitium and alveoli forms hyaline membranes (an eosinophilic substance), further decreasing compliance and increasing the hypoxemia as seen by a widening alveolar-arteriole O_2 gradient and hypoxemia that is unresponsive to increasing the FI_{O_2} (refractory hypoxemia). Table 20-13 correlates the clinical features of ARDS with x-ray and pulmonary function findings.

Assessment and Diagnosis

The clinical picture, depending on the precipitating event, may be one of acute full-blown pulmonary edema with frothy sputum, air hunger, tachypnea, tachycardia, and hypotension or one of gradually increasing respiratory insufficiency and hypoxemia. Generally, during the early phase of ARDS, the patient will exhibit hyperventilation, a normal compensatory mechanism to the hypoxemia. Crackles may

be present over the lung fields, and patchy infiltrates may be seen on chest x-ray. As the syndrome progresses, the patient will demonstrate a persistent low Pa_{O_2} despite high inspired oxygen concentrations. The Pa_{CO_2} will remain low at first, as a result of the hyperventilation. Eventually, however, Pa_{CO_2} retention will accompany the hypoxemia. Signs and symptoms of tissue hypoxia will be evident as the condition worsens. Increasing pulmonary vascular resistance has been found to be a poor prognostic sign.[64] With significant lung involvement, the clinical picture reflects severe respiratory failure. Chest x-ray evaluation reveals a "white out" of the lung.

Some patients will develop pulmonary fibrosis with permanent pulmonary disability if they survive the event.

Diagnosis of ARDS is based on clinical and laboratory criteria, as reviewed in the box below.

CRITERIA FOR DIAGNOSING ARDS

A compatible clinical history of a precipitating event
Hypoxemia—Pa_{O_2} less than 50 mm Hg on an FI_{O_2} of 0.6,[64] other authorities recommend a Pa_{O_2} less than 60 mm Hg at an FI_{O_2} of 0.50 or more[90]
Decreased pulmonary compliance of less than 50 ml/cm H_2O
Radiological evidence of diffuse bilateral alveolar infiltrates
Absence of underlying cardiogenic pulmonary edema and lung disease evidenced by a pulmonary capillary wedge pressure of no greater than 18 mm Hg[64]
Increased shunt fraction and increased dead space ventilation (Vd/Vt)[64]

Treatment

Currently, major therapy for ARDS involves treating the underlying cause, preventing further alveolar capillary membrane damage, and supporting tissue oxygenation through the use of positive pressure ventilation, with careful attention to perfusion.

Recognition of the patient at risk for developing ARDS should be part of any therapeutic approach. At this time, instituting prophylactic, positive pressure breathing modalities in patients has not prevented development of the syndrome, yet early recognition and aggressive treatment of hypoxemia is warranted.

Arterial blood gases should be closely monitored in at-risk patients (review the box on p. 426). Progressive deterioration in PaO_2 represents incipient respiratory failure requiring early ventilatory support. Criteria for establishment of ventilatory support in at-risk patients, as outlined by Norwood and Civetta,[71] include (1) respiratory rate >30 to 35 breaths per minute, and (2) PaO_2 <55 mm Hg with FIO_2 of 21%. Retention of CO_2 would be a further indication that ventilatory support is needed.[71]

Ventilatory support should be as physiological as possible to avoid gas exchange problems, alkalemia, and progressive respiratory muscle weakness. Norwood and Civetta[71] feel that controlled mandatory ventilation (CMV) should never be used alone, because it is not similar to normal breathing. They recommend intermittent mandatory ventilation (IMV) or synchronized IMV (SIMV). IMV/SIMV diminishes the side effects associated with CMV by permitting spontaneous ventilation in addition to intermittent mechanical support. When the IMV/SIMV modality is used, the mechanically delivered ventilations should be administered in one to two breath increments up to a level per minute that maintains a normal blood pH and $PaCO_2$. The tidal volume of the ventilator inhalation is usually equal to 5 ml/pound or 10 to 15 ml/kg of body weight.[71] Since the IMV/SIMV mode allows the patient to breathe spontaneously by means of a circuit that bypasses the machine, the patient's respiratory rate indirectly reflects adequacy of ventilation. Generally, the number of ventilator-derived breaths (IMV/SIMV) should be increased when the patient's spontaneous rates become tachypneic (>30/min) or if the patient's breathing becomes labored. Subjective complaints by the patient of difficulty breathing, breathlessness, or increasing anxiety may indicate need for an IMV/SIMV rate adjustment. The additional modality of PEEP with IMV/SIMV is one mode of respiratory support. Table 20-14 outlines methods of ventilator support used in ARDS.

Depending on the severity of the disease process, initiation of therapy to reverse the hypoxemia may initially necessitate an FIO_2 > 0.5 to achieve a satisfactory level of oxygenation (PaO_2 > 70 mm Hg). When this occurs, measures should be taken to recruit alveoli by the use of PEEP. PEEP is used to reduce the loss of functional residual capacity by opening alveoli. PEEP provides an airway pressure greater than atmospheric pressure at the end of exhalation and thus holds the alveoli open. This decreases pulmonary shunting, which reduces hypoxemia and allows for a reduction in FIO_2 to nontoxic levels (FIO_2 < 50%). Institution of PEEP should begin at 2 to 3 cm H_2O.[71,98] (PEEP as a

ventilator modality is explained in Chapter 21.)

Caution must be used in applying PEEP, because the intrathoracic pressure changes created can decrease cardiac output. Most authorities recommend a gradual increase in PEEP and use of the minimal PEEP pressure that will still allow for adequate oxygenation (PaO_2 > 70 mm Hg with FIO_2 < 0.5).[71,98]

Individual investigators have used different parameters to decide when PEEP is sufficient. Suter and others[98] adjusted PEEP levels to the point at which the greatest improvement in pulmonary compliance was experienced. They, as well as others,[11,71,98] do not recommend the use of PEEP > 15 cm H_2O. Optimal PEEP has been described as the amount that reduces intrapulmonary shunt fraction (Qsp/Qt) to less than 20%.[64] Regardless of the method used, the goal of ventilatory support is adequate oxygenation by means of nontoxic levels of FIO_2. A reduction of FIO_2 below 0.50% is desired as soon as the patient's condition permits. Maintaining higher levels of FIO_2 fosters absorption atelectasis, disruption of surfactant production, and oxygen toxicity.

Once PEEP has been instituted, the intrapulmonary shunt should be calculated every 10 to 15 minutes after each increase in the PEEP level until significant improvement in clinical status has been achieved. Hemodynamic monitoring of the cardiac output should be implemented in most patients to adequately assess cardiac function. Reductions in cardiac output associated with PEEP may be lessened by increasing preload and by the use of inotropic agents. Dobutamine has been found to be more useful than dopamine in increasing the cardiac output in ARDS, since it decreases the pulmonary capillary wedge pressure (PCWP), may lesson pulmonary water accumulation.[66] If a pulmonary artery catheter is not available for Qsp/Qt measurements, the PEEP can be increased until the PaO_2/FIO_2 ratio is 250 to 300:1. This ratio has been found to correspond to a 15% to 25% shunt fraction.

Ventilatory support should be maintained until correction of the cause has occurred and respiratory involvement has been corrected. Blood gas analyses and chest x-rays should be evaluated for attainment of normal values and resolutions of pulmonary congestion. Weaning before reaching these clinical goals will generally be unsuccessful. All parameters including FIO_2, IMV/SIMV rate, and PEEP should be serially reduced as opposed to sudden termination. Support is considered minimal when the FIO_2 is 0.4 or less, the IMV/SIMV rate is 2 per minute, and PEEP is about 5 cm.[64,71] At this point, with satisfactory arterial blood gases, weaning can begin.

If the patient does not require intubation on the basis of maintaining airway patency, extubation at the end of the weaning process can proceed. Successful weaning, according to Norwood and Civetta,[71] exists when the patient can maintain pH >7.35, $PaCO_2$ <45, respiratory rate <30/minute, a PaO_2 >55, and FIO_2 of 0.21 on a constant positive airway pressure of 5 cm H_2O without any supplemental IMV/SIMV breaths.

Other Therapeutic Approaches

No evidence shows that administration of glucocorticoids improves the outcome of ARDS. In animal studies, steroids

Table 20-14 Ventilator modes used during the treatment of ARDS

Ventilator modes	Application
Assist control (A/C) with PEEP	Allows for adjustment for varying volumes and high minute ventilation Decreases the work of breathing over IMV/SIMV With PEEP and effective tidal volume, recruits alveoli Generally, requires only mild sedation Commonly used, available on all models and generations of ventilators Patient can influence rate of ventilation, not tidal volume
IMV/SIMV	Control mode ventilator with a circuitry that permits uninhibited spontaneous ventilation by the patient For V̇E to increase the patient's spontaneous breaths must increase Is associated with lower mean airway pressure than A/C[64] Increases the work of breathing over A/C Usually requires only mild sedation SIMV—synchronizing the ventilator-delivered breath with the patient's own ventilation prevents competition between the patient's respiratory rhythm and the ventilator rhythm Allows for partial ventilator support; that is, the patient and ventilator provide a portion of the required ventilation
Pressure-controlled inverted ratio ventilation	Increases the inspiratory time of the ventilator to 50% of the respiratory cycle with an inspiratory pause of 20-30%[64] Has been shown to improve Pao_2 and $PaCo_2$ in ARDS patients Allows for more even gas distribution in lungs May require significantly more sedation than for A/C or IMV/SIMV
High-frequency jet ventilation (HFV)	Uses small volumes (less than dead space volume) at high-frequency rates to achieve gas exchange
High-frequency positive presure ventilation (HFPPV)	Creates lower peak and mean airway pressures than conventional volume ventilation
High-frequency oscillation (HFO)	Can be used with PEEP Bronchospasm unresponsive to medications can require termination of HFV Generally requires only mild sedation No proven benefits seen in ARDS
Differential lung ventilation (DLV)—selective PEEP	Useful for patients with severe unilateral lung disease when conventional means have failed Different rates, tidal volumes, and PEEP are selected for each lung Requires double-lumen endotracheal tube and two ventilators for manipulation of several parameters
Extracorporeal membrane oxygenation (EMO)	Used with conventional ventilator support for partial hypoxemia and hypercapnia Studies showed no long-term improvement in survival and therefore not recommended at this time[64]

have caused a reduction in free oxygen radicals, and use early in the syndrome may be efficacious but is still debatable.[18,105] Large doses of steroids have been effective in treating a small number of patients with ARDS associated with fat emboli, but only if administered early in the syndrome.[2,32] Investigation continues in the use of imidazole and indomethacin in the treatment of ARDS. These agents have been shown to reduce production of arachidonic acid, a cellular element believed to be a mediator of lung injury. Presently, the use of these agents is considered experimental.

Because protaglandins appear to play a role in the pathological changes associated with ARDS, experimental use of PGE_1 infusions is being studied.[64] Though the preliminary outcomes of using prostaglandin are encouraging, larger clinical trials need to be completed before it can be considered an appropriate part of ARDS management.

Fluid therapy is aimed at maintaining adequate intravascular volume to provide sufficient cardiac output and tissue perfusion, yet minimize contribution to lung edema. Hemodynamic monitoring is recommended as a way to accurately assess fluid needs. A pulmonary wedge pressure in the range of 10 to 12 mm Hg is desired, and the use of fluid challenges, or diuretics, depending on the direction of the pressure alteration, should be used to achieve this range.

Although disagreement exists about the use of crystalloids versus colloids, various studies fail to show that colloids are more advantageous. Supporting the cardiovascular system with crystalloid fluids is acceptable, unless severe protein depletion (50% of normal) exists.

Nursing Care

Throughout the course of ARDS, respiratory monitoring is an important nursing responsibility. Identification of patients at risk for developing ARDS should activate a plan of frequent purposeful respiratory assessment. Sophistication of the type of data achievable varies with the respiratory support being provided to patients, since the newer computer-operated ventilators can monitor multiple ventilatory function parameters.

Even when mechanical ventilatory support and intubation are not necessary, indirect data about gross lung compliance and hypoxemia can be obtained at the bedside. Ear or pulse oximetry measurements of SaO_2 and incentive spirometry measurements should be evaluated on all patients at risk for

ARDS (see the box on p. 426). Initial arterial blood gas values are essential. A complete physical examination of the patient's respiratory system should be performed initially and once each shift, with more frequent assessment of lung sounds and respiratory rate occurring every 2 hours. An elevated respiratory rate and falling PaO_2 should warn the nurse of a change in the patient's condition and the need for further assessment.

In ARDS, as the lungs "stiffen" from pathophysiological changes, incentive spirometer performance as it reflects functional residual capacity (FRC) will decline. Vital capacity measurements will decrease in ARDS and a vital capacity below 1.5 L or 20 ml/kg may indicate impending respiratory failure.[64,77]

Patients receiving ventilatory therapy should have additional parameters reflecting lung mechanics routinely monitored. Some ventilators have inline pneumotachographs available that constantly measure lung volume and pressures. These measurements are used to provide a pressure-volume curve that indicates lung compliance. A gas sample port may also be available for measuring exhaled carbon dioxide, which allows determination of adequacy of ventilation.

Tidal volume and airway pressures can be monitored by observing various ventilator dials and the spirometer. When automatic measurements of compliance are not available as

---

Nursing Diagnosis and Management
Adult respiratory distress syndrome

- Impaired Gas Exchange related to ventilation-perfusion inequality secondary to increased alveolar capillary membrane permeability, p. 487

- Ineffective Airway Clearance related to impaired cough secondary to loss of glottic closure with cuffed endotracheal/tracheostomy tube, p. 476

- Potential for Aspiration risk factors: presence of tracheostomy or endotracheal tube, p. 489

- Decreased Cardiac Output related to decreased preload secondary to mechanical ventilation with or without PEEP, p. 335

- Altered Nutrition: Less Than Body Protein-Calorie Requirements related to lack of exogenous nutrients and increased metabolic demand, p. 713. (See also discussion of metabolic results from carbohydrate overfeeding, Chapter 10.)

- Potential for Infection risk factor: invasive monitoring devices, p. 346

- Sensory-Perceptual Alterations related to sensory overload, sensory deprivation, sleep pattern disturbance, p. 601

- Hopelessness related to failing or deteriorating physical condition, p. 839

- Anxiety related to threat to biological, psychological, and/or social integrity, p. 852

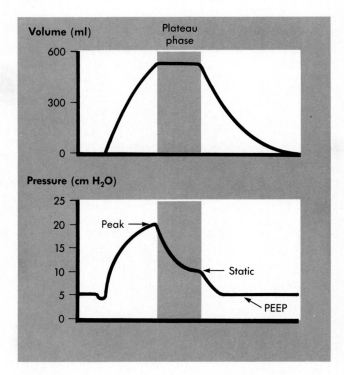

Fig. 20-1 Relationship between tidal volume and airway pressure in a patient requiring mechanical ventilation is plotted on the above curve. The inspiratory plateau in the volume tracing is achieved by temporary occlusion of the expiratory tubing. During this period, airway pressure falls from a peak of 20 cm H_2O to a static pressure of 10 cm H_2O. These readings allow calculation of static and dynamic compliance. (Printed with permission from Tobin MJ: Hosp Prac 21(6): 69, 1986. Illustration by Mr. Albert Miller.)

part of the ventilator data, manual measurements can be taken by the respiratory therapist. Static compliance (Cst) is measured by dividing the tidal volume by the inspiratory plateau pressure (Pplateau) minus PEEP (see Fig. 20-1). The normal static compliance is 70 ml/cm H_2O. Dynamic compliance (Cdyn), though more difficult to measure, can be estimated by dividing the tidal volume by inspiratory peak pressure. Normal dynamic flow compliance is 45 ml/cm H_2O. As with any measurement, it is the trend (as opposed to individual numbers) that should be used to determine improvement or deterioration in the patient's condition. Obviously, in the ARDS patient, decreasing compliance reflects a worsening of the syndrome.

Ongoing gas monitoring will be needed to manage the patient with ARDS. This includes arterial blood gases, oximetry, and mixed venous sampling if available. Continuous monitoring of the $PaCO_2$ is not as useful as continuous O_2 monitoring in ARDS victims.

During mechanical ventilation, the best oxygenation at lowest airway pressures is desired. The initial maximal inspiratory pressure (Pmax), except when severe pulmonary disease is present, is usually <50 cm H_2O. If higher pressures are generated, this can indicate that excessive flow rates or excessive tidal volumes have been established on the ventilator settings. High inspiratory pressures increase the risk of barotrauma. In severe ARDS the pressure needed to adequately ventilate the patient may be significantly above normal; however, if excessive pressure is the only means of ensuring adequate gas exchange, the risk of barotrauma must be accepted. Mean airway pressure is more important than peak pressure in considering risks for barotrauma. In some cases, especially during emergencies, the trachea is intubated with too small a tube, which creates unnecessary air flow resistance. The critical care nurse should consider this factor during initial evaluation of the patient's airway.

Automated mechanical ventilator systems generating a pressure-volume curve with each breath are helpful in assessing ventilatory setting and potential for barotrauma. Curves that flatten out (Figure 20-2) with a large pressure increase and little volume increase indicate a reduction in FRC and greater likelihood of overdistention and barotrauma.[64]

Alarm systems on mechanical ventilators alert the nurse of potential patient problems. The ventilator alarms should never be shut off or bypassed. In the interest of patient safety, in some newer computerized ventilators critical alarms are established in such a way that the computer will not allow them to be inoperative. Table 20-15 reviews common alarm situations and the nurse's response.

Attention to proper patient positioning is another nursing intervention utilized to relieve hypoxemia. Norton and Conforti[70] suggest measuring oxygenation in various patients 30 minutes after position changes to determine optimal oxygenation. Evidence also suggests that ARDS patients with bilateral lung involvement may benefit from a prone, Trendelenburg's position, because this promotes blood flow to the areas of lung that receive largest amount of tidal volume during mechanical ventilation.[45,70] Proper abdominal support as well as secure access to the airway should be provided. The diaphragm in patients pharmacologically paralyzed has been shown to be located in a more cephalad position at rest then in nonparalyzed patients.[87] This condition could lead to predominance of tidal volume being distributed to the apices of the lung and should impact on patient position.[87] When bilateral or unilateral lung involvement exists, positioning with the more normal lung down has shown to improve oxygenation.[7,28,103]

Suctioning the patient with ARDS on a PEEP modality may necessitate special consideration to technique and equipment. When possible, suctioning should occur by means of a closed suctioning system to avoid ventilator disconnection and loss of PEEP.[87] If this cannot be achieved as a result of the equipment available, use of a PEEP valve is recommended. When a manual resuscitation bag is used, it must be able to deliver a volume 1½ times the patient's Vt to assure hyperinflation and prevent alveolar collapse.

The nurse must titrate fluid replacements accurately to assure adequate cardiac output and avoid overhydration. All infusions should be delivered through a mechanical volume device. Hemodynamic lines require close monitoring, and, when several invasive pressures are being followed, the PA wave line should be chosen for continuous visualization.

Establishing a baseline patient weight and following the weight on a daily or alternate-day basis is an accurate and efficient way to evaluate fluid balance. Generally, weight gains of >0.5 kg (1.1 pounds)/day or >2.5 kg (5 pounds)/week indicate fluid retention.[53]

Complications can result from the ARDS syndrome itself or from the treatment modalities. Decreased cardiac output as a result of PEEP and pulmonary infarction from pulmonary artery catheterization are examples of the latter. Early recognition of complications allows for intervention and hopefully lessens the morbidity (see the box on p. 434).

Development of renal failure in the ARDS patient is an

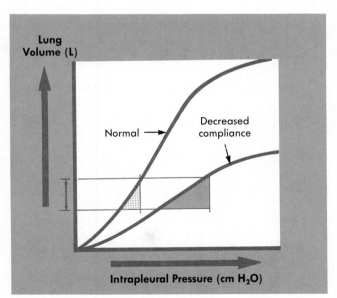

Fig. 20-2 Pressure-volume curves are plotted for a normal subject and a patient with decreased lung compliance. For a given change in lung volume (*delineated area*), change in intrapleural pressure is considerably greater than that in the patient with decreased lung compliance. (Printed with permission from Tobin MJ: Hosp Prac 21(6): 69, 1986. Illustration by Mr. Albert Miller.)

Table 20-15 Ventilator alarms and nursing actions

Tidal volume less than pre-set	Low-pressure alarm	High-pressure alarm	PEEP (low alarm)	Auto (intrinsic PEEP)	Apnea alarm
Partial or complete disconnection from ventilator Leak in patient breathing circuit (tubing) Malfunction in the exhaled Vt spirometer Lack of seal at tracheostomy or endotracheal tube Malfunction in the volume ventilator 1. If discrepancy between measured Vt and preset value is greater than 20%, or if there is an alteration in clinical state (agitation, obtundation, decrease BP), disconnect patient from ventilator. 2. Manually "hand bag" the patient. 3. If leaks persist with hand-bag system, endotracheal or tracheostomy tube is malfunctioning. Air may be felt or heard escaping, the patient may talk or make sounds.	Alarm indicates leak in system 1. Employ same schemas as low Vt state. 2. If patient is receiving CPAP, then the low-pressure alarm system is the only indication of a disconnection or major leak.	Indicates change either in "system" resistance (e.g., H_2O in breathing circuit or secretions, bronchospasm, or obstruction in the endotracheal tube) or change in lung compliance 1. Inspect tubing, check for kinks in tubing, patient clamping down on tube, and suction patient. 2. Observe ease or difficulty in passing catheter through the endotracheal or tracheostomy tube. 3. Listen for bilateral lung sounds, check level of tube for depth or insertion, if questions remain about tube placement, check chest x-ray film. 4. Patient may be "bucking" the ventilator, assess need to sedate, give support and reassurance. If anxiety and agitation exist, rule out hypercapnia and hypoxemia before sedating the patient.	Indicates leaks in system or mechanical failure of PEEP mechanism 1 Check "system" similar to Vt leak. 2. Call respiratory therapy.	Ventilator pressure manometer reads zero during exhalation; therefore must check during no-flow state. Occlude exhalation port at end exhalation; manometer should read zero. 1. If auto PEEP is present, allow more time for exhalation. "Stacking" (inhalation occurring while patient is still exhaling) can be detected if a volume displacement spirometer is in use.	Can be triggered by IMV/SIMV or CPAP modes when patient does not initiate breath within preset time unit. 1. Assess patient for fatigue or change in status. Frequent periods of apnea may necessitate more controlled breaths.

4. If leak is positional (i.e., seen with tracheal dilation), reposition tube and/or patient.

5. If not positional, recheck pilot balloon.

6. If leak remains, endotracheal tube should be replaced, contact physician and coordinate arrangements.

7. If leak resolves with "bagging," the problem is in ventilator system. Check all connections and tubing. Correct and reconnect patient to ventilator.

8. If malfunction cannot be easily corrected, contact respiratory therapy. Maintain patient ventilation.

Always ensure that an adequate FIo_2 is used; use $FIo_2$1.0 if in doubt. When in doubt, manual resuscitation should be used and ventilator replaced.

Modified from MacDonnell K, Fahey P, and Segal M: Respiratory intensive care, Boston, 1987, Little, Brown & Co.

COMPLICATIONS ASSOCIATED WITH ADULT RESPIRATORY DISTRESS SYNDROME

Pulmonary

Pulmonary emboli
Pulmonary barotrauma
Pulmonary fibrosis
Pulmonary complications of ventilatory and monitoring procedures
    Mechanical ventilation
        Right main stem intubation
        Alveolar hypoventilation
    Swan-Ganz catheter
        Pulmonary infarction
        Pulmonary hemorrhage
    Tracheal intubation
        Laryngeal injury
        Tracheal stenosis

Gastrointestinal

Gastrointestinal hemorrhage
Illeus
Gastric distension
Pneumoperitoneum

Renal

Renal failure
Fluid retention

Cardiac

Dysrhythmia
Hypotension
Low cardiac output

Infection

Sepsis
Nocosomial pneumonia

Hematological

Anemia
Thrombocytopenia
Disseminated intravascular coagulation

Other

Hepatic
Endocrine
Neurological
Psychiatric

---

ominous sign as mortality rises to the 60th percentile. Careful monitoring of urinary output, urine specific gravity, and body weights can alert the nurse to renal insufficiency and allow for prompt aggressive treatment that may prevent renal failure. Creatinine clearance should be used in place of the BUN or serum creatinine, since these may be normal in renal insufficiency. When the volume of urinary output per hour is relatively constant, a secondary urinary creatinine clearance measurement correlates well with 24-hour clearance and can be used.[64] Since it is known that inappropriate antidiuretic hormone (ADH) secretion can occur with mechanical ventilation, especially associated with PEEP > 10 cm H_2O, this complication should be considered.[39,64]

Nosocomial infections can be fatal for ARDS patients. Meticulous hand washing and use of aseptic techniques when suctioning and caring for any indwelling catheters are mandatory. Minimizing the number of invasive lines is recommended. Pneumonia is a frequent development among ARDS patients; self-colonization of the lower respiratory tract by organisms located in the oropharynx is a likely cause. Use of prophylactic antibiotics is not recommended, because this practice seems to encourage the growth of more virulent organisms. A major contributing factor in the development of infections is malnutrition, which should be avoided or corrected in ARDS patients as quickly as possible. In a majority of patients, enteral alimentation will generally suffice. When enteral feedings are contraindicated, parenteral hyperalimentation should be initiated.

THORACIC SURGERY

Surgery of the lung is performed to remove tumors, benign and malignant, for pleurodesis in repeated pneumothoraxes, and to resect abscesses or empyemas unresponsive to antibiotic therapy. Surgical resection of tumors is the most frequent reason for a thoracotomy (Table 20-16).

Description / Cause

Cancer of the lung represents 22% of all cancers in men and 10% of cancers in females.[39] In 1986, it was estimated that 149,000 new lung cancers were diagnosed. Because of the late stage at which many lung cancers are diagnosed, only 20% to 25% can be treated surgically.[39]

Surgical treatment may involve wedge resection, segmentectomy, lobectomy, or pneumonectomy depending on the site, extent of lung tissue involvement, and tumor cell type involved. A wedge resection indicates part of a lobe has been surgically removed, a lobectomy indicates an entire lobe has been removed, and a pneumonectomy indicates removal of an entire lung.

Assessment and Diagnosis

Before surgery, a complete evaluation of the patient is needed to determine the appropriateness of surgery as a treatment and to determine whether removal of lung tissue can be done without jeopardizing respiratory function. This is especially important when a lobectomy or pneumonectomy is being considered.

When resection is being undertaken for tumor treatment, preoperative evaluation of the type and extent of tumor must

Table 20-16 Tumors of the lung treated by surgery

Name	Cause/characteristics	Treatment
Hydatid cysts of lung	Caused by *Echinococcus* disease—usually seen in Mediterranean countries, South America, Australia, New Zealand	Thoracotomy with enuceation of cyst—if diffuse/infected, larger pulmonary resection
Solitary pulmonary nodule (coin lesion)	May be benign or malignant, requires excision to obtain diagnosis	If malignant, lung resection
Benign tumors—endobronchial	Polyp, fibroma, lipoma, chondroma, leiomyoma, osteoma, lymphoma	Remove by bronchoscopy, if unable remove by thoracotomy and partial resection
Hamartoma	Common, circumscribed, benign tumor as a result of malformation of organ, ususaly in periphery lung	Enuceation or local excision
Bronchial carcinoid	Slow-growing tumor found in large bronchi	Resection
Malignant tumor	Sarcoma—rare as primary neoplasm—usually secondary to Hodgkin's disease	Lobectomy
Carcinoma	Involves many cell types, which affects prognosis; squamous cell, epidermoid, undifferentiated, large cell, small cell, oat cell, adenocarcinoma	If no metastasis, lobectomy or pneumonectomy; when metastasis exists, chemotherapy and/or radiation therapy

be performed. Tumor type may be determined by cytology or tissue biopsy. Cytology of sputum or pleural fluid can reveal cell type in a significant number of patients. Early morning collection of sputum on 3 or more consecutive days will yield positive results in 40% to 90% of the patients.

Tissue biopsies may be obtained by cutaneous needle biopsy, bronchoscopy, mediastinoscopy or mediastinotomy, or direct thorocotomy. Bronchoscopy and associated mediastinoscopy are frequently performed to determine the extent of invasion when a tumor is cancerous. Surgical treatment should be used only for local, noninvasive tumors.

The preoperative evaluation should include pulmonary function tests to determine the patient's ability to lose lung tissue. Kirsh and others[51] have cited the following criteria as suitable for tolerating pulmonary resection:

$Pco_2 < 45$ mm Hg at rest or with exercise

$Pao_2 > 50$ mm Hg at rest or with exercise

FEV > 2000 ml, FVC > 2000 ml, or maximum FVC at 50% predicted value in patients requiring pneumonectomy

FEV > 1,500 ml in patients requiring lobectomy

Calculated FEV > 800 ml by preoperative spirometry with ventilatory perfusion scan

Treatment

A pneumonectomy is required when a tumor involves the lobar and hilar lymph nodes or when a lobectomy would not remove all of the tumor. Pneumonectomy permits a wide resection of the lymphatic drainage system, but it is also associated with higher morbidity, because the loss of such a large amount of lung tissue can result in inadequate lung capacity and pulmonary hypertension.

For a lobectomy to be performed, the tumor must be isolated to a lobe and the lymph nodes must be free from metastasis. Less lung tissue is resected with this procedure,

reducing the complications and morbidity and maintaining greater functional ability for the patient.

Segmentectomy and wedge resection remove the least amount of lung tissue. To be effective, the tumor must be peripherally located without chest wall involvement or other metastasis. These procedures are associated with a low operative mortality of about 2% to 5%.[92]

To provide adequate surgical exposure for lung resection, the patient is usually placed in a lateral decubitus position during surgery. A posterolateral incision is made to permit upward displacement of the scapula. When a pneumonectomy or upper lobectomy is planned, an incision is generally made in the area of the fifth or sixth rib bed. When a lower lobectomy is planned, approach through the seventh rib area is more usual. Removing a rib and entering the thorax through the rib bed is preferred, because a tighter air seal is possible at closure.

When significant lung secretions are present or a high risk of operative site bleeding exists, modification of the lateral decubitus position may be necessary. Special care is taken to avoid drainage of blood or secretions into the unaffected lung during surgery, because such an occurrence could cause dangerous, if not fatal, hypoxemia and cardiac dysfunction. In some cases, special double-lumen endotracheal tubes, such as a Carlens tube, can be used to protect the unaffected lung from secretions while surgery is in progress.

After pneumonectomy, the mediastinal position requires evaluation. This is done on closure of the operative site and involves manometric measurement and chest x-ray examination. With the patient lying supine, pressure in the empty chest cavity should be -4 to -6 cm of H_2O pressure. When it is abnormal, air or fluid can be added or withdrawn. A chest x-ray examination will show the location of the mediastinum.

Various complications are associated with pulmonary resection. The loss of parenchyma can result in respiratory insufficiency and pulmonary hypertension. Hemodynamic monitoring with balloon-tipped catheters is not routine in thoracotomy patients but should be implemented in patients with compromised cardiac function. Changes in pulmonary artery pressures can be used to evaluate cardiac function, fluid status, and intrathoracic changes.

Postoperative development of a bronchopleural fistula is a chief cause of mortality. This develops when a suture line fails to secure occlusion of the bronchial stump.[31] During surgery, careful attention is given to isolating and closing the bronchus in attempts to secure a lasting seal with subsequent stump healing.

Nursing Care

Nursing care of the post thoracotomy patient involves interventions aimed at (1) supporting ventilation and gas exchange, (2) monitoring the patient for signs and symptoms

---

Nursing Diagnosis and Management
Thoracic surgery

- Ineffective Breathing Pattern related to thoracic pain, p. 483

- Ineffective Airway Clearance related to thoracic pain, p. 477

- Impaired Gas Exchange related to ventilation-perfusion equality secondary to (specify), p. 487

- Acute Pain related to transmission and perception of noxious stimuli secondary to thoracic surgery, p. 594.

- Activity Intolerance related to knowledge deficit of energy-saving techniques, p. 344

- Knowledge Deficit: Activity Restrictions related to lack of previous exposure to information, p. 69

- Sleep Pattern Disturbance related to fragmented sleep, p. 88

- Altered Nutrition: Less Than Body Protein-Calorie Requirements related to lack of exogenous nutrients and increased metabolic demand, p. 713

- Potential for Infection risk factors: protein-calorie malnourishment, central intravenous line, pp. 346 and 720

- Body Image Disturbance related to actual change in body structure, function, and appearance, p. 833

- Altered Role Performance related to physical incapacity to resume usual or valued role, p. 836

- Ineffective Individual Coping related to situational crisis and personal vulnerability, p. 850

- Sexual Dysfunction related to activity intolerance secondary to chronic lung disease, p. 867

---

of complications, and (3) assisting the patient to return to an adequate activity level.

Postoperatively, strict attention must be given to avoidance of respiratory depression caused by narcotics used to control pain. The patient's rate may be normal, but the tidal volume can be depressed as a side effect of narcotic administration. This can be evaluated by periodic measurement of the tidal volume. Shortness of breath in the first few days following pneumonectomy or lobectomy is abnormal and may be related to hypoxemia, retained secretion, hypoventilation, or other causes.

Careful evaluation of the mediastinal position is required regularly in the postoperative period as an indication of intrathoracic pressure. As with a tension pneumothorax, deviation of the mediastinum can lead to cardiorespiratory insufficiency and failure. The mediastinal position can be determined by (1) palpating for tracheal deviation, (2) palpating and auscultating the position of the apex of the heart, and (3) chest x-ray examination. If a mediastinal shift occurs, correction by injecting or withdrawing air/fluid should be performed. Chest x-rays used to evaluate the mediastinal position must avoid any oblique proliferation of the x-ray, because this may cause erroneous interpretation.

Deep breathing exercises should be performed regularly with all post thoracotomy patients. These exercises help reexpand collapsed lung tissue, thus promoting early resolution of the pneumothorax in patients with partial lung resections. Coughing, which should only be encouraged when secretions are present, assists in mobilizing secretions for removal. Because of intraoperative positioning and preoperative and perioperative medications, atelectasis and secretion pooling are common during the postoperative period. Furthermore, as a result of postoperative pain, the patient's ventilations may be shallow, thereby encouraging the development of atelectasis and secretion stasis.[31] Respiratory infections can occur from retained secretions and incomplete lung expansion. Deep breathing and, when appropriate, coughing should be encouraged in the first few days after surgery.

Positioning the patient should take into account the surgical incision site, the surgery, and the perioperative position. Frequent turning helps to improve ventilation and perfusion in the lungs. The patient should not be turned directly onto the unaffected side during the initial period after a pneumonectomy, because the bronchial stump incision is fresh and there is an increased risk of disruption of the suture line. Tilting the patient slightly toward the unaffected side is possible, but the surgeon should indicate when free side-to-side positioning is safe.

Except following a pneumonectomy, chest tubes are placed to remove air and fluid. When auscultating lungs, air leaks should be evaluated. In the early phase, an air leak is commonly heard over the affected area, because the pleura has not yet tightly sealed. As healing occurs, this leak should disappear. An increase in an air leak or appearance of a new air leak should prompt investigation of the thoracic drainage system to discover whether air is leaking into the system from outside or whether the leak originates from the patient's incision. A significant air leak can result in a tension pneumothorax. Increased air leaks not related to the thoracic drainage system may indicate disruption of sutures.

Hemorrhage is an early life-threatening complication that can occur in thoracotomy. In all patients, except those with pneumonectomy, an increase in chest tube drainage can signal excessive bleeding. During the immediate postoperative period, chest tube drainage should be measured every 15 minutes and this frequency decreased as the patient stabilizes. When chest tube loss is >100 ml/hour, when fresh blood is noted, or when a sudden increase in drainage occurs, hemorrhage should be suspected.[31]

Resections of a large lung area or pneumonectomies may be followed by a rise in the central venous pressure. With the loss of one lung, the right ventricle must empty its stroke volume into a vascular bed that has been reduced by 50%. This means a higher pressure system is created, which may tax the limit of the right ventricle leading to right ventricular heart failure. Depending on previous heart function, acute decompensation of both ventricles can result. Measures are aimed at supporting cardiac function and avoiding intravascular volume excess.

Within a few days of surgery, range of motion to the shoulder on the operative side should be performed. The patient frequently splints the operative side and avoids shoulder movement because of pain. If immobility is allowed, stiffening of the shoulder joint can result. This is referred to as "frozen shoulder" and may require physical therapy and rehabilitation to regain satisfactory range of motion of the shoulder joint.

Usually on the day after surgery, the patient will be able to sit in a chair. Activity should be systematically increased, with attention to the patient's activity tolerance. With adequate pulmonary function present before surgery and a surgical approach designed to preserve respiratory function, full return to previous activity levels is possible. This may take as much as 6 months to 1 year, depending on tissue resected and the patient's general condition.

CHEST TRAUMA
Description

Chest trauma is a frequent cause of patient admission to critical care units. Depending on its severity, the chest injury may be immediately life threatening, create significant morbidity, or be associated with minimal problems. Approximately 50 million traumatic injuries occur annually in the United States.[64] Chest injury accounts for 25% of traumatic deaths and is a major factor in an additional 25% to 50% of all traumatic deaths.[88] Because of the improvement in out-of-hospital care by emergency medical technicians (EMTs), significant numbers of severely injured people are being treated in critical care units around the nation.

Although most chest injury victims are initially treated in emergency centers, it is possible that the critical care nurse will be the first caregiver to identify the injury.[4] Therefore the critical care nurse must be familiar with the signs and symptoms of chest trauma as well as with treatment modalities.

Adequate function of the pulmonary system depends on an (1) intact lung parenchyma, (2) functioning alveolar capillary gas exchange, (3) intact pleura, (4) intact thoracic wall, (5) patent laryngotracheobronchial tree, and (6) neural innervation. Any or all of these factors can be affected by penetrating or blunt chest trauma. Blunt trauma may not be visibly appreciated but can be severe enough to produce death. It is important to thoroughly assess patients for all possible causes of a condition or complaint.

Cause

The forces involved in blunt chest injury can result from high-speed traffic accidents, falls from great heights, or simple banging against tubs or other household appliances. When the chest receives a direct blow, as with a steering wheel impact, concussive forces may injure areas distant from the impact area, similar to results seen in blast injuries. When rapid deceleration occurs, shearing, stretching, and torsion of the great vessels can result in intimal tears with pseudoaneurysm or vessel rupture following.

Injuries of specific thoracic bony structures are frequently associated with underlying tissue damage. Fracture of the first rib has been associated with major chest, abdominal, and vascular injuries.[64,88] Because the first rib is well protected, a significant force must occur to produce fracture.[24,88] Likewise, fracture of ribs 7 through 10, especially posteriorly, is frequently accompanied by liver or spleen lacerations, depending on the side of fracture.[24,88] Sternal fractures are frequently associated with thoracic injuries such as ruptured esophagus, myocardial contusion, ruptured bronchus, or aortic injury.[24,64]

Assessment and Diagnosis

When initially assessing victims of chest injury or potential chest injury, the nurse should quickly evaluate the components of the respiratory process for manifestations of inadequate airway ventilation and/or gas exchange (see the box on p. 438). The specific traumatic event should direct the nurse to look for associated injuries. For the purpose of this presentation, chest trauma will be discussed as either impact or penetrating. Because of the high mortality associated with chest trauma, emergency treatment should be initiated simultaneous with assessment and diagnosis.

When the trauma victim is first seen, suctioning equipment should be available, two large-bore intravenous lines should be placed for transfusion therapy, and frequent monitoring of vital signs and respiratory parameters should be instituted.[64] Chest x-ray evaluations and other radiographic studies should be obtained immediately. Patients with impact injuries should always be treated as though a cervical spine injury exists until the potential of spinal injury has been ruled out. A complete assessment, as outlined in the box on p. 438, should be performed initially and periodically. Repeated monitoring for pulmonary complications is necessary, even in patients with few initial findings, because of the danger of associated lung contusion.

Impact Injuries/Rib Fractures

Rib fractures are the most common result of impact injuries. If they are uncomplicated, pain is the most significant sequela experienced by the patient.[100] In most cases, patients with rib fractures alone are not generally admitted to a critical care unit, but with fractures of certain ribs the po-

MANIFESTATIONS OF INADEQUATE RESPIRATORY PROCESS

INADEQUATE AIRWAY

Stridor
Noisy respirations
Supraclavicular and intercostal retractions
Flaring of nares
Labored breathing with use of accessory muscles

INADEQUATE VENTILATION

Absence of air exchange at nose and mouth (breathlessness)
Minimal/absent chest wall motion
Manifestations of obstructed airway
Central cyanosis
Decreased or absent breath sounds, (bilateral, unilateral)
Restlessness, anxiety, confusion
Paradoxical motion involving significant portion of chest wall
Decreased Pao_2, increased $Paco_2$, decreased pH

INADEQUATE GAS EXCHANGE

Tachypnea
Decreased Pao_2
Increased dead space
Central cyanosis
Chest infiltrates on x-ray evaluation

ASSESSMENT OF CHEST TRAUMA

1. Check airway for blood, secretions, or vomitus and clean away (protect airway in unconscious victim).
2. Observe patient's ventilations: are they normal, labored, absent; is splinting present?
3. Obtain vital signs: blood pressure, pulse, respiratory rate. Check for pulsus paradoxus, which could indicate cardiac tamponade.
4. Inspect chest wall movement for symmetry or lack of symmetry.
5. Palpate chest (front and back) for tenderness, rib or sternal fractures, crepitus; assess for wounds or evidence of wound.
6. Auscultate lung fields. Listen over mediastinum for Hammon's sign (mediastinal emphysema—high-pitched metalic sound).
7. Assess for hypovolemia, check neck veins for fullness or distension.
8. Assess signs/symptoms of tissue hypoxia.
9. Evaluate mental status.
10. Obtain Vt and forced vital capacity measurements if possible.
11. Evaluate peripheral pulses—carotid, brachial, radial, femoral.
12. Auscultate heart sounds, especially for murmur and friction rubs.
13. Review available laboratory data especially arterial blood gases, hemoglobin, and hematocrit levels.
14. Review chest x-ray examination results. If first rib fracture is present be especially suspicious of accompanying intrathoracic trauma. Posterior fracture involving seventh to tenth ribs is often associated with laceration of liver or spleen. Evaluate patient carefully for signs of bleeding.
15. Check for acute gastric distention. Listen for bowel sounds. Consider need for nasogastric tube to decompress stomach.

tential for complications may indicate admission to a critical care unit initially (see the box at bottom right). Because of the discomfort associated with inhalation, the patient may institute splinting breaths. This leads to decreased lung expansion, and if uncorrected, atelectasis and V/Q abnormalities. Shackford[88] recommends initial measurement of Vt and FVC in evaluating a patient's ability to ventilate. When Vt is <5 ml/kg or FVC <10 ml/kg, severe compromise exists and pain relief should be directed at increasing these values. Shackford further recommends intercostal nerve blocks for up to three rib fractures and epidural anesthesia for four or more fractures. Taping or binding rib fractures is not recommended, because increased splinting and decreased gas exchange will result.[64] Nursing attention should be focused on relief of pain while maintaining adequate tidal volume and minute ventilation.

Flail Chest

Flail chest is a type of complicated rib fracture that results when several ribs (three or more) are fractured in more than one location or in association with sternal fracture and costochondral separation. Flail chest is associated with paradoxical motion of the affected chest wall as a result of loss of chest wall stability. When the patient inhales, the fractured segment will suck in; during exhalation, it will bulge out. In most cases, this abnormality is readily apparent on inspection, however, both posterior and anterior inspection

RATIONALE FOR ADMISSION TO CRITICAL CARE UNIT IN RIB FRACTURES

Fracture of two or more ribs in elderly patient or in patient with compromised respiratory function
Fracture of first rib or seventh to tenth ribs because of likelihood of associated underlying injury
Persistent hypoventilation (Vt < 5 ml/kg) despite adequate pain control

is necessary to avoid overlooking a posterior flail.

The patient with a flail chest should be evaluated for ventilatory mechanics with attention given to effective ventilation and Vt. Since the patient fits a high-risk group for lung contusion, pulmonary compliance measures should be periodically assessed. Pain control should be implemented along with turning and deep breathing, because the contusion will decrease lung compliance. Gas exchange should be evaluated by arterial blood gases, and when the $PaCO_2$ excretion is adequate, oxygenation can then be periodically assessed by oximetry. In the past, the goal of treatment was stabilization of the flail chest, initially by mechanical means and later by volume ventilators. Today it is recognized that the extent of the underlying lung injury is more important than the flail itself. When flail chest is associated with significant hypoxemia or hypercapnia, intubation and mechanical ventilation may be required.

Lung Contusion Associated with Flail Chest

Since flail injury indicates a severe force of impact, it is not unusual to see associated lung contusion, hemothorax, and/or pneumothorax. Head trauma is also frequently associated with flail chest, because both are common sequelae of high-speed traffic accidents.[43] Lung contusion is the crush injury that occurs to the parenchyma as a result of impact and deceleration. The functional derangement seen in the parenchyma leads to decreased compliance, increased airway resistance and decreased diffusing capacity.[64] V/Q mismatching increases in the contused lung. Surfactant levels may decrease after the first 24 hours after the parenchymal injury and continue to do so for 48 hours.

Early examination of the patient may reveal crackles over the contused lung. Hemoptysis may be present. The chest should be examined for bruising, rib fracture, and paradoxical movement. Initial chest x-ray examination may not reveal a contusion, because it can take 4 to 6 hours[4] to develop following trauma, although 70% of victims do demonstrate abnormal findings. Chest x-ray changes appear as nonsegmental infiltrates that may worsen over the first 24 hours after injury. Depending on the severity of the contusion or whether associated aspiration of gastric contents occurred during the injury or resuscitation period, frank ARDS can develop.

When pulmonary pressure monitoring is in place, pulmonary vascular resistance and V/Q ratios can be monitored. Decreasing compliance and increasing resistance along with low V/Q ratios are highly suggestive of a contused lung.

It is worth noting that the contused lung, when possible, is best treated by conservative means. Mechanical ventilation associated with PEEP increases the parenchymal injury and should be used only when supplemental oxygen fails to correct hypoxemia or when severe hypercapnia occurs. When no evidence of respiratory distress exists, and the PaO_2 is >65 mm Hg, supplemental oxygen, tidal volume and vital capacity measurements, pain relief and pulmonary toilet measurements are instituted.[88] If the tidal volume or the vital capacity declines despite pain control, or if signs of respiratory distress occur, more aggressive therapy is indicated such as intubation and CPAP with IMV/SIMV initiated. Patients with tachypnea and hypoxemia from the onset require initial ventilatory support, because these findings indicate respiratory insufficiency. Stabilization of the chest is not necessarily a therapeutic concern.

Early mortality is associated with traumatic injuries and blood loss. Later mortality is related to bacterial pneumonia or other lung complications such as ARDS. Normal defenses to bacterial invasion are disrupted in the contused lung, making these patients susceptible to pneumonias. (See the discussion of lung defenses in pneumonia.) Prophylactic antibiotic therapy has not proved to be effective and may give rise to resistant organisms.[64] Steroids should not be given because they decrease the lungs' ability to clear bacteria.[32,106]

When lung contusion is present, careful fluid balance must be maintained to minimize vascular fluid leakage into the lung tissue. Volume replacement should be titrated to ensure adequate perfusion, as seen by cardiac output measurements or urinary output and vital signs if direct cardiac output information is unavailable.

Because of the complication of respiratory infection, protective measures should be implemented to reduce risks to these patients. Careful attention to pulmonary toilet is required to control secretion retention. Those patients with excessive secretion production require frequent position changes, effective coughing, and suctioning when secretions are evident to prevent the accumulation of secretions and to prevent the development of atelectasis and pneumonia.

Initial and periodic measurements of tidal volume and vital capacity are required to recognize early changes that may herald impending respiratory failure. Pain control is important, since pain can compromise the patient's ventilatory effort by eliciting voluntary splinting. The patient should be asked to use the pain-rating scale to quantify the pain. Pain rated as 7 or higher on a 0 to 10 scale indicates a narcotic analgesic should be given.[52]

Cardiovascular Involvement in Chest Trauma

Myocardial damage can occur with impact injuries. The damage may result from a steering wheel impact or from abrupt deceleration associated with traffic accidents. The injury may take the form of myocardial rupture, myocardial contusion, or pericardial laceration and hemorrhage. When the heart ruptures as a result of the force of impact, death often ensues from cardiac tamponade. If death is not immediate, an emergency pericardiocentesis must be performed.

Myocardial Contusion

Myocardial contusion is often present in chest trauma patients and should be suspected in all incidences of steering wheel impact. The right ventricle, because of its anatomical location within the mediastinum, is more often contused than the left. Definitive signs may be minimal, but can include nonspecific ST-T wave changes on ECG, right strain pattern on ECG (P wave changes, R wave amplitude changes in anterior leads), development of ECG signs associated with acute myocardial infarction, a pericardial friction rub, and positive CK-MB isoenzymes. Development of a new murmur is significant as it indicates valvular abnormalities. If the contused area affects cardiac output, heart failure can ensue. This may be confirmed by visualization of an increased cardiac size on chest x-ray examination and development of the typical clinical findings of congestive failure. Two-dimensional echocardiography is the best method available to diagnose myocardial contusion.[64,88]

Treatment for myocardial contusion is the same as if the patient had experienced an acute myocardial infarction. Dysrhythmias must be controlled, while overall therapy is aimed at decreasing the work of the heart and promoting its rest. Development of pericardial fluid should be assessed through echocardiograms, while pericardiocentesis may be necessary for fluid removal. Rupture of the myocardium can occur during the resolution of large full-thickness contusions. This may result in an acute cardiac tamponade. A narrow pulse pressure and decreasing systolic pressures associated with pulses paradoxsus herald the tamponade event. Increased neck vein distention and dysrhythmias can also occur. Emergency pericardiocentesis and surgery are required to save the patient's life. When myocardial rupture occurs, it can present as a sudden cardiac arrest unresponsive to therapy.

Vascular Injuries

Along with deceleration injuries to the heart and lung, shearing or rupture of major vessels may occur. In fatal automobile accidents, one of six victims was found to have a ruptured aorta, an event associated with immediate fatality in 80% of the cases.[24,88] When the patient survives a ruptured aorta, he or she usually presents with severe hypovolemia and shock. Chest x-ray evaluation in 92% of the cases shows a widened superior mediastinum.[24] Displacement of the trachea can be seen in association with a hemothorax. An ascending angiogram is the definitive method of diagnosis. These patients require prompt recognition of x-ray findings followed by immediate surgical correction of the rupture. If surgical correction must be delayed, the systolic blood pressure should be kept <120 mm Hg with antihypertensive drugs. When head injury also exists, some vasodilators, such as sodium nitroprusside, have been found to increase intracranial pressure, therefore trimethaphan camsylate or propranolol hydrochloride has been recommended.[88]

Penetrating Injuries

Penetrating injuries can be associated with impact injury or can occur as a result of a missile entering the thoracic or mediastinal cavity. Common missiles are bullets and stabbing weapons. In the course of impact accidents, mechanical parts or fractured ribs may become the penetrating object. These injuries can be associated with hemorrhage, foreign debris, and disruption of the external chest wall.

Disruption of the pressures within the pleural space is frequently seen in penetrating injuries. Depending on the cause of the injury, a closed pneumothorax, an open pneumothorax, a tension pneumothorax, a hemopneumothorax, or hemothorax can result.

Pneumothorax

Pneumothorax occurs in 15% to 40% of all patients with traumatic chest injury. When a pneumothorax is large, decreased chest excursion on the affected side may be noticed. Subcutaneous emphysema may be felt, and tracheal deviation away from the affected side is possible. Percussion reveals hyperresonance with loss of breath sounds, tactile fremitus, and voice sounds over the affected area. The patient should be assessed for mediastinal emphysema, which when present is heard as a high-pitched metallic sound that is synchronous with the heart beat. In stabbings of the chest, the wound is readily visible, whereas bullet wounds may be recognized only by hearing the swish of air with ventilation. Small pneumothoraces may be missed in trauma victims but can become noticeable if mechanical ventilation is instituted. In this situation, the ventilator may force air out of the pleural tear and create a tension pneumothorax.

Clinical findings associated with open pneumothorax are similar to those associated with closed pneumothorax.

A pneumothorax of less than 20% requires no treatment unless complications occur or underlying lung disease or injury is present.[24] Misaligned rib fractures have been known to cause repeated puncture of the pleura and subsequent pneumothorax. A large pneumothorax should have the air evacuated from the pleural space by chest tubes and, if a persistent air leak occurs, can require surgery to close the laceration. Chest tubes are usually placed in the second or third intercostal space (ICS) anteriorly for air evacuation. Sucking chest wounds (open pneumothoraces) require immediate treatment to prevent hypoventilation and profound tissue hypoxia. Open pneumothorax requires immediate placement of chest tubes, or a Heimlich valve, with simultaneous dressing of the wound.

Open chest wounds need debridement and surgical closure. In large wounds Marlex mesh or muscle flap may be needed for closure. Hemothorax often accompanies these wounds.

Tension Pneumothorax

A tension pneumothorax may often be associated with sucking chest wounds, as a flap of skin can act as a one-way valve allowing air to enter the wound during inhalation and trapping it during exhalation. This creates a tension pneumothorax, because air is forced into the pleural cavity without being able to escape. As air builds up, it compresses the lung and displaces the mediastinum toward the unaffected side. The mediastinal displacement along with hypoxemia creates significant cardiac instability and decreased cardiac output. The patient will become increasingly agitated, and hypoxemia, signs of tissue hypoxia, and gasping for air may be seen. If the tension pneumothorax is not relieved, blood flow to and from the heart will be significantly reduced and will eventually cease as a result of displacement and kinking of the great vessels. An uncorrected tension pneumothorax is fatal. Tension can be released quickly by inserting a large bore needle into the second anterior intercostal space on the affected side to allow the trapped air to escape.[4] Regular chest tube placement should follow emergency decompression. Closed chest tube drainage is indicated in any patient with a pneumothorax requiring mechanical ventilation to prevent the possibility of a tension pneumothorax occurring.

Hemothorax

Hemothorax, or blood in the pleural space, can be asymptomatic or it can be life threatening. When associated with significant bleeding, the patient may be in shock as a result of decreased cardiac output and have respiratory distress caused by a mediastinal shift. Breath sounds will be decreased or absent over the affected area along with dullness to percussion. A chest x-ray examination should demonstrate the presence of pleural fluid. Whenever possible, the chest x-ray examination should be taken in the upright position to afford the best visualization of pleural fluid.[100] If a question exists after a portable chest x-ray examination, a lateral or lateral/decubitus film should be obtained. A small hemothorax will result in blunting of the costophrenic angles, whereas larger hemothoraces will produce partial to complete opacification of the involved side.

Treatment is dictated by the size of the hemothorax. When the hemothorax is small and asymptomatic, no treatment may be needed. If symptoms exist or when the patient requires mechanical ventilation, chest tubes should be inserted. Serial x-ray films to track resolution are necessary, along with serial hematocrit and coagulation studies. Bleeding that spontaneously halts is probably venous in origin. When bleeding continues for 2 hours or more, systemic vessels and arterial sources are likely.

Moderate to large hemothoraces (500 to 1000 ml) require chest tube insertion and drainage. Frequently a 32 to 36 size chest tube will be used followed by suction up to 25 cm H_2O.[24] Chest tube placement is usually at the level of the sixth to eighth ICS posteriorly to promote fluid drainage. The flow of drainage should be monitored frequently (up to every hour) after chest tube insertion until stabilization of the flow occurs. In 85% of cases, a hemothorax will stop bleeding without surgical intervention.[24] Verification that bleeding has subsided cannot be accomplished by chest tube drainage alone, because obstruction of the chest tube is possible. Serial x-rays, hematocrits, and coagulation studies should be obtained. Adequate volume replacement is necessary to maintain cardiac output and tissue perfusion. Indications for thoracotomy exists when more than 200 ml blood loss per hour for 3 to 4 hours occurs or when bleeding increases over 3 to 5 hours or more than 300 to 500 ml blood loss occurs in a 2-hour period.[24,64] Significant blood loss requires blood transfusion with banked blood or by means of the autotransfusion technique. Autotransfusion when possible is recommended, since it eliminates the concerns of donor matching and possible transference of communical disease and reduces some of the complications associated with blood transfusions. When an infected hemothorax is present, surgical evacuation is generally required.

Hemopneumothorax

Hemothorax and pneumothorax commonly occur together in trauma patients. Presenting findings would reflect both conditions and vary in relation to the severity of the insult. Treatment considerations are the same, and when chest tube drainage is needed tubes will be placed to drain both the excess air and fluid.

Esophageal Injury

Although less common, esophageal perforation can occur during traumatic injury. Most often esophageal injury is associated with penetrating traumas as opposed to blunt injury, although the latter is possible. When associated with blunt trauma, esophageal injury is probably the result of the shearing forces associated with deceleration.

Clinically, the patient may complain of dysphagia and upper abdominal pain. Subcutaneous and mediastinal emphysema, pneumothorax, or hydropneumothorax are often seen in conjunction with esophageal injury. Hematemesis may be present along with bloody nasal discharges. Chest x-ray findings are nonspecific, reflecting air in the mediastinum or pneumothorax. If a chest tube is placed that reveals hydrothorax, methylene blue should be instilled into the esophagus.[24,64] The presence of methylene blue in chest tube drainage will then confirm perforation of the esophagus. Esophagoscopy and esophagograms can be performed in patients with suspected injury, however, injury has been present when these tests were negative.

Surgical intervention is required for esophageal perforation and is most successful if performed early. Thoracotomy is necessary with small wounds being treated by primary closure and larger wounds requiring diversion of drainage in association with cervical esophagostomy or esophagogastric junction ligation and gastrostomy.

REFERENCES

1. Abels LP: Acute respiratory failure, Crit Care Quart 1:4, 1978.
2. Alho A and others: Corticosteroids in patients with a high risk of fat embolism syndrome, Surg Gynecol Obstet 147:358, 1978.
3. Ali J and others: Consequences of postoperative alterations in respiratory mechanics, Am J Surg 128:376, 1974.
4. Asensio J and others: Trauma: a systematic approach to management, Am Fam Physician 38(3):97, 1988.
5. Ashbaugh DG and others: Acute respiratory distress in adults, Lancet 2:319, 1967.
6. Aubier M and others: Effect of hypophosphatemia on diaphragmatic contractility in patients with acute respiratory failure, N Engl J Med 313:420, 1985.
7. Baehrendtz S and Hedenstierns G: Differential ventilation and selective positive end-expiratory pressure: effects on patients with acute bilateral lung disease, Anesthesiology 61:511, 1984.
8. Balk R and Bone R: Adult respiratory distress syndrome, Med Clin North Am 62:551, 1983.
9. Bartlett RH: Respiratory therapy to prevent pulmonary complications of surgery, Resp Care 29(6):667, 1984.
10. Baum G and Wolinsky E: Textbook of pulmonary disease, ed 3, Boston, 1983, Little, Brown and Co.
11. Bernard G and Brigham K: The adult respiratory distress syndrome, Ann Rev Med 85:195, 1985.
12. Bone D and others: Aspiration pneumonia, prevention of aspiration in a patient with tracheostomies, Ann Thorac Surg 18:30, 1974.
13. Bone R: Adult respiratory distress syndrome, Clin Chest Med 3(1):42, 1982.
14. Boucher BA, Witt WO, and Foster TS: The postoperative adverse effects of inhaled anesthetics, Heart Lung 15(1):63, 1986.
15. Brandstetter R: The adult respiratory distress syndrome, Heart Lung 15(2):155, 1986.
16. Brigham K: Mechanisms of lung injury, Clin Chest Med 3:9, 1982.
17. Burton GG and Hodgkin JE: Respiratory care: a guide to clinical practice, Philadelphia, 1984, JB Lippincott Co.
18. Cadierno-Carpintero M and others: Adult respiratory distress syndrome, Cardiovasc Rev Rep 8(3):35, 1987.
19. Chase RA and Gordon J: Overwhelming pneumonia, Med Clin North Am 70(4):945, 1986.
20. Chokshi S, Asper R, and Khandheria B: Aspiration pneumonia: a review, Am Fam Physician 33:195, 1986.
21. Cole A, Weller S, and Sykes M: Inverse ratio ventilation compared with PEEP in adult respiratory failure, Intens Care Med 10:227, 1984.
22. Connors A, McCaffree D, and Gray B: Evaluation of right heart catheterization in the critically ill patient without myocardial infarction, N Engl J Med 308:263, 1983.
23. Cooper K and Wetstein L: Emergency management of acute infiltrative pulmonary disease, Emerg Decision 2:53, 1986.
24. Cowley RA and Dunham C: Initial assessment and management, Shock trauma/critical care manual, Baltimore, 1982, University Park Press.
25. Crocker P and Quick G: Acute respiratory failure, Emerg Med 18:26, 1986.
26. Dal Santo G: Acid aspiration: pathophysiological aspects, prevention and therapy, Int Anesthesiol Clin 24:49, 1986.
27. Didier EP: Some effects of anesthetics and the anesthetized state of the respiratory system, Resp Care 29(5):463, 1984.
28. East T, Pace N, and Westenskow D: Lateral position with differential lung ventilation and unilateral PEEP following unilateral acid aspiration in the dog, Acta Anesthesiol Scand 28:529, 1984.
29. Fahey P, Harris K, and Vanderwarf C: Clinical experience with continuous monitoring of mixed venous oxygen saturation in respiratory failure, Chest 85(5):748, 1984.
30. Fein A and others: The risk factors, incidence and prognosis of ARDS following septicemia, Chest 1:40, 1983.
31. Finkelmeier B: Difficult problems in postoperative management, Crit Care Quart 9(3):59, 1986.
32. Flick M and Murray J: High-dose corticosteroid therapy in the adult respiratory distress syndrome, JAMA 251:1054, 1983.
33. Frame P: Acute infectious pneumonia in the adult, Basic Resp Dis 10(3):2, 1982.
34. Fuchs P: Before and after chest surgery stay right on respiratory care, Nursing 83(13):46, 1983.
35. Fulmer JD and Snider GL: American college of chest physicians/ national heart, lung and blood institute national convergence on oxygen therapy, Heart Lung 13(5):550, 1984.
36. Gantz N: Respiratory infections in the elderly, Geriatr Med Today 6(12):13, 1987.
37. Glenn W and others: Thoracic and cardiovascular surgery, ed 4, Norwalk, Conn, 1983, Appleton-Century-Crofts.
38. Goodman N: Differential diagnosis of pulmonary alveolar infiltrates, Am Rev Resp Dis 95:681, 1967.
39. Great paradox of lung cancer: the most deadly yet the most preventable, Prim Care Cancer 36(1):8, 1986.
40. Griffin DE and Wallace RJ: Bacterial pneumonia in the adult: diagnosis and therapy, Hosp Med 24:188, 1988.
41. Guenter C and Welch M: Pulmonary medicine, ed 2, Philadelphia, 1982, JB Lippincott Co.
42. Guyton AC: Textbook of medical physiology, Philadelphia, 1986, WB Saunders Co.
43. Hart L: Hidden chest trauma in the head-injured patient, Crit Care Nurse 6(4):51, 1986.
44. Hodgkin JE and Petty TL: Chronic obstructive pulmonary disease: current concepts, Philadelphia, 1987, WB Saunders Co.
45. Hurst J and others: Combined use of high-frequency jet ventilation and induced hypothermia in the treatment of refractory respiratory failure, Crit Care Med 85:771, 1985.
46. Jacobs NF: Community acquired pneumonia in later life, Emerg Med 20(4):20, 1988.
47. Johnson MA: Bronchitis and common pneumonias: pathogenic causes and treatment, Fam Prac Recert 8(8):49, 1986.
48. Johnson W: Nosocomial infection of respiratory tract with gram negative bacillus, Ann Intern Med 77:701, 1972.
49. Johnson NT and Pierson DJ: The spectrum of pulmonary atelectasis: pathophysiology, diagnosis, and therapy, Resp Care 31(11):1107, 1986.
50. Kirilloff L and others: Does chest physical therapy work? Chest 88(3):436, 1985.
51. Kirsh MN and others: Major pulmonary resection for bronchogenic carcinoma in the elderly, Ann Thorac Surg 22(4):369, 1976.
52. Lane G, Cronin K, and Peirce A: Flow charts: clinical decision making in nursing, Philadelphia, 1983, JB Lippincott Co.

53. Lane G and Peirce A: When persistence pays off, Nursing 82(12):44, 1982.

54. Laszlo J: Understanding cancer, New York, 1987, Harper & Row Publishers.

55. Leedom JM and Yu VL: Pneumonia in compromised patients, Patient Care, p. 153, Feb 1988.

56. Levison M and others: Clindamycin compared with penicillin for the treatment of anaerobic lung abscess, Ann Intern Med 98:466, 1983.

57. Lockhart G: Thoracic trauma, Crit Care Quart 9(3):32, 1986.

58. Luce JM, Tyler ML, and Pierson DJ: Intensive respiratory care, Philadelphia, 1984, WB Saunders Co.

59. Luce JM: Clinical risk factors for postoperative pulmonary complications, Resp Care 29(5):484, 1984.

60. Mackenzie C and Shin B: Cardiorespiratory function before and chest physiotherapy in mechanically ventilated patients with post-traumatic respiratory failure, Crit Care Med 13(6):483, 1985.

61. MacNee W: Treatment of respiratory failure: a review, J R Soc Med 78:61, 1985.

62. Marini JJ: Postoperative atelectasis: pathophysiology, clinical importance and principles of management, Resp Care 29(5):516, 1984.

63. Martin L: Pulmonary physiology in clinical practice: the essentials for patient care and practice, St Louis, 1987, The CV Mosby Co.

64. McDonnell K, Fahey P, and Segal M: Respiratory intensive care, New York, 1987, Little, Brown and Co.

65. Methany N, Spies M, and Eisenberg P: Frequency of nasoenteral tube displacement and associated risk factors. Res Nurs Health 9:241, 1986.

66. Molloy D and others: Hemodynamic management in clinical acute hypoxemic respiratory failure. Dopamine vs. dobutamine, Chest 90:636, 1986.

67. Murray JF: The normal lung, Philadelphia, 1986, WB Saunders Co.

68. Murray HW: Pulmonary infection following aspiration, Emerg Decision 4(6), June 1988.

69. Neff TA and others: Indications for oxygen therapy, Heart Lung 13(5):553, 1984.

70. Norton L and Conforti C: The effect of body position on oxygenation, Heart Lung 14(1):45, 1985.

71. Norwood S and Civetta J: Ventilatory support in patients with ARDS, symposium on critical care, Surg Clin North Am 65(4):895, 1985.

72. O'Bryne C: Post-operative care and complications in the thoracotomy patient, Crit Care Quart 7:4, 1985.

73. O'Donohue WJ: National survey of the usage of lung expansion modalities for the prevention and treatment of postoperative atelectasis following abdominal and thoracic surgery, Chest 87(1):76, 1985.

74. Oakes R: Ventilatory failure, Prim Care Emerg Decisions 2(6):25, 1986.

75. Peitzman A and others: Pulmonary acid injury, effects of positive end-expiratory pressure and crystalloid vs. colloid fluid resuscitation, Arch Surg 117:662, 1982.

76. Petty T and Ashbaugh D: The adult respiratory distress syndrome—clinical factors influencing prognosis and principles of management, Chest 70:233, 1971.

77. Petty T: Adult respiratory distress syndrome: definition and historical perspective, Clin Chest Med 3(1):3, 1982.

78. Pontopidan H, Geffin B, and Lowenstein E: Acute respiratory failure in the adult, N Engl J Med 287:743, 1972.

79. Quick G: Beware! ARDS ahead: care history #75, Hosp Phys 21(11):17, 1985.

80. Roberts J and others: Diagnostic accuracy of fever as a measure of postoperative pulmonary complications, Heart Lung 17(2):166, 1988.

81. Robinson J: Giving emergency care competently, Horshans, Pennsylvania, 1978, Nursing Skillbook, Nursing 78 Books, Intermediate Communication.

82. Rogers R and Juer J: Physiologic considerations in the treatment of acute respiratory failure, Basic RD 3(4):61, 1975.

83. Rosenow E, Wilson V, and Cockerill F: Pulmonary disease in the immunocompromised host, Mayo Clin Proc 60:473, 1985.

84. Rossi A and others: Measurements of static compliance of the total respiratory system in patients with acute respiratory failure during mechanical ventilation, Am Rev Resp Dis 131:672, 1985.

85. Rossi A and others: Respiratory mechanics in mechanically ventilated patients with respiratory failure, New York, 1985, The American Physiological Society.

86. Sabiston D and Spencer F: Gibbon's surgery of the chest, ed 4, Philadelphia, 1983, WB Saunders Co.

87. Schumann L and Parsons G: Tracheal suctioning and ventilator tubing changes in adult respiratory distress syndrome: use of a positive end-expiratory pressure valve, Heart Lung 14(4):362, 1985.

88. Shackford SB: FACS: blunt chest trauma: the intensivist's perspective, J Intens Care Med 1(3):125, 1986.

89. Shapiro BA and others: Clinical application of respiratory care, Chicago, 1985, Year Book Medical Publishers.

90. Shapiro BA: Respiratory critical care: state of the art controversies—new horizons, vol 8, Chicago, 1988, Respiratory Care Seminars, Inc.

91. Shapiro BA, Harrison RA, and Walton JR: Clinical application of blood gases, Chicago, 1982, Year Book Medical Publishers.

92. Shields TW: Carcinoma of the lung. In Shields TW, editor: General thoracic surgery, Philadelphia, 1983, Lea & Febiger.

93. Snapper JR and Brigham KI: Pulmonary edema, Hosp Prac 2(5):87, 1986.

94. Spray SB, Zudema GD, and Cameron JL: Aspiration pneumonia, incidence of aspiration with endotracheal tubes, Am J Surg 131:70, 1976.

95. Steere AC and others: Handwashing practices for prevention of nosocomial infections, Arch Intern Med 83:683, 1975.

96. Stock CM and others: Prevention of postoperative pulmonary complications with CPAP, incentive spirometry, and conservative therapy, Chest 87(2):151, 1985.

97. Sukumarin M and others: Evaluation of corticosteroid treatment in aspiration of gastric contents: a controlled clinical trial. Mt Sinai J Med (NY) 47:335, 1980.

98. Suter PM, Fairly AB, and Isenburg MD: Optimum end-expiratory airway pressure in patients with acute pulmonary failure, N Engl J Med 292:284, 1975.

99. Tillman BF and Bernard GR: Pulmonary edema, Emerg Decisions 2:4, 1986.

100. Tillotson P, Tillotson C, and Deluca S: Radiography for chest trauma, Emerg Decisions 4:11, 1988.

101. Timberlake GA: Trauma in the golden hour, Emerg Med 18(20):78, 1986.

102. Tobin MJ: Physiology in medicine: update on strategies in mechanical ventilation, Hosp Prac 21(6):69, 1986.

103. Tyler ML: The respiratory effects of body position and immobilization, Resp Care 29(5):472, 1984.

104. Vasbinder-Dillon D: Understanding mechanical ventilation, Crit Care Nurse 8(7):42, 1988.

105. Warren P and others: Respiratory failure revisited: acute exacerbations of chronic bronchitis between 1961-1968 and 1970-1976, Lancet 1:467, 1980.

106. Weigelt JA and others: Early steroid therapy for respiratory failure, Arch Surg 120:536, May 1985.

107. West JB: Respiratory physiology, Baltimore, 1985, Williams & Wilkins.

108. West JB: Pulmonary pathophysiology, Baltimore, 1987, Williams & Wilkins.

109. Wolfe J, Bone R, and Ruth W: Effects of corticosteroids in the treatment of patients with gastric aspiration, Am J Med 63:719, 1977.

110. Wynne W: Aspiration pneumonitis: correlation of experimental models with clinical disease, Clin Chest Med 3(1):25, 1982.

111. Ziskind MM: The acute bacterial pneumonias in the adult, Basic RD 3(2):53, 1975.

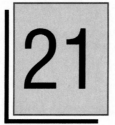

CHAPTER

21

Pulmonary Therapeutic Management

CHAPTER OBJECTIVES

- *Describe important aspects of the nursing care of a patient receiving oxygen therapy.*
- *List complications of the use of artificial airways and describe how nursing interventions can help prevent the complications*
- *Discuss the various modes of mechanical ventilation.*
- *Identify suctioning guidelines that will assist in preventing hypoxemia, atelectasis, and infection.*
- *Describe important aspects of the nursing care of a patient on mechanical ventilation and of a patient being weaned from mechanical ventilation*

OXYGEN THERAPY
Goals of Therapy

Normal cellular function depends on a supply of oxygen adequate to meet metabolic needs. Along with oxygen, all cells require energy to maintain their function or biochemical reactions, many of which are life sustaining. Cellular energy is derived from high-energy phosphate bonds such as those in adenosine triphosphate (ATP). Most cellular energy is used, transported, and stored in the form of these high-energy phosphate bonds, which, when broken, release their tremendous energy supply.

Energy is normally stored and released from the high-energy phosphate bonds by what is called oxidative metabolism. Oxygen must be available in the cell so that cellular processes continue to release the energy needed for biochemical processes. The level of cellular oxygen tension at which necessary cellular functions decrease is called the critical oxygen tension. Tissue hypoxia exists when cellular oxygen tensions are inadequate.

The primary indications for oxygen administration are hypoxemia and tissue hypoxia. As already discussed in Chapter 20, there are several causes of hypoxemia and tissue hypoxia. The goal of oxygen administration, in all cases, is to provide a sufficient concentration of inspired oxygen to permit full use of the oxygen-carrying capacity of the

arterial blood, thus ensuring adequate tissue oxygenation if the cardiac output is adequate and if the hemoglobin concentration and structure are normal. Restoring adequate tissue oxygen tension will eliminate the compensatory responses to hypoxia. Increased ventilatory work is a normal response to hypoxemia and/or tissue hypoxia, as is increased myocardial work. Both of these increased work loads can be decreased or prevented by the use of appropriate oxygen therapy.

Principles of Therapy

Oxygen is an atmospheric gas that must also be considered a drug because, like most other drugs, oxygen has detrimental as well as beneficial effects. Oxygen is one of the most commonly used and misused drugs. As a drug, it must be administered for good reason and in a proper, safe manner. Oxygen is generally ordered either in liters per minute or as a concentration of oxygen expressed as a percent, such as 40%, or as a fraction of inspired oxygen (FIO_2), such as 0.4.

The amount of oxygen administered depends on the pathophysiological mechanisms affecting the patient's oxygenation status and should ideally provide an arterial partial pressure of oxygen (PaO_2) of 70 to 100 mm Hg so that a hemoglobin saturation of greater than 90% is achieved. The concentration of oxygen given to an individual patient is a clinical judgment that is based on the many factors that influence oxygen transport such as hemoglobin concentration, cardiac output, and the arterial oxygen tension. Once oxygen therapy has begun, the patient should be continuously assessed for level of oxygenation and the factors affecting it. Arterial blood gas values should be evaluated several times daily until the desired PaO_2 is reached and has stabilized. If the desired response to the amount of oxygen delivered is not achieved, the oxygen supplementation should be adjusted and the patient's condition reevaluated. It is important to use this dose-response method so that the lowest possible level of oxygen is administered that will still achieve a satisfactory PaO_2.

More recently, alternatives to frequent arterial punctures or arterial line withdrawals have been developed, including continuous monitoring of arterial hemoglobin saturation

444

with an oximeter (various probe sites available) or monitoring of mixed venous oxygen saturation ($S\bar{v}O_2$) through a pulmonary artery catheter.[4] The introduction of the fiberoptic pulmonary artery catheter has provided continuous monitoring of $S\bar{v}O_2$.

Hazards of Oxygen

Oxygen is a colorless, tasteless, and odorless gas that, although seemingly innocuous, is actually quite hazardous. Oxygen does not burn but does support combustion, a matter of importance to its use in the hospital. A mere spark can become a large, hot flame in the presence of an oxygen-enriched environment, and the burning speed increases as the partial pressure of oxygen in the environment increases. Thus the higher the oxygen within the environment, the faster and hotter is the fire. The "No Smoking" signs that are posted are extremely important for this reason.

Methods of Delivery

Oxygen therapy can be delivered by many different devices. The devices most often seen in the hospital and home are nonrebreathing systems. These systems are either high flow or low flow and are of variable degrees of complexity. With a high-flow system, the gas flows out of the device into the patient's airways in amounts sufficient to meet all inspiratory volume requirements; and the concentration of the oxygen delivered is not affected by the ventilatory pattern of the patient. A low-flow system supplies a gas flow that is insufficient to meet all inspiratory volume requirements and is dependent on the existence of a reservoir of oxygen, its dilution with room air, and the patient's ventilatory pattern. The anatomical reservoir in this case is composed of the nasopharynx and the oropharynx. As the patient's ventilatory pattern changes, the inspired oxygen concentration varies because of the different amount of air used to mix with the reservoir gas and the constant flow of oxygen. A common misconception is that a low-flow system delivers only low concentrations of oxygen and a high-flow system delivers only high concentrations of oxygen.

Low-flow systems

Nasal cannula and catheter. Low concentrations of oxygen can be successfully delivered through a nasal cannula or prongs. The nasal cannula has the advantages of being lightweight, economical, disposable, and easily applied. Cannulas are generally well tolerated by patients and are one of the most commonly used devices for oxygen administration. Nasal cannulas do have the disadvantage of instability, resulting in displacement by a restless or unobservant patient. Pathological conditions such as deviated septum, mucosal drainage and edema, and nasal polyps can interfere with the oxygen intake.

The cannula is made of soft plastic and has two prongs that insert 1 cm into each nare. Oxygen flow from 1 to 6 L per minute can be delivered comfortably with the FIO_2 ranging from 24% to 44%. Higher flows such as 7 and 8 L per minute should be avoided because of the irritating and drying effect on the nasal mucosa.

Controversy exists about the efficacy of oxygen administration through a nasal cannula in mouth-breathing patients. Studies have shown that the final delivery of oxygen to the blood is not significantly affected by mouth breathing,[50,53] because the inspired ambient air flow in the oral pharynx entrains oxygen from the nasopharynx. Other studies, however, have shown tracheal concentration differences with mouth breathers.[53]

Since the nasal cannula is a low-flow system in which the oxygen concentration delivered relies on a mixture of ambient air and oxygen, the overall oxygen concentration will be altered by tidal volume and ventilatory pattern. For example, when a patient has a large tidal volume, the FIO_2 delivered to the alveoli will be low because more air from the atmosphere mixes with the oxygen. Conversely, when the tidal volume is small, the FIO_2 will be high. When a patient has a regular breathing pattern with consistent rate and tidal volume, cannulas can provide controlled oxygen therapy.

The nasal catheter is another low-flow device. It is inserted through the nasal passage until its tip lies in the oropharynx. It has several holes in its terminal 1 inch. More reliable control of FIO_2 can be achieved by using a nasal catheter, but its successful use depends on proper insertion and maintenance. There actually is little indication for catheter use because of its tendency to irritate the nasal passage and because of the need to move the catheter every day to the alternate nare so that pharyngeal damage is minimized.

Transtracheal oxygen catheters. Transtracheal oxygen therapy is a relatively new system that delivers oxygen directly into the trachea through a small hole in the neck called a tract. It is generally used for patients requiring chronic oxygen therapy who are admitted to the critical care unit with exacerbations of their lung disease.

In the 1980s Dr. Henry J. Heimlich originally developed the concept of transtracheal oxygen delivery.[29] Since that time there has been considerable research on the system and the development of improved catheters. Christopher and others[12] have developed a transtracheal oxygen program that uses three different catheter designs: stent, SCOOP 1, and SCOOP 2. Each catheter is used during a specific time in the healing process of the tract. Transtracheal catheters are pliable, plastic catheters that are inserted into the trachea through the tract in the neck. The catheter is held in place by a bead-chain necklace, but the oxygen tubing itself must also be secured so that it will not become disconnected or dislodged.

Some of the situations in which transtracheal oxygenation would be recommended include the following:
- Need for continuous, 24-hour oxygen
- PaO_2 ≤55 mm Hg
- Complications of nasal cannula use such as dry, sore, bleeding nose or ears
- Evidence of cor pulmonale
- Erythrocythemia
- Motivation and ability to care for the catheter

Benefits of transtracheal oxygen therapy include decreased oxygen flow rates (sometimes as much as one fourth to one half of the flow for nasal cannula oxygen), improved appearance and thus self-concept, decreased pulmonary hypertension, renewed sense of taste and smell, improved compliance with the oxygen therapy, greater mobility, and better general health.

Patients who are admitted to the critical care unit with a transtracheal catheter should continue to receive oxygen through their transtracheal catheter unless they require intubation. If a higher FIO_2 than can be achieved with the transtracheal method is needed, the transtracheal catheter can be used in conjunction with another method such as an oxygen mask. It is important to maintain the catheter in its tract because the tract can close within hours if the catheter is removed. If the tract closes, the procedure must be repeated, if appropriate. The catheter can be sutured in place if the bead chain must be removed.

Cleaning the catheter is a nursing responsibility while the patient is hospitalized and should be performed according to the protocol for the particular catheter. Several of the catheters are cleaned in place (Erie trachette and SCOOP 1) and one is removed for cleaning (SCOOP 2). It is especially important for the patient to receive oxygen through a nasal cannula or mask at the appropriate liter flow during cleaning of the transtracheal catheter. When a patient has increased production of mucus, the catheter may need cleaning more often than is normally done to prevent its becoming plugged with mucus. Signs of a plugged catheter include a "squealing" from the oxygen humidifier, which is caused by release of pressure from the pressure-limiting valve on the humidifier, and signs of decreasing blood oxygenation such as increased respiratory rate, increased heart rate, and agitation.

Experience has shown that having the transtracheal catheter in place does not interfere with intubation and mechanical ventilation. The catheter should be disconnected from the oxygen source and left in place during these therapies. Cleaning per protocol should still be performed. Mucous balls, which are a phenomenon inherent to transtracheal catheters, may be suctioned through the endotracheal tube if they are knocked loose from the catheter while it is being cleaned.

If a patient with a transtracheal catheter requires a tracheostomy, it is recommended that the tracheostomy be performed at the site of the transtracheal tract. Once the tracheostomy tube is no longer required as an airway, the stoma can be allowed to heal around a transtracheal stent or catheter.

Oxygen Masks

There are several different types of oxygen masks, which vary in construction and purpose. Most masks are made of soft plastic and are disposable. Masks can be uncomfortable because of the tight fit required on the face and because of the head strap that is necessary to hold the mask in place. Masks can also become hot because of the heat generated from the face around the nose and mouth. Some patients, especially those in severe respiratory distress, complain of claustrophobic feelings when wearing a mask. Despite the oxygen flow into the mask, patients feel "air hunger" because of the close fit of the mask and the heat trapped within it.

Care and close observation should be used when masks are on patients who are likely to vomit since the flow of vomitus can be blocked, thus increasing the chance of aspiration. Masks should also be used with care on the un-

conscious patient. An oral airway should always be in place to prevent airway obstruction by a flaccid tongue.

Simple masks. The usual simple, open-face mask is a disposable plastic unit that does not have any valves or reservoir bag. It covers the nose and mouth, has vents for exhaled air, and can deliver oxygen concentrations up to 60%. Oxygen flow rates at a minimum of 5 to 6 L per minute should be used to wash out the exhaled carbon dioxide that accumulates within the mask. Controlled oxygen therapy is difficult with an open-face mask because it does not provide precise inspired oxygen concentrations. However, this mask is a convenient and relatively comfortable device for delivering moderate oxygen concentrations over short periods and thus is widely used, especially in areas such as the recovery room. One of the main uses for simple masks is to deliver humidification or aerosol therapy. Limitations are similar to those of all masks and include discomfort and frequent removal of the mask for activities such as eating, expectorating, and coughing.

Partial rebreathing mask. The partial rebreathing mask is similar to the rebreathing mask that is used for delivery of anesthesia in the operating room. The partial rebreathing mask is a tight-fitting mask with a reservoir bag that is always open to the mask. The reservoir bag allows delivery of concentrations of oxygen greater than 60% to nonintubated patients. The purpose of the mask is to conserve oxygen by having the patient rebreathe some of his or her exhaled air. The oxygen source flows into the neck of the mask, allowing oxygen to flow directly into the mask during inhalation and into the bag during exhalation. A liter flow into the bag of at least 5 to 6 L per minute is required to prevent deflation of the reservoir bag. Because of the constant filling of the reservoir bag, only the first one third of the exhaled air volume enters the bag. This exhaled air is high in oxygen and low in carbon dioxide, because it is the volume of air that ventilated the anatomical dead space. Because minimal room air enters the mask, the concentration of delivered oxygen is fairly predictable, even if the patient's ventilatory pattern exceeds the flow rate of the oxygen source (see Chapter 19, Table 19-4, for the predicted oxygen concentrations of oxygen delivery systems).

Nonrebreathing masks. The nonrebreathing mask is another mask and reservoir bag system similar to the partial rebreathing system. With this mask, however, there is a one-way valve between the bag and mask, and no air enters the bag during exhalation. The exhaled air is diverted to the atmosphere through a flap valve in the facepiece. If the oxygen source fails or the patient's needs suddenly exceed the flow of oxygen, a flap or spring-loaded valve either in the neck or in the mask itself permits the intake of room air. When the nonrebreathing mask has a tight seal over the face, it is designed to deliver 90% to 100% oxygen. However, studies have shown that the mask delivers an average of 63% oxygen.[53] Factors responsible for this decreased concentration of oxygen include entrainment of room air because of a loose-fitting mask and open exhalation ports that allow room air to dilute the oxygen from the reservoir bag.

High-flow systems. High-flow systems provide a flow rate and reservoir capacity that are adequate to provide the total inspired volume required by the patient. Both high and low oxygen concentrations can be delivered by these systems; the oxygen concentrations are much more controlled and can be delivered in a range of 24% to 100%. One advantage of a high-flow system is that changes in the patient's ventilatory pattern do not affect the FIO_2 as long as the device is properly applied and a consistent oxygen flow can be delivered. The temperature and humidity of the gas can also be controlled since the entire inspired volume is being supplied.

Venturi mask. The most reliable control of FIO_2 can be achieved by using a Venturi mask, which controls the oxygen concentration by flowing 100% oxygen at high velocity through a narrowed orifice or "jet." This high velocity causes entrainment of air at the orifice. The higher the velocity, the more the air is entrained; this is what is referred to as the Bernoulli principle, and it is one of the most accurate means of delivering a prescribed concentration of oxygen. The FIO_2 can be varied by changing the orifice size without causing significant change in the FIO_2 as long as the minimal flow is achieved. Venturi masks currently in use can deliver 24%, 28%, 35%, and 40% oxygen. The recommended flow rates for these percentages are, respectively, 6 L, 6L, 10L, and 10 L per minute.

Venturi masks are especially efficacious in patients who are chronically hypoxemic and hypercapnic such as occurs with chronic obstructive pulmonary disease (COPD). An excessive concentration of oxygen could cause respiratory depression in these patients because their respiratory center is no longer responsive to hypercapnia and is dependent on a low PaO_2 for stimulation to breathe. The Venturi mask can provide a COPD patient with a precise oxygen concentration that does not change with ventilatory pattern and hence offers more control for an oxygen-sensitive patient.

Venturi masks cause all the discomfort of other masks and are also very wasteful of oxygen. The high air flow produced by the mask can be drying to the mucous membranes. Attempts to humidify the gas have not been very successful because of the large amount of entrained air.

Complications of Oxygen Therapy

Oxygen, like most drugs, has adverse effects and complications resulting from its use. The old adage, "if a little is good, a lot is better," does not apply to oxygen. The lung is designed to handle a concentration of 21% oxygen, with some adaptability to higher concentrations, but adverse effects and oxygen toxicity can result if a high concentration is administered too long.

Hypoventilation. The first adverse effect of oxygen administration is hypoventilation. The hypoxemic, hypercapnic patient who has chronic lung disease is at potential risk of hypoventilation with oxygen supplementation. In this type of patient and those patients with a depressed respiratory drive (such as a patient with drug-overdose), the administration of oxygen may actually cause abolition of the hypoxemia that is responsible for driving the ventilation, resulting in hypoventilation and an increase in the arterial partial pressure of carbon dioxide ($PaCO_2$). An elevated $PaCO_2$ will cause hyperventilation in most patients because carbon dioxide is the stimulus to breathe. But in patients who rely on hypoxemia as their main respiratory drive (for example, in patients who are chronically hypercapnic), the $PaCO_2$ may continue to rise as hypoventilation progresses. Eventually, the patient becomes somnolent and even obtunded because of carbon dioxide narcosis. Because of this risk of hypoventilation and carbon dioxide accumulation, all chronically hypercapnic patients require careful low-flow oxygen administration.

Absorption atelectasis. Another adverse effect of high concentrations of oxygen is absorption atelectasis. Breathing high concentrations of oxygen washes out the nitrogen that normally fills the alveoli. The higher the FIO_2 delivered to the alveoli, the lower will be the amount of nitrogen. Since nitrogen does not diffuse from an alveolus into the pulmonary capillary, it is responsible for holding open the alveolus. Therefore gradual shrinking of the alveolus can occur if a patient receives a high FIO_2 and is ventilating minimally. In this situation, oxygen in the alveolus is absorbed into the bloodstream faster than it can be replaced by ventilation, and collapse of the alveolus can result.

The effect high concentrations of oxygen have on surfactant also contributes to atelectasis. It has been postulated that surfactant, although not destroyed by hyperoxia, is redistributed and removed from close contact with the alveolar walls where it functions to keep the alveoli open.[53]

Oxygen toxicity. The most detrimental effect of breathing a high concentration of oxygen is the development of oxygen toxicity, which is dependent on the oxygen tension and the duration of exposure. No significant damage occurs to the lung exposed to an FIO_2 of 0.5 or less at sea level for extended periods,[7,59] and 100% oxygen can be breathed for 24 hours or less by healthy and even by cardiopulmonary-diseased patients with little evidence of pulmonary dysfunction[50] or clinical signs of oxygen toxicity.[59] However, there are wide variations to oxygen tolerance among individuals, and scientific study is lacking.[53] The patients most likely to develop oxygen toxicity are those that require intubation, mechanical ventilation, and high oxygen concentrations for extended periods.

The initial abnormality in oxygen toxicity apparently is impaired ciliary activity, which decreases mucociliary clearance. The first symptom is substernal chest pain that is exacerbated by deep breathing. A dry cough and tracheal irritation follow. Eventually, there is definite pleuritic pain on inhalation, followed by dyspnea. Upper-airway changes may include a sensation of nasal stuffiness, sore throat, and eye and ear discomfort. Chest radiographs and pulmonary function tests remain normal until symptoms are severe. Complete, rapid reversal of these symptoms will occur as soon as normal oxygen concentrations return. This stage in the development of oxygen toxicity can affect many organs other than the lungs, including the central nervous system, vascular system, hematopoietic system, and the heart (Table 21-1).

As oxygen toxicity progresses, objective pulmonary damage becomes evident. A chest radiograph reveals atelectatic streaks and patches of bronchopneumonia, and bronchoscopy reveals tracheobronchitis but no infection. There is also a definite decrease in vital capacity, decreased compliance, reduced functional residual capacity, and evidence

Table 21-1 Acute effects of high concentrations of normobaric oxygen*

Part affected	Site of action	Result	Outcome
Ear, sinuses	Air in body cavities	Replacement of air by oxygen, which is then absorbed	Sinus and ear pain
Airways	Mucosa of nose, throat, trachea, and bronchi	Irritation	Decreased mucociliary clearance; mucosal swelling and inflammation
Lung parenchyma	Poorly ventilated areas	Nitrogen is washed out and oxygen is absorbed	Atelectasis, microatelectasis
Ventilation	Peripheral chemoreceptors	Depressed ventilatory drive	Increased tissue carbon dioxide and $Paco_2$, which stimulate the ventilatory drive
	Deoxygenated hemoglobin—decreased	Decreased carbon dioxide carriage	Same as for peripheral chemoreceptors
	Hypoxic drive—abolished	Carbon dioxide narcosis	Hypoventilation, apnea
Pulmonary function	Airways and parenchyma	Decreased compliance	Reduced vital capacity
Heart	Vagal receptors	Slight bradycardia	Decreased cardiac output†
	Cardiac muscle	Slightly depressed	Decreased cardiac output†
Regional circulation	Coronary and cardiac vessels	Arteriolar constriction	Uncertain†
	Peripheral circulation	Arteriolar constriction	Slight hypertension†
	Retinal circulation	Arteriolar constriction	Impaired visual fields
	Conjunctival vessels	Vasodilation	Conjunctivitis
	Pulmonary circulation	Vasodilation	Improved ventilation/perfusion (V/Q) mismatch, decrease in pulmonary hypertension
Blood	Erythrocyte membrane	Damage	Hemolysis
	Kidneys	Fluid retention‡	Decreased serum albumin and hematocrit

Modified from Ziment I: Respiratory pharmacology and therapeutics, Philadelphia, 1978, WB Saunders Co.
*Time for the effects to develop is variable.
†Clinical significance is rare.
‡Initial fluid retention is usually followed by diuresis.

Table 21-2 Factors that modify the development of oxygen toxicity

Hasten onset or increase severity	Delay onset or decrease severity
Adrenocortical hormones	Acclimatization to hypoxia
Adrenocorticotropic hormone	Adrenergic-blocking drugs
Carbon dioxide inhalation	Anesthesia
Convulsions	Chlorpromazine
Dexamethasone	Gamma-aminobutyric acid
Dextroamphetamine	Ganglionic blocking drugs
Epinephrine	Hypothermia
Hyperthermia	Hypothyroidism
Insulin	Intermittent exposure
Norepinephrine	Reserpine
Thyroid hormones	Starvation
Vitamin E deficiency	Vitamin E

Modified from Spearman C and Sheldon R: Egan's fundamentals of respiratory therapy, ed 4, St Louis, 1988, The CV Mosby Co.

of pulmonary shunting. These abnormalities are reversible several days after return to normal oxygen concentrations. If high oxygen concentrations are still needed, permanent damage may occur. There are individual susceptibilities to oxygen toxicity and even variances within an individual (Table 21-2).

The pathological features of oxygen toxicity can be divided into an early exudative stage and a late proliferative stage. Within 24 to 48 hours of oxygen exposure, exudative changes appear. Initially, the capillary endothelial cells become damaged, and they leak serum protein and fluid into the interstitial space of the alveolar wall. This fluid is collected by the lymphatic system, which empties it into the general circulation.

As the capillary damage progresses, the flow of fluid out of the capillaries increases and may exceed the lymphatic system's ability to drain it. There is minimal gas exchange impairment at this point; however, with continued exposure to hyperoxia, the type I alveolar cells become damaged, allowing the escaped alveolar capillary fluid to pass directly into the alveolar spaces and causing "flooding" of the alveoli and severe gas exchange impairment.

Oxygen-induced damage to the cells of the alveolar wall initiates a self-sustaining process of ongoing injury. The by-products of the injured cells attract inflammatory cells, especially the polymorphonuclear leukocytes (PMNs). While PMNs ingest the inflammatory debris, they release proteolytic enzymes and oxygen free radicals that further damage the alveolar tissue.

The lung will respond with cellular proliferation if it survives the aforementioned process and the disease process originally responsible for the hypoxemia. Cellular proliferation occurs as an attempt to repair the alveolar damage, and the alveolar walls become filled with fibroblasts. Alveolar type II cells, which are relatively tolerant to hyperoxia,[7] replicate and reestablish the damaged alveolar wall. Endothelial cell repair and replacement occurs, and the pulmonary edema is reabsorbed. The final result is irregular scarring. Clinically, other complications such as infection must also resolve.

Summary. Oxygen is an extremely beneficial drug if used correctly, but it is sometimes taken for granted. Oxygen administration requires close patient observation and continuous application of the oxygen device to ensure controlled oxygen therapy. Use of supplemental oxygen is especially important during activities that will decrease the blood oxygen level such as turning, dangling, coughing, walking, eating, and even just talking.

Other modalities of therapy may also be used along with oxygen therapy for the hypoxemic patient, including aerosol therapy, chest physiotherapy, medications, and assisted-breathing techniques (for example, intermittent positive pressure breathing). By using these other measures, the concentration of oxygen necessary to provide adequate oxygenation may be decreased to a minimum, thus reducing the chances of oxygen toxicity.

Hyperbaric Oxygen Therapy

Hyperbaric oxygen therapy is a medical intervention whereby 100% oxygen is breathed at increased atmospheric pressure in an enclosed pressure chamber. Hyperbaric chambers date back 300 years when Henshaw built the first chamber, in which air was compressed using a bellows.[34] Previously, there was no sound physiologic basis for hyperbaric oxygen therapy nor was there any animal or clinical research to direct its use. However, since the 1930s there have been studies establishing the appropriate indications and guidelines for the use of hyperbaric oxygen therapy.

The Undersea and Hyperbaric Medical Society (UHMS) was founded in 1967 and initially used its specialized talents for the support of persons engaged in undersea activities. UHMS is the one body of scientists and physicians with the combined expertise to guide hyperbaric medicine activities. In 1983, the Hyperbaric Medical Committee of UHMS developed a report on hyperbaric oxygen therapy.[20] The committee organized disorders for which hyperbaric oxygen therapy is effective into two categories (Table 21-3). Category 1 conditions are disorders for which hyperbaric oxygen therapy is the primary mode of treatment. Also in this category are conditions in which it is an important adjunct to other primary therapy measures. The efficacy of hyperbaric oxygen therapy in these disorders has been shown through research and clinical experience. Category 2 con-

Table 21-3 Conditions known to be effectively treated by hyperbaric oxygen (category 1) or for which such treatment is considered experimental (category 2)

Category 1	Category 2
Radiation necrosis: osteoradionecrosis, soft-tissue radiation necrosis	Head and spinal cord injury (traumatic)
Decompression sickness	Bone grafts
Carbon monoxide poisoning (acute): smoke inhalation	Carbon tetrachloride poisoning (acute)
Gas embolism (acute)	Cerebrovascular accident, either thrombotic or embolic (acute): stroke; frostbite
Gas gangrene	Fractures
Osteomyelitis (refractory)	Hydrogen sulfide poisoning
Soft-tissue infection and tissue necrosis caused by mixed aerobic and anaerobic organisms; Bacteroides infection	Abscess, either intraabdominal or intracranial
Crush injury with traumatic ischemia	Lepromatous leprosy
Compromised skin grafts or flaps; selected problem wounds	Meningitis
Selected mycotic infections (refractory: mucormycosis, actinomycosis, canibolus coronato)	Pseudomembranous colitis (antimicrobial agent-induced)
Cyanide poisoning (acute)	Radiation, myelitis, cystitis, enteritis, proctitis
Cerebral edema (acute)	Sickle cell crisis and/or hematuria (sickle cell anemia)
Thermal burns	Mutliple sclerosis
Anemia from exceptional blood loss	Retinal arterial insufficiency (acute)
	Retinopathy adjunctive to scleral buckling procedures in patients with sickle cell peripheral retinopathy and retinal detachment
	Pyoderma gangrenosum
	Selected anaerobic infections (refractory): actinomycosis

From the Hyperbaric Medicine Committee of the Undersea Medical Society, Revised classification, 1986, Bethesda, Md, The Committee.

ditions represent disorders for which hyperbaric oxygen therapy is considered experimental. This category concerns life-threatening or limb-threatening cases in which evidence is strong that hyperbaric oxygen may be of value.

Although hyperbaric chambers are not in many medical centers, the number of chambers in the United States, as well as the number of patients being treated, is growing. Two types of chambers are in use—the monoplace and the multiplace. The monoplace chamber holds only one patient and is compressed with 100% oxygen. The maximal compression depth is approximately 66 feet of sea water. The multiplace chamber can hold multiple patients, as well as staff, with the number dependent on the chamber size. The chamber is compressed with air, and the patients breathe 100% oxygen by mask or hood or by ventilator through an artificial airway. A multiplace chamber can reach a depth of 165 feet of sea water, which is the maximal depth needed to treat decompression sickness (bends) or air embolism.

Hyperbaric oxygen therapy works in many ways to provide its therapeutic effects. The hyperbaric state improves the oxygen-carrying capacity of the blood, possibly improving the oxygenation of ischemic tissue. The increased barometric pressure in the chamber greatly increases the amount of oxygen that is dissolved into plasma. At sea level (1 atmosphere) there is normally 0.3 cc of oxygen dissolved per 100 ml blood; at 3 atm 6 cc of oxygen will be dissolved per 100 ml blood. Thus a low hemoglobin count is compensated by the increased oxygen dissolved in plasma. During treatment, a patient's PaO_2 may be as high as 800 to 2000 mm Hg. As well as increasing oxygen delivery to the tissues, hyperbaric oxygen therapy treatments enhance leukocyte function and cause neovascularization, which is the growth of new blood vessels. All of these processes promote wound healing, especially in diabetic ulcers, osteoradionecrosis (damage and death to tissue and bone as a result of radiation therapy), nonhealing wounds, or traumatic injuries. Further, the increased pressure within the hyperbaric chamber reduces the size of gas emboli, possibly accounting for restoration of blood flow to anoxic areas.

High oxygen levels in the tissues will prevent toxin production and eventually kill bacteria such as *Clostridium perfringens* (gas gangrene). Hyperbaric oxygen therapy also shortens the half-life of carboxyhemoglobin (with carbon monoxide poisoning) and provides sufficient tissue oxygenation for normal aerobic metabolism despite a high carboxyhemoglobin level.

Each disorder treated by hyperbaric oxygen therapy has a specific protocol that uses the Navy's hyperbaric treatment tables to determine depth, time at depth, and decompression time. Most routine treatments such as for wound healing compress or "dive" to 45 to 60 feet of sea water and stay at that depth for approximately 90 to 120 minutes.

The chamber is staffed by specially trained technicians, nurses, and doctors. A well-trained staff is essential because the chamber presents some situations that are unique to the hyperbaric state. The multiplace chamber must always have a technician or a nurse inside with the patient(s). This person is responsible for monitoring the patient, as well as for monitoring those items that are affected by pressure such as air volume in the cuff of an endotracheal tube, intravenous

(IV) drip chambers, and blood pressure cuffs. The physical status of the patient must be closely observed. Problems such as respiratory difficulty, ear pain, decreasing blood sugar (specifically in diabetics), bradycardia, and symptoms of oxygen toxicity may arise that result from the hyperoxic state or from the pressure changes the patient undergoes while in the chamber.

Some risks and adverse effects of hyperbaric oxygen therapy are inherent with the therapy. Barotrauma to the middle ear and paranasal sinuses is probably the most frequently seen problem that occurs when care is not taken to equalize the pressure in these areas during descent. Administering vasoconstrictor sprays or pills may help. Presence of sinus problems or an upper respiratory infection (URI) may preclude diving. Performing bilateral myringotomies may be necessary to prevent ear trauma to a patient who is unable to clear his ears or sinuses, especially when the patient is unconscious.

A major concern during hyperbaric therapy is the development of oxygen toxicity. Hyperbaric oxygen toxicity has some distinguishing features from normal barometric toxicity and is actually an acceleration in the development of various syndromes of normobaric oxygen toxicity. Clinical pulmonary oxygen toxicity is not a threat during hyperbaric oxygen therapy as long as standard Navy hyperbaric treatment tables are used. Central nervous system (CNS) oxygen toxicity is of concern at oxygen partial pressures greater than 3 atm. The effects of CNS toxicity are dose related and almost always reversible. Therefore patients must have air breaks interspersed with breathing the 100% oxygen in a multiplace chamber to prevent oxygen toxicity at depth. Generally, CNS oxygen toxicity is manifested by signs of CNS hyperexcitability, with the most dramatic symptom oxygen convulsion. The seizure may even be the first sign of oxygen toxicity. The treatment of CNS oxygen toxicity includes removal of the oxygen, use of a bite block, seizure precautions, and protection of the patient. Conditions that affect the development of oxygen toxicity at normobaric oxygen levels (see Table 21-2) also apply to the hyperbaric oxygen therapy setting.

Nursing care for patients undergoing hyperbaric therapy. The severity of illness requiring a patient to undergo hyperbaric therapy may range from chronic illness to acute critical illness; thus patients undergoing hyperbaric oxygen therapy may be on any nursing unit within the hospital, including critical care areas. Although not involved in care of the patient undergoing hyperbaric oxygen therapy while in the chamber, it is important that the critical care nursing staff be aware of the precautions taken in the chamber and the unique needs of that patient. Because of the oxygen-enriched environment, there is an increased risk of fire in the chamber; thus certain precautions must be taken. No electricity can be used in the chamber, and specially adapted or battery-operated, pressure-tested equipment such as cardiac monitors and infusion pumps must be used. Further, the pressure in the chamber can affect equipment (for example, by decreasing battery life). While in the chamber, 100% cotton clothing is provided for the patients because it decreases the chance that lint, static electricity, and hydrocarbons will be brought into the chamber. Makeup, hair creams or sprays, skin creams, or any oily substances must be removed before treatment. Perfumes and other odorous compounds should not be used because of the close quarters in the chamber and sharing the same air throughout the treatment.

Any IV bottles that enter the chamber must be plastic or have an air vent. Cuffs or balloons on tubes should be filled with water or saline solution, or they will need adjustment during compression and decompression.

Before therapy, it is advisable for the patient undergoing hyperbaric oxygen therapy to refrain from smoking to decrease irritation to the lungs. Hard contact lenses should be removed, since an air bubble can develop underneath a lens and cause damage to the eye during decompression. If there is any nasal stuffiness or symptoms of upper respiratory infection, the physician should be notified. Some patients will require administration of an antihistamine, decongestant, or vasoconstrictor spray before therapy to prevent barotrauma of the ears or sinuses. Patients should be adequately medicated for pain before therapy so that they will remain comfortable while in the chamber. Light sedation may be required for some patients to decrease the claustrophobic feeling while in the chamber.

Most patients do very well in the hyperbaric chamber, provided they are informed before therapy about the effects of pressure, ear-clearing maneuvers, benefits of the treatments, and the routine. An elevated temperature may preclude hyperbaric therapy because fever increases the chance of developing oxygen toxicity. A fasting blood sugar should also be obtained before therapy if a patient is diabetic, since the hyperbaric treatment may alter the patient's blood sugar.

Patients should refrain from smoking for several hours after a dive, again to decrease lung irritation but also because the high oxygen environment may linger for several hours in a patient's hair or clothing. It is normal for a patient to feel tired after a dive. Temporary visual changes, including blurred vision, may also occur. These and any other untoward symptoms should be reported to the physician.

Most patients requiring hyperbaric oxygen therapy have a chronic medical problem with which they are trying to cope. Their emotional needs are generally quite high, and they require support, understanding, and patience.

ARTIFICIAL AIRWAYS
Endotracheal Intubation

An endotracheal tube is the most commonly used artificial airway for providing short-term airway management. The endotracheal airway may be placed through the orotracheal or nasotracheal route. In most situations involving emergency placement the orotracheal route is used since the approach is simpler and affords use of a larger diameter endotracheal tube.[63,65] Nasotracheal intubation provides greater patient comfort over time and is preferred in situations in which the patient has suffered a jaw fracture or when it is anticipated that the endotracheal tube may be needed for more than 48 hours[51,65] (Tables 21-4 and 21-5).

Indications for endotracheal intubation are as follows: (1) respiratory insufficiency or failure,[63] (2) airway maintenance in patients who develop obstruction despite the presence of a pharyngeal airway,[63] (3) prevention of massive aspiration of stomach contents in a compromised patient, (4) removal of airway secretions,[63] and (5) need to provide a fraction of inspired oxygen (FIO_2) >60% (relative indication).

Endotracheal intubation should not be performed in the alert, conscious patient because of the risk of inducing vomiting; instead, the patient should be sedated to facilitate tube placement. When intubation is elective, neutralization of gastric contents should be undertaken, which can be done by using histamine H_2 receptor antagonists such as cimetidine or clear antacids such as sodium citrate.[40] The intubation process should be limited to less than 45 to 60 seconds. Successful intubation should result in (1) auscultation of breath sounds in both lungs, (2) warm, exhaled air felt at the end of the exhalation port in spontaneously breathing patients, and (3) bilateral movement of the upper chest wall when mechanical ventilation is instituted.

Tube placement should be verified by a chest x-ray. The tip of the endotracheal tube should be 2 cm above the carina to achieve equal bilateral ventilation.[65] After the chest x-ray, tube placement may need adjustment. Once final adjustment of the position is complete, the level of insertion (marked in centimeters on side of tube) should be noted and the tube securely anchored.

Tracheal Intubation

Tracheostomy is a life-saving procedure used only when other choices are not feasible, and it is preferred in patients in whom long-term problems contraindicate the use of an endotracheal tube. The following are indications for its use: (1) to prevent or reverse upper airway obstruction,[39] (2) to prevent aspiration in a patient with anticipated long-term swallowing problems, (3) to facilitate secretion removal in a patient with long-term pulmonary problems,[39] (4) to provide a closed system for mechanical ventilation, (5) for a patient with intolerance for an endotracheal tube, and (6) for a patient in whom passage of endotracheal tube is undesirable or impossible (laryngeal or pharyngeal obstruction).[28]

A tracheostomy provides the best route for long-term airway maintenance and avoids the oral, nasal, pharyngeal, and laryngeal complications of endotracheal intubation.[39,63] The tube is shorter, wider, and less curved than the endotracheal tube; thus the resistance to airflow is less, and breathing is easier. The tracheostomy has other advantages over endotracheal intubation, including (1) easier secretion removal, whether by suctioning or by patient cough, (2) increased patient acceptance and comfort, (3) the possibility of the patient's eating and talking, and (4) the facilitation of ventilator weaning since a tracheostomy tube is easier to breathe through when the patient is off the ventilator (Table 21-6).

Problems Associated with Artificial Airway Placement

Significant problems can be associated with tracheostomy or endotracheal tube placement. The tubes impair the respiratory defense system by bypassing the upper airway system; thus the warming and humidifying of air must be

Table 21-4 Advantages and disadvantages of orotracheal intubation

Advantages	Disadvantages
No surgical procedure required for insertion	Requires skilled person to insert
No damage to nasal passage	May not be well tolerated, requiring more patient sedation
Not associated with sinusitis	More difficult to stabilize than nasotracheal tube
Larger and shorter tube usually used, resulting in less resistance and mucous plugging	May need oral airway to prevent tube biting
Tracheobronchial suctioning easier than through nasotracheal tube	Patient may "tongue out" tube
Easier to pass than nasotracheal tube during an emergency	Impaired oral hygiene
	Cannot be used after major dental or mandibular surgery
	May cause laryngeal damage (vocal cord injury or paralysis) or subglottic stenosis
	Subglottic stenosis
	Patient cannot speak, making communication difficult
	Endobronchial intubation possible

Modified from MacKenzie C: Heart Lung 12(5):485, 1983.

Table 21-5 Advantages and disadvantages of nasotracheal intubation

Advantages	Disadvantages
No surgical procedure required for insertion	Required skilled person to insert
Tube easily fixed	Needs a smaller diameter and longer tube than is used for orotracheal intubation; therefore there is greater resistance, and a fiberoptic bronchoscope may not pass
Well tolerated	
Easy swallowing	Mucus plugging more likely than with orotracheal tube
Less sedation required	Possible sinusitis
Unimpaired oral hygiene	Tracheobronchial suctioning not as effective as through orotracheal tube or tracheostomy
Self-extubation less likely	Cannot be used with nasal cerebrospinal fluid leaks or with sinus or nasal fractures
	Vocal cord injury or paralysis; subglottic stenosis; patient cannot speak, making communication difficult
	Abnormal bleeding times or bleeding abnormalities may preclude use
	Endobronchial intubation possible
	May cause necrosis of intranasal septum

Modified from MacKenzie C: Heart Lung 12(5):485, 1983.

Table 21-6 Advantages and disadvantages of a tracheostomy

Advantages	Disadvantages
No damage to the larynx; no endobronchial intubation	Surgical procedure and anesthesia necessary
Unimpaired oral hygiene and sinus drainage	If extubation occurs during first 24 hours, possibly difficult to reinsert the tube
Speech possible if cuff deflated or speaking attachment used	Possible creation of false passage anterior to trachea in patients with thick necks
Minimal resistance from short, wide tube and little mucous plugging during ventilation	Possible tearing of posterior tracheal membrane during tracheostomy tube insertion
Suctioning easier and more effective	Erosion of innominate artery with tip of tube or with low tracheostomy stoma
Better tolerated than orotracheal and nasotracheal tubes	Increased likelihood of infection
Easily stabilized	Possible ugly scar or persistent tracheocutaneous fistula after healing
In spontaneously breathing patient, easy attachment of ventilator if acute respiratory distress occurs	
After 48 hours, replacement of accidentally extubated tube by nonanesthesiologist without use of sedation or muscle relaxants	

Modified from MacKenzie C: Heart Lung 12(5):485, 1983.

performed by external means. Cleansing or filtering the air is not feasible, but suctioning and tracheostomy care remove some particles. There is great potential for tracheobronchial tree infection after the placement of an artificial airway.[39] Studies show that once an artificial airway is placed, contamination of the lower airways will follow within 24 hours.[28,50,63] This results from colonization of the lower airways with bacteria commonly found in the upper airways. The patient's general condition and the presence or absence of pulmonary trauma or disease significantly affect the likelihood that an infection will ensue.

Other consequences of artificial airway placement include an altered body image and loss of independence. Nutrition is impaired during the acute stage of airway placement because of loss of oral feeding. Supplemental enteral or parenteral nutrition is mandatory. Verbal communication is impaired until the trachea can be plugged or a talking trach is inserted. Endotracheal tubes preclude talking; further, tube movement when patients attempt to talk increases local irritation and should be discouraged. Careful attention must be given to minimize tracheal damage resulting from tube movement. Flexible mounts and swivels should be used to lessen the transmission of ventilator tube movement to the airway. The patient's tracheal tube requires adequate support during turning, positioning, and suctioning. When necessary, sedation should be used to control prolonged coughing, agitation, or uncontrolled movements.[39]

Types of Airway Tubes Available

Many different materials and tube styles have been used through the years. Most tubes are made of a plastic material and have an inflatable cuff attached. Tube materials are constantly evaluated in a search for a substance that is non-irritating and flexible, sheds secretions, and is stable in the body. Some currently available tubes include these characteristics, and each generation of development results in progress toward an ideal design and substance.

Metal tubes have been used for many years and are still made of sterling silver or silver plate. Because of their inflexibility, patient discomfort, and the high risk of associated pressure necrosis and because metal stimulates mucus production and tissue irritation, they are no longer widely used. If used, metal tubes are generally used for the patient with a permanent tracheostomy after laryngectomy. Polyvinyl chloride (PVC) is used most often for endotracheal tubes because it has a low tissue toxicity factor and is pliable at body temperatures. Silastic (silicone rubber) tubes have gained popularity because of their relatively low tissue toxicity and their flexibility and because they can be autoclaved. However, Silastic tubes are expensive, and PVC tubes are more often used in short-term situations. Nylon tubes are rigid but lightweight and are easily cleaned; however, the material can be irritating to the mucous membranes and also breaks down in moist heat. Generally, synthetic tube materials (1) have a longer shelf life than rubber, (2) are softer than metal and therefore less traumatic, (3) weigh less than metal tubes, (4) conduct less heat or cold than metal tubes, (5) can be cut to length, and (6) have a strong cuff-to-tube attachment.

Tracheostomy tubes may be single-lumen or double-lumen tubes. Single-lumen tubes consist of two parts: (1) the tube and a built-in cuff, which is connected to an air line for inflation purposes, and (2) an obturator, which is used during tube insertion. The double-lumen tubes consist of the tube with the attached cuff, the obturator, and an inner cannula that can be removed for cleaning and reinserted or, if disposable, replaced by a new sterile inner cannula. The inner cannula can be quickly removed if it becomes obstructed, making the system safer for patients with significant secretion problems. Debate exists about the need for the inner cannula because of the development of newer tube materials and improved humidification systems. These advances decrease secretion adherence to the inside of the tube and may eliminate the need for a removable inner cannula. Single-lumen tubes provide a larger inside diameter for air flow than double-lumen tubes, thus reducing air-flow resistance and allowing the patient to ventilate through the tube with greater ease.

Artificial Airway Cuffs

The cuff on an airway tube is a small balloonlike device that is attached or built into the bottom section of the tube. When inflated, it prevents leakage of inhaled air past the tube into the upper airway; thus a closed system is maintained during cuff inflation. When the patient is mechanically ventilated and, in most cases, during and after feeding, the cuff should be inflated. At other times, unless indicated, it should be deflated.

Cuff performance characteristics are critical. Ideally, the cuff should gently conform to the trachea without permitting significant air leakage past it during ventilation. The cuff should inflate evenly, center itself in the trachea, allow intracuff pressure monitoring, and provide a system to indicate when it is inflated or deflated. The most common complication of cuffed airway tubes results from pressure exerted against the tracheal wall by the cuff. Pressure >20 to 30 mm Hg can break down the trachea if exerted over a significant period of time.[5] Cuff pressures >50 mm Hg can destroy the outer lining of the trachea if maintained more than 15 minutes.[5,42] Cuffs on endotracheal and tracheostomy tubes are of two types—high pressure–low volume cuffs (hard cuffs) and low pressure–high volume cuffs (soft cuffs).

Hard cuffs (first generation) were the first developed and are the least satisfying. When a hard cuff is filled, it exerts a pressure against the tracheal wall greater than the capillary filling pressure of the trachea, leading to necrosis. A hard cuff can exert pressure in excess of 300 mm Hg against the trachea.[50] The tracheal capillary filling pressure is approximately 30 mm Hg, venous pressure is approximately 18 mm Hg, and lymphatic pressure is 5 mm Hg.[5,50] This means that when a cuff is filled, arterial circulation and venous and lymphatic drainage virtually cease in that area.

Soft cuffs (second generation) are designed to seal the trachea at a pressure minimal enough to allow capillary filling at the site of cuff inflation. When properly filled, a soft cuff exerts <30 mm Hg pressure against the surrounding trachea. Soft cuffs (high volume) are larger than hard cuffs when filled and distribute their volume throughout more of the trachea, thus effecting a seal at a lower pressure. Recently, high volume–low pressure cuffs have been further refined to thinner cuff walls and smaller diameters. These third generation cuffs reduce the contact area of the trachea and eliminate the folds and invaginations of second generation cuffs that lead to aspiration.[50]

The following example illustrates the advantage of a soft cuff over a hard cuff. Assume that to seal a patient's trachea it takes an air volume of 3 cc. Two balloons are available— one with a 3-cc capacity and one with a 10-cc capacity. The first balloon will seal the trachea only when it is fully inflated. The second balloon will seal the trachea when it is partially inflated. A partially inflated balloon feels "soft"; a fully inflated balloon feels "hard." This is, in effect, the difference between the two types of airway cuffs.

A hard cuff does not conform to the natural contours of the trachea; in fact, it forces the trachea to conform to its shape. A soft cuff conforms to the natural contour, thus causing less tracheal distortion.

When a patient is ventilated mechanically, inflation of the cuff should be done by the "minimal occlusion" technique; with the cuff inflated, air is removed in 0.2-cc amounts until an air leak can be heard or felt. The cuff is then reinflated with 0.2 cc of air until the inspiratory leak stops, as determined by listening with a stethoscope placed over the larynx. This is the best assurance that the cuff is not overinflated and the patient is protected from aspiration. The respiratory therapist should assist with or perform cuff inflation. Overfilling a cuff is of no value and is a great detriment to the patient, as demonstrated by Snowberger.[52] If the trachea is sealed at 3 cc, instilling additional volume will not improve the seal; it will only increase the pressure in the cuff, potentially damaging the trachea. The object of cuff inflation is to place the minimal amount of air in the cuff that will allow sealing of the airway and prevent aspiration.[50,52]

One cuff on the market, made of foam, is self-inflating. It is deflated during tube insertion, after which the air line is opened to room air and the cuff self-inflates. It maintains a constant pressure of 20 mm Hg.[5] Removal can be complicated if the plastic sheath covering the form is perforated. When perforation occurs, the foam may not be deflatable because the air cannot be totally aspirated. Other cuff systems are designed to maintain constant pressure, not exceeding 20 to 25 mm Hg during peak inhalation and exhalation. In a 1985 study, Bernhard and others[5] found that three cuffed endotracheal tubes (NCC hi-lo, Portex Profile XL, and Sheridan HVT) achieved low pressures (<25 mm Hg). The Bivona Fome-cuff and NCC hi-lo were two tracheostomy tube cuffs that achieved pressures <20 mm Hg in Bernhard's study.[5]

Each airway tube's size in millimeters is recorded on the outside edge of the tube. It is important for the physician to select the correct size tube for the dimensions of the patient's trachea. Should the tube be too small, the volume of air needed in the cuff for a proper seal may lead to tracheal damage. A common rule is that the tube should be approximately two thirds the inside diameter of the trachea.[65] To accommodate secretion removal and breathing, the tube should be as large as possible without exceeding the two-thirds rule.

Complications Resulting from Use of Artificial Airways

Tracheal damage from cuff pressure is a frequent complication of endotracheal or tracheal intubation. Research studies have demonstrated superficial lesions occurring less than 12 hours after tube placement, with more severe erosion occurring over time.[63] Mackenzie[39] summarized the factors that precipitate laryngotracheal damage and the complications seen in artificial airways (Table 21-7). The box on p. 455 outlines general measures that can be taken to decrease the complications of intubation.

Tracheal necrosis. Cuffed artificial airway tubes that have been in place as few as 3 to 5 days have caused early necrosis in the tracheal cartilage.[52] When this necrosis occurs in the posterior tracheal mucosa, a tracheoesophageal fistula results. The fistula allows air to escape into the stomach, causing distention. It also allows gastric aspiration of stomach contents into the trachea. This complication occurs more commonly when both an artificial airway and a standard size nasogastric tube are present. Using small gastric feeding tubes decreases chances of formation of tracheoesophageal fistula.

Anterior wall tracheal necrosis may cause erosion of the tracheal tube into the innominate artery, a rare but life-threatening complication.[42] It is suspected when a pulsating tracheostomy tube is observed or if bright red blood is expelled. Immediate intervention is necessary since exsanguination can occur. Continuous bleeding through a tracheostomy tube may be an early sign of innominate artery erosion, and it should be evaluated by the physician.

Tracheal dilation. A prolonged intubation period may allow pressure from an artificial airway cuff to distort and dilate the tracheal wall. Suspicions should arise when increasing amounts of cuff air are needed to create a seal or when bulging of the tracheal wall is seen at the cuff site on an x-ray.

Tracheal stenosis. Tracheal stenosis is a narrowing of the trachea that occurs 1 week to 2 years after endotracheal intubation or tracheostomy. It results from healing of the inflamed area in which the tube cuff was located.

Stenosis is more common with a tracheostomy than with an endotracheal intubation, with the incidence 65% and 19%, respectively.[28,52,65] Symptoms occur when 50% or more of the tracheal diameter is reduced and include dyspnea, loss of exercise tolerance, stridor, and recurrent pulmonary infections. The severity of stenosis can be reduced by tube choice, maintenance of proper cuff pressure, using shorter intubation periods, and prevention of respiratory infection and excessive tube movement.[63]

Infections. Tracheostomy requires an open incision into the trachea, which is associated with risk of wound infection and possible sepsis. Aseptic care of the site and proper suction technique reduce the infection risks.

Airway obstruction. Airway obstruction is a potential complication associated with the kinking of an endotracheal tube, secretion buildup, or slippage of a soft cuff over the end of the artificial airway. If obstruction is suspected, repositioning the patient's head, neck, or tube should be attempted. Other methods to reduce the obstruction include deflating the cuff, attempting to pass a suction catheter, or

Table 21-7 Factors that predispose damage to the airways by artificial tubes

General factors	Site-specific factors
Duration of intubation Duration of mechanical ventilation Inadequate patient sedation Repeated flexion and extension of the neck Decerebrate or decorticate movements Patient out of phase with controlled mechanical ventilation ("bucking" the ventilator) Traction on the tube during turning, suctioning, and ventilator connection and disconnection Previous prolonged intubation Chronic airway or lung disease (especially sputum-producing disease) requiring frequent suctioning procedures Airway infection Hypotension	**LARYNGEAL** Multiple orotracheal or nasotracheal intubations Inexperienced laryngoscopist, an emergency intubation, or self-extubation Too large a translaryngeal tube Tube material **TRACHEAL** Cuff overinflation Combination of high positive end-expiratory pressure (PEEP) and low lung compliance Too small or large a cuff in relation to the tracheal size Noncircular cross-sectional tracheal shape Cuff material

Modified from MacKenzie C: Heart Lung 12(5):485, 1983.

NURSING INTERVENTIONS TO MINIMIZE TRACHEAL DAMAGE RESULTING FROM ARTIFICIAL AIRWAY PLACEMENT

- Stabilize the tube as much as possible to prevent movement within the larynx.
- Avoid frequent retaping since this involves unnecessary manipulation of tube.
- Note the depth of the tube at placement and periodically thereafter to avoid displacement.
- Avoid overinflation of the cuff—maintain pressure <25 mm Hg.
- Do not engage in periodic deflation or inflation of cuff.
- Do not use high pressure–low volume cuffs; use only high volume–low pressure cuffs.
- When nasotracheal intubation is present, inspect nares every day for signs of septal ischemia.
- Provide frequent mouth cleansing to decrease infection.
- Take measures to avoid traumatic extubation by patient (sedate or restrain).
- Follow strict aseptic technique when giving artificial airway care and when suctioning (use proper universal blood and body secretion precautions; gloves, and goggles should be worn by the nurse(s)).
- Avoid excessive negative pressure during suctioning; use only amount necessry to remove secretions (keep below 120 mm Hg).
- Support ventilator tubing to avoid traction on the patient's airway tube.
- Take measures to avoid excessive movement by patient (i.e., repeated flexion and extension of head, coughing, chewing, tonguing the tube).

removing the inner cannula. If none of the maneuvers are successful and the patient cannot breathe through the tube, it must be removed.

Subcutaneous emphysema. Subcutaneous emphysema, or mediastinal emphysema, occurs when air escapes from the tracheostomy incision into the tissues, dissects fascial planes under the skin, and accumulates around the face, neck, and throat. These areas may then appear puffy, and slight finger pressure reveals a crackling sensation (crepitation) under the skin where the air is present. Subcutaneous emphysema can occur immediately after the tracheostomy tube is inserted or anytime later, particularly if the tube is too short. Generally, this is not a serious complication because the air will eventually be reabsorbed. Rarely, mediastinal subcutaneous emphysema is associated with pneumothorax.

Other known complications are presented in the box on p. 456.

AIRWAY MANAGEMENT
Humidification

Humidification of air is normally performed by the mucosal layer of the upper respiratory tract. When this area is bypassed such as occurs in endotracheal intubation and tracheostomy or when supplemental oxygen is used, humidification by external means is necessary. Various humidification devices add water to inhaled gas to prevent drying and irritation of the respiratory tract, to prevent undue loss of body water, and to facilitate secretion removal by expectoration or by suctioning.

Bubble diffusion humidifiers are commonly used to provide moisture to inhaled gas. They may be warm or cold humidifiers. With a cold humidifier, the gas diffuses out of a stem submerged in water. The gas breaks into small bubbles and vaporizes. At room temperature, the gas provides only approximately 50% of the humidification needed by

---

COMPLICATIONS OF ARTIFICIAL AIRWAYS

TUBE (OROTRACHEAL AND NASOTRACHEAL)-RELATED COMPLICATIONS

Trauma during insertion
Sinusitis (nasotracheal)
Supraglottic and epiglottic edema
Laryngeal unlcerations or granuloma
Inability to vocalize
Vocal cord paralysis or immobility
Laryngitis, stridor, or hoarseness on extubation
Subglottic stenosis
Tracheal erosion from the tip of the tube
Tracheal granuloma
Endobronchial intubation
Airway infection
Necrosis of nasal septum (nasotracheal)
Pneumothorax[47]
Posterior laryngeal abscess with obstruction[48]

TRACHEOSTOMY STOMAL COMPLICATIONS

Incorrect position—too low, too high, or not in midline
Surgical complications during and after stomal creation
Rupture of the posterior tracheal membrane during insertion of the tracheostomy tube through the stoma
False passage of the tube into the subcutaneous tissue anterior to the tracheal stoma
Innominate artery erosion from an incorrectly positioned stoma or erosion from the tip of the tracheostomy tube
Persistent fistula or scarring on healing
Stenosis at the level of the stoma because of granuloma formation
Infection

CUFF-RELATED COMPLICATIONS

Trauma during insertion through larynx or during accidental extubation (orotracheal and nasotracheal)
Tracheal wall erosion
Tracheomalacia
Tracheoesophageal fistula
Tracheal stenosis
Tracheal granuloma
Tracheitis
Cuff leak with loss of airway seal, leading to inadequate ventilation
Aspiration past an improperly sized or inflated cuff

---

the body; hence this method of humidification can lead to drying and irritation of mucous membranes when used for a significant time period. Diffusion humidifiers are unable to adequately humidify gas at higher rates of flow, making them more suitable for low-flow oxygen delivery over short time spans. Cold humidifiers are relatively simple and reliable devices and are available as disposable units, thus decreasing maintenance time and eliminating potential infections associated with reusable equipment.

Warm humidifiers provide better humidification than cold humidifiers since warm humidification supplies heat as well as moisture and breaks gas into smaller particles at higher flow rates. Heated cascade humidifiers are preferred for use with intubated patients since 100% humidification of inhaled gas can be assured.

Aerosol Therapy

An aerosol is a liquid particle suspended in a gas. Often, distilled water or saline solutions are used as the liquid aerosol, but other solutions may be used. The inhalation of aerosols increases secretion clearance and liquifies mucus, but continuous administration of water aerosol can lead to water retention and fluid overload. Aerosol therapy should be used cautiously in patients with heart failure, respiratory distress, or decreased ability to clear secretions.

The effects of aerosols on the respiratory tract are dependent on the level into which the aerosol penetrates the lungs. Penetration is related to particle size so that particles >30 μm in diameter are deposited in the upper airway, whereas particles <5 μm can reach the smaller airways.[26]

The patient's breathing pattern can affect penetration. Slower breathing will result in more fallout deposition in the upper airways, whereas larger tidal volumes and mouth breathing can encourage deeper aerosol penetration.[26] Aerosol deposition increases with momentary breath holding at peak inhalation.

Aerosols are cleared from the lungs by the mucociliary blanket or by phagocytosis. Nebulizers are used to deliver aerosols to many patients with a respiratory disease involving mucus production. Nebulizers are classified by power source, aerosol production, and water production. The two most commonly used nebulizers are the jet nebulizer and the ultrasonic nebulizer. They have a potential for becoming a source of bacterial contamination of the respiratory tract and require a careful program of disinfection between patient use.

Suctioning

Tracheal suctioning is a method of clearing secretions from the airways and is performed through an artificial airway (endotracheal or tracheal tube) either nasotracheally or orotracheally. Suctioning through the oral or nasal passages is difficult and is limited to clearance of the upper airway.

Tracheal suctioning is a frequently performed procedure for removing secretions from the trachea in patients with a compromised cough reflex. It involves the use of sterile technique and is performed in a manner that is effective yet minimizes associated complications (see the box, "Complications of Tracheal Suctioning"). Although no standard procedure exists, certain common techniques of tracheal suctioning are described in the literature and include the following: (1) preoxygenation of the patient,[3,13,16,46,51] (2) use of sterile, disposable suction trays equipped with gloves, catheter, and solution, (3) limiting the suctioning period to 15 seconds or less, (4) periodic instillation of sterile saline solution to liquify secretions, and (5) wearing masks and goggles as part of universal precaution techniques. Three

---

COMPLICATIONS OF TRACHEAL SUCTIONING

HYPOXEMIA

Suctioning removes oxygen from the airways and may lead to hypoxemia. Hypoxemia can be minimized by preoxygenation and by keeping the wall suction pressure as low as possible while still allowing effective mucus removal. Many techniques of preoxygenation exist—manual resuscitator bagging, ventilator sighing, and providing a ventilator with regular tidal volume. Currently hyperinflation (1½ times the usual tidal volume) and high FIo_2 (0.6-1.0) are recommended for the ventilator-dependent patient. Manual resuscitator bagging may not deliver an FIo_2 of 1.0.[13]

TRAUMATIC AIRWAY ULCERATION

Traumatic airway is directly related to the amount of wall suction pressure used. The wall suction should be set at a level that allows easy removal of secretions but not so high that trauma to the airways is induced. Suction should be kept below 120 mm Hg. Excessively high suction does not mean better secretion clearance.

CARDIAC DYSRHYTHMIAS

Cardiac dysrhythmias include premature ventricular contractions, tachycardia, bradycardia, and sudden death. The dysrhythmias result from hypoxemia and/or vagal receptor stimulation that can occur with suctioning. Preoxygenation may lessen dysrhythmia formation. The cardiac monitor should be observed during suctioning, and suctioning should be interrupted if significant dysrhythmias occur (as per unit protocol).

BRONCHOSPASMS

Bronchospasms are associated with catheter irritation of the tracheal membranes and with coughing,; use of bronchodilators may be effective.

INFECTION

Infection is related to placement of an artificial airway and/or a break in sterile technique while suctioning.

ATELECTASIS

Atelectasis is created by excessive wall suction pressure and/or by suctioning too long and/or by using a catheter too large. The suction catheter should be no greater than one half of the internal diameter of the tracheal tube, and wall suction should be kept at the lowest level (<120 mm Hg) that will still support effective suctioning.

---

of these practices require further scrutiny to apply a suctioning technique based on tested clinical rationale.

Preoxygentation. Hypoxemia is a serious side effect of tracheal suctioning and, if not minimized, can lead to tissue hypoxia. Many studies have explored ways to lessen hypoxia associated with tracheal suctioning. Barnes and Kirchhoff[3] concluded that preoxygenation should be provided to all ventilated patients and that the methodology used to provide oxygen should be tailored to the patient's clinical situation, whether by hyperinflation, hyperventilation, hyperoxygenation, or insufflation (see the box on p. 458). They further concluded that spontaneously breathing patients may require only a few breaths of room air or supplemental oxygen before suctioning and that no single procedure is beneficial for all patients.

Preventing hypoxemia has also led to the development of suctioning equipment and techniques that avoid removing the patient from ventilator support. This is referred to as closed system suctioning. The benefits include maintaining pressure ventilation, maintaining oxygenation, and continuation of positive end-expiratory pressure (PEEP).[49,57] Care must be taken to ensure that proper ventilator settings are selected to prevent negative airway pressure from occurring during closed system suctioning, leading to mucosal injury and airway collapse.[57] Carlon, Fox and Ackerman[10] found no clinically significant improvement of oxygenation results when they compared closed and open suction methods.

Since closed suction systems are many times more expensive than regular systems, cost effectiveness should be considered when deciding about generalized use, as should the fact that closed suction systems prevent dissemination of contaminated secretions—an important factor when choosing equipment and technique.

Duration of suctioning. The effect of limiting the duration of suctioning is not as clear-cut as it once seemed. Medical personnel have been admonished to limit suctioning to 10-second periods, but some studies have indicated little change in the fall of the Pao_2 after the initial 5 seconds of suctioning, even when periods ranging from 10 to 45 seconds in duration were used.[3] Recent advances in fiberoptic pulmonary catheters allow continuous measurements of mixed venous oxygen saturations; when available, the effects of suctioning duration can be readily monitored, allowing moment-to-moment variation of suctioning time. When mixed venous oxygen saturation monitoring is unavailable, oximetry can be used, even though its response to changes in oxygenation is somewhat delayed.

Saline solution instillation. One practice commonly used to manage tenacious secretions is the instillation of 2 to 5 ml of sterile saline solution through an artificial airway into the tracheobronchial tree. Hanley[25] found normal saline solution instillations resulted in an unpredictable distribution of saline solution within the lungs and that blind suctioning removed little of the instilled saline solution from the airways. Because mucus and saline solution do not easily mix, instilling saline solution acts more as a lavage.[51] The concept of bronchial lavage during suctioning has further been explored by Muto.[43] He also found saline solution injected at the opening of the endotracheal or tracheostomy tube did not result in liquefying secretions and was not all retrieved

TECHNIQUES TO PREVENT HYPOXEMIA RESULTING FROM SUCTIONING

INSUFFLATION

Insufflation refers to supplemental oxygen delivered by a double-lumen suctioning catheter or by the side arm on the endotracheal or tracheal adapter. It provides simultaneous oxygen delivery during suctioning.

HYPEROXYGENATION

Hyperoxygenation refers to increasing the fraction of inspired oxygen (FIO_2), usually to 100%, before, during, and after suctioning. This may be achieved by turning the ventilator oxygen setting to 100% or by using a resuscitation bag to provide the patient with 100% oxygen. If increasing the oxygen is accomplished by changing the ventilator setting, sufficient time must elapse to achieve that oxygen concentration in the system. The time lapse varies with the type of ventilator used.

HYPERINFLATION

Hyperinflation refers to increasing the patient's tidal volume, usually by 150%. This can be achieved by using the sigh component of the ventilator or by using some resuscitation bags. When the patient is being ventilated at high tidal volumes, regular resuscitation bags may not be able to provide the volume necessary to achieve hyperinflation. Hyperinflation does not refer to changes in FIO_2, although increasing the FIO_2 frequently accompanies hyperinflation.

HYPERVENTILATION

Hyperventilation refers to an increase in ventilatory rate without necessarily changing the tidal volume or oxygen level delivered.

SUCTIONING GUIDELINES

1. Determine if suctioning is warranted by evaluating the patient for the presence of Jacquette's 15 symptoms; six indicate suctioning is necessary.
2. Always use universal precautions against contamination by blood and body fluids. Use gloves, goggles, and a mask when performing or assisting with suctioning.
3. Preoxygenate all ventilated patients and at-risk patients when planning to suction (methodology remains controversial), and, when possible, monitor patient's oxygenation status through continuous mixed venous display or oximetry, altering supplemental oxygen technique according to results.
4. Use sterile disposable equipment for each suctioning procedure. Choose catheter size one half the internal diameter of the artificial tube. When possible, use a closed-suction system to avoid removing the patient from the ventilator, especially when postive end-expiratory pressure (PEEP) modality is in use. Newer generation ventilators allow preoxygenation with 100% oxygen and hyperinflation by selecting special functions.
5. Use the lowest amount of wall suction pressure necessary to remove secretions.
6. Base the duration of each suctioning pass on the necessity of secretion removal and the displayed oxygen levels (mixed venous or oximetry). Fewer passes may be less detrimental to oxygenation and less damaging to mucosa than many short-duration suctioning attempts.
7. Suction secretions in the oropharynx and from the top of the tube cuff after tracheal suctioning is complete.
8. Stop suctioning if bradycardia occurs, and provide supplemental oxygenation. Reevaluate the patient for need of suctioning before reinstituting procedure. Evaluate the effectiveness of the preoxygenation routine used.
9. Interrupt suctioning if ventricular ectopy occurs or increases, and provide supplemental oxygen before reinstituting the suction procedure.
10. Interrupt suctioning if the saturated arterial oxygen (Sao_2) drops below 85%, and provide supplemental oxygen until the Sao_2 returns to more than 90%.
11. No set approach suits every patient situation; vary the suctioning procedure according to the clinical response of the patient.

by regular suctioning methods. In an attempt to improve suctioning technique, he developed Irri-Cath™, a double-lumen catheter that irrigates and suctions simultaneously.[43] Muto and his colleagues have used this technique on intubated patients at Massachusetts General Hospital and believe the Irri-Cath reduces the tracheobronchial irritation associated with suctioning, significantly decreases the incidence of bronchoscopy for retained secretions, and speeds the recovery of patients who have secretion problems.[43] This technique has not been widely adopted as of this writing, and further investigation by other practitioners is needed to determine its efficacy versus that of saline solution instillations.

Suctioning guidelines. The use of suctioning can be hazardous in unstable critically ill patients. Factors that signal a higher risk for side effects from suctioning are the presence of a PaO_2 <70 mm Hg, a wide alveolar to arterial (A-a) gradient, and shock, dysrhythmias, or acid-base imbalances (see the following box for suctioning guidelines).

Since, at best, no clear procedure exists to eliminate the hazards of tracheal suctioning, the procedure should be performed only when necessary. Routine suctioning should be avoided because it increases respiratory tract trauma, stimulates secretion production, increases the risk of infection, and exposes the patient to other complications previously outlined.

MECHANICAL VENTILATION

Mechanical ventilation is used to treat hypoxemia and tissue hypoxia, to maintain positive pressure in the airways throughout the respiratory cycle, to lessen the work of breathing, and to provide ventilation for patients who cannot, themselves, effectively ventilate. The most common indication for mechanical ventilation is impending or actual acute ventilatory failure defined as an arterial partial pressure of carbon dioxide ($PaCO_2$) >50 mm Hg with a pH less than 7.25. Reversal of this process is desired while minimizing the complications of mechanical ventilation. Mechanical ventilators work through either negative or positive pressure applied to the chest.

Negative Pressure Ventilators

Negative pressure ventilators were the first type developed. The iron lung, or tank ventilator, fits over the patient's entire body except for his or her head and generates a negative pressure gradient that moves air into the lung. These ventilators prohibit access to the patient and are not practical for this reason. However, negative pressure therapy can benefit patients with (1) hypoventilation caused by mechanical (chest wall or neuromuscular) abnormalities, (2) hypoventilation caused by central respiratory system abnormalities, and (3) hypoxemic respiratory failure.[6]

Some of the benefits of negative pressure ventilation include the following[6]:

* Avoidance of an artificial airway—especially advantageous when long-term ventilation is needed

* Improved arterial oxygenation in spontaneously breathing adults with progressive pulmonary disease
* Decreased need for sedation and muscle relaxants
* Decreased work of breathing when used as intermittent therapy
* Alternative to electrophrenic pacing for some patients with primary alveolar hypoventilation

Positive Pressure Ventilators

Positive pressure ventilators achieve lung inflation by applying intermittent positive pressure ventilation (IPPV) or continuous positive pressure ventilation (CPPV) to the airway. This requires a relatively airtight seal between the patient and the ventilator, which is usually achieved by a balloon-cuffed tracheal or endotracheal tube. Positive pressure ventilators may be subdivided into volume-cycled, pressure-cycled, and time-cycled machines. Some newer generation ventilators can vary the cycling mechanism.

Volume ventilators are designed to deliver a preset volume of gas to the patient. The machine can deliver the volume of gas despite changes in pressure within the patient's lungs. To avoid barotrauma to the lungs, pressure limits can be programmed into the ventilator. When the pressure limit is exceeded, the ventilator will "spill" the remaining volume of gas out of the system, but barring this situation, the ventilator will deliver the set volume throughout considerable pressure ranges.

Pressure ventilators deliver gas until a preset pressure is reached; thus the volume delivered varies when the pressure

Table 21-8 Types of high-frequency ventilation (HFV)

Type of HFV	Apparatus	Rate	Physiological mechanism	Uses
High-frequency positive pressure ventilation (HFPPV)	Pneumatic valve	50-150 breaths per minute (bpm)	Convection Augmented, facilitated, or enhanced diffusion	Laryngoscopy Bronchoscopy Neonates and infants during surgical procedures and in the postoperative period Some types of thoracic surgery Adults and infants in respiratory failure. Neonates with hyaline membrane disease
High-frequency jet ventilation (HFJV)	Solenoid or fluidic-controlled ventilator	100-1000 bpm Gas delivered under 10-50 lb of pressure per square inch	Convection Augmented, facilitated, or enhanced diffusion Central cone of advancing jet stream reaches the conducting airways	Laryngoscopy Bronchopleural fistula Tracheal reconstruction (stenosis) Acute respiratory failure
High-frequency oscillation (HFO)	Oscillating mechanism: piston-driven or radio loudspeaker	180-2400 cycles per minute (3-40 Hz units)	Coaxial flow associated with laminar flow	Neonates with severe respiratory distress syndrome

From Gruden M: Crit Care Nurs 5(1):37, 1985.

within the patient's lungs increases or decreases for any reason. Pressure ventilators are not useful for ventilation of critically ill patients because pressure ventilators do not adapt well to changes in lung compliance and resistance. Also, many pressure-cycled ventilators cannot deliver positive end-expiratory pressure (PEEP), limiting their application.

Time-cycled ventilators deliver gas during a preset time interval. They are less popular because of the difficulty in delivering consistent tidal volumes in the presence of changing respiratory dynamics.

Newer generation ventilators are equipped with computers, internal mechanisms that allow the choice of various modes of ventilation, and built-in features that provide continuous compliance measurements and display of volume pressure curves. Most modern ventilators allow application of various modes of therapy and fine adjustment of inspired

oxygen. Oxygen delivery can vary precisely from 21% (room air) to 100%.

High-frequency ventilation, a new addition to the positive pressure family, delivers small tidal volumes at a high ventilatory rate in an effort to reduce the barotrauma and the cardiac complications associated with normal-frequency mechanical ventilation. Three systems have evolved using high-frequency ventilation—high-frequency jet ventilation, high-frequency positive pressure ventilation, and high-frequency oscillation (Table 21-8).

Modes of Application

The term ventilator mode refers to how the machine ventilates for the patient. Selection of a particular mode of ventilation determines how much the patient will participate in his own ventilatory pattern (see the box, "Modes of Mechanical Ventilation"). Choice depends on the patient's sit-

---

MODES OF MECHANICAL VENTILATION

CONTROLLED MECHANICAL VENTILATION (CMV)

Delivery of a preset number of breaths per minute at a preset volume. Breathing cannot be triggered by the patient. *Use:* apneic patient secondary to brain damage, muscle paralysis, sedation.

ASSISTED MECHANICAL VENTILATION (AMV)

Ventilator triggered by the patient's inspiratory effort. Patient controls the rate of breathing while the ventilator controls the tidal volume (V_T) and performs the work. The patient continues to perform a significant amount of the work of breathing (WOB) rather than passively inhaling; excessive inspiratory effort can occur.

ASSIST-CONTROL VENTILATION (ACV)

Delivery of a breath triggered by the inspiratory effort of the patient after a preselected time interval has elapsed. A back-up rate is set, which will support the patient if his respiratory efforts fall below the set ventilator rate. *Use:* wide range of patients who are spontaneously breathing but who have ventilatory failure or gas exchange inefficiency.

INTERMITTENT MANDATORY VENTILATION (IMV) AND SYNCHRONIZED INTERMITTENT MANDATORY VENTILATION (SIMV)

Receipt by spontaneously breathing patient of periodic positive pressure breaths at a selected rate. SIMV is a modification that synchronizes the mechanical breath and patient's spontaneous breathing. *Uses:* wide range of patients with need for ventilator support and as a method of systematic weaning.

PRESSURE SUPPORT VENTILATION (PSV)

Also called inspiratory flow assistance. To decrease the WOB, PSV combines the features of assisted ventila-

tion and continuous positive airway pressure (CPAP). When triggered, the ventilator applies a small amount of positive pressure to the airways. It is intended to overcome resistance and thereby decrease the WOB, improve mixed venous oxygen saturation (Sv_{O_2}), and lower minute ventilation ($\dot{V}_E$), respiratory rate, and oxygen consumption ($\dot{V}_{O_2}$). *Uses:* spontaneously breathing patient and weaning.[42]

PRESSURE-CONTROLLED INVERTED RATIO VENTILATION (PC-IRV) AND INVERSE INSPIRATORY TO EXPIRATORY VENTILATION (IVR)

Also called prolonged inspiratory time ventilation. *Uses:* inspiratory:expiratory (I:E) ratios as high as 3:1 or 4:1 in treating hypoxemic patients not responding to other mechanical ventilatory forms; adult respiratory distress syndrome (ARDS); limited study—still considered experimental.

DIFFERENTIAL LUNG VENTILATION (DLV)

Also known as independent lung ventilation and selective PEEP. A modified technique of one-lung ventilation is used in surgery. DLV requires intubation with a double-lumen endotracheal tube (Carlen, Ravanian, Robertshaw, Univent, or Broncho-cath) and allows establishment of separate ventilator parameters for each lung. It can be arranged by using (1) one ventilator with adjustable circuits, (2) two asynchronous ventilators independently delivering ventilation, (3) two synchronized ventilators using separate circuits, (4) one volume ventilator and one high-frequency ventilator, (5) two CPAP circuits, or (6) one ventilator and one CPAP circuit. *Uses:* severe unilateral asymmetric lung disease such as in patients with trauma, bronchopleural fistula, pneumonia, or an aspiration lung disorder.[42]

uation, as well as the personal biases and experiences of the clinicians.

Intermittent mandatory ventilation (IMV) has many advocates. This mode allows the spontaneously breathing patient to continue breathing while the ventilator periodically gives a selected breath. Proponents of IMV argue that it reduces the need for muscle paralysis and sedation, prevents a patient's "bucking" the ventilator, and achieves a more normal ventilation/perfusion (V/Q) matching.

IMV may relieve the detrimental reduction in cardiac output associated with positive pressure ventilation. This is more likely true if the patient is not exposed to significant increases in the work of breathing as a result of IMV. Synchronized intermittent mandatory ventilation (SIMV) was developed to prevent "stacking" of respirations, which could occur when random periodic breaths were given by the ventilator to spontaneously breathing patients. The SIMV system depends on a demand valve, which senses a fall in airway pressure as the patient begins to inhale and opens to allow spontaneous inhalation. Some demand valves require

---

DEFINITIONS OF BASIC VENTILATOR SETTINGS

RESPIRATORY RATE

Number of breaths the ventilator will deliver per minute. It may be exceeded by a spontaneously breathing patient in assist-control and intermittent mandatory ventilation (IMV) modes. Total respiratory rate equals patient rate plus ventilator rate. Common starting rate is 12 to 14 per minute. Adjust rate to pH and $Paco_2$.

TIDAL VOLUME

Volume delivered to patient during a normal ventilator breath. Usual volume is selected 5 to 15 cc/kg.

INSPIRATORY:EXPIRATORY (I:E) RATIO
Peak flow rate

Maximal flow rate that machine delivers during tidal breath.

Inspiratory flow rate

Some machines allow separate adjustment of flow rate, whereas in other machines, flow rate is determined by tidal volume, respiratory rate, and I:E ratio. Majority of ventilators deliver a square flow wave pattern (⎍), with a rapid rise in flow that remains constant throughout inhalation. Some ventilators have tapered flow patterns (⁀). The I:E ratio should be 1:1.5 or 1:2 to allow complete exhalation and to avoid air trapping.

I:E ratio

Adjusted directly on time-cycled ventilators. It is determined by tidal volume and rate of inspiratory flow on volume-regulated ventilators. Usually a 1:2 ratio is sought unless inverse ratio ventilation is in use.

SENSITIVITY

A control that adjust the ventilatory response to patient respiratory effort. In the control mode, sensitivity is off, so the machine does not respond to spontaneous patient effort. Otherwise, sensitivity is adjusted to allow the patient to initiate a ventilator (AC mode) breath or to breathe spontaneously (IMV mode).

SIGHS

Allows periodic selection of a larger-than-normal tidal volume. This feature substitutes for the normal sighing reflex. It is purported to prevent microatelectasis and intrapulmonary shunting. Usually sigh volumes are 1½ to 2 times tidal volume. Frequency can be individualized. If regular tidal volume is >than 7 cc/kg, sighing may not be necessary.

POSITIVE END-EXPIRATORY PRESSURE (PEEP)

Available on most ventilators. PEEP maintains greater than atmospheric pressure in airways at the completion of exhalation, serving to increase the functional residual capacity (FRC). It is adjusted up to 20 cm H_2O. Greater amounts are not recommended because of adverse effect on cardiac output.

PRESSURE LIMITS

Adjustable setting to regulate the maximal pressure the machine can generate to deliver the tidal volume. Once the pressure limit is reached, ventilator will spill undelivered tidal or sigh volume to the atmosphere to protect the patient from barotrauma. Limit is usually established as 12 to 20 cm H_2O above the normal ventilating pressure. Audible and visual alarms are used to signal excess pressure.

OXYGEN CONCENTRATION (FIo₂)

Selects delivery of oxygen between 21% and 100%. The concentration of oxygen should be kept at the lowest possible level to prevent oxygen toxicity. Concentrations <50% are desirable.

MONITORS/ALARMS

Devices on ventilators to track the volumes and FIo_2 delivered. Many ventilators have a spirometer to monitor tidal volumes. Audible and visual alarms signal improper amounts.

RESEARCH ABSTRACT
Patient perceptions of the mechanical ventilation experience

Gries ML and Fernsler J: Focus Crit Care 15:52, 1988.

PURPOSE

The purpose this study was to ascertain patients' perceptions of the mechanical ventilation experience in a critical care unit.

FRAMEWORK

Although reports document nurses' perceptions of a need for research related to mechanical ventilation, few published accounts of systematic research on patients' perceptions of the ventilation experience appear in the literature. Neuman's model of nursing provided the framework for this study. Patients in critical care units are open systems receiving input from extrapersonal and interpersonal factors in their environment. They strive to maintain a steady state by adjusting themselves to the environment or the environment to themselves. Mechanical ventilation is frequently used for a patient when overwhelming physical stressors disrupt the steady state. Although it sustains life, mechanical ventilation constitutes an environmental disturbance and therefore constitutes a stressor. The personal feelings that patients associate with the experience of mechanical ventilation influence their reactions and their ability to reconstitute or reach a steady state.

METHOD

An interview schedule of 14 fixed-alternative and open-ended questions was constructed and administered to the subjects. Subjects were nonrandomly selected from two small community acute care hospitals in the Mid-Atlantic region, were more than 18 years of age, alert, and oriented, and had received mechanical ventilation by a Bear I or MA1 ventilator through nasotracheal or endotracheal intubation. Patients who had tracheostomies or who had prior working experience with mechanical ventilation were excluded from the study. Tape recorded interviews were conducted 1 to 7 days after extubation, and interview times ranged from 10 to 35 minute. Responses were transcribed verbatim within 2 days of the interview.

RESULTS

The sample consisted of nine patients who ranged in age from 35 to 81 years. Patients reported 11 different negative experiences associated with mechanical ventilation therapy. Women identified fewer stressors than did men. Reported negative experiences were categorized into four categories. Intrapersonal physiological stressors included activity restrictions and positive pressure ventilation, (e.g., "gagging" feelings). Intrapersonal psychosociocultural stressors included insufficient explanations, vivid dreams, inability to cope, and extubation experiences. Communication was the major source of stress in the interpersonal category—both the inability to communicate by the patient and the lack of patience on the part of the nurses. The negative experiences most frequently reported were the extrapersonal stressors of the endotracheal tube and suctioning.

IMPLICATIONS

The high number of subjects who experienced stress related to the presence of the endotracheal tube indicates a need to investigate measures that may reduce the physical discomfort from the tube and suctioning. Since activity restrictions are a source of stress, patients must be carefully assessed for activity, which should be initiated as soon as possible. Both sensory and procedural information must be provided by the nurse to the patient, and a mechanism for the patient to communicate must be established. The small sample size limits generalizing the study, and the need for other research designs that incorporate the results of this study are indicated.

too much inspiratory effort on the part of the patient and greatly increase the work of breathing to the patient's detriment.

Various settings on the ventilator allow individualizing the parameters to a patient requiring support. The basic group of settings found on most modern ventilators is outlined in the box, "Definitions of Basic Ventilator Settings."

Positive End-Expiratory Pressure

One of the most controversial areas of ventilator setting is the positive end-expiratory pressure (PEEP) adjustment.[32] When PEEP is used it maintains an airway pressure greater than atmospheric pressure at the end of exhalation. This pressure increases alveolar volume and/or recruits previously collapsed alveoli. The overall effect is to increase the FRC. In patients with diffuse infiltrative pulmonary disease, application of PEEP decreases hypoxemia and often allows reduction of FIO_2 to less toxic levels. Statements about PEEP's reducing or redistributing lung fluid in patients with noncardiogenic edema have not been supported by current studies.[42] In some circumstances, PEEP has been effective in improving oxygenation and reducing intrapulmonary shunts.

PEEP indicates positive airway pressure at the end of exhalation. Various forms of breathing circuits achieve this state (see the box, "Forms of Positive Expiratory Pressure").

FORMS OF POSITIVE EXPIRATORY PRESSURE

CONTINUOUS POSITIVE AIRWAY PRESSURE (CPAP)

Used in the spontaneously breathing patient who may or may not be intubated.

Advantages

Keeps airway pressure greater than ambient pressure throughout inhalation and exhalation

Provides patient with alternative to mechanical ventilatory support; may be useful in treating cardiac pulmonary edema because CPAP improves oxygenation and decreases venous return

Does not require intubation

Disadvantages

Aerophagia and gastric distention

Aspiration of stomach contents

Decreased cardiac output

Barotrauma

Facial erosion and irritation from CPAP mask

Patient discomfort and poor tolerance[24]

The CPAP mask requires a light, airtight seal; its recommended time for use is 6 to 12 hours. The CPAP mask is used intermittently as a postoperative treatment and as a nighttime prevention of acute respiratory failure in the patient with neurological disease.[32]

Expiratory positive airway pressure (EPAP)

Used in spontaneously breathing patients. It has greater swings in airway pressure and thus increases the work of breathing significantly over that with CPAP and for that reason is not widely used.

Continous positive pressure breathing (CPPB)

Term used when the patient is in the assist-control mode. CPPB triggers inhalation by creating ventilator sub-PEEP pressure rather than subatmospheric pressure.

CPPB implies a small decrease in positive pressure before inhalation, but airway pressure remains above atmospheric pressure.

Continuous positive pressure ventilation (CPPV)

Patient ventilated throughout controlled mechanical ventilation mode. It allows application of PEEP without a fall in airway pressure.

Disadvantages

■ Cardiac output can fall more than with other forms of mechanical support associated with PEEP.

POSITIVE END-EXPIRATORY PRESSURE (PEEP)

Maintains pressure in the airway above atmospheric pressure at end of exhalation, therefore adding to FRC with PEEP up to 15 cm H_2O. PEEP increases alveolar diameter and improves arterial oxygenation. Most popular methods of application involve the following:

1. Best PEEP (best compliance as seen by pressure-volume curve)[42]
2. Optimal PEEP (lowest shunt fraction [Qs/Q_T])[32,42]
3. Least PEEP (lowest pressure in cm H_2O that provides arterial partial pressure of oxygen [Pa_{O_2}] >60 mmHg with Fl_{O_2} <0.60)[32,42]

Advantages

■ Increases FRC
■ *Decreases shunting*
■ Allows use of lower levels of Fl_{O_2}

Disadvantages

■ Increases risk of barotrauma
■ Reduces cardiac output
■ Generally contraindicated in patients with unilateral lung disease[32]

When PEEP is used with intermittent mandatory ventilation, the patient receives continuous positive pressure ventilation (CPPV) with ventilator breaths and continuous positive airway pressure (CPAP) with spontaneous breaths.

PEEP should be instituted and discontinued in a planned, systematic manner in which (1) PEEP is the only variable manipulated, (2) adjustments in PEEP are made at 3 to 5 cm H_2O at a time, and (3) the time interval between change and evaluation is held at more than 20 minutes to judge responses adequately.[42]

The patient response to PEEP is evaluated in various ways. Some clinicians use changes in shunt fraction, some use level of FI_{O_2}, whereas others use mixed venous oxygen (see box, "Bases for Selection of Best Level of PEEP").

Abrupt institution or withdrawal of high levels of PEEP can create problems associated with cardiac output and hypoxemia.

When PEEP is used, the risk of barotrauma is increased, especially in patients with unilateral lung disease or emphysema. It is not generally used in patients with chronic obstructive pulmonary disease (COPD), but improper adjustment of ventilator settings can result in "auto-PEEP." Auto-PEEP occurs with incomplete emptying of a lung area, which can occur when the respiratory rate is fast and the I:E ratio is too short. The presence of auto-PEEP can be evaluated by occluding the exhalation port at the end of exhalation and reading the pressure dial. A positive pressure reading indicates auto-PEEP is occurring.

BASES FOR SELECTION OF BEST LEVEL OF PEEP

1. Greatest oxygenation as determined by Pao_2 or Pao_2/Fio_2 fraction
2. Best compliance as seen by pressure volume curve
3. Lowest dead space/tidal volume ratio ($V_D:V_T$); lowest V_D/V_T occurs at greatest compliance
4. Lowest pulmonary vascular resistance
5. Lowest shunt fraction (Qs/Q_T); a shunt of 15% or a Pao_2 to Fio_2 ratio of 300 or more is frequently chosen
6. Lowest $PAco_2$-$Peco_2$ gradient; when dead space increases, cardiac output decreases
7. Least amount of PEEP to provide Pao_2 >60 mm Hg, with Fio_2 <0.6

Modified from Hess D: Crit Care Nurs Q11(3):62, 1988; and from MacDonnell K, Fahey P, and Segal M: Respiratory intensive care, Boston, 1987, Little, Brown & Co, Inc.

COMPLICATIONS ASSOCIATED WITH MECHANICAL VENTILATION

UPPER AIRWAY TRAUMA CAUSED BY INTUBATION

Dental damage
Nasal damage
Vocal cord hematoma
Laryngeal edema
Tracheal ulcers
Tracheal dilation
Tracheal stenosis
Tracheoesophageal fistula
Laryngeal stenosis
Tracheomalacia

INCREASED WORK OF BREATHING

Caused by decreased lumen size of artificial airways
Caused by breathing through synchronized intermittent mandatory ventilator circuitry or by presence of auto-PEEP

INFECTION

From equipment contamination
From colonization of lower tract through artificial airway tube

BAROTRAUMA

Pneumomediastinum
Subcutaneous emphysema
Pneumothorax
Pneumoperitoneum

REDUCED CARDIAC OUTPUT

Caused by decreased venous return
Caused by increased right-ventricular afterload
Caused by decreased left-ventricular distensibility
Leads to subsequent alteration in renal, hepatic, cerebral function

---

Nursing Care for the Patient on Mechanical Ventilation

Routine assessments. Routine monitoring of ventilator function is important to patient safety. This task is generally performed by respiratory therapists on an hourly or as-needed basis. Even so, the nursing staff needs to verify respiratory settings, monitors, and alarms as part of patient assessment and care.

Monitoring should also encompass evaluation of the patient's status in relationship to desired outcomes of ventilation and to prevent or minimize complications associated with respiratory therapy. Bedside evaluation of vital capacity, minute ventilation, arterial blood gas (ABG) values, and other pulmonary function tests may be warranted, according to the patient's condition.

Static and dynamic compliance should be monitored. Some newer generation ventilators give a continuous display of volume-pressure curves and exhaled carbon dioxide, allowing moment-to-moment evaluation of respiratory function and immediate intervention as needed. Compliance and resistance can be approximated on older ventilators by excluding the exhalation port at the end of expiration.

Assessment for complications of mechanical ventilation. Mechanical ventilation is often lifesaving, but like other interventions, it is not without its own complications. Some complications are preventable, whereas others can be minimized but not eradicated (see the box, "Complications Associated With Mechanical Ventilation," for common side effects).

Changes in cardiac output become more pronounced in hypoxemic patients. Ensuring adequate vascular volume will negate the decreased cardiac output in some patients. Continuous positive pressure ventilation (CPPV) or positive pressure ventilation with PEEP has the most dramatic effect on decreasing cardiac output. This decrease in cardiac output relates to the positive pressure that is maintained in the thoracic cavity throughout the respiratory cycle, which serves to decrease venous return and cardiac filling. PEEP also increases right-ventricular afterload, which causes dilation of the right ventricle and subsequent shifting of the intraventricular septum leftward.[42]

The displaced septum, in addition to compression of the left ventricle by distended lungs, further reduces cardiac output. Decreased cardiac output is not always associated with impaired tissue perfusion and hypoxemia. Adequacy of cardiac output can be monitored by evaluating the mixed venous oxygen and by assessing the patient. Retarded venous return to the heart has been implicated as a causative factor in hepatic dysfunction and in increased intracranial

RESEARCH ABSTRACT

Effects of two methods of preoxygenation on mean arterial pressure, cardiac output, peak airway pressure, and postsuctioning hypoxemia

Preusser BA and others: Heart Lung 17(3):290, 1988.

PURPOSE

The purpose of this study was to determine which method of preoxygenation—manual resuscitation bag (MRB) or ventilator—produced the least change in mean arterial pressure, cardiac output, and peak airway pressure and prevented postsuctioning hypoxemia during preoxygenation at two different lung inflation volumes.

FRAMEWORK

Preoxygenation with 100% oxygen at volumes greater than tidal volume (lung hyperinflation) before endotracheal suctioning has been shown to prevent postsuctioning hypoxemia. The MRB and the ventilator are two methods of delivering preoxygenation that are commonly used; however, problems are associated with both methods. Although preoxygenation prevents the serious complication of hypoxemia, strong evidence indicates that lung hyperinflation itself may have deleterious effects. It has been suggested that the increase in intrathoracic pressure associated with lung hyperinflation, which is indirectly reflected in airway pressure, may cause the hemodynamic alterations.

METHODS

An experimental design was used in which subjects served as their own controls. The independent variables included two randomly ordered methods of administering the lung inflation volumes, the Hope II MRB with an 800-cc reservoir and the MA1 ventilator, and two randomly ordered preoxgenation volumes calculated at 12 and 14 cc/kg of lean body weight. Each subject received one of the two lung-inflation volumes through either the MRB or the ventilator once an hour for 4 consecutive hours, followed by 10 seconds of continuous endotracheal suctioning. Subjects who had undergone coronary bypass graft surgery with no history of chronic obstructive pulmonary disease or chronic renal failure and who had endotracheal tubes and arterial and pulmonary artery catheters were evaluated 3½ hours after surgery. Baseline mean arterial pressure, cardiac output, and arterial blood gas values were obtained 1 minute before the onset of protocol.

RESULTS

Ten subjects, ranging in age from 44 to 73 years, with a mean of 3.7 grafts were studied. Endotracheal tube size was 8.0 or 8.5, thereby ensuring an inner diameter of endotracheal tube to outer diameter of suction catheter ratio of 2:1 when using a size 14 Fr suction catheter. The MRB produed a greater (12 mm Hg) increase in mean arterial pressure than the ventilator (9 mm Hg), which was not statistically significant ($p < 0.09$), MRB caused a larger increase in cardiac output than the ventilator, but this was not statistically significant ($p < 0.10$). The MRB generated significantly higher ($p < 0.001$) mean airway pressures (45 mm Hg) than the ventilator (23 mm Hg); the larger the volume, the higher was the pressure. Both methods effectively prevented postsuctioning hypoxemia; the larger the volume, the higher was the Pao_2.

IMPLICATIONS

On the basis of this study it is recommended that nurses use smaller volumes delivered through the ventilator when preoxygenating before endotracheal suctioning. Although both the MRB and the ventilator effectively prevented postsuctioning hypoxemia, the MRB caused a greater increase in peak airway pressure. Lung preoxygenation using larger volumes caused greater increase in mean arterial pressure and cardiac output. If the MRB is used, it is strongly recommended that the practitioner turn the oxygen flowmeter to flush, use a MRB with a large reservoir, and prime the bag slowly, using a two-handed compression followed by a slow refill. When possible, a test of the MRB's Flo_2 with an oxygen analyzer should be performed. The patient should receive preoxygenation breaths with smaller volumes, and the breaths should be syncronized with the patient's own ventilatory effort. It is essential to record the patient's mean arterial pressure before the preoxygenation-suctioning episode and to observe the patient, noting the mean arterial pressure for at least 10 minutes after the procedure. Limitations of this study include the small sample size and that the subjects were relatively healthy, aside from their cardiovascular disease. The study needs replication and the population expanded to include patients with a variety of pulmonary, renal, and neurological problems.

pressure associated with mechanical ventilation. Further studies must focus on these complications to determine if mechanical ventilation is the only cause involved.

Weaning from mechanical ventilation. Weaning should begin only after the acute disease(s) requiring ventilator support for the patient have been corrected and patient stability has been achieved.[33] Once this stage of illness has been reached, spontaneous breathing mechanics should be evaluated.

Patients who can maintain an arterial oxygen saturation at 90% on an FIO_2 of 0.21 while breathing spontaneously with a continuous positive airway pressure (CPAP) of <5 cm H_2O have a 94% success rate for weaning.[42] Many physiological parameters are followed during the course of mechanical ventilation to gauge the patient's readiness for weaning.

The box, "Criteria for Weaning," lists the parameters and described values most authorities believe are necessary before weaning from mechanical ventilation can be attempted.

General principles of weaning. The success of weaning is dependent on the underlying disease of the patient and the length of ventilator support. Patients with several underlying diseases, with severe chronic obstructive pulmonary disease (COPD), or who have been ventilated in excess

---

CRITERIA FOR WEANING

DEGREE OF SHUNT

Less than 0.20 or P(A-a) O_2 gradient <350 mm Hg (or 100%)[7]

DEAD SPACE TO TIDAL VOLUME

Dead space less than 0.6 of tidal volume (V_D/V_T ratio <0.6)[55]

VITAL CAPACITY (VC)

VC >10 cc/kg or 20% to 25% of predicted normal [33,55]

MAXIMAL VOLUNTARY VENTILATION (MVV)

Patient able to double minute ventilation on demand, generally indicating a reserve for breathing independently[55]

INSPIRATORY FORCE

Patient able to generate at least −20 to −25 cm H_2O pressure for adequate spontaneous ventilation[37]

FORCED EXPIRATORY VOLUME IN ONE SECOND (FEV₁)

Needs to move 10 cc/kg for successful weaning[7]

RESPIRATORY RATE (RR)/MINUTE VENTILATION ($\dot{V}_E$)

Resting, spontaneous RR <30/minute and resting, spontaneous $\dot{V}_E$ <10 L/minute

---

Nursing Diagnosis and Management
Controlled mechanical ventilation

- Ineffective Breathing Pattern related to respiratory muscle deconditioning secondary to mechanical ventilation, p. 482.

- Ineffective Airway Clearance related to impaired cough secondary to loss of glottic closure with cuffed endotracheal/tracheostomy tube, p. 476.

- Potential for Aspiration Risk Factors: Tracheostomy or endotracheal tube, impaired swallowing, facial/oral/neck surgery or trauma, wired jaws, p. 489.

- Decreased Cardiac Output related to decreased preload secondary to mechanical ventilation with or without PEEP, p. 335.

- Sleep Pattern Disturbance related to fragramented sleep, p. 88.

- Body Image Disturbance related to functional dependence on life-sustaining technology, p. 834.

- Powerlessness related to health care environment or illness-related regimen, p. 837.

- Ineffective Individual Coping related to situational crisis and personal vulnerability, p. 850.

- Anxiety related to threat to biological, psychological, or social integrity, p. 852.

---

of 30 days can pose special problems during weaning.[42] However, before attempting to discontinue mechanical ventilation, certain factors should be considered.

The patient should be stable without support of vasopressors for 12 to 24 hours before weaning. Some clinicians may use low-dose dopamine to augment renal blood flow or low-dose nitroglycerin to prevent cardiac decompensation resulting from a sudden increase in venous return, which will occur when positive pressure ventilation is discontinued.[42] The patient should be clear of any significant infection before weaning proceeds.

Special attention should be given to the patient's nutritional status. Often, ventilator patients, because of their overall condition and inability to take food orally, are receiving parenteral or enteral feedings. Studies have demonstrated excessive carbon dioxide production from carbohydrate calories can create hypercapnia during weaning.[18] Recent studies suggest critically ill hospitalized patients require approximately 2000 cal/day, which is much less than previously believed. Some sources recommend reducing caloric intake by 50% once weaning is instituted.[18]

The patient's pH, $PaCO_2$, and PaO_2 should be comparable to baseline, preintubation levels before weaning is undertaken.

RESEARCH ABSTRACT

Biofeedback and progressive relaxation in weaning the anxious patient from the ventilator: a brief report

Acosta F: Heart Lung 17(3):299, 1988.

PURPOSE

The purpose of this case study was to determine the effect of biofeedback and relaxation on a patient with chronic obstructive pulmonary disease (COPD) who had apprehension during aerosol "T-piece" weaning trials.

FRAMEWORK

Patients with COPD are tense and anxious because they must live with chronic shortness of breath. The tension created by anxiety and fear produces a tightening of the chest muscles, making the process of breathing more difficult than need be. Removal of these patients from ventilators is often a long and difficult process. Progressive relaxation produces decreased muscle tension; biofeedback has been used to decrease respiratory rate and stress in patients with COPD. Biofeedback has been reported to improve breathing performance of patients during ventilator weaning trials.

METHODS

A case study approach was used to examine the experience of one patient during weaning trials. The patient was a 58-year-old man with a history of COPD who had been admitted through the emergency room and was intubated with ventilatory assistance for respiratory failure. He required 1½ months of ventilatory support, and weaning was begun on the forty-sixth day and was continued for 25 days. Toleration time was limited to 5 minutes during the first day because of his shortness of breath and was gradually increased to a total of only 4 hours because of his fear of suffocation. At this time, the patient was approached about and he consented to the use of biofeedback and progressive relaxation. The patient was taught biofeedback and progressive relaxation in a relatively darkened room while he was reclining in an easy chair. Ear oximetry was monitored before, during, and after the procedure. Each session lasted approximately 30 minutes.

RESULTS

On the twenty-sixth day of weaning trials, biofeedback and progressive relaxation were begun and were continued for 12 days. With each session, the weaning tolerance time gradually increased from ½ hour at the first session to 13 hours by the last session. The patient's heart rate and respiratory rate decreased after the sessions. The lowering of both these parameters coincided with an increased in oxygen saturation after the relaxation session. With the introduction of relaxation therapy, the patient was able to tolerate weaning trials for longer periods of time, eventually leading to successful weaning from ventilation.

IMPLICATIONS

It can be inferred from this study that an anxious patient who has pulmonary dysfunction will respond more favorably to the stress of ventilator weaning when taught to achieve a relaxed state. The limitation of this study is the fact that it examined only one patient; therefore the results may not be generalized to other patients. The implication for research is for designing studies that use other research designs (i.e., experimental or quasi-experimental) that examine a larger number of subjects and control extraneous and intervening variables.

Weaning difficult patients such as those with COPD or on long-term ventilator support should be a systematic purposeful process that takes advantage of the patient's best energy level and allows rest and sleep because sleep deprivation interferes with weaning. Early daytime weaning will probably be more successful.

Weaning difficult patients requires their cooperation. Discrete, attainable goals should be set to avoid overexertion and respiratory muscle fatigue on the part of the patient. Failure at weaning attempts may result in patient depression or despondency.

While weaning is in process, the patient should be monitored for signs of fatigue, hypoxemia, and tissue hypoxia.

Once the patient has been weaned, the endotracheal or tracheal tube should be removed unless some condition is present that contraindicates this action.

CHEST TUBES

Chest tubes are inserted into the pleural space to remove fluid or air from it and thus reinstate the negative intrapleural pressure and reexpand collapsed lungs or portions of the lungs. The box, "Indications for Chest Tube Drainage," outlines the major indications for chest tubes.

When chest tubes are needed for removal of air, insertion is at the second or third intercostal space of the anterior thoracic wall. This location best removes air which rises to the top of the pleural space, as opposed to the fluid, which gravitates to the lowest level of the space. Placement of chest tubes to drain fluid is low in the thoracic cavity at the sixth, seventh, or eighth intercostal space. Some patient situations call for placement of tubes at both locations to evacuate both air and fluid. Once the chest tube is placed, it is connected to a water-seal drainage system.

INDICATIONS FOR CHEST TUBE DRAINAGE

Pneumothorax >20%
   Traumatic
   Spontaneous
   Tension pneumothorax
Hemothorax >500 cc
Pneumohemothorax
   Surgically induced
   After chest surgery
   Traumatic
Pleural effusion
Mechanically ventilated patients with any size pneumothorax or hemothorax

Water-seal drainage systems have evolved from separate glass bottles of one, two, or three containers into a self-contained disposable plastic unit that can be used in various modes.

The drainage system is aseptically prepared for use, with sterile water placed in the water seal and suction control chambers. Usually the water-seal chamber is filled at the 2-cm to 3-cm level, and the suction-control chamber is filled with 15 to 25 cm of water. When only air is being evacuated, lower levels of suction can be used. Connection points of the drainage tubing should be sealed with tape and an occlusive dressing applied at the chest tube sight. Petroleum (Vaseline) gauze, once used at all chest tube insertion sites, has been eliminated from use except when the tube is inadvertently removed, and the use of only a dry sterile gauze with tape is necessary because the suction is believed to remove any air leak from around the chest tube insertion point.

Once the chest tubes are placed, efforts are directed at maintaining the patency and sterility of the system. The one-unit disposable system improves the maintenance of sterility. When drainage occurs in excess of the system's capacity, a new setup is used, or, in the case of some systems, the drainage container can be easily removed and replaced. The disposable systems also have self-sealing sampling ports that allow obtaining drainage for examination without interruption of the integrity of the unit.

Maintaining drainage involves careful attention to the suction applied and to maintenance of unobstructed drainage tubes. Kinks and large loops of tubing should be avoided because they prevent drainage and air evacuation, which may prevent timely lung reexpansion or may result in a tension pneumothorax. Retained drainage also becomes an excellent medium for multiplication of bacteria.

The water-seal chamber must be routinely observed for unexpected bubbling caused by an air leak in the system. When suspicious bubbling is present, the source must be identified. To determine if the source is within the system or within the patient, systematic brief clamping of the drainage tube should be performed. Staying as close to the oc-

clusive dressing as possible, the nurse should place a padded clamp on the drainage tubing. If the air bubbling stops, the air leak is located between the patient and the clamp. The leak can be within the patient or at the insertion site. Therefore the clamp is removed and the chest tube site exposed. The tube is inspected as it enters the chest to make sure all the eyelets are within the patient. If an eyelet port is outside the chest, it can be a source of air leaking into the system and must be occluded, possibly requiring the attention of the physician. When the insertion site has been eliminated as a leakage source, the chest dressing is reapplied, with it completely and securely covering the site.

If the air bubbling does not stop when a clamp is placed on the chest tube, the leak is located between the clamp and the drainage collector. By releasing the clamp and moving down the tubing a few inches at a time until the bubbling stops, the leak is located. If this action is practical, the area of the leak can be taped to reestablish a seal. If this technique proves unreliable or impossible, the system or tubing should be replaced.

Padded clamps and sterile petroleum gauze should be kept at the patient's bedside at all times. If the chest tube or system is inadvertently interrupted, the clamp is applied to the chest tube as close to the insertion site as possible while the drainage system is reestablished. Sterile petroleum gauze is applied to the chest wall if the chest tube is accidentally removed. Implementing both these techniques immediately in such cases will minimize or prevent the formation of a pneumothorax and avoid greater complications.

When a hemothorax is present, drainage must be carefully assessed and measured to avoid the presence of unrecognized bleeding. When the chest tubes are placed after surgery or traumatic injury, fresh blood may be expected immediately. Both the amount and characteristics of the blood should change within a few hours if the bleeding has stopped. Drainage of more than 100 ml/hour for 2 consecutive hours or a sudden change in amount of bloody drainage requires further investigation.[15] The patient should be completely assessed and the physician consulted. In some cases

Nursing Diagnosis and Management
Chest tubes

- Ineffective Breathing Pattern related to modifiable chest wall restrictions secondary to pneumothorax and/or pleural effusion, p. 481

- Ineffective Breathing Pattern related to thoracic pain, p. 483

- Ineffective Airway Clearance related to thoracic pain, p. 477

- Impaired Gas Exchange related to ventilation-perfusion inequality secondary to (specify), p. 487

- Body Image Disturbance related to actual change in body structure, function, or appearance, p. 833

surgical intervention may be necessary. Routine milking or stripping of chest tubes is not recommended because excessive negative pressure can be generated in the chest.[11,38] Pressures as high as -350 cm H_2O have been recorded using chest strippers, a manual device.[11] If blood clots are present in the drainage tubing or obstruction is present, careful milking of the chest tubes may be performed.

Throughout the duration of chest tube placement, the patient should be periodically assessed for reexpansion of the lung and for complications of chest tube drainage. The nurse should assess the thorax and lungs, paying particular attention to any tracheal deviation, asymmetry of chest movement, presence of subcutaneous emphysema, characteristics of breathing, quality of lung sounds, and presence of tympany or percussion sounds, which are indicative of pneumothorax.

Proper care of the system and monitoring of the patient will prevent iatrogenic complications of chest tube drainage.

CHEST PHYSIOTHERAPY

Historically, chest physiotherapy (CPT) has been used to supplement the patient's coughing effort or to substitute for it in absent cough states. CPT is directed at improving mucus and sputum clearance and airway function and includes all or various combinations of chest percussion, chest vibration, postural draining, coughing, or suctioning.

Recently, the efficacy of these techniques has been questioned. In an effort to evaluate their overall and specific usefulness in clinical situations, Kirilloff and others[36] completed an extensive review of the investigative studies involving CPT interventions. Their findings and conclusions

Table 21-9   Effects of chest physiotherapy on patients with respiratory complications[36]

Acutely ill patients	Intervention	Outcomes
With chest radiograph changes and increased secretions	Postural drainage Percussion, deep breathing, coughing, or suctioning	Increased Pao₂ 30 minutes after chest physiotherapy (CPT) and at 1 hour Increased sputum expectoration
With scant secretions	Same	No improvement in arterial blood gas (ABG) values or volume of sputum No improvement in VC, FEV, FRC Decrease in Pao₂ after chest percussion and greater decrease 30 minutes after CPT No improvement in chest radiograph or length of hospital stay

CONCLUSIONS

Beneficial to acutely ill patients with increased volume of secretions
Beneficial to patients with lobar atelectasis
No benefit to patients with status asthmaticus
May cause bronchospasm and hypoxemia in acutely ill patients

With a large volume of secretions (e.g., with cystic fibrosis or bronchiectasis)	CPT versus coughing alone or with forced expiration technique	Coughing and CPT produced approximately equal results in sputum amount and radioaerosol clearance Sputum and radioaerosol clearance increased with forced exhalation techniques over that with cough alone or in combination with postural drainage
	CPT	Increased FRC
With small volume of secretions	CPT	No improvement in FVC, FEV, or sputum production

CONCLUSIONS

CPT improves mucous clearance in chronic patients with copious sputum production; directed, coached coughing may be as beneficial as postural drainage in these patients.
Forced exhalation techniques may increase sputum clearance with or without postural drainage in patients with chronic copious sputum production.
Patients with chronic lung disease who are producing small amounts of sputum show no beneficial changes with CPT.

*VC, Vital capacity; FEV, forced expiratory volume; FRC, functional residual capacity; FVC, forced vital capacity.

are briefly summarized in Table 21-9. The reader is encouraged to refer to their original work for a more detailed discussion. The outcomes of their review are pertinent to the nurse clinician because they indicate CPT is not appropriate in every patient population or situation.

Proper application of CPT requires knowledge of the anatomical arrangement of lung segments so that positioning for gravity drainage will result. When positioning a patient, the area of lung to be drained should be uppermost, with the airway as vertical as possible. Because the patient's condition affects his or her ability to tolerate postural drainage, the length of percussion or vibration time will vary. In critically ill patients, CPT may be required every 2 to 4 hours, but often a routine of performing early morning and late evening CPT is established.[58] CPT should not be performed within 1 hour of eating because of patient discomfort and the possibility of regurgitation and aspiration.[58]

Percussion and vibration, along with postural drainage, comprise CPT. Percussion and vibration help dislodge mucus from airway walls, making its removal by postural drainage and coughing more effective. Percussion uses the nurse's hands in a cupped configuration to clap rhythmically on the patient's chest wall. Percussion (or clapping, as it is also called) is performed for approximately 2 minutes over the thorax of the lung segment requiring drainage.[64] The chest should be covered with a towel during percussion.

Vibration can be performed manually or with the aid of a mechanical vibrator or percussor. When manual vibration is performed, the nurse's flat hands are placed firmly against the chest wall. As the patient exhales, the nurse shakes her arms while pressing on the patient's chest, creating a gentle vibratory sensation in the patient's chest. This technique is repeated two to three times in an area. Vibration or percussion can be used alone or with postural drainage. Vibration is as effective as percussion and may be better tolerated in some critically ill patients.

CPT may be contraindicated in patients with recent hemoptysis or severe hypertension and in patients with unstable hemodynamics. Central nervous system problems such as cerebral aneurysm and edema contradict the use of CPT.[23]

REFERENCES

1. Albert R: Least PEEP: Primum non nocere, Chest 87(1):2, 1987.
2. Aubier M and others: Effect of hypophosphatemia on diaphragmatic contractility in patients with acute respiratory failure, N Engl J Med 313(7):420, 1985.
3. Barnes CA and Kirchhoff KT: Minimizing hypoxemia due to endotracheal suctioning: a review of the literature, Heart Lung 15(2):164, 1986.
4. Bernard G and Bradley R: Adult respiratory distress syndrome: diagnosis and management, Heart Lung 15(3):250, 1986.
5. Bernhard W and others: Intracuff pressures in endotracheal and tracheostomy tubes: related cuff physical characteristics, Chest 87(6):720, 1985.
6. Blaufuss J and Wallace C: Two negative pressure ventilators: current clinical application and nursing care, Crit Care Nurs Q 9(4):14, 1987.
7. Burton G and Hodgkin J: Respiratory care: a guide to clinical practice, ed 2, Philadelphia, 1984, JB Lippincott Co.
8. Cane RD and Shapiro BA: Mechanical ventilatory support: concepts in emergency and critical care, JAMA 254(1):87, 1985.
9. Capps J and Schade K: Work of breathing: clinical monitoring and considerations in the critical care setting, Crit Care Nurs Q 11(3):1, 1988.
10. Carlon G, Fox S, and Ackerman N: Evaluation of a closed-tracheal suction system, Crit Care Med 15(5):522, 1987.
11. Carroll P: The ins and outs of chest drainage systems, Nursing 16(2):86, 1986.
12. Christopher K and others: Transtracheal oxygen therapy for refractory hypoxemia, JAMA 256(4):494, 1986.
13. Chulay M and Graeber G: Efficacy of a hyperinflation and hyperoxygenation suctioning intervention, Heart Lung 17(1):15, 1988.
14. Cosenza JJ and Norton LC: Secretion clearance: state of the art from nursing perspective, Crit Care Nurse 6(4):23, 1986.
15. Cowley RA and Dunham CM: Shock trauma/critical care manual: initial assessment and management, Baltimore, 1982, University Park Press.
16. Crabtree GS: Reducing tracheal injury and aspiration, Dimens Crit Care Nurs 7(6):324, 1988.
17. Crabtree-Goodnough SK: The effects of oxygen and hyperinflation on arterial oxygen tension after endotracheal suctioning, Heart Lung 14(1):11, 1985.
18. Dark D, Pingleton M, and Kerby G: Hypercapnia during weaning: a complication of nutritional support, Chest 88(1):141, 1985.
19. Davidson L and Brown S: Continuous SvO_2 monitoring: a tool for analyzing hemodynamic status, Heart Lung 15(3):287, 1986.
20. Davis J: Hyperbaric oxygen therapy: a committee report, Bethesda, Md, 1983, Undersea Medical Society, Inc.
21. Fuchs P: Before and after chest surgery: stay right on respiratory care, Nursing 83 13(5):46, 1983.
22. Fuchs-Carroll P: The ins and outs of chest drainage systems, Nursing 86 16(12):26, 1986.
23. Gaskell DV and Webber BA: The Brompton hospital guide to chest physiotherapy, ed 4, Oxford, 1980, Blackwell Scientific Publications, Ltd.
24. Gruden MA: High-frequency ventilation: an overview, Crit Care Nurse 5(1):36, 1985.
25. Hanley MV: Normal saline intratracheal instillation in intubated patients and dogs, master's thesis, Seattle, 1977, University of Washington.
26. Harper R: A guide to respiratory care, Philadelphia, 1981, JB Lippincott Co.
27. Heffner JE, Miller KS, and Sahn S: Tracheostomy in the intensive care unit: part I, Chest 90(2):269, 1987.
28. Heffner JE, Miller KS, and Sahn S: Tracheostomy in the intensive care unit: part II, Complications, Chest 90(3):430, 1987.
29. Heimlich H: Respiratory rehabilitation with transtracheal oxygen system, Ann Otol Rhinol Laryngol 91(6):643, 1982.
30. Heimlich H and Carr G: Transtracheal catheter technique for pulmonary rehabilitation, Ann Otol Rhinol Layngol 94(5):502, 1985.
31. Herve P and others: Hypercapnic acidosis induced by nutrition in mechanically ventilated patients: glucose versus fat, Crit Care Med 13(7):537, 1986.
32. Hess D: Controversies in respiratory critical care, Crit Care Nurs Q 11(3):62, 1988.
33. Hess D: Perspectives on weaning from mechanical ventilation: with a note on extubation, Respir Care 32(3):167, 1987.
34. Jacobson J, Morsch J, and Rendell-Baker L: The historical perspective of hyperbaric therapy, Ann NY Acad Sci 117:651, 1965.
35. Jacquette G: To reduce hazards of tracheal suctioning, AJN 71(12):2362, 1971.
36. Kirilloff LH and others: Does chest physical therapy work? Chest 88(3):436, 1985.
37. Kline JL and others: The use of calculated relative inspiratory effort as a predictor of outcome in mechanical ventilation weaning trials, Respir Care 32(1):870, 1987.
38. Lane G, Cronin K, and Pierce A: Flow charts: clinical decision making in nursing, Philadelphia, 1983, JB Lippincott Co.
39. MacKenzie C: Compromises in the choice of orotracheal or nasotracheal intubation and tracheostomy, Heart Lung 12(5):485, 1983.

40. Manchikanti L and others: Bicitra^R (sodium citrate) and metoclopramide in outpatient anesthesia for prophylaxis against acid pneumonitis, Anesthesiology 63(4):378, 1985.
41. Massaro D: Oxygen: toxicity and tolerance, Hosp Pract 21(7):95, 1986.
42. McDonnell K, Fahey P, and Segal M: Respiratory intensive care, Boston, 1987, Little, Brown & Co, Inc.
43. Muto R: Personal communication, November, 1988.
44. Pepe P and Marini J: Occult positive end-expiratory pressure in mechanically ventilated patients with airflow obstruction, Am Rev Respir Dis 126(1):166, 1982.
45. Petty TL: Intensive and rehabilitative respiratory care, Philadelphia, 1982, Lea and Febiger.
46. Preusser B and others: Effects of two methods of preoxygenation on mean arterial pressure, cardiac output, peak airway pressure and post-suctioning hypoxemia, Heart Lung 17(3):290, 1988.
47. Rashkin M and Davis T: Acute complications of endotracheal intubation, Chest 89(2):165, 1986.
48. Ritz R and others: Contamination of a multiple-use suction catheter in a closed-circuit system compared to contamination of a disposable, single-use suction catheter, Respir Care 31(11):1086, 1986.
49. Schumann L and Parsons G: Tracheal suctioning and ventilator tube changes in adult respiratory distress syndrome: use of a positive end-expiration pressure valve, Heart Lung 14(4):362, 1985.
50. Shapiro B and others: Clinical application of respiratory care, ed 3, Chicago, 1985, Year Book Medical Publishers, Inc.
51. Skelton M and Nield M: Ineffective airway clearance related to artificial airway, Nurs Clin North Am 22(1):167, 1987.
52. Snowberger P: Prevention of complications: decreasing tracheal damage due to excessive cuff pressures, Dimens Crit Care Nurs 5(3):136, 1986.
53. Spearman C and Sheldon R: Egan's fundamentals of respiratory therapy, ed 4, St Louis, 1982, The CV Mosby Co.
54. Spofford B and others: Transtracheal oxygen therapy: a guide for the respiratory therapist, Respir Care 32(5):345, 1987.
55. Sporn P and Marganroth M: Discontinuation of mechanical ventilation, Clin Chest Med 9(1):113, 1988.
56. Suter PM, Fairly AB, and Isenburg MD: Optimum end-expiratory airway pressure in patients with acute pulmonary failure, N Engl J Med 292(6):284, 1975.
57. Taggart J, Dorinsky N, and Sheahan J: Airway pressures during closed system suctioning, Heart Lung 17(5):536, 1988.
58. Tecklin JS: Positioning, percussing and vibrating patients for effective bronchial drainage, Nursing 79 9(3):64, 1979.
59. Tisi G: Pulmonary physiology in clinical medicine, ed 2, Baltimore, 1983, Williams & Wilkins Co.
60. Toben B and Lewandowski V: Nontraditional and new ventilatory techniques, Crit Care Nurs Q 11(3):12, 1988.
61. Tobin MJ: Physiology in medicine: update on strategies in mechanical ventilation, Hosp Pract 21(6):69, 1986.
62. Traver GA: Ineffective airway clearance: physiology and clinical application . . . cough effectiveness, Dimens Crit Care Nurs 4(4):198, 1985.
63. Trout C: Artificial airways: tubes and tracks, Respir Care 21(6):513, 1976.
64. Waterson M: Teaching your patients postural drainage, Nursing 78 8(3):51, 1978.
65. Wu W and Huang S: Tracheal intubation, Consultant 26(5):34, 1986.

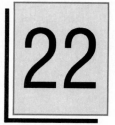

Pulmonary Care Plans

THEORETICAL BASIS AND MANAGEMENT

CHAPTER OBJECTIVES

- *Discuss the theoretical concepts related to ineffective airway clearance.*
- *Identify and describe nursing interventions that are essential in the treatment of ineffective airway clearance.*
- *Discuss the theoretical concepts related to ineffective breathing pattern.*
- *Identify and describe nursing interventions that are essential in the treatment of ineffective breathing pattern.*
- *Discuss the theoretical concepts related to impaired gas exchange.*
- *Identify and describe nursing interventions that are essential in the treatment of impaired gas exchange.*
- *Identify and describe nursing interventions that are essential in the treatment of potential for aspiration.*

INEFFECTIVE AIRWAY CLEARANCE

Ineffective airway clearance is defined as, "A state in which an individual is unable to clear secretions or obstructions from the respiratory tract to maintain airway patency."[23]

Causes of Ineffective Airway Clearance

Clearance of tracheobronchial secretions occurs through the mucociliary system within the airways. This system is a combination of mucus and cilia, which work to move mucus, other secretions, and foreign matter up from the lower airways into the segmental, lobar, and main-stem bronchi from which they can be expectorated or swallowed. Normal amounts of mucus are transported through the larynx and swallowed without notice, but excessive amounts stimulate the cough reflex.[29] Sometimes, pathological conditions occur within the pulmonary system that impair and/or overload the functioning of the mucociliary system, resulting in

an accumulation of mucus. Disorders commonly seen in critical care units that are known to fit this description include acute and chronic bronchitis, chronic obstructive pulmonary disease (COPD) (with or without an exacerbation), and acute lower airway infections. As a result of the ineffective functioning of the mucociliary system in these patients, mucus clearance and other foreign matter clearance are insufficient and must be augmented by coughing. When coughing becomes ineffective in clearing the airways, interventions must be planned that will assist the patient in maintaining normal airway clearance. Coughing is vital to airway clearance, and when it becomes impaired, ineffective airway clearance may result.

Medical interventions assisting with airway clearance include administration of drugs such as bronchodilators, mucolytics, and expectorants. Additionally, drug therapy can be augmented by bronchial drainage and/or chest physiotherapy.

The focuses of this discussion and the succeeding nursing care plans are the nursing care of patients with difficulty clearing mucus and how the application of effective nursing interventions assists in resolving ineffective airway clearance. Relevant interventions include teaching effective coughing, proper patient positioning that will augment coughing and ventilation, effective hydration and/or humidification, and removal of mucus through other means such as bronchial drainage, chest physiotherapy, or suctioning.

Defining Characteristics of Ineffective Airway Clearance

The specific signs and symptoms of ineffective airway clearance include the following:
- Congested lung fields (crackles and wheezes)
- Elevated arterial partial pressure of carbon dioxide ($Paco_2$)
- Hypoxemia
- Thick, tenacious mucus
- Weak, ineffectual cough

Congested lung fields, or the presence of crackles and wheezes during lung auscultation, indicate excessive mucus in the airways, collapsed alveoli, and/or of airway narrowing. These adventitious sounds may occur generally throughout the lung or in a specific area such as in a lobe or in an area defined by thoracic landmarks. It is vital that the examiner record accurately where the crackles and wheezes occur because some nursing interventions such as chest physiotherapy, bronchial drainage, or positioning for rest or sleep will be directed at the specific lung area.

Hypercapnia and hypoxemia occur as a result of ineffective airway clearance when mucus is in such a great volume that significant alveolar hypoventilation and ventilation/perfusion inequality are produced,[17,47] Patients with COPD and chronic bronchitis who evidence hypercapnia and hypoxemia do so partly or wholly because excessive mucus in the airways is not cleared.[47]

Thick, tenacious mucus can be extremely difficult to expectorate and thus easily results in ineffective airway clearance. Thinning of thick mucus requires hydration and, when an artificial airway is in place, humidification of the system.

A weak, ineffectual cough does little to remove mucus. Patients who are at risk for weak coughing include those (1) with COPD, especially those with a strong emphysemic component to their COPD because emphysema compromises exhalation, (2) with emphysema, (3) who have had abdominal or thoracic surgery since coughing may exacerbate incisional or surgical pain, (4) who are confined to bed rest or who spend an inordinate amount of time positioned in bed in such a way that natural diaphragmatic descent and/or chest expansion is compromised, (5) who have artificial airways, and (6) who have an absent cough as a result of coma or a high cervical spine injury.

General signs and symptoms. Signs and symptoms that are more general and that are found in clinical situations in addition to those which define ineffective airway clearance include dyspnea, cyanosis, tachypnea, restlessness, and anxiety. Although they cannot effectively define ineffective airway clearance by themselves, when identified along with the specific sign and symptoms listed previously, they further confirm the diagnosis.

Nursing Interventions for Ineffective Airway Clearance

The care plans that follow list many nursing interventions for treating ineffective airway clearance. Although some of the interventions require no detailed explanations or rationale (for example, to administer oxygen to correct hypoxemia or to suction and clear oral secretions), others need their theoretical basis explained.

Teaching an effective cough technique. Coughing is sometimes necessary, even in a healthy individual, for the removal of mucus from the tracheobronchial tree. To be effective, however, the cough must be a composite of several distinct and necessary phases, which are listed in Table 22-1. Effective coughing depends on (1) a deep inhalation, (2) strong contraction of the muscles of exhalation, in particular the abdominal muscles, (3) a functioning glottis, and (4) airways that remain open during the terminal exhalatory phase of the cough. Abnormal functioning of any of the above mechanisms will decrease the effectiveness of coughing. Inability to take a deep breath, weak abdominal muscles, unwillingness to use the abdominal muscles because of pain or poor positioning, and chronic diffuse small airway collapse such as can occur with COPD can significantly reduce cough effectiveness. A reduction of cough effectiveness in the presence of mucus production will lead to ineffective airway clearance (see Table 22-1).

Patients with excessive mucus production often exhaust themselves coughing in an inefficient manner. Teaching a controlled cough technique that results in the effective production of mucus can be instrumental in assisting the patient to control this aspect of his or her illness. Cough instruction is useful in conjunction with all respiratory therapy modal-

Table 22-1 Factors that interfere with production of an effective cough

Components of a normal cough	Factors that interfere with normal coughing	Nursing action
Inhalation to near-total lung capacity	General weakness	Consider teaching huff or quad coughing*
	Inability to take a deep breath	
	Positioning that impairs the deep breath	Position for effective cough
Closure of the glottis	Bypass of the glottis by artificial airway	—
Contraction of the abdominal muscles	Weak abdominal muscles	Huff cough
	Painful use of muscles	Analgesics
	Positioning that impairs use of the abdominal muscles	Position for effective cough
Sudden opening of the glottis with explosive exhalation	Inability to exhale with force	Quad coughing
	Diffuse small airway collapse on exhalation	Huff coughing
	Bypass of the glottis by artificial airway	

*Huff and quad cough techniques are discussed on p. 474.

ities and with patients who have had abdominal or thoracic surgery.[47] However, only those patients who have documented mucus or who are strongly suspected of having retained mucus should be encouraged to cough. Coughing causes airway irritation and fatigue[14]; further, it promotes airway and alveolar collapse, particularly in the absence of secretions.[4]

The reader should be aware that the cough procedure presented here is not a scientifically studied technique but is one that has been received quite successfully by patients, respiratory therapists, and nurses in both the acute and rehabilitative settings.[36] This technique involves the steps listed in the box below.

There may be patients who cannot follow the controlled cough technique. Other types of coughing that successfully remove mucus such as huff or quad coughing can be encouraged.

Huff coughing is a series of coughs produced with the glottis held open while saying the word, "huff." The sharp sound of a cough should not be produced with a huff cough, but the sound should be that of forced exhalation.[53] Huff coughing may be helpful for COPD patients who have significant airway collapse on forced exhalation, because huff coughing is associated with higher flow rates in these patients than in the normal closed-glottis approach to coughing. Furthermore, huff coughing may assist in moving secretions from the smaller airways into the main-stem bronchi

---

CONTROLLED COUGH TECHNIQUE

1. *Maximal inhalation*—an effective cough is contingent on filling the lungs and airways distal to the mucus so that the succeeding forced exhalation will propel the mucus up to the airways. Maximal inhalation also increases airway caliber; as a result, it is more likely that the air will pass distal to partially obstructing mucus or foreign matter.[53]
2. *Hold breath 2 seconds*—this step permits the patient to prepare for exhalation and allows distribution of the inhaled air to the lung's periphery.[47]
3. *Cough twice*—the first cough will loosen mucus, the second will propel the mucus. Further coughing may use excessive oxygen and energy at a time when the lung volume has already been expelled with the first two coughs, and the effort is thus wasted.
4. *Pause*—just long enough to regain control.
5. *Inhale by sniffing*—sniffing is recommended, because a deep inhalation through the mouth may drive loose mucus back down into the airways.
6. *Rest*.

Adapted from Moser KM and others: Shortness of breath: a guide to better living and breathing, St. Louis, 1983, The CV Mosby Co.

---

or trachea where the controlled cough technique can be used for effective expectoration.

Quad coughing is helpful in patients who have flaccid or weakened abdominal musculature. The most obvious example is the patient with paralysis or weakness caused by neuromuscular disorders. Quad coughing calls for the nurse to push upward and inward on the abdomen, toward the diaphragm, while the patient exhales.

Proper patient positioning. The most effective position for coughing is upright and flexed forward at the waist. Lying supine or even in a semi-Fowler's position does not allow total lung inflation, diaphragmatic descent, or intercostal muscle action and thus decreases the efficiency of the cough.[29] Additionally, patients who have abdominal incisions may experience less incisional pain when coughing while drawing their knees up toward the chest[29] and/or by splinting the incision against a pillow. The feet should be supported rather than allowed to dangle; in this way the support can be used as a brace against which to generate greater abdominal muscle tension, producing a stronger cough. The brace will also help prevent muscular strain of the lower back.[9]

When a head-up position is contraindicated, the side-lying position with knees bent is preferable to the supine recumbent position.[9,14]

Effective hydration and airway humidification. Shapiro and associates[47] consider adequate systemic hydration as the second most important factor in mobilizing secretions from the airways (an effective cough is first). Hydration decreases mucus viscosity and enhances mucociliary effectiveness and cough.[53] In the nonintubated patient, hydration can be accomplished systematically with oral or intravenous fluids. Sources recommend that 1½ to 3 L of decaffeinated fluid per day are necessary to prevent thick mucus and to facilitate cough.[14,36] However, although almost all authorities on pulmonary disease agree that adequate systemic hydration is necessary to mobilize secretions, there is no evidence that overhydration will further assist in mucus mobilization.[17] Cardiovascular and renal function should be considered before hydration orders are implemented; further, patients with COPD who are also hypercapnic tend to retain fluid even in the absence of cardiac decompensation.[17]

Chest physiotherapy. Chest physiotherapy (CPT) is the general title for a group of airway clearance therapies consisting of bronchial drainage, chest percussion, and chest vibration. Effective coughing is an essential aspect of each of these techniques. Although CPT may be initially ordered by a physician, thereby placing it in the category of medical interventions, it is often performed or supervised by the nurse, moving it into the category of a collaborative intervention. In cases of suspected ineffective airway clearance for which coughing alone is insufficient in removing secretions, CPT must be considered. It is often a nursing responsibility to evaluate the need for CPT and to inform the physician that an order should be written.

The specifics about CPT, including recent research findings, are discussed in Chapter 21.

Ineffective Airway Clearance related to excessive secretions

DEFINING CHARACTERISTICS
- Congested lung fields, audible mucus in airways
- Arterial partial pressure of oxygen (Pa_{O_2}) <predicted for age and a given fraction of inspired oxygen concentration (FI_{O_2})
- Pa_{CO_2} >45 mm Hg

OUTCOME CRITERIA
- Cough produces thin mucus.
- Lungs are clear to auscultation.
- Pa_{O_2} is equal to predicted for age.
- Pa_{CO_2} of 35 to 45 mm Hg indicates adequate depth and rate of ventilation.

NURSING INTERVENTIONS *AND RATIONALE*

1. Continue to monitor the assessment parameters listed under "Defining Characteristics."
2. In the absence of cardiac or renal dysfunction, hydrate the 24-hour fluid requirements per body surface area (BSA) (see Appendix C for BSA formula) *to thin secretions. Adequate hydration is the most effective mucolytic. Avoid caffeinated beverages, because caffeine is a mild diuretic and can contribute to fluid loss.*
3. Monitor serum osmolality, *considering that an elevation may indicate need for further hydration.*
4. Provide humidification to airways through mask, room vaporizer, other means *to assist in thinning secretions.* When artificial airway is present, ensure that humidification to airway is available and functioning properly. *Thick, tenacious secretions may mean insufficient fluid intake and/or insufficient external humidification.*
5. Instruct and supervise controlled cough technique. If controlled cough technique is not possible, consider huff coughing or quad coughing techniques.
6. Position for optimal coughing by placing patient either in high-Fowler's position with knees drawn up and a brace for his or her feet or on side with knees drawn up. *High-Fowler's position promotes best diaphragmatic descent and maximal inhalation, which allow maximal cough. Drawn-up knees assist in abdominal muscle contraction, resulting in a stronger expulsive force and cough velocity.*
7. Assess sputum for color, consistency, and amount.

Yellow or green may mean chest infection; an increase in amount may mean a worsening condition.

8. Assess for signs or symptoms of chest infection such as fever, tachycardia, yellow or green mucus (culture and sensitivity may be necessary), leukocytosis, increase in pulmonary crackles or wheezes on chest auscultation, and chest radiograph consistent with alveolar infiltrates.
9. If patient is hypoxemic, administer oxygen, observing the following principles:
   - Without physician's collaboration, liter flow should be no greater than 2 L/min in patients whose pulmonary history is unknown or reveals a pattern of chronic carbon dioxide retention, *because, a high FI_{O_2} in these patients may depress ventilatory drive.*
   - Oyxgen should be administered with the goal of achieving a Pa_{O_2} no greater than 100 mm Hg. *A higher Pa_{O_2} is of little value and may necessitate using an FI_{O_2} higher than 40%, which can precipitate oxygen toxicity (see Chapter 21, "Oxygen Toxicity".*
   - With physician's collaboration, consider the application of mechanical ventilation with positive end-expiratory pressure (PEEP) in patients whose hypoxemia is refractory to high concentrations of oxygen through mask or nasal prongs.
10. Reposition frequently (at least q2 hr) and dynamically *to mobilize secretions and to match ventilation with perfusion.*
11. With physician's collaboration, teach and supervise bronchial drainage with or without chest physiotherapy *to assist with the expulsion of retained secretions.*
12. Consider suctioning nasopharyngeal airway or artificial tracheal airway when secretions are audible.
13. Allow rest periods between coughing sessions, chest physiotherapy, or other demanding activities.
14. Consider breathing exercise sessions that incorporate sustained maximal inhalation of at least 10 per hour with or without the use of an incentive spirometer *to prevent atelectasis.*

Ineffective Airway Clearance related to impaired cough secondary to loss of glottic closure with cuffed endotracheal or tracheostomy tube

DEFINING CHARACTERISTICS

- Impaired cough resulting from bypass of glottis with artificial airway
- Retained lung secretions, lung field congestion

OUTCOME CRITERIA

- Cough is productive of thin mucus.
- Lung auscultation reveals mobilization of secretions with cough.

NURSING INTERVENTIONS *AND RATIONALE*

1. Continue to monitor the assessment parameters listed under "Defining Characteristics."
2. Ensure that the inspired air source (at *any* FIo_2) is humidified, *because the artificial airway bypasses the body's normal humidification system.*
3. In the absence of cardiac or renal disease, hydrate to 24-hour fluid requirements per BSA *to thin secretions.*
4. In patients with reduced vital capacity resulting from weak abdominal and/or diaphragmatic musculature, teach and supervise abdominal muscle-tightening exercises and diaphragmatic breathing.
5. Position for optimal coughing by placing patient either in high-Fowler's position with knees drawn up or on side with knees drawn up. *High-Fowler's position promotes best diaphragmatic descent and maximal inhalation, which allow maximal cough. Drawn-up knees assist in abdominal muscle contraction, resulting in a stronger expulsive force and cough velocity.*
6. Practice coughing, simulating glottis effect:
    - Have patient take deep breath.
    - Place gloved finger over end of airway tube.
    - Have patient contract abdominal muscles.
    - Immediately remove finger.
7. Suction artificial airway as necessary per unit standards. Consider airway lavage, instilling 2 to 4 ml sterile sodium chloride solution during inhalation.
8. Suction oropharyngeally and obtain frequent cuff pressure measurements *to prevent aspiration of oropharyngeal secretions* (see "Potential for Aspiration").

Ineffective Airway Clearance related to knowledge deficit of controlled cough and hydration techniques

DEFINING CHARACTERISTICS

- Frequent hospitalizations for exacerbations of underlying chronic lung disease
- Weak, ineffectual cough
- Congested lung fields on auscultation
- Thick, tenacious mucus

OUTCOME CRITERIA

- Lung auscultation reveals mobilization of secretions with cough.
- Patient demonstrates correct controlled-cough technique.
- Cough is productive of thin mucus.

NURSING INTERVENTIONS *AND RATIONALE*

1. Continue to monitor the assessment parameters listed under "Defining Characteristics."
2. Have patient demonstrate usual technique of airway clearance *to ascertain method of coughing and to point out to the patient why his or her cough is ineffective.*
3. Teach controlled-cough technique. Emphasize the principles of cough physiology discussed on pp. 473-474.
4. In the absence of cardiac or renal dysfunction, teach patient to increase fluid intake to at least his 24-hour fluid requirements per BSA *to keep secretions thin and easily expectorated.* Beverages should be decaffeinated and nonalcoholic.

Ineffective Airway Clearance related to respiratory muscle dysfunction and impaired cough secondary to quadriplegia, paraplegia, Guillain-Barré syndrome, myasthenia gravis, and others

DEFINING CHARACTERISTICS

■ Weak, ineffectual cough
■ Lung fields congested to auscultation
■ Observed weakness of respiratory muscle groups

OUTCOME CRITERIA

■ Cough is productive.
■ Secretions are thin and clear.

NURSING INTERVENTIONS *AND RATIONALE*

1. Continue to monitor the assessment parameters listed under "Defining Characteristics."
2. If hypoxemic, administer oxygen, observing principles detailed under "Ineffective Airway Clearance related to excessive secretions."
3. In the absence of cardiac or renal dysfunction, teach and provide hydration to 24-hour fluid requirements per BSA *to thin secretions and facilitate airway clearance.*
4. Assist with quad coughing, *since weakened or flaccid abdominal muscles will prevent effective cough.*
5. Position patient for most effective cough.
6. Consider chest physiotherapy (bronchial drainage and chest percussion) three to four times per day *to assist with the expulsion of retained secretions.*
7. Change position at least q2 hr *to prevent stasis of secretions and to match ventilation with perfusion.*

Ineffective Airway Clearance related to abdominal or thoracic pain

DEFINING CHARACTERISTICS

■ Congested lung fields, audible mucus in airways
■ Weak, ineffectual cough
■ Presence of pain

OUTCOME CRITERIA

■ Lungs are clear to auscultation.
■ Cough produces thin mucus.

NURSING INTERVENTIONS *AND RATIONALE*

1. Continue to monitor the assessment parameters listed under "Defining Characteristics."
2. Treat pain according to its etiology. See "Acute Pain" in Chapter 28.
3. If hypoxemic, administer oxygen, observing the following principles:
   ■ Without physician's collaboration, liter flow should be no greater than 2 L/min in patients whose pulmonary history is unknown or reveals a pattern of chronic carbon dioxide retention, *because a high FIO_2 in these patients can depress ventilatory drive.*
   ■ Oxygen should be administered with the goal of achieving a PaO_2 no greater than 100 mm Hg. *A higher PaO_2 is of little value and may necessitate using an FIO_2 higher than 40%, which can precipitate oxygen toxicity (see Chapter 21, "Oxygen Toxicity").*
4. In the absence of cardiac or renal dysfunction, hydrate to 24-hour fluid requirements per BSA *to thin secretions and improve airway clearance.*
5. Emphasize deep breathing exercises with sustained maximal inhalation. *They will stimulate an effective cough if, in fact, secretions are present in the airways. Additionally, a more effective cough will be achieved because the high volumes of deep breathing will result in an increased velocity of expired air.*
6. Teach and provide incisional splinting, if appropriate, during breathing exercises in anticipation of cough stimulation and during coughing episodes.

INEFFECTIVE BREATHING PATTERN

Ineffective breathing pattern is defined by the North American Nursing Diagnosis Association as "the state in which an individual's inhalation and exhalation do not enable adequate pulmonary inflation or emptying." Larson and Kim[27] define ineffective breathing patterns as "states in which the individual's inspiratory and/or expiratory pattern does not provide adequate ventilation."

Causes of Ineffective Breathing Pattern

Ineffective breathing pattern results when the muscles of ventilation (the diaphragm and the intercostal muscles) are used *inadequately* for ventilation and/or when the accessory muscles of ventilation are used *improperly* for ventilation. The normal function of these muscles has been discussed in Chapter 17, "Pulmonary Anatomy and Physiology." Ineffective breathing pattern has many causes, which vary significantly in the ways they mediate the disturbance in breathing pattern. These causes include respiratory muscle weakness or fatigue, chronic airflow limitation, abdominal and thoracic pain or surgery, and modifiable or unmodifiable chest wall restrictions.

Respiratory muscle weakness or fatigue. Respiratory muscle fatigue occurs when the normal muscles of ventilation cannot generate or maintain the force required for ventilation. Respiratory fatigue can limit exercise tolerance, magnify dyspnea, alter arterial blood gases, alter the breathing pattern, and may eventually lead to ventilatory failure.

In the hospitalized patient, respiratory muscle *fatigue* is indicated by an abrupt rise in $PaCO_2$, by rapid, shallow ventilations, or by paradoxical abdominal wall motion (abdomen moves in during inhalation and out during exhalation).[24,40,45] Rapid, shallow ventilations are inefficient because they increase physiological dead space and tend to exhaust the patient while not providing ventilation effective enough to meet the metabolic needs of the body (demonstrated by the rising $PaCO_2$).

The ineffective breathing pattern resulting from respiratory muscle fatigue can be a serious complication of failure to wean from mechanical ventilation and, when diagnosed, will only respond to complete rest of the respiratory muscles. Thus the patient must resume mechanical ventilation, and weaning attempts must temporarily halt. Another example of respiratory muscle fatigue occurs in the patient who is admitted with severe cardiogenic pulmonary edema and who progresses quickly from a state of tachypnea to a state of apnea as the work of breathing exhausts him or her and as compromise of his or her oxygen supply continues. Treatment is the institution of mechanical ventilation. Other treatments for respiratory muscle fatigue include pharmacological bronchodilation and continued treatment of any acute illness contributing to the muscle fatigue. Under no circumstances should the patient with respiratory muscle fatigue be instructed in muscle training exercises, fatigued muscles require rest, not more exercise.[1]

Respiratory muscle *weakness* is indicated by a chronic reduction in muscle strength and by a chronic rise in $PaCO_2$. It occurs most commonly in the critical care unit or in the step-down units as a result of prolonged mechanical ventilation (7 days or more) in patients with (1) a chronic lung disease exacerbated by an acute infection, (2) an overwhelming acute pulmonary disease such as adult respiratory distress syndrome, (3) ventilatory failure resulting from extensive extrapulmonary multiorgan failure, or (4) a neuromuscular disease such as Guillain-Barré syndrome.[51] Respiratory muscle weakness and/or respiratory muscle atrophy is more common in patients who have been on *controlled* mechanical ventilation (CMV), rather than in patients who have been on assisted mechanical ventilation (AMV) or synchronized interimittent mandatory ventilation (SIMV), because these methods apparently allow enough use of the muscles of ventilation to prevent respiratory muscle atrophy and to preclude serious weakness.[32,33] Controlled mechanical ventilation, on the other hand, does not allow patient effort during the ventilatory period; thus, it can allow some beginning muscle atrophy, depending on the length of time the patient is mechanically ventilated.

Respiratory muscle weakness and fatigue can result from other causes related to critical illness, including the following:

- Overuse of opiates or muscle relaxants
- Protein-calorie malnutrition[28,52]
- Improper nutritional support (wherein the volume of infused carbohydrate results in a rise in the $PaCO_2$ above that which the patient can reduce through ventilation[35])
- Cor pulmonale because of its tendency to decrease the blood supply to the diaphragm[52]
- Inadequate correction of or inability to correct cardiovascular disease
- Hypophosphatemia, because it impairs diaphragmatic contractility[1,28]
- Other electrolyte abnormalities such as hypokalemia, hypocalcemia, and hypomagnesemia, each of which contributes to poor muscle contractility[1,28]
- Chronic poor patient positioning, which does not facilitate diaphragmatic descent, thus hindering the best use of the diaphragm and/or requiring the use of accessory muscles of ventilation
- Chronic pulmonary disease that causes use of the accessory muscles of ventilation at rest and compromises the normal pattern of ventilation
- Hypoxemia and hypercapnia[8,52]
- Pain, particularly abdominal or thoracic pain

Chronic airflow limitations. Chronic airflow limitations occur most often with those diseases which alter airflow dynamics throughout the tracheobronchial tree; examples include chronic bronchitis, emphysema, and asthma. Although chronic bronchitis, emphysema, and asthma are very different in pathophysiology and clinical manifestations, they share the common characteristics of airflow limitation, dyspnea, and changes in breathing pattern.[25] Patients with these diseases are often admitted to critical care units during an exacerbation of the disease. The *exacerbation* can simply mean a worsening of the disease, or it can mean the patient has developed an acute chest infection that has worsened the disease process and magnified symptoms.

The most common changes in breathing pattern in patients with chronic airflow limitation include the use of the accessory muscles of ventilation at rest as well as during activity, an increase in ventilatory rate, and sometimes a decrease in tidal volume. This altered breathing pattern is detrimental for several reasons.

First, the accessory muscles of ventilation are not efficient at moving the thoracic cage, and lungs, and to do so to provide ventilation, require a significant amount of oxygen. Thus consistent use of the accessory muscles of ventilation, particularly at rest, will increase the patient's oxygen requirements. At the same time, chronic lung disease can limit the amount of oxygen available to a patient. The resulting situation is one of increased oxygen demand with, perhaps, no ability or a limited ability to meet the demand, often resulting in activity intolerance and dyspnea.

Another reason the altered breathing pattern is detrimental involves the decreased tidal volume and increased ventilatory rate consistent with chronic pulmonary disease. This pattern increases the ventilation of dead space. Dead space ventilation does not contribute to oxygenation since air does not reach the alveoli—it reaches only the conducting airways (dead space). Therefore, although the increased ventilatory rate requires more oxygen (because an increased rate is more work), the decreased depth impairs oxygen uptake since less air reaches the alveoli. This altered breathing pattern can result in activity intolerance in the chronically ill pulmonary patient.

Abdominal or thoracic pain. Abdominal or thoracic pain can lead to an ineffective breathing pattern manifested by shallow rapid ventilations and splinting of the anatomical area in which the pain is located. Shallow ventilations alone, even when occurring in a person with healthy lungs, put the person at risk for development of atelectasis.

Patients who have had upper-abdominal surgery frequently display a marked reduction in lung volumes, bilateral diaphragmatic elevation and lower-lobe atelectasis. This diaphragmatic dysfunction is believed caused by inhibition of phrenic nerve output related to stimulation of visceral or somatic efferent pathways during the upper-abdominal surgery.[52] (See the section, "Atelectasis," in Chapter 20.)

Modifiable or unmodifiable chest wall restrictions. Chest wall restrictions cause an ineffective breathing pattern because of the propensity of the restrictions to decrease tidal volume, increase ventilatory rate, and cause a sensation of dyspnea. Modifiable chest wall restrictions are those which can be corrected with treatment or time and result from pneumothorax, pleural effusion, surgery, or trauma involving the chest wall. Unmodifiable chest wall restrictions are permanent, at least in the short run, and include those which result from obesity, kyphoscoliosis, ascites, or neuromuscular disorders.

The ineffective breathing patterns related to modifiable chest wall restrictions, especially those resulting from chest or abdominal surgery or trauma, have a high likelihood of causing atelectasis. The low tidal volume and high ventilatory rate generally caused by splinting and pain are the direct causes of the atelectasis.

Defining Characteristics of Ineffective Breathing Pattern

Defining characteristics of an ineffective breathing pattern include dyspnea, tachypnea, decreased tidal volume, use of the accessory muscles of ventilation at rest or with activity, auscultation of abnormal breath sounds, and changes in arterial blood gas values, specifically changes in the $PaCO_2$. Other defining characteristics reported in the literature include shortness of breath,[57] orthopnea, bradypnea, splinted-guarded respirations, and hyperpnia.[10]

Nursing Interventions of Ineffective Breathing Pattern

Methods of treating ineffective breathing pattern are related to the cause. The nursing assessment should reveal data that directs interventions to a specific area. For example, when ineffective breathing pattern results from pain caused by chest trauma or surgery, nursing interventions should be directed toward pain relief. The nursing care plans included with this chapter list many specific nursing interventions that can be used to treat ineffective breathing pattern. Some interventions are discussed in more detail.

Pursed-lip and diaphragmatic breathing. Pursed-lip and diaphragmatic breathing are techniques that can help improve the control of ventilation and prolong pulmonary emptying time.[9] The objectives of these breathing techniques include (1) promoting greater use of the diaphragm while decreasing use of the chest and neck accessory muscles of ventilation, (2) allowing the patient to suppress the tendency for hurried, gasping ventilations, (3) improving the effectiveness of alveolar ventilation by increasing tidal volume, prolonging pulmonary emptying time, and improving the relationship between ventilation and perfusion within the lungs and possibly, and (4) improving the strength and endurance of the inspiratory muscles.

Pursed-lip breathing is an expiratory maneuver often adopted by dyspneic patients in an effort to control their dyspnea. This maneuver stimulates positive end-expiratory pressure (PEEP), prevents premature airway collapse, and is believed to provide internal stability of the airways during exhalation.[25]

The pursed-lip breathing technique is easily learned (see box, "Pursed Lip Breathing"). However, patients with severe shortness of breath, depending on its cause, may not benefit from instruction of this technique until their condition improves enough to allow a learning experience.

Diaphragmatic breathing (see box, "Diaphragmatic Breathing") is a method through which the patient tones his or her diaphragm. It may be particularly helpful to the patient with emphysema or to the patient with an emphysemic component to another obstructive pulmonary disease.

Emphysema will inevitably lead to an ineffective breathing pattern, because progression of emphysema produces severe hyperinflation of the lungs, which compresses and flattens the diaphragm, rendering the diaphragm useless for ventilation. As the diaphragm becomes less functional, patients compensate by using their neck and chest accessory muscles to provide the ventilation that was previously the function of the diaphragm. Designed for use only during exercise, the accessory muscles use excessive amounts of oxygen when, to the exclusion of the diaphragm, they provide ventilation at rest. The patient with emphysema may benefit from education in diaphragmatic breathing so that this muscle can be toned and be once again functional.[13]

PURSED-LIP BREATHING

- With mouth closed, inhale through nose.
- Exhale through mouth with lips "pursed" (lips in a whistling or kissing position).
- Make exhalation at least twice as long as inhalation (2 seconds in, 4 seconds out).

RATIONALE

Explain to the patient that this maneuver keeps airways open longer during exhalation and evacuates trapped air. The procedure for pursed-lip breathing can be used, along with diaphragmatic breathing, during episodes of shortness of breath.

DIAPHRAGMATIC BREATHING

Have the patient place two fingers just below the xiphoid process and push in with his or her fingers while sniffing gently. Explain that the movement felt at the fingertips is the diaphragm moving as he or she sniffs and that this muscle requires exercise so that it can increase the efficiency of breathing.

TECHNIQUE

- Place one hand on chest, one hand on abdomen.
- Inhale, pushing abdominal hand outward.
- Exhale slowly (through pursed lips), allowing abdominal hand to fall inward.
- Chest hand should remain still.

RATIONALE

Explain that this maneuver saves energy because the diaphragm uses oxygen more efficiently than the accessory muscles and that this technique retrains the diaphragm to assume the work of breathing. Diaphragmatic breathing is useful in terminating episodes of acute shortness of breath but should also be incorporated into a regular routine of muscle retraining.

Diaphragmatic breathing, when practiced in conjunction with pursed-lip breathing, can decrease respiratory rate and increase tidal volume.[17] It has long been thought, although research has yet to prove it true, that diaphragmatic breathing allows the patient to tone and retrain his or her diaphragm so that it can once again be used as the primary muscle of inhalation,[13] whereas pursed-lip breathing prevents further air trapping responsible for the lung hyperinflation associated with emphysema.

Correcting respiratory muscle weakness. Although strength training of weakened respiratory muscles may be necessary, it is hardly advisable for a patient to begin a full program during recovery from acute illness or during weaning from mechanical ventilation. Weaning requires increased use of the respiratory muscles, which, if already weakened, may not be able to function consistently if such a program is begun during an acute illness.

When studies of respiratory muscle strength training show positive results (and many studies show no positive results), it is only after weeks of training with patients who are not hospitalized. Since it is not advisable for respiratory muscle training to proceed during mechanical ventilation or weaning or during acute illness and since respiratory muscle weakness does exist, the critical care nurse must use other approaches to assist the patient with respiratory muscle weakness.

Included in these approaches is the assessment for and correction of, when possible, each of the conditions listed previously that can exacerbate respiratory muscle weakness such as electrolyte disturbances or patient positioning that does not allow free diaphragmatic descent or chest wall expansion (see p. 478). Additionally, it is important that any source that might increase the *work of breathing* (WOB) be identified and eliminated. In the mechanically ventilated patient, this includes eliminating extra dead space from within the system or from an unnecessarily long endotracheal tube. The WOB can increase because of added inspiratory work from ventilator circuitry used during intermittent mandatory ventilation (IMV) or SIMV. Because of the manner in which some of the older ventilators were designed, use of IMV or SIMV causes extra work on the part of the patient because spontaneous breathing requires the patient to overcome the intrinsic pressure and flow resistant characteristics of the ventilator circuitry.[7,33,34,51] For this reason, newer ventilators should be used when weaning is begun, or T-piece weaning may be considered. Ventilators that offer pressure support can decrease the WOB enough to provide sufficient rest of the ventilatory muscles.[21,30]

Aminophylline or theophylline administration may be suggested to the physician because therapeutic doses of these drugs both improve the contractility of the diaphragm[3,16,17] and protect against diaphragmatic fatigue, although significant controversy exists in the literature.[2,3,37,51] Further, theophylline will ease the WOB by relaxing smooth muscle, most notably the bronchial smooth muscle.

Ineffective Breathing Pattern related to chronic airflow limitations

DEFINING CHARACTERISTICS

- Use of accessory muscles of ventilation
- Reported and/or observed episodes of respiratory panic
- Chest breathing

OUTCOME CRITERIA

- Patient demonstrates pursed-lip and diaphragmatic breathing regularly and during episodes of respiratory panic.

NURSING INTERVENTIONS *AND RATIONALE*

1. Continue to monitor the assessment parameters listed under "Defining Characteristics."
2. Teach and supervise pursed-lip breathing. *Explain that this maneuver keeps airways open longer during exhalation and evacuates trapped air.* The procedure for pursed-lip breathing should be used along with diaphragmatic breathing during episodes of shortness of breath.
3. Teach and supervise diaphragmatic breathing. *Explain that this maneuver saves energy (the diaphragm uses oxygen more efficiently than the accessory muscles) and retrains the diaphragm to assume its normal percentage of the work of breathing.* Diaphragmatic breathing is useful in terminating episodes of acute shortness of breath but should *also* be incorporated into an hourly routine of muscle retraining.
4. During episodes of acute shortness of breath or respiratory panic, it is useful for the nurse to actually *breathe with* the patient, using pursed-lip and diaphragmatic breathing techniques. It is *not* useful during such an episode to instruct or encourage the use of these techniques. Statements such as, "Now slow down your breathing" or "Take nice big breaths for me," *do little to assist the patient in regaining control of his breathing pattern. Additionally, concentration on techniques of breathing may serve the very beneficial function of distracting the patient from fear and panic.*

Ineffective Breathing Pattern related to modifiable chest wall restrictions secondary to pneumothorax or pleural effusion

DEFINING CHARACTERISTICS

- Shallow tachypnea
- Atelectatic crackles
- Diminished breath sounds
- Asymmetrical chest expansion

OUTCOME CRITERIA

- Respiratory rate at rest is <20.
- Atelectatic crackles are minimal or absent.
- Breath sounds are full and equal bilaterally.
- Chest expands symmetrically.

NURSING INTERVENTIONS *AND RATIONALE*

1. Continue to monitor the assessment parameters listed under "Defining Characteristics." Additionally, check serial chest radiographs *to monitor resolution of underlying disorder.*
2. Treat pain, if present, according to cause. See "Acute Pain" in Chapter 28.
3. If hypoxemic, administer oxygen, observing the principles detailed under "Ineffective Breathing Pattern related to abdominal or thoracic pain."
4. Teach and supervise deep breathing with sustained maximal inspiration. *In the patient with a pneumothorax and a chest tube, this maneuver reexpands the lung and evacuates air (and fluid) from the pleural space into the chest drainage system. In the patient with a pleural effusion, this maneuver may reexpand atelectatic portions of the lung overlying the pleural effusion.*
5. Reposition the patient q2 hr, observing the "good lung down" principle *to limit pain, as well as to better match ventilation with perfusion* (see pp. 485-486). Favor a head-of-bed up position *to facilitate diaphragmatic descent.*
6. Avoid coughing exercises unless there are audible secretions in the airways. *Coughing is painful and, if performed unnecessarily (as in the absence of secretions), may promote airway collapse or atelectasis.*
7. For assessment and maintenance of chest tubes and closed chest drainage systems, see Chapter 21.

Ineffective Breathing Pattern related to respiratory muscle deconditioning secondary to mechanical ventilation

DEFINING CHARACTERISTICS

- Hypercapnia
- Atelectatic crackles
- Use of accessory ventilatory muscles
- Anxious behaviors
- During spontaneous breaths, tidal volume less than predicted, diminished basilar breath sounds, decreased chest excursion, and tachypnea

OUTCOME CRITERIA

- Tidal volume is greater than or equal to predicted.
- Breath sounds are clear from apices to bases.
- Normocapnia.

NURSING INTERVENTIONS *AND RATIONALE*

Continue to monitor the assessment parameters listed under "Defining Characteristics."

For mechanically ventilated patients

1. Assist the patient to distinguish spontaneous breaths from mechanically delivered breaths by helping him or her to identify the sensation of breathing *(this is lost when air bypasses the nasooropharynx)* through simple kinesthetic feedback: "The machine is giving you six breaths per minute; you are breathing on your own in between the machine breaths. Feel the difference between the machine's breaths and your own. You are working to make your own breaths as deep and full as the machine's."
2. Carefully snip excess length from the proximal end of the endotracheal tube *to decrease dead space and thereby decrease the work of breathing. Similarly, ensure that ventilator circuit tubings impose no excess dead space.*
3. Collaborate with physician about the application of pressure support to the mechanical ventilator or about the use of a ventilator which will not increase the work of breathing during the IMV or SIMV breaths. *There should be no excessive work of breathing on the part of the patient because of ventilator circuitry. Pressure support may decrease the work of breathing.*
4. Position patient in semi-Fowler's position *for best use of ventilatory muscles and to facilitate diaphragmatic descent.*
5. Confront patient's fear and support his or her confidence; provide progress reports frequently: "The volume of your breaths is steadily increasing and this has made your lungs clearer. Your hard work is paying off."
6. Avoid pharmacological sedation if possible. Consult with physician in selecting a sedative drug with minimal muscle relaxant effects.
7. With physician's collaboration, ensure that at least 50% of the diet's nonprotein caloric source is in the form of lipid (fat) versus carbohydrates to prevent excess carbon dioxide accumulation. *Carbon dioxide is an end product of carbohydrate metabolism, and its excess accumulation in the bloodstream falsely suggests a reduction in the patient's alveolar ventilation. Additionally, excess carbon dioxide increases the patient's ventilatory work load.*

Ineffective Breathing Pattern related to abdominal or thoracic pain

DEFINING CHARACTERISTICS

- Atelectatic crackles
- Asymmetrical chest expansion caused by splinting
- Hypocapnia
- Diminished basiliar breath sounds, shallow breathing
- Presence of pain

OUTCOME CRITERIA

- Breath sounds are clear and equal bilaterally.
- Chest expands symmetrically.
- $Paco_2$ is 35 to 45 mm Hg.

NURSING INTERVENTIONS *AND RATIONALE*

1. Continue to monitor the assessment parameters listed under "Defining Characteristics."
2. Treat pain according to its cause. See "Acute Pain" in Chapter 28.
3. If patient is hypoxemic, administer oxygen, observing the following principles:
   - Without physician's collaboration, liter flow should be no greater than 2 L/min in patients whose pulmonary history is unknown or reveals a pattern of chronic carbon dioxide retention *because a high Flo_2 in these patients may depress ventilatory drive.*
   - Oxygen should be administered with the goal of achieving a Pao_2 no greater than 95 mm Hg.
   - Observe caution when administering oxygen at Flo_2 greater than 40% *in view of the higher risk for oxygen toxicity.* With physician's collaboration, consider the application of mechanical ventilation with PEEP in patients whose hypoxemia is refractory to high concentrations of oxygen.

For thoracic pain

1. Carefully distinguish between chest wall pain and the pain of myocardial ischemia. For example, ask the patient if this pain is his "usual" chest wall or incisional pain, palpate the chest wall to elicit the pain, and have the patient take a deep breath to elicit the pain. *These maneuvers will reasonably confirm the existence of chest wall or incisional pain versus the pain of myocardial ischemia. If any doubt exists, a 12-lead electrocardiogram (ECG) should be obtained.*
2. Teach and supervise deep breathing or incentive spirometry with sustained maximal inhalation. The emphasis with these modalities should be on the *diaphragmatic breathing technique* (see box on p. 480 and care plan "Ineffective Breathing Pattern related to knowledge deficit of pursed-lip and diaphragmatic breathing") *to increase abdominal expansion and decrease chest wall expansion, thereby decreasing pain.*
3. Reposition patient at least q2 hr, observing the "good lung down" principle (see pp. 485-486). *This will result in decreased incidence of pain and better matching of ventilation with perfusion.*
4. Treat impaired coughing. See "Ineffective Airway Clearance related to abdominal and thoracic pain."

For abdominal pain

1. Teach and supervise deep breathing or incentive spirometry with sustained maximal inspiration. *The emphasis for these maneuvers should not be diaphragmatic breathing but chest breathing to decrease the incidence of abdominal pain.*
2. Reposition patient frequently and dynamically. Favor semi-Fowler's to high-Fowler's position *to maximize chest expansion.*

Ineffective Breathing Pattern related to unmodifiable chest wall restrictions secondary to kyphoscoliosis or obesity

DEFINING CHARACTERISTICS

- Activity intolerance (i.e., heart rate elevations 30 beats above baseline with activity [15 beats above baseline for patients on beta or calcium channel blockers]; heart rate elevations above baseline 5 minutes after activity; dyspnea)
- Shallow tachypnea

OUTCOME CRITERIA

- Patient has subjective and objective activity tolerance.

NURSING INTERVENTIONS *AND RATIONALE*

1. Continue to monitor the assessment parameters listed under "Defining Characteristics."
2. Prevent unnecessary exertion *because the patient's ventilatory reserve is limited.* Grade all activity to within the patient's tolerance as measured by heart rate elevations less than 30 beats above baseline with activity. Heart rate elevations less than 15 beats above baseline with activity indicates activity tolerance in patients receiving beta or calcium channel blockers.
3. If patient is hypoxemic, administer oxygen, observing the principles detailed under "Ineffective Breathing Pattern related to abdominal or thoracic pain." Ensure that oxygen is administered, especially during activity.
4. Teach and supervise energy-saving techniques (see Care Plan on p. 344).
5. Teach and supervise diaphragmatic breathing. *Diaphragmatic breathing is especially effective in patients with unmodifiable chest wall restrictions because it allows an increase in the tidal volume through diaphragmatic descent, which is otherwise impossible through chest wall expansion.* Incorporate the sustained maximal inspiration maneuver when possible.
6. Reposition patient dynamically q2 hr, favoring semi-Fowler's to high-Fowler's position *to facilitate diaphragmatic descent.*
7. Ideally, position the patient sitting at the bedside with arms resting on a pillow on the overbed table. *This position eliminates splinting of the chest wall against any surface and thereby decreases chest wall restriction and work of breathing.*

IMPAIRED GAS EXCHANGE

The North American Nursing Diagnosis Association (NANDA) defines impaired gas exchange as "a state in which the individual experiences a decreased passage of oxygen and/or carbon dioxide between the alveoli of the lungs and the vascular system."

Causes of Impaired Gas Exchange

Many medical disorders can result in impaired gas exchange. Some most commonly seen in critical care units are acute respiratory failure (ARF), adult respiratory distress syndrome (ARDS), acute pneumonia, acute exacerbations of chronic obstructive pulmonary disease (COPD), end-stage emphysema, pneumothorax, and atelectasis. These disorders result in impaired gas exchange because of the intrapulmonary pathology for which they are responsible, including ventilation-perfusion imbalance, pulmonary shunting, and alveolar hypoventilation. Treatment of the medical disorders and, consequently, the intrapulmonary pathology associated with impaired gas exchange may or may not be possible, and the success of treatment varies greatly with the individual and with the extent of his or her illness. Bronchodilators, mucolytics, antibiotics, intermittent positive pressure breathing (IPPB), chest physiotherapy, and incentive spirometry are all directed at increasing alveolar ventilation, treating infection, or removing mucus from the airways. Oxygen therapy is used because of its direct effect on increasing the PaO_2.

Impaired gas exchange can result secondarily from the need for a specialized pulmonary hygiene regimen and/or specialized patient positioning. Treatment of the secondary causes of impaired gas exchange rests strictly within the realm of nursing and is discussed further under "Nursing Interventions."

Defining Characteristics of Impaired Gas Exchange

The most important defining characteristics of impaired gas exchange are *hypoxemia*, defined as a PaO_2 <80 mm Hg or less than predicted for the patient's age and/or *hypercapnia*, defined as an $PaCO_2$ >45 mm Hg. Impaired gas exchange can only be definitively diagnosed by assessing arterial blood gas values. Other defining characteristics of impaired gas exchange listed in the literature may be presumptive of it, but none is definitive. Presumptive defining characteristics include confusion, somnolence, lethargy, restlessness, irritability, inability to move secretions, cardiac dysrhythmias, polycythemia, inability to concentrate,[44] tendency to assume a three-point breathing position, increased anterior-posterior chest diameter, increased pulmonary vascular resistance, and cyanosis.

Hypoxemia and hypercapnia are vital to the diagnosis of impaired gas exchange. Critical care nurses should be aware of the physical signs and symptoms that portend hypoxemia or hypercapnia, because it is often their presence that prompts the drawing of blood for arterial blood gas analysis. A review of these indicators reveals how closely they relate to the presumptive signs and symptoms of impaired gas exchange.

Hypoxemia, before it progresses to tissue hypoxia, has

no physical signs or symptoms. The clinical effects are a direct result of tissue hypoxia. (See the discussion of hypoxemia and hypoxia in Chapter 20.) Early indicators of tissue hypoxia can be very subtle. Slight hyperventilation, minor visual disturbances, and impairment of intellectual function often are present.[53] Many of the more commonly cited signs and symptoms do not occur until the PaO_2 falls below 40 to 50 mm Hg.[29,53,55] They include tachycardia, increased cardiac output, headache, lethargy, somnolence, and confusion. Although these signs and symptoms are indicative of tissue hypoxia, they may also portend other events such as neurological, cardiac, or metabolic disease. For this reason, they cannot be considered definitive of *impaired gas exchange.*

Exclusive of assessment of an elevated $PacO_2$, the signs and symptoms of hypercapnia include headache (usually occipital), asterixis, lethargy, and confusion. High levels of $PacO_2$ are narcotic and cause clouding of consciousness.[55] Headache results from the increased cerebral blood flow mediated by the elevated $PacO_2$. Because the pH will fall as the $PacO_2$ rises, the signs and symptoms of hypercapnia are as much related to the depressed pH as they are to the elevated $PacO_2$.

Nursing Interventions for Impaired Gas Exchange

In considering the diagnosis impaired gas exchange, many nurses are tempted to relate the diagnosis to COPD, ARDS, or ARF, for example, Impaired Gas Exchange related to ARDS. The problem with this approach is that nurses do not treat these causes—physicians do. Nurses, on the other hand, treat aspects of these diseases (for example, ineffective breathing pattern or ineffective airway clearance), and nurses also collaborate to institute and monitor the progression of the medical interventions associated with these diseases. (The medical interventions for these and other pulmonary diseases, as well as the nursing care associated with pulmonary disease and their medical interventions, have been discussed previously in this text.) Because impaired gas exchange is a nursing diagnosis that often refers to the dysfunction of the alveolar-capillary membrane, few *independent* nursing interventions will treat impaired gas exchange. Indeed, the medical community has difficulty treating diseases that affect the alveolar-capillary membrane, hence the high degree of morbidity and mortality from ARDS. As a result, impaired gas exchange differs significantly from ineffective airway clearance and ineffective breathing pattern, diagnoses in which there are many more independent or collaborative nursing interventions with which to treat the patient. However, impaired gas exchange can result partially from a need for pulmonary hygiene and improper patient positioning, both of which are amenable to nursing interventions.

Pulmonary hygiene. As a cause of impaired gas exchange, the need for pulmonary hygiene is not difficult to assess. All patients with excessive mucus within their airways need either a program of pulmonary hygiene or need their present program reevaluated. Pulmonary hygiene is a broad term having various meanings throughout the country. For this discussion it includes maintenance of airways free from mucus through chest physiotherapy, incentive spirom-

etry, instruction in cough technique, hydration, and suctioning. All these treatments should be considered when evaluating a program for treating impaired gas exchange. However, impaired gas exchange often results from mucus or secretions within the small airways in which coughing and suctioning are of no value.

Although the use of chest physiotherapy and incentive spirometry may require a physician's order, the nurse either performs or supervises the treatments. Chest physiotherapy is aimed at augmenting the removal of mucus within the airways through percussion of the chest, assumption of Trendelenberg's position by the patient (when he or she can tolerate it), and effective coughing on the part of the patient. Incentive spirometry is aimed at providing lung inflation that will prevent atelectasis. Critically ill patients who are not on mechanical ventilation will benefit from incentive spirometry, because atelectasis is one of the major complications of critical illness and prolonged hospitalization.

Cough and hydration will treat impaired gas exchange by augmenting mucus removal. Hydration is thought to decrease the viscosity of mucus, thus easing expectoration. However, many critically ill patients require fluid restrictions that disallow effective hydration. In these cases, collaboration with the physician about alternative treatment such as the administration of mucolytic or bronchodilator drugs may be of benefit. Increasing the humidification through the ventilator tubing may be one method of thinning secretions, although it should be remembered that humidification will also add to the patient's fluid volume and may be contraindicated when a diagnosis of fluid volume excess is present or possible. Instruction in effective cough technique is essential when mucus is present within the airways. When a patient appears too weak to generate an effective cough alone, the use of huff coughing or quad coughing should be considered.

Suctioning the airways is effective only in removing mucus from the trachea and possibly from the upper portion of the main-stem bronchi. Suctioning through a tracheostomy tube allows the catheter to reach farther than suctioning through an endotracheal tube or through the nasopharynx. However, Luce, Tyler, and Pierson[29] maintain that, "even when suctioning through a tracheostomy tube, suctioning cannot be counted on to clear secretions from any portion of the airway distal to the trachea." For these reasons, suctioning is not a treatment that should be used alone. The effectiveness of suctioning as a treatment for impaired gas exchange will only be apparent when combined with cough, hydration, and perhaps, chest physiotherapy.

Since a depressed PaO_2 may already exist in patients with impaired gas exchange, the suctioning procedure should be accomplished with as little further depression of the PaO_2 as possible. Methods to achieve this include preoxygentation and postoxygentation of the airway, hyperinflation of the lungs with preoxygenation and postoxygenation of the airway, or use of an oxygen insufflation suction catheter.

Patient positioning. Patient positioning has recently been implicated in altering the PaO_2.[12,38,54] Many studies have researched the effects of body position on PaO_2 and lung volumes. Extensive literature reviews published by Tyler[54] and Norton and Conforti[38] have revealed the efficacy of

Table 22-2 Results of research on the effects of the lateral position on oxygenation

Author	Date	N	Subjects	Description	Pao$_2$	Q̇s/Q̇t	CO	V̇o$_2$	AaDo$_2$	Paco$_2$	Vd/Vt
Zach and others	1974	38	Unilateral	SB*	↑ GLD					↔	
			Bilateral	SB	↑ RLD					↔	
			Normal	SB	↔					↔	
Katz and Barash	1977	1	Multiple trauma	PPB	↑ GLD	↓	↔				
Seaton and others	1979	12	Lobectomy via thoracotomy incision (all had chronic lung disease)	SB preoperatively	↔					↔	↔
				SB	↑ GLD	↓			↓		
Dhainaut and others	1980	4	Unilateral pneumonia	SB	↑ GLD	↓	↔	↔			
Remolina and others	1981	9	Unilateral lung disease	8 SB	↑ GLD					↔	
				1 PPB							
Ibanez and others	1981	10	Unilateral disease	PPB and PEEP	↑ GLD				↓	↔	

From Norton LC and Conforti CG: Heart Lung 14(1):45, 1985.
*Key: SB, spontaneous breathing; PPB, positive pressure breathing; GLD, good lung down; RLD, right lung down; ↔, no change.

Table 22-3 Effects of position on arterial oxygenation—the results of nine studies

			Patient position		
Author	Factor affecting lung	Variable measured	Supine	Sick lung dependent	Healthy lung dependent
Zack and others	Unilateral infiltrate	Pao$_2$*		77	86
Remolina and others	Unilateral infiltrate	Pao$_2$	67	59	106
Tyler (unpublished master's thesis)	Unilateral infiltrate	ΔPao$_2$		−23 mm Hg	−1 mm Hg
Seaton and others	Thoracotomy	Pao$_2$ preoperatively	69	68	69
		Pao$_2$ postoperatively†	98	100	106
Syracuse	Unilateral consolidation	ΔPao$_2$		−19%	+17%
Dhainaut	Unilateral pneumonia	Pao$_2$‡	149		254
Heaf	Unilateral infiltrate (in infants)	Pao$_2$	78	82	73
Sonnenblick	Unilateral pleural effusion	Pao$_2$		67	72
Rindfleisch	Asymmetric pleural effusion	Sao$_2$	94.3%	93.4%	94.7%

Modified from Tyler ML: Respir Care 29(5): 472, 1984.
*In mm Hg; values shown are means.
†Flo$_2$ 0.40.
‡Flo$_2$ 1.00.

positioning the good lung down in patients with unilateral lung disease and of positioning the right lung down in patients with bilateral lung disease (Table 22-2). Tyler[54] writes,

The successful use of body position to enhance lung function is based on the recognition of the gravity-dependent nature of perfusion and ventilation in the lung. Because perfusion is greater in whatever part of the lung is dependent, it is possible to selectively increase or decrease blood flow to various areas of the lung. The patient is simply positioned so that the area in which increased blood flow is desired is dependent.

Most of the published research has shown Pao$_2$ elevations with these positioning maneuvers. Table 22-3 shows the change in the Pao$_2$ that occurs when the healthy lung is placed dependent versus placing the sick lung dependent.

The good lung down position favors oxygenation because ventilation/perfusion (V/Q) matching is improved. However, the effect of position on the Pao$_2$ is modified by age and lung disease. Further, a very few pathologies do exist that benefit from having the sick lung dependent, including unilateral interstitial pulmonary emphysema and lung abscess.[12] In cases of doubt about the benefit of position on oxygenation, arterial blood gas values should be evaluated so that any increase or decrease in the Pao$_2$ resulting from the position change may be recorded on the patient's plan of care.

Impaired Gas Exchange related to ventilation-perfusion inequality secondary to (specify)

DEFINING CHARACTERISTICS

Definitive

- $Pao_2 <$ predicted for age
- $Paco_2 > 45$ mm Hg (hypercapnia)

Presumptive

- Confusion
- Somnolence
- Restlessness
- Irritability
- Inability to move secretions

OUTCOME CRITERIA

- Pao_2 is equal to predicted for age.
- $Paco_2$ is 35 to 45 mm Hg or back to baseline for patient.
- Airways are clear of mucus.

NURSING INTERVENTIONS *AND RATIONALE*

1. Continue to monitor the assessment parameters listed under "Defining Characteristics." Additionally, observe for physical signs and symptoms of tissue hypoxia (increased respiratory rate, visual disturbances, impairment of intellectual function, headache, lethargy, tachycardia, dysrhythmias) and hypercapnia (headache [usually occipital], asterixis, lethargy, confusion).

2. Administer oxygen, observing the following principles:
   - Without physician's collaboration, liter flow should be no greater than 2 L/min in patients whose pulmonary history is unknown or reveals a pattern of chronic carbon dioxide retention, *because high a Flo_2 in these patients may depress ventilatory drive.*
   - Oxygen should be administered with the goal of achieving a Pao_2 no greater than 100 mm Hg. *A higher Pao_2 is of little value and may necessitate an Flo_2 higher than 40% which can precipitate oxygen toxicity (see "Oxygen Toxicity" in Chapter 21).*
   - With physician's collaboration, consider the application of CPAP or mechanical ventilation with PEEP in patients whose hypoxemia is refractory to high concentrations of oxygen. *CPAP and PEEP accomplish alveolar hyperinflation, thereby increasing the surface area for gas exchange.*

3. In the absence of cardiac or renal dysfunction, hydrate to 24-hour fluid requirements per body surface area (BSA) (see Appendix C for BSA formula) *to thin secretions. Adequate hydration is the most effective mucolytic. Avoid caffeinated beverages because caffeine is a mild diuretic and can contribute to fluid loss.*

4. Monitor serum osmolality, *considering that an elevation may indicate need for further hydration.*

5. Provide humidification to airways through mask, room vaporizor, or other means *to assist in thinning secretions.* When artifical airway is present, ensure that humidification of airway is available and functioning properly. *Thick, tenacious secretions may indicate insufficient fluid intake and/or, a need for external humidification.*

6. Consider suctioning if mucus is suspected within the trachea. If mucus is suspected within the main-stem or segmental bronchi, assist in its passage into the trachea through cough or chest physiotherapy. *Most studies have shown suctioning is effective only in evacuating mucus from the tracheal level; therefore every effort should be made to move mucus into the trachea before suctioning is attempted.* Always preoxygenate and postoxygenate the patient's airways as part of the suctioning technique *to prevent further decrease of the Pao_2 as a result of suctioning.*

7. For a patient with unilateral lung disease, position him or her with the good lung down because *this will best match ventilation with perfusion and result in improved Pao_2.* (Exception: place sick lung down in cases of lung abcess or unilateral interstitial pulmonary emphysema.)

8. For patient with bilateral lung disease, position with right lung down because *this lung is larger than the left lung and affords a greater area for ventilation and perfusion. Further, the cardiac output may be enhanced in the right lateral position.*

9. Evaluate arterial blood gas values obtained with the patient in various positions so that the position that results in the best oxygenation may be revealed.

10. Change the patient's position at least q2 hr, favoring those positions that allow the best oxygenation. Limit the time the patient spends in a position that compromises oxygenation. Avoid any position that seriously decreases the Pao_2.

11. When appropriate, instruct patient in controlled-cough technique or huff or quad cough techniques, depending on the patient's cough ability.

12. Obtain order for incentive spirometry and instruct in its proper use *as a means to prevent atelectasis, which can further complicate or worsen impaired gas exchange.*

13. Evaluate need for chest physiotherapy.

Impaired Gas Exchange related to alveolar hypoventilation secondary to (specify)

DEFINING CHARACTERISTICS

- Pao_2 <predicted for age
- Hypercapnia

OUTCOME CRITERIA

- Pao_2 is within limits of norm for age.
- $Paco_2$ is 35 to 45 mm Hg.

NURSING INTERVENTIONS *AND RATIONALE*

1. Continue to monitor the assessment parameters listed under "Defining Characteristics." Additionally, observe for physical signs and symptoms of tissue hypoxia (increased respiratory rate, visual disturbances, impairment of intellectual function, headache, lethargy, tachycardia, dysrhythmias) and hypercapnia (headache [usually occipital], asterixis, lethargy, confusion).
2. Administer oxygen, observing the following principles:
   - Without physician's collaboration, liter flow should be no greater than 2 L/min in patients whose pulmonary history is unknown or reveals a pattern of chronic carbon dioxide retention *because a high Flo_2 in these patients may depress ventilatory drive.*
   - Oxygen should be administered with the goal of achieving a Pao_2 no greater than 100 mm Hg. *A higher Pao_2 is of little value and may necessitate an Flo_2 higher than 40% which can precipitate oxygen toxicity (see "Oxygen Toxicity" in Chapter 21).*
   - With physician's collaboration, consider the application of continuous positive airway pressure (CPAP) or mechanical ventilation with positive end-expiratory pressure (PEEP) in patients whose hypoxemia is refractory to high concentrations of oxygen. *CPAP and PEEP accomplish alveolar hyperinflation, thereby increasing the surface area for gas exchange.*
3. Intervene deliberately to resolve the specific cause of the alveolar hypoventilation.

Potential for Aspiration

Definition: The state in which an individual is at risk for entry of gastrointestinal secretions, oropharyngeal secretions, or solids or fluids into tracheobronchial passages.

RISK FACTORS

- Reduced level of consciousness
- Depressed cough and gag reflexes
- Presence of tracheostomy or endotracheal tube
- Incomplete lower esophageal sphincter
- Gastrointestinal tubes
- Tube feedings
- Medication administration
- Situations hindering elevation of upper body
- Increased intragastric pressure
- Increased gastric residual
- Decreased gastrointestinal motility
- Delayed gastric emptying
- Impaired swallowing
- Facial/oral/neck surgery or trauma
- Wired jaws

DEFINING CHARACTERISTICS OF AN ACTUAL PROBLEM

Early
- Hypoxemia

Later (6 hours after aspiration)
- Dyspnea
- Wheezing, crackles
- Cough with pink, frothy exudate, resembling cardiogenic pulmonary edema
- Fever

- Tachycardia
- Hypotension
- Radiological: patchy alveolar infiltrates in portions of lung dependent at time of aspiration
- Evidence of gastric contents in lung secretions

OUTCOME CRITERIA

- Lungs are clear to auscultation.
- Pao_2 is proportional to that predicted for age and Flo_2.
- Lung secretions show no evidence of gastric contents.
- Patient is afebrile.

NURSING INTERVENTIONS *AND RATIONALE*

1. Continue to monitor the assessment parameters listed under "Defining Characteristics."
2. Auscultate bowel sounds and assess abdominal contour and girth. *Rule out hypoactive peristalsis and abdominal distention with gastric contents, thereby avoiding the heightened risk of esophageal reflux.*
3. Position patient with 30-degree elevation of head of bed (lying on side ideally) *to prevent gastric reflux through gravity.* Whenever head elevation is contraindicated, a right lateral decubitus position is recommended *because it facilitates passage of gastric contents across the pylorus.*

Potential for Aspiration—cont'd

4. Suction and clear oropharyngeal secretions. For patients with cuffed tracheostomy or endotracheal tubes, suction oropharyngeally and obtain cuff pressure measurements *to limit aspiration of oropharyngeal secretions.*

5. Maintain patency and functioning of nasogastric suction apparatus.

6. Treat nausea promptly; consider obtaining physician's order for antiemetic *to prevent vomiting and resultant aspiration.*

7. With physician's collaboration, consider administration of oral antacids and H_2 receptor antagonists *to increase gastric pH and thereby limit chemical burn to lung tissue should aspiration occur.*

Additional interventions for patients receiving continuous or intermittent enteral tube feedings

1. Position patient with 45-degree head elevation at all times *to prevent gastric reflux across an epiglottis held open by the gastric tube.* If a head-down position becomes necessary at any time, interrupt the feeding 30 minutes to 1 hour before position change.

2. Check placement of feeding tube either by auscultation or radiographically at regular intervals (e.g., before administering intermittent feedings, after position changes, and after suctioning, coughing episodes, or vomiting). *The feeding tube can migrate without demonstrating a change in its external position.*

3. Instill blue food coloring to feeding solutions *to assist identification of gastric contents in pulmonary secretions. Green, red, or yellow food dye is unacceptable because each resembles other body substances.*

4. If possible, aspirate enteral contents through feeding tube and measure residual amounts before intermittent feedings and at regular intervals during continuous feedings. Consider withholding intermittent feedings for residuals greater than 100 to 150 ml and interrupting continuous feedings for residuals greater than 20% of the hourly rate.

5. With physician's collaboration, consider administering metoclopramide (Reglan) *to increase upper gastrointestinal motility and gastric sphincter tone and to decrease gastric volume.*

Additional interventions for patients with impaired swallowing

1. Assess for classic indicators of impaired swallowing—drooling (especially persistence of drooling with head reclined), food retained in mouth, poor head and neck control, tongue pumping or excess mouth movement before swallowing, coughing during or after eating, breathy or "gurgly" voice, and slurred speech.

2. Initiate consult with in-house "swallowing team." This team may consist of a speech pathologist, occupational therapist, physical therapist, dietitian, and/or physical rehabilitation nursing and medical staff members. *Swallowing is not a reflex but a patterned response involving both voluntary and non-volitional components. It may, in some instances, be retrained after injury.*

3. Predict the patient's swallowing competence by assessing the symmetry and dynamics of tongue mobility. *The swallowing response consists of coordinated movements of the tongue, palate, pharynx, larynx, and esophagus. This response is initiated by the tongue; therefore competence in initiating the swallow may be partially predicated.*

4. Predict airway protection by asking the patient to cough and clear the throat. *A cough that is weak, "gurgly," or unobtainable indicates reduced airway closure, which is the reason for aspiration during the swallow.*

5. For the patient who is either being evaluated for swallowing difficulty or in whom swallowing is being reinitiated (e.g., after tracheal extubation or prolonged nothing-by-mouth status), observe swallowing competence by placing 3 ml of water on the patient's tongue. The swallow should be initiated within one second of introducing water to the oral cavity. If response is delayed or no response occurs after three attempts, consider formal evaluation by "swallowing team" and initiate NPO status. *Water is hardest to swallow and easiest to aspirate; if swallowing is impaired sufficiently to result in pulmonary aspiration, the 3 ml of water is a safe medium with which to demonstrate this impairment.*

6. When reasonable swallowing competence has been established, provide foods with the consistency of yogurt, ice cream, pudding, or custard. *Semisolids are more easily swallowed than either liquids or solids.*

7. Avoid introducing fluids into the patient's mouth with the use of a syringe. *This maneuver partially bypasses the tongue, interfering with the swallowing response and therefore increasing the risk of aspiration.*

POTENTIAL FOR ASPIRATION

The nursing diagnosis Potential for Aspiration describes a state of high risk for the development of the medical problem, pulmonary aspiration. The nursing management of the potential problem is presented here, whereas the pathophysiological basis for the actual event is discussed in the section, "Aspiration Lung Disorder," p. 419, in Chapter 20.

REFERENCES

1. Aldrich TK: Respiratory muscle fatigue, Clin Chest Med 9(2):225, 1988.
2. Aubier M: Pharmacotherapy of respiratory muscles, Clin Chest Med 9(2):311, 1988.
3. Aubier M and others: Aminophylline improves diaphragmatic contractility, N Engl J Med 305:249, 1981.
4. Bartlett RH: Respiratory therapy to prevent pulmonary complications of surgery, Respir Care 29(6):667, 1984.
5. Bodai BI and others: A clinical evaluation of an oxygen insufflation/suction catheter, Heart Lung 16(1):39, 1987.
6. Bostick J and Wendelglass ST: Normal saline instillation as part of the suctioning procedure: effects on PaO$_2$ and the amount of secretions, Heart Lung 16(5):532, 1987.
7. Boysen PG: Respiratory muscle function, Respir Care 32(7):572, 1987.
8. Braun N: Respiratory muscle dysfunction, Heart Lung 13(4):327, 1984.
9. Burton GG and Hodgkin JE: Respiratory care: a guide to clinical practice, Philadelphia, 1984, JB Lippincott Co.
10. Carpenito LJ: Nursing diagnosis: application to clinical practice, Philadelphia, 1983, JB Lippincott Co.
11. Dantzker DR and Martin JT: Monitoring respiratory muscle function, Respir Care 30(6):422, 1985.
12. Demers RR: Down with the good lung—(usually) (editorial), Respir Care 32(10):849, 1987.
13. Derenne JP, Macklem PT, and Roussos CH: The respiratory muscles: mechanics, control and pathophysiology, Am Rev Respir Dis 118:119, 1978.
14. Hanley MV and Tyler ML: Ineffective airway clearance related to airway infection, Nurs Clin North Am 22(1):135, 1987.
15. Herala M and Gislason T: Chest physiotherapy: evaluation by transcutaneous blood gas monitoring, Chest 4:801, 1988.
16. Hodgkin JE: Non-ventilator aspects of care for ventilator-assisted patients, Respir Care 31(4):334, 1986.
17. Hodgkin JE and Petty TL: Chronic obstructive pulmonary disease: current concepts, Philadelphia, 1987, WB Saunders Co.
18. Hoffman LA: Ineffective airway clearance related to neuromuscular dysfunction, Nurs Clin North Am 22(1):151, 1987.
19. Hopp LJ and Williams M: Ineffective breathing pattern related to decreased lung expansion, Nurs Clin North Am 22(1):193, 1987.
20. Hurley ME: Classification of nursing diagnoses: proceedings of the sixth conference, St Louis, 1986, The CV Mosby Co.
21. Kacmarek RM: The role of pressure support ventilation in reducing the work of breathing, Respir Care 22(2):99, 1988.
22. Kim MJ: Respiratory muscle training: implications for patient care, Heart Lung 13(4):333, 1984.
23. Kim MJ and Larson JL: Ineffective airway clearance and ineffective breathing patterns: theoretical and research base for nursing diagnosis, Nurs Clin North Am 22(1):125, 1987.
24. Kreiger BP and Ershowsky P: Noninvasive detection of respiratory failure in the intensive care unit, Chest 94(2):255, 1988.
25. Lareau S and Larson JJ: Ineffective breathing pattern related to airflow limitations, Nurs Clin North Am 22(1):179, 1987.
26. Larson JL and Kim MJ: Ineffective airway clearance and ineffective breathing pattern: theoretical and research base for nursing diagnosis, Nurs Clin North Am 22(1):125, 1987.
27. Larson JL and Kim MJ: Ineffective breathing pattern related to respiratory muscle fatigue, Nurs Clin North Am 22(1):207, 1987.
28. Lewis MI and Belman MJ: Nutrition and the respiratory muscles, Clin Chest Med 9(2):337, 1988.
29. Luce JM, Tyler ML, and Pierson DJ: Intensive respiratory care, Philadelphia, 1984, WB Saunders Co.
30. MacIntyre NR: Pressure support ventilation—1987 (preface), Respir Care 33(2):98, 1988.
31. MacIntyre NR: Weaning from mechanical ventilatory support: volume assisting intermittent breaths versus pressure-assisting every breath, Respir Care 33(2):121, 1988.
32. Marini JJ: Exertion during ventilator support: how much and how important? Respir Care 31(5):385, 1986.
33. Marini JJ: Mechanical ventilation: taking the work out of breathing, Respir Care 31(8):695, 1986.
34. Marini JJ: The role of the inspiratory circuit in the work of breathing during mechanical ventilation, Respir Care 32(6):419, 1987.
35. Moore MC: Pocket guide to nutrition and diet therapy, St Louis, 1988, The CV Mosby Co.
36. Moser KM and others: Shortness of breath: a guide to better living and breathing, St Louis, 1983, The CV Mosby Co.
37. Moxham J: Aminophylline and the respiratory muscles: an alternative view, Clin Chest Med 9(2):325, 1988.
38. Norton LC and Conforti CG: The effects of body position on oxygenation, Heart Lung 14(1):45, 1985.
39. Openbrier DR and Covey M: Ineffective breathing pattern related to malnutrition, Nurs Clin North Am 22(1):225, 1987.
40. Pardy RL, Reid DW, and Belman MJ: Respiratory muscle training, Clin Chest Med 9(2):287, 1988.
41. Pierce JB and Piazza DE: Difference in postsuctioning arterial blood oxygen concentration values using two postoxygenation methods, Heart Lung 16(1):34, 1987.
42. Preusser BA and others: Effects of two methods of preoxygenation on mean arterial pressure, cardiac output, peak airway pressure, and postsuctioning hypoxemia, Heart Lung 17(3):290, 1988.
43. Riegel B and Forshee T: A review and critique of the literature on preoxygenation for endotracheal suctioning, Heart Lung 15(5):507, 1985.
44. Roberts SL: Physiologic nursing diagnoses are necessary and appropriate for critical care, Focus Crit Care 15:42, 1988.
45. Rochester DF: Respiratory effects of respiratory muscle weakness and atrophy, Am Rev Respir Dis 134(5):1083, 1986.
46. Rochester DF: Respiratory muscle function in health, Heart Lung 13(4):349, 1984.
47. Shapiro BA and others: Clinical application of respiratory care, Chicago, 1985, Year Book Medical Publishers, Inc.
48. Sharp JT: The respiratory muscles in chronic obstructive pulmonary disease, Respir Dis 134(5):1089, 1986.
49. Shekleton ME and Nield M: Ineffective airway clearance related to artificial airway, Nurs Clin North Am 22(1):167, 1987.
50. Smith RM, Benson MS, and Schoene RB: The efficacy of oxygen insufflation in preventing arterial oxygen desaturation during endotracheal suctioning of mechanically ventilated patients, Respir Care 32(10): 865, 1987.
51. Sporn PH and Morganroth ML: Discontinuation of mechanical ventilation, Clin Chest Med 9(1):113, 1988.
52. Tobin MJ: Respiratory muscles in disease, Clin Chest Med 9(2):263, 1988.

53. Traver GA: Respiratory nursing: the science and the art, New York, 1982, John Wiley & Sons, Inc.
54. Tyler ML: The respiratory effects of body positioning and immobilization, Respir Care 29(5):472, 1984.
55. West JB: Pulmonary pathophysiology: the essentials, Baltimore, 1987, Williams & Wilkins.
56. West JB: Respiratory physiology: the essentials, Baltimore, 1985, Williams & Wilkins.
57. York KA and Martin PA: Clinical validation of respiratory nursing diagnosis: a model. In Hurley ME: Classification of nursing diagnoses: proceedings of the sixth conference, St Louis, 1986, The CV Mosby Co.

NEUROLOGICAL ALTERATIONS

23

Neurological Anatomy and Physiology

CHAPTER OBJECTIVES

- *List the four protective mechanisms of the central nervous system.*
- *Describe the functions of the three portions of the brainstem.*
- *State two major functions of each of the four lobes of the cerebrum.*
- *Trace anterior and posterior cerebral circulation.*
- *Identify the major motor and sensory tracts of the spinal cord.*
- *Discuss the vascular supply to the spinal cord.*

The nervous system is a unique, complex, and still somewhat mysterious network of fibers running throughout the body that has the task of directing body systems and functions. Receiving thousands of bits of information each second from different sensory organs, this system transmits, analyzes, interprets, and integrates responses throughout the billions of nervous system cells. A basic understanding of the anatomy and physiology of the nervous system is essential to the delivery of quality critical care nursing. Although the roles and functions of the nervous system are diverse, a few principles and concepts apply to all. This chapter reviews the divisions of the nervous system and its microstructure or cellular level and functions. Mechanisms devised to provide protection to the nervous system also are presented. Finally, the anatomy and physiology of all components of the central nervous system are outlined.

DIVISIONS OF THE NERVOUS SYSTEM

The nervous system is the most highly organized system of the body, with all of its parts functioning as an inseparable unit. For review, this system may be classified in terms of location or according to function.

Anatomical Divisions

1. The central nervous system (CNS) comprises all the portions of the brain and spinal cord.
2. The peripheral nervous system (PNS) comprises the 12 pairs of cranial nerves plus the 32 pairs of spinal nerves and the peripheral nerves that connect the CNS with the body wall and the viscera.

Physiological Divisions

1. The *somatic, or voluntary, nervous system* is composed of fibers that connect the CNS with structures of the skeletal muscles and the skin.
2. The *autonomic, or involuntary, nervous system* is composed of fibers that connect the CNS with smooth muscle, cardiac muscle, internal organs, and glands. It includes its sympathetic and parasympathetic branches.

Most activities of the nervous system originate from sensory receptors such as visual, auditory, or tactile receptors. This sensory information is transmitted to the CNS by *afferent fibers* (sensory fibers). *Efferent fibers* (motor fibers) transmit the CNS response to the periphery to produce a motor response such as contraction of skeletal muscles, contraction of the smooth muscles of organs, or secretion by endocrine glands. Transmission of both afferent (sensory) and efferent (motor) information in the CNS is performed by *internuncial fibers*. To better understand the macrostructure and functions of the nervous system it is essential to look first at the microstructure, or cellular level.[3]

MICROSTRUCTURE OF THE NERVOUS SYSTEM

The cellular units of the nervous system are the neurons and the neuroglia.[6,7] The neurons are the functional units of the nervous system and are responsible for conduction of nerve impulses, and the neuroglial cells provide support, repair, and protection for the delicate neurons.

Neurons. More than 10 billion neurons are in the CNS alone. The cellular appearance of a neuron varies, depending on its specific function, but each cell contains three basic

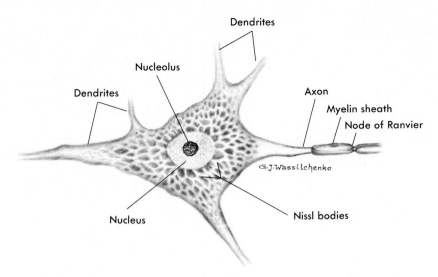

Fig. 23-1 Diagram of the neuron with composite parts.

components (Fig. 23-1). The first component is the *cell body* (soma), which controls the metabolic activity of the cell. Inside the cell body is the nucleus, which stores ribonucleic acid (RNA) and deoxyribonucleic acid (DNA) and also contains the nucleolus for synthesis of RNA. Nissl bodies for storage of RNA and synthesis of protein, Golgi apparatus for storage of protein and synthesis of cell membranes, neurofibrils for support, and lysosomes, which function as intracellular scavengers, are also contained in the cell body. An intact, well-nourished cell body is essential to the life of the neuron as a whole. If the cell body dies, the rest of the neuron also dies and cannot be replaced. These specialized cells cannot reproduce themselves; therefore cell bodies are grouped together in relatively protected areas. Cell bodies form the gray matter in the brain, the brainstem, and the spinal cord. Ganglia, small nodules of nervous tissue lying close to the CNS, are cell bodies in the peripheral nervous system. The structural classification of neurons is as follows:

1. Unipolar: cell body with one process, which divides into a central branch—the axon—and a peripheral branch—the dendrite
2. Bipolar: cell body with two processes, one axon, and one dendrite
3. Multipolar: cell body with one axon and several dendrites

Dendrites, the second component of a neuron, are branched fibers extending only a short distance from the cell body. Each neuron may have several dendrites, which carry impulses to the cell body. The third component of a neuron is the *axon.* Each neuron contains only one axon, which carries information away from the cell. Axons can be microscopic in length or extend up to 4 feet. Many axons are protected by a *myelin sheath,* which is a white protein-lipid complex laid down by Schwann cells in the PNS and by oligodendrocytes in the CNS. Myelin sheath acts as insulation for the conduction of nerve impulses. Fibers enclosed in the sheath are called myelinated fibers; those not enclosed are called unmyelinated fibers. The white matter of the CNS is composed of myelinated fiber tracts.

Myelin is not a continuous layer but has gaps called *nodes of Ranvier.* Nerve impulses are conducted from node to node; therefore conduction is more rapid. Loss of myelin sheath integrity disrupts nerve impulse transmission. Multiple sclerosis, for example, is a disease that causes degeneration of myelin.

Neuroglia. Neuroglial cells are the support cells to the neuron. There are four types of neuroglial cells: astroglia, oligodendroglia, ependyma, and microglia (Fig. 23-2). These cells provide structural support, nourishment, and protection for the neurons (Table 23-1). In the nervous system there are 6 to 10 times more neuroglial cells than neurons. The clinical significance of neuroglia is its ability to retain mitotic abilities, as compared to neurons, which do not retain them. Therefore neuroglia can become the source of nonmetabolic CNS primary neoplasms.

Physiology of Nervous Tissue

The nervous system consists of chains of neurons with no actual anatomical continuity. Each neuron is a separate unit in contact with another neuron or target cell through *synapses* (Fig. 23-3).

The generation of a nerve impulse, as with other cells of the body, begins with the depolarization of the cell membrane (see Chapter 11). The speed of the impulse conduction depends on whether the nerve is myelinated or unmyelinated. In an unmyelinated nerve, depolarization must travel the entire length of the fiber. In myelinated nerves, impulses "jump" from one node of Ranvier to another. This node-to-node conduction, called *saltatory transmission,* increases the velocity of impulse transmission and decreases energy demands. Impulses are transmitted away from cell bodies by axons and pass from the axon of one cell body to the dendrite or cell body of another neuron through the synapse.

Actual synaptic transmission is a chemical process involving the release of neurotransmitters. Anatomically, a synapse travels from the *presynaptic terminal or knob* at the end of an axon, across the *synaptic cleft,* and to the *postsynaptic membrane.*

Neurotransmitters. Neurotransmitters, chemical sub-

Ependymal cell   Astrocyte

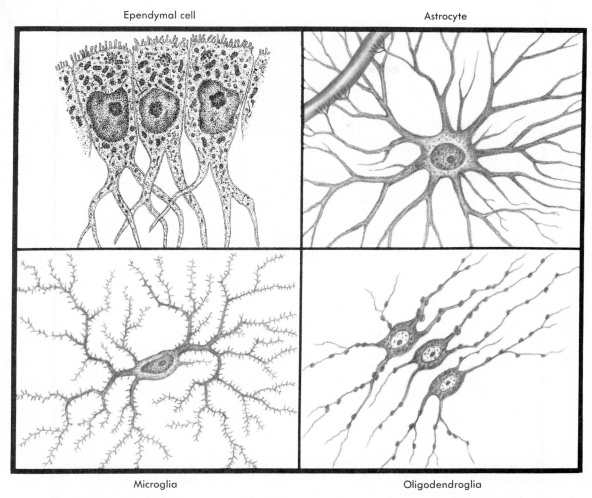

Microglia   Oligodendroglia

Fig. 23-2 Types of neuroglial cells. (From Thompson JM and others: Mosby's manual of clinical nursing, ed 2, St Louis, 1989, The CV Mosby Co.)

Table 23-1 Types of neuroglial cells

Cell type	Function
Astroglia (astrocyte)	Supplies nutrients to neuron structure and to support framework for neurons and capillaries; forms part of the blood-brain barrier
Oligodendroglia	Forms the myelin sheath in the CNS
Ependyma	Lines the ventricular system; forms the choroid plexus, which produces CSF
Microglia	Occurs mainly in the white matter; phagocytizes waste products from injured neurons

stances secreted by the presynaptic terminal, provide the connection from axon to dendrite for transmission of the nerve impulse.[4] As a nerve impulse reaches the presynaptic terminal, neurotransmitters are secreted into the microscopic synaptic cleft, causing a change in the permeability of the postsynaptic membrane and therefore passage of the impulse across the synaptic cleft.

More than 30 different chemical substances have been identified as neurotransmitters and can be divided into two types—*excitatory* and *inhibitory*. Excitatory neurotransmitters promote the conduction of the impulse from one cell to the next. When inhibitory neurotransmitters are released, the neuron's internal charge becomes more negative and the resistance to depolarization is increased. The most common known neurotransmitters are acetylcholine, dopamine, norepinephrine, serotonin, γ-aminobutyric acid, glycine, and glutamic acid.

After synaptic transmission, binding of the neurotransmitters to the postsynaptic membrane continues until the neurotransmitter is inactivated by an enzyme (acetylcholine is inactivated by acetylcholinesterase), reabsorbed by the presynaptic terminal, or diffused away from the postsynaptic membrane.

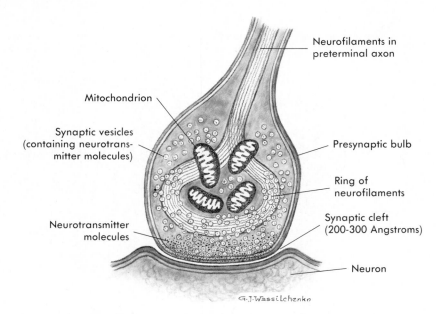

Neurofilaments in
preterminal axon

Mitochondrion

Synaptic vesicles
(containing neurotrans-
mitter molecules)

Presynaptic bulb

Ring of
neurofilaments

Synaptic cleft
(200-300 Angstroms)

Neurotransmitter
molecules

Neuron

G.J.Wassilchenko

Fig. 23-3 Schematic diagram of a synapse.

Dysfunction of synaptic pathways results in poor or absent transmission of the nerve impulse. Parkinson's disease, resulting from the lack of dopamine in the basal ganglia, allows excitatory neurotransmitters to go unchecked. Symptoms of Parkinson's disease include tremors, rigidity of limbs, and difficulty initiating movement. Myasthenia gravis, a disease characterized by generalized weakness and fatigability of voluntary muscles, is caused by a reduction of acetylcholine receptors on the postsynaptic membrane.

CENTRAL NERVOUS SYSTEM

The CNS, composed of the spinal cord, brainstem, and brain, is the control unit for all physiological functions. Review of the anatomy and physiology of the CNS begins with the most basic functions of the brainstem and progresses through the diencephalon to the highly developed cerebrum. The spinal cord is reviewed at the end of this section. Maintaining a healthy CNS is challenged by the delicateness of the nerves and tissues involved. Therefore, several mechanisms are in place to provide protection and support to these fragile structures.

Protective Mechanisms

The brain and spinal cord have similar protective mechanisms,[1,2,8] but because of the distinct anatomical differences of these two portions of the CNS, each is discussed separately (see Spinal Cord section).

Bony structures. The outermost protective measures underneath the integument are the bony structures that encase the CNS. The skull (Fig. 23-4), or cranium, forms the bony container that surrounds the brain. Composed of eight flat, irregular bones fused through suture lines, the skull provides the brain protection from direct force or superficial trauma. Excessive force causing fracture of the skull can destroy this protective mechanism and push bony fragments into the fragile brain tissue.

Viewing the skull from the inside, the superior surfaces form a smooth inner wall, whereas the base of the skull, or basilar skull, contains ridges and folds with sharp edges, which provide structure for the support of different portions of the brain (Fig. 23-5). Sharp blows to the head that cause shifting of intracranial contents can lead to brain tissue laceration and contusion across these sharp edges.

The cranium is an enclosed vault except for one large opening at the base called the *foramen magnum,* through which the brainstem projects and connects to the spinal cord. Several other very small openings in the base of the skull allow entrance and exit of blood vessels and cranial nerves.

Meninges. Beneath the skull lies the second layer of intracranial protection, the meninges. The three layers of meninges are the dura mater, the arachnoid, and the pia mater (Fig. 23-6).

Dura mater. The first meninges beneath the skull is the dura mater. Consisting of two layers, this tough, fibrous membrane provides several functions. The outermost layer comprises the periosteum for the cranial bones and therefore adheres to the skull. The inner, meningeal layer of the dura extends into the cranial space. The four extensions of the dural layer are the falx cerebri, tentorium cerebelli, falx cerebelli, and diaphragma sellae.

The *falx cerebri* divides the right and left hemispheres of the brain vertically through the longitudinal fissures extending from the frontal lobe to the occipital lobe. The *tentorium cerebelli* forms a tent between the occipital lobes and the cerebellum and separates the cerebral hemispheres from the brainstem and cerebellum. Intracranial terminology labels all structures above the tentorium as supratentorial and all structures below as infratentorial. Structures below the tentorium are also located in the area referred to as the posterior fossa.

The *falx cerebelli* forms the division between the two lateral lobes of the cerebellum. The final compartment of the dura mater is the *diaphragm sellae,* which forms a roof

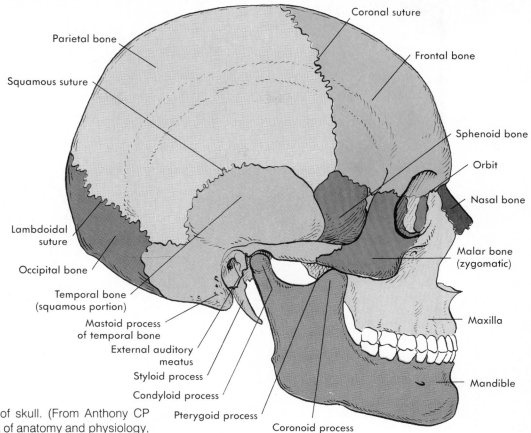

Fig. 23-4 Lateral view of skull. (From Anthony CP and Kolthoff NJ: Textbook of anatomy and physiology, St Louis, 1975, The CV Mosby Co.)

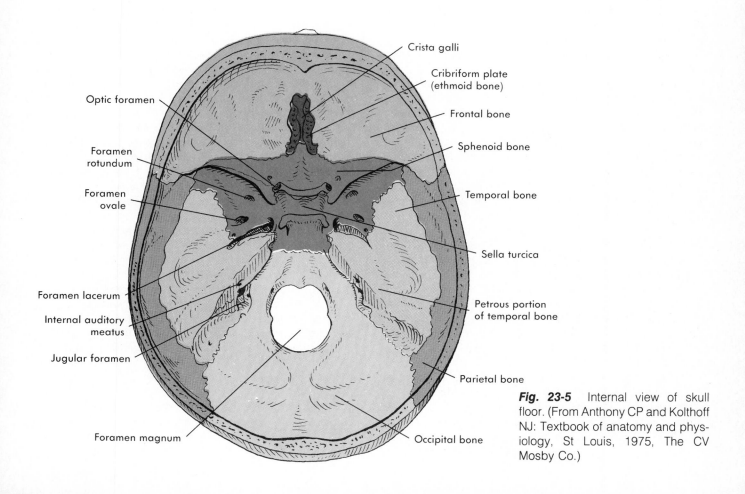

Fig. 23-5 Internal view of skull floor. (From Anthony CP and Kolthoff NJ: Textbook of anatomy and physiology, St Louis, 1975, The CV Mosby Co.)

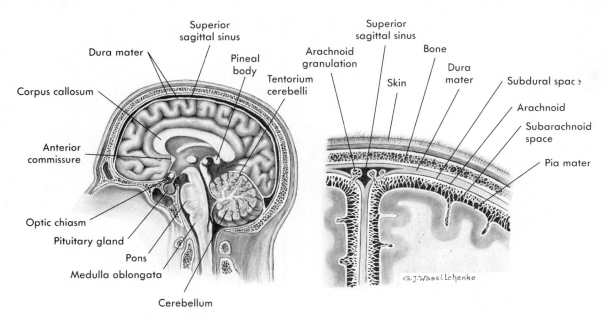

Fig. 23-6 Meningeal layers of the brain.

over the sella turcica. Inside the sella turcica is the pituitary gland.

Further dural separations form the venous sinuses located throughout the intracranial space. These venous sinuses, which collect blood from intracerebral and meningeal veins, drain into the internal jugular vein to return venous blood to the heart.

Between the dura mater and the next meninges, the arachnoid, lies the subdural space. This narrow space has a large number of unsupported small veins connecting the arachnoid and dura, so this area is highly susceptible to injury. When the small vessels are stretched and torn, a subdural hematoma is formed.

Arachnoid membrane. The arachnoid membrane, the second meninges, is a delicate, fragile membrane that loosely surrounds the brain. Fine threads of elastic tissue called *trabeculae* connect the arachnoid to the pia mater, creating a spongy, weblike structure called the subarachnoid space. Located in the subarachnoid space are cerebrospinal fluid (CSF) and a variety of cerebral arteries and veins.

At the base of the brain, widened areas of subarachnoid space form cisterns, or pools of CSF. The largest of these cisterns, the *cisterna magna,* lies between the medulla and the cerebellum and communicates with the fourth ventricle.

Tufts of arachnoid membrane, called *arachnoid villi,* or granulations, project into the superior sagittal and transverse venous sinuses. This communication between arachnoid villi and sinuses allows reabsorption of CSF from the subarachnoid space into the venous space. Several conditions such as meningitis or subarachnoid hemorrhage can obstruct these arachnoid villi and decrease the rate of CSF reabsorption. This arachnoid villi obstruction is termed *communicating hydrocephalus.*

Pia mater. The innermost delicate meninges is known as the pia mater. Rich in small blood vessels that supply a large volume of arterial blood to cerebral tissues, this membrane closely follows all folds and convolutions of the brain's surface. Tufts or folds of the pia mater in the lateral, third, and fourth ventricles form a portion of the choroid plexus that is responsible for the production of CSF.

Ventricular system. A central CSF-filled core of the brain is called the ventricular system (Fig. 23-7). Made of four connected chambers lined with ependymal cells, the ventricles provide the anatomical structure around which the brain and brainstem are formed.

The two largest ventricles, one within each of the cerebral hemispheres, are called the lateral ventricles. Extending from the frontal lobe to the occipital lobe, they consist of a body and a frontal, temporal, and occipital horn. When cannulation of the ventricular system is required for drainage of CSF, that is, placement of an intracranial pressure monitor or CSF shunt, the frontal horn of the lateral ventricle is most often selected.

Connecting through the foramen of Monro, the two lateral ventricles interface with a central cavity, the third ventricle. Located directly above the midbrain, the third ventricle lies between the structures of the thalamus in the diencephalon.

The cerebral aqueduct (aqueduct of Sylvius) communicates with the fourth ventricle, which lies between the brainstem and the cerebellum. At the base of the fourth ventricle, two openings, the foramen of Luschka and the foramen of Magendie, open the ventricular system into the subarachnoid space. Any blockage of CSF flow in the ventricular system such as a blood clot in the cerebral aqueduct or a mass pressing against the cerebral aqueduct causes dilation of the ventricles, termed *noncommunicating hydrocephalus.*

Cerebrospinal fluid. CSF fills the ventricular system and surrounds the brain and spinal cord in the subarachnoid space. Protection of the CNS is thereby accomplished because the CSF system acts as a "shock absorber" and participates in the removal of waste products from cerebral tissue.

CSF is normally a clear, colorless, odorless solution secreted by the choroid plexuses (95%) located in all four

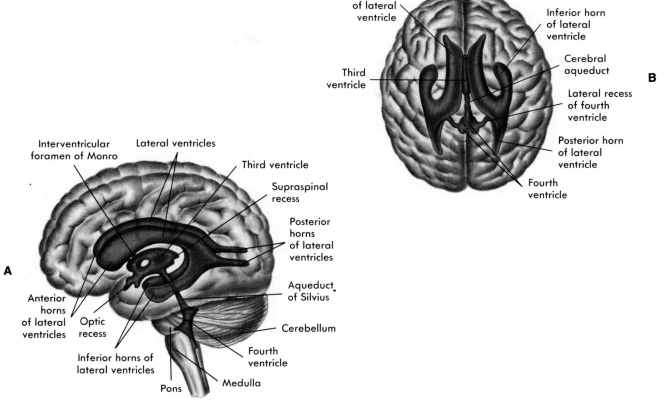

Fig. 23-7 Cerebral ventricles. **A,** Lateral view. **B,** Superior view. (From Thompson JM and others: Mosby's manual of clinical nursing, ed 2, St Louis, 1989, The CV Mosby Co.)

Table 23-2 Normal CSF

Property	Values
pH	7.35-7.45
Specific gravity	1.007
Appearance	Clear and colorless
Cells	0 white blood cells (WBCs)
	0 red blood cells (RBCs)
	0-10 lymphocytes
Glucose	50-75 mg/dl (two thirds blood sugar)
Protein	5-25 mg/dl
Volume	135-150 cc
Pressure	70-200 mm H_2O (lumbar puncture)
	3-15 mm Hg (ventricular)

ventricles and also in small amounts by ependymal cells and capillaries of the pia mater. Believed to be a filtrate of blood, CSF contains some unique properties that make the actual secretion process still a mystery (Table 23-2).

The production of CSF occurs at a rate of approximately 20 ml/hour or 500 ml/day. With a circulating volume of 135 to 150 ml, CSF must be reabsorbed daily to prevent development of hydrocephalus. The CSF system does not have any feedback mechanism for volume regulation; therefore CSF is continually produced at the rate of 20 ml/hour, regardless of the total circulating volume. Since CSF is essentially a filtrate of blood and occurs by diffusion, blood pressure is an important component in the overall CSF-production process. Cerebral metabolism and serum osmolality also affect CSF production.

Flow of CSF occurs through a closed system between the ventricles and the subarachnoid space (Fig. 23-8). CSF formed in the lateral ventricles flows through the foramen of Monro into the third ventricle. This fluid, plus the additional CSF formed by the choroid plexus of the third ventricle, flows through the cerebral aqueduct and joins the CSF produced by the fourth ventricle. Exit from the ventricular system occurs medially through the foramen of Magendie and laterally through the two foramina of Luschka. Once out of the ventricles, CSF flows in the subarachnoid space, down around the spinal cord, and up over the surface of the brain, where it is reabsorbed into the venous circulation through the arachnoid villi.

Blood-brain barrier. The final protective mechanism is a physiological mechanism that helps maintain a delicate balance in the brain's internal environment. The blood-brain barrier regulates the transport of nutrients, ions, water, and

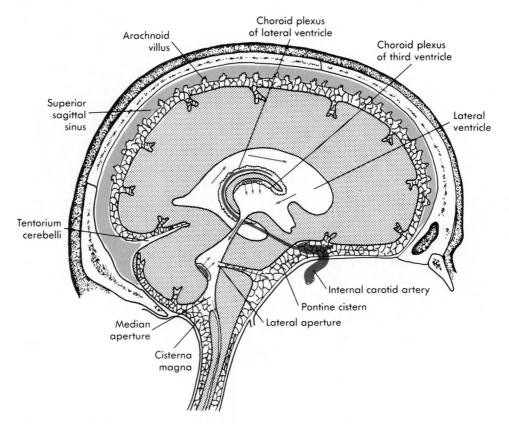

Arachnoid villus

Choroid plexus of lateral ventricle

Choroid plexus of third ventricle

Superior sagittal sinus

Lateral ventricle

Tentorium cerebelli

Internal carotid artery

Pontine cistern

Lateral aperture

Median aperture

Cisterna magna

Fig. 23-8 Path of circulation of cerebrospinal fluid from its formation in the ventricles to its absorption into the superior sagittal sinus. (From Nolte J: The human brain, ed 2, St. Louis, 1987, The CV Mosby Co.)

waste products through selective permeability.[3,6] Stabilization of the physical and chemical environment surrounding the neurons of the CNS is the goal of the blood-brain barrier. Many substances such as metabolites or toxic compounds cannot cross the blood-brain barrier. Other substances such as antibiotics cross slowly, thus having a lesser concentration in the brain than in other areas of the body.

The blood-brain barrier operates on the concept of "tight junctions" between capillary endothelium and astrocytes of the CNS. In contrast to other capillaries in the body, cerebral capillaries are surrounded by astrocyte end feet. One function of the astrocyte is to supply nutrients to the neuron. The selective permeability of the blood-brain barrier keeps out toxic or harmful compounds and protects the fragile, irreplaceable neuron.

Passage of substances across the blood-brain barrier is a function of particle size, lipid solubility, and protein-binding potential. Most drugs or compounds that are lipid soluble and stable at body pH rapidly cross the blood-brain barrier. The blood-brain barrier is also very permeable to water, oxygen, carbon dioxide, and glucose.

The blood-brain barrier exists only in certain areas of the CNS. The areas in which it does not exist, the pineal region, the hypothalamus, and the floor of the fourth ventricle, require contact with plasma to sense changes in concentration of glucose, carbon dioxide, and serum osmolality. Initiation of feedback mechanisms by the hypothalamus in response to these changes regulates the internal environment of the rest of the body.

Of clinical significance, disruption or alteration of blood-brain barrier permeability occurs with injury to cerebral tissue. This injury could be mechanical from trauma, chemical from toxins or drugs, or functional from intracranial tumors. Brain irradiation also may alter the permeability of the blood-brain barrier. Systemic chemotherapeutic agents can be administered because they do not cross the blood-brain barrier, thus preventing destruction of the neuronal tissue by these harsh agents. The obvious disadvantage is that use of chemotherapy in CNS neoplasms is often ineffective.

Two other weaker barrier systems also exist. The *blood-CSF barrier* existing in the capillary endothelium, pial membranes, and ependymal cells of the choroid plexus permits selective transport of substances into the CSF. Finally, the *brain-CSF barrier* is a weak barrier between CSF and interstitial fluid. Because this barrier is weaker, drugs placed directly into CSF (intrathecal injection) will pass into interstitial CNS fluid.

Brainstem

Medulla oblongata. As the spinal cord extends through the foramen magnum of the skull, it becomes the lowermost portion of the brainstem, the medulla oblongata. In the caudal portion of the medulla, decussation (crossing) of the motor fibers occurs. Below the point of decussation, stimuli from the right side of the brain control movement in the left side of the body and vice versa.[3,5]

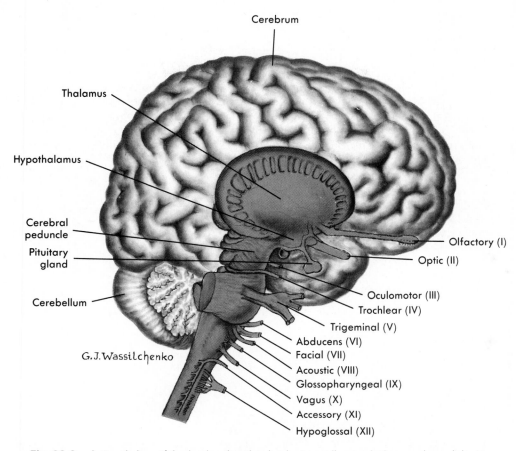

Fig. 23-9   Lateral view of the brain, showing brainstem, diencephalon, and cranial nerves.

The medulla also contains groups of neurons or "centers" that control such involuntary functions as swallowing, vomiting, hiccoughing, coughing, vasoconstriction, and respirations. The medullary respiratory center works in conjunction with the apneustic and pneumotaxic centers of the pons to control respirations. It is responsible for the basic involuntary rhythm of respirations but cannot maintain a smooth, life-sustaining respiratory pattern without stimuli from other higher centers of the brain (Fig. 23-9).

Also located in the medulla are the origins of cranial nerves IX (glossopharyngeal), X (vagus), XI (spinal accessory), and XII (hypoglossal) (Table 23-3). The *reticular formation* begins in the medulla.

Pons. Located above the medulla, the pons continues to relay information to and from the brain and spinal cord along fiber tracts. The ventral surface of the pons contains fibers that connect to the cerebellum. These pathways allow the transmission of influences from the cerebellum to the cerebral cortex, ensuring efficiency and smoothness of movement. Located in the pons are two respiratory control centers—the apneustic and the pneumotaxic—which communicate with the medullary respiratory center. The apneustic center controls the length of inspiration and expiration, and the pneumotaxic center controls the rate of respirations. Behind the pons lies the fourth ventricle.[3,5]

The origins of cranial nerves V (trigeminal), VI (abdu-

cens), VII (facial), and VIII (acoustic) are in the pons.[6] The medial longitudinal fasciculus is an important fiber tract in the pons. In a normally functioning brainstem, the medial longitudinal fasciculus connects cranial nerves III, IV, and VI with the vestibular and pontine paramedian reticular formation, allowing coordinated and appropriate movements of the eyes in response to noise, motion, position, or arousal. Portions of the reticular formation are also in the pons.

Midbrain. The midbrain forms the junction between the pons and diencephalon. Cranial nerves III and IV originate in this region. The aqueduct of Sylvius, which connects the third and fourth ventricles, is in the midbrain. Again, fibers of the reticular formation are present.

The major function of the midbrain is to relay stimuli involved in voluntary motor movement of the body. Also arising in the midbrain are the tectospinal and rubrospinal tracts of the extrapyramidal (involuntary) motor functions. The tectospinal tract controls reflex motor movements in response to visual and auditory stimuli, and the rubrospinal tract controls tone of flexor muscles.[3,5]

Reticular Formation

The reticular formation is a diffuse set of neurons, both gray matter nuclei and white matter fiber tracts, that extend from the upper level of the spinal cord, through the medulla, pons, and midbrain into the thalamus and cerebral cortex.[2,4]

Table 23-3 Cranial nerves, origins, course, and functions

Cranial nerve	Origin and course	Function
I OLFACTORY		
Sensory	Mucosa of nasal cavity; only cranial nerve with cell body located in peripheral structure (nasal mucosa). Pass through cribriform plate of ethmoid bone and go on to olfactory bulbs at floor of frontal lobe. Final interpretation is in temporal lobe.	Smell. However, system is more than receptor/interpreter for odors; perception of smell also sensitizes other body systems and responses such as salivation, peristasis, and even sexual stimulus. Loss of sense of smell is termed *anosmia.*
II OPTIC		
Sensory	Ganglion cells of retina converge to the optic disc and form optic nerve. Nerve fibers pass to optic chiasm, which is above pituitary gland. Some fibers decussate, others do not. The two tracts then go to the lateral geniculate body near the thalamus and then on to the end station for interpretation in the occipital lobe.	Vision (Fig. 23-10).

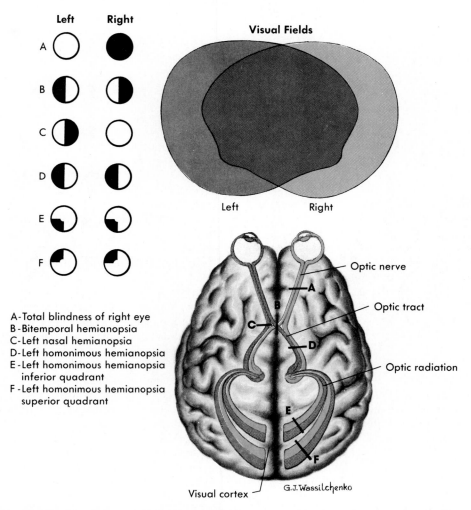

A - Total blindness of right eye
B - Bitemporal hemianopsia
C - Left nasal hemianopsia
D - Left homonimous hemianopsia
E - Left homonimous hemianopsia inferior quadrant
F - Left homonimous hemianopsia superior quadrant

G.J. Wassilchenko

Fig. 23-10 Visual fields showing optic nerve, optic chiasm, optic tracts, and optic radiations. Examples of various visual field defects.

From Rudy E: Advanced neurological and neurosurgical nursing, St Louis, 1984, The CV Mosby Co.

Table 23-3   Cranial nerves, origins, course, and functions—cont'd

Cranial nerve	Origin and course	Function
III OCULOMOTOR		
	Originates in midbrain and emerges from brainstem at upper pons.	Extraocular movement of eyes (Fig. 23-11).
Motor	Motor fibers to superior, medial, inferior recti, and inferior oblique for eye movement; levator muscle of the eyelid.	Raise eyelid.
Parasympathetic	Parasympathetic fibers to ciliary muscles and iris of eye.	Constric pupil; changes shape of lens.

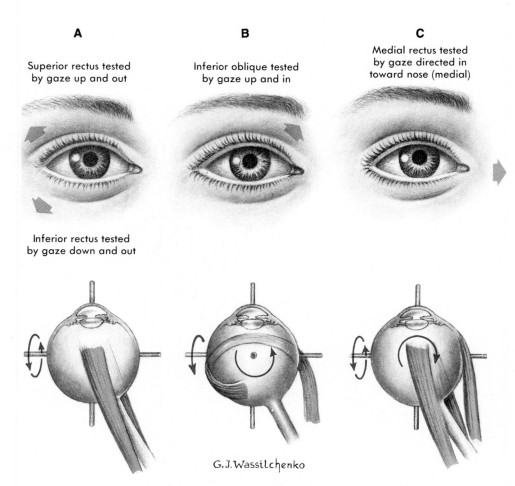

A

Superior rectus tested by gaze up and out

B

Inferior oblique tested by gaze up and in

C

Medial rectus tested by gaze directed in toward nose (medial)

Inferior rectus tested by gaze down and out

G.J.Wassilchenko

Fig. 23-11   **A,** Superior and inferior rectus muscles. Superior rectus moves eye upward; inferior rectus moves eye down and in. **B,** Inferior oblique muscle elevates and abducts the eye. **C,** Medial rectus muscle adducts eye toward the nose.

Cranial nerve	Origin and course	Function
IV TROCHLEAR		
Motor	Midbrain origin near oculomotor, emerges at upper pons near cerebral peduncle. Motor fibers to superior oblique muscle of eyeball.	Extraocular movement of eyes (Fig. 23-12).

Continued.

Table 23-3   Cranial nerves, origins, course, and functions—cont'd

Cranial nerve	Origin and course	Function

Superior oblique tested
by gaze down and in

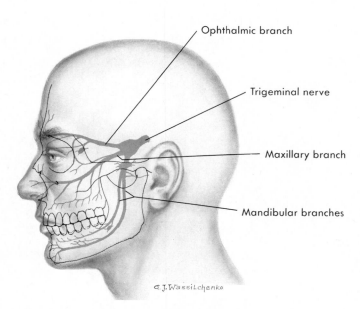

G.J.Wassilchenko

Fig. 23-12   Superior oblique muscle, which rotates the eye down and out at the same time it causes intorsion or inward rotation of the eyeball. The strongest primary action of this muscle is adduction; thus the gaze for testing this muscle is in and down.

V TRIGEMINAL

Cranial nerve	Origin and course	Function
Sensory	Originates in fourth ventricle and emerges at lateral parts of pons. Has three branches to face: ophthalmic, maxillary, and mandibular.	*Ophthalmic branch:* Sensation to cornea, ciliary body, iris, lacrimal gland, conjunctiva, nasal mucosal membranes, eyelids, eyebrows, forehead, and nose. *Maxillary branch:* Sensation to skin of cheek, lower lid, side of nose and upper jaw, teeth, mucosa of mouth, sphenopolative-pterygoid region, and maxillary sinus. *Mandibular branch:* Sensation to skin of lower lip, chin, ear, mucous membrane, teeth of lower jaw and tongue.
Motor	Goes to temporalis, masseter, pterygoid gland, anterior part of digastric muscles (all for mastication), and the tensor tympani and tensor veli palatini muscles (clench jaws).	Muscles of chewing and mastication and opening jaw (Fig. 23-13).

Ophthalmic branch

Trigeminal nerve

Maxillary branch

Mandibular branches

G.J.Wassilchenko

Fig. 23-13   Trigeminal nerve with innervation to face by ophthalmic, maxillary, and mandibular branches.

Table 23-3 Cranial nerves, origins, course, and functions—cont'd

Cranial nerve	Origin and course	Function
VI ABDUCENS		
Motor	Posterior part of pons goes to lateral rectus muscle for eye movement.	Extraocular eye movement; rotates eyeball outward (Fig. 23-14).

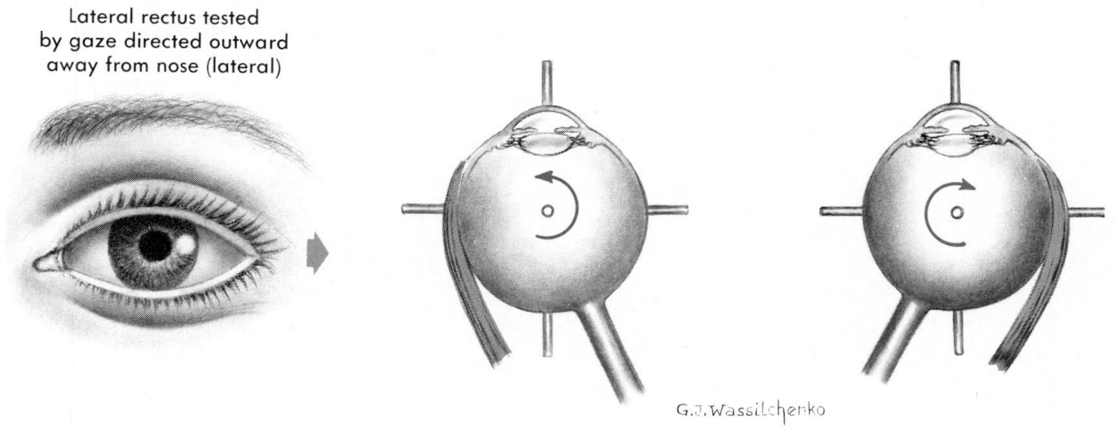

Lateral rectus tested
by gaze directed outward
away from nose (lateral)

G.J.Wassilchenko

Fig. 23-14 Lateral rectus muscle, which abducts the eye away from the nose to the temporal side of the head.

Cranial nerve	Origin and course	Function
VII FACIAL		
Sensory	Lower portion of pons goes to anterior two thirds of tongue and soft palate.	Taste anterior two thirds of tongue. Sensation to soft palate.
Motor	Pons to muscles of forehead, eyelids, cheeks, lips, ears, nose, and neck.	Movement of facial muscles to produce facial expressions, close eyes.
Parasympathetic	Pons to salivary gland and lacrimal glands.	Secretory for salivation and tears.
VIII ACOUSTIC	Two divisions:	
Sensory	*Cochlear division:* Originates in spinal ganglia of the cochlea, with peripheral fibers to the organ of Corti in the internal ear. Goes to pons, and impulses transmitted to the temporal lobe.	Hearing.
	Vestibular division: Originates in otolith organs of the semicircular canals in the inner ear and in the vestibular ganglion. Terminates in pons, with some fibers continuing to cerebellum. The only cranial nerve that originates wholly within a bone, the petrous portion of the temporal bone.	Equilibrium.
IX GLOSSOPHARYNGEAL		
Sensory	Posterior one third of tongue for taste sensation and sensations from soft palate, tonsils, and opening to mouth in back of oral pharynx (fauces). Fibers go to medulla and then to the temporal lobe for taste and sensory cortex for other sensations.	Taste in posterior one third of tongue. Sensation in back of throat; stimulation elicits a gag reflex.
Motor	Medulla to constrictor muscles of pharynx and stylopharyngeal muscles.	Voluntary muscles for swallowing and phonation.
Parasympathetic	Medulla to parotid salivary gland via otic ganglia.	Secretory, salivary glands. Carotid reflex.

Continued.

Table 23-3 Cranial nerves, origins, course, and functions—cont'd

Cranial nerve	Origin and course	Function
X VAGUS		
Sensory	Sensory fibers in back of ear and posterior wall of external ear go to medulla oblongata and on to sensory cortex.	Sensation behind ear and part of external ear meatus.
Motor	Fibers go from medulla oblongata through jugular foramen with glossopharyngeal nerve and on to pharynx, larynx, esophagus, bronchi, lungs, heart, stomach, small intestines, liver, pancreas, kidneys.	Voluntary muscles for phonation and swallowing. Involuntary activity of visceral muscles of heart, lungs, and digestive tract.
Parasympathetic	Medulla oblongata to larnyx, trachea, lungs, aorta, esophagus, stomach, small intestines, and gallbladder.	Carotid reflex. Autonomic activity of respiratory tract, digestive tract including peristalsis and secretion from organs.
XI SPINAL ACCESSORY		
Motor	This nerve has two roots, cranial and spinal. Cranial portion arises at several rootlets at side of medulla, runs below vagus, and is jointed by spinal portion from motor cells in cervical cord. Some fibers go along with vagus nerve to supply motor impulse to pharynx, larynx, uvula, and palate. Major portion to sternomastoid and trapezius muscles, branches to cervical spinal nerves C2-C4.	Some fibers for swallowing and phonation. Turn head and shrug shoulders.
XII HYPOGLOSSAL		
Motor	Arises in medulla oblongato and goes to muscles of tongue.	Movement of tongue necessary for swallowing and phonation.

Composed of both motor and sensory tracts, the reticular formation is closely tied to functions of the basal ganglia, thalamus, cerebellum, and cerebral cortex. This formation of neural fibers has many excitatory and some inhibitory capabilities, achieving the capacity to regulate the activity from the sources mentioned and to enhance, suppress, or modify impulse transmission. The main role of the reticular formation is to provide a balance between the excitatory and inhibitory stimuli to maintain normal muscle tone, which supports the body against gravity. Damage to the inhibitory areas above the reticular formation (cerebellum and basal ganglia) leads to an excitatory response of the body. Decorticate (abnormal flexion) or decerebrate (abnormal extension) posturing is a result of such an injury. Also located in the reticular formation are centers for blood pressure, respiration, and heart rate function.

Reticular activating system. Located within the same region as the reticular formation is the reticular activating system (RAS) (Fig. 23-15). Also a diffuse network of fibers extending from the lower brainstem to the cerebral cortex, the RAS has two main levels. The lower portion of the RAS in the brainstem assists with the control of wake-sleep cycles and consciousness. The upper portion in the thalamus region allows the ability to focus attention on a specific task. When the upper RAS is damaged, the patient exhibits a vegetative state, exhibiting sleep-wake cycles and other brainstem functions but no upper levels of cerebration. Although the RAS is not the "center" of consciousness, communication between the cerebral cortex of the RAS is apparently necessary for consciousness to occur.[2,4]

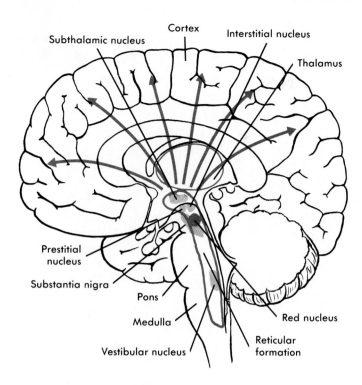

Subthalamic nucleus — Cortex — Interstitial nucleus — Thalamus — Prestitial nucleus — Substantia nigra — Pons — Medulla — Vestibular nucleus — Red nucleus — Reticular formation

Fig. 23-15 Reticular activating system. (From Thompson JM and others: Mosby's manual of clinical nursing, ed 2, St Louis, 1989, The CV Mosby Co.)

Cerebellum

The cerebellum, separated from the cerebrum by the tent-like structure of the tentorium cerebelli, has also been called the "little brain" or the "hind brain." Approximately one fifth the size of the brain, the cerebellum is composed of two lateral hemispheres and a central portion called the vermis. As is the cerebrum, the cerebellum is composed of a thin outer layer of gray matter or cortex and a core of white matter or fiber tracts. Four pairs of nuclei are located deep in the white matter.

The cerebellum influences muscle tone associated with equilibrium, orientation in space, locomotion, and posture to ensure synchronization of muscle action. Input is received from sensory pathways of the spinal cord, the brainstem, and the cerebrum. Output is through descending motor pathways such as the corticospinal, vestibulospinal, and reticulospinal tracts.

Cerebellar influences work through continual excitatory and inhibiting stimuli from deep nuclei of the white matter. The balancing of these two opposing forces results in smooth motor movements instead of rapid, jerky, erratic movements. This complex system in the cerebellum monitors and adjusts motor activity simultaneously with the performance of the activity.

Diencephalon

The diencephalon, the lowest structure of the cerebrum, lies at the top of the brainstem surrounding the third ventricle.[3,6,8] It is divided into four regions: the thalamus, hypothalamus, epithalamus, and subthalamus (see Fig. 23-9). Also located in this area are the pituitary gland and the internal capsule. The first two cranial nerves, I (olfactory) and II (optic), originate in the diencephalon region.

Thalamus. The largest region of the diencephalon, the thalamus, consists of two connected ovoid masses of gray matter forming the lateral walls of the third ventricle deep in the cerebral hemispheres. The thalamus is a relay station for both motor and sensory activity, basic neuronal activity such as processing of brain activity (measured by electroencephalogram) and memory, thought, emotion, and complex behavior (Fig. 23-16).

The thalamus's role as a relay station for sensory input is a complex function coordinated with the parietal lobe of the cerebrum. All sensory pathways, except olfactory, communicate with some area of the thalamus. With the assistance of stimuli from the cerebral cortex, the thalamus sorts and sends sensory impulses to the appropriate area of the cerebral cortex for final processing.

The role of the thalamus in motor activity is one of co-

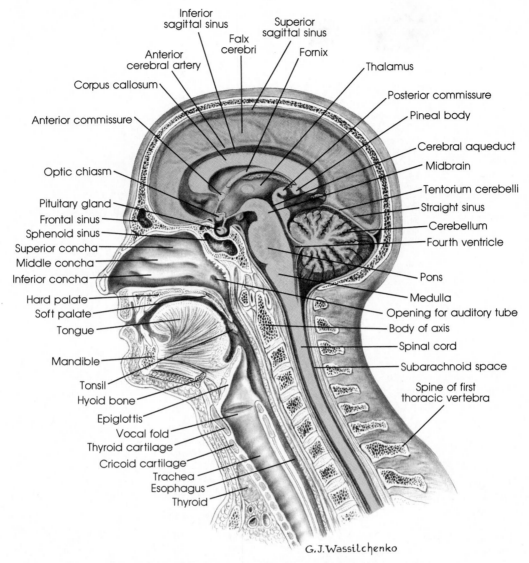

Fig. 23-16 Schematic drawing of sagittal section of head.

ordination and integration. It assists the cerebrum and cerebellum in providing a smooth, integrated motor response.

Hypothalamus. The hypothalamus, located below the thalamus, forms the floor and anterior lateral walls of the third ventricle. Other landmarks around the hypothalamus are the optic chiasm, which is located behind the hypothalamus, and the pituitary gland, sitting below the hypothalamus in the sella turcica. The pituitary stalk connects the hypothalamus to the pituitary gland.

Functions of the hypothalamus include regulating and maintaining internal body environment and interacting with the limbic system to generate actual physical responses to emotions, such as blushing when embarrassed. Areas of the internal environment regulated and maintained by the hypothalamus include (1) temperature regulation, (2) autonomic nervous system responses, (3) regulation of food and water intake, (4) control of hormonal secretions of the pituitary, and (5) behavioral responses.

Temperature regulation. Temperature regulation is

achieved by the anterior and posterior parts of the hypothalamus. As blood with increased temperature flows through the anterior region of the hypothalamus, stimuli travel to sweat glands to produce perspiration, to peripheral vessels to cause vasodilation, which allows heat loss through the skin, and to respiratory centers to increase respiratory rate. Low blood temperature stimulates the posterior region of the hypothalamus and causes vasoconstriction, piloerection or "goose bumps," and shivering, which increases cell metabolism and produces heat.

Autonomic nervous system responses. The hypothalamus serves as the "brain" for the autonomic or involuntary nervous system. The parasympathetic (resting) system response is elicited by stimulation of the anterior region of the hypothalamus. The sympathetic (fight or flight) system responds when the posterior region of the hypothalamus is stimulated.

Regulation of food and water intake. Food intake is regulated by two centers: the *hunger center,* which causes the sensation of hunger when stimulated, and the *satiety center,* which decreases the desire for food when the stomach is full or blood glucose is high. Water intake is regulated through the secretion of *antidiuretic hormone* (ADH). A change in serum osmotic pressure is the stimulus for ADH response. An increase in serum osmotic pressure stimulates the release of ADH, and decreases in serum osmotic pressure depress the release of ADH (see Chapter 39).

Control of hormonal secretions by the pituitary gland. The interrelationships between the hypothalamus and the pituitary in the production, storage, and secretion of hormones are discussed in the section on the pituitary gland.

Behavioral responses. Behavioral responses influenced by the hypothalamus and interacting with the limbic system include behaviors associated with aggression, pleasure, punishment, and sexual activities.

Epithalamus. Located in the dorsal portion of the diencephalon, the epithalamus contains the pineal gland, which is believed to play a role in physical growth and in sexual development. This gland often calcifies in early adulthood and can be identified on computed tomographic scan or radiographic films.

Subthalamus. The subthalamus is located below the thalamus. It is integrated with extrapyramidal tracts of the autonomic nervous system and the basal ganglia.

Pituitary gland. The pituitary gland, also known as the hypophysis, has been called the "master gland" because of its role in the regulation of hormone production of all other endocrine organs. Lying in the sella turcica, the pituitary gland is connected to the hypothalamus by the pituitary or hypophyseal stalk. The pituitary gland itself is divided into two lobes, the anterior (adenohypophysis) and the posterior (neurohypophysis). The anterior and posterior lobes of the pituitary are different and are described individually.

Anterior lobe. The anterior lobe constitutes 75% of the pituitary gland and is responsible for regulation of the majority of endocrine function. Hormone and other electrolyte levels in the blood are sensed by the hypothalamus. The hypothalamus then sends neurosecretory substances (releasing or inhibiting factors) through the blood supply of the pituitary stalk portal vein to the anterior pituitary. These neurosecretory substances cause the anterior pituitary gland to release or inhibit specific hormones. The seven major hormones of the anterior pituitary are adrenocorticotropic hormone (ACTH), thyroid-stimulating hormone (TSH), growth hormone (GH), prolactin (PRL), follicle-stimulating hormone (FSH), luteinizing hormone (LH), and melanocyte-stimulating hormone (MSH). Hormones are produced, stored, and then secreted from the pituitary when stimulated by the hypothalamus. Once the anterior pituitary hormone is released, it travels to the target endocrine gland and stimulates secretion of endocrine hormone, which then circulates through the blood supply back to the hypothalamus where an increased hormonal level is sensed. The hypothalamus stops the release of neurosecretory substances and the stimulating cycle is broken. See the box below for an example of this cycle, using the thyroid gland and thyroxin.

Posterior lobe. The posterior lobe constitutes the other 25% of the pituitary gland and is directly connected to the hypothalamus by the pituitary stalk. The posterior lobe does

---

HORMONE-STIMULATING CYCLE

Thyroxin level is low in blood
↓
Hypothalamus senses low level
↓
Hypothalamus releases thyrotropin-releasing factor (TRF)
↓
TRF travels through portal venous system to anterior pituitary
↓
Anterior pituitary secretes thyroid-stimulating hormone (TSH) into blood
↓
TSH travels to thyroid gland and stimulates production of thyroxin
↓
Hypothalamus senses circulating amount of thyroxin
↓
TRF is not released

---

not produce any hormones. However, the posterior lobe does secrete two hormones, ADH and oxytocin, which are produced by cells in the hypothalamus and trickle down fiber tracts through the pituitary stalk for storage in the posterior pituitary. When ADH or oxytocin release is required, the hypothalamus stimulates the pituitary to release these hormones rapidly in response to a variety of stimuli.

Internal capsule. Fiber tracts from many portions of each half of the cerebrum converge in the area of the diencephalon on their way to the brainstem and spinal cord to form the internal capsule. The internal capsule contains both afferent and efferent fibers but is mainly considered a motor, or efferent, pathway (Fig. 23-17). All afferent (sensory) fibers traveling to the cortex travel through the internal capsule in the following succession: brainstem to thalamus to internal capsule to cerebral cortex. All efferent (motor) fibers leaving the cortex also pass through the internal capsule. Because of the collection of all major motor and sensory fibers through this small area, a tiny area of damage to the internal capsule causes major loss of motor and some sensory function on the opposite side of the body.

Basal Ganglia

The main role of the basal ganglia is associated with motor function.[2,8] It provides a pathway and assists in processing information from the cerebral motor cortex and the thalamus. The basal ganglia is composed of several subcortical nuclei located deep within the white matter of the cerebral hemispheres. These paired sets of nuclei include the corpus striatum (composed of the caudate nuclei, the putamen, and the globus pallidus), the amygdala, the claustrum, the subthalamic nuclei, and the substantia nigra (see Fig. 23-17).

Much of the basal ganglia's function is through the extrapyramidal (involuntary) motor pathways. It influences

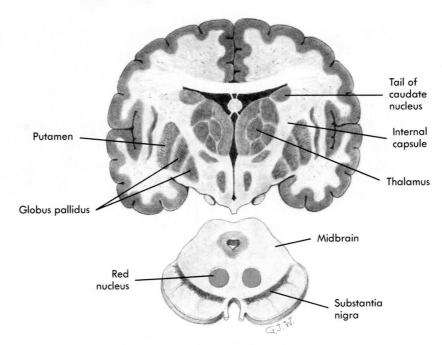

Fig. 23-17 Coronal section of brain.

motor activity to integrate voluntary movement with associated movements and postural adjustments and suppresses skeletal muscle tone and postural reflexes. The basal ganglia also processes input from visual, labyrinthine, and proprioceptive sources, resulting in smooth coordinated movements of the body without loss of balance.

Cerebrum

The cerebrum is the largest portion of the brain, comprising 80% of its weight. It is composed of two cerebral hemispheres (right and left) incompletely divided by the longitudinal fissure. The cerebral hemispheres are connected at the base of the longitudinal fissure by the corpus callosum. The corpus callosum is a large tract of transverse or commissural fibers that provide a communication link between the two hemispheres.

The outside of the cerebrum is covered with a thin layer of gray matter (multiple layers of unmyelinated cell nuclei) called the cerebral cortex. Underneath the cerebral cortex are the white matter (myelinated) tracts, which communicate impulses from the cerebral cortex to other areas of the brain. Three types of fibers—commissural (transverse), projection, and association—are in the white matter and are named for the role they play in communication of information. *Commissural fibers* are tracts that communicate between corresponding parts of the two hemispheres. The corpus callosum is the largest of these fiber tracts. *Projection fibers* communicate between the cerebral cortex and lower regions of the brain and spinal cord. *Association fibers* communicate between various regions of the same hemisphere.

The cerebral hemispheres are divided into four surface lobes, based on anatomical divisions or fissures. The four paired lobes are the *frontal lobes,* the *parietal lobes,* the *temporal lobes,* and the *occipital lobes* (Fig. 23-18). An-

other area deeper inside the cerebrum can also be classified as a lobe and is called the *limbic lobe.*

Classification of different areas of the cerebral cytoarchitecture, based on minute histological differences of the cell, is credited to Brodmann. More than 100 of these numbered areas have been identified (Fig. 23-19). See Table 23-4 for a summary of the cerebral lobes and their major functions.

Frontal lobe. The largest of the four lobes of the cerebral hemispheres is the frontal lobe. The frontal lobe lies underneath the frontal bone of the skull and is separated posteriorly from the parietal lobe by the central fissure (fissure of Rolando) and inferiorly from the temporal lobe by the lateral fissure (Sylvian fissure). The major functions of the frontal lobe are voluntary motor function, higher mental functions, cognition, memory, personality, and language. Some of the higher control centers for autonomic nervous system function also lie in the frontal lobe.

The prefrontal area of the frontal lobe (areas 9 to 12) is concerned with the process of cerebration (or thought), affect, feeling, and emotion, as well as autonomic nervous system response in relation to emotional changes. The rationale behind the use of biofeedback techniques and relaxation techniques correlates with the prefrontal area's influence on the autonomic nervous system.

The premotor area (areas 6 and 8) is an association area for the motor area lying adjacent to it. When stimulated, the prefrontal area provides general body movements such as turning the eyes and head and turning the trunk with the head. A connection exists between the premotor area and cranial nerves III, IV, VI, IX, X, and XII to allow coordination of the movements described (Fig. 23-20).

The motor area, or motor strip (area 4), contains the cells for voluntary (pyramidal) motor functions of the opposite

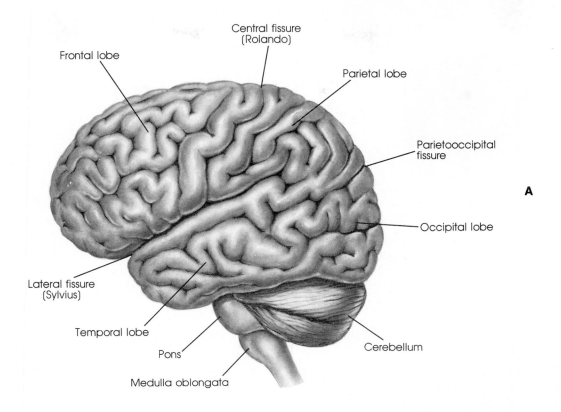

A

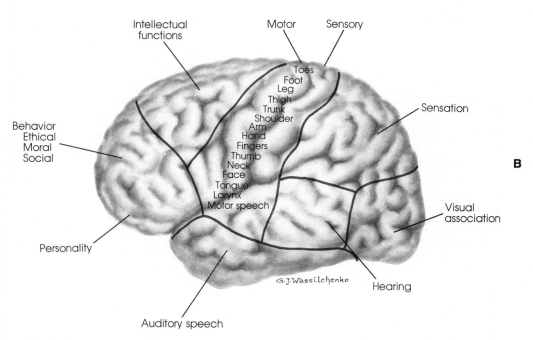

B

Fig. 23-18 **A,** Lateral view of cerebral hemisphere (showing lobes and pricipal fissures), cerebellum, pons, and medulla oblongata. **B,** Principal functional subdivisions of cerebral hemisphere.

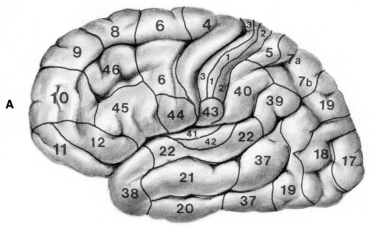

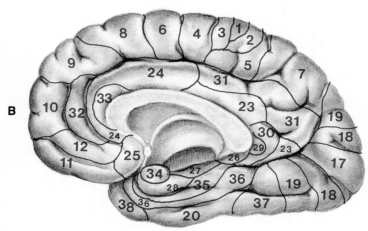

G.J.Wassilchenko

Fig. 23-19 Cytoarchitectural map of the lateral and medial surface of the human cortex according to Brodmann's map. **A,** Lateral surface. **B,** Medial surface.

Table 23-4 Cerebral lobes and their major functions

Cerebral lobes	Major functions
Frontal	Personality
	Moral, ethical, and social values
	Abstract thought
	Long-term memory
	Motor strip for opposite side of body
Parietal	Sensory strip for opposite side of body
	Two-point discrimination
	Recognition of object by size, shape, weight, or texture
	Body part awareness
Temporal	Hearing
	Special senses of taste and smell
	Interpretive area—integrates sounds, thoughts, and emotions
Occipital	Vision
	Visual recognition of objects
	Reading comprehension

side of the body. The motor-strip functions are drawn spatially by the homunculus (Fig. 23-21, *A*). The appearance is of an upside-down man with a foot on the medial aspect of the frontal lobe. The knees, hips, trunk, and shoulders extend over the outer surface of the cortex and the hands, thumb, head, face, and tongue down the side to the lateral fissure, which is the border of the frontal lobe. The size of the area for each body part along this strip is proportional to the amount of dexterity associated with the body part's function. Therefore the large surface area of the trunk occupies a relatively small part of the motor strip. The smaller areas such as the thumb or tongue that involve a great deal of dexterity and fine motor movement occupy a larger area of this strip.

Broca's area (areas 44 and 45) is located at the inferior frontal gyrus. Part of the speech center, this area is responsible for the motor aspects of speech and is involved in coordination of activities for the formulation of verbal speech. Damage to this area results in an *expressive* or *nonfluent aphasia.*

Parietal lobe. The parietal lobe is directly posterior to the frontal lobe on the other side of the central fissure. The posterior border of the parietal lobe is the parietooccipital fissure, which separates it from the occipital lobe. The in-

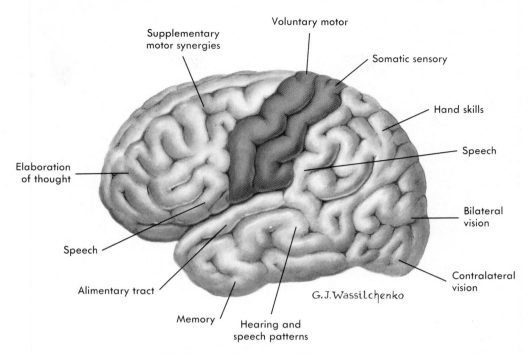

Fig. 23-20   Functions of specific cortical areas.

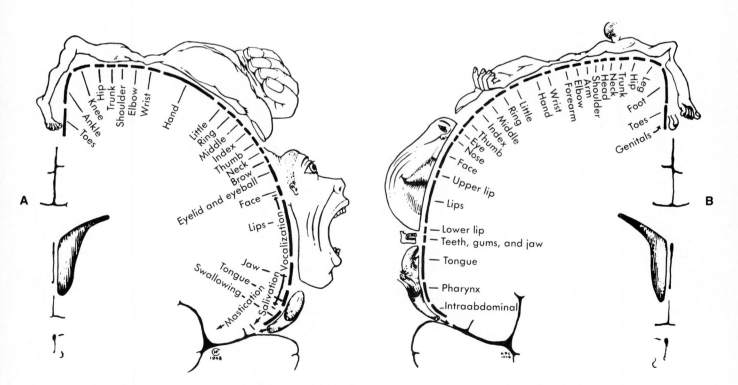

Fig. 23-21   Classic drawing of **A,** motor homunculus and, **B,** sensory homunculus. (From Penfield W and Rasmussen T: The cerebral cortex of man, 1950, Macmillan, Inc; renewed 1978 by Theodore Rasmussen.)

ferior border is incompletely defined by the posterior portion of the lateral fissure. The main function of the parietal lobe is sensory, including integration of sensory information, awareness of body parts, interpretation of touch, pressure, and pain, and recognition of object size, shape, or texture.

The parietal lobe contains a sensory strip (areas 1, 2, and 3) that lies adjacent to the motor strip of the frontal lobe. Similar to the homunculus of the motor strip, the sensory homunculus re-creates a caricature of an upside-down man (Fig. 23-21, *B*). Sensory areas of body parts lie close to motor areas of the same parts. Also, areas of the body with greater tactile response occupy larger areas on the sensory strip. Fibers going to the sensory strip bring stimuli associated with cutaneous and deep sensibility sensations, as well as cutaneous sensation of touch, pressure, position, and vibration. Input from the thalamus also reaches the sensory strip.

Associative areas of the parietal lobe (areas 5 and 7) interpret sensory input in terms of size, shape, texture, and weight. The parietal lobe provides the ability to localize a sensation and define it in terms of pressure, temperature, or vibration. Interpretive aspects of the parietal lobe's response to stimuli include awareness of body parts, orientation in space, and recognition of environmental spatial relationships.

A portion of the sensory aspect of speech and the understanding of the written word is located in the anterior-inferior area of the parietal lobe. Along with a portion of the temporal lobe, this area is called Wernicke's area (area 22).

Temporal lobe. The temporal lobe lies beneath the temporal bone in the lateral portion of the cranium. The anterior, lower border of the temporal lobe is encased in the sphenoid wing. With a strong blow to the head the temporal lobe is easily contused and lacerated as it moves against this hard, irregular surface. Separated from the frontal and parietal lobes by the lateral fissure, the primary functions of this lobe include hearing, speech, behavior, and memory.

The primary auditory areas (areas 41 and 42) receive sound impulses and assist in determining the source of the sound and interpreting the meaning of the sound. These areas are closely linked with Wernicke's area, which is located in both the parietal and temporal lobes. Responsible for the comprehension of both spoken and written language, Wernicke's area, in the dominant hemisphere, is called an associative area. Disruption of this area leads to *receptive (fluent) aphasia*—the individual can hear but is unable to interpret the message.

In the superior portion of the temporal lobe where the frontal, parietal, and temporal lobes meet is an essential *interpretive area* in which auditory, visual, and somatic association areas are integrated into complex thought and memory. Seizures in this region of the temporal lobe cause auditory, visual, or sensory hallucinations.

Occipital lobe. The occipital lobe of the cerebrum forms the most posterior portion. It is separated from the cerebellum by the tentorium. Primary responsibility of the occipital lobe is vision and the interpretation of visual stimuli.

The primary visual cortex (area 17) receives impulses from projections of the optic tract. These impulses are then referred to the visual associative areas (areas 18 and 19) for interpretation and integration.

Limbic lobe. One other cerebral section, which is anatomically part of the temporal lobe, is often separated from the temporal lobe for discussion of function and is called (although sometimes controversially) the limbic lobe. Also called the rhinencephalon, this lobe forms the border of the lateral ventricles and contains the hippocampus, the uncus, primary olfactory cortex, and the amygdaloid nucleus. The functions of the limbic lobe are self-preservation, primitive behavior, moods, the visceral processes associated with emotion, short-term memory, and the interpretation of smell.

Cerebral Circulation

The brain constitutes 2% of the body's weight but uses 20% of the body's cardiac output. It requires approximately 750 ml of cerebral blood flow per minute. The role of cerebral circulation is to provide enough blood to supply oxygen, glucose, and nutrients to the cerebral tissues. There is no reserve of either oxygen or glucose in the cerebral tissues, and a lack or inadequate amount of either one rapidly disrupts cerebral function and produces irreversible damage. Two pairs of arteries, the internal carotids and the vertebral arteries, are responsible for supplying blood to the brain. Anatomically they can be separated into the arteries of the anterior circulation and the posterior circulation (Fig. 23-22).[1,2,8] These two circulations are connected at the base of the brain by the circle of Willis.

Anterior circulation. The anterior circulation begins with the common carotid arteries (Fig. 23-23). The left common carotid originates from the arch of the aorta, and the right common carotid originates from the innominate artery. At the level of the crycothyroid junction, the common carotid splits to form the external and internal carotid arteries. The external carotid feeds the face, the scalp, and the skull and includes the branch called the *middle meningeal artery,* which lies between the skull and the dura. When torn or lacerated, blood from the middle meningeal artery can develop into an epidural hematoma.

The internal carotid artery continues upward through the carotid siphon and enters the base of the skull through an opening in the petrous bone. At the base of the brain the internal carotid connects with the circle of Willis and then branches into the anterior and middle cerebral arteries, which are primarily responsible for anterior circulation. One major branch of the internal carotid, the *ophthalmic artery,* exits before the circle of Willis and supplies blood to the optic nerve and eye.

Posterior circulation. Posterior circulation begins with the two vertebral arteries, which originate from the subclavian arteries and travel posteriorly through small openings in the lateral spinous processes of the cervical spine. They enter the skull through the foramen magnum and at the level of the pons the two vertebrals join to form the *basilar artery.* Branches of the basilar artery feed the brainstem and the cerebellum. The basilar artery continues upward into the posterior portion of the circle of Willis and into the two posterior cerebral arteries.

Circle of Willis. The circle of Willis is a vascular supply

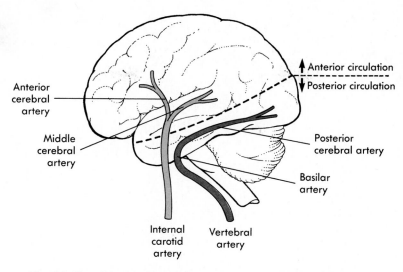

Fig. 23-22   Arteries of anterior and posterior cerebral circulation.

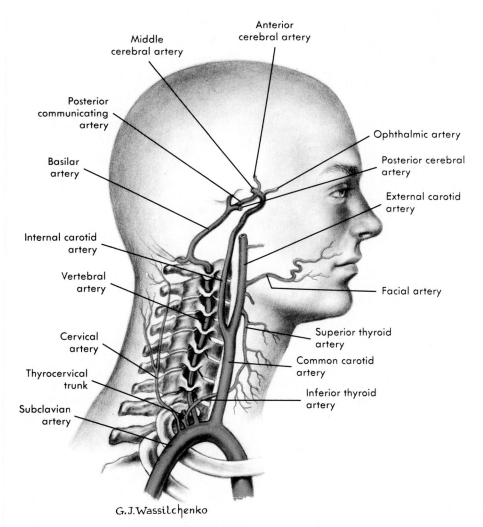

G.J.Wassilchenko

Fig. 23-23   Feeder arteries to the brain.

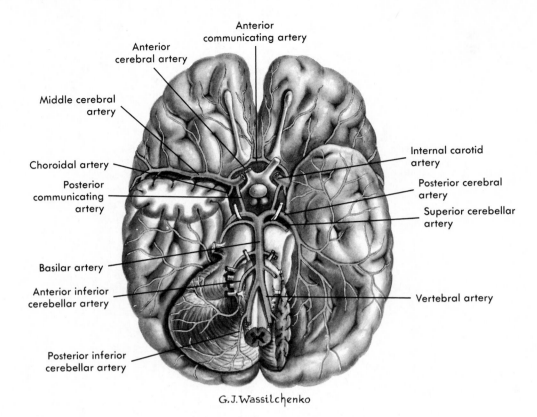

G.J.Wassilchenko

Fig. 23-24 Blood supply of the brain.

system unique to cerebral circulation (Fig. 23-24). Located in a small area above the optic chiasm in the subarachnoid space, the circle is fed by the internal carotid and basilar arteries. The three cerebral arteries (anterior, middle, and posterior) supplying each hemisphere are connected by communicating arteries to form a complete circle. The anterior communicating artery connects the right and left anterior cerebral arteries, and the two posterior communicating arteries connect the middle cerebral and posterior cerebral artery in each of the hemispheres.

In a normal situation the left internal carotid artery supplies blood to the left anterior and middle cerebral arteries, and the right internal carotid artery supplies blood to the right anterior and middle cerebral arteries, thus constituting anterior circulation. In the posterior circulation the basilar artery feeds both posterior cerebral arteries.

When an artery such as the right internal carotid is blocked with atherosclerotic material so that an inadequate amount of blood is flowing to the right anterior and middle cerebral arteries, blood from the left internal carotid will flow across the anterior communicating artery and assist with the vascular supply to the right hemisphere. Also, blood flow from the right posterior cerebral artery will flow through the right posterior communicating artery to supply blood to the right middle cerebral artery. Thus supply of oxygen and nutrients to the brain is not disrupted.

It is not unusual to have an anatomically incomplete circle of Willis. Autopsy and angiographic studies have supplied evidence that up to 50% of individuals have absent or hy-

poplastic communicating vessels.[2]

Anterior cerebral artery. The anterior cerebral artery runs anteriorly along the base of the brain and supplies the longitudinal fissure and therefore the medial surfaces of the frontal and parietal lobes. It also feeds the basal ganglia, portions of the internal capsule, and the corpus callosum.

Middle cerebral artery. The middle cerebral artery is the largest of the cerebral arteries. As a direct branch from the internal carotid, it travels laterally and feeds the surface of the frontal, parietal, and temporal lobes and the internal capsule.

Posterior cerebral artery. The posterior cerebral artery, a branch of the basilar artery, runs along the tentorium and feeds the occipital lobes and the medial and lateral aspects of the temporal lobe (Fig. 23-25).

Venous circulation. Venous drainage is accomplished by the venous sinuses of the dura. Capillary flow moves to venules and then to cerebral veins, which empty into the sinuses located throughout the cranium. Blood from these sinuses empties into the internal jugular vein, which empties into the superior vena cava and then back into the right atrium.

Spinal Cord

The spinal cord is the extension of the medulla after its exit from the foramen magnum.[5,7] It is a long ropelike structure composed of white and gray matter. The spinal cord itself tapers down to an end or *conus medullaris* at the level of the first or second lumbar vertebra. Exiting from the spinal cord are 31 pairs of spinal nerve roots, which travel through the intervertebral foramina. Since the spinal cord ends at L1 and the final nerve roots do not exit until the coccyx, long lengths of nerve roots called the *cauda equina* extend through the space in the lumbar and sacral regions. Most of the protective mechanisms for the cranium also exist, with slight modification, for the spinal cord.

Protective mechanisms

Bony structures. The bony structure that encases the spinal cord is the vertebral column. Comprising 33 vertebrae and 24 intervertebral disks, this column, held together by ligaments and tendons, provides support and protection for the spinal cord plus structure and flexibility for body movement. The vertebrae are divided into sections in relation to their appearance (Fig. 23-26). There are 7 cervical vertebrae, 12 thoracic vertebrae, 5 lumbar vertebrae, 5 sacral vertebrae (fused as 1), and 4 coccygeal vertebrae (fused as 1).

Although differences in vertebral appearance exist, the basic structure includes a vertebral body connected by two pedicles to the transverse processes (Fig. 23-27). Two laminae connect the transverse processes to the posterior segment of the vertebra, the spinous process, forming a ring. In the center of the spinal foramen is the canal, which houses the spinal cord.

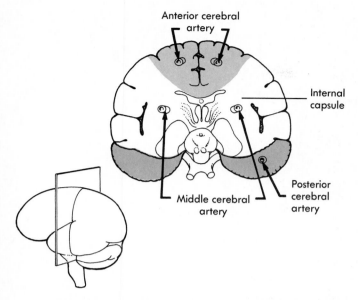

Fig. 23-25 Distribution of arterial blood supply.

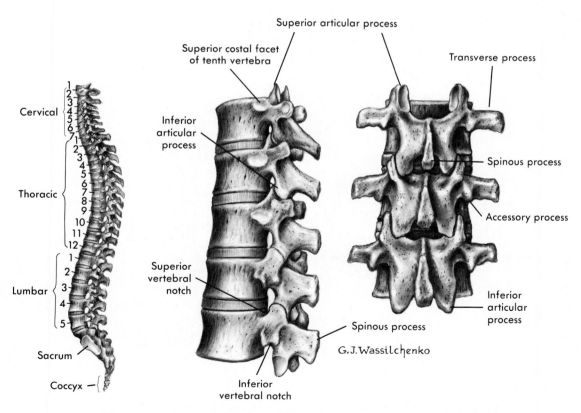

Fig. 23-26 Vertebral column and anatomical structures of vertebrae.

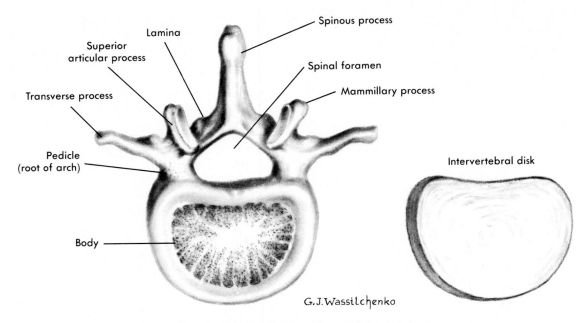

G. J. Wassilchenko

Fig. 23-27   Vertebra and intervertebral disk.

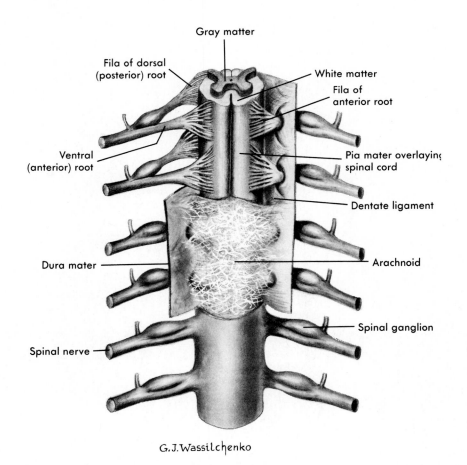

G. J. Wassilchenko

Fig. 23-28   Meningeal layers of the spinal cord. Segment of spinal cord is viewed from behind with portions of dura mater and arachnoid removed.

Intervertebral disk. The bodies of the vertebrae are separated by an intervertebral disk. These fibrocartilaginous structures are between each vertebral body from the first cervical vertebrae to the beginning of the sacrum. The intervertebral disk is composed of two layers. The inner core, the nucleus pulposus, is a soft gelatinous material, which assists in shock absorbancy along the spinal column. Surrounding the nucleus pulposus is the annulus fibrosus. This thick, tough outer layer provides firmer structure to assist the spinal column in supporting the weight of the body when upright.

When a patient suffering from severe back and leg pain is diagnosed as having a herniated disk, the annulus fibrosus has usually torn and a portion of the nucleus pulposus has herniated into the spinal foramen, pressing against the spinal nerve root as it exits the spinal cord across the pedicle. If surgery is required, a *laminectomy* or *diskectomy* is performed. It involves removal of one lamina to gain entrance to the spinal foramen. The herniated portion of the disk is then removed and pressure relieved.

Meninges. The meninges of the spinal cord are similar to those in the cranium (Fig. 23-28). The first meninges, the dura, is a continuation of the inner layer of the intracranial dura. Dura of the spinal cord encases the cord, the nerve roots, and the spinal nerves until they exit from the vertebral column. The dura extends to the level of the second

sacral vertebra, even though the spinal cord itself ends at the L1 or L2 level.

The arachnoid membrane is the same weblike delicate tissue that is in the cranium. Cerebrospinal fluid (CSF) flows in the subarachnoid space of the spinal cord also. Because the spinal cord terminates at L2 and the meninges continue to S2, a volume of CSF is contained in this space and can be tapped through a lumbar puncture procedure. The pia mater of the spinal cord is a thicker, firmer, less vascular membrane than that in the cranium.

Spinal nerves. There are 31 spinal nerve pairs: 8 cervical, 12 thoracic, 5 lumbar, 5 sacral, and 1 coccygeal (Fig. 23-29).

In the cervical region the first seven pairs of nerves exit the cord above the corresponding vertebrae. The C8 nerve pair exits the spinal cord below the C7 vertebra. From this point on, all thoracic, lumbar, and sacral nerves exit below the corresponding vertebrae.

The spinal nerve has two roots: the dorsal root and the ventral root. The dorsal root is an afferent pathway and carries sensory impulses from the body into the spinal cord. The ventral root is an efferent pathway and carries motor information from the spinal cord to the body. The dorsal and ventral roots join together as they exit the spinal foramen and become a spinal nerve. Distribution of the sensory components of the spinal nerve has been well defined. Displayed

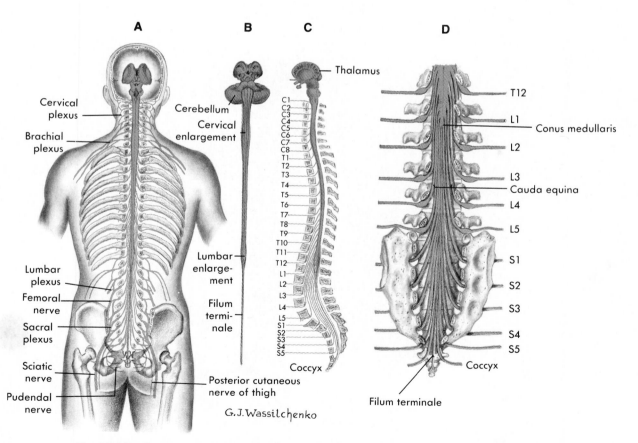

Fig. 23-29 Spinal cord within vertebral canal and exiting spinal nerves. **A,** Posterior view in situ. **B,** Anterior view. **C,** Lateral view. **D,** Cauda equina.

ANTERIOR VIEW

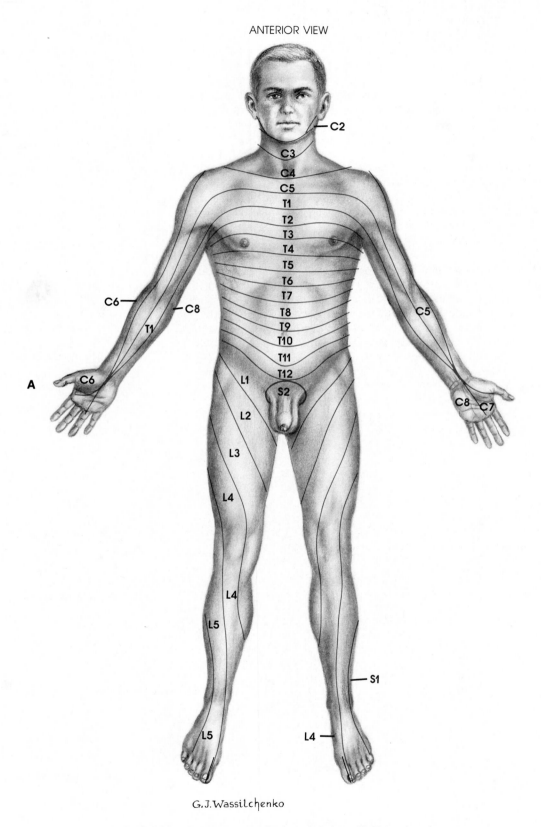

C2
C3
C4
C5
T1
T2
T3
T4
T5
T6
T7
T8
T9
T10
T11
T12
L1
S2
L2
L3
L4
L4
L5
L5

C6   C8
T1
A   C6

C5

C8 C7

S1

L4

G.J.Wassilchenko

Fig. 23-30   Dermatomes. **A,** Anterior view. **B,** Posterior view.

POSTERIOR VIEW

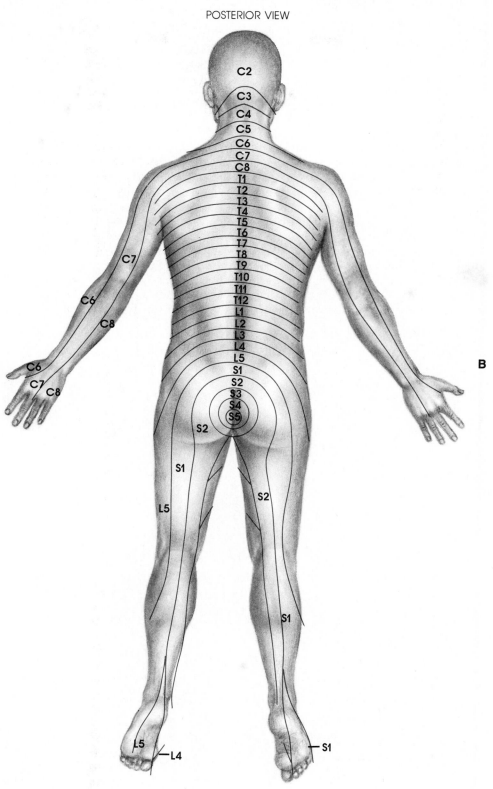

G.J.Wassilchenko

as sensory dermatomes, these diagrams allow identification of sensory innervation in the peripheral nervous system (Fig. 23-30).

Cross section. The spinal cord is composed of both gray matter and white matter.[2,6] The central gray matter, which appears in the shape of an H, consists of cell bodies, small projection fibers, and glial support cells. The gray matter has been divided into areas based on the cell body type located within their boundaries. The three basic divisions are the anterior horn, the lateral horn, and the posterior horn. The anterior horn contains motor cells and is the final junction of motor information before it exits the CNS. The lateral horn contains preganglionic fibers of the autonomic nervous system: sympathetic fibers T1 to L2 and parasympathetic fibers S2 to S4. The posterior horn contains axons from the peripheral sensory neurons.

The white matter, which surrounds the gray matter, contains the myelinated ascending and descending tracts, which carry information to and from the brain (Fig. 23-31). Spinal tracts are named so that the *prefix denotes the origin of the tract and the suffix is the destination,* thus allowing easy identification of sensory or motor tracts. Sensory tracts begin with the prefix *spino* and motor tracts end with the suffix *spinal.*

Ascending or sensory tracts	Descending or motor tracts
Lateral spinothalamic tract: ascension of pain and thermal sensations	Ventral and lateral corticospinal tracts: descending voluntary motor tracts
Anterior spinothalamic tract: ascension of light touch and pressure sensation	Rubrospinal tract: originates in the nucleus of the midbrain; receives fibers from cerebellum and descends in the lateral and anterior funiculi; conveys impulses to control muscle synergy and tone
Posterior white columns: ascension of discriminatory touch	

Many other motor and sensory tracts are within the spinal cord, but only those presented here can be clinically tested.

Vascular supply. Supply of arterial blood to the spinal cord comes from branches of the vertebral arteries plus small radicular arteries that enter at the intervertebral foramina. They combine to form the anterior spinal and two posterior spinal arteries. These three arteries, along with some additional radicular arterial flow from cervical, intercostal, lumbar, and sacral arteries, feed the entire length of the spinal cord (Fig. 23-32).

Arterial supply to the spinal cord is segmented at best;

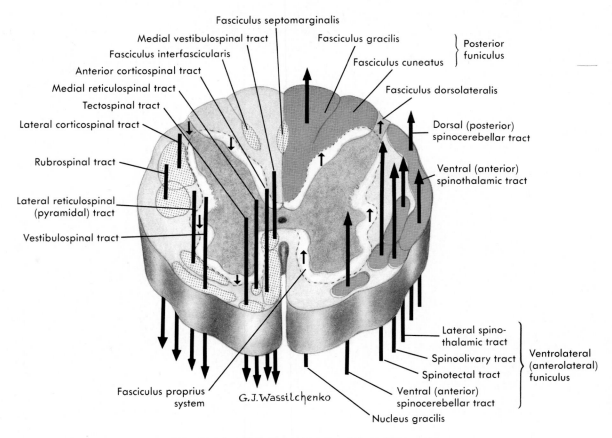

Fig. 23-31 Spinal cord tracts of the white matter.

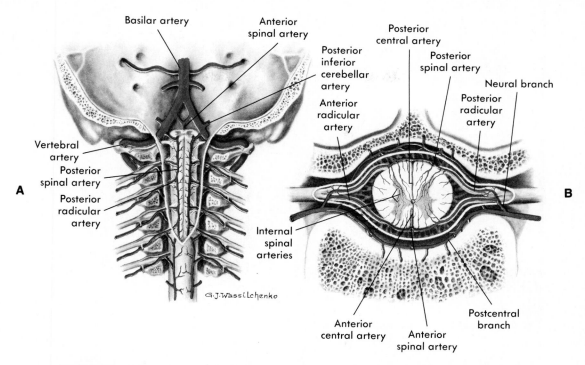

Fig. 23-32   Arteries of spinal cord. **A,** Cervical cord arteries. **B,** Vascular distribution in spinal cord.

therefore certain portions of the spinal cord that receive their blood supply from two separate sources are vulnerable areas. These vulnerable areas are C2 to 3, T1 to 4, and L1 to 2. Evidence of this tenuous blood supply can occasionally be noted in a patient after open heart surgery or abdominal aortic aneurysm repair who becomes paraplegic because of loss of the small arterial feeders from the aorta responsible for spinal cord circulation.

REFERENCES

1. Chusid JG: Correlative neuroanatomy and functional neurophysiology, ed 19, Los Altos, Calif, 1985, Lange Medical Publications.
2. Gilman S and Winans S: Manter and Gatz's essentials of clinical neuroanatomy and neurophysiology, ed 6, Philadelphia, 1982, FA Davis Co.
3. Guyton A: Textbook of medical physiology, ed 7, Philadelphia, 1986, WB Saunders Co.
4. Hickey JV: The clinical practice of neurological and neurosurgical nursing, ed 2, Philadelphia, 1986, JB Lippincott Co.
5. Ricci MM: American Association of Neuroscience Nurses core curriculum for neuroscience nursing, ed 2, Chicago, 1984, AANN.
6. Rudy EB: Advanced neurological and neurosurgical nursing, St Louis, 1984, The CV Mosby Co.
7. Snell R: Clinical neuroanatomy for medical students, Boston, 1980, Little, Brown & Co, Inc.
8. Williams PL and Warwick R, editors: Gray's anatomy, ed 36, New York, 1980, Churchill Livingstone, Inc.

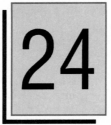

24

Neurological Clinical Assessment

CHAPTER OBJECTIVES

- List the five components of the neurological assessment.
- Discuss the acceptable and unacceptable methods of applying noxious stimuli.
- Describe the pathway of pupillary response.
- Define the respiratory patterns associated with neurological deterioration.
- State the changes in vital sign changes associated with neurological deterioration.
- Define brain death and persistent vegetative state.

Assessment of the patient with actual or potential neurological dysfunction is the essential beginning point in the nursing process and forms the basis for nursing diagnosis. Only if the nurse is aware of all components of a patient's physiological dysfunction can appropriate diagnosing, planning, intervention, and evaluation take place. This chapter presents a basic introduction to a neurological examination in the critical care environment.

COMPONENTS OF NEUROLOGICAL ASSESSMENT

Neurological assessment encompasses a wide variety of applications and a multitude of techniques. This chapter focuses on the type of assessment that would be performed in a critical care environment. The one factor common to all neurological assessments is the need to obtain a comprehensive history of events preceding hospitalization. If the patient is incapable of providing this information, family members or significant others should be contacted as soon as possible. Frequently, valuable information is gained from this knowledge, which directs the caregiver to focus on certain aspects of the patient's clinical assessment.

There are five major components of neurological assessment in the critically ill patient. They are evaluation of (1) level of consciousness, (2) motor movements, (3) pupils and eye signs, (4) respiratory patterns, and (5) vital signs.

Until all five of these parameters have been assessed, a complete neurological examination has not been performed.

Level of Consciousness

Assessment of the level of consciousness is the most important aspect of the neurological assessment. In most situations a patient's level of consciousness will deteriorate before any other changes in neurological assessment are noted. These deteriorations are often subtle and must be monitored carefully.

Components of consciousness. There are two major components of consciousness: *arousal or alertness* and *content of consciousness or awareness*.[7]

Arousal. Assessment of the arousal component of consciousness is an evaluation of the reticular activating system and its connection with the thalamus and the cerebral cortex. Arousal is the lowest level of consciousness, and observation is centered around the patient's ability to respond to verbal or noxious stimuli in an appropriate manner.

Awareness. Content of consciousness is a higher level function and is concerned with assessment of the patient's orientation to person, place, and time. Assessment of content of consciousness requires the patient to give appropriate answers to a variety of questions. Changes in the patient's answers indicating increasing degrees of confusion and disorientation may be the first sign of neurological deterioration.

Categories of consciousness. The following categories, though vague, are often used to describe the patient's level of consciousness[7]:

Alert—Patient responds immediately to minimal external stimuli.

Lethargic—State of drowsiness or inaction in which the patient needs an increased stimulus to be awakened.

Obtunded—A duller indifference to external stimuli exists and response is minimally maintained.

Stuporous—The patient can be aroused only by vigorous and continuous external stimuli.

Comatose—Vigorous stimulation fails to produce any voluntary neural response.

Patients are frequently difficult to categorize under these descriptions. Also, the levels of consciousness are not defined in enough detail, and communication of patient condition is often misinterpreted. For example, one clinician might describe a patient's response as obtunded, whereas the next clinician might describe the same response as stuporous. Because of this difficulty in communicating level of consciousness, a variety of assessment tools have been devised to assist in this evaluation.

Tools for assessment of consciousness. The general rule for evaluation of an altered level of consciousness is to systematically determine the type and degree of noxious stimuli required to produce a response. This concept is incorporated into a variety of clinical assessment tools.

Table 24-1   Glasgow coma scale

Category	Score	Response
Eye opening	4	Spontaneous—eyes open spontaneously without stimulation
	3	To speech—eyes open with verbal stimulation but not necessarily to command
	2	To pain—eyes open with noxious stimuli
	1	None—no eye opening regardless of stimulation
Verbal response	5	Oriented—accurate information about person, place, time, reason for hospitalization, and personal data
	4	Confused—answers not appropriate to question, but correct use of language
	3	Inappropriate words—disorganized, random speech, no sustained conversation
	2	Incomprehensible sounds—moans, groans, and mumbles incomprehensibly
	1	None—no verbalization despite stimulation
Best motor response	6	Obeys commands—performs simple tasks on command; able to repeat performance
	5	Localizes to pain—organized attempt to localize and remove painful stimuli
	4	Withdraws from pain—withdraws extremity from source of painful stimuli
	3	Abnormal flexion—decorticate posturing spontaneously or in response to noxious stimuli
	2	Extension—decerebrate posturing spontaneously or in response to noxious stimuli
	1	None—no response to noxious stimuli; flaccid

The most widely recognized level of consciousness assessment tool is the Glasgow Coma Scale (GCS).[8] This scored scale is based on evaluation of three categories: eye opening, verbal response, and best motor response (Table 24-1).

The best possible score on the GCS is 15, and the lowest score is 3. Generally a score of 7 or less on the GCS indicates coma.

Originally the scoring system was developed to assist with general communication of the severity of neurological injury. Adapted and modified, this scale has become the basis of many neurological assessment flow sheets. When using the GCS for serial assessment, several points should be kept in mind. The GCS is a level of consciousness assessment tool only and should never be considered a complete neurological examination. It is not a sensitive tool for evaluation of an altered sensorium. The GCS does not account for possible aphasia. The GCS is not a good indicator of lateralization of neurological deterioration. Lateralization involves decreasing motor response on one side or changes in pupillary reaction.

Whatever the choice of level of consciousness assessment tools, the goal of assessment of this parameter is to identify subtle changes in consciousness responses. Communication of small signs of deteriorating consciousness may allow early intervention and prevent neurological disaster.

Motor Movements

Levels of motor movements. A simple way of organizing the assessment of motor movements is to use the categories defined in the Glasgow Coma Scale[8] as a guide. The difference in this part of the assessment is that now each extremity is evaluated and recorded individually.

Obeys commands—Performs simple tasks on command. Able to repeat performance.

Localizes to pain—Organized attempt to localize and remove painful stimuli.

Withdraws from pain—Withdraws extremity from source of painful stimuli.

Abnormal flexion—Decorticate posturing spontaneously or in response to noxious stimuli (Fig. 24-1).

Extension—Decerebrate posturing spontaneously or in response to noxious stimuli (see Fig. 24-1).

Flaccid—No response to noxious stimuli; flaccid.

Additionally a comparison of function is made with that of the opposite extremity. If evaluating a patient with spinal cord injury or dysfunction, a separate scale should be used with more detail about motor strength of particular muscle groups (Fig. 24-2).

Motor assessment techniques

Obeys commands. Next to the assessment of orientation and awareness, the assessment of the patient's ability to follow commands is one of the highest levels of functioning evaluated. In assessing the ability to follow commands, there are several points that must be recognized. Commands given to a patient with an altered level of consciousness must be simple and direct statements such as, "Show me your thumb." A common error made by clinicians in assessing the patient's ability to respond to commands is to include the simple command along with other verbal communica-

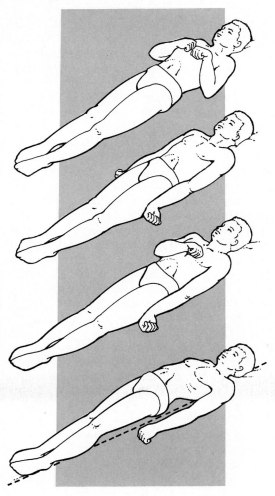

Fig. 24-1 Abnormal motor responses. **A,** Decorticate posturing. **B,** Decerebrate posturing. **C,** Decorticate posturing on right side and decerebrate posturing on left side of body. **D,** Opisthotonic posturing.

tion. To prevent sensory overload and therefore the patient's inability to respond to command, the command should not be included as part of any other verbal conversation. An example of the inappropriate use of a simple command is: "Robert, your mother is here. Let's show her how much better you are doing. Robert, show her your thumb. Come on Robert, you did it for me an hour ago. Robert, show your mother your thumb. She will be very excited if she could see you do this. Robert, I know you can do it. Don't be stubborn." As a patient is emerging from an unconscious state, the brain is less capable of processing and sorting multiple stimuli simultaneously. The key to assessment of the patient's ability to follow commands is to reduce surrounding stimuli or distractors and to keep the command simple and direct.

Another error commonly made in the assessment of the patient's ability to follow commands involves the type of command given. Appropriate commands are those not calling for random or reflex responses. "Squeeze my hand" is a common command used by caregivers and family alike.

In the low levels of consciousness, the reflex of hand grasp may be present and is initiated when the assessor's hand is placed within the patient's hand. If this is the case, it is often difficult to accurately assess whether the patient is responding to command or exhibiting a reflex response. Asking the patient to "Let go of my hand" after hand grasp is also difficult to accurately assess. Relaxation of the reflex can mimic the command: "Let go." Use of hand grasp in assessment of patient's motor strength is separate from this discussion.

Acceptable commands include "Show me your thumb" or "Stick out your tongue." When using these commands, care must be taken that the command is not followed by visual or tactile stimuli. It is not uncommon to observe an assessment in which the nurse asks the patient "show me your thumb" while the nurse is tapping the thumb. With this scenario it is impossible to determine whether the patient is following a verbal command or withdrawing from tactile stimuli.

Noxious stimuli. Once it has been determined that the patient is incapable of comprehending and following a simple command, the use of noxious stimuli is required to determine the motor responses of the body. There are a variety of acceptable ways of administering painful stimuli that will be presented here. There are also several commonly used but unacceptable means of delivering noxious stimuli that will also be discussed.

ACCEPTABLE

1. *Nail bed pressure* is an acceptable form of noxious stimuli. It requires use of an object such as a pen to apply firm pressure to the nail bed. Pressure applied to each extremity allows for evaluation of individual extremity function. The patient's movement must not be interrupted while the nurse is applying the nail bed pressure. Although this pressure is classified as noxious stimuli, if no response is elicited from nail bed pressure other noxious stimuli measures should be employed.

2. *Trapezius pinch* is another acceptable method of delivering noxious stimuli. Performed by squeezing the trapezius muscle, this method allows for observation of total body response to stimuli. Trapezius pinch is often difficult to perform on large or obese adults.

3. *Pinching of the inner aspect of the arm or leg* is the final acceptable form of administering noxious stimuli. A small portion of the patient's tissue on the sensitive inner aspect of the arm or leg is pinched firmly and each extremity is evaluated independently. Although this form of noxious stimuli is the most apt to cause bruising, it is also the most sensitive for eliciting a movement response.

UNACCEPTABLE

1. *Sternal rub* is often used as a form of noxious stimuli. Firm pressure is applied to the sternum in a rubbing motion usually with the assessor's knuckles. When used repeatedly the sternum could become excoriated, open, and infected. Open/handed firm patting of the sternal area to arouse the patient is acceptable.

2. *Supraorbital pressure* is another form of noxious stimuli that should be avoided. Patients with head injuries, frontal craniotomies, or facial surgeries should not be evaluated with this method because of the possibility of underlying

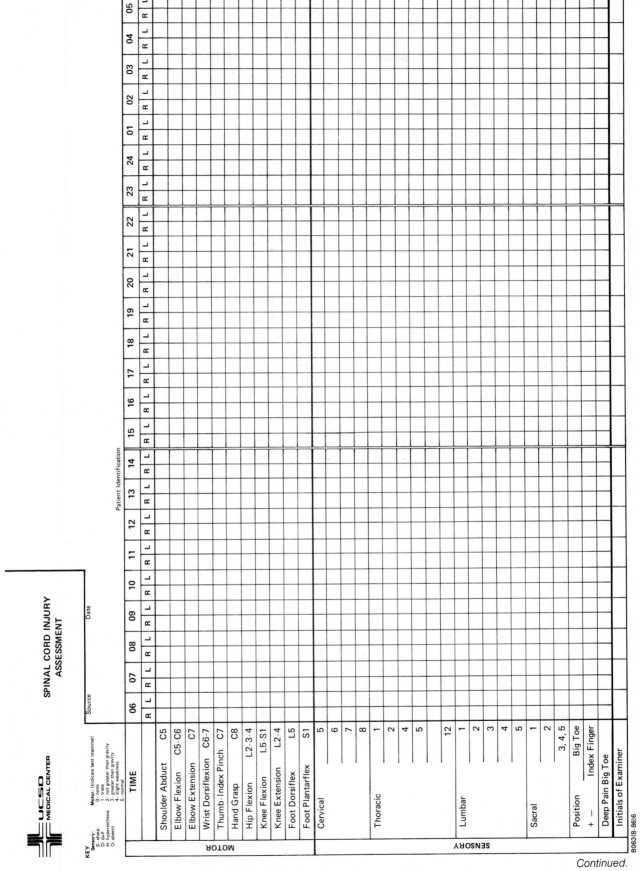

Fig. 24-2   Spinal cord assessment sheet.

Continued.

CUTANEOUS INNERVATION FOR SENSORY ASSESSMENT

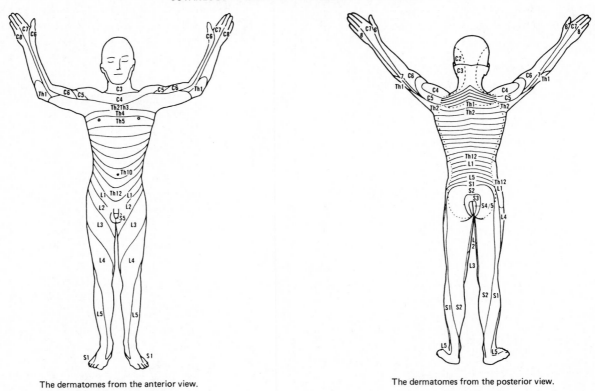

The dermatomes from the anterior view.

The dermatomes from the posterior view.

METHOD OF STABILIZATION

Tongs _____ Weights _____

Halo Brace _____

Cervical Collar _____

Other _____

COMMENTS _____

_____

_____

_____

_____

_____

_____

INITIAL	PRINT NAME AND TITLE	SIGNATURE

Fig. 24-2 Spinal cord assessment sheet—cont'd

fractured or unstable cranium. Therefore it is better not to develop the habit of applying supraorbital pressure to deliver noxious stimuli.

3. *Nipple pinching* and *testicle pinching* has been used for many years. Although never described in texts as an acceptable method for delivering noxious stimuli, it can often be observed in the clinical setting. For obvious reasons this type of noxious stimuli is inappropriate and unnecessary.

Assessment of lateralizing signs. Lateralizing signs are a difference in neurological assessment findings on one side of the body and include unilateral deterioration in motor movements or changes in pupillary response. Lateralizing signs help to localize the lesion to one side of the brain. For example, a patient who was withdrawing to painful stimuli with both arms at the last examination is now withdrawing on the right but exhibiting abnormal flexion on the left. This change in response on the left side points to an expanding intracranial lesion on the right.

The occurrence of lateralizing signs indicate an emergency situation. Unilateral deterioration of motor movements and pupillary response may herald herniation. Notification of the physician and immediate intervention is imperative.

Pupils and Eye Assessment

The assessment of pupillary function and eye movement is an important component of the neurological assessment.[11] Especially in the unconscious patient or the patient receiving neuromuscular blocking agents and sedation, pupillary response is one of the few neurological signs that can be assessed. Serial evaluation, appropriate technique, recognition of abnormalities, and good documentation are all important.

Anatomy of pupil response. Pupil reaction is a function of the autonomic nervous system. Parasympathetic control of pupil reaction occurs through innervation of the oculomotor nerve (CN III), which exits from the brainstem in the midbrain area. When the parasympathetic fibers are stimulated, the pupil constricts. Sympathetic control of the pupil originates in the hypothalamus and travels down the entire length of the brainstem. When the sympathetic fibers are stimulated, the pupil dilates (Table 24-2).

Pupil changes provide a valuable tool to assessment because of pathway location (Fig. 24-3). The oculomotor nerve lies at the junction of the midbrain and the tentorial notch. Any increase of pressure that exerts force down through the tentorial notch compresses the oculomotor nerve. Oculomotor nerve compression results in a dilated, nonreactive pupil. Sympathetic pathway disruption occurs with involvement in the brainstem. Loss of sympathetic

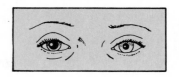
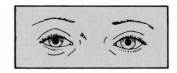
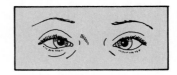
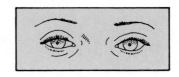
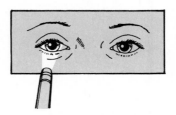

Fig. 24-3 Abnormal pupillary responses.

control leads to pinpoint, nonreactive pupils. Pupillary reactivity is also affected by medications, particularly sympathetic and parasympathetic agents, direct trauma, and eye surgery. Pupil reactivity is relatively resistant to metabolic dysfunction and can be used to differentiate between metabolic and structural causes of decreased levels of consciousness.

Anatomy of eye movement. Control of eye movements occurs with interaction of three cranial nerves: oculomotor (CN III), trochlear (CN IV), and abducens (CN VI). The pathways for these cranial nrves provide integrated function through the internuclear pathway of the medial longitudinal fasciculus (MLF) located in the brainstem. The MLF provides coordination of eye movements with the vestibular and reticular formation (Fig. 24-4).

Assessment of pupillary response. Evaluation of pupillary response includes assessment of size, shape (round, irregular, or oval), and degree of reactivity to light. Comparison should be made between the two pupils for equality. Any of these components of the pupil assessment could change in response to increasing pressure on the oculomotor nerve at the tentorium.

The technique for evaluation of direct pupillary response

Table 24-2 Pathways of pupillary response

Sympathetic	Parasympathetic
Brainstem	CN III
Dilates	Constricts

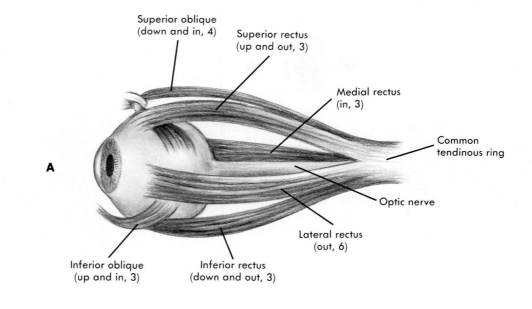

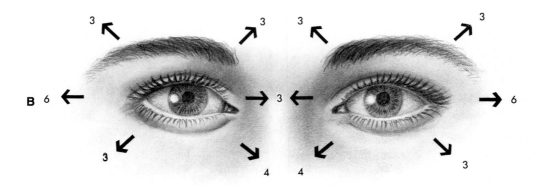

G. J. Wassilchenko

Fig. 24-4 Extraocular eye movements. **A,** Extraocular muscles. **B,** The six cardinal directions of gaze with the associated cranial nerve supply.

involves use of a narrow-beamed bright light shone into the pupil from the outer canthus of the eye. If the light is shone directly onto the pupil, glare or reflection of the light may prevent the assessor proper visualization. Concensual pupillary response is the constriction of the pupil in response to a light shone into the opposite eye.

Assessment of eye movements

Extraocular movements. In the conscious patient, the function of the three cranial nerves of the eye and their innervation with the MLF can be assessed by the nurse's asking the patient to follow a finger through the full range of eye motions. If the eyes move together into all six fields, extraolcular movements (EOM) are intact.[2]

Oculocephalic reflex (doll's eyes). In the unconscious patient assessment of ocular function and the innervation of the MLF is done by eliciting the doll's eyes procedure. If the patient is unconscious as a result of trauma, the nurse should ascertain that there is no cervical injury before performing this examination.

To assess the oculocephalic reflex, the nurse should hold the eyelids open and briskly turn the head to one side while observing the eye movements, then briskly turn the head to the other side and observe. If the oculocephalic reflex is intact, doll's eyes are present. The eyes deviate to the opposite direction in which the head is turned. If the oculocephalic reflex is not intact, doll's eyes are absent. This lack of response in which the eyes remain midline and move with the head indicates significant brainstem injury. If the oculocephalic reflex is abnormal, doll's eyes are abnormal. In this situation the eyes rove or move in opposite directions. Abnormal oculocephalic reflex indicates some degree of brainstem injury (Fig. 24-5).

Oculovestibular reflex (cold caloric test). The oculovestibular reflex is usually performed by a physician as one of the final clinical assessments of brainstem function. Twenty to 50 ml of ice water is injected into the external auditory canal. The normal eye movement response is a rapid nystagmus/like deviation toward the irrigated ear. This response indicates brainstem integrity. This test is an extremely noxious stimulation and may produce a decorticate

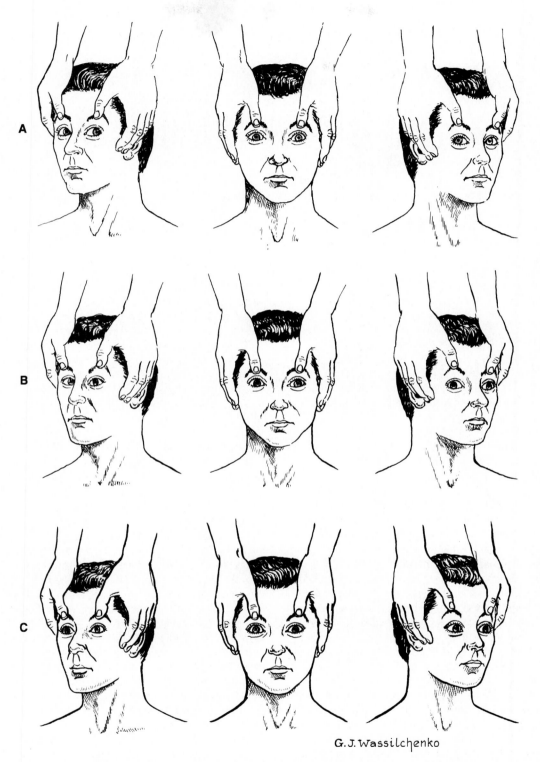

G.J.Wassilchenko

Fig. 24-5 Oculocephalic reflex (doll's eyes). **A,** Normal. **B,** Abnormal. **C,** Absent.

A   B   C

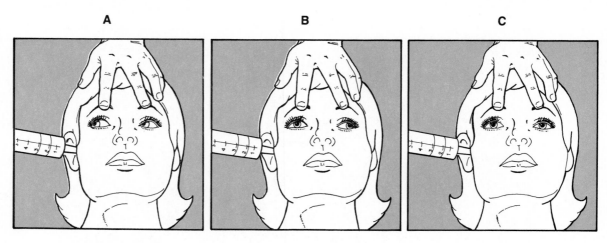

Fig. 24-6 Oculovestibular reflex (cold caloric test). **A,** Normal. **B,** Abnormal. **C,** Absent.

or decerebrate posturing response in the comatose patient. It is not recommended to perform this procedure on a conscious patient (Fig. 24-6).

An abnormal response would be dysconjugate eye movement, which indicates a brainstem lesion, or no response, which indicates little to no brainstem function.

Respiratory Patterns

Control of respirations. The activity of respirations is a highly integrated function receiving input from the cerebrum, brainstem, and metabolic mechanisms. There is a close correlation in clinical assessment between altered levels of consciousness, the level of brain or brainstem injury, and the respiratory pattern noted (Fig. 24-7).

Under the influence of the cerebral cortex and the diencephalon, three brainstem centers control respirations. The lowest center, the medullary respiratory center, sends impulses through the vagus nerve to innervate muscles of inspiration and expiration. The apneustic and pneumotaxic centers of the pons are responsible for the length of inspiration and expiration and the underlying respiratory rate.

Respiratory patterns. Changes in respiratory patterns assist in identifying the level of brainstem dysfunction or injury. The respiratory patterns are defined in Table 24-3.

Evaluation of respiratory pattern must also include evaluation of the effectiveness of gas exchange in maintaining adequate oxygen and carbon dioxide levels. Hypoventilation is not uncommon in the patient with an altered level of consciousness. Alterations in oxygenation or carbon dioxide levels can result in further neurological dysfunction. Intracranial pressure (ICP) will increase with hypoxemia or hypercapnia.

Finally, assessment of the respiratory function in a patient with neurological deficit must also include assessment of airway maintenance and secretion control. Cough, gag, and swallow reflexes responsible for protection of the airway may be absent or diminished.

There are also several respiratory patterns that have been noted as occurring with metabolic disorders, such as Kussmaul respirations. These respiratory patterns are initiated in the cerebral cortex in response to metabolic alterations and are a compensatory mechanism. Respiratory patterns of metabolic disorders are not identified in the same terms as the level of dysfunction of a structural injury.

Vital Signs

The final portion of the neurological examination is the evaluation of vital signs. As a result of the brain and brainstem influences on cardiac, respiratory, and body temperature functions, changes in vital signs can be an indicator of deterioration in neurological status.

Cardiac. The brain's tremendous metabolic demand requires an adequate supply of blood to continually perfuse the brain. Evaluation of the cardiovascular system identifies inappropriate supply for the known cerebral demand.

Decreased cardiac output. For whatever the reason (vasodilitation, bradycardia, tachycardia, hypovolemia, or inadequate pump), decreased cardiac output will lead to decreased perfusion of cerebral tissue, hypoxia, and neurological injury. In the presence of increased ICP, decreased cardiac output is even more detrimental because low blood pressure must overcome the additional resistance of intracranial pressure to provide blood to the brain.

Hypertension. A common manifestation of the intracranial injury is systemic hypertension. Cerbral autoregulation, responsible for the control of cerebral blood flow, is frequently lost with any type of intracranial injury. After cerebral injury, the body is often in a hyperdynamic state (increased heart rate, blood pressure, and cardiac output) as part of a compensatory response. With the loss of autoregulation, as blood pressure increases, cerebral blood flow increases, cerebral blood volume increases, and therefore intracranial pressure increases. Control of systemic hypertension is necessary to stop this cycle.

Bradycardia. The medulla and the vagus nerve provide parasympathetic control to the heart. When stimulated, this lower brainstem system produces bradycardia. Increasing intracranial pressure frequently causes bradycardia. Abrupt intracranial pressure changes can also produce dysrhythmias, such as premature ventricular contractions (PVC), atrioventricular (A-V) block, or ventricular fibrillation.

Cushing's triad is a set of three signs/symptoms (bradycardia, systolic hypertension, and bradypnea) that are related to pressure on the medullary area of the brainstem. These signs often occur in response to intracranial hypertension or a herniation syndrome.

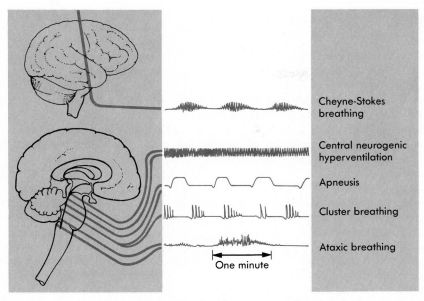

Fig. 24-7 Abnormal respiratory patterns with corresponding level of central nervous system activity.

Table 24-3 Respiratory patterns

Pattern of respiration	Description of pattern	Significance
Cheyne-Stokes	Rhythmic crescendo and decrescendo of rate and depth of respiration, includes brief periods of apnea	Usually seen with bilateral deep cerebral lesions or some cerebellar lesions
Central neurogenic hyperventilation	Very deep, very rapid respirations with no apneic periods	Usually seen with lesions of the midbrain and upper pons
Apneustic	Prolonged inspiratory and/or expiratory pause of 2-3 seconds	Usually seen in lesions of the mid to lower pons
Cluster breathing	Clusters of irregular, gasping respirations separated by long periods of apnea	Usually seen in lesions of the lower pons or upper medulla
Ataxic respirations	Irregular, random pattern of deep and shallow respirations with irregular apneic periods	Usually seen in lesions of the medulla

The appearance of Cushing's triad is a *late* finding that may be absent in neurological deterioration. Attention should be paid to alteration in each component of the triad and intervention initiated accordingly.

Neurological Changes Associated with Intracranial Hypertension

Assessment of the patient for signs of increasing intracranial pressure is an important function of the critical care nurse. Increasing ICP can be identified by changes in level of consciousness, pupillary reaction, motor response, vital signs, and respiratory patterns.

Level of consciousness. As ICP increases, the level of consciousness deteriorates. Increased restlessness and confusion, agitation, or decreased responsiveness could all be indicators of deterioration in neurological status. For the most part, level of consiousness is the first sign of deterioration in a conscious patient. Subtle changes that are identified and acted upon may prevent the serious consequences associated with neurological decline.

Pupillary reaction. Any changes in pupillary size, shape, or reactivity are ominous signs. In the unconscious patient, pupils are the most sensitive indication that deterioration is in progress.

Motor response Deterioration in motor strength or the appearance of lateralizing signs may indicate increasing ICP. Even subtle changes in motor response can be highly predictive of neurological deterioration.

Vital signs. As described, vital signs play a variable role in the evaluation of deteriorating neurological status. Increasing systolic blood pressure and/or development of bradycardia should signal the evaluator to further assess for potential deterioration in function.

Respiratory patterns. Change in respiratory patterns can be a sensitive indicator of decreasing levels of function. The assessment of this parameter is usually lost, because most patients with critical neurological injury are intubated and ventilaled to prevent the serious neurological damage caused by hypoxia and hypercapnia.

RAPID NEUROLOGICAL ASSESSMENT
The Conscious Patient

An adequate neurological assessment should focus on covering all major areas of neurological control. Any abnormalities identified can then be further evaluated and investigated. A neurological assessment should be organized, thorough, and simple so that it can be accurately and easily performed at each assessment point. The following is an example of a rapid neurological assessment that can be performed in the critical care unit on a conscious patient with known or potential neurological deficit.

1. Level of consciousness—Address the patient and ask a variety of orientation questions. Avoid the obvious, overused questions about name, date, and place and focus on questions about recent and past events from the patient's experiences, such as spouse's name, home address, what was eaten at the previous meal. Be sure that as examiner you are aware of the correct answers to all questions asked.
2. Observation of facial movements—During the level of consciousness assessment, observe the patient's facial movements for symmetry. Listen to speech patterns for evidence of slurred speech.
3. Perform pupil check and assess extraocular eye movements.
4. Motor assessment—Instruct patient to close eyes and to extend arms with palms upturned. Check for evidence of arm drift. This is a relatively sensitive evaluation of upper extremity weakness. Check hand grasp strength by placing two fingers in the palm of each of the patient's hands and instructing him or her to squeeze. (This hand grasp assessment is done to test upper extremity strength not the patient's ability to follow simple commands.) Both hand grasps should be evaluated simultaneously for comparison of strength. Place hand on patient's thigh and instruct him or her to raise the leg straight up against resistance. Assess both lower extremities for movement and strength. Ask the patient to plantar flex (step on the gas) and dorsiflex (pull his or her toes toward his or her nose) against resistance.
5. Sensory—With a finger, stroke the patient bilaterally on the face, upper arm, hand, leg, and foot. Ask the patient to identify what is touched and whether there is any difference in sensation between the two sides.
6. Check vital signs—Note any increases in blood pressure, decreases in heart rate, or change in respiratory patterns.
7. Finally, ask the patient if he or she feels any differently than at the last assessment.

This assessment, which usually takes less than 4 minutes, is meant to be a starting point. If any neurological deficit is identified that is new or different from that of the last assessment, attention must be focused in more detail on that abnormality.

The Unconscious Patient

In assessment of the unconscious patient, initial efforts are directed at achieving maximal arousal of the patient. Calling the patient's name, patting him or her on the chest, or shaking his or her shoulder accomplishes this task. Once the patient has been stimulated, the examiner can proceed with the neurological assessment.

1. Level of consciousness—Perform the Glasgow Coma Scale assessment.
2. Pupillary assessment—Perform pupillary assessment with special attention focused on size, reactivity, and shape of pupil in comparison to the opposite eye.
3. Motor examination—Assess each extremity individually by means of a predetermined coding score of motor movement.
4. Respiratory pattern—If the patient is not being mechanically ventilated, observe respiratory patterns for evidence of deteriorating level of function.
5. Vital signs—Observation of vital signs should include comparison of preassessment vital signs to postassessment vital signs. Special attention should be paid to arterial blood prerssure and ICP if these parameters are being monitored.

As in the assessment of the conscious patient, if any abnormalities or changes from previous assessment are noted, further investigation must occur. This assessment takes 3 to 4 minutes.

BRAIN DEATH AND PERSISTENT VEGETATIVE STATE

The subjects of brain death and patients in a persistent vegetative state (coma) remain controversial. Brief review of some of the issues surrounding both of these topics will be discussed.

Brain Death

The issue of brain death first became a consideration in the early 1960s when technological advancements permitted the maintenance of respirations, blood pressure, and heart rate through mechanical and pharmaceutical means. As skill in using these new technologies progressed, it became apparent that irreversible loss of brain function could occur, but death, as defined by cessation of heart beat and respirations, did not occur. Advances in the critical care environment paralleled the technological advances so that "life" could be supported almost indefinitely provided the proper mechanical support was accompanied by physical care.

At the same time, advances in organ transplantation techniques were occurring. The lack of necrosis and autolysis in the organs (except for the brain) of artificially maintained comatose patients made them ideal donor subjects.[10]

As awareness of the legal, medical, and ethical dilemmas surrounding the issue of brain death grew, it became apparent that a redefining of the term "death" was required. In the process of this definition, the term "brain death" evolved. Brain death is defined as an irreversible loss of all brain function. In 1968, the Harvard Medical School defined the first set of clinical criteria to aid in the diagnosis of brain death.[1] These critera included unresponsive coma, apnea, absent brainstem reflexes, absent spinal reflexes, two isoelectric electroencephalograms 24 hours apart, absence of drug intoxication, and absence of hypothermia. In the years following 1968, the Harvard Criteria as well as other proposed groups of critera were developed and researched in the clinical setting. Although no one set of criteria exists for all patients, an array of acceptable methods for establishing brain death have been described.

The legal issue involves the recognition of cessation of brain function as an equal definition with the cessation of cardiopulmonary function in the determination of death. California and Alaska were two states that first adapted the definition of death to include brain death. Since then, virtually all states developed some statutory change in law to recognize the existence of brain death.

In 1979, the American Medical Association House of Delegates passed a bill concerning the definition of brain death.

An individual who has sustained either (a) irreversible cessation of circulatory and respiratory functions, or (b) irreversible cessation of all functions of the entire brain, should be considered dead. A determination of death shall be made in accordance with accepted medical standards.[10]

In 1980, the Uniform Determination of Death Act, identical to the AMA bill, was passed by the National Conference of Commissioners of Uniform State Laws. Even those states that have not changed statutes to recognize the existence of brain death accept the existence of the phenomena.

The actual criteria used in any health care setting is usually developed by an agency-based ethics committee. Review of the criteria at the institution in which the critical care nurse is employed allows a better understanding of the process and procedures of the institution.[6]

Persistent Vegetative State

From the advancing technology of modern medicine came another entity described as persistent vegetative state. This comatose condition does not result in death if mechanical support is withdrawn but also does not include any recovery of consciousness. In brain death, all functions of the brain including the brainstem have ceased. In persistent vegetative state the higher cortical functions of the cerebral hemisphere have been irreversibly damaged, but the lower functions of the brainstem remain intact.[5] With brainstem function comes spontaneous respirations, as well as cardiovascular control. Also seen are some of the brainstem signs such as involuntary chewing, lip-smacking, and roving eye movements.

The issue of persistent vegetative state first gained national attention in the early 1970s with the case of Karen Ann Quinlan. Efforts by the parents to get ventilatory support removed from their irreversibly brain damaged child became a highly publicized legal case. When legal permission was finally obtained to remove ventilatory support, Karen Quinlan continued to survive in a persistent vegetative state for several years.

The emotional and financial strain to both family and society for a patient in a persistent vegetative state is enormous. Although the laws are now generally supportive of brain death, the issue of withdrawing support from a patient in a persistent vegetative state or even withholding additional support, is still controversial. Several courts have ruled that it is lawful to reduce care for patients in persistent vegetative state but have described differing standards and procedures for implementing such decisions.[3]

It is generally an easier task to decide not to treat any future infections, seizures, or clinical signs of deterioration in a patient with persistent vegetative state than it is to withdraw care. Questions about withdrawal of support such as nourishment or fluids have been widely discussed. In a landmark decision, the Supreme Judicial Court of Massachusetts ruled that a feeding tube could be removed from a patient in a persistent vegetative state if this was consistent with his previously expressed wishes.[9] The court did not compel the hospital to terminate treatment but permitted any hospital to comply with the patient's wishes.[4] This in effect strengthened the legal base of such documents as living wills. Living wills or other similar documents allow for the previously expressed wishes of the patient not to be maintained on life support if there is no reasonable expectation for recovery to be honored.

For the nurse caring for patients in a persistent vegetative state, the situation is often physically and emotionally draining. These patients are totally dependent on continuous, labor-intensive care for maintenance of normal bodily function. Nutrition is usually provided by tube feeding or occasionally by hyperalimentation. Pulmonary care includes frequent suctioning, chest physiotherapy, and repositioning. Skin care involves frequent turning, positioning, and bathing to reduce the incidence of decubitus ulcers. At the same time the nurse expends a large amount of emotional energy dealing with family and friends of the patient.

When confronted with the challenge of caring for a patient in a persistent vegetative state, the nurse should use all resources available for support. Patient care conferences, physician-nurse discussions, and family meetings with physician, nurse, and social services should be a standard of care. It is important that all those surrounding the patient have a realistic understanding of the prognosis of the patient. If family, nursing staff, and physician are all aware of the severity of the illness and the limited potential for recovery, at least some of the stress and anxiety may be decreased.

REFERENCES

1. Ad Hoc Committee of the Harvard Medical School to Examine the Definition of Brain Death: A definiton of irreversible coma, JAMA 205:337, 1968.
2. Bates B: A guide to physical exam, ed 2, Philadelphia, 1984, JB Lippincott Co.
3. Beresford HR: Severe neurologic impairment: legal aspects of decision to reduce care, Ann Neurol 15(5):409, 1984.
4. Brophy vs New England Sinai Hospital, Inc., J Am Geriatr Soc 35(7):669, 1987.
5. Cranford R: The persistent vegetative state: the medical reality (getting the facts straight), Hastings Cent Rep 18:27, 1988.
6. Davis KM and others: Brain death: nursing roles and responsibilities, J Neurosci Nurs 19(1):36, 1987.
7. Plum F and Posner J: The diagnosis of stupor and coma, ed 3, Philadelphia, 1980, FA Davis Co.
8. Teasdale G and Jennett W: Assessment of coma and impaired consciousness: a practical scale, Lancet 2:81, 1974.
9. Steinbrook R: Artificial feeding—solid ground not a slippery slope, N Engl J Med 318(5):286, 1988.
10. Ventura MG and Masser PG: Defining death: developments in recent law. In Rogers MC and Traystman RJ, editors: Critical Care Clinics: symposium on Neurologic Intensive Care, vol 1, no. 2, Philadelphia, 1985, WB Saunders Co.
11. Wilson SF and others: Determining interater reliability of nurses' assessment of pupillary size and reaction, J Neurosci Nurs 20(3):189, 1988.

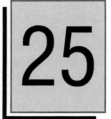

25

Neurological Diagnostic Procedures

CHAPTER OBJECTIVES

- *Discuss the role of the nurse in diagnostic testing.*
- *State the complications associated with cerebral angiography.*
- *Describe the differences in cerebral angiography and digital subtraction angiography.*
- *State the differences in the two types of dye used in myelography.*
- *Explain the differences in electroencephalography and evoked potentials.*
- *Discuss the patient positioning required for lumbar puncture.*

There is a wide array of diagnostic tests available to assist the clinician in identification of the cause of neurological dysfunction. Improved technology has raised the sophistication of assessment, especially in the area of radiographical procedures and electrophysiology studies. Neurodiagnostic testing is performed as an adjunct to a thorough neurological examination. When clinical findings are identified on examination, the clinician begins the process of diagnosing the problem. The type of diagnostic testing performed on the patient should provide the examiner the ability to further refine and locate the cause of the abnormality identified during the neurological assessment. Management of the patient is based on clinical symptoms, pathological conditions, and the results of the diagnostic tests.

The role of the nurse in neurological diagnostic testing is varied, but three functions are always present: (1) patient/family education, (2) physical preparation, and (3) awareness of potential complications.

It is essential that the patient be aware of the reason for a procedure, the procedural process, and any preprocedure preparation. There should also be a discussion of the sensations and the level of discomfort involved. Once the physician has discussed the risks of the procedure with the patient, the nurse is available to listen to the patient's fears and attempt to lessen anxiety.

The nurse assists in the physical preparation by providing medications, scrubs, or dye solutions. During the procedure, the nurse might also assist in maintaining patient position or compliance with procedure.

Besides being able to discuss concerns about risk factors with the patient, the nurse assesses the patient for development of any complications associated with the procedure. Proper observation and intervention, if necessary, is a nursing responsibility.

The goal of this chapter is not to attempt to review all diagnostic studies available but to focus on the tests frequently performed on the critically ill patient. Discussion of each test will include a definition and purpose of the test, a review of the procedure, and the patient care needs both before and after the procedure.

RADIOLOGICAL PROCEDURES
Skull and Spine Films

The purpose of radiographs of the skull or spine are to identify fractures, anomalies, or possibly tumors. The role of skull radiographs in trauma has diminished with the advent of computerized axial tomography (CT scan). If the patient is to be sent for CT scan during the initial assessment process, a skull radiograph may not be necessary.

The procedure for obtaining skull and spine radiographs is a relatively painless process. Proper patient positioning is essential, especially for spine radiographs. In searching for spine fractures it is frequently difficult to obtain a clear view of C1 to C2 and C6 to C7. C1 to C2 is obtained by taking the x-ray through the open mouth of the patient (Water's view). If the patient is intubated this is usually impossible. Therefore spinal precautions, that is, cervical collar and strict maintenance of head alignment, must be maintained until the patient's conditon allows for open mouth views. To obtain C6 to C7 views it is often necessary that the nurse or technician pull down firmly on the patient's arms while the film is being taken to allow visualization.

Nursing care involves positioning of the patient to obtain adequate films. Any situation in which traumatic injury, especially head injury, is the cause of the patient's admission to the critical care unit, the cervical spine should be treated as unstable until proved otherwise.

Computerized Axial Tomography

Computerized axial tomography (CT scan) provides the clinician with a mathematically reconstructed view of multiple sections of the head and body. This is accomplished by passage of intersecting x-ray beams through the examined area and measurement of the density of substances through which the x-ray beam passes. The more dense the substance the x-ray beam passes through, the whiter it will appear on the finished film. The less dense a substance, the blacker it will appear. Therefore in a normal CT scan of the head, bone appears white, blood appears off-white, brain tissue appears shaded gray, CSF appears off-black, and air appears black (Fig. 25-1).

The purpose of the CT scan is to obtain rapid, noninvasive visualization of structures. CT scan is indicated in the diagnostic work-up of severe headache, head trauma with associated loss of consciousness, seizures, hydrocephalus, suspicion of space-occupying lesions, hemorrhage, or vascular lesions and edema. There are two types of CT scans—contrast and noncontrast scans. The noncontrast scan is noninvasive, requires no premedication of the patient, and is good for analysis and location of normal brain structures. Noncontrast CT scans of the head are appropriate in trauma patients in whom the goal is to view the intracranial area for evidence of intracranial hemorrhage, cerebral edema, or shift of structures. Noncontrast CT scan is also appropriate in the diagnosis of hydrocephalus.[2,4]

Contrast CT scan involves the use of an intravenously injected contrast medium. The use of contrast enhances the vascular areas and allows for detection of vascular lesions or the further definition of lesions noted on a noncontrast scan.

Nursing care of the patient receiving a CT scan can be divided into two areas of focus: observation of patient tolerance of procedure and observation of patient reaction to the dye in contrast scanning. Because of the associated activity and positioning, transporting and scanning of a crit-

ically ill patient with known or suspected intracranial hypertension can cause a deterioration in the patient's condition. The nurse must always remain with the patient during CT scan and closely observe the neurological status, vital signs, and intracranial pressure, if monitored.

If the patient is to receive a contrast CT scan, questions about possible sensitivity to iodine-based dye should be ascertained beforehand if at all possible. During the infusion of the dye and for 10 to 30 minutes after, the patient should be closely observed for anaphylactic reaction. Less than 1% per year of all patients receiving contrast CT scans have severe anaphylactic reactions, shock, or cardiac arrest.

Magnetic Resonance Imaging

Magnetic resonance imaging (MRI) is a relatively new procedure. The patient is placed in a large magnetic field. The nuclei of the atoms of the body are stimulated and momentarily absorb some of the energy generated by the magnetic field. Different tissue densities absorb and subsequently release differing amounts of energy. The release of the energy (resonance frequency) is then measured and plotted (Fig. 25-2).[1]

In MRI small tumors that have tissue densities different from those of the surrounding cells can be identified before they would be visible by any other radiographic test. MRI can also identity small hemorrhages deep in the brain that are invisible on CT scan. Finally, MRI is able to identify areas of cerebral infarct within a few hours of the incident, as well as small areas of plaque in patients with multiple sclerosis.

Nursing care of these patients involves patient teaching and preparation. The procedure is lengthy and requires the

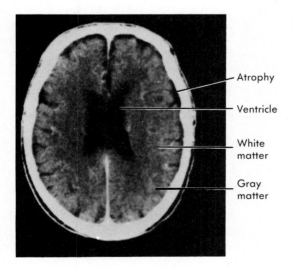

Fig. 25-1 CT scan image. (From Ballinger PW: Merrill's atlas of radiographic positions and radiologic procedures, ed 5, St. Louis, 1982, The CV Mosby Co.)

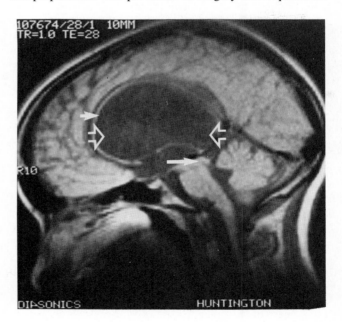

Fig. 25-2 Magnetic resonance image of the brain. Sagittal section demonstrating marked enlargement of the lateral ventricle *(open arrow)* with stretching of the corpus callosum *(arrowhead)* as a result of aqueductal stenosis *(arrow)* (SE 1000/28). (From Stark D and Bradley WG: Magnetic resonance imaging, ed 1, St. Louis, 1988, The CV Mosby Co.)

patient to lie motionless. The neurologically impaired patient may not be able to comprehend these instructions, and sedation will be required. Removal of all metal from the patient's body and clothing is essential, as the basis of MRI is a magnetic field. In the past it was believed that any metal material such as dental filling, prostheses, or internal clips or staples, would prevent the scanning of the patient. Further study and changes in the type of metals used for many procedures has made the test safer. Any questions about specific devices or metals should be directed to the neuroradiologist before testing. The test is considered relatively safe and noninvasive, but the procedure is still too new to have all risks identified.

Cerebral Angiogram

Cerebral angiogram[4] involves the injection of radiopaque contrast medium into the intracranial or extracranial vasculature. With the use of serial radiological filming, angiography traces the flow of blood from the arterial circulation through the capillary bed to the venous circulation. Cerebral angiography allows visualization of the lumen of vessels to provide information about patency, size (narrowing or dilation), any irregularities, or occlusion. Angiography is necessary in the diagnosis of cerebral aneurysm, arteriovenous malformation, carotid artery disease, and some vascular tumors. Information obtained from angiography guides the surgeon in choosing the operative approach or provides information on which to make medical management decisions other than surgery.

The procedure involves placement of a catheter in the femoral artery and threading it up the aorta and into the origin of the cerebral circulation. Other injection sites include a direct carotid or vertebral artery puncture or placement of a catheter in the brachial, axillary, or subclavian artery. Several views of vessels can be studied on angiogram. A four-vessel angiogram involves injections into the right and left internal carotid arteries and the right and left vertebral arteries. If the area of suspected disease has already been identified, a single vessel study may be all that is required. This is particularly true when angiography is used as a follow-up in the evaluation of intracranial vascular surgery. Also, if carotid artery disease is a working diagnosis, angiogram may include views of the arch of the aorta, plus the external and internal carotid arteries.

Once the catheter is appropriately placed, the contrast medium is injected. Following this, a rapid succession of radiographs are taken as the contrast medium progresses through the cerebral circulation. Separate contrast medium injections occur for each vessel being studied.

Nursing care associated with this invasive procedure is comprehensive. In patient preparation, patient instruction and education are essential. The patient's complete understanding of the role this procedure plays in diagnosis plus the process of the procedure relieves anxiety about the unknown and also ensures cooperation in what is frequently an uncomfortable procedure. Discomfort in the procedure involves lying still on a cold, hard table and possible pain during preparation and insertion of the groin catheter. A hot, burning sensation is often experienced when the contrast medium is injected. This is especially true if the contrast is injected into the external carotid system. Preparation of patients for this burning sensation assures them that it is not an abnormal occurrence. Finally, the patient must be aware of the postprocedure assessment that will be performed.

Before and after the procedure the patient must be well hydrated to assist the kidneys in clearing the heavy dye load. Inadequate hydration may lead to an acute nephrotic tubular necrosis (ATN) and renal shutdown. If the patient is unable to tolerate oral fluids, an intravenous line should be placed before the procedure is begun.

Complications associated with a cerebral angiogram include (1) cerebral embolus caused by the catheter dislodging a segment of atherosclerotic plaque in the vessel, (2) hemorrhage or clot formation at the insertion site, (3) vasospasm of a vessel caused by the irritation of catheter placement, (4) thrombosis of the extremity distal to the injection site, or (5) allergic reaction to the contrast medium.

Post procedure assessment involves vital sign measurement every 15 minutes, neurological evaluation, observation of the injection site, and assessment of neurovascular integrity distal to the injection site. Any abnormalities noted must be immediately reported.

Digital Subtraction Angiography

Digital subtraction angiography[4] is a newer method of visualizing the arteriovenous circulation of the intracranial space. Radiographic dye is injected either into the venous or the arterial circulation, but significantly less dye is necessary for this procedure than for arterial angiography. Films taken before and after dye injection are superimposed on each other and all matching images are subtracted. This leaves only the dye enhanced cerebral vessels present for study and evaluation. Digital subtraction angiography eliminates the shadows and distortions of bone or other material that sometimes block the viewing of the cerebral vessels.

The major disadvantage of digital subtraction angiography involves the patient's ability to remain motionless during the entire procedure. Even swallowing interferes significantly with the imaging process. With venous injection of dye for the digital subtraction angiography, intracranial and extracranial vessels are enhanced. With arterial injection of dye, the same complications are possible as with cerebral angiography.

Myelography

Myelography[2] is the radiography of the spinal cord and vertebral column following injection of a contrast material into the subarachnoid space by lumbar or cisternal puncture. Myelography allows visualization of the spinal canal, the subarachnoid space around the spinal cord, and the spinal nerve roots through the use of radiograph. Indications for myelography include identification of spinal canal blockage caused by herniated intervertebral discs, spinal cord tumors, bony fragments or growths, or congenital anomalies (Fig. 25-3).

The procedure involves a lumbar or cisternal puncture followed by an injection of contrast medium. Done under fluoroscopy, the infusion of the dye is observed and radiographic films are taken. Two basic types of contrast medium

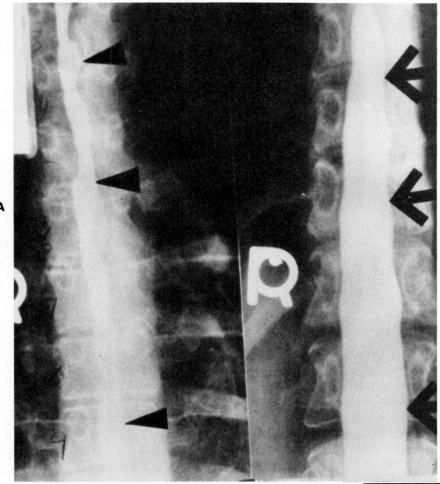

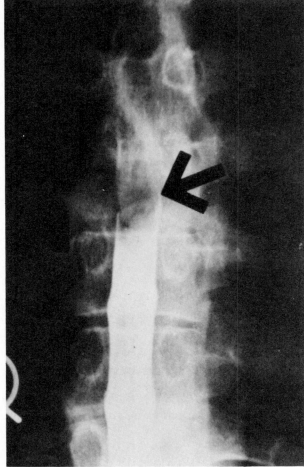

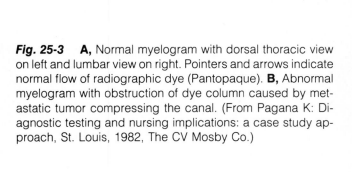

Fig. 25-3 **A,** Normal myelogram with dorsal thoracic view on left and lumbar view on right. Pointers and arrows indicate normal flow of radiographic dye (Pantopaque). **B,** Abnormal myelogram with obstruction of dye column caused by metastatic tumor compressing the canal. (From Pagana K: Diagnostic testing and nursing implications: a case study approach, St. Louis, 1982, The CV Mosby Co.)

are used—an oil-based preparation (Pantopaque) or a water-based preparation (metrizamide). Use of an oil-based preparation, which is heavier than the cerebrospinal fluid (CSF), allows the radiologist to place the patient in a variety of positions while observing the flow of dye through the spinal subarachnoid space. Disadvantages of the oil-based preparation include the lack of absorption of the dye from the subarachnoid space. Pantopaque must be removed at the end of the procedure. Use of an oil-based preparation is associated with a higher incidence of severe postprocedure headache as a result of loss of cerebrospinal fluid. Postprocedure care of a patient with a Pantopaque myelogram involves keeping the patient flat in bed for 4 to 6 hours to prevent headache and CSF leak from the puncture site.

Use of the water-based preparation, which is lighter than CSF, allows for better visualization of nerve roots and projections off the spinal cord. Metrizamide is absorbed by the arachnoid system and therefore does not require removal after the procedure. Disadvantages to use of a water-based preparation include rapid dissolution of the dye into the subarachnoid space. The patient cannot be rolled into different positions to observe dye flow. Because of the potential toxicity of water-based preparations to the cerebral tissue, care must be taken to ensure that a large dye load does not reach the surface of the brain. This is accomplished by keeping the patient's head elevated 30 to 45 degrees after the procedure. Toxicity is evidenced by grand mal seizures. Patients receiving a metrizamide myelogram should be kept well hydrated to assist in clearing of the dye through the urine. Use of phenothiazines is to be avoided after metrizamide myelography because of the increase in symptoms of toxicity.

Possible risks involved with myelography include injection of the dye outside of the subarachnoid space, arachnoiditis as a result of irritation of the arachnoid membranes from a foreign material, allergic reactions to the dye that may cause confusion, disorientation or an anaphylactic reaction, headache, or grand mal seizure.[3]

CEREBRAL BLOOD FLOW STUDIES

The goal of cerebral blood flow studies[4] is to measure the amount of blood flow overall or in regions of the brain to detect areas of increased or decreased cerebral circulation. Normal cerebral blood flow values average 50 to 55 ml of flow per 100 g of cerebral tissue per minute. Studies to determine the actual amount of cerebral blood flow in the injured brain would be a valuable addition to the planning of interventions. Some techniques are available, but as yet none of the procedures have achieved wide acceptance in clinical practice.

Uses of cerebral blood flow studies include evaluation of cerebral vasospasm after subarachnoid hemorrhage, evaluation of cerebral blood flow during operative procedures that require extreme hypotension such as aneurysm clipping, and evaluation of the changes in cerebral blood flow after cerebral vascular surgery such as carotid endarterectomy, cerebral revascularization (superficial temporal artery–middle cerebral artery bypass), or arteriovenous malformation excision.

Methods of determining cerebral blood flow range from intracarotid injection of radioisotopes to intravenous injection to inhalation of isotopes or nitrous oxide. The most clinically acceptable method of cerebral blood flow analysis involves inhalation of xenon-133 for 3 to 5 minutes. Clearance of this isotope from brain tissue is then monitored from 16 to 32 probes that are placed externally around the head. Information from the probes is passed to a computer that calculates regional cerebral blood flow. This is the least invasive of all techniques. The difficulty with this method is that all body tissues take up xenon and then clear it, including the skin and muscles of the scalp under detectors. Although mathematical calculations are factored in, cerebral blood flow results are an estimated value at best. Further research and development are necessary to make this valuable diagnostic tool clinically acceptable and accurate.

ELECTROPHYSIOLOGY STUDIES

There are two basic electrophysiological studies used in the critical care setting. Both of these studies can be done intermittently to evaluate symptoms or review progress, or they can be performed continuously to assist the clinicians in ongoing assessment of neurological function.

Electroencephalography

Electroencephalography (EEG)[1,5] is the recording of electrical impulses, commonly called brain waves, generated by the brain. This test has been in existence for many years and is well known to the general public. It is important for the nurse caring for a patient with a neurological dysfunction to be aware of the appropriate indications for use of this testing procedure. The purpose of the EEG is to detect and localize abnormal electrical activity. This abnormal activity can be defined as slowing, which occurs in areas of injury or infarct, or spikes and waves seen in irritated tissue. Indications for the use of an EEG include seizure focus identification, infarct, metabolic disorders, confirmation of brain death (electrocerebral silence), and some head injuries.

Electrodes are placed noninvasively on the head and the electrical impulses detected are transferred to a central recording device that records the information in wave form. There are five types of waves or rhythms that may be present.

Alpha	8 to 13 cycles/second	Normal, relaxed state with eyes, closed, seen often in occipital leads
Theta	4 to 7 cycles/second	Less common in adults than in children, characteristic of coma in brain injury
Beta	12 to 40 cycles/second	Fast waves indicating mental or physical activity
Sleep spindles	12 to 14 cycles/second	Seen in stage 2 sleep, not REM
Spike and wave	Variable	Seen in irritable brain tissue such as seizure

For further discussion on EEG, see Chapter 6, "Sleep Physiology and Assessment."

In preparing the patient for an EEG, teaching should stress the noninvasive aspects of this procedure. The awake patient may be asked to perform certain simple tasks during the procedure, such as blinking, closing the eye, or swallowing. Occasionally, testing needs to be performed during sleep or after a period of sleep deprivation.

Continuous monitoring of the EEG is becoming more common in the critical care environment. The goal of continuous EEG monitoring is to identify changes in electrical activity that could indicate inadequate vascular supply to an area or provide evidence of subclinical seizures. Subclinical seizures are evidenced by sharp spike and wave electrical activity that is not in evidence by visual observation of the patient. Subclinical seizures increase cerebral metabolic rate in response to the greatly increased cellular activity. This increased metabolic rate requires increasing supply of oxygen and nutrients to an already compromised vascular supply system. Detection and treatment of subclinical seizures may prevent secondary brain injury.

Evoked Potentials

Evoked potentials[1,2] involve the recording of electrical impulses generated by a sensory stimulus as it travels through the brainstem and into the cerebral cortex. Measuring evoked potentials is a sophisticated way of observing the status of sensory pathways as they enter the central nervous system, travel through the brainstem, and reach the cerebral cortex. Evoked potentials can also be used during therapeutically induced comas, such as barbiturate coma, since these sensory pathways are unaffected by the depressive activity of such drugs. Another use of evoked potentials is in the determination of the existence of brainstem or spinal cord injury in the traumatically injured patient.

There are three types of evoked potential tests: (1) visual evoked responses (VER), (2) brainstem auditory evoked responses (BAER), and (3) somatosensory evoked responses (SSER). VER involves monitoring of the visual pathways through the brainstem and cortex in response to viewing a shifting geometric pattern on a screen or placing a mask over the eye that sends a flashing light stimulus. BAER involves monitoring the auditory pathway through the brainstem and cortex in response to a rhythmic clicking sound sent through earphones placed over the patients ears. SSER involves monitoring of sensory pathways from the extremities ascending the spinal cord through the brainstem and into the cortex. This is done by administering a small electrical shock to a nerve root in the periphery such as the ulnar or radial nerve.

Preparation of awake patients involves appropriate teaching so that they cooperate with the instructions for the procedure. No pain or discomfort is involved in the administration of these tests, except for the irritation of the small electrical shock used for SSER.

LUMBAR PUNCTURE

The main purpose of lumbar puncture (LP) is to enter the subarachnoid space to obtain diagnostic information or provide therapeutic intervention. Diagnostic information comes from samples of cerebrospinal fluid evaluated for the presence of subarachnoid blood, infection, or laboratory analysis. Pressure readings are also obtained for use diagnostically. Therapeutic modalities of an LP include removal of bloody or purulent CSF that the arachnoid villi are unable

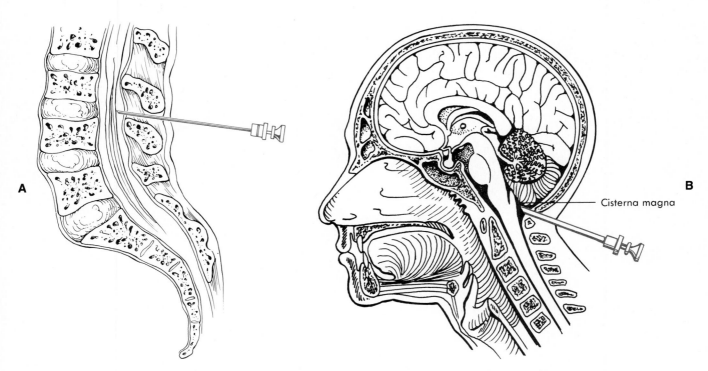

A

B

Cisterna magna

Fig. 25-4 **A,** Lumbar puncture. **B,** Cisternal puncture. (From Long BC and Phipps WJ: Medical-surgical nursing: a nursing process approach, ed 2, St. Louis, 1989, The CV Mosby Co.)

to clear, injection of medications into the subarachnoid space to bypass the blood-brain barrier (antibiotics or analgesics), or the introduction of spinal anesthesia.

An LP involves the introduction of an 18 to 22 gauge hollow needle into the subarachnoid space at L4 to L5 below the end of the spinal cord that is usually at L1 to L2. The patient can be placed either in the lateral recumbent position with the knees and head tightly tucked or in the sitting position leaning over a bedside table or some other support (Fig. 25-4).

Risks associated with a lumbar puncture include possible brainstem herniation if intracranial pressure is elevated or respiratory arrest associated with neurological deterioration. During the procedure the nurse must monitor the patient's neurological and respiratory status. Also, if the patient is not fully alert and cooperative, the nurse may need to assist the patient in maintaining the position necessary for performance of the LP.[5]

Cisternal puncture which is the introduction of a needle into the cisterna magna at the C1 to C2 level is another method for obtaining access to the subarachnoid space. Risks of cisternal puncture are slightly higher than those associated with an LP but necessary if there is inability to enter the lumbar space because of scar tissue or some other physical barrier or if there is a total blockage of the CSF pathway somewhere along the spinal column.

REFERENCES

1. Borel C and Hanley D: Neurologic intensive care unit monitoring. In vol 1, Symposium on neurologic intensive care, Rogers MC and Traystman RJ, editors: Philadelphia 1985, WB Saunders Co.
2. Hickey JV: The clinical practice of neurologic and neurosurgical nursing, ed 2 Philadelphia, 1986, JB Lippincott Co.
3. Jones AG: Side effects following metrizamide myelography and lumbar laminectomy, Neurosci Nurs 19(2):90, 1987.
4. Ricci MM: Core curriculum for neuroscience nursing, Chicago, 1984, American Association of Neuroscience Nurses.
5. Rudy EB: Advance neurological and neurosurgical nursing, St Louis, 1984, The CV Mosby Co.

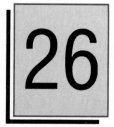

CHAPTER

26

Neurological Disorders

CHAPTER OBJECTIVES

- *Discuss the mechanisms of injury for head trauma and spinal cord trauma.*
- *Define the treatment dilemmas of aneurysm rupture associated with vasospasm and rebleeding.*
- *Define the concept of "malignant tumors" in the intracranial space.*
- *Describe the pathophysiology of epidural, subdural, and intracerebral hematomas.*
- *State the difference between complete and incomplete injury in spinal cord trauma.*
- *Discuss the pathophysiology of Guillain-Barré syndrome.*

An understanding of the pathology of a disease, the areas of assessment on which to focus, and the usual medical management allow the critical care nurse to more accurately anticipate and plan nursing interventions. Although there is a wide array of neurological disorders, only a few routinely require care in the critical care environment. This chapter presents a review of cerebral trauma, central nervous system tumors, cerebral vascular disease, spinal cord injury, and Guillan-Barré syndrome.

CEREBRAL TRAUMA

Cerebral trauma is a growing problem as society develops technology that allows for increasing speed in transportation, increasing mobility, and increasing sophistication in weaponry. Nothing but prevention can reduce the incidence of cerebral trauma.

Incidence

It is estimated that one in 12 deaths in the United States, greater than 160,000 deaths per year, results from some injury or trauma.[5] The overall incidence of injury is 200 per 100,000 population per year. Of these injury-related deaths, it is estimated that 44% are deaths related to brain injury.[22] Therefore the annual death rate from overall injury is 71

per 100,000 population per year, and the incidence of death from brain injury is 30 per 100,000 population per year.[25] Trauma is the fourth leading cause of death in the United States and is the leading cause of death in persons aged 1 to 44 years.[28]

Variations in the definitions of brain (or head) injuries make an evaluation of the incidence of brain injury difficult. In some classifications, head injury includes skull fractures and scalp lacerations without concurrent brain injury. Based on the 1984 United States population of 235 million, there are approximately 470,000 cases of brain injury annually. Of the patients sustaining head trauma, 80% to 90% have mild to moderate trauma, while only 10% have severe life-threatening injuries.

The incidence of brain injury is highest among young people. Studies show a peak incidence between the ages of 15 to 24. Secondary peaks occur in infancy and childhood as well as in the elderly. The male to female ratio is greater than 2:1, with the greatest difference in ratio occurring in the 15 to 24-year-old age group.

Cause

In descending order of occurrence, the causes of head trauma include motor vehicle accidents, falls, assault including those with firearms, sports and recreation, and other. The incidence of each of these causes varies depending on geographical location. For example, in one study of San Diego County, California, 52% of the head injuries were from motor vehicle accidents, and 15% from assault or firearms.[22] In a study of Bronx, New York, 25% of the head injuries were from motor vehicle accidents, and 30% from assault or firearms.[8]

Pathophysiology

Mechanism of injury. The pathophysiology of head trauma depends somewhat on the mechanism of injury.[24] Impact injuries, such as motor vehicle accidents, deal with acceleration-deceleration forces and rotational forces. Missile injuries result in a different type of tissue damage. The degree of injury depends on the forces involved.

Acceleration-deceleration. Acceleration and deceleration forces are always a factor to some extent in impact

543

injuries. As the skull hits or is hit by a force, the semisolid substance of the brain continues to move and the brain tissue hits the skull at the point of impact, reverses direction, and hits the other side of the skull. This can occur repeatedly until all the force or energy generated at impact is dissipated. Injury to brain tissue caused by acceleration-deceleration includes contusion, laceration, and shearing or tearing of tissue.

Rotation. Rotation of intracranial contents also occurs with impact injury and is usually associated with acceleration-deceleration mechanisms. In rotation, brain tissue rotates or turns resulting in distortion or tearing of tissue.

Missile injury. Missile or penetrating injuries cause direct damage to cerebral tissue. In the case of missile injury, further damage occurs as cerebral tissue responds to the high-energy release in the missile (bullet, shrapnel, etc.)

Pathogenesis

Review of the pathophysiology of head injury can be divided into two categories: primary injury (that which occurs on impact) and secondary injury (that which occurs as a result of insult after the original trauma.[13]

Primary injury. The primary injury is that which occurs at the time of impact. Caused by the dynamic forces of acceleration-deceleration or rotation, primary injuries include contusion, laceration, shearing injuries, or hemorrhage.

Primary injury may be considered mild with little or no neurological damage identified on computerized axial tomography (CT scan) to severe with major tissue damage. In addition to the actual tissue damage that occurs, dysfunction of some of the normal intracranial physiological mechanisms also occurs secondarily. Loss of autoregulation and increased permeability of the blood-brain barrier frequently occur. These dysfunctions may lead to hyperemia (increased blood volume) and vasodilation of cerebral vessels as well as an increase in the extracellular fluid space. As a result, the volume of the intracranial contents increases.

If the swelling is great enough to cause significantly increased pressure inside the intracranial vault, secondary injury may occur.

Secondary injury. Secondary injury results from physiological insults to an already damaged brain. Insults that cause secondary injury are hypoxia, hypercapnia, hypotension, cerebral edema, or sustained hypertension. Beyond causing injury to tissue, each of these factors also contributes to significant increases in intracranial pressure (ICP).

Hypoxia produces secondary injury through two mechanisms. Tissue ischemia occurs in the area not adequately oxygenated, and the cells of the ischemic area become edematous. Extreme vasodilation of the cerebral vasculature occurs in an attempt to supply O_2 to the cerebral tissue. This increase in blood volume increases intracranial volume and therefore intracranial pressure.

Hypercapnia is a powerful cerebral vasodilator. Most often caused by hypoventilation in an unconscious patient, hypercapnia leads to increased blood volume and increased intracranial pressure (ICP).

Significant hypotension prevents adequate perfusion of O_2 and nutrients to neural tissue. It is important to note that

hypotension is rarely associated with head injury. If a trauma patient is unconscious and hypotensive as the result of severe head injury, assessment of the chest, abdomen, and pelvis for indications of internal bleeding should be aggressive.

Cerebral edema occurs as a result of the changes in the cellular environment caused by contusion, loss of autoregulation, and increased permeability of the blood-brain barrier. Cerebral edema can be focal as it localizes around an area of contusion (just as tissue edema occurs in other parts of the body in response to injury) or diffuse as a result of hypotension or hypoxia. The extent of cerebral edema can be minimized by controlling the other aspects of secondary injury, such as oxygenation, ventilation, and blood pressure.

Hypertension is commonly seen initially in the patient with severe head injury. As a result of the loss of autoregulation, increased blood pressure results in increased intracranial blood volume and ICP. Every effort should be made to maintain a normal blood pressure to prevent the secondary injury caused by increased ICP.

The effects of increases in intracranial pressure may be varied. As pressure increases inside the enclosed vault of the skull, cerebral perfusion decreases, which leads to further compromise of the intracranial contents. The effects of increasing pressure and decreasing perfusion precipitate a downward spiral of events. (For a more extensive discussion of intracranial pressure, see Chapter 5.)

Classification of head injuries. Injuries of the brain are described by the functional changes or losses that occur. Some of the major functional abnormalities seen in head injury will be described in the following section.

Concussion. A concussion is a mild form of diffuse brain injury, occurring as the consequence of the acceleration-deceleration and rotational motion of the head. They are associated with a global disruption but have no macroscopically visible lesion.

A concussion syndrome involves a temporary reversible disturbance of neurological function with or without loss of consciousness. If loss of consciousness occurs, it may last for seconds to an hour. The neurological dysfunctions present as confusion, disorientation, and sometimes a period of posttraumatic amnesia.

Other symptoms seen after concussion are headache, dizziness, irritability, inability to concentrate, impaired memory, and fatigue.[9] Not all postconcussion patients complain of these symptoms, and a majority reported no symptoms after a month. A few patients develop postconcussion syndrome and continue to complain of the headaches, dizziness, inability to concentrate, and memory difficulties for more than a year. This indicates that a concussion may not be as benign an injury as previously believed.

Contusion. Cerebral contusion is the most frequently encountered lesion of all head injuries.[12] Cerebral contusion is described as bruising of the brain without puncture or tearing of the *pia membrane.* The"bruised" area is made up of edematous cells of the gray matter with petechiae or hemorrhage as well as necrosis. Underlying white matter is affected to a varying degree depending on the severity of the contusion. Contusion occurs from the absorption of energy into the cerebral tissue upon impact. Two forms of lesions are noted (Fig. 26-1). *Coup injury* is injury to the

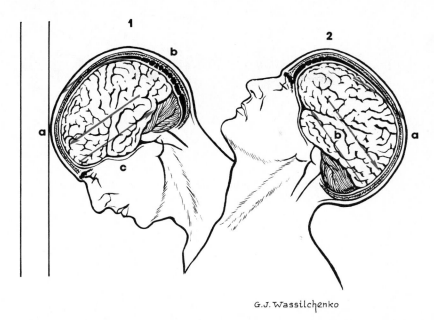

G.J. Wassilchenko

Fig. 26-1   Coup and contrecoup head injury following blunt trauma. *1*, Coup injury: impact against object. *a*, Site of impact and direct trauma to brain; *b*, Shearing of subdural veins; *c*, Trauma to base of brain. *2*, Contrecoup injury: impact within skull. *a*, Site of impact from brain hitting opposite side of skull; *b*, Shearing forces throughout brain. These injuries occur in one continuous motion—the head strikes the wall (coup), then rebounds (contrecoup).

cerebral tissue directly under the point of impact. *Contrecoup injury* is distant from the site of impact and occurs because of the motion of the cerebral contents inside the skull.

Contusions occur most often at the base of the frontal and temporal lobes as the brain is impacted against the irregular bony floor of the frontal bone and sphenoid wing. Contusions may also occur in the inner aspects of the cerebral hemispheres as a result of acceleration of the brain against the falx cerebri.

The signs and symptoms of contusion are related to the location of the contusion, the degree of contusion, and the presence of other associated lesions. Contusions can be small, localized areas of dysfunction resulting in a focal neurological deficit or they can be larger, in which case over 2 to 3 days following the impact injury the area increases in size as a result of edema and further hemorrhages. This large contusion produces a mass effect that causes significant increases in ICP.

Contusions of the tips of the temporal lobe are a common occurrence and are of particular concern. Because the inner aspects of the temporal lobe surround the opening in the tentorium where the midbrain enters the cerebrum, edema and mass effect in this area can cause rapid deterioration of the patient's condition and lead to herniation. Because of the location, this deterioration can occur with little or no warning at deceptively low intracranial pressure.

Diagnosis of contusion is made by CT scan. If the CT scan indicates contusion, especially in the temporal area, the nurse must pay particular attention to neurological assessment and look for subtle changes in pupillary signs or vital signs irrespective of a stable ICP.

Treatment of cerebral contusion is controversial. Since contusion continues to progress over 3 to 5 days after the primary injury, contusions, particularly large ones, can be a significant factor in secondary injury. If contusions are small, focal, or multiple, they are treated medically with serial assessments, ICP monitoring, and treatment for increased intracranial pressure as described in Chapter 27. Larger contusions that produce considerable mass effect are surgically removed early to prevent the increased edema and intracranial pressure found as contusion matures.[42]

Outcome from cerebral contusion varies also depending on the location and the degree of contusion. Mortality from contusion may be as high as 45% as a result of the potential for late deterioration and death that is as significant as the initial injury.[27]

Hematomas. Hematomas resulting from head injury form a mass lesion and lead to increased intracranial pressure. Three types of hematomas will be discussed here (Fig. 26-2). The first two hematomas, epidural and subdural, are extraparenchymal (outside of brain tissue) and produce injury by pressure effect and displacement of intracranial contents. The third type of hematoma, intracerebral, directly damages neural tissue as well as producing injury from pressure effects and displacement of intracranial contents.

EPIDURAL HEMATOMA. Epidural hematoma (EDH) is a collection of blood between the inner table of the skull and the outermost layer of the dura. Epidural hematoma is frequently associated with injury to the middle meningeal artery. A blow to the head that causes a linear skull fracture on the lateral surface of the head may tear the middle meningeal artery. As the artery bleeds, it pulls the dura away from the skull, creating a pouch that expands into the intracranial space.

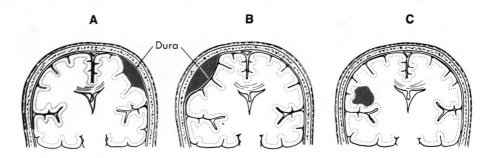

Fig. 26-2 Different types of hematomas.

The incidence of EDH is relatively low. Approximately 2.8% of patients admitted to the hospital for head injury have EDH.[31] In the severely injured or comatose patient the incidence may be as high as 9%.[36]

EDH may occur as a result of low-impact injuries such as falls or high-impact injuries such as motor vehicle accidents. EDH occurs from trauma to the skull and meninges, not the acceleration-deceleration forces seen in other head trauma. Patients with EDH make up a significant percentage of the "talk and die" or "talk and deteriorate" population. These groups are composed of patients whose primary injury was not severe enough to disrupt cerebral functioning but with time and the development of secondary injury may deteriorate or die.

The "classic" signs and symptoms of a patient with EDH include brief loss of consciousness at time of impact followed by a period of lucidity that may last up to 12 hours. This lucid period is followed by rapid deterioration in neurological status from confusion to coma, with changes in pupillary reaction and onset of decerebrate or decorticate posturing. These are all signs of herniation. Rapid neurological intervention is required to save the patient's life.

Diagnosis of EDH is based on clinical symptoms and evidence of a collection of epidural blood identified on CT scan. Treatment of EDH involves surgical intervention to remove the blood and cauterize the bleeding vessels.

Outcome after EDH varies from excellent outcome with no neurological sequelae to a persistent vegetative state or death. Outcome is almost completely dependent on the timing of surgical intervention. The earlier the surgical intervention in the course of deterioration, the better the outcome.

SUBDURAL HEMATOMA. Subdural hematoma (SDH) is the accumulation of blood between the dura and arachnoid membrane in the subdural space. Most subdural hematomas occur over the surface of the brain and result from the tearing of the bridging veins between the brain and the dura. The acceleration-deceleration and rotational forces associated with trauma are the major causes for SDH development. Subdural hematoma is often associated with underlying cerebral contusion as a result of the nature of the impact injury. Outcome or recovery after SDH is lower than that after EDH because of the increased forces and motion of the brain involved in all types of SDH except those that are chronic.

There are three types of SDH based on the timeframe during which symptoms are first identified. The three categories are acute, subacute, and chronic. Acute subdural hematomas are those hematomas which are clinically symptomatic in the first 24 to 48 hours after impact injury. Often the degree of underlying cerebral contusion or damage is so significant that unconsciousness occurs at the moment of impact and is never regained. In other situations, the patient has a lucid period before deterioration. Careful observation for deterioration in level of consciousness or lateralizing signs such as inequality of pupils or motor movements is essential. Although it is difficult to identify the type of mass lesion (EDH versus SDH versus intracerebral hematoma), without CT scan, rapid identification, testing, and surgical intervention prevent further neurological deficit.

Subacute subdural hematomas are hematomas that develop symptomatically 3 to 20 days after trauma. In subacute hematomas the expansion of the hematoma occurs at a rate slower than that in acute SDH; therefore it takes longer for symptoms to become obvious. Clinical deterioration with subacute SDH is usually slower than that with acute SDH, but treatment by surgical intervention, when appropriate, is the same.

Chronic subdural hematoma is the term used when symptomatology occurs 20 or more days after injury. The majority of patients with chronic SDH are elderly or in late middle age. Many have a history of alcoholism, and some are on anticoagulation therapy. In up to 50% of the patients, no history of head injury exists. If a history of head injury does exist, it is often mild.[13]

The pathophysiology of chronic SDH is slightly different from that of acute SDH. The inital hemorrhage may be quite small, or, as in the case of elderly or alcoholic patients, the cerebral volume may be decreased as a result of atrophy. Whatever the cause, the space occupied by the initial hemorrhage is not sufficient to manifest clinical signs of increasing pressure. Within one week after the hemorrhage, fibroblasts that invade the hematoma have formed an outer membrane that encapsulates the clot. Further expansion of the encapsulated mass occurs through seepage of capillary fluid into the clot or additional small hemorrhages inside the membrane. Once the hematoma becomes large enough to exert pressure on cerebral contents, symptoms appear.

Signs and symptoms of chronic SDH are insidious. Since history of trauma is often absent or not significant enough to be recalled, chronic SDH is seldom an initial diagnosis. SDH patients, often elderly, have a variety of symptoms, such as lethargy, absentmindedness, headache, vomiting, stiff neck, photophobia, symptoms of transient ischemic attack (TIA), or seizures.

Evaluation of the patient with CT scan will confirm the diagnosis of chronic SDH. If the SDH has been present for longer than 2 weeks, the fluid visualized within the membranes is either isodense (same density as brain tissue) or hypodense (less dense than brain tissue).

If surgical intervention is requried, evacuation of the chronic SDH may occur by craniotomy, burr holes, or catheter drainage. A craniotomy for removal of the chronic SDH allows for visualization and removal of the outer membranes of the clot. This procedure is highly invasive and requires administration of general anesthetic. The two other approaches can be accomplished with local anesthetic in a cooperative patient. Both procedures, burr hole placement or catheter drainage, involve drilling a hole in the skull over the site of the chronic SDH and draining out fluid. Drains or catheters are left in for at least 24 hours to facilitate total drainage.

Outcome after chronic SDH evacuation is variable. Return of neurological status is often dependent on the degree of neurological dysfunction before removal. Since this pathology is most common in the elderly or debilitated patient, recovery is a slow process. Recurrence of chronic SDH is not infrequent.

INTRACEREBRAL HEMATOMA. Intracerebral hematoma (ICH) is a homogenous collection of blood within the parenchyma. This is contrasted by the appearance of blood as well as contused and edematous cerebral cells in hemorrhagic contusion.

Traumatic causes of ICH include depressed skull fractures, penetrating injuries (bullet, knife, pointed objects), or sudden acceleration-deceleration motion. In sudden acceleration-deceleration, ICH occurs as the brain is lacerated across the under surfaces of the frontal bone and the sharp edges of the sphenoid wing.

Medical treatment of ICH is controversial in terms of surgical or nonsurgical management. It is generally believed that hemorrhages that are not causing significant ICP problems should be treated nonsurgically. Over time the hemorrhage will be reabsorbed. If significant problems with ICP occur as a result of the ICH producing a mass effect, surgical removal is necessary.

Late ICH into the necrotic center of a contused area is possible. Sudden clinical deterioration of a patient, 6 to 10 days after trauma, may be the result of ICH.

Outcome from ICH depends greatly on the location of the hemorrhage. Size, mass effect, and displacement of other intracranial structures also affect the outcome.

Missile injuries. Missile injuries are caused by objects that produce significant focal damage but little acceleration-deceleration or rotational injury. The injury may be depressed, penetrating, or perforating. Depressed injuries are caused by fractures of the skull with penetration of the bone into cerebral tissue. Penetrating injury is caused by a missile that enters the cranial cavity but does not exit. A low-velocity penetrating injury may involve only focal damage and no loss of consciousness. A high-velocity injury, such as a bullet, may involve severe injury as a result of the ricocheting of the bullet through the brain. The shock waves from the high-velocity missile also cause significant cerebral disruption. Perforating injuries are missile injuries that enter and then exit the brain. Perforating injuries have much less ricochet effect but are still responsible for significant injury. (Fig. 26-3).

Risk of infection and cerebral abcess is a concern in missile injuries. If fragments of the missile are embedded within the brain, careful consideration of the location and risk of increasing neurological deficit is weighed against the risk of abscess or infection. Outcome from missile injury is based on the degree of penetration and the location of the injury, as well as the velocity of the missile.

Diffuse axonal injury. Diffuse axonal injury (DAI) covers a wide range of brain dysfunction caused by acceleration-deceleration and rotational forces. This term or diagnosis is usually reserved for the most severe dysfunction. Cerebral concussion is the least severe form of diffuse axonal injury. DAI describes prolonged coma from the time of injury that is not the result of mass lesions or ischemia.

The pathophysiology of DAI is related to the stretching and tearing axons that occur with the motion of the brain inside the cranium at the time of impact.[13] Disruption of axonal transmission of impulses results in loss of conscious-

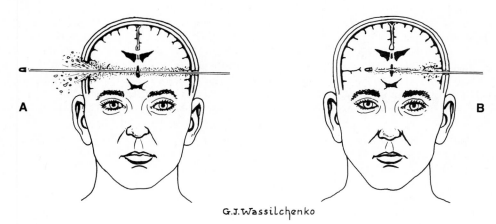

G.J.Wassilchenko

Fig. 26-3 Bullet wounds of the head. Bullet wound or other penetrating missile will cause an open (compound) skull fracture and damage to brain tissue. Shock wave effects are transmitted throughout the brain. **A,** Perforating injury. **B,** Penetrating injury.

ness. Unless surrounding tissue areas were significantly injured to cause small hemorrhages, DAI is not visible on CT scan. These injuries are usually deep within cerebral tissue and at the base of the cerebrum. Other areas of cerebral contusion may also occur with DAI.

Treatment of DAI includes support of vital functions and maintenance of ICP within normal limits. Outcome from severe DAI is poor because of the extensive dysfunction of cerebral pathways.

Assessment and Diagnostics

Rapid assessment and triaging of patients with head injury is critical to a favorable prognosis. To assist with the inital assessment, head injuries have been divided into three descriptive categories based on the patient's Glasgow Coma Scale (GSC) and length of the unconscious state. The three categories are mild, moderate, and severe injury.

Degree of injury

Mild injury. Mild head injury is described as a GCS of 13 to 15 with loss of consciousness for 0 to 15 minutes. Patients with mild injury are often seen in the emergency room and discharged home with a family member who is instructed to routinely evaluate the patient and return the patient to the hospital if any further symptoms appear. A small number of this group makes up the "talk and die" population. A CT scan is seldom performed unless deterioration occurs.[27,33]

Moderate injury. Moderate head injury is described as GCS of 9 to 12 with loss of consciousness up to 6 hours. Patients with this type of head injury are usually hospitalized. They are at high risk for deterioration from increasing cerebral edema and increasing ICP and require close observation. Hemodynamic and ICP monitoring along with ventilatory support is often not required in this group unless other systemic injuries make it necessary. Therefore constant clinical assessment is an important function of the nurse. A CT scan is usually performed initially, but otherwise only if deterioration occurs.

Severe injury. Severe head injury is described as GCS of 3 to 8 with loss of consciousness for longer than 6 hours. Patients with severe head injury often receive ventilatory support along with ICP and hemodynamic monitoring. A CT scan is performed to rule out any mass lesions that should be surgically removed. Patients are placed in a critical care setting for continual assessment, monitoring, and management.

Initial assessment.
As in all traumatic injuries, the evaluation of the ABCs (airway, breathing, and circulation) should be the first step in assessment. These assessments are particularly important in head injury because of the known deleterious effects of hypoxia, hypoventilation, and hypoperfusion on head injury. These conditions greatly contribute to the development of secondary injury. Usually, even when a patient with severe head injury is breathing spontaneously, endotracheal or nasotracheal intubation with mechanical ventilatory support is performed to reduce the risk of hypoxia and hypercapnia. Remember, hypotension is seldom caused by severe head injury.

After stabilization of the ABCs is accomplished, a neurological assessment is performed. Level of consciousness,

motor movements, pupillary response, respiratory function, and vital signs are all part of a complete neurological assessment in the patient with severe head injury.

Serial assessment.
Once the patient is admitted to the critical care unit, serial assessments of neurological function as well as monitoring of hemodynamic and ICP parameters become the main focus of the nurse. Thorough, systematic evaluation is required at least hourly to detect subtle deteriorations in neurological function. Frequently neurological signs are masked in the patient with severe head injury because of the use of muscle relaxants and sedation for ICP control. In these situations observations for changes in pupils and vital signs become even more important. Also, appropriate evaluation and troubleshooting of the intracranial pressure monitoring system is an essential role of the nurse.

Diagnostics
CT scan. The advent of CT scan has greatly enhanced the diagnosis and evaluation of patients with head trauma. With a rapid, noninvasive procedure, invaluable information about the presence of mass lesions or cerebral edema can be obtained. The critical care nurse should always remain with a head injury patient during CT scan to provide continued observation and monitoring during transport and scanning. ICP monitoring should be maintained constantly during this process in order to detect spikes or steady increases in ICP. Transporting, moving the patient from bed to CT table, and putting the head flat in the CT scan are all stressful events and could cause severe increases in ICP. Continuous monitoring allows for rapid intervention.

Evoked potentials. Evoked potentials are becoming more widely used in the head-injured population to assess function and improvement and as a predictor of outcome.

EEG. EEG is also used either intermittently or continuously to monitor the status of cerebral function.

For further discussion of each of these diagnostic tests, see Chapter 25.

Medical Management

Surgical management.
If a mass lesion has been identified on CT scan and is causing a shift of intracranial contents or increasing intracranial pressure, surgical intervention is necessary. A craniotomy is performed to remove the EDH, SDH, or large ICH. Occasionally, if an area of contusion is large and hemorrhagic and associated with an elevated ICP, a craniotomy for removal of the contused area is performed to relieve pressure and prevent herniation.[42]

Nonsurgical management.
Nonsurgical management revolves around management of ICP, maintenance of vital sign parameters, and treatment of any complications such as pneumonia or infection that may occur. For review of the treatments for increased ICP and complications, see Chapter 27.

Nursing Care

Care of the patient with head injury involves continual, systematic assessments of neurological function as well as rapid intervention when deterioration is noted. The critical care nurse must accurately assess the patient's condition. Observation of ICP responses to any nursing care or other interventions should be noted so that appropriate planning of nursing care can occur.

Most of the care of these patients centers around maintenance of normal hemodynamic parameters and intervention for increases in ICP. These critically ill patients who have such a complex disorder require careful planning of care and continued evaluation of ICP response. Many nursing research studies have been conducted to evaluate a patient's ICP response to turning, positioning, suctioning, noise, family visitation, and other nursing care. These studies indicate that increases in ICP are possible from all these interventions. Incorporation of the results of these research studies into planning of the care of the patient with severe head injury may result in fewer spikes in ICP.

CENTRAL NERVOUS SYSTEM TUMORS

In the central nervous system (CNS), most primary neoplastic growths are a result of irregular mitosis of the support cells, the neuroglia. Neurons themselves have little ability to regenerate and minimal to no mitotic capability. Primary CNS tumors are classified as benign or malignant, but the definition of these terms varies from the tumor classification system of the rest of the body. Benign CNS tumors are those growths lying in accessible areas of the CNS with slow growth and lack of invasiveness. These can be completely removed without significant neurological deficit. Malignant tumors are neoplasms such as glioblastoma multiforme, which have multiple fingerlike projections into normal tissue. Attempts to completely remove all of the tumor would cause unacceptable neurological damage. Another type of CNS malignancy is the presence of a usually benign growth that lies deep in vital structures of the CNS where attempt at removal would cause severe neurological deficit. It is malignant by location not by histological classification.

Generally, CNS tumors do not metastasize outside of the CNS. Metastatic cells from the body do reproduce in the CNS. Primary lesions of the lung, breast, and prostate contribute most significantly to metastatic lesions in the brain.

Incidence

The overall incidence of CNS tumors in the United States is 10,000 cases of brain tumors and 4,000 cases of spinal cord tumors per year.[23] The majority of tumors occur in two age peaks. One peak is in childhood (ages 3 to 12) and the other in the later years (ages 50 to 70).

Cause

Pediatric tumors vary in histology and other characteristics from tumors in the adult. A fairly common neoplastic disease in childhood, CNS tumors rank second only to the leukemias. More than two thirds of the pediatric lesions are in the posterior fossa (the cerebellum, midbrain, and brainstem region). The most common tumor in children is the medulloblastoma that accounts for a quarter of the primary intracranial tumors in this age group.[10] Other tumors of childhood are astrocytomas of the cerebellum, astrocytomas of the brainstem, and the malignant glioblastoma multiforme of both the cerebellum and the brainstem.[4]

In the adult population, the most common tumor is glio-

> ## Nursing Diagnosis and Management
> ### *Cerebral trauma*
>
> ■ Altered Cerebral Tissue Perfusion related to increased intracranial pressure secondary to brain trauma, hemorrhage, edema, p. 581
> ■ Potential for Aspiration risk factors: reduced level of consciousness, depressed cough and gag reflexes, presence of tracheostomy or endotracheal tube, gastrointestinal tube, tube feedings, delayed gastric emptying, p. 489
> ■ Ineffective Airway Clearance related to impaired cough secondary to loss of glottic closure with cuffed tracheostomy or endotracheal tube, p. 476.
> ■ Ineffective Breathing Pattern related to respiratory muscle deconditioning secondary to mechanical ventilation, p. 482
> ■ Impaired Gas Exchange related to ventilation-perfusion inequality secondary to stasis of secretions, p. 487
> ■ Altered Nutrition: Less Than Body Protein-Calorie Requirements related to lack of exogenous nutrients and increased metabolic demand, p. 713. (See also discussion of metabolic results from carbohydrate overfeeding, Chapter 10.)
> ■ Potential for Infection risk factors: protein-calorie malnourishment, invasive monitoring devices, pp. 346 and 720
> ■ Potential Impaired Skin Integrity risk factors: reduced mobility, nutritional deficit, enteral tube feedings, stool incontinence, p. 725
> ■ Sensory-Perceptual Alterations related to sensory overload, sensory deprivation, sleep pattern disturbance, p. 601
> ■ Body Image Disturbance related to actual change in body structure, function, and appearance, p. 833
> ■ Altered Role Performance related to physical incapacity to resume usual or valued role, p. 836

---

blastoma multiforme, followed by meningioma and astrocytoma. Glioblastomas represent more than one half of all primary intracranial lesions.[35]

Pathophysiology

Basic to understanding the pathophysiology associated with any tumor of the brain or spinal cord is the accurate identification of the cell of origin and assessment of the aggressiveness of the cells of the tumor. A variety of classification systems have been developed over the years to categorize CNS tumor cells. For discussion here, tumors will be grouped by the "cell of origin" and order of frequency.[43]

It must be remembered that tumors of the CNS are competing with normal tissue for space inside the enclosed environment of the cranium or spinal column. Malignancy of intracranial tumors can be thought of in terms of cytological and biological malignancy. Cytological malignancy is based on cellular morphology, necrosis, mitosis, and invasiveness. Biological malignancy is the likelihood that a tumor will cause the death of a patient.[23] Most cytologically malignant brain tumors are also biologically malignant. Because of the brain's sensitivity to increased pressure, some cytologically benign tumors are biologically malignant.

Classification

Gliomas. Gliomas arise from the four neuroglial cells: astrocytes, oligodendroglia, ependymal cells, and microglia. Also considered a cause for gliomas histologically are neuroglial precursors. Gliomas compose more than 50% of all primary tumors of the CNS.

ASTROCYTOMAS. Astrocytomas are the largest group of neuroglial cells. They are believed to provide support and nutrients to the neuron. A range of tumors from benign to highly malignant arise from the astrocyte cell. These tumors are graded from I to IV. Astrocytoma grade I is a slow-growing tumor with a life expectancy for the patient of up to 15 years. Astrocytoma grade II is a less well-differentiated cell that grows more rapidly, and the patient has a life expectancy of 8 to 10 years. Astrocytoma grade III has increasing malignant cytological features. Life expectancy of the patient with this tumor group is 2 to 5 years. The final most severe astrocytoma, grade IV, is also known as glioblastoma multiforme. It is characterized by grossly undifferentiated cells, significant necrosis, and a high incidence of hemorrhage into the lesion. Life expectancy of the patient with glioblastoma multiforme is 6 to 18 months.[23]

Astrocytomas of the cerebellum and posterior fossa are most commonly seen in childhood and can range from grades I to IV. Because this is usually a slow-growing cystic tumor, the patient's life expectancy may be 10 years or longer with incomplete excision. Complete excision of these tumors is often possible.

OLIGODENDROGLIOMAS. Oligodendrogliomas arise from oligodendrocytes, which are responsible for myelination of nerve fibers in the CNS. Oligodendrogliomas are usually benign but are occasionally malignant. They are slow growing, fairly solid, and discrete from surrounding brain tissue. Oligodendrogliomas are likely to have calcification as part of the mass. Frequently oligodendroglioma cells are found mixed with astrocytoma cells. The presence of a significant number of oligodendroglioma cells in an astrocytoma is a good prognostic sign.

EPENDYMOMAS. Ependymomas arise from the cells that line the ventricular cavities and the central canal of the spinal cord. Tumors arising from these cells are situated deep within the CNS. Usually a tumor of childhood, these tumors range from slow to rapid growth. Morbidity and mortality in this group of tumors is related to the rate of growth but also to the deep CNS location that makes accessibility to the lesion difficult.

Neuron tumors. Tumors arising from neuronal tissue are extremely rare because of the lack of mitotic ability of the neuron. Neuroblastoma, rarely a primary CNS lesion, and ganglioblastoma, tumors of ganglion cells, are two types most noted. These tumors occur in children and range from benign to malignant.

Meningiomas. Meningiomas arise from the cells of the pia and arachnoid, especially the arachnoid granulations. The majority of meningiomas are noninvasive and considered benign. They are encapsulated and well demarcated from surrounding tissue. Meningiomas are most often found around the venous sinuses, over the convexities of the brain, or on the sphenoid ridge. These extremely slow-growing tumors can become quite large before symptoms appear. Meningiomas are the most common extramedullary CNS tumor.

Acoustic neuromas or Schwannomas. These tumors arise around cranial nerves, particularly the acoustic (VIII) nerve. They are from Schwann cells, which are responsible for producing myelin in the peripheral nervous system. These tumors are frequently small and considered benign, but they grow in the brainstem area that is difficult to access. Morbidity and mortality of these tumors is usually associated with pressure and damage to surrounding brainstem structures.

Pituitary tumors. Pituitary tumors are made up of three types that arise from the adenohypophysis or anterior lobe of the pituitary. These three tumor types are chromophobic, eosinophilic, and basophilic adenomas.

The chromophobe adenoma responsible for 90% of pituitary tumors is a nonsecretory space-occupying tumor. These tumors produce their effect by putting pressure on surrounding secretory cells, which causes decreased production of stimulating hormones. This produces symptoms of hypopituitarism: irregular menses, amenorrhea, decreased libido, impotence, decreased body hair, and decreased production of other stimulating hormones.

There are two recognized hormone-secreting pituitary tumors. Eosinophilic adenomas secrete growth hormone (GH) that results in *giantism* before puberty and *acromegaly* after puberty. Basophilic adenomas secrete adrenocorticotropic hormone (ACTH), which results in Cushing's syndrome. Further alteration of this classification system is required because it has become clear that other pituitary hormone–producing tumors, such as prolactin-secreting adenoma, also occur.

Two types of surgery are available for the removal of a pituitary tumor: transcranial hypophysectomy and transsphenoidal hypophysectomy (Fig. 26-4). The transsphenoidal approach has gained wide acceptance and is the surgery of choice unless the pituitary tumor has extended into the intracranial vault. Overall, the prognosis for pituitary tumors that have not invaded surrounding structures of the CNS is excellent.

Craniopharyngiomas. Craniopharyngiomas are tumors derived from remnants of embryonic tissue. They are found primarily in children. These tumors are frequently cytologically benign but biologically malignant because of the location or invasive potential.

Craniopharyngiomas are made of epithelial-type cells that secrete a cholesterol-containing viscous fluid that is an irritant to the CNS. Frequently, the tumor portion is only a small part of the lesion, with the larger portion being composed of a fluid-filled cyst.[23]

Vascular tumors. Vascular tumors of the CNS include hemangioma, hemangioblastoma, and, in some classifica-

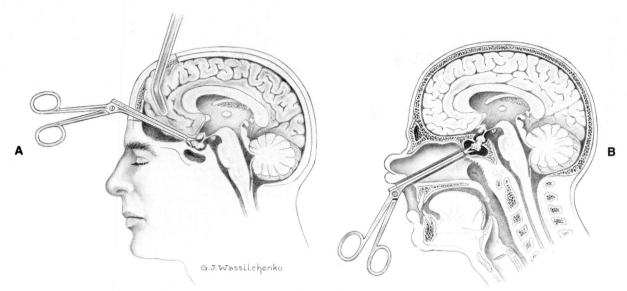

G.J.Wassilchenko

Fig. 26-4 **A,** Transcranial hypophysectomy. **B,** Transsphenoidal hypophysectomy.

tions, the arteriovenous malformation (AVM). A heman-gioma is a closely packed group of abnormally dilated blood vessels. The hemangioblastoma contains a mixture of cap-illaries and large stromal cells. Both tumors are usually small and considered benign unless hemorrhage occurs. These lesions are found in both the brain and spinal cord.

The arteriovenous malformation is a tangled mass of ar-terial and venous vessels that may present as a mass lesion or CNS hemorrhage. AVMs will be discussed in the section on cerebral vascular disease in this chapter.

Metastatic lesions. Lesions that most commonly give rise to metastases in the CNS are lung and breast lesions. Tumor cells are spread by blood or the lymphatic system. Metastatic lesions are generally well circumcised with a defined mar-gin. However, lesions are usually multiple. The incidence of metastatic tumors of the CNS is on the increase as therapy for limiting growth at other tumor sites improves.[23] Gen-erally the blood-brain barrier remains intact with metastatic lesions so treatment with chemotherapeutic agents is diffi-cult.

Assessment and Diagnosis

Assessment of a patient with suspected CNS tumor is focused around the specific neurological abnormalities pre-sented by the patient. Possible neurological dysfunctions are as varied as the different protions of the CNS. Patients may initially have focal neurological deficit, history of increasing headaches that are worse in the morning than in the evening, seizure activity, hormonal changes, or personality changes.

Physical examination serves to further define the focal neurological deficit. If the tumor is large enough to create a mass effect, papilledema may be found. Papilledema is present in 70% to 75% of all brain tumors.

Depending on the suspected pathology, diagnostic work-up may include a CT scan, MRI, EEG, neuroendocrine tests, cerebral angiogram, chest x-ray examination, or bone scan. After a specific lesion has been identified a biopsy is fre-quently performed for a histological diagnosis. Once the type of tumor has been diagnosed, medical management can be planned.

Medical Management

Medical management of CNS tumor is centered around surgery, radiation, and chemotherapy. Depending on the type and location of the tumor, any or all of these treatment modalities may be employed.

If there is a major component of cerebral edema associated with the identified tumor, steroids are often the beginning point of medical management. The use of steroids, partic-ularly dexamethasone (Decadron), can result in a significant reversal of neurological symptoms temporarily. Steroids, believed to reduce cerebral edema by strengthening the cell membrane, reduce neurological deficit by reducing intra-cranial pressure.

Surgery. Surgical removal of the entire lesion is the goal but not always the outcome. In benign, well-defined lesions, surgical removal may be the only treatment necessary. In invasive, poorly defined lesions, surgery is the beginning point of treatment. Even though it is well recognized that a craniotomy will not remove 100% of an invasive tumor, "debulking" of the tumor mass reduces pressure on sur-rounding structures and may slow the growth process.

Radiation. With incompletely excised tumors, radiation is often the next step of medical management. Some tumors that occur in functionally critical areas, such as the brain-stem, hypothalamus, or thalamus, are not surgically acces-sible without resulting in significant neurological deficit. Radiation may be the primary medical management of these tumors. The goal of radiation is to destroy or retard the growth of tumor cells without damaging normal tissue. His-tological diagnosis of the tumor cell is essential in planning the type of radiation to be used. The total dose of radiation varies depending on the tumor type, location, size of the field, and prior or concurrent chemotherapy. Generally it is not recommended to give more than 3500 to 5000 rads in total radiation treatment.

Use of stereotaxically placed radioactive-loaded catheters implanted into the tumor bed is a method currently being investigated. The patient undergoes catheter placement in the operating room and is managed overnight in the critical care unit. The next day the catheters are loaded with radioactive material and the patient is transferred to a room equipped for handling radiation implants.

Chemotherapy. Until recently, chemotherapy treatment was unavailable to patients with malignant brain tumors because it was believed that chemotherapeutic agents *did not cross the blood-brain barrier.* Although that is still of primary concern, other factors also limit the effects of chemotherapy on brain tumors. Tumors of the CNS are small by nature. Although mitosis of abnormal cells in the tumor bed is occurring, it may not occur at a fast enough rate for a course of chemotherapy to be effective.[37] Also, with further study it appears that the microenvironment of the tumor area is not heterogeneous and therefore not 100% sensitive to any one chemotherapeutic agent.[37]

In all considerations of chemotherapy, attention must be focused on protection of the normal delicate cerebral tissue.

Future treatment modalities. Research and investigation in improved treatment of malignant CNS tumors continue in all the areas previously discussed. Microsurgical techniques and the use of laser surgery may allow access to previously inoperable tumors and improved excision of invasive tumors. A variety of approaches in radiation therapy, including radionuclide seed implantation and the concurrent use of a variety of chemotherapeutic agents in conjunction with radiation, are under investigation. Advances in chemotherapy include the continued development of agents with greater specificity for CNS tumor cells.

A new concept in CNS tumor management is currently under clinical investigation. It involves the use of regional hyperthermia to destroy tumor cells. Hypoxia, poor blood flow, and acidic pH, common features in inner regions of many brain tumors, all enhance sensitivity to hyperthermia. Further clinical trials are needed to evaluate the efficacy of this therapy.[40]

Whatever the focus of the future, continued research for the treatment of malignant CNS tumors can only improve the outcome of this often tragic disease.

Nursing Care

Most nursing management of the patient with a CNS tumor does not occur in the critical care environment. Generally, patients are in the critical care unit during the postoperative stage of craniotomy. With the advent of steroids, the cerebral edema associated with brain tumors and craniotomy has virtually been eliminated. Patients with an uncomplicated craniotomy for removal of a brain tumor often remain in the critical care unit only overnight, if at all. Patients who have had excision of a cervical or high thoracic spinal cord tumor will be in the unit postoperatively for close observation of respiratory status and motor/sensory function of the extremities.

The psychosocial aspects of a patient with a CNS tumor must never be ignored, even in the immediate postoperative period. Support must be offered to the family or significant others as well as the patient.

Nursing Diagnosis and Management
Cerebral tumors

- Altered Cerebral Tissue Perfusion related to increased intracranial pressure secondary to brain tumor, edema, p. 581
- Unilateral Neglect related to stroke involving the right cerebral hemisphere, p. 590.
- Impaired Verbal Communication: Aphasia related to cerebral speech center injury, p. 598
- Potential for Aspiration risk factors: depressed cough and gag reflexes and decreased gastrointestinal motility secondary to anesthesia, impaired swallowing, p. 489
- Potential for Infection risk factor: invasive monitoring devices, p. 346
- Potential Impaired Skin Integrity risk factors: steroid therapy, reduced mobility, p. 725.
- Sleep Pattern Disturbance related to fragmented sleep, p. 88
- Sensory-Perceptual Alterations related to sensory overload, sensory deprivation, sleep pattern disturbance, p. 601
- Anxiety related to threat to biological, psychological, and/or social integrity, p. 852
- Ineffective Individual Coping related to situational crisis and personal vulnerability, p. 850
- Body Image Disturbance related to actual change in body structure, function, and appearance, p. 833
- Altered Role Performance related to physical incapacity to resume usual or valued role, p. 836
- Knowledge Deficit: Prognosis, Medications, Activity Restrictions, Reportable Symptoms related to lack of previous exposure to information, p. 69
- Hopelessness related to perceptions of failing or deteriorating physical condition, p. 839

CEREBROVASCULAR DISEASE
Cerebrovascular Accident

Cerebrovascular accident, commonly known as stroke, is a descriptive term for the onset of neurological symptoms caused by the interruption of blood flow to the brain. There are two basic types of stroke: ischemic and hemorrhagic. Ischemic stroke is a stroke that produces symptoms resulting from an occlusion of a blood vessel. This can be either thrombotic or embolic in nature. The majority of thrombotic strokes are the result of the accumulation of atherosclerotic plaque in the vessel lumen, especially at bifurcations or curves of the vessel. An embolic stroke occurs when a small embolus from the heart or lower cerebral circulation travels distally and lodges in a small vessel resulting in loss of blood supply. Hemorrhagic strokes are divided into intracerebral hemorrhage and subarachnoid hemorrhage. Intracerebral hemorrhage is most often caused by hypertensive rupture of a cerebral vessel. Subarachnoid hemorrhage can be caused by aneurysm rupture or arteriovenous malformation (AVM) rupture. In a prospective study of 694 patients hospitalized for stroke, 53% had thrombotic strokes, 31% had embolic strokes, 10% had intracerebral hematoma, and 6% had subarachnoid hemorrhage from aneurysm or AVM.[17]

Incidence. Stroke is the third leading cause of death in the United States, preceded only by heart disease and cancer. Along with the high mortality rate associated with stroke, there is significant morbidity in patients who survive. The Framingham study, an extensive 20-year follow-up of survivors of stroke in the 45 to 74 year age range, found that 31% needed assistance in self-care, 20% required assistance in ambulation, 71% had impaired vocational capacity 7 years after stroke, and 16% were institutionalized.[14] It is estimated that 1.6 million Americans have had strokes; 40% require special services and 10% total care.[41]

Risk factors. The risk of having a stroke before reaching age 70 is one in 20.[18] The major risk factors related to stroke are associated with factors that lead to the development of atherosclerosis. The major risk factors include hypertension, cardiac impairments, or diabetes mellitus.

Hypertension. By far the greatest risk factor of stroke is hypertension. The risk of stroke is equal in men and women with comparable blood pressure. Hypertension is a factor in both ischemic and hemorrhagic stroke.

Hypertension leads to structural changes in cerebral arteries and accelerated atherogenesis. It also impairs cerebral autoregulation over time.

Cardiac impairments. Cardiac abnormalities such as atrial fibrillation, coronary artery disease, or enlarged heart exist in 75% of stroke patients. Atrial fibrillation, in particular, is associated with a high incidence of stroke. Blood pools in the poorly emptying atria of the heart. Tiny clots form in the left atrium which then move through the heart and out into the cerebral circulation to cause embolic stroke.

Diabetes mellitus. Vascular disease in general is more prevalent in patients with diabetes mellitus. Thrombotic stroke from the accumulation of atherosclerotic plaque is the most common type of stroke in diabetic patients.

Minor risk factors. Other factors that have been linked less consistently with stroke are elevated blood lipids, obesity, smoking, stress, and family history.

The discussion of assessment, pathophysiology, diagnosis, and management of the above-mentioned cerebral vascular disease processes is too large an undertaking for this chapter. Instead, focus will be directed on the three pathological conditions of hemorrhagic disease: aneurysm, arteriovenous malformation, and spontaneous hemorrhage. Because of the sudden onset and potential for mass effect of these hemorrhagic diseases, a critical care environment for stabilization and support is required more often than in the care of other types of cerebrovascular disease.

Cerebral Aneurysm

An aneurysm is an outpouching of the wall of a blood vessel that results from weakening of the wall of the vessel. Aneurysms can occur in vessels in other parts of the body from a variety of causes, but in this section the focus will be on cerebral aneurysms. Most cerebral aneurysms are saccular or berrylike with a stem and neck. Aneurysms are usually small, 2 to 6 mm in diameter, but may be as large as 6 cm. Clinical concern arises if an aneurysm ruptures or becomes large enough to exert pressure on surrounding structures.

Incidence. It is estimated that approximately 6% of strokes are caused by aneurysm rupture. The incidence of cerebral aneurysm has been estimated at 9.6 per 100,000 population.[26] It is possible for an individual to live a full lifespan with an unruptured cerebral aneurysm.

Subarachnoid hemorrhage (SAH) is the result of aneurysm rupture. Although there are other causes of SAH, aneurysm rupture is responsible for 70%.[26] Subarachnoid hemorrhage is a serious phenomenon with a mortality rate of 40% to 50%. The peak incidence of aneurysm rupture is between 40 to 65 years of age. Few aneurysms rupture in persons under the age of 20.[39]

Cause. Ninety percent of aneurysms are congenital. The other 10% can be a result of traumatic injury (that stretches and tears the muscular middle layer of the arterial vessel), infectious material (most often from infectious vegetation on valves of the left side of the heart after subbacterial endocarditis) that lodges against a vessel wall and erodes the muscular layer, or of undetermined cause. Multiple aneurysms occur in 20% to 25% of the cases and are often bilateral, occurring in the same location on both sides of the head.

Aneurysms frequently occur at the base of the brain on the circle of Willis. The distribution is anterior communicating artery, 30%; posterior communicating artery, 25%; branching of the middle cerebral artery, 13%; and all other locations, 32% (Fig. 26-5). Most cerebral aneurysms, especially those which are congenital, occur at the bifurcation of blood vessels.

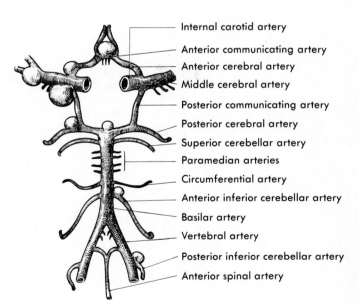

Internal carotid artery
Anterior communicating artery
Anterior cerebral artery
Middle cerebral artery
Posterior communicating artery
Posterior cerebral artery
Superior cerebellar artery
Paramedian arteries
Circumferential artery
Anterior inferior cerebellar artery
Basilar artery
Vertebral artery
Posterior inferior cerebellar artery
Anterior spinal artery

Fig. 26-5 The common sites of berry aneurysms. The size of the aneurysm in the drawing is proportional to the frequency of occurrence at the various sites. (From Wyngaarden JB and Smith LH, editors: Cecil textbook of medicine, ed 16, Philadelphia, 1982, WB Saunders.)

Pathophysiology. The cause of the vessel development defect that occurs in the congenital aneurysm is unknown. A small portion of the inner muscular or elastic layer of the vessel is poorly developed, leaving a thin vessel wall. As the individual matures, blood pressure rises and more stress is placed on this thin vessel wall. Ballooning out of the vessel occurs, which gives the aneurysm its berrylike appearance.

The aneurysm becomes clinically significant when the vessel wall becomes so thin that it ruptures, sending arterial blood at a high pressure into the subarachnoid space. For a brief moment of aneurysm rupture, intracranial pressure is believed to approach mean arterial pressure and cerebral perfusion falls.[29] In other situations, the aneurysm expands and places pressure on surrounding structures. This is particularly true with the posterior communicating artery aneurysm that puts pressure on the oculomotor nerve (CN III) causing ipsilateral pupil dilation and ptosis.

Assessment and diagnosis

Initial presentation. The initial presentation of a patient with an aneurysm is usually following subarachnoid hemorrhage. SAH becomes the working diagnosis until the cause of the hemorrhage is determined. Signs and symptoms of SAH range from sudden onset of "worst headache of my life" to coma or death.

Subarachnoid hemorrhage has been divided into five grades for classification of severity of the neurological deficits associated wtih the bleed.[15]

Grade I   Asymptomatic, minimal headache, slight nuchal rigidity
Grade II   Moderate to severe headache, nuchal rigidity, minimal neurological deficit
Grade III   Drowsiness, confusion, mild focal neurological deficit
Grade IV   Stupor, moderate to severe hemiparesis, early decerebrate posturing
Grade V   Comatose, decorticate or decerebrate posturing, moribund appearance

Forty-five percent of the patients who survive SAH report sudden brief loss of consciousness followed by severe headache, 45% report severe headache associated with exertion but no loss of consciousness, and in 10% the bleeding was severe enough to cause loss of consciousness for up to several days.[11] Vomiting, nuchal rigidity (stiff neck), photophobia, seizure, hemiplegia, or other focal neurological deficits are also common.

A review of histories shows that the patient often reports one or more incidences of sudden onset of headache with vomiting in the weeks preceding major SAH. These are "warning leaks" of the aneurysm in which small amounts of blood ooze from the aneurysm into the subarachnoid space. The presence of blood is an irritant to the meninges, particularly the arachnoid membrane. This irritation causes headache, stiff neck, and photophobia. These small "warning leaks" are seldom detected because the condition is not severe enough for the patient to seek medical attention. If a neurological deficit, such as third cranial nerve palsy, develops before aneurysm rupture, medical intervention is sought and the aneurysm may be surgically secured before the devastation of rupture can occur.

Diagnostic tests. Diagnosis of subarachnoid hemorrhage is based on clinical presentation as well as CT scan and lumbar puncture. When SAH is suspected, a CT scan is performed to identify subarachnoid blood. Seventy-five percent of the cases demonstrate blood in the basal cisterns if CT scan is done within 48 hours of the hemorrhage. Based on the appearance and the location of the SAH, diagnosis of cause such as aneurysm or AVM may be made from the CT scan.

If CT scan is unequivocal, a lumbar puncture is performed to obtain CSF for analysis. Cerebrospinal fluid after SAH is bloody in appearance with a red cell count >1,000. If lumbar puncture is performed more than 5 days after the SAH, CSF fluid is xanthochromic (dark amber) as blood products are broken down. Cloudy CSF usually indicates some type of infectious process such as bacterial meningitis, not subarachnoid hemorrhage.

Once the SAH has been documented, a cerebral angiogram is necessary to identify the exact cause of the SAH. If a cerebral aneurysm rupture is the cause, angiogram is also essential to define the exact location of the aneurysm in preparation for surgery (Fig. 26-6).

Medical management. Medical management of patients with SAH is complex. Decisions about surgical intervention and the timing of that intervention are based on the patient's clinical presentation.

The two major complications following a subarachnoid hemorrhage from aneurysm rupture are rebleeding and vasospasm.

Rebleeding. Rebleeding is another major subarachnoid hemorrhage that may occur at any time in an unsecured aneurysm. The incidence of rebleeding is as great as 50% in the first few months, with the highest incidence being in the first few days after hemorrhage.[16] Mortality rate with rebleeding has been reported to be as high as 70%.[20] Definitive treatment for prevention of rebleeding is surgical clipping of the aneurysm. Because of the patient's clinical condition and the technical difficulty of the surgery, early surgical repair of the aneurysm is not always possible. Early surgery (within the first 48 hours after hemorrhage) is recommended for patients with a grade I or grade II SAH.[1] In these patients, the initial hemorrhage did not produce significant neurological deficit, but the risk of rebleeding with a tragically high incidence of mortality is present until the aneurysm is secured.

For years the use of antifibrinolytic agents (aminocaproic acid) has been suggested in situations in which early surgery is not an option. Antifibrinolytic agents act by preventing the production of fibrin responsible for resolving the clot at the tip of the aneurysm. Controversy continues to surround the use of these agents. Studies reporting the actual reduced incidence of rebleeding have been mildly positive. The main issue with the use of antifibrinolytic agents is the tendency of this drug to increase the incidence and severity of the other common SAH complication—vasospasm. Clinical trials continue to evaluate the efficacy of this treatment.[6,19]

Cerebral vasospasm. The presence or absence of cerebral vasospasm has a significant effect on the outcome of a patient after SAH. Vasospasm is the narrowing of the lumen of the vessel either from actual spastic constriction of the vessel or an inflammatory swelling of the vessel wall that narrows the lumen. Vasospasm is a critical issue because

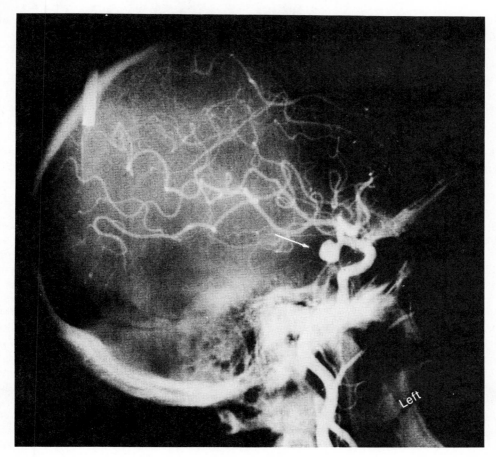

Fig. 26-6 Cerebral angiography showing location of aneurysm at posterior communicating artery. (From Tortorici M: Fundamentals of angiography, St. Louis, 1982, The CV Mosby Co.)

of its location in the cerebral vasculature. Because aneurysms occur at the circle of Willis, the major vessels responsible for feeding cerebral circulation are affected by vasospasm. Decreased arterial flow occurs in large areas of the cerebral hemispheres depending on the arterial vessels involved in the vasospasm reaction. Ischemic stroke is the outcome of this decreased flow. The peak period for vasospasm is 7 to 14 days after rupture. Vasospasm begins around the third day after rupture and can last for 3 to 4 weeks. Over 30% to 40% of SAH patients develop vasospasm. In grades III and IV SAH vasospasm has been reported in >65% of the patients.[30]

Treatment. A variety of therapies have been evaluated in an attempt to reverse or overcome the vasospasm. To date, two treatments seem to have potential benefit: induced hypervolemic hypertension and calcium channel blockers.

Hypervolemic hypertension involves increasing the patient's blood pressure and cardiac output through the use of fluid and volume expanders such as plasma. Systolic blood pressure is maintained between 150 and 160. This increase in volume and pressure forces blood at higher pressures through the vasospastic area. Many anecdotal reports exist of patient's neurological deficits improving as systolic pressure increases from 130 to between 150 and 160. The obvious deterrent to use of induce hypertension is the risk of

rebleed in an unsecured aneurysm. This therapy can be used safely only after surgery for aneurysm clipping. The second complication associated with hypervolemic hypertension therapy is the risk of pulmonary edema associated with fluid overload. Careful monitoring of pulmonary artery wedge pressure, cardiac output, oxygenation, and chest x-ray examination is important.

The second therapy for the treatment of vasospasm is the use of calcium channel blockers. Although the exact role of calcium channel blockers in the prevention of vasospasm is not known, evidence is mounting in clinical research trials of its effectiveness if begun immediately after the initial hemorrhage.[1,6,30] Results of ongoing clinical trials should soon identify the efficacy of this therapy along with the most effective drug and dosage.

Timing of surgery is a key medical management issue. Historically, aneurysm patients were placed in a dark, quiet room for 10 to 14 days following subarachnoid hemorrhage. Blood pressure was kept low and sedation was used. If the patient survived the risk of rebleed and the course of vasospasm, surgery was performed. The surgical outcome from this procedure was good, but many patients did not survive until the time of the surgery.

Since the introduction of microsurgery and improved surgical techniques, patients are frequently taken to the operating room within the first 48 hours after rupture. This early surgical intervention to secure the aneurysm eliminates the risk of rebleeding and allows hypertensive therapy to be used in the postoperative period for the treatment of vasospasm. Early surgery also allows the neurosurgeon to flush out the excess blood and clots from the basal cisterns (reservoir of CSF around the base of the brain and circle of Willis) to reduce the risk of vasospasm.

Early surgery is not recommended for all patients. Especially in those patients with grades IV to V SAH, early surgery may contribute to the morbidity or mortality. Careful consideration of each patient's clinical situation is necessary in determination of the timing of surgery.

Aneurysm clipping is the surgical procedure that is performed for repair of the aneurysm. This procedure involves a craniotomy to expose the area of aneurysm. The aneurysm itself is isolated and a clip is placed over the neck of the aneurysm to eliminate the area of weakness. As stated earlier, this is a technically difficult procedure that requires the skill of an experienced neurosurgeon. It is not uncommon, particularly in early surgery, for the clot to break away from the aneurysm as it is surgically exposed. Extensive hemorrhage into the craniotomy site is the result, and cessation of the hemorrhage often causes increased neurological deficits.

Development of hydrocephalus is a late complication that frequently occurs after SAH. Blood that has circulated in the subarachnoid space and has been absorbed by the arachnoid villi may obstruct these villi and reduce the rate of CSF absorption. Over time, increasing volumes of CSF in the intracranial space produce communicating hydrocephalus.

Treatment for this is placement of a drain to remove CSF. This can be temporary with a catheter placed into the lateral ventricle and attached to an external drainage bag or permanent with the placement of a ventriculoperitoneal shunt.

Arteriovenous Malformation

Arteriovenous malformation (AVM) is a tangled mass of arterial and venous blood vessels that shunt blood directly from the arterial side into the venous side, bypassing the capillary system. AVMs may be small, focal lesions or large lesions that occupy almost an entire hemisphere.

Incidence. Although the incidence of AVM is not great, the management of a patient with an AVM is a medical challenge. Ten percent of all subarachnoid hemorrhages are caused by AVM.[26] In contrast to the middle-aged population with SAH from aneurysm, the AVM tends to bleed at a younger age. The peak age for bleed of an AVM is 15 to 35. The mortality rate of the initial hemorrhage is approximately 20%. Risk of recurrent hemorrhage is about 20%, with an increase in mortality of 10% with each rebleed.[39]

Cause. The cause of an AVM is always congenital. The exact embryonic reason for the development of this malformation is unknown. AVMs are not confined to the cerebral circulation. AVMs can be found in the spinal cord and in the renal, gastrointestinal, or integumentary system; Port wine stains of the skin may be caused by small superficial AVMs.

Pathophysiology. Once the embryonic dysfunction that resulted in the AVM has occurred, the pathophysiology is related to the size and location of the malformation. The AVM can be fed by one or more cerebral arteries. Called feeders, these arteries tend to enlarge over time and increase the volume of blood shunted through the malformation as well as increase the overall mass effect. Large, dilated tortuous draining veins also develop as a result of the increasing flow of blood. Blood flowing into the venous side of the AVM does so at a higher than normal pressure. In a normal vascular flow, mean arterial presure is 70 to 80 mm Hg, mean arteriole pressure is 35 to 45 mm Hg, and mean capillary pressure drops from 35 to 10 mm Hg as it connects with the venous side. Lack of this capillary bridge allows blood with a mean pressure of 35 to 45 mm Hg to flow into the venous system. Because there is no muscular layer in the vein as there is in the artery, veins become extremely engorged.

As a result of the shunting of blood through the AVM and away from normal cerebral circulation, poor perfusion occurs in the underlying cerebral tissues. This decreased perfusion produces a chronic ischemic state that results in cerebral atrophy.

Assessment and diagnosis. Initial assessment of the patient depends on the presenting symptoms. Although subarachnoid hemorrhage is one of the most common and severe presenting symptoms, there are other signs and symptoms that also may occur before subarachnoid hemorrhage.

The onset of seizures is frequently a reason for the patient with an AVM to seek medical attention. As the mass of the AVM enlarges and the flow of blood increases, the pulsation of the blood vessel against the cerebral tissue surface causes a disturbance of the electrical activity of the area. Seizures can be focal or generalized.

Headaches are another common symptom of patients with an AVM. Headache may occur as a result of the increasing mass effect of the lesion or be associated with vascular changes in response to the shunted blood. Headaches alone do not often trigger the suspicion of AVM, since there is a wide variety of reasons for headache.

A very small percentage of the patients demonstrate a bruit and will report a constant swishing sound in the head with each heart beat. In other patients, the bruit can be auscultated with a stethoscope placed over the skull.

Other symptoms of AVM may include motor/sensory defects, aphasia, dizziness, or fainting. Since a majority of patients are under the age of 30, symptoms such as these would not likely be attributed to atherosclerotic vascular disease.

Diagnostic evaluation includes CT scan, EEG, and angiogram. CT scan is performed initially as a noninvasive study to begin the diagnostic process. If an AVM is suspected from the results of the noncontrast scan, a contrast scan is performed. EEG is done to attempt to localize any seizure focus or to define areas of cortical injury caused by cerebral ischemia or atrophy.

Finally, for confirmation and definition of the AVM, an angiogram is performed. If surgical intervention is planned, an angiogram is required to identify the feeding arteries and draining veins of the AVM.

Medical management

Surgical excision. Medical management of the patient has traditionally involved surgical excision of the AVM or conservative management of the symptoms such as seizures and headache. The decision for surgical excision depends on the location and size of the AVM. Some malformations are located so deep in cerebral structures (the thalamus or midbrain) that attempts to remove the AVM would cause severe neurological deficits. The history of previous hemorrhage, the age, and general condition of the patient are also taken into account in the decision about surgical intervention.

Reperfusion bleeding. Surgical excision of large AVMs include the risk of reperfusion bleeding. As feeding arteries of the AVM are clamped off, the arterial blood that usually flowed into the AVM is now diverted into the surrounding circulation. In many cases the surrounding tissue has been in a state of chronic ischemia and the arterial vessels feeding these areas are maximally dilated. As arterial blood begins to flow at a higher volume and pressure into these dilated arteries, seeping of blood from the vessels may occur. The evidence of reperfusion bleeding in the operating room is an indication that no more arterial blood can be diverted from the AVM without risk of serious intracerebral hemorrhage. In the postoperative phase, low blood pressure is maintained to prevent further reperfusion bleeding. In large AVMs, two to four stages of surgery might be required over a 6 to 12 month period.

Embolization. Embolization is another method of reducing the size of an AVM. It may also be used on surgically inaccessible AVMs. Embolization is an interventional radiology technique in which a catheter is placed in the groin or other site, similar to that done in an angiogram. Under fluoroscopy, the catheter is threaded up to the internal carotid artery. Small silastic beads or a variety of other materials such as glue are then slowly introduced through the catheter. The increased flow to the AVM should carry the blocking material into the AVM. The purpose of this procedure is to block the feeding arterial portion of the AVM and therefore eliminate the AVM. Frequently, embolization and surgery are combined. The patient receives one to three sessions of embolization to reduce the size of the lesion and then has a craniotomy for total excision.

Risks to the procedure include lodging of the substance in a vessel feeding normal tissue. This creates an embolic stroke. Onset of neurological symptoms occurs immediately. Another risk involves passage of the embolic substance right through the lesion out the venous system and into the lung. If that should occur the patient experiences a pulmonary embolus.

Radiation therapy, particularly proton beam radiation, is occasionally used for large lesions that are not surgically accessible. The overall success of radiation therapy is unknown.

Intracerebral Hemorrhage

Intracerebral hemorrhage is the escape of blood into cerebral tissue. Causes of intracerebral hemorrhage are aneurysm or AVM rupture, trauma, or hypertensive hemorrhage. This section will concentrate on hypertensive hemorrhage. Hemorrhage destroys cerebral tissue, causes cerebral edema, and increases intracranial pressure.

Incidence. The incidence of hypertensive hemorrhage accounts for 2% of all deaths in the United States and is responsible for about 10% of the strokes and 15% of all intracranial hemorrhages.[17]

Cause. The cause of hypertensive stroke is largely a long-standing history of hypertension. Blood dyscrasia (leukemia, hemophilia, sickle cell disease), anticoagulation therapy, and hemorrhage into brain tumors are other possible causes of intracerebral hemorrhage. Frequently on questioning, the patient with a hypertensive hemorrhage will admit to having discontinued antihypertensive medication 2 to 3 weeks before the hemorrhage.

Pathophysiology. The pathophysiology of intracerebral hemorrhage is caused by continued elevated blood pressure exerting force against smaller arterial vessels that have become damaged from arteriosclerotic changes. Eventually this artery breaks, and blood bursts from the vessel into the cerebral tissue, creating a hematoma. Intracranial pressure rises precipitously in response to the increased overall intracranial volume.

Assessment and diagnosis. Initial assessment usually reveals a critically ill patient. They are often unconscious and require ventilatory support. History from a relative or significant other describes a sudden onset of severe headache with rapid neurological deterioration.

Vital signs usually reveal a severely elevated blood pressure (200/100 to 250/150), slow pulse, and deep, labored respirations. The patient arrives in the emergency room with many of the signs of increased intracranial pressure. ABCs should be addressed first to make sure airway is adequate, breathing patterns are acceptable, and circulation is present.

Administration of an antihypertensive medication is usually begun immediately to reduce the blood pressure to relatively normal pressure. If the hemorrhage is significant enough to cause incased ICP, the blood pressure should not be allowed to drop rapidly or too low. If blood pressure drops below 140 systolic and ICP remains high, cerebral perfusion may be compromised.

Medical management. Medical management of a hypertensive hemorrhage is similar to that of a traumatic hemorrhage. Surgical removal of the clot is dependent on the size and location of the clot, the patient's ICP, and other neurological symptoms. If the hematoma is large and causes a shift in structures or ICP is elevated despite routine methods to lower it, a craniotomy for removal of the hematoma is performed. Nonsurgical management includes measures to maintain the ICP within normal limits and support of all other vital functions until the patient regains consciousness.

Nursing Care

Nursing management of the previously discussed cerebrovascular diseases requires that the nurse have a thorough knowledge of the pathophysiology of the disease as well as a good understanding of the treatment plan. Accurate, detailed assessment is essential. Frequently the first sign of clinical deterioration is evidenced through subtle changes in the neurological examination.

Adequate blood pressure is necessary to continue to supply the brain with the appropriate amount of oxygen and nutrients. However, when damage or disease of the cerebrovascular system is the cause of the patient's hospitalization, the actual level of blood pressure that is most appropriate for the patient is dependent on the underlying pa-

---

Nursing Diagnosis and Management
Cerebral vascular disease

- Altered Cerebral Tissue Perfusion related to increased intracranial pressure secondary to brain hemorrhage, edema, stroke, hydrocephalus, p. 581

- Altered Cerebral Tissue Perfusion related to vasospasm secondary to subarachnoid hemorrhage after ruptured intracranial aneurysm or arteriovenous malformation, p. 579

- Unilateral Neglect related to right cerebral hemisphere stroke, p. 590

- Impaired Verbal Communication: Aphasia related to cerebral speech center injury, p. 598

- Potential for Aspiration risk factors: reduced level of consciousness, presence of endotracheal tube, gastrointestinal tube, tube feedings, situation hindering elevation of upper body (vasospasm after subarachnoid hemorrhage), decreased gastrointestinal motility secondary to anesthesia, impaired swallowing, p. 489

- Potential Altered Peripheral Tissue Perfusion risk factor: vasopressor therapy (vasospasm after cerebral artery aneurysm rupture), p. 341

- Impaired Gas Exchange related to alveolar hypoventilation secondary to decreased level of consciousness, p. 488

- Ineffective Breathing Pattern related to respiratory muscle deconditioning secondary to mechanical ventilation, p. 482

- Ineffective Airway Clearance related to impaired cough secondary to loss of glottic closure with cuffed endotracheal tube, p. 476

- Activity Intolerance related to postural hypotension secondary to prolonged immobility, p. 344

- Altered Nutrition: Less Than Body Protein-Calorie Requirements related to lack of exogenous nutrients and increased metabolic demand, p. 713. (See also discussion of metabolic results from carbohydrate overfeeding, Chapter 10.)

- Potential for Infection risk factors: invasive monitoring devices, p. 346

- Potential Impaired Skin Integrity risk factors: reduced mobility protein-calorie malnourishment, steroid therapy, altered cutaneous sensation, p. 725

- Anxiety related to threat to biological, psychological, and/or social integrity, p. 852

- Ineffective Individual Coping related to situational crisis and personal vulnerability, p. 850

- Sensory-Perceptual Alterations related to sensory deprivation, sensory overload, sleep pattern disturbance, p. 601

- Sleep Pattern Disturbance related to fragmented sleep, p. 88

- Body Image Disturbance related to actual change in body structure, function, and appearance, p. 833

- Powerlessness related to health care environment and illness-related regimen, p. 837

- Altered Role Performance related to physical incapacity to resume usual or valued role, p. 836

- Self-Esteem Disturbance related to feelings of guilt over physical deterioration, p. 835

- Knowledge Deficit: Physical Rehabilitation, Medications, Reportable Symptoms related to lack of previous exposure to information, p. 69

---

thology. For example, after spontaneous intracerebral hemorrhage or initial subarachnoid hemorrhage, it is important to keep the blood pressure relatively low. In vasospasm after subarachnoid hemorrhage, relatively high blood pressures are required for adequate perfusion. The nurse's role is to monitor blood pressure constantly, administer medications as necessary, and observe the patient's activities and interactions in response to blood pressure.

If the patient is comatose after the cerebrovascular insult, all interventions for caring for the immobile patient should be initiated. Immobility is implicated in many patient complications so intervention to reduce the effects of immobility should occur as soon as possible.

Emotional support to the patient and family is, as always, important. Especially if the patient is dealing with a neu-

rological deficit such as hemiplegia, aphasia, or any significant neurological deficit, fear of dependency and of becoming a burden are issues that must be faced. Both the patient and family should be involved in all aspects of planning of care.

TRAUMA OF THE SPINAL CORD

Injury to the spinal cord that causes permanent damage and disability is a devastating illness. Although strides have been made in reducing the number and severity of complications associated with spinal cord injury, little has been found effective in reversing the dysfunction as a result of injury. Nothing but prevention can reduce the incidence of permanent disability from spinal cord injury.

Incidence

The incidence of acute spinal cord trauma resulting in permanent injury is approximately 12,000 annually in the United States. Of these 12,000, 4,000 die before reaching the hospital and about 1,000 die during hospitalization.[34] One half of these injuries result in quadriplegia and one half in paraplegia.

Spinal cord injury occurs in five of every 100,000 persons, with the incidence of injury to males 3:1 over that to females.[32] Most patients (62%) range in age from 15 to 35 years, with another slight increase in incidence in the elderly as the result of falls.

Cause

In decreasing order of incidence, the causes of injury are vehicular accidents, falls on or off the job, sports injuries, and penetrating or missile injuries.[3]

Significant to consideration of spinal cord injury are the personal, family, and society costs associated with permanent injury to the spinal cord. Recently, the estimated first year cost of caring for one individual with spinal cord injury exceeded $250,000.[38] The estimated annual cost to society is greater than $2 billion per year.

Mechanism of Injury

The type of injury sustained is dependent on the mechanism of injury. Review of the mechanism of injury includes the velocity, momentum, angle of impact, and degree of abnormal motion involved in sustaining the injury. The most common mechanisms of injury are hyperflexion, hyperextension, rotation, axial loading (vertical compression), and missile or penetrating injuries.

Hyperflexion. Hyperflexion injury is most often seen in the cervical area especially at the level of C5 to C6, the most mobile portion of the cervical spine. This type of injury is most often caused by sudden deceleration motion as in head-on collisions. Injury occurs from compression of the cord as a result of fracture fragments or dislocation of the vertebral bodies. Instability of the spinal column occurs because of rupture or tearing of the posterior muscles and ligaments.

Hyperextension. Hyperextension injuries involve backward and downward motion of the head often seen in rear-end collisions or diving incidents. In this type of injury the spinal cord itself is stretched and distorted. Disruption of intervertebral discs occur as well as compression or fracture of the posterior elements of the vertebral column. Neurological deficits associated with this injury are often caused by contusion and ischemia of the cord without significant bony involvement. A mild form of hyperextension injury is the "whiplash" injury.

Rotation. Rotation injuries often occur in conjunction with a flexion or extension injury. Severe rotation of the neck or body results in tearing of the posterior ligaments and displacement (rotation) of the spinal column. The condition termed *locked facets* is a result of rotation and involves displacement of the facet junction of one or more vertebral elements, thereby producing cord compression. Cervical traction or surgery is required to return these facets to normal positions and reduce cord compression.

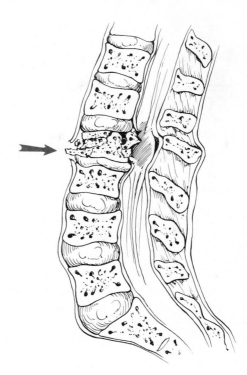

Fig. 26-7　Burst fracture of vertebral body causing damage to spinal cord. (From Long BC and Phipps WJ: Medical-Surgical Nursing: a Nursing Process Approach, ed 2, St. Louis, 1989, The CV Mosby Co.)

Axial loading. Axial loading or compression injuries occur from vertical force along the spinal cord. This is most commonly seen in a fall from a height in which the person lands on feet or buttocks. Compression injuries cause burst fractures of the vertebral body that often send bony fragments into the spinal canal or directly into the spinal cord (Fig. 26-7).

Missile or penetrating injuries. Missile or penetrating injury to the spinal cord is caused by bullet, knife, or any other object that penetrates the cord. These types of injury cause permanent damage by anatomically transecting the spinal cord.

Pathophysiology

Injury to the vertebral column can occur without accompanying injury to the spinal cord, and, conversely, injury to the spinal cord can occur without radiographic or surgical evidence of vertebral column injury. Primary injury to the spinal cord occurs from direct damage to neural tissue and vascular supply at the time of trauma. As a result of primary injury a chain of events resulting in ischemia, hypoxia, edema, and, ultimately, infarction and hemorrhage necrosis of the cord leads to significant secondary injury.[2]

Much of the study of the dynamics of spinal cord injury has been done through the use of experimental models. Injury to the spinal cord simultaneously involves the meninges, blood vessels, and neurological tissues. Though multiphasic in nature, there are four basic areas that contribute to secondary injury:

1. Morphological damage is caused by stretching, tear-

ing, cutting, or displacement of normal spinal cord tissues. This damage often leads to edema of the cord.

2. Vascular damage and hemorrhage occur as perfusion pressure to the damaged area drops significantly. This decreased perfusion results in decreased tissue oxygenation, ischemia, and necrosis. Small hemorrhagic areas are seen early (within minutes) in the gray matter and later in the white matter.

3. Structural changes of white and gray matter (injury at the cell level) cause opening of the tight vascular endothelial junctions. This leads to electrophysiological alteration causing sodium to leak from the cell and results in a negative resting membrane potential.

4. Biochemical reactions to trauma result in an accumulation of vasoactive amines such as norepinephrine, serotonin, and histamines. These substances produce a toxic vasospasm that further impedes microcirculation and tissue oxygenation.[34]

Much of the current research in spinal cord injury is directed toward arresting or reversing these secondary processes of injury. Local cryotherapy to reduce metabolic demands may provide a protective effect in limiting hemorrhage and edema. Use of steroids has been proposed to reduce the cell membrane degeneration. Calcium channel blockers and adrenergic blockers have been tried to reduce the production or interaction of vasoactive amines. Naloxone (Narcan) has been tried to block the effects caused by the release of neural endorphins into a damaged area. To date no definitive therapy has proved effective and research continues.

Functional Injury of the Spinal Cord

Whatever the mechanism of injury or the type of vertebral column injury, the main focus of attention and intervention is toward the functional injury of the spinal cord. Functional injury refers to the degree of disruption of normal spinal cord function. Functional injuries are divided into two injury categories: complete and incomplete. Complete injuries are divided into quadriplegia and paraplegia. Incomplete injuries are further subdivided into central cord syndrome, anterior cord syndrome, Brown-Sequard syndrome, posterior cord syndrome, and cauda equina syndrome.

Complete injury. A complete injury of the spinal cord results in total sensory, motor, and autonomic nervous system dysfunction below the level of injury. This injury could be a result of anatomical dissection of the spinal cord or physiological dissection as a result of disruption of neurochemical pathways. More than 50% of all patients diagnosed initially as having complete injury obtain some return of function with the resolution of spinal shock (see the section entitled "Spinal Shock").

A complete injury in the cervical region results in quadriplegia. The degree of arm dysfunction is dependent on the level of injury. A complete injury in the thoracolumbar region results in paraplegia. Both quadriplegia and paraplegia involve loss of normal bowel and bladder function.

Incomplete injury. Incomplete injury to the spinal cord involves damage or dysfunction of one portion of the cord with normal pathways and function intact in the other portions of the cord.

Central cord syndrome. Resulting from contusion, compression, or hemorrhage of the central gray matter of the cord, central cord syndrome is generally a cervical region injury. Because of the damage to gray matter, cell bodies, and nuclei at the level of injury, motor loss of the upper extremities is significant. Flaccidity, as characterized by a lower motor neuron injury (LMN), is seen. The lower extremities may exhibit upper motor neuron (UMN) injury with spasticity. Accompanying this motor injury is a varying degree of sensory loss, as well as a varying degree of bowel and bladder dysfunction (Fig. 26-8).

Hyperextension injuries, particularly if the patient has bony spurs from a preexisting degenerative disease, are the most common cause of central cord syndrome.

Anterior cord syndrome. Anterior cord syndrome is caused by injury to the anterior gray horn cells (motor), the spinothalamic tracts (pain perception), and the corticospinal tracts (temperature perception). This injury results in loss of motor function below the level of the lesion. Also lost are the sensations of pain and temperature. Sensations of touch, position sense, pressure, and vibration are maintained.

Anterior cord syndromes are most often caused by flexion injuries or acute herniation of the intervertebral disc.

Brown-Sequard syndrome. Brown-Sequard syndrome is caused by a transverse hemisection of the cord. Because of the anatomy of motor and sensory pathways of the spinal cord, Brown-Sequard syndrome results in (1) ipsilateral loss of motor function, either paralysis or paresis, (2) ipsilateral loss of touch, vibration, pressure, and position sensation, and (3) contralateral loss of pain and temperature sensation. For example, a patient with a right-sided hemisection of the cord would exhibit right-sided loss of motor function as well as right-sided loss of touch and position sense. The right side would retain the ability to sense pain and temperature. On the left side below the level of injury, the patient would lose sensation of pain and temperature but retain motor function, touch, and position sense.

Brown-Sequard syndrome is caused by open, penetrating injuries such as knife or gunshot wounds or an acute ruptured intervertebral disc.

Posterior cord syndrome. Posterior cord syndrome is rare. This injury results in loss of light touch and proprioception below the level of injury. Motor function and the sensation of pain and temperature remain intact. Posterior cord syndrome is usually associated with cervical hyperextension.

Cauda equina lesion. Injury at the levels below the end of the spinal cord at L1 are referred to as cauda equina lesions. Deficits from injury to the cauda equina vary according to the particular nerve roots involved. Damage can be bilateral or unilateral and involve both motor and sensory function. LMN lesions of the S1 to S4 area lead to flaccid bowel and bladder functions. All other lesions of the spinal cord that affect bowel and bladder function lead to UMN injury that allows for spastic control of bowel and bladder function.

Spinal shock. Spinal shock is a term applied to a condition that occurs immediately after an acute spinal cord injury. Spinal shock is the complete loss of all reflex activity

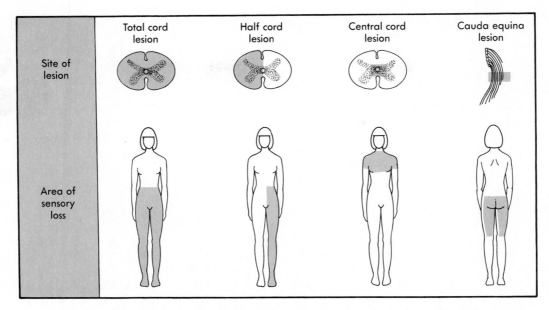

Fig. 26-8 Common patterns of sensory abnormality. *Upper diagrams*, site of lesion; *lower diagrams*, distribution of corresponding sensory loss.

below the level of injury. This includes not only loss of deep tendon reflexes but also loss of vasomotor tone, temperature control, and bowel and bladder tone. Loss of these reflexes results clinically in bradycardia, hypotension, hypothermia, urinary retention, and paralytic ileus.

The pathophysiology of spinal shock is incompletely understood; however, it is thought to result from a sudden loss of impulses from the higher centers of the brain that normally maintain the spinal cord neurons in a state of excitement. Sudden loss of this excitability stimulus reduces significantly the resting excitability potential of the spinal cord reflexes below the level of the lesion.

Over a period of hours to months, reflex activity returns to normal. Often the first reflex activity to return is in the perianal area with the bulbocavernosus reflex (contraction of the anal orifice with genital stimulation). Actually the reappearance of any reflex that has been lost in spinal shock is a signal that the shock state is receding. As reflexes return they demonstrate a hyperactive response. Loss of higher center control leaves all reflexes below the level of injury with an UMN spasticity.

Because of the immediate onset of spinal shock, the actual degree or permanence of any spinal cord injury is difficult to predict in the early hours after the injury. Up to 50% of all patients who appear to have complete spinal cord injury on initial evaluation regain some degree of spinal cord function after spinal shock ends.[3]

Assessment and Diagnosis

Assessment of the patient with a known or suspected spinal cord injury begins at the scene of the trauma. All trauma victims should be treated for spinal cord injury until proved otherwise. This involves stabilization of the neck and back through the use of cervical collars, backboard, sand bags, or tape to prevent motion of the spine. In the unconscious patient, stabilization of the spine at the scene is even more critical since the patient is unable to relay any signs or symptoms of spinal cord injury. Once the patient is transported to the emergency department, further and more detailed spinal cord assessment will occur.

As in all trauma assessments, evaluation of the ABCs (airway, breathing, and circulation) is vital to the outcome of the patient with spinal cord injury. Particularly if the patient has sustained a high cervical injury (C1 to C4) evaluation of breathing is critical to survival. As spinal shock sets in, circulation also becomes a problem. Loss of vasomotor tone results in hypotension.

Neurogenic shock. Neurogenic shock is another symptom seen in patients with cervical injury. A portion of the sympathetic nervous system lies in the thoracolumbar region of the spinal cord and receives continuous information from the brainstem down through the cervical cord. Injury in the cervical region disrupts the pathway and leads to loss of sympathetic control. This loss results in vasodilatation of the vascular beds, bradycardia resulting from the lack of sympathetic balance to parasympathetic stimuli from the vagus nerve (CN X), and loss of the ability to sweat below the level of injury.

In assessment of a patient who presents with manifestations of shock, it is important to remember that in hypovolemic shock the patient is hypotensive and *tachycardic*. In neurogenic shock the patient is hypotensive but *bradycardic*.

Initial evaluation. Once the ABCs of assessment are performed and the patient has an adequate airway, respirations, and viable blood pressure, assessment of the level and degree of spinal column or spinal cord injury begins.

Motor-sensory examination. A detailed motor and sensory examination is performed in all patients with suspected spinal cord injury. It is important to assess all 32 spinal nerves for evidence of dysfunction. Carefully mapped out pathways for the sensory portion of the spinal nerves, called dermatomes, assist the examiner in localizing the functional level of injury.

It is essential that the initial examiner describe motor and sensory function in detail so that subsequent serial examinations can rapidly identify deterioration as a result of the onset of edema or secondary injury. The easiest way to accomplish this is through the use of a spinal cord injury assessment sheet (Fig. 24-2). Motor strength is graded from 1 to 5. Sensation is described as normal, diminished, absent, or hyperesthetic. Frequently the examiner uses a pen to draw a line on the patient to indicate areas of sensory change.

Serial evaluation. Ongoing assessment of the patient with spinal cord injury should occur at least hourly, or more frequently if needed, in the first 48 to 72 hours after injury. This assessment, performed by the nurse, needs to include detailed evaluation of muscle group function and sensory function. Again, use of a spinal cord injury assessment sheet aids in the standardization of these assessments. Any evidence of deterioration in either motor or sensory function should be immediately communicated to the physician. Especially in the cervical region, a small increase in the level of injury has tremendous impact in the patient's overall rehabilitation potential.

Diagnostic evaluation. Along with the clinical evaluation of spinal cord function, diagnostic tests are performed to identify spinal column injury as well as electrophysiological dysfunction.

Radiographic evaluation. Radiographic evaluation of the spine includes anterioposterior and lateral views for all area of the spinal column. CT scan, tomograms, myelography, and MRI may also be used in the diagnostic process. For further review of these procedures see Chapter 25. Strict immobilization of the neck and back of the SCI patient during transfer and movement for radiographic procedures is essential.

Medical Management

After diagnosis and assessment of the type of spinal cord or spinal column injury, medical management decision making occurs. Justification for immediate surgical intervention includes radiographic evidence of bony fragments or disc material in the spinal canal producing pressure on the spinal cord. This potentially reversible dysfunction causes progressive neurological deficit and indicates increasing compression of the spinal cord.

Surgical management. Surgical intervention is performed to provide spinal column stability in the event of an unstable injury. Unstable injuries are defined as disrupted ligaments and tendons, particularly the posterior ligamentous complex, or the inability to maintain normal alignment of the vertebral column. Identification and immobilization of unstable injuries is particularly important in the patient with incomplete neurological deficit. Without adequate stabilization, movement and dislocation of the vertebral column could cause a complete neurological deficit.

A variety of surgical procedures may be performed to achieve decompression and stabilization.

Laminectomy—Removal of the lamina of the vertebral ring to allow decompression and removal of bony fragments or disc material from the spinal canal.

Spinal fusion—Surgically fusing 2 to 6 vertebral elements together to provide stability and prevent motion. Fusion is done through the use of bone plugs or bone chips taken from the iliac crest, wire, or acrylic glue.

Rodding—Stabilization and realignment of larger segments of the spinal column by means of a variety of rodding procedures such as Harrington rods or Leuke rods. The rods are attached by screws and glue to the posterior elements of the spinal column. These types of procedures are most often done to stabilize the thoracolumbar area.

Nonsurgical management. If the injury to the spinal column is believed to be stable, nonsurgical management of the injury is the treatment of choice. Nonsurgical management will be discussed separately for cervical and thoracolumbar injuries.

Cervical injuries. Management of the cervical injury involves immobilization of the fracture site and realignment of any dislocation. This is accomplished through skeletal traction that involves the use of tongs inserted into the skull and connected to traction weights. There are several types of cervical tongs used. Gardner-Wells and Crutchfield tongs are the most common. These tongs can be applied at the bedside with the use of local anesthetic.

After the insertion of the tongs, the patient is immobilized on a kinetic treatment table, a Stryker frame, a Circ-o-lectric bed, or a regular hospital bed. The kinetic treatment table is the most popular method of cervical immobilization, since it maintains spinal column alignment while providing constant turning motion to reduce pulmonary and skin breakdown complications so often associated with spinal cord injury patients. The Stryker frame and Circ-o-lectric bed are becoming less acceptable because of the amount of movement that occurs in the neck as the patient is moved from back to stomach. Use of cervical skeletal traction on a regular bed causes great difficulty in providing adequate care to the pulmonary system and skin because of the extensive degree of immobility.

After adequate realignment of the spinal column has occurred through skeletal traction, a halo traction brace is often applied. The halo traction brace allows for the maintenance of cervical spine immobility as well as increasing mobility of the patient. The ability to place the patient in a sitting position, as well as get him or her out of bed and possibly out of the acute care hospital, contributes to reduced complications and shortened length of hospital stay. With the increased mobility provided by the halo brace, the patient can also become involved in the rehabilitation process more quickly.[7]

Thoracolumbar injury. Nonsurgical management of the patient with a thoracolumbar injury also involves immobilization. Skeletal traction may also be used in high thoracic injury. For the most part, stable injuries of the thoracolumbar spine are injuries causing no misalignment of the spinal canal. Immobilization to allow for healing of fractures is accomplished by flat bed rest with the use of a plastic or fiberglass jacket, a body cast, or a brace. Rotorest beds and Stryker frames may also be used to increase the mobility of these patients.

Nursing Diagnosis and Management
Spinal cord injury

■ Dysreflexia related to excessive autonomic response to noxious stimuli secondary to spinal cord injury (T-6 or above), p. 587

■ Hypothermia related to spinal cord injury, p. 585.

■ Decreased Cardiac Output related to vasodilation and bradycardia secondary to sympathetic blockade of neurogenic (spinal) shock following spinal cord injury (T-6 or above), p. 339

■ Impaired Gas Exchange related to alveolar hypoventilation secondary to loss of accessory muscle function, p. 488

■ Impaired Gas Exchange related to ventilation-perfusion inequality secondary to stasis of secretions, p. 487

■ Ineffective Breathing Pattern related to respiratory muscle deconditioning secondary to mechanical ventilation, p. 482

■ Ineffective Airway Clearance related to impaired cough secondary to loss of glottic closure with tracheostomy or endotracheal tube, p. 476.

■ Ineffective Airway Clearance related to respiratory muscle dysfunction and impaired cough secondary to quadriplegia, p. 477

■ Potential for Aspiration risk factors: depressed cough reflex (T-6 and above), presence of tracheostomy tube, gastrointestinal tube, tube feedings, situation hindering elevation of upper body, increased intragastric pressure, increased gastric residual, decreased gastrointestinal motility, delayed gastric emptying, p. 489

■ Activity Intolerance related to prolonged immobility and loss of vasomotor tone, p. 344

■ Potential Impaired Skin Integrity risk factors: immobility, loss of sensation, enteral tube feedings, stool and urine incontinence, p. 725

■ Body Image Disturbance related to actual change in body structure, function, and appearance, p. 833

■ Altered Role Performance related to physical incapacity to resume usual or valued role, p. 836

■ Self-Esteem Disturbance related to feelings of guilt over physical deterioration, p. 835

■ Powerlessness related to health care environment and illness-related regimen, p. 837

■ Ineffective Individual Coping related to situational crisis and personal vulnerability, p. 850

■ Hopelessness related to perceptions of failing or deteriorating physical condition, p. 839

■ Knowledge Deficit: Dysreflexia, Urinary Tract Infections, Upper Respiratory Infections, Skin Care, Mobility Strategies related to lack of previous exposure to information, p. 69

■ Altered Health Maintenance related to lack of perceived threat to health, p. 67

Nursing Care

Nursing management of the patient with spinal cord injury centers around both the physical and psychosocial aspects of the injury.

Physical care

Respiratory. In all patients with cervical injury careful attention must be paid to the respiratory status. In a complete injury or an injury such as anterior cord syndrome, in which motor function has been lost, all control of respiratory accessory muscles in the thorax is lost. Therefore the patient is using diaphragmatic breathing. At the level of C4 the phrenic nerve exits to innervate the diaphragm for respirations. Injury at the level of C4 or above will result in a loss of the function of phrenic nerve causing cessation of respiratory effort. If mechanical ventilation has not been established, careful assessment of the patient's respiratory effectiveness and identification of any ascension of the functional level of injury is essential.

Secretions and the ability to clear them are a significant problem in the patient with cervical injury. Because of loss of the intercostal muscle intervention, the patient's ability to cough is greatly diminished. Suctioning or assisted coughing (quad coughing) are needed to prevent pneumonia or atelectasis.

Immobility. All other care of the spinal cord–injured patient centers around prevention of further complications as a result of the effects of immobility. Skin care becomes a critical element in these patients, because there is no sensation of pressure or pain to indicate the development of decubitus ulcers.

Vital signs. If spinal shock or neurogenic shock is present, close observation of blood pressure and temperature are essential. Hypotension is more appropriately treated with the use of vasoactive agents versus fluids. Remember the patient is not hypovolemic but has a dilated vascular bed. Injudicious use of fluids can lead to overload and pulmonary edema.

Bradycardia caused by the loss of sympathetic innervation to the SA node may be treated with a parasympathetic blocker such as atropine if cardiac output is compromised. The patient should be kept warm and covered to prevent the loss of body heat passively through the dilated vascular bed.

Bowel and bladder. Initially after spinal cord injury, bowel and bladder tone is flaccid. Urinary retention occurs, and the insertion of an indwelling Foley catheter should be one of the first procedures performed. Use of an indwelling catheter prevents bladder stretching and overdistention that could permanently injure the muscular wall of the bladder and prevent the return of spastic bladder control.

A bowel program to prevent fecal impaction and encourage normal, regular bowel function should begin immediately.

Psychological aspects of nursing management.
The psychosocial aspects of nursing care are important parts of the patient's care. This devastating injury is disruptive to both the patient and the family. Both can be expected to go through the stages of grieving because of loss of lifestyle and life roles. The nurse should focus on assisting all individuals to effectively move through these stages of grieving to acceptance.

GUILLAIN-BARRÉ SYNDROME

Guillain-Barré syndrome (GBS), also known as Landry-Guillain-Barré syndrome, is a postinfectious peripheral polyneuritis characterized by a rapidly progressive ascending peripheral nerve dysfunction leading to paralysis. It is 90% to 100% reversible and is one of the most common peripheral nervous system diseases. Becuase of the ventilatory support required for these patients, GBS is one of the few peripheral neurological diseases requiring a critical care environment.

Incidence

The incidence of GBS is 1.7 per 100,000 population. It occurs equally in all ages and both sexes. The incidence of GBS increased slightly for a period of time after the 1977 swine flu vaccinations.[21]

Cause

The cause of GBS is unknown, but more than 50% of patients reported a mild febrile illness, either respiratory or gastrointestinal, 1 to 3 weeks before the onset of signs and symptoms. The result is a possible autoimmune response of the peripheral nervous system.

Pathophysiology

This disease affects the motor and sensory pathways of the peripheral nervous system as well as the autonomic nervous system functions of the cranial nerves. The major finding in GBS is a segmental demyelination process of the peripheral nerves. Inflammation around this demyelinate area causes further dysfunction.

The myelin sheath of the peripheral nerves is generated by the Schwann cells and acts as an insulator for the peripheral nerve. Myelin promotes rapid conduction of nerve impulses by allowing the impulses to jump along the nerve via nodes of Ranvier. Disruption of the myelin fiber slows and may eventually stop the conduction of impulses along the peripheral nerves. In GBS, the more thickly myelinated fibers of motor pathways and the cranial nerves are more severely affected than the thinly myelinated sensory fibers of cutaneous pain, touch, and temperature. Symptoms of GBS include motor weakness, paresthesias and other sensory changes, cranial nerve dysfunction (especially the oculomotor, facial, glossopharyngeal, vagus, spinal accessory, and hypoglossal), and some autonomic nervous system dysfunction.

GBS is believed to be an autoimmune response to antibodies formed against the recent febrile illness. Immune reactions from the T cells and B cells of the lymphatic system set up a local inflammatory reaction that triggers further inflammation.

Once the temporary inflammatory reaction stops, myelin-producing cells begin the process of reinsulating the demyelinated portions of the peripheral nervous system. When remyelination occurs, normal neurological function should return. In some instances the axon may be damaged during the inflammatory process. The degree of axonal damage is responsible for the degree of neurological dysfunction which persists after recovery.

Assessment and Diagnosis

Clinical signs and symptoms. The usual course of GBS begins with an abrupt onset of lower extremity weakness that progresses to flaccidity and ascends over a period of hours to days. Motor loss is usually symmetrical. In the most severe cases, complete flaccidity of all peripheral nerves, including spinal and cranial nerves, occurs.

Admission to the hospital occurs when lower extremity weakness prevents mobility. Admission to the critical care unit occurs when progression of the weakness threatens respiratory muscles. As the patient's weakness progresses, close observation is essential. Frequent assessment of the respiratory system, including ventilatory parameters such as inspiratory force and tidal volume, are necessary. The most common cause of death in GBS patients is from respiratory arrest.

As the disease progresses and respiratory effort weakens, intubation and mechanical ventilation are necessary. Continued, frequent assessment of neurological deterioration occurs until the patient reaches the peak of the disease and plateaus.

Diagnostic findings. The diagnosis of GBS is based on clinical findings plus CSF analysis and nerve conduction studies. CSF analysis demonstrates a normal protein initially that elevates in the fourth to sixth week. No other changes in CSF occur. Nerve conduction studies that test the velocity at which nerve impulses are conducted are significantly reduced as would be expected with the demyelinating process of the disease.

Medical Management

The medical management of GBS is limited. No curative treatment exists for this disease. It simply must run its course. The course of GBS is characterized by ascending paralysis that plateaus for 1 to 4 weeks. This is followed by descending paralysis and return to normal or near-normal function. The main focus of medical management is the support of bodily functions and the prevention of complications.

Some physicians support the use of steroids for their antiinflammatory effect. The effectiveness of steroids are difficult to assess. If steroids are prescribed, all usual precautions associated with steroid use should be followed.

The use of plasmapheresis has also been attempted. Plasmapheresis involves plasma exchanges or washes that remove the antibodies causing the GBS. Plasmapheresis has achieved minimal acceptance in treatment, and studies to determine the effectiveness of this therapy continue.

Nursing Care

The nursing management of the patient with GBS is extensive. The goal of nursing management is to support all normal body functions until such time as the patient can do so on his or her own. Nursing management focuses on immobility, pulmonary care, nutritional support, pain management, and, very importantly, emotional support.

Immobility. In patients with GBS, immobility may last for months. The usual course of GBS involves an average of 10 days for symptom progression and 10 days at maximum level of dysfunction followed by 2 to 48 weeks of recovery. Although reversible, recovery from GBS is a long process.

Pulmonary care. Total ventilatory support and pulmonary toilet are required at the peak level of the illness. As the patient's symptoms recede, weaning from the ventilator and initiation of coughing and deep breathing exercises will be important in prevention of pulmonary complications.

Nutritional support. Implementing nutritional support should occur early in the course of the disease. Since it is known that GBS recovery is a long process, adequate nutritional support will be a problem for an extended period of time. Nutritional support is usually accomplished through the use of enteral feeding. The less invasive method of providing nutrition is preferable to the use of total parenteral nutrition because it reduces the risk of infection in a patient who is highly vulnerable.

Pain control. Pain control is an important component in the care of patients with GBS. Although the patient has minimal to no motor function, most sensory functions are maintained. The patient feels considerable muscle ache and pain. Because of the lengthy nature of this illness, it is important to work closely with the physician and patient to identify a safe, effective long-term solution to pain management.

Emotional support. The emotional support required by these patients is extensive. Although the illness is almost 100% reversible, the total helplessness of the patient, the constant pain or discomfort, plus the length of the course of the disease makes this a difficult experience to deal with. It is important to remember that GBS does not affect the level of consciousness or cerebral function. Interaction and communication are necessary elements of the nursing plan of care.

> ## Nursing Diagnosis and Management
> ### Guillain-Barré syndrome
>
> - Ineffective Airway Clearance related to respiratory muscle dysfunction and impaired cough secondary to Guillain-Barré syndrome, p. 477
> - Sensory-Perceptual Alterations related to sensory overload, sensory deprivation, sleep pattern disturbance, p. 601
> - Acute Pain related to transmission and perception of noxious stimuli secondary to reestablishment of myoneural activity, p. 594
> - Ineffective Airway Clearance related to impaired cough secondary to loss of glottic closure with tracheostomy or endotracheal tube, p. 476
> - Impaired Gas Exchange related to alveolar hypoventilation secondary to respiratory muscle paralysis, p. 488
> - Potential for Aspiration risk factors: depressed cough and gag reflexes, presence of tracheostomy or endotracheal tube, gastrointestinal tube, tube feedings, decreased gastrointestinal motility secondary to immobility, impaired swallowing, p. 489
> - Ineffective Breathing Pattern related to respiratory muscle deconditioning secondary to mechanical ventilation, p. 482
> - Altered Nutrition: Less Than Body Protein-Calorie Requirements related to lack of exogenous nutrients, p. 713. (See also discussion of metabolic results from carbohydrate overfeeding, Chapter 10.)
> - Potential for Infection risk factors: protein-calorie malnourishment, invasive monitoring devices, pp. 346 and 720
> - Potential Impaired Skin Integrity risk factors: protein-calorie malnourishment, immobility, steroid therapy, stool and urine incontinence, p. 725
> - Activity Intolerance related to postural hypotension secondary to prolonged immobility, p. 344
> - Body Image Disturbance related to functional dependence on life-sustaining technology, p. 834.
> - Powerlessness related to health care environment and illness-related regimen, p. 837
> - Anxiety related to threat to biological, psychological, and/or social integrity, p. 852
> - Ineffective Individual Coping related to situational crisis and personal vulnerability, p. 850
> - Knowledge Deficit: Course of Treatment, Prognosis related to lack of previous exposure to information, p. 69

REFERENCES

1. Adams HP: Early management of the patient with recent aneurysmal subarachnoid hemorrhage, Stroke 17(6):1068, 1986.
2. Adornato BT and Glasberg MR: Disease of the spinal cord. In Rosenberg RN, editor: Neurology, New York, 1988, Grune & Stratton.
3. Albin MS: Acute cervical spinal injury. In Rogers MC and Traystman RJ, editors: Critical care clinics: neurologic intensive care, Philadelphia, 1985, WB Saunders Co.
4. Albright AL, Price RA, and Guthkelch AN: Brainstem gliomas of children: a clinicopathological study, Cancer 52:2313, 1983.
5. Baker SP, O'Neill B, and Karpf RS: The injury fact book, Lexington, Mass, 1984, DC Heath & Co.
6. Beck DW and others: Combination of aminocaproic acid and nicardipine in treatment of aneurysmal subarachnoid hemorrhage, Stroke 19(1):63, 1988.
7. Browner CM: Halo immobilization brace care: an innovative approach, J Neurosci Nurs 19(1):24, 1987.
8. Cooper JD, Tabaddor K, and Hauser WA: The epidemiology of head injury in the Bronx, Neuroepidemiology 2: 70, 1983.
9. Dacey RG and Dikmen SS: Mild head injury. In Cooper PR, editor: Head injury, Baltimore, 1987, Williams & Wilkins.
10. Farwell JR, Dohrmann GJ, and Flannery JT: Medulloblastoma in childhood: an epidemiological study, J Neurosurg 61:657, 1984.
11. Fisher CM: Clinical syndromes in cerebral thrombosis, hypertensive hemorrhage and ruptured aneurysm, Clin Neurosurg 22:117, 1975.
12. Fretag E: Autopsy findings in head injuries from blunt forces: statistical evaluation of 1367 cases, Arch Path 75:402, 1963.
13. Graham DI, Adams JH, and Gennarelli TA: Pathology of brain damage

in head injury. In Cooper PR, editor: Head injury, Baltimore, 1987, Williams & Wilkins.

14. Gresham GE and others: Epidemiologic profile of long-term stroke disability: the Framingham study, Arch Phys Med Rehab 60:487, 1979.

15. Hunt WE and Hess RM: Surgical risks as related to time of intervention in the repair of intracranial aneurysms, J Neurosurg 28:14, 1968.

16. Jane JA, Winn HR, and Richardson AE: The natural history of intracranial aneurysms; rebleeding rates during acute and long-term period and implication for surgical management, Clin Neurosurg 24:176, 1977.

17. Jankovic J: Differential diagnosis of stroke. In Meyer JS and Shaw T, editors: Diagnosis and management of stroke and TIAs, Menlo Park, Calif. 1982, Addison-Wesley Pub. Co.

18. Kannel WB and others: Components of blood pressure and risk of atherothrombotic brain infarction: the Farmingham study, Stroke 7:327, 1976.

19. Kassell NF and others: Treatment of ischemic deficits from vasospasm with intravascular volume expansion and induced arterial hypertension, Neurosurgery 11(3):337, 1982.

20. Kassell NF, Haley EC, and Torner JC: Antifibrinolytic therapy in the treatment of aneurysmal subarachnoid hemorrhage, Clin Neurosurg 33:137, 1986.

21. Keenlyside R and Brezman D: Fatal Guillian-Barré syndrome after the national influenze immunization program, Neurology 30:929, 1980.

22. Klauber MR, Marshall LF, and Barrett-Conner E: Prospective study of patients hospitalized with head injury in San Diego county, 1978, Neurosurgery 9:236, 1981.

23. Kornblith PL, Walker MD, and Cassady JR: Neurologic oncology, Philadelphia, 1987, JB Lippincott Co.

24. Kraus JF: Epidemiology of head injury. In Cooper PR, editor: Head injury, Baltimore, 1987, Williams & Wilkins.

25. Kraus JF and others: The incidence of acute brain injury and serious impairment in a defined population, Am J Epidemiol 119:186, 1984.

26. Locksley HB: Natural history of subarachnoid hemorrhage, intracranial aneurysm and AVM. In Sachs AL and others: Intracranial aneurysms and subarachnoid hemorrhage: a cooperative study, Philadelphia, 1969, JB Lippincott Co.

27. Marshall LF, Toole BM, and Bowers SA: The national traumatic coma data bank. Part 2. Patients who talk and deteriorate: implications for treatment, J Neurosurg 59:285, 1983.

28. National Center for Health Statistics: monthly Vital Statistics Report. Advanced Report of Final Mortality Statistics, 1982, Hyattsville, Md, Public Health Service. Dec. 20, 1984. 33(9):Supp DHHS Pub. No. (PHS) 85-112.

29. Normes H and Magnaes B: Intracranial pressure in patients with ruptured saccular aneurysm, J Neurosurg 36:536, 1972.

30. Petruk KC and others: Nimodipine treatment in poor-grade aneurysm patients: results of a multicenter double blind placebo-controlled trial, J Neurosurg 68(4):505, 1988.

31. Phonprasert C and others: Extradural hematoma: analysis of 138 cases, J Trauma 20:679, 1980.

32. Piepmeier JM: Cervical fracture. In Long DM, editor: Current therapy in neurological surgery, St Louis, 1985, The CV Mosby Co.

33. Rimel RW and others: Disability caused by minor head injury, Neurosurgery 9:221, 1981.

34. Sances A and others: The biomechanics of spinal injuries, CRC Crit Rev Biomech Eng 11:1, 1984.

35. Schoenberg BS: Epidemiology of primary nervous system neoplasms. In Schoenberg BS, editor: Advances in neurology, vol 19, New York, 1978, Raven Press.

36. Seelig JM and others: Traumatic acute epidural hematoma: unrecognized high lethality in comatose patients, Neurosurgery 15:617, 1984.

37. Shapiro WR and others: Heterogeneous response to chemotherapy of human gliomas grown in mice, Cancer Treat Rep 65(suppl 2):55, 1981.

38. Spinal Cord Injury, No. 81-160. Bethesda, 1981, US Dept. of Health and Human Services, National Institutes of Health.

39. Tindall RSA: Cerebrovascular disease. In Rosenberg RN, editor: Neurology, New York, 1980, Grune & Stratton.

40. Welsh DM: Volumetric insterstitial hyperthermai: nursing implications for brain tumor treatment, J Neurosci Nurs 20(4):229, 1988.

41. Wolf P and Kannel W: Controllable risk factors for stroke: preventive implications of trends in stroke mortality. In Meyer JS and Shaw T, editors: Diagnosis and management of stroke and TIAs, Menlo Park, Calif., 1982, Addison-Wesley Publishing Co.

42. Wrobel CJ and Marshall LF: Closed head injury management dilemmas. In Long DM, editor: Current therapy in neurological surgery, St Louis, 1985, The CV Mosby Co.

43. Zulch DJ: Principles of the New World Health Organization (WHO) Classification of Brain Tumors, Neuroradiology 19:59, 1980.

27

Neurological Therapeutic Management

CHAPTER OBJECTIVES

- Discuss the concept of cerebral autoregulation.
- Diagram the volume-pressure curve.
- Calculate cerebral perfusion pressure.
- Describe the therapies commonly used to treat intracranial hypertension.
- Discuss the complications associated with high-dose barbiturate therapy.
- List the four supratentorial herniation syndromes.

Despite the diversity of neurological pathologies, one aspect of the critical care management of the neurosurgical patient is common to a wide variety of these pathological conditions. This chapter focuses on the concepts of intracranial pressure (ICP) and the types of ICP monitoring. Also discussed are the therapies for management of intracranial hypertension.

ASSESSMENT OF INTRACRANIAL PRESSURE
Monro-Kellie Hypothesis

The intracranial space comprises three components: brain substance (80%), cerebrospinal fluid (CSF) (10%), and blood (10%). Under normal physiological conditions, the ICP is maintained below 15 mm Hg mean pressure. Basic to understanding the pathophysiology of ICP is the Monro-Kellie hypothesis.[11] This hypothesis proposes that an increase in volume of one intracranial component must be compensated by a decrease in one or more of the other components so that total volume remains fixed. This compensation, although limited, includes displacing CSF from the intracranial vault to the lumbar cistern, increasing CSF absorption, and compressing the low-pressure venous system.

Volume-Pressure Curve

When the brain is capable of compliance, significant increases in intracranial volume can be tolerated without much

increase in ICP. However, the amount of intracranial compliance is limited. Once this limit has been reached, a state of decompensation with increased ICP results. As the ICP rises, the relationship between volume and pressure changes, and small increases in volume may cause major elevations in ICP (Fig. 27-1). The exact configuration of the volume-pressure curve and the point at which the steep rise in pressure occurs vary with individual patients.[16] The configuration of this curve is also influenced by the cause and the rate of volume increases within the intracranial vault; for example, a patient with an acute epidural hematoma will neurologically deteriorate more rapidly than the patient with a meningioma of the same size. Monitoring these changes

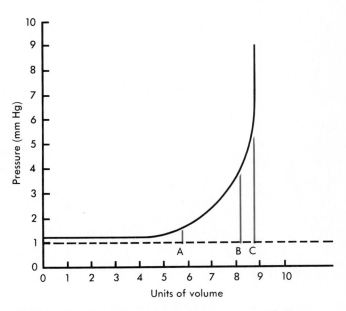

Fig. 27-1 Intracranial volume-pressure curve. **A,** Pressure is normal, and increases in intracranial volume are tolerated without increase in intracranial pressure. **B,** Increases in volume may cause increases in pressure. **C,** Small increases in volume may cause large increases in pressure.

567

in intracranial dynamics and continuous clinical assessment of the patient's neurological status have proven beneficial in diagnosing and treating sustained rises in ICP. Such elevations of ICP often precede evidence of neurological deterioration obtained through the clinical assessment.

Cerebral Blood Flow and Autoregulation

Cerebral blood flow is proportional to meet the metabolic demands of the brain. Although the brain is only 2% of body weight, it requires 15% to 20% of the resting cardiac output and 15% of the body's oxygen demands.[17] In the past it was believed that cerebral blood flow depended passively on arterial pressure. However, the normal brain has a complex capacity to maintain a constant blood flow despite wide ranges in arterial pressure—an effect known as autoregulation (Fig. 27-2). Mean arterial pressure (MAP) of 50 to 150 mm Hg does not alter cerebral blood flow when autoregulation is present.[17] Outside the limits of this autoregulation, cerebral blood flow becomes passively dependent on the perfusion pressure. Other factors besides arterial blood pressure that affect cerebral blood flow are conditions that result in acidosis, alkalosis, and changes in metabolic rate.[9] Conditions that cause acidosis (hypoxia, hypercapnia, and ischemia) result in cerebral vascular dilation. Conditions causing alkalosis (hypocapnia) result in cerebral vascular constriction. Normally, a reduction in metabolic rate (for example, from hypothermia or barbiturates) decreases cerebral blood flow, and increases in metabolic rate (for example, from hyperthermia) result in an increase in cerebral blood flow.

Cerebral Perfusion Pressure

Currently, it is difficult to measure cerebral blood flow in the clinical setting. Cerebral perfusion pressure (CPP), an estimated pressure, is the blood pressure gradient across the brain and is calculated as the difference between the incoming MAP and the opposing ICP on the arteries[6,17]:

$$CPP = MAP - ICP$$

The CPP in the average adult is approximately 80 to 100 mm Hg, with a range of 60 to 150 mm Hg. The CPP should be maintained near 60 mm Hg to provide adequate blood supply to the brain. If the CPP drops below this point, ischemia may develop. A sustained CPP of 30 mm Hg or less usually will result in neuronal hypoxia and cell death. When the mean systemic arterial pressure equals the ICP, cerebral blood flow may cease.

Assessment Techniques

Monitoring techniques. Continuous measurement of ICP was first pioneered by Guillaume and Janny[5] in 1951 and was applied systematically to neurologically injured patients by Lundberg[10] in 1960. Lundberg also outlined criteria for the ideal ICP monitor. These criteria called for a procedure that would minimize the risk of trauma, intracranial infection, and CSF leakage, as well as provide continuous reliable pressure recording during diagnostic and therapeutic measures.

Since that time, much has been learned through the monitoring of ICP. However, there is still no agreement among neurosurgeons about which method is most appropriate. The common sites for monitoring ICP are the intraventricular space, the subarachnoid space, the epidural space, and the parenchyma.

The type of monitor placed in the ventricular system is usually a small catheter known as a ventriculostomy catheter. It is inserted through a burr hole with the patient under local anesthesia and is usually placed in the anterior horn of the lateral ventricle. If at all possible, the side chosen for placement of the ventriculostomy is the nondominant hemisphere (Fig. 27-3, *A*).

The second type of monitor frequently used is the subarachnoid bolt or screw. This small, hollow device is placed in a patient under local anesthesia through a burr hole, with the distal end lying in the subarachnoid or subdural space. The insertion of this device is easier than insertion of the ventriculostomy (Fig. 27-3, *B*).

Another type of device commonly used is the epidural monitor. It too is placed through a burr hole while the patient is under local anesthesia. It is essential for the physician to strip the dura away from the inner table of the skull before inserting the epidural monitor. The most common type of epidural monitor is the fiberoptic or pneumatic sensor, although there are other implantable epidural transducers that are often used for long-term monitoring (Fig. 27-3, *C*).

A new type of ICP monitoring system is the fiberoptic transducer-tipped catheter (Fig. 27-3, *D*). This small (4 Fr) catheter can be placed intraventricularly, intraparenchymally, in the subarachnoid space, or in the subdural space.

There are advantages and disadvantages to each of these systems.[7] The type of monitor chosen depends on both the suspected pathology and physician's preference. Table 27-1 lists the specific advantages and disadvantages of these methods for monitoring ICP.

Intracranial pressure waves. Since the beginning of ICP

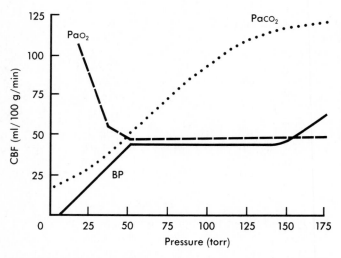

Fig. 27-2 Effects of arterial blood pressure, oxygen, and carbon dioxide on cerebral blood blow.

RESEARCH ABSTRACT

Effects of conversation on intracranial pressure in comatose patients

Johnson SM, Omery A, and Nikas D: Heart Lung 18(1): 56, 1989.

PURPOSE

The purpose of this study was to examine the effects of emotionally referenced conversations on intracranial pressure (ICP).

FRAMEWORK

The dynamics of ICP provide the theoretical framework for this study. The concepts of emotional stress and its potential effects on cerebral blood flow are also of importance. A mechanism of particular importance to this study is the ability of the brain to autoregulate cerebral blood flow. Researchers have investigated the effects of various activites on ICP such as body positioning, hygienic measures, suctioning, environmental stimuli, and passive range of motion. The descriptions of emotionally referenced conversation's influencing ICP have been mentioned only anecdotally. The questions and controversies about the effects of conversation on ICP have not been resolved by the studies heretofore conducted. There is significant evidence from them to support the assumption that increased mentation and emotional arousal have increased cerebral blood flow. In the injured brain that has lost autoregulation functions, increase in blood flow will usually cause an increase in ICP. The literature also clearly describes the correlation between the stress response (either physical or mental) and increases in arterial blood pressure, which can potentially result in an increase in ICP.

METHODS

A time series design was used, with subjects serving as their own control. Eight subjects were selected by convenience sampling. The subjects were in critical care units and had continuous ICP monitoring devices (either a subdural fiberoptic catheter or a ventriculostomy catheter) in place, had a Glasgow Coma Score (GCS) of 10 or less, and had had no nursing or medical interventions within 15 minutes of the baseline data collection period. Two conversation types were used, and continuous measurements of ICP were recorded. Type 1 conversation was an emotionally referenced conversation that reflected an actual nursing report on the patient's current condition. Type 2 conversation was a predetermined dialogue unrelated to the patient. Two nurses performed the conversation, and the investigator recorded the ICP from the digital monitor at 15-second intervals. During the 3-minute conversation, there was no physical contact with the bed, patient, or any equipment. After a 15-minute rest period, the other conversation was presented.

RESULTS

Demographic variables were analyzed using descriptive statistics. There were six men and two women, and their average age was 30.6 years. Trauma was the most frequent source of neurological insult, and five of the eight had endotracheal tubes in place. T-tests were performed between the mean scores of the minimal, maximal, and average ICP measurements before, during, and after both conversations. There were no significant differences between the ICP at baseline and during any conversation. There were also no significant differences between the ICP during type 1 and type 2 conversations. There was, however, a statistically significant decrease in ICP when minimal ICP measurements before type 2 conversations were compared with measurements recorded during type 2 conversation. There were also individual patient fluctuations in both directions during the two conversations.

IMPLICATIONS

The data demonstrated a wide variation of individual patient responses. The results of the current study suggest that the influence of conversation on the ICP is individual and may be influenced by the patient's level of consciousness, and it must be considered on an individual basis. In patients with a GCS less than 5, verbal language in general may not be interpreted and may therefore have no effect on the ICP. Because of the many variables that were impossible to control and the small sample, the findings need further validation. There is need to scrutinize the content of conversation at the patient's bedside and to continue research to identify environmental influences on ICP. Further studies investigating a variety of conversational situations such as family and therapeutic dialogue or gentle tactile stimulation may be beneficial to the field of neuroscience nursing.

monitoring, clinicians have been interested in the waveforms associated with intracranial dynamics. As with arterial and pulmonary artery waves, the ICP wave has a systolic and a diastolic component (Fig. 27-4). Except in the research setting, little is being done in pulse-wave analysis of ICP waves, although recent reports have indicated that intracranial compliance may be assessable through the analysis of pulse waves. Instead, attention has focused on the ICP wave form *trend* or the trend of ICP over time. The three waves identified were first described by Lundberg[10] in the 1960s as A, B, and C waves (Fig. 27-5). These waves reflect spontaneous alterations in ICP associated with respiration, systemic blood pressure, and deteriorating neurological status.

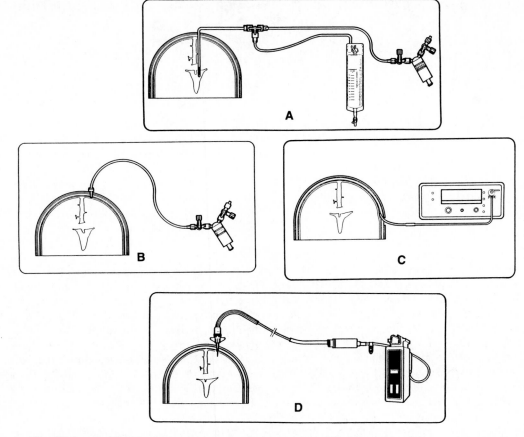

Fig. 27-3 **A,** Ventricular pressure monitoring system. **B,** Subarachnoid pressure monitoring system. **C,** Epidural pressure monitoring system. **D,** Intraparenchymal pressure monitoring system. (Courtesy Camino Laboratories, San Diego, Calif.)

Table 27-1 Comparison of ICP monitoring systems

System	Advantages	Disadvantages
Ventricular catheter	Reliable measurement within CSF Access for CSF drainage and sampling Access for determination of volume-pressure curve	Difficulty locating lateral ventricle Risk of intracerebral bleeding or edema at cannula track Risk of infection Need for transducer repositioning with head movement
Subarachnoid bolt/ screw	Useful if ventricles are small No penetration of brain Decreased risk of infection	Unable to drain CSF Unreliable pressure when high ICP herniates brain into bolt Requires intact skull Need for transducer repositioning with head movement
Epidural sensor	Ease of insertion No dural penetration Lower risk of infection No adjustment of transducer needed with head movement	Unable to drain CSF Unable to recalibrate or rezero after placement Questionable accuracy of sensing ICP through dura Separate large monitoring system required
Fiberoptic transducer-tipped catheter	Versatile system Able to be placed in three different areas of cerebrum Able to monitor intraparenchymal pressure Access for CSF drainage with ventricular system No adjustment of transducer needed with head movement	Catheter relatively fragile Unable to recalibrate or rezero after placement Separate monitoring system required

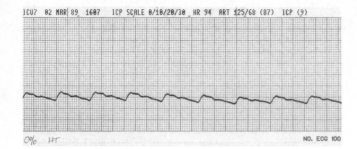

ICU7 02 MAR 89 1607 ICP SCALE 0/10/20/30 _ HR 94 ART 125/68 (87) ICP (9)

0% HT   NO. ECG 100

Fig. 27-4 Intracranial pressure waveform.

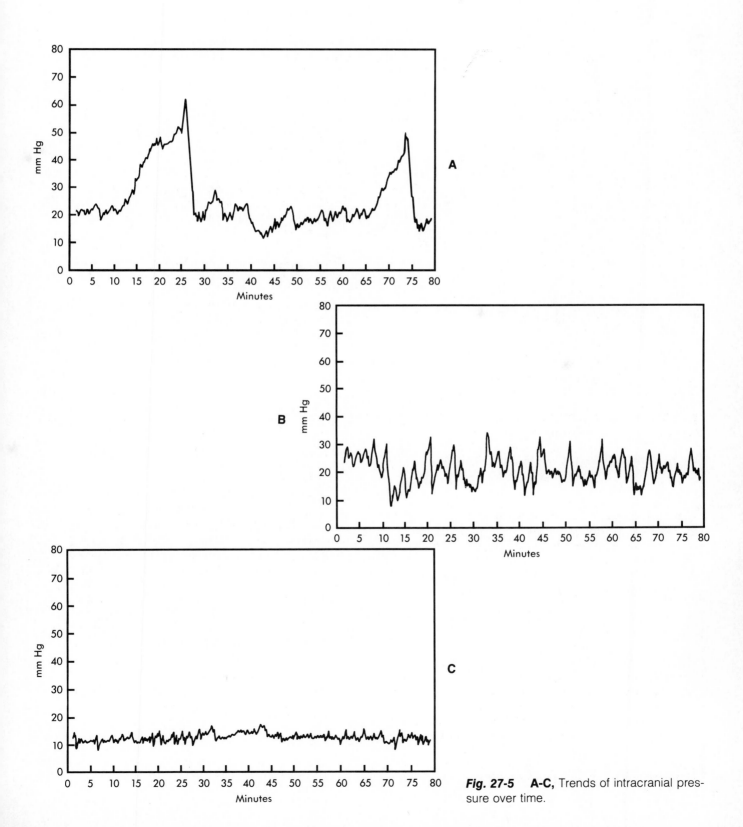

A

B

C

Fig. 27-5 **A-C,** Trends of intracranial pressure over time.

A waves, also called plateau waves because of their distinctive shape, are the most clinically significant of the three types. A waves usually occur in an already elevated baseline ICP (>20 mm Hg) and are characterized by a sudden transient increase of ICP of 50 to 100 mm Hg that lasts for 5 to 20 minutes before this pressure wave returns to its previous baseline. Plateau waves are believed significant because of the reduced cerebral perfusion pressure associated with ICP in the 50 to 100 mm Hg range. Transient signs of intracranial hypertension such as a decreased level of consciousness, bradycardia, pupillary changes, or respiratory changes may accompany these waves. It has been suggested that prolonged increases in ICP associated with plateau waves could result in transient as well as permanent cell damage from ischemia. Management of A waves is directed at the reduction of the high pressure and prevention of other plateau waves.

B waves are sharp, rhythmic oscillations with a sawtooth appearance that occur every 30 seconds to 2 minutes and can raise the ICP up to 50 mm Hg. Although the significance of B waves has not been determined, they are usually associated with fluctuating or "unstable" ICP and are frequently a precursor to plateau waves.

C waves, smaller rhythmic waves that occur every 4 to 8 minutes, occur at normal levels of ICP. C waves are related to normal fluctuations in respirations and systemic arterial pressure.

MANAGEMENT OF INTRACRANIAL HYPERTENSION

Once intracranial hypertension is documented, therapy must be prompt to prevent secondary insults. All therapies are directed toward reducing one or more of the components (blood, brain, CSF) that lie within the intracranial vault. A major goal of therapy is to determine the cause of the elevated pressure and, if possible, remove the cause.[26] Com-

---

MANAGEMENT OF INTRACRANIAL HYPERTENSION

1. Keep patient's head elevated 30-45 degrees and in neutral plane.
2. Maintain controlled ventilation to an arterial partial pressure of carbon dioxide (Paco₂) of 25-30 torr with adequate sedation and muscle relaxants.
3. Maintain arterial partial pressure of oxygen (Pao₂) >70 torr.
4. Maintain systemic arterial pressure between 100 and 160 mm Hg systolic.
5. Maintain normothermia.
6. Use prophylactic anticonvulsants.
7. Perform ventricular drainage if possible.
8. Administer lidocaine intravenous (IV) bolus as pretreatment for suctioning.
9. Administer mannitol (0.25-1 mg/kg) as needed.
10. Administer high-dose barbiturate therapy as needed.

---

puted tomography becomes invaluable in identifying mass lesions that can be surgically evacuated.[3] In the absence of a surgically treatable mass lesion, intracranial hypertensionis treated medically. Nurses play an important role in rapid assessment and implementation of appropriate therapies for reducing ICP (see the box in the previous column).

Patient Positioning

Positioning of the patient is a significant factor in both the prevention and treatment of elevated ICP. Positions that allow proper venous return are ones that maintain the head and neck elevated 30 to 45 degrees and in a neutral position at all times. In these positions, gravity enhances venous drainage from the brain and head.[15,24]

Positions that impede venous return from the brain cause spikes in ICP. Obstruction of jugular veins or an increase in intrathoracic or intraabdominal pressure is communicated as increased pressure throughout the open venous system, thereby impeding drainage from the brain and increasing ICP. Positions that decrease venous return from the head (that is, Trendelenburg, prone, extreme flexion of the hips, and angulation of the neck) should be avoided. Other impediments to cerebral venous drainage are positive end-expiratory pressure (PEEP) >5 to 10 cm H₂O pressure, coughing, suctioning, tight tracheostomy tube ties, and the Valsalva maneuver.

Controlled Ventilation

Controlled hyperventilation is an important adjunct of therapy for the patient with increased ICP. If the carbon dioxide pressure (Pco₂) can be reduced from its normal level of 35 to 40 mm Hg to a range of 25 to 30 mm Hg in the patient with intracranial hypertension, vasoconstriction of cerebral arteries, reduction of cerebral blood flow, and increased venous return will result. Reducing the intracranial blood volume results in a general reduction in ICP.[26] It is well documented that high levels of Pco₂ cause cerebral vasodilation and contribute to elevated ICP. For this reason, Pco₂ levels greater than 40 mm Hg are considered dangerous.

The brain requires a constant supply of oxygen adequate to meet the demands of cerebral metabolism. Therefore maintaining uninterrupted oxygenation is of utmost importance in the management of the brain injured. In addition, hypoxia is a profound stimulus to increase cerebral blood flow and cerebral blood volume; therefore inadequate oxygenation in the presence of poor intracranial compliance will increase ICP.[18]

Although it is evident that hypoxemia should be avoided, no benefits can be gained from excessively high levels of oxygen. In fact, increasing inspired oxygen concentrations (FIo₂) above 60% may lead to toxic changes in lung tissue. With the increasing use of devices that monitor oxygen saturation (that is, pulse oximeter and mixed venous oxygen saturation [Svo₂] monitors), there is greater awareness of the circumstances such as suctioning and restlessness that can cause oxygen desaturation and, therefore, elevate ICP.

Sedation and Muscle Relaxants

Any treatment modality that increases the incidence of noxious stimulation to the patient carries with it the potential for increasing ICP. Such noxious stimuli include pain secondary to injuries sustained with the initial trauma, the presence of an endotracheal tube, coughing, suctioning, repositioning, bathing, and many routine nursing care procedures. Even patients who do not seem to move may respond to paralysis with decreased ICP, presumably because of improved chest wall compliance.[21]

To ensure adequate ventilation (PCO$_2$ of 25 to 30 and oxygen pressure [PO$_2$] >70) and in anticipation of the deleterious effects of noxious stimuli on ICP, sedatives alone or in combination with muscle relaxants may be used. Their use is only recommended in patients who have an ICP monitor in place, since sedation and especially muscle relaxants make a neurological assessment unreliable. Although sedation of the unconscious patient can obscure portions of the neurological examination, its benefit may outweigh the risks.

The use of muscle relaxants without sedation is not recommended. Agents such as pancuronium bromide, for example, have no analgesic effect and do not adequately protect patients from pain and the physiological responses that can occur from pain-producing procedures and, most importantly, from stimulation originating in the larynx. The need to have an endotracheal tube in place for long periods of time makes it necessary to sedate most and paralyze many of these patients.[12]

Temperature Control

Cerebral metabolic rate is directly proportional to body temperature, and it increases 5% to 7% per degree centigrade of increase in body temperture.[13] This fact is significant because as the cerebral metabolic rate increases, blood flow to the brain must increase to meet the tissue demands. To avoid the increase in blood volume that is associated with an increased cerebral metabolic rate, hyperthermia must be prevented in the brain-injured patient. Antipyretics and cooling devices should be used when appropriate while the source of the fever is sought. Conversely, hypothermia reduces cerebral metabolic rate. At 30° C cerebral metabolic rate is decreased 50%. Maintenance of body temperature between 30° and 37° C may be beneficial if full cardiopulmonary support is given and if shivering, which greatly increases the body's metabolic requirements, is prevented. Sedation and neuromuscular blocking agents or phenothiazines are used to control shivering when hypothermia is used. Because of problems with intravascular hypovolemia, metabolic acidosis, and brain swelling associated with rewarming, the use of hypothermia for ICP control has not found wide acceptance.[18]

Persistent fluctuation and/or hypothermia or hyperthermia in conjunction with head injury is a grave prognostic sign and has usually been associated with death or a persistent vegetative state. These patients may represent a group with severe hypothalamic injury.[13]

Blood Pressure Control

Sustained systolic arterial hypertension (>160 mm Hg) in conjunction with elevated ICP should be vigorously treated. Control of systemic arterial hypertension may require nothing more than the administration of a sedative agent. Small, frequent doses may be sufficient to blunt noxious stimuli and prevent their triggering rises in blood pressure. In cases in which sedation has proven inadequate in controlling systemic arterial hypertension, primary antihypertensive agents are used. Care must be taken in choosing antihypertensive agents because many of the peripheral vasodilators are also cerebral vasodilators (for example, nitroprusside and nitroglycerin). It is believed, however, that all antihypertensives cause some degree of cerebral vasodilation. To reduce this vasodilating effect, it has been suggested that cotreatment with beta blockers (for example, propranolol and labetalol) may be beneficial.[18]

Seizure Control

The incidence of posttraumatic seizures has been estimated at 5% in the head-injured population. Because of the risk of a secondary ischemic insult associated with seizures, many physicians prescribe anticonvulsant medications prophylactically. Seizures cause metabolic requirements to increase, resulting in elevated cerebral blood flow, cerebral blood volume, and ICP even in paralyzed patients. If blood flow cannot match demand, ischemia will develop, cerebral energy stores will be depleted, and irreversible neuronal destruction will occur.[18]

The usual anticonvulsant regimen for seizure control includes phenytoin and/or phenobarbital in therapeutic doses. The loading dose for phenytoin is 15 to 18 mg/kg, and the loading dose for phenobarbital is 4 to 8 mg/kg. Maintenance doses of phenytoin are administered to achieve a therapeutic blood level of 10 to 20 μg/ml. Maintenance doses of phenobarbital are administered to keep the blood level at 2 to 3 mg%.[2]

When administering phenytoin intravenously, it must be given with normal saline solution and administered slowly (less than 50 mg/minute). Rapid IV administration has caused hypotension and heart block. Intramuscular injection of phenytoin is not recommended because of its poor absorption from the tissues. Finally, when administering phenytoin orally in conjunction with tube feedings, therapeutic levels should be closely monitored because absorption apparently is erratic. One recommendation to improve the absorption of phenytoin when given with enteral feedings is to discontinue the tube feeding 1 hour before the dose and reinstitute the feeding 1 hour after the dose. The effectiveness of this method in promoting the steady reabsorption of phenytoin needs substantiation through research. When administering the phenobarbital loading dose, careful monitoring of the patient's vital signs is necessary to avoid a precipitous drop in blood pressure.

The question of the need for anticonvulsants after cerebral trauma remains unanswered. Studies of this issue, including the risks and benefits of anticonvulsant therapy, are currently being undertaken.

Lidocaine

Various forms of sensory stimulation (including tracheal intubation, laryngoscopy, and endotracheal suctioning) may provoke marked increases in ICP and MAP. One therapy used to prevent cerebral ischemia and acute intracranial hypertension has been the administration of lidocaine through an endotracheal tube or intravenously before nasotracheal suctioning.[26]

Lidocaine was initially introduced as a local anesthetic in 1948, and it is believed that its anesthetic properties make it efficacious in blunting ICP spikes secondary to tracheal stimulation. Studies have found that peak lidocaine concentrations are linearly related to the administered dose and that the rate of absorption depends on the vascularity of the site of administration.[18,26] It has also been documented that lidocaine is initially distributed to the lungs, then to the heart and kidneys, and then to muscle and adipose tissue.

Administering lidocaine prophylactically before endotracheal suctioning has been widely practiced. In most cases, 50 to 100 mg is administered intravenously approximately 2 minutes before suctioning the patient. If the endotracheal route is chosen, 2 cc of 4% lidocaine is the preferred dose, and suctioning must be completed within 5 minutes of administering the drug. It is believed that adherence to this procedure protects the patient from the associated increases in ICP that occur with suctioning. A number of studies are in progress investigating the usefulness of lidocaine in this area.

Cerebrospinal Fluid Drainage

CSF drainage for intracranial hypertension may be used along with other treatment modalities. CSF drainage is accomplished by the insertion of a pliable catheter into the anterior horn of the lateral ventricle, preferably on the nondominant side. Such drainage can help support the patient through periods of cerebral edema by controlling spikes in ICP. One of the major advantages of the ventriculostomy is its dual role as both a monitoring device and a treatment modality. Because CSF provides a favorable medium for the development of infection, it is essential that flawless aseptic technique be followed during insertion and maintenance of the system. The ventricular system is connected to a drainage bag and is then maintained as a closed system for the period of time the ventriculostomy remains in place—usually 3 to 5 days.

When using this system for treatment, there are two ways to accomplish removal of CSF: it can be removed intermittently when ICP becomes elevated, or it can be removed continuously, with the ventriculostomy bag at a predetermined level above the lateral ventricle. Intermittent drainage involves draining CSF for brief periods (30 to 120 seconds) when ICP exceeds the upper limits of normal. Frequent periods of drainage (more than four times per hour) should be reported to the physician. Continuous drainage is most often ordered when the patient has significant amounts of blood in the subarachnoid space (for example, with a subarachnoid hemorrhage). The ventricular drainage bag is placed 10 to 15 cm above the level of the third ventricle so that if ICP exceeds 10 to 12 mm Hg, CSF will be shunted into the drainage bag. One very important concept to keep in mind is that when intracranial hypertension or a mass lesion is suspected, a lumbar puncture is contraindicated because of the risk of downward herniation.

Diuretics

Osmotic agents. The effectiveness of osmotic agents in the reduction of ICP has been known for decades. The mechanism by which these diuretics reduce ICP continues as a subject of investigational interest. One belief is that these agents act by remaining relatively impermeable to the blood-brain barrier, thereby drawing water from normal brain to plasma.[8,12] The direction of flow is from the hypoconcentrated tissue to the hyperconcentrated cerebral vasculature. If the situation becomes reversed and the tissue becomes hyperconcentrated in relation to the cerebral vasculature, a *rebound phenomenon* could occur. These agents have little direct effect on edematous cerebral tissue situated in an area of defective blood-brain barrier; instead, they require an intact blood-brain barrier for osmosis to occur.

The three best-known osmotic diuretics are urea, mannitol, and glycerol. Urea, the first osmotic diuretic widely accepted in the treatment of intracranial hypertension, was introduced by Javid[8] in the late 1950s. Although urea is still used in some clinical settings, mannitol has gained wide acceptance as the osmotic diuretic of choice. Mannitol, a larger molecule than urea, is retained almost entirely in the extracellular compartment and has little to none of the rebound effect noted with urea. It has also been suggested that mannitol in particular improves perfusion to ischemic areas of the brain, producing cerebral vasoconstriction and resulting in a reduction of ICP.[12] Glycerol, the effect of which is similar on the brain to that of mannitol, has the advantage of oral administration. It also apparently is a safe drug for long-term use. The fact that glycerol can be administered orally has no real benefit in the medical treatment of the severely brain-injured patient.

Perhaps the most frequent difficulty associated with the use of osmotic agents is the production of electrolyte disturbances. Careful attention should be paid to body weight and fluid and electrolyte stability. Serum osmolality should be kept between 300 to 320 mOsm/L. Hypernatremia and hypokalemia are frequently associated with repeated administration of osmotic agents. Central venous pressure readings should be monitored to prevent hypovolemia. The usual dose of mannitol is 0.5 to 1.5 g/kg. Recent data suggest that small doses (0.25 g/kg) decrease ICP as rapidly and profounding as higher doses (1 g/kg), but the effect is somewhat less prolonged (4 to 6 hours).[18] Smaller doses of mannitol simplify fluid and electrolyte management, and their use is encouraged whenever possible.[12,26]

Nonosmotic agents. Nonosmotic diuretics have also been used to decrease ICP. Furosemide, one such nonosmotic diuretic, may act differently from osmotic agents by pulling sodium and water from edematous areas and, perhaps, by decreasing CSF production. One advantage of furosemide administration over the use of osmotic diuretics is that its effect is not generally associated with increases in serum osmolality. Therefore electrolyte imbalances may not be as severe with the use of nonosmotic diuretics.

Another diuretic in this category is acetazolamide. The action of this drug is to reduce the rate at which CSF is produced in the choroid plexus. Generally, the use of acetazolamide in head-injured patients is contraindicated because of its cerebral vasodilative effect.

High-Dose Barbiturate Therapy

Barbiturate therapy is a treatment protocol developed for the management of uncontrolled intracranial hypertension that has not responded to the conventional treatments previously described. Uncontrolled ICP is described in the literature as follows:[13,14,20]

1. ICP >20 mm Hg for 30 minutes or more, with unresponsiveness to aggressive use of conventional therapies
2. ICP >40 mm Hg for 15 minutes or more, CPP <50 mm Hg, or both

In the early 1970s barbiturate therapy consisting of administering large doses of short-acting barbiturates to induce and maintain coma was introduced.[22] Although the specific action of barbiturates in the reduction of ICP is unclear, several theories exist to explain their effect on the central nervous system and the subsequent cerebral protection they provide. Barbiturates increase the cerebral vascular resistance and therefore decrease cerebral blood flow, resulting in a reduction in intracranial volume. Systemic blood pressure is also lowered, reducing hydrostatic pressure in the damaged cerebral tissue and helping arrest edema formation.[25] Barbiturates also slow cerebral metabolism by reducing the functional electrical generation of the neurons. This decreased cerebral metabolism thus lessens the glucose and oxygen demands of the brain.[1,23] Barbiturates are also effective anticonvulsants and may suppress subclinical seizure activities. Finally, it has been postulated that barbiturates are scavengers of free radicals and thereby prevent cell membrane damage and destruction.[23,25]

The two most commonly used drugs in high-dose barbiturate therapy are pentobarbital and thiopental. Pentobarbital, a longer-acting barbiturate, is administered in a loading dose of 3 to 5 mg/kg of body weight over a 15-minute period, with a maintenance dose of 1 to 2 mg/kg/hour. Thiopental, a shorter-acting barbiturate, is administered in a loading dose of 1 to 5 mg/kg of body weight and a maintenance dose of 1 to 3 mg/kg/hour. The goal with either of these drugs is a reduction of ICP to 15 to 20 mm Hg while maintaining a MAP of 70 to 80 torr. A therapeutic serum blood level for high-dose barbiturate therapy is 3 to 5 mg%. Patients are maintained on high-dose barbiturate therapy until ICP has been controlled within the normal range for 24 hours. Barbiturates should never be stopped abruptly but should be tapered slowly over approximately 4 days.[12]

The success of barbiturate therapy is directly proportional to the aggressiveness of the previously used conventional therapy. Therefore if hyperventilation, blood pressure control, and osmotic diuretics have not been used to their fullest extent, the addition of barbiturates will create a larger number of good outcomes in patients who might have done as well without their addition.[18] Because of the extensive resources required (extensive invasive monitoring and qualified medical and nursing personnel) and the risks of hypotension and infection, the indiscriminate use of barbiturates is not recommended.[25]

Complications of high-dose barbiturate therapy. Complications of high-dose barbiturate therapy can be disastrous unless a specific and organized approach is used. The complications most frequently encountered are hypotension, hypothermia, and decreased cardiac output. If any occur and are allowed to persist unchecked, the consequences may lead to secondary insults to an already damaged brain. Hypotension, the most common complication, is a result of

---

Nursing Diagnosis and Management
Increased intracranial pressure

- Altered Cerebral Tissue Perfusion related to increased intracranial pressure secondary to brain trauma, hemorrhage, edema, infection, tumor, stroke, or hydrocephalus, p. 581
- Altered Cerebral Tissue Perfusion related to vasospasm secondary to subarachnoid hemorrhage after ruptured intracranial aneurysm or arteriovenous malformation, p. 579
- Potential for Infection risk factors: invasive monitoring devices, p. 346
- Potential for Aspiration risk factors: reduced level of consciousness, depressed cough and gag reflexes, presence of tracheostomy or endotracheal tube, gastrointestinal tube, tube feedings, delayed gastric emptying, and decreased gastrointestinal motility secondary to immobility, p. 489
- Ineffective Airway Clearance related to impaired cough secondary to loss of glottic closure with cuffed tracheostomy or endotracheal tube, p. 476
- Ineffective Breathing Pattern related to respiratory muscle deconditioning secondary to mechanical ventilation, p. 482

---

peripheral vasodilation and can be compounded in an already dehydrated patient who has received large doses of an osmotic diuretic in an attempt to control ICP. Careful monitoring of fluid status by central venous pressure or a pulmonary artery catheter can help in preventing this complication. Hypothermia results from a decrease in basal metabolic rate. This problem can lead to cardiac irritability and arrest if not reversed. To avoid these sequelae, the patient's temperature should be maintained between 33° to 37° C, and warming devices should be used if necessary. Decreased cardiac output results from hypotension or cardiac muscle suppression. It can be avoided by frequent monitoring of fluid status, cardiac output, and serum drug levels. If an adequate cardiac output cannot be maintained in the presence of normothermia, barbiturates must be reduced, regardless of serum levels.

The major unresolved issue in the use of high-dose barbiturates is their effect on outcome after head injury. Several laboratory and clinical trials have been undertaken to address this issue. Results of a multicenter randomized trial of barbiturates found that most elevations of ICP could be controlled with aggressive use of standard therapies of ICP managment. The small subset of patients who fail to achieve ICP control with standard therapy does benefit from the judicious, carefully monitored and administered high-dose barbiturate therapy.[4]

HERNIATION SYNDROMES

The goal of neurological evaluation, ICP monitoring, and treatment of increased ICP is to prevent herniation. Her-

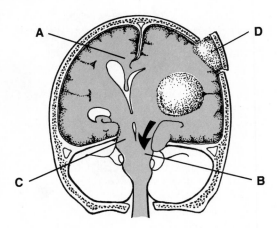

Fig. 27-6 Supratentorial herniation. **A,** Cingulate. **B,** Uncal. **C,** Central. **D,** Transcalvarial.

niation of intracerebral contents results in the shifting of tissue from one compartment of the brain to another and places pressure on cerebral vessels and vital function centers of the brain. If unchecked, herniation rapidly causes death as a result of the cessation of cerebral blood flow and respirations.

Supratentorial Herniation

There are four types of supratentorial herniation syndromes: Central or transtentorial, uncal, cingulate, or transcalvarial (Fig. 27-6).

Uncal herniation. Uncal herniation is the herniation syndrome most often noted. In uncal herniation, a unilateral, expanding mass lesion, usually of the temporal lobe, increases ICP, causing the tip of the temporal lobe (uncus) to displace laterally. Lateral displacement pushes the uncus over the edge of the tentorium, puts pressure on the oculomotor nerve (cranial nerve III) and posterior cerebral artery ipsilateral to the lesion, and flattens the midbrain against the opposite side.

Signs and symptoms of uncal herniation include ipsilateral pupil dilation, respiratory pattern changes leading to respiratory arrest, and contralateral hemiplegia leading to decorticate or decerebrate posturing. If no intervention occurs, uncal herniation results in fixed and dilated pupils, flaccidity, and respiratory arrest.

Central or transtentorial herniation In central herniation an expanding mass lesion of the midline, frontal, parietal, or occipital lobes results in downward displacement of the hemispheres, basal ganglia, and diencephalon through the tentorial notch. Central herniation is often preceded by uncal and cingulate herniation.

Signs and symptoms of central or transtentorial herniation include loss of consciousness, small, reactive pupils progressing to fixed, dilated pupils, respiratory changes leading to respiratory arrest, and decorticate posturing progressing to flaccidity. In the late stages, uncal and central herniation syndromes are similar in their effects on the brainstem.

Cingulate herniation. Cingulate herniation occurs when an expanding lesion of one hemisphere shifts laterally and

forces the cingulate gyrus under the falx cerebri. Cingulate herniation occurs frequently. Whenever a lateral shift is noted on a computed tomographic (CT) scan, cingulate herniation has occurred. Little is known about the effects of cingulate herniation, and there are no signs and symptoms that assist in its diagnosis. Cingulate herniation is not life-threatening on its own, but if the expanding mass lesion that caused cingulate herniation is not controlled, uncal or central herniation will follow.

Transcalvarial herniation. Transcalvarial herniation is the extrusion of cerebral tissue through the cranium. In the presence of severe cerebral edema, transcalvarial herniation occurs through an opening from a skull fracture or craniotomy site.

Infratentorial Herniation

There are two infratentorial herniation syndromes: upward transtentorial herniation and downward cerebellar herniation.

Upward transtentorial herniation. Upward transtentorial herniation occurs when an expanding mass lesion of the cerebellum causes protrusion of the vermis (central area) of the cerebellum and the midbrain upward through the tentorial notch. Compression of the third cranial nerve and diencephalon occur. Obstruction of CSF flow occurs with blockage of the central aqueduct and distortion of the third ventricle. Deterioration occurs rapidly.

Downward cerebellar herniation. Downward cerebellar herniation occurs when an expanding lesion of the cerebellum exerts pressure downward, sending the cerebellar tonsils through the foramen magnum. Compression and displacement of the medulla oblongata occurs, rapidly resulting in respiratory and cardiac arrest.

The best treatment of any of these herniation syndromes is prevention. The goal of accurate assessment, evaluation, and intervention is the prevention of increasing pressure forces inside the cranium that would lead to herniation.

REFERENCES

1. Anderson BJ: The metabolic needs of head trauma victims, J Neurosci Nurs 19(4):211, 1987.
2. Commission for the Control of Epilepsy and Its Consequences: Plan for nationwide action on epilepsy, vol 4, DHEW Pub No (NIH) 78-279, Bethesda, Md, 1978, National Institutes of Health.
3. Eisenberg HM, Weiner RN, and Tabaddor K: Emergency care: initial evaluation. In Cooper PR, editor: Head injury, ed 2, Baltimore, 1987, The Williams & Wilkins Co.
4. Eisenberg HM and others: High-dose barbiturate control of elevated intracranial pressure in patients with severe head injury, J Neurosurg 69:15, 1988.
5. Guillaume J and Janny P: Monometrie intracranienne continue; interet physio-pathologique et clinique de la methode, Presse Med 59:953, 1951.
6. Hickey JV: The clinical practice of neurological and neurosurgical nursing, ed 2, Philadelphia, 1986, JB Lippincott Co.
7. Hopkins CC: Infection: pathogenesis, prevention, and treatment. In Ropper AH, Kennedy SK, and Zervas NT, editors: Neurological and neurosurgical intensive care, Baltimore, 1983, University Park Press.
8. Javid M: Urea in intracranial surgery: a new method, J Neurosurg 18:51, 1961.
9. Jennett B and Teasdale G: Management of head injuries, Philadelphia, 1981, FA Davis Co.

10. Lundberg N: Continuous recording and control of ventricular fluid pressure in neurosurgical practice, Acta Psychiatr Neurol Scand Suppl 149:1, 1960.

11. Marmarou A and Tabaddor K: Intracranial pressure: physiology and pathophysiology. In Cooper PR, editor: Head Injury, ed 2, Baltimore, 1987, The Williams & Wilkins Co.

12. Marshall LF and Marshall SB: Medical management of intracranial pressure. In Cooper PR, editor: Head injury, ed 2, Baltimore, 1987, The Williams & Wilkins Co.

13. Marshall LF, Smith RW, and Shapiro HM: The outcome with aggressive treatment in severe head injuries, J Neurosurg 50:20, 1979.

14. Miller JD: Barbiturates and raised intracranial pressure, Ann Neurol 6(3):189, 1979.

15. Mitchell PH: Intracranial hypertension: influence of nursing care activities, Nurs Clin North Am 21(4):563, 1986.

16. Mitchell PH, Amos D, and Astley C: Nursing and ICP: studies of two clinical problems. In Miller JD, editor: Intracranial pressure VI, New York, 1986, Springer-Verlag.

17. Rockoff MA and Kennedy SK: Physiology and clinical aspects of raised intracranial pressure. In Ropper AH, Kennedy SK, and Zerfas NT, editors: Neurologic and neurosurgical intensive care, Baltimore, 1983, University Park Press.

18. Rockoff MA and Ropper AH: Treatment of intracranial hypertension. In Ropper AH, Kennedy SK, and Zervas NT, editors: Neurologic and neurosurgical intensive care, Baltimore, 1983, University Park Press.

19. Rockoff MA, Marshall LF, and Shapiro HM: High dose barbiturate therapy in humans: a clinical review of 60 patients, Ann Neurol 3:83, 1979.

20. Rudy EB: Advanced neurological and neurosurgical nursing, St Louis, 1984, The CV Mosby Co.

21. Shapiro HM: Intracranial hypertension: therapeutic and anesthetic considerations, Anesthesia 43:445, 1975.

22. Shapiro HM, Wyte SR, and Loeser J: Barbiturate-augmented hypothermia for reduction of persistent intracranial hypertension, J Neurosurg 40:90, 1974.

23. Siesjo BK and others: Brain metabolism in the critically ill, Crit Care Med 4:283, 1976.

24. Snyder M: Relation of nursing activities to increases in intracranial pressure, J Adv Nurs 8:273, 1983.

25. Swann KW: Management of severe head injury. In Ropper AH, Kennedy SK, and Zervas NT, editors: Neurological and neurosurgical intensive care, Baltimore, 1983, University Park Press.

26. Wrobel CJ and Marshall LF: Closed head injury management dilemmas. In Long DM, editor: Current therapy in neurological surgery, vol 2, St Louis, 1985, The CV Mosby Co.

CHAPTER

28

Neurological Care Plans

THEORETICAL BASIS AND MANAGEMENT

CHAPTER OBJECTIVES

- Discuss the theoretical basis for such neurological phenomena as altered cerebral tissue perfusion, ineffective thermoregulation, dysreflexia, and unilateral neglect.
- Develop nursing diagnoses for critical care patients with neurological alterations.
- Identify measurable outcome criteria for critical care patients with neurological alterations.
- Formulate nursing management strategies for critical care patients with such neurological phenomena as altered cerebral tissue perfusion, ineffective thermoregulation, dysreflexia, and unilateral neglect.
- Develop comprehensive nursing management approaches for critical care patients experiencing pain or sensory-perceptual alterations.

ALTERED CEREBRAL TISSUE PERFUSION
Theoretical Basis and Management

Altered cerebral tissue perfusion does not account for all of the pathological processes in the brain that cause neurological dysfunctions. However, the terminology is consistent with the North American Nursing Diagnosis Association (NANDA) list of approved nursing diagnoses that, at the time of this publication, best describe the patient with failure of the normal intracranial compensatory mechanisms that maintain adequate cerebral perfusion.

Alterations in cerebral tissue perfusion can occur in very localized or widespread areas of the brain and can lead to neuronal ischemia and dysfunction. Localized areas of decreased cerebral perfusion can be caused by embolic or thrombotic strokes. Brain injuries from trauma, tumor, or hemorrhage result in localized or widespread swelling and edema, which also lead to decreased cerebral tissue perfusion. Cerebral ischemia can occur from vasospasm, the abnormal narrowing of cerebral arteries that often occurs after intracranial aneurysm rupture. This vasospasm can occur in vessels local or distant to the site of rupture, resulting in focal, segmental, or diffuse areas of decreased cerebral tissue perfusion.[32]

Increased intracranial pressure (ICP), a major cause of widespread decreased cerebral perfusion, represents a primary concern of neuroscience nurses caring for patients with neurological problems. It and its nursing management are the focus of this discussion.

To enable the reader to better understand the physiological mechanisms that can lead to decreased cerebral tissue perfusion, normal cerebral homeostasis is reviewed. Normal cerebral homeostasis is a function of cerebral spinal fluid (CSF) dynamics, cerebral blood flow and metabolism, and ICP.[48]

CSF dynamics. Under normal circumstances there is a balance between the rate of CSF production and the rate of CSF absorption, with the rate of absorption being pressure dependent. As ICP increases, a compensatory mechanism of the brain attempts to maintain normal ICP and cerebral homeostasis by increasing the rate of CSF absorption. Further compensation, leading to a reduction in ICP, occurs through displacement of some of the CSF from the cerebral subarachnoid spaces into the more distensible spinal subarachnoid space. Any block in the circulation or absorption of CSF can lead to failure of this cerebral homeostatic mechanism and result in increased ICP.

Cerebral blood flow and metabolism. The brain demands a constant and generous supply of oxygen, glucose, and other metabolic substances to maintain physiological functioning. Adequate cerebral blood flow is essential to supply these substrates. When cerebral blood flow falls below 18 to 20 ml/100 g brain tissue/minute, ischemic brain damage can occur. Major factors affecting cerebral blood flow include systemic blood pressure, arterial blood gases, metabolic demands of the brain, and ICP.[48]

Normally, cerebral autoregulation maintains adequate cerebral blood flow in the presence of varying systemic blood pressures. In the presence of central nervous system (CNS) injury, cerebral autoregulation is disrupted, and cerebral blood flow will change passively with systemic blood pres-

578

sure. Hypotension can thus lead to decreased cerebral blood flow.

Cerebral perfusion pressure (CPP) represents the difference between the mean systemic arterial pressure (MSAP) and the ICP (MSAP − ICP = CPP). This simple formula is readily adapted to the clinical setting if the patient has an ICP monitoring device in use. To avoid ischemic damage, the brain requires a CPP of 60 to 80 mm Hg.[42] Decreased blood pressure (BP) and/or increased ICP can thus lead to decreased CPP, resulting in cerebral ischemia. For instance, if the MSAP equals 80 mm Hg and the ICP equals 30 mm Hg, then MSAP − ICP = 50 mm Hg, a dangerously low CPP.

Arterial blood gases exert a profound effect on CBF. Carbon dioxide, which affects the pH of the blood, is a potent vasoactive substance. Carbon dioxide retention (hypercarbia) leads to cerebral vasodilation, with increased cerebral blood volume, whereas hypocarbia leads to cerebral vasoconstriction and a reduction in cerebral blood volume. Hyperventilation therapy to induce hypocarbia is often used as a means of reducing ICP by reducing cerebral blood volume within the cranium. Prolonged hypocarbia, however, especially at an arterial partial pressure of carbon dioxide ($PaCO_2$) less than 20 mm Hg, can produce cerebral ischemia.[48]

Low arterial partial pressure of oxygen (PaO_2), especially below 50 mm Hg, leads to cerebral vasodilation, which increases the intracranial blood volume and can contribute to increased ICP. The brain is thus exposed to ischemia directly through arterial hypoxemia, as well as through increased ICP. High PaO_2 has not been shown to affect cerebral blood flow in either direction.

Cerebral blood volume may further be reduced through compression of the intracranial veins, expressing blood out of the brain. This is another compensatory mechanism of the brain for maintaining normal ICP.

Metabolic activity in the brain significantly influences cerebral blood flow. Normally, when cerebral metabolic activity increases, there is a corresponding increase in cerebral blood flow to meet the demand.[48] Any pathological process that decreases cerebral blood flow could lead to a mismatch between metabolic demand and blood supply,

resulting in cerebral ischemia. Barbiturate therapy is based on the principle of reducing cerebral metabolic rate in the presence of uncontrolled intracranial hypertension (prolonged increased ICP).

Intracranial pressure. ICP refers to the pressure within the cranium. It is determined by the amounts of CSF, brain substance with its associated intracellular and extracellular fluid, and intracranial blood volume contained in venous, capillary, and arterial vessels that are present within the cranium at any one time and by the relationship of these components to the capacity of the cranium. The amounts of the three components vary from time to time. If there is an increase in volume in any one of the components or the addition of a volume such as a tumor, there must be a reciprocal decrease in the volume of another component or ICP will rise. This concept is known as the modified Monro-Kellie hypothesis.[42]

ICP is measured directly by monitoring CSF pressure in the ventricles of the brain or in the cerebral subarachnoid space or by monitoring intraparenchymal pressure. Indirect monitoring of CSF pressure can be performed with extradural or subdural fiberoptic sensors. Normal ICP is approximately 0 to 15 mm Hg.

Increased ICP (>15 mm Hg) is present in several pathological states, including closed head injury, meningitis, and Reye's syndrome. Sustained increased ICP for longer than 15 to 30 minutes produces secondary ischemic damage to the brain beyond that produced by the primary brain pathology.[32]

As previously discussed, CSF and cerebral blood volume can change to maintain normal ICP. Aside from cerebral atrophy which takes time, the brain tissue itself has little capacity to compensate for increased intracranial volume. Since the brain is locked within its rigid cranial vault, the only compensation an edematous and swollen brain has is to move from a compartment of high pressure to a compartment of lower pressure—a phenomenon termed herniation.[42] This life-threatening event represents the ultimate ischemic brain insult. Medical and nursing measures are directed toward early detection and treatment of increased ICP and prevention of brain herniation. See Chapter 27 for a discussion of brain herniation.

Altered Cerebral Tissue Perfusion related to vasospasm secondary to subarachnoid hemorrhage after ruptured intracranial aneurysm or arteriovenous malformation

NOTE: Vasospasm takes place in two phases. The acute phase occurs within minutes or hours of aneurysm rupture and serves as a protective mechanism by decreasing blood flow to the site and lessening the chance of rebleeding. Chronic vasospasm begins approximately 3 to 4 days after aneurysm rupture and persists for days to weeks.[34,47] Early management of subarachnoid hemorrhage also includes aggressive treatment to prevent or combat vasospasm. Therefore this care plan addresses the simultaneous management of subarachnoid hemorrhage and vasospasm.

DEFINING CHARACTERISTICS
Subarachnoid hemorrhage
■ Aneurysm grading system according to Hunt and Hess[24]
Grade I: minimal bleed
    Asymptomatic or minimal headache
    Slight nuchal rigidity
Grade II: mild bleed
    Moderate-to-severe headache
    Nuchal rigidity
    Minimal neurological deficit (e.g., possible cranial nerve palsies—oculomotor [cranial nerve III] most

Continued.

Altered Cerebral Tissue Perfusion related to vasospasm secondary to subarachnoid hemorrhage after ruptured intracranial aneurysm or arteriovenous malformation—cont'd

common; unilateral pupillary dilation, ptosis, and dysconjugate gaze)

    Grade III: moderate bleed

        Drowsiness

        Confusion

        Nuchal rigidity

        Possible mild focal neurological deficits

    Grade IV: moderate-to-severe bleed

        Very decreased level of consciousness, stupor

        Possible moderate-to-severe hemiparesis

        Possible early posturing (decorticate or decerebrate)

    Grade V: severe bleed

        Profound coma

        Posturing

        Moribund appearance

- Pathological reflexes resulting from meningeal irritation
  Kernig's sign: resistance to full extension of the leg at the knee when the hip is flexed
  Brudzinski's sign: flexion of the hip and knee during passive neck flexion
- Photophobia
- Nausea and vomiting

Vasospasm related to subarachnoid hemorrhage
- Worsening headache
- Confusion and decreasing level of consciousness
- Focal motor deficits such as unilateral weakness of extremities
- Speech deficits such as slurring, receptive or expressive aphasia
- Increasing BP

OUTCOME CRITERIA

- Patient is oriented to time, place, person, and situation.
- Pupils are equal and normoreactive.
- BP is within patient's norm.
- Motor function is bilaterally equal.
- Headache, nausea, and vomiting are absent.
- Patient has no signs or symptoms of increased ICP and herniation as evidenced by ICP 0-15 mm Hg and by above criteria.
- Patient verbalizes importance of and displays compliance with reduced activity.

NURSING INTERVENTIONS *AND RATIONALE*

1. Continue to monitor the assessment parameters listed under "Defining Characteristics." Additionally, assess for indicators of increased ICP and brain herniation (see care plan, "Altered Cerebral Perfusion related to increased ICP"). *ICP will increase during vasospasm only when caused by the edema resulting from brain infarction.*

2. Anticipate early surgical intervention for patients with grade I or II symptoms.
3. Maintain patent airway and adequate ventilation, and supply oxygen as ordered *to prevent hypoxemia and hypercarbia.*
4. Monitor ABG values and maintain Pao_2 >80 mm Hg and $Paco_2$ <45 mm Hg.
5. If hypertensive-hypervolemic therapy is prescribed, administer crystalloid and colloid IV fluids and monitor pulmonary capillary wedge pressure (PCWP), pulmonary artery diastolic pressure (PAD), systemic vascular resistance (SVR), and BP to achieve and maintain prescribed parameters. Systolic blood pressure is usually maintained at 150-160 mm Hg.
6. Monitor lung sounds and chest x-ray reports *because of the risk of pulmonary edema associated with fluid overload.*
7. Anticipate administration of calcium channel blockers such as nifedipine *to decrease peripheral vascular resistance and cause vasodilation.*
8. For patients in severe vasospasm, anticipate barbiturate administration *to decrease cerebral metabolic rate.*
9. Keep head of bed flat *to optimize cerebral perfusion.*
10. Rebleeding is a potential complication of aneurysm rupture; to PREVENT REBLEEDING, the following interventions constitute subarachnoid precautions:
    - Ensure bed rest in a quiet environment *to lessen external stimuli.*
    - Maintain darkened room *to lessen symptoms of photophobia.*
    - Restrict visitors and instruct them to keep conversation as nonstressful as possible.
    - Administer prescribed sedatives as needed *to reduce anxiety and promote rest.*
    - Administer analgesics as prescribed *to relieve or lessen headache.*
    - Provide a soft, high-fiber diet and stool softeners *to prevent constipation, which can lead to straining and increased risk of rebleeding.*
    - Assist with activities of daily living (feeding, bathing, dressing, toileting).
    - Avoid any activity that could lead to increased ICP; ensure that the patient does not flex the hips beyond 90 degrees and avoids neck hyperflexion, hyperextension, or lateral hyperrotation *that could impede jugular venous return.*

Altered Cerebral Tissue Perfusion related to increased intracranial pressure secondary to brain trauma, hemorrhage, edema, infection, tumor, stroke, hydrocephalus

DEFINING CHARACTERISTICS

- ICP >15 mm Hg, sustained for 15-30 minutes
- Headache
- Vomiting, with or without nausea
- Seizures
- Decrease in Glasgow Coma Scale of two or more points from baseline
- Alteration in level of consciousness, ranging from restlessness to coma
- Change in orientation: disoriented to time and/or place and/or person
- Difficulty or inability to follow simple commands
- Increasing systolic BP of more than 20 mm Hg with widening pulse pressure
- Bradycardia
- Irregular respiratory pattern (e.g., Cheyne-Stokes, central neurogenic hyperventilation, ataxic, apneustic)
- Change in response to painful stimuli (e.g., purposeful to inappropriate or absent response)
- Signs of impending brain herniation, which, in addition to the above, may include the following:
    Hemiparesis or hemiplegia
    Hemisensory changes
    Unequal pupil size (1 mm or more difference)
    Failure of pupil to react to light
    Dysconjugate gaze and inability to move one eye beyond midline if third, fourth, or sixth cranial nerves involved
    Loss of oculocephalic or oculovestibular reflexes
    Possible decorticate or decerebrate posturing

OUTCOME CRITERIA

- ICP is ≤15 mm Hg.
- CPP is >60 mm Hg.
- Clinical signs of increased ICP as described above are

NURSING INTERVENTIONS *AND RATIONALE*

1. Continue to monitor the assessment parameters listed under "Defining Characteristics."
2. Maintain adequate CPP.
   a. With physician's collaboration, maintain BP within patient's norm by administering volume expanders, vasopressors, or antihypertensives.
   b. Reduce ICP.
      - Elevate head of bed 30 to 45 degrees *to facilitate venous return*.
      - Maintain head and neck in neutral plane (avoid flexion, extension, or lateral rotation) *to enhance venous drainage from the head*.
      - Avoid extreme hip flexion.
      - With physician's collaboration, administer steroids, osmotic agents, and diuretics.

- Drain CSF according to protocol if ventriculostomy in place.
- Assist patient to turn and move self in bed (instruct patient to exhale while turning or pushing up in bed) *to avoid isometric contractions and Valsalva maneuver.*

3. Maintain patent airway, adequate ventilation, and supply oxygen *to prevent hypoxemia and hypercarbia.*
4. Monitor arterial blood gas (ABG) values and maintain Pao_2 >80 mm Hg, $Paco_2$ at 25-35 mm Hg, and pH at 7.35-7.45.
5. Avoid suctioning beyond 10 seconds at a time; hyperoxygenate and hyperventilate before and after suctioning.
6. Plan patient care activities and nursing interventions around the patient's ICP response. Avoid unnecessary additional disturbances and allow patient up to 1 hour of rest between activities as frequently as possible. *Studies have shown the direct correlation between nursing care activities and increases in ICP.*[33]
7. Maintain normothermia with external cooling or heating measures as necessary. Wrap hands, feet, and male genitalia in soft towels before cooling measures *to prevent shivering and frostbite.*
8. With physician's collaboration, control seizures with prophylactic and as necessary (PRN) anticonvulsants. *Seizures can greatly increase the cerebral metabolic rate.*
9. With physician's collaboration, administer sedatives, barbiturates, or paralyzing agents *to reduce cerebral metabolic rate.*
10. Counsel family members to maintain calm atmosphere and to avoid disturbing conversation (e.g., condition, pain, prognosis, family crisis, financial difficulties).
11. If signs of impending brain herniation are present, do the following:
    - Notify physician at once.
    - Be sure head of bed is elevated 45 degrees and patient's head is in neutral plane.
    - Slow mainline intravenous (IV) infusion to keep open rate.
    - If ventriculostomy catheter in place, drain CSF as ordered.
    - Prepare to administer osmotic agents and/or diuretics.
    - Prepare patient for emergency computed tomographic (CT) head scan and/or emergency surgery.

INEFFECTIVE THERMOREGULATION
Theoretical Basis and Management

Body temperature represents a balance between heat production and heat loss. Heat production varies in accordance with skeletal muscle activity, type of food eaten, the temperature of the environment, and the condition of certain endocrine glands such as the thyroid. In addition, sympathetic stimulation with the release of epinephrine and norepinephrine can directly affect the metabolic rate and cause an increase in heat production. Most of the body's heat loss occurs through the skin and is regulated by the amount of blood flowing through the cutaneous vessels and by the activity of the sweat glands.[12]

The hypothalamus acts as the thermostat to maintain body temperature. The "set point" of this thermostat can be changed in the following two ways. First, pyrogens, activating substances that produce fever, are released from damaged body tissues, from the destruction of leukocytes, or from invading pathogens themselves. These pyrogens in the bloodstream cause the hypothalamic thermostat set point to rise. With the thermostat fixed on a higher-than-normal temperature, the rate of energy heat production is increased until the body temperature reaches this new set point.[42] Second, the hypothalamic thermostat can also lower the set point in response to strong stimulation of skin temperature sensors. If the skin becomes overheated, the thermostatic set point is reduced a few tenths of a degree. The heat-losing activities of the hypothalamus are brought into play quickly before the excessive heat sensed by the skin can be transmitted to the interior of the body.[19]

The body temperature of humans is maintained within a narrow range despite extremes in environmental conditions and physical activity.[38] The hypothalamus also maintains body temperature by stimulating or inhibiting autonomic responses to changes in internal temperature. The hypothalamus senses the temperature of the blood passing through it and receives impulses from receptors for both warmth and cold located in the skin. In response to elevated body temperature, impulses go out from the hypothalamus to cause heat loss and inhibit heat production. Sweat glands are stimulated to produce perspiration, allowing evaporative heat loss. Vasodilation of peripheral vessels causes additional heat loss through the skin. Increased respirations also enhance evaporative heat loss.[43] Body temperatures exceeding 41° to 42.2° C (105.8° to 108° F) cause depression of the control mechanism in the hypothalamus, resulting in decreased sweating. Temperatures greater than 41° C for more than a short time cause increased cerebral metabolism and increased ICP and irreparable damage to brain cells, as well as to other body systems.[42]

Responses to cooler body temperatures sensed by the hypothalamus include vasoconstriction, abolition of sweating, and piloerection, or "goose bumps," all of which decrease heat loss. Heat production is increased by shivering.

The temperature-regulating centers in the hypothalamus can be damaged by toxic agents, trauma, tumors, infection, or vascular disease, leading to body temperature shifts above or below normal. Other abnormal conditions affecting body temperature include failure of autonomic responses because of disorders of the spinal cord, peripheral nerves, or skin.

Of course, extremes of environmental temperatures can overwhelm the normal temperature-controlling mechanisms.[42]

Elderly people are more susceptible to extremes of hyperthermia or hypothermia because of decreased metabolic rates and decreased effectiveness of thermoregulatory mechanisms.

Hyperthermia. Lesions of the more anterior portion of the hypothalamus lead to hyperthermia, which is often resistant to antipyretic drugs. Increased heat production, for example, from thyrotoxicosis, and impaired heat loss that occurs in decreased cardiac output states are some of the other causes of hyperthermia. In addition, extremes of environmental temperatures can lead to heat exhaustion or worse (heatstroke).

Malignant hyperthermia represents an extremely critical disorder of temperature regulation related to the use of potent anesthetic agents and depolarizing muscle relaxants that induce a hypermetabolic condition. It is an inherited disorder that affects males more often than females.[10] The triggering anesthetic releases calcium from the sarcoplasmic reticulum of muscle cells; for the muscle fibers to relax, calcium must be pumped back into the sarcoplasmic reticulum. This mechanism does not occur in malignant hyperthermia, and myoplasm calcium levels rise. Increased muscular contraction occurs, along with rigidity, and it and chemical events lead to increased heat production and oxygen consumption.[38] Temperatures can rise as high as 46° C (115° F). Potassium, magnesium, and phosphate leak into the extracellular fluid, and sodium moves into the cell. Creatine phosphokinase (CPK) and myoglobin leak out of the muscle membrane and are excreted by the kidneys. Myoglobin can accumulate in the kidneys, leading to renal failure. In addition, altered platelet function can result in disseminated intravascular coagulation (DIC).[10]

Malignant hyperthermia should be suspected if intense muscle fasciculations and rigid masseter muscles are observed during anesthesia induction. Further clinical signs of malignant hyperthermia and its management are discussed in the nursing care plan.

Hypothermia. Lesions in the more posterior parts of the hypothalamus may lead to hypothermia or poikilothermia (body temperature varies with that of the environment). Acute illnesses such as congestive heart failure, uremia, diabetes mellitus, drug overdosage, and acute respiratory failure can cause acute failure of thermoregulation and lead to hypothermia. Hypothermia can also occur in a patient with a spinal cord injury that interrupts normal sympathetic outflow, but this hypothermia is not related to hypothalamic dysfunction. A more well-known cause of hypothermia occurs from accidental exposure to excessively low environmental temperatures in which body heat is lost through conduction, convection, and radiation. In fact, 50% of the body's heat production can be lost through radiation from an uncovered head. Accidental hypothermia has been associated with myxedema, pituitary insufficiency, Addison's disease, hypoglycemia, cerebrovascular disease, cirrhosis, pancreatitis, and ingestion of drugs or alcohol.[38] A common scenario for hypothermia is to find an unconscious patient lying on the ground in wintertime. Immersion in cold water creates an even more dramatic hyothermia because thermal conductivity of water is estimated to be 32 times that of thermal conductivity of air.[29]

Somnolence and hypotension often accompany hypothermia. At core body temperatures near 30° C, ventricular dysrhythmias occur, particularly ventricular fibrillation. At core temperatures below 26.7° C, unconsciousnss occurs, and below 24° C, apnea is common, followed by asystole.[10,38] Treatment is aimed at preventing further heat loss and performing rewarming measures and advanced cardiac life support measures.

For the management of hyperthermia or hypothermia caused by primary brain pathology affecting hypothalamic thermoregulation, cautiously try to maintain normothermia, monitoring closely for rapid variations in body temperature. Refer to the neurological care plans that follow on hyperthermia related to pharmacogenic hypermetabolism and hypothermia related to environmental exposure to guide nursing interventions.

Hyperthermia related to pharmacogenic hypermetabolism (malignant hyperthermia)

DEFINING CHARACTERISTICS

Early signs
- BP >140/90
- Profuse diaphoresis
- Pulse rate >100
- Masseter and general skeletal muscle rigidity and fasciculations
- Tachypnea
- Decreased level of consciousness

Late signs
- Increasing core body temperature up to 42°-43° C (107.6°-109.4° F)
- Hot skin
- High-output left-ventricular failure
    - Systemic blood presure <90
    - Pulse rate >100 and ventricular dysrhythmias
    - Cardiac index >4.0
    - PCWP and PAD >15 mm Hg; possible pulmonary edema
- Continued skeletal muscle rigidity and fasciculations
- Pao_2 <80 mm Hg
- Respiratory and metabolic acidosis
- Fixed, dilated pupils
- Seizures/coma/decerebrate posturing
- Urinary output <30 ml/hr; reddish-brown (myoglobinuria)
- Prolonged bleeding (DIC)

OUTCOME CRITERIA

- Core body temperature is below 38.3° C (101° F).
- Muscle rigidity and fasciculations are absent.
- Patient is alert and oriented.
- Pupils are normoreactive.

NURSING INTERVENTIONS *AND RATIONALE*

1. Continue to monitor assessment parameters listed under "Defining Characteristics."
2. Rapidly decrease metabolism.
    - It is recommended that health care institutions have an emergency malignant hyperthermia kit available that contains the items indicated below.
    - Administer dantrolene (Dantrium), *which relaxes skeletal muscles by reducing the release of calcium from the sarcoplasmic reticulum.*
    - Observe for infiltration into surrounding tissues. *Dantrolene is very alkaline and irritating to tissues.*
3. Initiate cooling measures.
    - Administer cold IV solutions (IV bag has been soaked in ice bath before administration).
    - Provide cool water sponge bath.
    - Apply cooling blanket until temperature within 1° to 3° F of desired level *to avoid "overshoot" in which excessive cooling lowers the body temperature below the desired range.*
    - Institute iced saline solution lavages of stomach, rectum, and bladder.
    - Monitor core temperature continuously *to avoid overcooling.*
4. Reverse metabolic and respiratory acidosis.
    - With physician's collaboration, administer sodium bicarbonate as necessary *to treat metabolic acidosis.*
    - Initially hyperventilate patient with 100% oxygen; then ventilate with 15-20 ml/kg tidal volume at 15-20 breaths/min.

Continued.

Hyperthermia related to pharmacogenic hypermetabolism (malignant hyperthermia)—cont'd

- Assess ABG values frequently and make ventilatory adjustments as necessary *to remedy hypoxemia and hypercarbia.*
5. Provide adequate nutrients to the tissues and correct electrolyte imbalances.
   - With physician's collaboration, administer 50% dextrose and regular insulin *to increase glucose uptake into liver to meet hypermetabolic needs of body and enhance the movement of potassium from extracellular fluid back into the cells.*
   - Monitor serum electrolytes *to assess efficacy of above action.*
   - Monitor blood urea nitrogen (BUN) and creatinine levels *to evaluate for renal failure.*
   - Monitor serum enzyme levels, particularly CPK elevations, *for indication of degree of muscle hyperactivity.*
6. Correct cardiovascular instability and dysrhythmias.
   - Titrate vasoactive and inotropic drips per protocol to desired systemic blood pressure, PCWP, and/or PAD.
   - Follow critical care emergency standing orders about the administration of antidysrhythmic agents.

7. Maintain a high urinary output (≥50 ml/hour). With physician's collaboration, perform the following:
   - Administer osmotic agents (mannitol) *for excretion of excess fluid load and to increase urinary output to prevent renal failure.*
   - Administer diuretics (furosemide) *to enhance secretion of myoglobin, potassium, sodium, and magnesium.*
   - Administer supplemental potassium chloride as indicated by serum potassium levels.
   - Possibly administer steroid (e.g., Solu-Cortef) *for its mineralocorticoid effect of potassium excretion, to increase glomerular filtration rate, and to reduce cerebral edema.*
8. Correct hematological abnormalities.
   - With physician's collaboration, administer heparin if DIC suspected.
   - Monitor coagulation studies *for indications of DIC and for efficacy of heparin therapy.*
   - Assess stool/urinary/nasogastric (NG) drainage for occult blood.
9. Weigh patient daily *to assist in assessment of hydration status.*

Hypothermia related to exposure to cold environment, illness, trauma (including spinal cord trauma), or damage to the hypothalamus

DEFINING CHARACTERISTICS

- Core body temperature below 35° C (95° F)
- Skin cold to touch
- Slurred speech, incoordination
- At temperature below 33° C (91.4° F):
    Cardiac dysrhythmias (atrial fibrillation, bradycardia)
    Cyanosis
    Respiratory alkalosis
- At temperatures below 32° C (89.6° F):
    Shivering replaced by muscle rigidity
    Hypotension
    Dilated pupils
- At temperatures below 28°-29° C (82.4-84.2° F):
    Absent deep tendon reflexes
    Hypoventilation (3 to 4 breaths/min to apnea)
    Ventricular fibrillation possible
- At temperatures below 26°-27° C (78.8-80.6° F):
    Coma
    Flaccid muscles
    Fixed, dilated pupils
    Ventricular fibrillation to cardiac standstill
    Apnea

OUTCOME CRITERIA

- Core body temperature is greater than 35° C (95° F).
- Patient is alert and oriented.
- Cardiac dysrhythmias are absent.
- Acid-base balance is normal.
- Pupils are normoreactive.

NURSING INTERVENTIONS *AND RATIONALE*

NOTE: Rapid rewarming of a chronically hypothermic patient by active external measures can lead to peripheral vasodilation, resulting in further loss of body temperature, mobilization of blood containing high potassium, low pH, high PCO_2, and low PO_2, profound hypotension, and fatal ventricular fibrillation. Keep in mind that children have been successfully resuscitated after immersion in cold water for 20 to 40 minutes.

1. Continue to monitor the assessment parameters listed under "Defining Characteristics." Additionally, continuously monitor core body temperature with a low-reading thermometer.
2. Intubation and mechanical ventilation may be needed. Heated air or oxygen can be added *to help rewarm the body core.* Because carbon dioxide production is low, do not hyperventilate the hypothermic patient, *because this action may induce severe alkalosis and precipitate ventricular fibrillation.*
3. Apply cardiopulmonary resuscitation (CPR) and advanced cardiac life support until core body temperature is up to at least 29.5° C before determining that patient cannot be resuscitated.

4. Monitor ABG values to direct further therapy, and be sure that the pH, PaO_2, $PaCO_2$ are corrected for temperature.
5. For abrupt-onset hypothermia (for example, immersion in cold water, exposure to cold, wet climate, collapse in snow) rewarming can take place rapidly *because the pathophysiological changes associated with chronic hypothermia have not had time to evolve.*
   - Institute rapid, active rewarming by immersion in warm water (38°-43° C).
   - Apply thermal blanket at 36.6°-37.7° C. Some researchers suggest rewarming only the torso or trunk first, leaving the extremities exposed to room temperature. *This is to prevent early peripheral vasodilation with abrupt redistribution of intravascular volume. This also prevents colder blood trapped in the extremities from returning to the body core before the heart is rewarmed.*[29]
   - Perform rapid core rewarming with heated (37°-43° C) IV infusion, hemodialysis, peritoneal dialysis, and colonic or gastric irrigation fluids.
6. Electrical defibrillation is usually successful in terminating ventricular fibrillation if the temperature is greater than 28° C.
7. Administer cardiac resuscitation drugs sparingly *because as the body warms, peripheral vasodilation occurs. Drugs that remain in the periphery are suddenly released, leading to a "bolus effect" that may cause fatal dysrhythmias.*
8. Monitor peripheral circulation *because gangrene of the fingers and toes is a common complication of accidental hypothermia.*
9. For chronic hypothermia, how aggressive the treatment is will depend on the setting, the underlying disease, and the body temperature. Concurrent treatment of the underlying disease processes is indicated.
   - Core temperatures greater than 33° C may be rewarmed either slowly or rapidly.
   - Coma in a patient with a temperature greater than 28° C is probably not caused by hypothermia. Look for other causes such as hypoglycemia, alcohol, narcotics, and head trauma and treat accordingly.
   - If patient is hyperglycemic, remember that insulin is ineffective at body temperatures below 30° C.
   - Restore intravascular volume cautiously *to avoid circulatory overloading of the hypothermic heart and to avoid precipitating pulmonary edema.* As circulation and a more normal temperature are restored, the patient may require large volumes of crystalloid and colloid fluids *to refill the dilated vascular bed.*

DYSREFLEXIA
Theoretical Basis and Management

Dysreflexia (autonomic dysreflexia, autonomic hyperreflexia, mass reflex phenomenon) is a life-threatening, exaggerated response of the autonomic nervous system that occurs in patients with cervical or high thoracic (T6 or above) spinal cord lesions. It is associated with a massive, uninhibited sympathetic cardiovascular response to a noxious stimulus such as a distended bladder, distended bowel, or a skin irritation. It is characterized by paroxysmal hypertension, pounding headache, pallor followed by facial flushing, sweating above the level of cord injury, engorgement of the temporal and neck vessels, nasal congestion, blurred vision, pilomotor erection (goose bumps), chills without fever, nausea, and occasionally bradycardia. Dysreflexia is recognized as a medical emergency because the unrelieved, excessive hypertension can lead to left-ventricular failure, myocardial infarction, seizures, and intracranial or retinal hemorrhages.[42,43,47]

Pathogenesis. Normally, the sympathetic and parasympathetic divisions of the autonomic nervous system are under the control of higher brain centers in the cerebral cortex and hypothalamus. Spinal cord injury causes a functional transection of the cord with a sudden loss of ascending impulses and impulses from the descending pathways, which normally maintain the cord neurons in a ready state of excitability.[43]

Initially, all autonomic and sensory-motor function of the isolated spinal cord is abolished, and the temporary syndrome of spinal shock ensues.[3] Spinal shock is characterized by paralysis and loss of all sensation below the level of injury; by cardiovascular instability such as hypotension, bradycardia, loss of body temperature control, and lack of sweating; by paralytic ileus and fecal retention; and by paralysis of the bladder.

After spinal shock dissipates (days to months), reflex activity and autonomic functions below the level of injury return but without the modulating control of the higher centers in the brain. These changes result in hyperactive reflexes and inappropriate autonomic responses to stimuli. Sensory impulses that would normally travel up to and be interpreted by the cerebral cortex are blocked at the level of the spinal cord lesion. Consequently, the sensations of a full bladder, a full bowel, or a skin lesion are never really "felt" by the spinal cord injury patient. Since the afferent and efferent autonomic connections with the isolated spinal cord are intact, the neurons of the sympathetic nervous system, located in the lateral horns of the thoracic and lumbar cord, are stimulated. Without higher level interpretation of a stimulus, a mass reflex may occur. The spinal sympathetic response is the release of norepinephrine, causing severe sustained vasoconstriction of splanchnic arterioles, which increases the resistance to blood flow. Severe systemic hypertension results and cannot be relieved by the action of the vasomotor center in the brainstem. Uncontrolled hypertension can reach systolic blood pressure levels of 240 to 300 mm Hg. The parasympathetic nerves are unable to inhibit the action of the sympathetic nerves because of the level of the spinal cord lesion. But the vagus nerves arising from the brainstem can inhibit cardiac rate through the baroreceptor reflexes.[23,42]

Stimuli that can precipitate dysreflexia most often come from the bladder and include distention (often from an occluded indwelling catheter), infection, calculi, and manipulation from a cystoscopy. Other stimuli come from the bowel and include fecal impaction, rectal examination and suppository insertion or come from the skin and include sores, areas of broken skin, temperature extremes, or tight clothing or sheets.[47]

Treatment. Treatment of dysreflexia is directed toward immediate elimination of the precipitating stimuli. Until this occurs, other therapies such as antihypertensive drugs and ganglionic blocking agents may be ineffective. In extreme cases, low spinal anesthesia may be necessary.[42]

Education of the patient and prevention of precipitating stimuli remain the primary goals of treatment, with susceptible individuals maintained on long-term oral ganglionic blocking agents or drugs that alter sympathetic outflow.

Dysreflexia related to excessive autonomic response to certain noxious stimuli (i.e., distended bladder, distended bowel, skin irritation) occurring in patients with cervical or high thoracic (T-6 or above) spinal cord injury

DEFINING CHARACTERISTICS

Major

- Paroxysmal hypertension (sudden periodic elevated BP in which systolic pressure is greater than 140 mm Hg and diastolic pressure is greater than 90 mm Hg); for many spinal cord injury patients, a normal BP may be only 90/60
- Bradycardia (most common; pulse rate <60 beats per minute) or tachycardia (pulse rate >100 beats per minute)
- Diaphoresis (above the injury)
- Facial flushing
- Pallor (below the injury)
- Headache (a diffuse pain in different portions of the head and not confined to any nerve distribution area)

Minor

- Nasal congestion
- Engorgement of temporal and neck vessels
- Conjunctival congestion
- Chills without fever
- Pilomotor erection (goose bumps)
- Blurred vision
- Chest pain
- Metallic taste in mouth
- Horner's syndrome (constriction of the pupil, partial ptosis of the eyelid, enophthalmos, and sometimes loss of sweating over the affected side of the face)

OUTCOME CRITERIA

- Systolic BP is <140 mm Hg, and diastolic blood pressure is <90 mm Hg (or within patient's norm).
- Pulse rate is >60 or <100 beats per minute (or within patient's norm).
- Headache is absent.
- Nasal stuffiness, sweating, and flushing above level of injury are absent.
- Chills, goose bumps, and pallor below level of injury are absent.
- Patient verbalizes causes, prevention, symptoms, and treatment of condition.

NURSING INTERVENTIONS *AND RATIONALE*

1. Continue to monitor the assessment parameters listed under "Defining Characteristics."
2. Place on cardiac monitor and assess for bradycardia, tachycardia, or other dysrhythmias. *Disturbances of cardiac rate and rhythm can occur because of autonomic dysfunction associated with dysreflexia.*
3. Do not leave patient alone. One nurse monitors the blood pressure and patient status every 3 to 5 minutes while another provides treatment.
4. Place patient's head of bed to upright position *to decrease BP and promote cerebral venous return.*
5. Investigate for and remove offending cause of dysreflexia.

a. Bladder
   - If catheter not in place, immediately catheterize patient.
   - Lubricate catheter with lidocaine jelly before insertion.
   - Drain 500 ml of urine and recheck BP.
   - If BP still elevated, drain another 500 ml of urine.
   - If BP declines after the bladder is empty, serial BP should be monitored closely *because the bladder can go into severe contractions causing hypertension to recur.* With physician's collaboration, instill 30 ml tetracaine through the catheter *to decrease the flow of impulses from the bladder.*
   - If indwelling catheter in place, check for kinks or granular sediment that may indicate occlusion.
   - If plugged catheter is suspected, irrigate it gently with no more than 30 ml of sterile normal saline solution. If the bladder is in tetany, fluid will go in but will not drain out.
   - If unable to irrigate catheter, remove it, reinsert a new catheter, and proceed with its lubrication, drainage, and observation as stated above.
   - Atropine is sometimes administered *to relieve bladder tetany.*

b. Bowel
   - Using glove lubricated with anesthetic ointment, check rectum for fecal impaction.
   - If impaction is felt, *to decrease flow of impulses from bowel,* insert anesthetic ointment into rectum 10 minutes before manual removal of impaction.
   - A low, hypertonic enema or a suppository may be given *to assist bowel evacuation.*

c. Skin
   - Loosen clothing or bed linens as indicated.
   - Inspect skin for pimples, boils, pressure sores, and ingrown toenails and treat as indicated.

6. If symptoms of dysreflexia do not subside, have available the IV solutions, and antihypertensive drugs of the physician's choosing (e.g., hydralazine, phentolamine, diazoxide, sodium nitroprusside). Administer medications and monitor their effectiveness. Assess BP, pulse, and subjective and objective signs and symptoms.
7. Instruct patient about causes, symptoms, treatment, and prevention of dysreflexia.
8. Encourage patient to carry informational card to present to medical personnel in the event dysreflexia may be developing.

UNILATERAL NEGLECT
Theoretical Basis and Management

Unilateral neglect, or *hemi-inattention*, is a perceptual neurological defect characterized by an unawareness or denial of an affected half of the body. This neglect may also extend to extrapersonal space. This defect most often results from right-hemispheric brain damage that causes left hemiplegia. Such a disorder of perception may also include disturbances of body image, spatial judgment, and sensory interpretation. Perceptual defects are not as readily noticeable as are motor deficits but may be more debilitating to the patient and can lead to the inability to perform skilled or purposeful tasks.[36] In addition to unilateral neglect, several other sensory-perceptual alterations that can occur with hemispheric damage are discussed here.

Lesions in the nondominant or right parietal lobe cause unilateral neglect more often than left-hemispheric lesions.[11] In most people the left side of the brain is dominant for speech, analytical abilities, and verbal and auditory memory, and the right side specializes in spatial relations, perception, creativity, and nonverbal memory. It is believed that the right hemisphere also has some influence on speech by conveying meaning beyond actual words through the use of gesture, body language, and facial expressions.[39]

Stroke is a common cause of right-hemispheric damage that can result in unilateral neglect. The blood supply to the parietal lobe is provided by all three major cerebral arterial distributions. The middle cerebral artery supplies the major portion of the parietal lobe, with the anterior cerebral artery supplying the anterior and medial parts and the posterior cerebral artery supplying a small posterior portion. Stroke in any of these vessels can damage the parietal lobe, resulting in perceptual impairments.[36]

Through the thalamus the parietal lobe receives sensory fibers that convey cutaneous and deep sensations arising from the opposite side of the body. Kinesthetic alterations in sensory perception include *hemianesthesia*, the loss of sensation in the affected side, and *paresthesias,* feelings such as heaviness, numbness, tingling, prickling, and a heightened sensitivity in the affected side. The loss of muscle-joint sense can lead to a loss of *proprioception* or position sense, which affects the patient's balance and ability to ambulate.[26]

Some sensory data for vision are interpreted and integrated within the parietal lobe to establish an awareness of the body and its parts and a sense of spatial relationships. Defects in spatial orientation can interfere with the patient's ability to judge position, distance, movement, form, and the relationship of his or her body parts to surrounding objects. Patients may confuse such concepts as up and down and forward and backward. They may have difficulty following a route from one place to another and may even get lost in areas that were once familiar. Stroke patients may also experience reading and writing problems related to visual perception and visual-spatial deficits. One type of spatial dyslexia is related to unilateral spatial neglect. The patient may not look at the beginning of a line of written material that appears on the left. Instead the patient fixes attention on a point to the right of the beginning of the line and reads to the end of the line. If asked to draw a design,

only half of a design or drawing is completed.[36]

Some of these spatial-neglect problems are related to visual field defects. Visual field defects may accompany the unilateral neglect syndrome, although they do not cause it. A hemispheric lesion can interrupt the visual pathways, with the resulting visual defect dependent on the location and extent of the lesion. Fig. 23-10 demonstrates that, at the optic chiasm, nerve fibers coming from the nasal half of each retina cross to the opposite side, whereas fibers coming from the temporal half of each retina do not cross. This partial crossing allows binocular vision. In the optic chiasm, fibers from the nasal half of each retina join the uncrossed fibers from the temporal half of the retina to form the optic tract. Impulses conducted to the right hemisphere by the right optic tract represent the left field of vision, and those conducted to the left hemisphere by the left optic tract represent the right field of vision. Optic radiations extend back to the occipital lobes. Visual defects restricted to a single field, right or left, are called *homonymous*.[36] For example, a right-hemispheric lesion resulting in the loss of the left half of the visual field of each eye is called *homonymous hemianopsia.*

It is not uncommon for the patient experiencing unilateral neglect to have a significant visual field loss. The nurse may be the first person to detect that the patient has this defect. The patient with hemianopsia may neglect all sensory input from the affected side and may initially appear unresponsive if approached from the affected side. If the nurse approaches the patient from the healthy side, the patient may actually be quite alert. Another clue to hemianopsia may appear when the patient is seen to eat food only from one half of the tray.

Hemianopsia often recedes gradually with time. Many patients can learn to scan their environment visually to compensate for the defect, although in the acute stage of stroke the patient may be too lethargic to follow instructions in methods of visual scanning. This visual defect can lead to fear and confusion for the patient. The nurse can lessen the detrimental effects of hemianopsia by making sure that the patient's bed is positioned so that the patient can see the door of the room and can see people coming and going. If the patient's "blind" side faces the door, the tendency to neglect the affected side will be accentuated.[15,36] Once the patient is learning to scan visually, it may be advantageous to reverse this bed position so that the patient must scan visually to interract with his or her environment.

Other specific syndromes resulting from right-hemispheric lesions and associated with unilateral neglect include language problems such as difficulty understanding concepts such as proverbs and idioms. Patients may talk excessively but have difficulty getting to the point. Their voice and facial expressions may lack emotion (flat affect), and they may have difficulty understanding facial expressions and emotions in others.[39]

Body image is often disturbed after stroke. *Anosognosia* is the term used to denote varying degrees of denial of the affected side of the body. This denial may range from inattention to actual refusing to acknowledge a paralysis by neglecting the involved side or by denying ownership of the side, attributing the paralyzed arm or leg to someone else.

This denial may cease as the acute cerebral pathology and the patient's sensorium clear, although decreased motor ability or paralysis and decreased sensation in the affected side may persist.[15,36]

Perceptual disorders often include various *agnosias,* which are disturbances of the recognition or identification of objects that have been perceived by a single sense function—either vision, hearing, or touch.[36] Auditory agnosia and aphasia are discussed in detail in the section, "Impaired Communications."

In addition to experiencing visual field defects, some patients may also have visual agnosias. Some patients are unable to recognize objects or pictures of objects, whereas others cannot recognize faces and may have to rely on the voice or characteristic mannerisms of a familiar person to identify that person.[36]

Tactile agnosia, or *astereognosis,* is a perceptual disorder in which a patient is unable to recognize by touch alone an object that has been placed in his or her hand. This may occur even in the presence of an intact sense of touch. If allowed to see or hear the object, the patient is very likely to recognize it.[36]

Lesions in the parietal lobe, as well as in other cortical structures, can result in *apraxia,* which is an inability to perform a learned movement voluntarily. Even though the patient may understand the task to be performed and may have intact motor ability, he or she is unable to perform the task and often fumbles and makes mistakes. The patient suffering from dressing apraxia, for example, may not be able to orient clothing in space and becomes tangled in the clothing when attempting to dress. In unilateral neglect, the patient may actually fail to dress or groom the neglected half of the body.[36]

Patients with right-hemispheric pathological conditions may also exhibit emotional lability with periods of euphoria, impulsiveness, and inattention. A short attention span, lack of insight, and poor judgment may lead to injuries as the patient attempts to perform activities beyond his or her capabilities.[11,15,36]

Nurses tend to have higher expectations of patients with right-hemispheric strokes because of their ability to speak. However, these patients do in fact have a poorer prognosis than patients who are aphasic from left-hemispheric strokes.[15]

The previous discussion has touched on some, but certainly not all, of the sensory-perceptual alterations that may accompany stroke. Clinically, the stroke patient often has diffuse cerebrovascular disease and has perhaps experienced prior strokes. Perceptual defects are not always as readily apparent or as clear-cut as described here, underscoring the importance of ensuring that a comprehensive multidisciplinary neurological evaluation of the stroke patient occurs within the critical care unit, using such team members as social workers, physical therapists, speech therapists, and occupational therapists. After this evaluation and with the physician's collaboration, a realistic determination of the patient's potential level of recovery should be made. This step is followed by formulating a multidisciplinary plan for comprehensive rehabilitation that can and should begin within the critical care unit.

Unilateral Neglect related to perceptual disruption secondary to stroke involving the right cerebral hemisphere

DEFINING CHARACTERISTICS

Major (must be present)
- Neglect of involved body parts and/or extrapersonal space
- Denial of the existence of the affected limb or side of body

Minor (may be present)
- Denial of hemiplegia or other motor and sensory deficits
- Left homonymous hemianopsia
- Difficulty with spatial-perceptual tasks
- Left hemiplegia

OUTCOME CRITERIA

- Patient is safe and free from injury.
- Patient is able to identify safety hazards in the environment.
- Patient recognizes disability and describes physical deficits present (e.g., paralysis, weakness, numbness).
- Patient demonstrates ability to scan the visual field to compensate for loss of function or sensation in affected limb(s).

NURSING INTERVENTIONS *AND RATIONALE*

1. Continue to monitor the assessment parameters listed uner "Defining Characteristics."
2. Maintain patient safety: *because of the patient's usually brief stay within the critical care unit, the emphasis is placed on patient safety. Therefore the environment is adapted to the patient's deficit.*
   - Position the patient's bed with the unaffected side facing the door.
   - Approach and speak to the patient from the unaffected side. If the patient must be approached from the affected side, announce your presence as soon as entering the room *to avoid startling the patient.*[11]
   - Position the call light, bedside stand, and personal items on the patient's unaffected side.
   - If the patient will be assisted out of bed, simplify the environment *to eliminate hazards* by removing unnecessary furniture and equipment.
   - Provide frequent reorientation of the patient to the environment.
   - Observe the patient closely and anticipate his or her needs. In spite of repeated explanations, the patient may have difficulty retaining information about the deficits.
   - When patient is in bed, elevate his or her affected arm on a pillow *to prevent dependent edema and support the hand in a position of function.*
3. Assist the patient to recognize the perceptual defect.
   - Encourage the patient to wear any prescription corrective glasses or hearing aids *to facilitate communication.*
   - Instruct the patient to turn the head past midline to view the environment on the affected side.
   - Encourage the patient to look at the affected side and to stroke the limbs with the unaffected hand.

Encourage handling of the affected limbs *to reinforce awareness of the affected side.*
- Instruct the patient to always look for the affected extremity or extremities when performing simple tasks *to know where it is at all times.*
- After pointing to them, have the patient name the affected parts.
- Encourage the patient to use self-exercises (e.g., lifting the affected arm with the good hand).
- If the patient is unable to discriminate between the concepts of "right" and "left," use descriptive adjectives such as "the weak arm," "the affected leg," or "the good arm" to refer to the body. Use gestures not just words, to indicate right and left.

4. Collaborate with the patient, physician, and rehabilitation team to *design and implement a beginning rehabilitation program for use during critical care unit stay.*
   - Use adapative equipment (braces, splints, slings) as appropriate.
   - Teach the patient the individual components of any activity separately, then proceed to integrate the component parts into a completed activity.[36]
   - Instruct the patient to attend to the affected side, if able, and to assist with the bath or other tasks.
   - Use tactile stimulation *to reintroduce the arm or leg to the patient.* Rub the affected parts with different textured materials *to stimulate sensations (warm, cold, rough, soft).*[11]
   - Encourage activities that required the patient to turn the head toward the affected side and retrain the patient to scan the affected side and environment visually.
   - If patient is allowed out of bed, cue him or her with reminders to scan visually when ambulating. Assist and remain in constant attendance *because the patient may have difficulty maintaining correct posture, balance, and locomotion.* There may be vertical-horizontal perceptual problems, with the patient leaning to the affected side to align with the perceived vertical. Provide sitting, standing, and balancing exercises before getting the patient out of bed.
   - Feeding: see "Potential for Aspiration, risk factors: impaired swallowing," p. 488.
     a. Avoid giving patient any very hot food items that could cause injury.
     b. Place the patient in an upright sitting position if possible.
     c. Encourage the patient to feed himself or herself; if necessary, guide the patient's hand to the mouth.
     d. If the patient is able to feed himself or herself, place one dish at a time in front of the patient. When the patient is finished with the first, add another dish. Tell the patient what he or she is eating.[36]

Unilateral Neglect related to perceptual disruption secondary to stroke involving the right cerebral hemisphere—cont'd

e. Initially place food in the patient's visual field; then gradually move the food out of the field of vision and teach the patient to scan the entire visual field.[11]

f. When the patient has learned to visually scan the environment, offer a tray of food with various dishes.

g. Instruct the patient to take small bites of food and to place the food in the unaffected side of the mouth.

h. *To eliminate retained food in the affected side of the mouth,* teach the patient to sweep out these pockets of food with the tongue after every bite.[11]

i. After meals or oral medications, check the patient's oral cavity for pockets of retained material.

5. Initiate patient and family health teaching.
   - Assess to ensure that both the patient and the family understand the nature of the neurological deficits and the purpose of the rehabilitation plan.
   - Teach the proper application and use of any adaptive equipment.
   - Teach the importance of maintaining a safe environment and point out potential environmental hazards.
   - Instruct family members how to facilitate relearning techniques (e.g., cueing, scanning visual fields).

ACUTE PAIN
Theoretical Basis and Management

Pain is defined by NANDA as "a state in which an individual experiences and reports the presence of severe discomfort or an uncomfortable sensation."[11] Pain is a protective mechanism for the body. It occurs when tissues of the body are damaged, causing an individual to take some action to relieve it. Both humans and animals are subject to feeling pain throughout their lives, so it becomes a universally distressing feeling, whether acute or chronic. Relief of pain remains one of the major aspects of medical and nursing practice because fear of pain is second only to fear of death.

Critically ill patients, experiencing the acute pain of their disease process or surgical procedure, are particularly vulnerable to pain. In addition, they are often subjected to painful invasive procedures for the purposes of monitoring, diagnosing, or treating their illness.

Acute pain is usually associated with body injury of some kind, with the pain disappearing when the injury heals. Chronic pain, on the other hand, persists beyond the expected healing time, lasts longer than 6 months, and often cannot be attributed to a specific injury.[4]

Signs of acute pain. Acute pain begins at a specific time and is usually accompanied by objective physical signs, which include the autonomic (sympathetic) responses of tachycardia, hypertension, diaphoresis, mydriasis, and pallor. Skeletal muscle reactions associated with acute pain include grimacing, clenching fists, pacing the floor, writhing, guarding, or splinting the affected part. Psychic reactions may include distinct verbalizations of suffering and pleas for help and expressions of anger and crying. The person may also appear anxious, apprehensive, and fearful.

These objective physical signs are not always the most reliable indicators of the presence of pain. Pain has been described as a subjective experience, with the patient the only authority about the pain being experienced. McCaffery[31] defines pain as "whatever the experiencing person says it is, existing when he/she says it does." The nurse has the responsibilities of believing the patient and of seeking more information about the pain.[31]

Pain theories. Several complex theories of pain perception have been offered over the last 20 years. Current views are that pain has a sensory component and a reactive component.[40]

The *specificity theory,* in brief, describes the transmission of pain impulses through special fibers to specific pain centers in the brain. Some afferent fibers go to motor fibers of the reflex arc in the spinal cord so that muscles respond immediately, for example, by pulling the hand away quickly when a finger has touched a hot object. Other afferent fibers ascend through the spinothalamic tract to the thalamus where impulses are relayed to the cerebral cortex for processing. The spinothalamic tract is believed to carry sensory discriminative aspects of pain.[40]

The reticulospinal tract carries noxious sensations to the medullary and pontine reticular formation and terminates in the midbrain, thalamus, and hypothalamus. This tract is primarily responsible for poorly localized burning pain and visceral sensations.[40]

The phenomenon of phantom limb pain, postherpetic neuralgia, and causalgia are explained by the *pattern theory* of pain. The key concept of this theory is that after tissue injury, circuits that act as pattern-generating mechanisms can be established in the dorsal horns and possibly in other places along the sensory system, causing pain perception even though the stimuli that initiated pain are no longer present. Nonpainful stimuli such as light touch or a breath of wind can cause these reverberating pattern circuits to send impulses to the brain that are interpreted as pain. These same circuits sometimes fire spontaneously, even in the absence of peripheral stimulation.[35]

The specificity and the pattern theories do not adequately explain the pain process, however, because recent findings indicate that pain transmission can be modulated.

The *gate control theory* presented by Melzack and Wall in 1965 implies that these transmitted pain impulses can be modulated or altered through cortical and spinal influences.[44] The potential blocking ability of certain cells along the transmission route can result in little or no pain perception, regardless of the intensity of the pain stimulus.[44]

Small-diameter fibers of peripheral nerves conduct excitatory pain signals to the substantia gelatinosa in the dorsal horns of the spinal cord. If nothing blocks these impulses, they are transmitted to the ascending tracts that travel up the spinal cord to the brain where the pain is perceived. Large-diameter afferent fibers on the surface of the skin carry innocuous information that can, in effect, close the "gate" in the substantia gelatinosa, blocking the transmission of pain. These cutaneous large fibers can be stimulated by touch, vibration, rubbing, and scratching. Simply stated then, the gate is opened by activation of the small fibers but can be closed by stimulation of the large fibers. This excitation-inhibition is called the gating mechanism.[44]

Information from the brain can also increase or decrease the transmission of pain by relaying impulses that can open or close the gate down to the substantia gelatinosa. Information such as memories, emotions, and situations influence not only the perception of but the meaning attached to the pain impulse.[21]

The gate control theory helps explain the effects of pain therapies such as relaxation techniques and cutaneous stimulation such as heat, cold, massage, and transcutaneous electrical nerve stimulation (TENS).

Other pain theories support the concept that pain impulses are mediated in the spinal cord before they reach the brain. The *endogenous opioid system* consists of biochemical substances known as endorphins. Three major groups of endorphins (β-endorphins, enkephalins, and dynorphin) are morphinelike peptides produced naturally in the body at various sites along neural synapses in the CNS. They modulate the transmission of pain perceptions by attaching to specific opioid receptors found in various regions of the brain and in the substantia gelatinosa of the dorsal horns of the spinal cord. Many of these opioid receptors in the brain are in areas associated with emotions. In addition to raising pain thresholds, endorphins, much like morphine, also produce sedation and feelings of euphoria. Like morphine, the pain-relieving actions of endorphins can be blocked by naloxone.[7]

It is believed that pain activates the endogenous opioid system. Other factors may also activate this system and include elevations of BP, fear, stress, restraint, and hypoglycemia.[40] Endorphin levels have also been found elevated with exercise, noxious states, labor, and delivery. Endorphin release may also explain why many individuals do not initially feel pain at the time of an accident or why a painful injury may be rendered painless during the heat of battle or sport. These persons experience a "stress analgesia." Endorphins might help explain the phenomenon of pain relief in some individuals following administration of placebos. Acupuncture and TENS use may also cause the release of endorphins, which add to the pain-relieving properties of these techniques. There is increasing evidence, too, that people who experience chronic high levels of pain may be deficient in endorphins.[21,40]

Although endorphins are associated with pain inhibition, other neuropeptides are associated with pain transmission. The level of many neuropeptides fluctuates throughout the day, possibly explaining why pain sensitivity seems higher (lower pain threshold) in the afternoon than in the morning. This fluctuation will influence an individual's analgesic requirements at different times of the day.[26]

Psychosocial influences. Most body pain is a combination of mental events and physical stimuli. In fact, sustained anxiety, fear, and anger can even produce painful alterations in physiology such as muscle contractions and tension headaches.[11,26]

Pain is evaluated in higher brain centers in the cortex. People can experience different levels of pain in response to the same injury or insult. Physiological differences such as endorphin levels help explain the phenomenon but not entirely. Pain tolerance differs among individuals and can vary within any individual in different situations. Personal factors such as knowledge of pain, its meaning, and its cause, the ability to control pain, a person's stress level, as well as energy or fatigue levels influence pain tolerance.[11,26]

Social and environmental factors such as interactions with others, responses of family and friends, stressors, and sensory overload or deprivation influence pain. A person's cultural background, beliefs, and past experiences can also influence pain. The situation in which pain occurs is also significant. For instance, the pain associated with elective surgery may be perceived as more severe than that occurring from wounds incurred in battle, even if the latter involves a greater degree of tissue injury.[11,26]

Stress contributes to the severity of perceived pain. Persons who receive explanations of what they will feel in advance of painful procedures experience less stress than those who receive little or no explanation. A consequence of less stress may be an actual reduction in the severity of perceived pain.[11,26]

Cultural and societal influences on peoples' expression of pain are great. For example, people with stoic backgrounds tend to avoid verbal and nonverbal expressions of pain. Other cultures encourage outward displays of discomfort such as moaning and crying. These factors have great implications for nurses responsible for assessing and treating pain. The stoic individual is actually at risk for receiving inadequate pain relief measures. Health care workers must remember that these cultural differences affect only the expression of pain and not the differences in sensitivity to pain.[26]

Types of acute pain. Pain arising from different locations in the body and from underlying pathophysiological processes accounts for some characteristic pain patterns. Superficial structures such as subcutaenous tissue, fascia, periosteum, ligaments, tendons, and parietal pleura are richly supplied with small pain fibers. Hence, pain resulting from stimulation of these regions is relatively well localized and is often pricking and burning in nature. Conversely, visceral pain is poorly localized and is often referred to other areas, because the viscera and deeper somatic structures are more sparsely innervated with small pain fibers. Pain of visceral origin is usually felt somewhere within the segmental distribution of several nerve roots. For example, the most common sites of pain from myocardial ischemia include behind the sternum, in the left pectoral region and shoulder, along the inner aspect of the left arm to the elbow, and occasionally in the back. All these sites are within the distribution of T1 to T3 nerve roots. Visceral pain is usually described as aching but may be sharp and penetrating (knifelike). Rarely, it is burning such as in the heartburn of esophageal irritation.[1,27]

When pain arises from a nerve root or trunk its distribution follows the afferent distribution of the nerve. For example, the pain of a herniated intervertebral disk compressing the fifth lumbar nerve root will cause deep as well as superficial pain extending down the lateral thigh and leg.[27]

Muscle cramps or spasms can provoke severe pain, and the muscles may be visibly and palpably taut. Massage and vigorous stretch are the most effective ways to stop the spasms. Muscle cramps can be caused by motor system disease, tetany, and dehydration after excessive sweating and salt loss. Metabolic diseases such as uremia, hypocalcemia, and hypomagnesemia can also cause muscle spasms. Exactly why the muscle spasms cause pain is debatable, but it is probably because the overactive muscles demand more oxygen than can be supplied, resulting in ischemia with a buildup of ischemic metabolites.[2,50]

The pain of muscle injury is similar to visceral pain in type, localization, and referral because deep skeletal pain and visceral pain are mediated through common deep sensory systems. In fact, chest wall pain can often mimic the pain of myocardial ischemia.[1]

Acute ischemic pain causes burning or aching pain in the tissues distal to a vascular occlusion. The pain is possibly caused by the release of metabolic factors related to tissue hypoxia and anoxia. Since exercise increases the metabolic demands of the tissues, pain from ischemia characteristically builds with the use of the involved muscles and is initially relieved by rest. Eventually, the ischemic pain is felt at rest, increases in intensity, and becomes aggravated by movement.[26,46]

Often the pain of an ischemic leg will be aggravated by elevating the leg and lessened by dangling or lowering the leg. In addition, the extremity distal to the occlusion will experience a loss of pulses, delayed capillary filling, and a decrease in skin temperature, eventually becoming cold and pale. Loss of skin sensation occurs within the first hour, with feelings of numbness reported. After approximately 6 hours, painful, ischemic muscle contractures develop.[26,46]

Evaluating pain. Evaluating a patient's pain can be a difficult endeavor because pain is a subjective experience. If the adage that *pain is whatever the experiencing person says it is* is followed, then that person should be believed. Rather than spending time determining if someone actually has pain, the nurse can use time wisely by assessing the situation, determining the possible causes of the pain, and instituting measures to alleviate it.

Determining the cause of pain when it is not obvious can be critical to the patient's well-being. For instance, it is vital that a differential diagnosis can be made for a patient's complaint of chest pain to confirm or deny the possibility of myocardial ischemia. Such a differential diagnosis is heavily influenced by the location, character, duration, and severity of the pain; what provokes it and makes it worse or better; the risk factor profile for coronary artery disease; and a past history of cardiovascular disease.[28] The need for a differential diagnosis of chest pain occurring in the postoperative open heart surgery patient also occurs with frequency. In these instances, the presence of increased pain intensity during deep breathing and coughing helps distinguish chest wall pain from myocardial ischemic pain.

The nurse also assesses the behavioral aspects of pain such as moaning, crying, grimacing, restlessness, pacing, guarding, or withdrawal. These behavioral manifestations cannot be used as the only clues to the existence of or the severity of pain, however, because some people will try hard not to show pain.

One of the best attempts to objectify the subjective is to ask the patient (if he or she is able) to rate the pain on a scale of 1 to 10. Explain to the patient that a 0 means the absence of pain, 1 represents the least pain, and 10 represents the worst pain the patient has ever experienced. Pain should be rated this way at its best, at its worst, and after pain relief measures to evaluate their effectiveness. This recorded response is used as a frame of reference to compare future episodes of pain.[11]

Children and ill adults with impaired verbal communication may not clearly communicate the psychic reactions associated with acute pain. The nurse may then have to rely on the physical clues that can indicate pain such as elevated BP and pulse rate and changes in activity level.[7,22]

The nursing care plan that follows explains in more detail the parameters for pain assessment, as well as nursing measures to alleviate pain.

Acute Pain related to transmission and perception of cutaneous, visceral, muscular, or ischemic impulses secondary to (specify)

DEFINING CHARACTERISTICS

Subjective
- Patient verbalizes presence of pain
- Patient rates pain on scale of 1 to 10

Objective
- Increase in BP, pulse, and respirations
- Pupillary dilation
- Diaphoresis, pallor
- Skeletal muscle reactions (grimacing, clenching fists, writhing, pacing, guarding or splinting affected part)
- Apprehensive, fearful appearance

OUTCOME CRITERIA

NOTE: Outcome is highly variable, dependent on individual patient and pain circumstance factors.
- Patient verbalizes that pain is reduced to a tolerable level or is removed.
- Patient's pain rating on scale of 1 to 10 is lower.
- BP, heart rate, and respiratory rate return to baseline 5 minutes after administration of IV narcotic or 20 minutes after administration of intramuscular (IM) narcotic.

NURSING INTERVENTIONS *AND RATIONALE*

1. Continue to monitor the assessment parameters listed under "Defining Characteristics." Additionally, monitor postural vital sign changes; determine hydration status and manage fluid volume deficit, if indicated, before administering narcotic analgesic.
2. Modify variables that heighten the patient's experience of pain.
   - Explain to the patient that frequent, detailed, and seemingly repetitive assessments will be conducted *to allow the nurse to better understand the patient's pain experience, not because the existence of pain is in question.*
   - Explain the factors responsible for pain production in the individual. Estimate the expected duration of the pain if possible.
   - Explain diagnostic and therapeutic procedures to the patient in relation to sensations the patient should expect to feel.
   - Reduce the patient's fear of addiction by explaining the difference between drug tolerance and drug addiction. Drug tolerance is a physiological phenomenon in which a drug dose begins to lose effectiveness after repeated doses; drug dependence is a psychological phenomenon in which narcotics are used regularly for emotional, not medical reasons.[11]
   - Instruct patient to ask for pain medication when pain is beginning and not to wait until it is intolerable.
   - Explain that the physician will be consulted if pain relief is inadequate with the present medication.
   - Instruct patient in the importance of adequate rest,

especially when it reduces pain, *to maintain strength and coping abilities and to reduce stress.*
3. Pharmacological interventions.
   - For postsurgical or posttraumatic cutaneous, muscular, or visceral pain, perform the following:
     a. Medicate with narcotic maximally to break the pain cycle as long as level of consciousness and vital signs are stable: check patient's previous response to similar dosage and narcotic.

NOTE: First dose received postoperatively is usually reduced by one half *to evaluate patient's individual response to medication.*

   b. Continuous pain requires continuous analgesia.
      (1) Establish optimal analgesic dose that brings optimal pain relief.
      (2) Offer pain mediation at prescribed regular intervals rather than making patient ask for it.
   c. If administering medication on prn basis, give it when patient's pain is just beginning, rather than at its peak. Advise patient to intercept pain, not endure it, or it may take several hours and higher doses of narcotics to relieve pain, leading to a cycle of undermedication and pain alternating with overmedication and drug toxicity.
   d. Perform rehabilitation exercises (turn, deep breathe, leg exercises, ambulate) shortly before peak of drug effect *because this will be the optimal time for the patient to increase activity with the least risk of increasing pain.*
   e. In making the transition from IM or IV to by mouth (po) medications, try alternating them in the following pattern: IM, IM, po, IM, po, po, IM, po, po, po, IM, po . . . or IV, IV, IM, IV, IM, IM, IV, IM, IM, IM, IV, IM . . . .
   f. To assess effectiveness of pain medication, do the following:
      (1) Reevaluate pain 5 minutes after IV and 20 minutes after IM medication administration, observe patient's behavior, and ask patient to rate pain on scale of 1 to 10.
      (2) Collaborate with physician to add or delete other medications such as antiemetics, hypnotics, sedatives, or muscle relaxants that potentiate the action of analgesics.
      (3) Observe for indicators of undertreatment: report of pain not relieved; observed restlessness, sleeplessness, irritability, and anorexia; decreased activity level.
      (4) Indicators of overtreatment: hypotension or bradycardia; respiratory rate <10/min; excessive sedation.

g. IF IV patient-controlled analgesia (PCA) is used, perform the following:

(NOTE: *Patient-controlled analgesia allows patients to administer small doses of their prescribed medication when they feel the need. Constant levels of the drug in the bloodstream mean lower doses can be used to obtain analgesia. Pain control is improved because the patient is in control and experiences less fear of unrelieved pain. Reduced net narcotic use is noted as is less sedation. Critical care patients appropriate for patient-controlled analgesia are those who are alert such as burn patients, trauma patients without head injury, and some postoperative patients.*)

(1) Instruct the patient as follows[18]: "When you have pain, instead of ringing for the nurse to receive pain medicine, push the button that activates the machine, and a small dose of pain medicine will be injected into your IV line. Give yourself only enough medicine to take care of your pain but do not activate the machine for a dose if you start to feel sleepy. Try to balance the pain relief against sleepiness. If your pain medicine seems to stop working despite pushing the button several times, call the nurse to check your IV. If this is still a problem, the nurse will call your doctor."

(2) Monitor vital signs, especially BP and respiratory rate, every hour for the first 4 hours and assess postural heart rate and BP before initial ambulation.

(3) Monitor respirations every 2 hours while patient is on patient-controlled analgesia.

(4) If patient's respirations decrease to <10/min or if patient is overly sedated, anticipate IV administration of naloxone.

h. If epidural narcotic analgesia is used, do the following:

(NOTE: *The delivery of narcotics such as morphine by epidural route to specific receptors in the spinal cord selectively blocks pain impulses to the brain for up to 24 hours. Effective analgesia can be obtained without many of the negative side effects or serum narcotic concentrations. Critical care patients appropriate for epidural analgesia include postsurgical and trauma patients.*)

(1) Keep patient's head elevated 30 to 45 degrees after injection *to prevent respiratory depressant effects.*

(2) Observe closely for respiratory depression up to 24 hours after injection. Monitor respiratory rate every 15 minutes for 1 hour every 30 minutes for 7 hours, and every 1 hour for the remaining 16 hours.

(3) Assess for adequate cough reflex.

(4) Avoid use of other CNS depressants such as sedatives.

(5) Observe for reports of pruritis, nausea, or vomiting.

(6) Anticipate administration of naloxone for respiratory depression (and smaller doses of naloxone for pruritis).

(7) Assess for and treat urinary retention.

(8) Assess epidural catheter site for local infection. Keep catheter taped securely.

- For peripheral vascular ischemic pain (hypothetical vascular occlusion of leg), do the following:

a. Correctly identify and differentiate ischemic pain from other types of pain.

NOTE: *Ischemic pain is usually a burning, aching pain made worse by exercise and lessened or relieved by rest. Eventually the pain occurs at rest. Coldness and pallor of extremity may be noted, especially if the limb is elevated above the heart level. Rubor and mottling of the skin may be evident from prolonged tissue anoxia and inability of damaged vessels to constrict. Eventually cyanosis and gangrenous tissue will be evident. Chronic ischemia leads to trophic changes in the limb such as flaking skin, brittle nails, hair loss, leg ulcers, and cellulitis.*

b. Administer pain medications and evaluate their effectiveness as previously described. Remember that the pain of ischemia is chronic and continuous and can make the patient irritable and depressed.

c. Treat the cause of the ischemic pain and institute measures to increase circulation to the affected part (see Altered Peripheral Tissue Perfusion care plans, p. 341).

4. Nonpharmacological interventions.

- Treat contributing factors (see "Theoretical Basis and Management"); provide explanations (see intervention number 2 at beginning of this care plan).

- Apply comfort measures, using gate control theory.

a. See Appendix D for methods of therapeutic touch.

b. Use relaxation techniques such as back rubs, massage, warm baths. Use blankets and pillows *to support the painful part and reduce muscle tension.* Encourage slow, rhythmic breathing.

c. Encourage progressive muscle relaxation techniques.

(1) Instruct patient to inhale and tense (tighten) specific muscle groups, then relax the muscles as exhalation occurs.

(2) Suggest an order for performing the tension-relaxation cycle (e.g., start with facial muscles and move down body ending with toes).

d. Encourage guided imagery.[30]

(1) Ask patient to recall an experienced image that is very pleasurable and relaxing and involves at least two senses.

(2) Have patient begin with rhythmic breathing and progressive relaxation, then travel mentally to the scene.

Continued.

Acute Pain related to transmission and perception of cutaneous, visceral, muscular, or ischemic impulses secondary to (specify)—cont'd

(3) Have the patient slowly experience the scene—how it looks, sounds, smells, feels.

(4) Ask patient to practice this imagery in private.

(5) Instruct the patient to end the imagery by counting to three and saying, "Now I'm relaxed." If person does not end the imagery and falls asleep, the purpose of the technique is defeated.

e. If TENS unit is prescribed by physician, do the following:

(NOTE: *TENS is a battery-operated unit that serves as a nerve stimulator. It produces mild, tingling sensations as it blocks incisional pain messages to the brain. It is sometimes used as part of the pain relief program for the postsurgical patient.*)

(1) Take the TENS unit, patient pamphlet, and teaching electrodes to the patient before surgery to explain the process.

(2) Apply electrodes to skin and instruct patient in proper use of unit. Let patient experience how the TENS unit should feel when activated. Refer to manufacturer's directions for proper application and operation of TENS unit.

(3) Electrodes are usually placed by the physician on the skin alongside the operative incision at the close of the surgical procedure in the operating room. The unit is usually used for 3 to 5 days as an adjunct to medications.

(4) When the patient is awake and alert, readjust the amplitude or output of the TENS unit to the patient's comfort as necessary. Keep the TENS unit on continuously unless ordered otherwise. Occasionally, percutaneous epidural nerve stimulation is used when more than one nerve root is involved in producing pain. Again, patients are able to control their pain by adjusting the rate and frequency of a millivoltage electrical current stimulator affixed externally.

f. Assist with biofeedback, which represents a wide range of behavioral techniques that provide the patient with information about changes in body functions of which the person is usually unaware. For example, information used to reduce muscle contraction is obtained by an electromyogram recorded from body surface electrodes. Changes in blood flow are produced by monitoring skin temperature changes. The person using biofeedback tries to change the display of information in the desired direction by actions such as reducing muscle tension or reducing or altering blood flow to a particular area. The critical care nurse should be familiar with the theoretical concepts of biofeedback and should support the patient in maximizing pain control through whatever techniques are successful for that patient.

IMPAIRED COMMUNICATION: APHASIA
Theoretical Basis and Management

Impaired communication is the state in which an individual has difficulty exchanging thoughts, ideas, or desires. Critical care nurses are acutely aware of the difficulties encountered in caring for patients with impaired communication. It is challenging enough to manage effective communication with intubated patients. But what of the brain-injured aphasic patient who may be unable to understand what is being said or written and/or who may be unable to express himself or herself verbally or in writing or even by gestures? Communication with such a patient can be frustrating and emotionally draining for the nurse as well as the patient. Humans operate primarily through the spoken and written word. It is said that when speech and language functions are disturbed as a consequence of brain disease, the resultant functional loss exceeds all others—even blindness, deafness, or paralysis—in gravity.[3]

Anatomy of language function. The posterior temporoparietal area contains the receptive speech center known as *Wernicke's area* (Fig. 28-1). The center for the perception of written language lies anterior to the visual receptive areas. Located at the base of the frontal lobe's motor strip and slightly anterior to it is *Broca's area,* also known as the motor speech center. These sensory and motor areas are connected by a large bundle of nerve fibers. Rather than receptive and motor language functions being entirely within discrete areas, it is believe that language is an integrated sensorimotor process, roughly located in these areas in the dominant cerebral hemisphere. It is also recognized that the elaborately complex functions of speech and language depend on other associative areas of the cerebrum and their thalamic connections. Consequently, there is much inconsistency in the degree of communication impairment among patients with lesions located in the same area of the brain.[3,36,39]

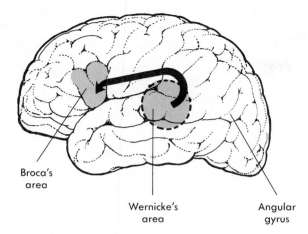

Fig. 28-1 Major areas of the cerebral cortex associated with speech. Arrow indicates interconnective fibers between the two speech areas.

Broca's area

Wernicke's area

Angular gyrus

Aphasia. Aphasia is a loss of language abilities caused by brain injury, usually to the dominant hemisphere. The left hemisphere is dominat for language function in 90% to 99% of right-handed individuals and in 50% to 75% of left-handed individuals. The most common cause of aphasia is vascular disease involving the left middle cerebral artery.[39] Other causes may be intracranial tumor or trauma in the frontal-parietal-temporal area.

Aphasia involves more than just understanding speech or expressing oneself through verbal means. Language is a much broader term, referring to what the individual is attempting to interpret or convey through listening, speaking, reading, and writing.[39] Most aphasias are partial rather than complete. The severity of the disorder depends on the area and the extent of the cerebral damage.

Fluent aphasia. Fluent aphasia, also referred to as sensory, Wernicke's, or receptive aphasia, occurs when the connection between the primary auditory cortex in the temporal lobe and the angular gyrus in the parietal lobe is destroyed. The patient's comprehension of speech is impaired, but he or she can still talk if the motor area for speech, Broca's area, is intact. The patient may in fact talk excessively, with many errors in the use of words. The patient is able to hear the examiner but cannot comprehend what is being said and cannot repeat the examiner's words. Such patients may talk nonsense, with rambling speech that gives little information. Patients with fluent aphasia also cannot read words, although they can see them. They cannot understand the symbolic content of printed or written symbols, a condition called alexia.[26,36,39]

Fluent aphasia usually improves in time to varying degrees. Some individuals improve to the point that it is difficult to detect the receptive deficit without special verbal and written tests. The most favorable outcomes are in those patients with the mildest forms of fluent aphasia.[3]

Nonfluent aphasia. Nonfluent aphasia, also known as motor, Broca's, or expressive aphasia, is primarily a deficit in language output or speech production. Depending on the lesion's size and exact location, there can be a wide variation in the motor deficit that results. Nonfluent aphasia can range from a mild dysarthria (imperfect articulation as a result of weakness or lack of coordination of speech musculature), to incorrect tonation and phrasing, and, in its most severe form, to complete loss of all ability to communicate through verbal and written means. In this severe form of aphasia, there is also a loss of ability to communicate through conventional gestures such as nodding or shaking the head for "yes" or "no." In most cases of nonfluent aphasia, the muscles of articulation are intact. If speech is possible at all, occasionally the words "yes" or "no" are uttered, sometimes appropriately. In some cases the words of well-known songs may be sung. Other patients, when excited or angered, may utter expletives.[3,39]

Some patients with nonfluent aphasia struggle or hesitate in trying to express words. They struggle to form words while using motor musculature (verbal apraxia), an articulatory disorder that is a feature of some nonfluent aphasias.[39] All of these difficulties lead to exasperation and despair for the patient.

Most patients with nonfluent aphasia also have severely impaired writing ability. Even though penmanship may be intact, they are unable to express themselves through writing—a deficit termed agraphia. If the right hand is paralyzed, as is often the case, the patient still cannot write or print with the left hand.[3]

In the recovery phase of severe nonfluent aphasia, patients become able to speak aloud to some degree, although words are uttered slowly and laboriously. However, many patients are able to learn to communicate ideas to some extent.[3]

Global aphasia. Global aphasia results when a massive lesion affects both the motor and sensory speech areas. The patient is unable to transform sounds into words and is unable to comprehend spoken words. All language modalities are affected, and impairment may be so severe that the patient may be unable to communicate on any level. These patients generally have severe hemiplegia and homonymous hemianopsia also. In these patients, language function rarely recovers to a significant degree unless the lesion is caused by some transient disorder such as cerebral edema or a metabolic derangement.[3,36]

Conduction aphasia. Conduction aphasia occurs when a lesion disrupts the connection between Broca's and Wernicke's areas, although the anatomical basis is poorly defined. The features of conduction aphasia often resemble those of fluent aphasia. The patient may produce speech, but little of it conveys meaning. The patient's use of written language reflects the same problems as speech. These patients may be well aware of their deficit. They may be alert and able to comprehend everything they see and hear but remain incapable of self-initiated speech or repetition of words. They will also have problems reading aloud, even though they may comprehend written words.[36]

Many other lesser-known and uncommon disorders of communication exist. This discussion explains only the most common forms of aphasia that the critical care nurse may encounter.

Impaired Verbal Communication: Aphasia related to cerebral speech center injury

DEFINING CHARACTERISTICS

Major (must be present)
- Inappropriate or absent speech or responses to questions

Minor (may be present)
- Inability to speak spontaneously
- Inability to understand spoken words
- Inability to follow commands appropriately through gestures
- Difficulty or inability to understand written language
- Difficulty or inability to express ideas in writing
- Difficulty or inability to name objects

OUTCOME CRITERIA

- Patient is able to make basic needs known.

NURSING INTERVENTIONS *AND RATIONALE*

1. Continue to monitor the assessment parameters listed under "Defining Characteristics."
2. Obtain a speech pathology evaluation (if available) *to determine the extent of the patient's communication deficit (e.g., if fluent, nonfluent, or global aphasia is involved).*
3. Have the speech therapist post a list of appropriate ways to communicate with the patient in the patient's room *so that all nursing personnel can be consistent in their efforts.*
4. Assess the patient's ability to comprehend, speak, read, and write.
   - Ask questions that can be answered with a yes or a no. If a patient answers yes to a question, ask the opposite (e.g., "Are you hot?" "Yes." "Are you cold?" "Yes."). *This may help determine if in fact the patient understands what is being said.*
   - Ask simple, short questions and use gestures, pantomime, and facial expressions to give the patient additional clues.
   - Stand in the patient's line of vision, giving a good view of your face and hands.
   - Have the patient try to write with a pad and pencil. Offer pictures and alphabet letters at which to point.
   - Make flash cards with pictures or words depicting frequently used phrases (e.g., glass of water, bedpan).[11]
5. Maintain an uncluttered environment and decrease external distractions that could hinder communication.
6. Maintain a relaxed and calm manner and explain all diagnostic, therapeutic, and comfort measures before initiating them.
7. Do not shout or speak in a loud voice. *Hearing loss is not a factor in aphasia, and shouting will not help.*
8. Have only one person talk at a time. *It is more difficult for the patient to follow a multisided conversation.*
9. Use direct eye contact and speak directly to the patient in unhurried, short phrases.
10. Give one-step commands and directions, and provide cues through pictures or gestures.
11. Try to ask questions that can be answered with a yes or a no, and avoid topics that are controversial, emotional, abstract, or lengthy.
12. Listen to the patient in an unhurried manner and wait for his or her attempt to communicate.
    - Expect a time lag from when you ask the patient something until the patient responds.
    - Accept the patient's statement of essential words without expecting complete sentences.
    - Avoid finishing the sentence for the patient if possible.
    - Wait approximately 30 seconds before providing the word the patient may be attempting to find (except when the patient is very frustrated and needs something such as a bedpan quickly).
    - Rephrase the patient's message aloud *to validate it.*
    - Do not pretend to understand the patient's message if you do not.[36]
13. Encourage the patient to speak slowly in short phrases and to say each word clearly.
14. Ask the patient to write the message, if able, or draw pictures if only verbal communication is affected.
15. Observe the patient's nonverbal clues for validation (e.g., answers "yes" but shakes head "no").
16. When handing an object to the patient, state what it is, *since hearing language spoken is necessary to stimulate language development.*
17. Explain what has happened to the patient and offer reassurance about the plan of care.
18. Verbally address the problem of frustration over inability to communicate and explain that patience is needed for both the nurse and the patient.
19. Maintain a calm, positive manner, and offer reassurance (e.g., "I know this is very hard for you, but it will get better if we work on it together").
20. Talk to the patient as an adult. Be respectful and avoid talking down to the patient.
21. Do not discuss the patient's condition or hold conversations in the patient's presence without including him or her in the discussion. *This may be the reason some aphasic patients develop paranoid thoughts.*
22. Do not exhibit disapproval of emotional utterances or spontaneous use of profanity; instead, offer calm, quiet reassurance.
23. If the patient makes an error in speech, do not reprimand or scold but try to compliment the patient by saying, "That was a good try."
24. Delay conversation if the patient is tired. *The symptoms of aphasia worsen if the patient is fatigued, anxious, or upset.*
25. Be prepared for emotional outbursts and tears in patients who have more difficulty in expressing themselves than with understanding. The patient may become depressed, refuse treatment and food, ignore relatives, and push objects away. Comfort the patient with statements such as, "I know it's frustrating and you feel sad, but you are not alone. Other people who have had strokes have felt the way you do. We will be here to help you get through this."[11,36,39]

SENSORY-PERCEPTUAL ALTERATIONS
Theoretical Basis and Management

Sensory-perceptual alterations is defined by NANDA as "a state in which an individual experiences a change in the amount or patterning of incoming stimuli accompanied by a diminished, exaggerated, distorted or impaired response to such stimuli."[11] Although a similar acute delirious state can occur as the result of idiosyncratic effects of medications, electrolyte imbalances, metabolic disturbances, and tissue hypoxia, the diagnosis is applied in this discussion to describe an acute, transient, *nonorganic* syndrome experienced by the critical care or critical care step-down patient in whom there is an altered response to sensory stimulation.

Fig. 28-2 depicts the usual pattern in which humans process environmental stimulation. The first step is to *perceive* by way of the *senses*. In the awake state, humans continuously receive information through stimulation of the five senses: auditory, visual, gustatory, olfactory, and tactile information.

The next step is to formulate a *feeling* state based on the processing of stimuli. Feelings of peace, safety, fear, desire, and anger result from sensory perceptions. Memory has a strong influence on the feeling state that follows sensory perceptions. Certain smells, sounds, and tactile sensations generate feeling states, pleasant and unpleasant, based on past associations. Similarly, sensory perceptions that are continually new or unfamiliar to the individual give rise to feelings of anxiety.

Following the feeling state is a *thinking* state in which thoughts are developed in relation to that which is sensed and felt: "I must move"; "I will stay"; "I want more."

Finally, *behavior* is motivated by the thought content or, in the individual acting on impulse, by the feeling. Behavior such as mobilization, immobilization, retreat, or advance is the enactment of a person's thoughts and/or feelings.

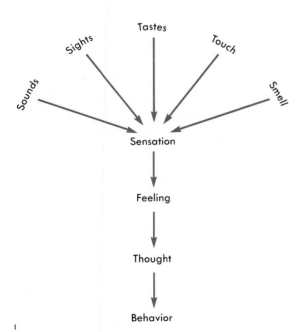

Fig. 28-2 Processing of environmental stimulation.

The nursing diagnosis sensory-perceptual alterations describes a situation in which there is *sensory misperception or misinterpretation;* consequently, feeling states, thought content, and behavior are often *nonreality based.*

Etiological/Related Factors. The diagnosis sensory-perceptual alterations has as its contributing factors sensory overload, sensory deprivation, and sleep-pattern disturbance.

Sensory overload. For the acutely ill patient in the critical care environment, there is an intense amount of sensory stimulation, which tends to be alien, unpleasant or assaultive, and continuous. Moreover, this stimulation is *comprehensive,* in that all five senses—taste, smell, touch, sight, and sound—are stimulated.

This *pansensory* stimulation of the critical care patient affects him or her in the following ways.

GUSTATORY. Because of fluid restrictions, nothing-by-mouth (NPO) status, impaired swallowing because of endotracheal tube, mouth breathing associated with shortness of breath, and the effects of certain drugs, the tastes experienced by critical care patients are often extremely unpleasant.

OLFACTORY. The odors associated with critical illness and the critical care environment are at times alien and/or unpleasant. The openness of the unit intensifies the pervasiveness of olfactory stimulation. Episodes of incontinence, emesis, gastrointestinal bleeding, and tracheal suctioning become public events for the sensory experience of many.

TACTILE. The tactile sensations of invasive lines and their bulky dressings, indwelling bladder catheters and rectal probes, artificial airway tubes, and the singularly uncomfortable sensation of being suctioned compose a sizeable fraction of the sensory experience of critically ill patients.

Pain, be it visceral, cutaneous, ischemic, or from muscle spasm, is a perennial concomitant to critical illness. However, what is particularly assaultive is the experience of human touch being nearly always accompanied by a painful procedure such as injections, placement of invasive lines, or position changes.

VISUAL. The patient in a critical care unit is a visual witness to resuscitation efforts (successful and unsuccessful), body removals, distraught families, and the hyperkinetic activity of scores of unfamiliar clinicians. He or she is a victim of constant lighting. From the patient's perspective, usually supine and looking up, the sights confer little meaning other than to suggest the intensity and urgency of the environment.

AUDITORY. Noise is a pollutant. In the critical care environment, random, nonmeaningful, alarming, and high-intensity noise constitutes the greatest source of sensory stimulation.[20] Table 28-1 lists noise levels of common events in the critical care unit measured at distances from the patient's head. When compared to noise levels in decibels (dB) designated as "acceptable" by the International Noise Council (day—45 dB, evening—40 dB, and night—20 dB), a case for there being excessive auditory stimulation in the critical care environment is readily made.

Not only the intensity of the noise but its nature and quality influence how it is perceived by the patient. The multiple-alarm conditions that are signalled by startling, high-frequency noises reinforce the patient's perception of physiological instability or deterioration and doom.

Table 28-1 Noise levels in critical care environment

Sound source	Noise in decibels (dB)
AT HEAD OF BED	
Dialysis alarm	63
Cooling blanket	67
Endotracheal suctioning	70
Cardiac rate alarm	71
AVCO Balloon Pump	74
Ice machine	75
MA-1 tidal volume	77
Chest percussion	83
MA-1 disconnect alarm	92
AT DISTANCE OF 10 FEET	
MA-1 tidal volume	66
Telephone ring	67
MA-1 sigh	68
Telephone dropped onto cradle	71
Closing of emergency cart drawer	74
Squeaking chair	76
MA-1 pressure alarm	76
Electrocardiogram electrode disconnect alarm	80
Bed screen moved	81
MA-1 disconnect alarm	83
AT DISTANCE OF 15 FEET	
Three physicians talking	68
Five physicians talking	74

Modified from Hansell HN: Heart Lung 13:62, 1984.

A consistent finding of research studies examining noise in patient care areas is that noise levels produced by clinical personnel are above those levels designated as acceptable and often greater than those generated by technological devices.[20]

Sensory deprivation. Amid the overload of *nonmeaningful* stimuli just described, the critical care patient at the same time is deprived of *meaningful,* familiar sensory stimulation necessary for psychic integration.

Familiar sights, sounds, and voices, textures, silence, and darkness are for the most part absent. *Touch* for the express purpose of human-to-human contact as opposed to therapeutic manipulation can be largely nonexistent in the critical care environment.

Sleep pattern disturbance. Discussed in detail in Unit II, "Sleep Alterations," the disturbed sleep pattern of the patient in critical care consists of sleep deprivation in general and deprivation of rapid eye movement (REM) sleep specifically. REM sleep integrates the individual's cognitive operations through dream states and increases adaptive capacity in the waking state.

Clinical manifestations. The net human response to the effects of sensory overload, sensory deprivation, and sleep

pattern disturbance is one of *sensory misperception or misinterpretation* and retreat into an inner reality.

Using the paradigm from Fig. 28-2, it is evident that the environment as perceived through the senses ceases to hold meaning for the individual; thus his or her perception of it becomes altered, giving rise to altered feeling states such as fear, danger, alienation, and lack of safety. Correspondingly, the content of thoughts becomes altered and often nonreality based as the individual attempts to derive meaning from his or her perceptions and feelings. The influence of memory and past association on both feelings and thoughts is appreciated when the patient discloses them. Persecutory, "prisoner-of-war" delusions are commonly revealed by patients with a history of armed service. Finally, behavior is motivated by these thoughts and feelings, and the patient is observed attempting to flee, resist, accuse, or defend.

Defining characteristics most commonly associated with the diagnosis sensory-perceptual alterations in the critical care patient are hallucinations, delusions, illusions, disorientation, short-term memory deficits, and impaired abstraction.[16]

Hallucinations. Hallucinations are sensory misperceptions that occur with *no* external stimulus[17]. As a sensory experience, a hallucination can be auditory, visual, tactile, or, less frequently, gustatory or olfactory. For example, a patient might report hearing voices or messages, seeing insects, or feeling spiders crawling over his or her skin. In the absence of organic causes, hallucinations experienced by critical care patients are thought to arise from deprivation of REM sleep (dream sleep) and can be thought of as *dreaming in the awake state.*

Another source for the development of hallucinations in this context is sensory deprivation.[16] In the absence of meaningful external stimulation, the individual partially dissociates from reality and engages in *autostimulation.* Autostimulation is the creation of an internal world consisting of private thoughts, ideas, and meanings incongruent with reality.[17]

Hallucinations cause a feeling of fright and, because they are experienced by the patient and no one else in the environment, represent a "betrayal" of the patient by the environment. This can lead to feelings of *suspicion* and *mistrust* and a belief that staff members are colluding in their denial of the patient's experiences.

Delusions. A delusion is a fixed, false belief that cannot be changed with logic and is one that the individual has not always held.[17] Occasionally, a delusion will evolve out of an auditory hallucination. For example, a patient hears voices telling him he is in great danger, the object of a plot. On this hallucination is fashioned a delusional system in which the patient believes himself or herself a prisoner of some revolutionary or persecutory endeavor.

One type of delusion (there are several) that merits distinction is *ideas of reference,* or *delusions of reference,* a situation in which the patient believes he or she is the object of all discussions and activity taking place around him or her. These ideas of reference stem not from an esteemed self-view but one of personal powerlessness, and they closely approximate paranoid, suspicious beliefs.

The environment of the critical care unit—open, busy, populated—presents a situation of high suggestibility for ideas of reference. There are, in fact, many discussions *about* the patient that do not *include* the patient. This external stimulation that excludes the patient from its boundaries can invoke feelings of detachment and suspiciousness. Such feelings are the precursors to the unrealistic persecutory beliefs that become the delusion. In a paradoxical sense, the delusion itself is the ego's attempt to defend against the patient's powerlessness and anxiety.

Illusions. An illusion is a misinterpretation of a real, external stimulus. This external stimulus is usually visual or auditory.[25] For example, patients may misinterpret their caregivers as significant others, living or deceased. Patients may also view those around them as benevolent spirits who have come to help them or, conversely, as demons who mean them harm.

Easton and MacKenzie[16] report about a critical care patient who believed himself tied inside a playpen in a supermarket. He told of shoppers selecting items from the shelves but not paying for the merchandise. His attempts at soliciting the attention of the shoppers were met only with shrugged shoulders. The patient, in reality, was restrained in his bed with the side rails up and was positioned facing the linen and medication carts.

Illusions invoke feelings of confusion and anxiety in the patient, and these feelings become the focus of nursing intervention.

Disorientation, short-term memory deficit, and impaired abstraction. These cognitive impairments are commonly associated with sensory-perceptual alterations in the critically ill adult.[16] They are primarily the result of sensory deprivation and REM sleep disturbance.

Sensory-Perceptual Alterations related to sensory overload, sensory deprivation, and sleep pattern disturbance

DEFINING CHARACTERISTICS

- Hallucinations
- Delusions
- Illusions
- Disorientation
- Short-term memory deficits
- Impaired abstraction

OUTCOME CRITERIA

- Patient has no evidence of hallucinations, delusions, or illusions.
- Results of reality testing are appropriate.
- Short-term memory is intact.
- Abstract reasoning is intact.

NURSING INTERVENTIONS *AND RATIONALE*

1. Continue to monitor the assessment parameters listed under "Defining Characteristics." Determine and document the patient's dominant spoken language, his or her literacy, and the language(s) in which he or she is literate. Determine and document his or her premorbid degree of orientation, cognitive capabilities, and any sensory-perceptual deficits. *It is sometimes the case that people are not literate in their spoken language or, less frequently, that they are literate only in their second language. These situations can result in unfortunate errors in the appraisal of patients' ability to communicate in writing and in estimating the extent of their orientation. Similarly, assuming that the patients were or were not fully oriented before critical care admission bases the nurse's assessment on possibly erroneous assumptions.*

For sensory overload

1. Initiate each nurse-patient encounter by calling the patient by name and identifying yourself by name. *This fosters reality orientation and assists the patient in filtering irrelevant or impersonal conversation.*
2. Assess the patient's immediate physical environment from his or her viewpoint and explain equipment, its sounds, and its therapeutic purpose. Demonstrate audible and visual alarms and explain the possible alarm conditions. *This decreases alienation of the patient from the technological environment and reduces the inherent sense of fear and urgency accompanying alarm conditions.*
3. For each procedure performed, provide "preparatory sensory information," i.e., explain procedures in relation to the sensations the patient will experience, including duration of sensations. *Preparatory sensory information enhances learning and lessens anticipatory anxiety.*
4. Limit noise levels. Certainly, audible alarms cannot and should not be silenced, and many critical, albeit noisy, activities must take place in the critical care area. It has been shown, however, that noise levels produced by clinical personnel exceed those levels designated as "acceptable" and are often greater than those generated by technological devices.[20] Staff conversations should be kept soft enough that they are inaudible to the patient whenever possible. Critical care personnel should assume that everything said at or around a patient's bedside is intended for that patient's awareness and that it will be interpreted as

Continued.

Sensory-Perceptual Alterations related to sensory overload, sensory deprivation, and sleep pattern disturbance—cont'd

pertaining to him or her. *As discussed below, conversations about the patient but not to him or her foster depersonalization and delusions of reference.*

5. Well-enforced noise limits should exist for nighttime.

6. Readjust alarm limits on physiological monitoring devices as the patient's condition changes (improves or deteriorates) to *lessen unnecessary alarm states.*

7. Consider use of head phones and audio cassette with patient's favorite and/or subliminal or classical music. *This can effectively filter out assaultive noise of the critical care environment and supplant it with familiar, soothing sounds and rhythms.*

8. Modify lighting. Day-night cycles should be simulated with environmental lighting. At no time should overhead fluorescent lights be abruptly turned on without either warning the patient, assisting him or her out of the supine position, and/or shielding his or her eyes with gauze or a face cloth. *Continuous bright lighting sustains anxiety and promotes circadian rhythm desynchronization.*

9. To the extent possible, shield patients from viewing urgent and emergent events in the critical care unit. *Resuscitation efforts, albeit difficult to conceal, engender fear in the patient and a sense of instability and vulnerability (e.g., "I'm next").* When such an event occurs, the nurse should endeavor to elicit the patient's cognitive and emotional reaction; thoughts, impressions, and feelings should be shared and misconceptions clarified. A useful approach for the nurse in this interchange is that of emphasizing the differences between the patient at hand and the one resuscitated (e.g., "He was considerably older," "more unstable," "had serious lung disease").

10. Ensure patients' privacy, their modesty and, at the very least, their dignity. Physical exposure and nudity, although seeming to pale in importance alongside such priorities as physiological assessment and stabilization, are primal indignities in all individuals. Patients should be kept minimally exposed. When, in the course of assessment and intervention, it becomes necessary to expose the patient, the nurse should first verbally apologize for this necessity. *To be naked is to feel vulnerable; to be vulnerable is to feel fearful. In this regard, fear is an emotional concomitant to critical care that is preventable through nursing intervention.*

For sensory deprivation

1. Provide reality orientation in four spheres (person, place, time, and situation) at more frequent intervals than when testing. Convey this information in the context of routine conversation. SAMPLE STATEMENTS: "Mr. Clark, this is Tuesday morning and you're in University Hospital. Your heart surgery was yesterday morning and you're doing well. My name is Joe, and I'm your nurse today." *The patient is made to feel patronized by repetitions such as, "Do you know where you are?"* Given the effects of general anesthesia, narcotic analgesics, sedatives, and sleep, it is fully expected that some degree of disorientation will exist normally.

2. Ensure the patient's visual access to a calendar. (Interestingly, the design of most state-of-the-art critical care units now reflects many of the principles of sensory stimulation. One such coronary care unit was designed with a large wall clock facing the patient. A patient who had spent more than a week in this unit later reflected that one of the most "distressing, frustrating" aspects of his stay in the coronary care unit was the monotonous, inescapable attention to the clock and its painfully slow documentation of the passing of time.)

3. Apprise the patient of daily news events and the weather.

4. Touch patients for the express purpose of communicating caring. Hold their hands, stroke their brows, rub the skin on an aspect of their arms. *Touch is the universal language of caring. In the setting of critical care, in which there is considerable physical body manipulation, it is useful and important to contrast assaultive touch with comforting touch.* Touch can be used as a technique for distraction from painful stimuli when used in conjunction with uncomfortable procedures. See Appendix D, "Therapeutic Touch." (IMPORTANT: See discussion of the use of touch in "Management of the Patient Experiencing Hallucinations.")

5. Foster liberal visitation by family and significant others. Encourage significant others to touch the patient as consistent with their individual comfort level and cultural norms.

6. Structure and identify opportunities for the patient to exercise decision-making skills, however small. *Although not so designated, patients with sensory alterations experience a type of "cognitive deprivation" as well.* (See "Powerlessness," Chapter 47).

Continued.

Sensory-Perceptual Alterations related to sensory overload, sensory deprivation, and sleep pattern disturbance—cont'd

7. Assist patients to find meaning in their experiences. Explain the therapeutic purpose of all that they are asked to do for themselves and all that is done with them and for them. Avoid statements such as, "Will you turn to that side for me?" or "I need you to swallow this medication." *These statements implicitly convey that the maneuver has some value for the nurses versus the patients.* Similarly, use "thank you" judiciously. *This simple salutation, when used indiscriminately, suggests something was done to benefit the nurses and not the patients.* Patients need to find meaning and to identify their roles in the experience of critical illness and critical care. The sensations that constitute this experience and those that do not are made bearable and intelligible when attached to the larger picture of their conditions, treatment, and progress.

For sleep pattern disturbances. For excellent management strategies of sleep pattern disturbance, refer to Chapter 8, "Sleep Care Plans: Theoretical Basis and Management."

For management of the patient experiencing hallucinations

1. Approach the patient with a calm, matter-of-fact demeanor. *The goal of this interaction is for the nurse to demonstrate external control. This helps decrease the anxiety and fear that generally accompany hallucinations and allows the patient to feel safe. Anxiety is transferable.*

2. *Address the patient by name. This is a useful presentation of reality because self-identity is the last sphere of orientation to vanish.*

3. In responding to the patient's description of the hallucination, DO NOT deny, argue, or attempt to disprove the existence of the perceived event. *Statements such as, "There are no voices coming from that air vent" or, "Look, I'm brushing my hand across the wall, and there are no bugs" confuse the patient further, because the hallucination, although frightening, is his or her perceived reality.*

4. Express to the patient that your experiences are dissimilar, and acknowledge how frightening his or hers must be. SAMPLE STATEMENT: "I don't hear (see, etc.) what you do, but I know how frightening such an experience must be to you. I'm Joe, your nurse, and I'm going to stay with you until the voices (etc.) go away." Remain with the patient, any patient, who is experiencing a hallucination. *Feelings of fear and anxiety often accelerate when a patient is left alone. He or she needs someone to represent a non-threatening reality. Additionally, validating the patient's feelings demonstrates acceptance and sensitivity to the experience and promotes trust.*

5. DO NOT explore the content of the hallucination with the patient by asking about its nature or character. *The nurse is the patient's link with reality. Pursuit of a detailed description of a hallucination may signify to the patient that the nurse accepts his or her sensory distortion as factual. This may further confuse the patient and distance him or her more from reality.** The nurse can help bridge the gap between the patient's misperception and reality by addressing the feelings (e.g., fear, anxiety) and/or meanings (e.g., danger, death) engendered by the hallucination. Determination of how the misperception affects the patient emotionally, acknowledgment of those feelings, and a calm, controlled, matter-of-fact approach will provide the trust and comfort he or she needs to tolerate this frightening experience. In other words, deal with the intent more than the content of the hallucination. *The resultant decrease in anxiety will enable the patient to focus more accurately on his immediate environment.*

6. Talk concretely with the patient about things that are really happening. SAMPLE STATEMENTS: "How does your chest incision feel this afternoon, Mr. Clark?" "Your sister Kate was here to see you, but you were sleeping. She went down to the cafeteria and will be back." "Your secretions are a little easier for you to cough up today." *Interpretation of reality-based stimuli by the nurse encourages the patient to focus on actual circumstances and discourages a preoccupation with sensory misperceptions.*

7. There may be circumstances in which it is appropriate for the nurse simply to distract the patient by changing the topic. This tactic is useful in situations of escalating anxiety and confusion or when all else fails. Topics should consist of basic themes that are universally understood and culturally congruent such as music, food, or weather. They may also be topics of special

---

*An exception is the patient who the nurse suspects is experiencing auditory hallucinations, i.e., hearing "voice commands." To ascertain that the voices are not telling the patient to harm himself, it is appropriate for the nurse to ask simply and concretely, "What are the voices saying?"

Continued.

Sensory-Perceptual Alterations related to sensory overload, sensory deprivation, and sleep pattern disturbance—cont'd

interest to the patient such as hobbies, crafts, or sports. Topics that evoke strong emotions such as politics, religion, or sexuality should be avoided with most patients. *This is especially true of the patient with reality distortions; sometimes hallucinations and delusions are expressions of repressed conflicts associated with religious, sexual, or aggressive issues. Pursuit of such subjects could increase confusion and anxiety.*

8. The use of touch: *Touch presents a nonthreatening external reality and can therefore be useful in the management of patients with sensory alterations. However, in the patient experiencing hallucinations (as well as delusions and illusions), touch can be readily misinterpreted as, for instance, aggression or pain, or it can actually provide the basis for a tactile illusion.* Therefore the use of touch as an intervention strategy should be avoided in any patient who evidences escalating anxiety or paranoid, suspicious, or mistrustful thoughts.

9. Types of hallucinations include the following: auditory—voices or running commentaries, with self-destructive messages; visual—persons or images that appear threatening; olfactory—smells that may be interpreted as poisonous gases; gustatory—tastes that seem peculiar or harmful; and tactile—touch that feels unusual or unnatural.

10. Specific management strategies for patients experiencing hallucinations.
    - Auditory hallucinations
      a. Patient behaviors: Head cocked as if listening to an unseen presence; lips moving.
      b. Therapeutic nurse responses: "Mr. Clark, you appear to be listening to something." *If patient acknowledges voices:* "I don't hear any voices, but I know this is troubling you. The voices will go away. Nothing is going to harm you. I'm Joe, your nurse, and I'll be here with you."
      c. Nontherapeutic nurse responses: "Tell me about your conversations with these voices." "To whom do the voices belong—anyone you know?"
    - Visual hallucinations
      a. Patient behaviors: Staring into space as if focused on an unseen object; startled movements and anxious facial expression.
      b. Therapeutic nurse responses: "Mr. Clark, something seems to be troubling you. Tell me what it is." *If patient states he visualizes people,*

images, or the devil in his environment and implies a sense of danger, respond, "There are only nurses and doctors here, Mr. Clark. I know this must be upsetting, but these images will go away. We're here with you in the hospital. Nothing will happen to you."

c. Nontherapeutic nurse responses: "Describe the people you see. What are they wearing?" "What does the devil mean in your life? What about God?"

For management of the patient experiencing delusions

1. Explain all unseen noises, voices, and activity simply and clearly. *They readily feed a delusional system.* SAMPLE STATEMENTS: "That is Dr. Smith. He's come to see you and other patients here in the hospital." "The voices and activity you hear are from the bedside of the patient behind this curtain. He's being helped by one of the nurses."

2. Avoid the "negative challenge" (for example, "Nobody here stole your belongings" or "Doctors and nurses do not harm people") of the patient's delusion. Similarly, avoid defending the referents of the patient's belief: "Nurses are good" and "Doctors mean well." *Remember, a delusion is a belief, albeit false, that cannot be changed with logic. To attempt this change is to challenge the patient's belief system and thereby escalate his or her anxiety, further blurring the boundaries between reality and the patient's internally based "logic."*

3. For the patient with persecutory delusions who refuses food, fluids, or medications because of a belief they have been poisoned or tainted, permit the refusal unless it is a life-threatening event. Try again in 20 minutes; allow the patient to choose an alternate selection of food or to read the label on the unit's medication. Coercion, show of force, or engaging in complicated, logical justifications will only heighten the patient's suspiciousness and possibly reinforce the delusional belief. *When the patient feels more in control, he or she need not rely on the "paradoxical" quality of the delusion to equip him or her with a false sense of power. His or her power instead is derived from making reality-based decisions.*

4. Staff members should be particularly careful not to engage in unnecessary laughter or whispering among themselves within view of the delusional patient. *The delusional patient is hypervigilant, scanning the en-*

Continued.

Sensory-Perceptual Alterations related to sensory overload, sensory deprivation, and sleep pattern disturbance—cont'd

vironment for evidence to corroborate or confirm his or her belief that staff members are colluding against him or her clearly, laughter and whispers easily suggest this belief, this delusion of reference. This rationale pertains to the patient experiencing hallucinations and/or illusions as well.

5. Observe the principles detailed in the third intervention under "Management of the Patient Experiencing Hallucinations."

For management of the patient experiencing illusions

1. As with the management of delusions, the nurse should simply and briefly interpret reality-based stimuli for the patient in a calm, matter-of-fact manner. *Seen and unseen noises, voices, activity, and people can provide the stimulus for a sensory misinterpretation, an illusion.*

2. The immediate environment of the patient should provide as low a level of stimulation as possible. Nursing interventions detailed previously under "Sensory Overload" are especially relevant here.

3. The theme of the nurse's verbal approach to the patient experiencing illusions is similar to that outlined for hallucinations and delusions: address the feelings and meanings associated with the experience, not the content of the sensory misinterpretation.

- Patient behaviors: Eyes darting, startled movements; frightened facial expression. "I know who you are. You're the devil come to take me to hell."
- Therapeutic nurse responses: "I'm Joe, your nurse, I know this experience is troubling for you. You're in the hospital, and no one here will harm you."
- Nontherapeutic nurse responses: "There are no such things as devils or angels." "Do you think the devil would be dressed in white?" *The first nontherapeutic nurse response carries a parental tone (i.e., "you know better than that"), thus infantilizing the patient and adding to his or her feelings of powerlessness over the environment. The second nontherapeutic response reflects obvious logic, which is not in the patient's sensory domain; therefore it cannot be processed and only adds to his or her confused state.*

4. Observe the principles detailed under the fifth item in "Management of the Patient Experiencing Hallucinations."

REFERENCES

1. Adams RD: Pain: general considerations. In Isselbacher KJ and others, editors: Harrison's principles of internal medicine, ed 9, New York, 1980, McGraw-Hill Book Co.
2. Adams RD and Brady WG: Other major muscle syndromes. In Isselbacher KJ and others, editors: Harrison's principles of internal medicine, ed 9, New York, 1980, McGraw-Hill Book Co.
3. Adams RD and Victor M: Principles of neurology, ed 3, New York, 1985, McGraw-Hill Book Co.
4. American Pain Society: Pain, Am J Nurs 88(6):816, 1988.
5. American Psychiatric Association: Diagnostic and statistical manual of mental disorders, ed IIIR, Washington DC, 1987, American Psychiatric Association.
6. Benson H: The relaxation response, New York, 1976, Avon Books.
7. Beyerman K: Flawed perceptions about pain, Am J Nurs, 82:302, 1982.
8. Bohachick P: Progressive relaxation training in cardiac rehabilitation: effect on physiologic variables, Nurs Res 33:283, 1984.
9. Bootz-Marx R: Factors affecting intracranial pressure: a descriptive study, J Neurosci Nurs 17(2):89, 1985.
10. Caine R, Molla K, and Reynolds R: Malignant hyperthermia: a critical care challenge, Dimens Crit Care Nurs 5(3):144, 1986.
11. Carpenito L: Nursing diagnosis: application to clinical practice, ed 3, Philadelphia, 1989, JB Lippincott Co.
12. Chaffee EE and Lytle IM: Basic physiology and anatomy, ed 3, Philadelphia, 1980, JB Lippincott Co.
13. Cunha BA and Tu RP: I. Fever in the neurosurgical patient, Heart Lung 17(6):608, 1988.
14. Davis C and Cunningham SG: The physiologic response of patients in the coronary care unit to selected music, Heart Lung 14:291, 1985.
15. Dudas S: Nursing diagnosis and interventions for the rehabilitation of the stroke patient, Nurs Clin North Am 21(2):350, 1986.
16. Easton C and MacKenzie F: Sensory-perceptual alterations: delirium in the intensive care unit, Heart Lung 17(3):229, 1988.
17. Fortinash KM: Assessment of mental status. In Malasanos L and others: Health assessment, St Louis, 1989, The CV Mosby Co.
18. Grossmont District Hospital: Patient controlled analgesia, La Mesa, Calif, 1988.
19. Guyton AC: Basic human physiology: normal function and mechanisms of disease, Philadelphia, 1971, WB Saunders Co.
20. Hansell HN: The behavioral effects of noise on man: the patient with "intensive care psychosis," Heart Lung 13(1):59, 1984.
21. Harrison M and Cotanch P: Pain: advances and issues in critical care, Nurs Clin North Am 22(3):691, 1987.
22. Heidrich G and Perry S: Helping the patient in pain, Am J Nurs p. 1828, Dec 1982.
23. Hickey JV: The clinical practice of neurological and neurosurgical nursing, ed 2, Philadelphia, 1986, JB Lippincott Co.
24. Hunt WE and Hess RM: Surgical risks as related to time of intervention in the repair of intracranial aneurysms, J Neurosurg 28:14, 1968.
25. Kaplan HF and Saddock BJ: Comprehensive textbook of psychiatry/IV, Baltimore, 1985, Williams & Wilkins.
26. Luckmann J and Sorensen KC: Medical-surgical nursing: a psychophysiologic approach, ed 3, Philadelphia, 1987, WB Saunders Co.
27. MacBryde CM and Blacklow RS: Signs and symptoms, ed 5, Philadelphia, 1970, JB Lippincott Co.

28. Mantle JA et al: Cardiovascular evaluation and therapy of unstable patients. In Kinney MR and others: AACN's clinical reference for critical-care nursing, ed 2, New York, 1989, McGraw-Hill Book Co.

29. Matz R: Hypothermia: mechanisms and countermeasures, Hosp Pract 21(1):45, 1986.

30. McCaffery M: Nursing management of the patient with pain, ed 2, Philadelphia, 1979, JB Lippincott Co.

31. McCaffery M: Understanding your patient's pain, Nurs 80 10:26, 1980.

32. Mitchell PH: Decreased adaptive capacity, intracranial: a proposal for a nursing diagnosis, J Neurosci Nurs 18(4):170, 1986.

33. Mitchell PH: Intracranial hypertension: influence of nursing care activities, Nurs Clin North Am 21(4):563, 1986.

34. Mitchell SK and Yates RR: Cerebral vasospasm: theoretical causes, medical management, and nursing implications, J Neurosci Nurs 18(6):315, 1986.

35. Numbers L: Pain: an introduction, Nursing (Oxford) 3(9):358, 1986.

36. O'Brien MT and Pallett PJ: Total care of the stroke patient, Boston, 1978, Little, Brown & Co.

37. Peach SC: Some implications for the clinical use of music facilitated imagery, J Music Ther 21:27, 1984.

38. Petersdorf RG: Disturbances of heat regulation. In Isselbacher KJ and others, editors: Harrison's principles of internal medicine, ed 9, New York, 1980, McGraw-Hill Book Co.

39. Pimental PA: Alterations in communication: biopsychosocial aspects of asphasia, dysarthria, and right hemisphere syndromes in the stroke patient, Nurs Clin North Am 21(2):321, 1986.

40. Puntillo KA: The phenomenom of pain and critical care nursing, Heart Lung 17(3):262, 1988.

41. Quinless FW, Cassese M, and Atherton N: The effect of selected preoperative, intraoperative, and postoperative variables on the development of postcardiotomy psychosis in patients undergoing open heart surgery, Heart Lung 14(4):334, 1985.

42. Raimond J and Taylor JW: Neurological emergencies: effective nursing care, Rockville, MD: 1986, Aspen Publishers, Inc.

43. Rudy EB: Advanced neurological and neurosurgical nursing, St Louis, 1984, The CV Mosby Co.

44. Siegele D: The gate control theory, AM J Nurs 74(3):498, 1974.

45. Stewart SMB: Controlling pain with epidural narcotics: nursing implications, Crit Care Nurse 6:50, 1986.

46. Strandness DE: Vascular diseases of the extremities. In Isselbacher KJ and others, editors: Harrison's principles of internal medicine, ed 9, New York, 1980, Mcgraw-Hill Book Co.

47. Swearingen PA, Summers MS, and Miller K: Manual of critical care: applying nursing diagnoses to adult critical illness, St Louis, 1988, The CV Mosby Co.

48. Ward JD and others: Cerebral homeostasis and protection. In Wirth FP and Ratcheson RA, editors: Neurosurgical critical care, vol 1, Concepts in neurosurgery, Baltimore, 1987, Williams & Wilkins.

49. Wittington HG: The biopsychosocial model applied to chronic pain, J Operational Psych 16(2):1, 1985.

50. Young RR, Bradley WG, and Adams RD: Approach to clinical myology. In Isselbacher KJ and others, editors: Harrison's principles of internal medicine, ed 9, New York, 1980, McGraw-Hill Book Co.

51. Zimmerman LM, Pierson MA, and Marker J: Effects of music on patient anxiety in coronary care units, Heart Lung 17(5):560, 1988.

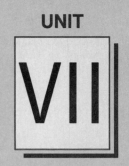

UNIT VII

RENAL AND FLUIDS ALTERATIONS

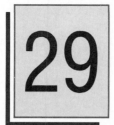

29

Renal and Fluids Anatomy and Physiology

CHAPTER OBJECTIVES

- *Identify and briefly describe the physiology of the normal anatomical structures of the kidney.*
- *Discuss important aspects of the following dynamics of fluid movement: osmosis, tonicity, diffusion, active transport, and filtration.*
- *Describe the clinical signs and symptoms that result when patients have deficiencies or excesses of serum electrolytes.*
- *Identify the pathway of renal filtrate.*
- *List and describe the functions of the kidneys.*

Take a moment to stop and think about how many glasses of water you have consumed today. Estimating your water intake may be difficult. Water, the single most important compound to human existence, is often taken for granted. On the other hand, it is lauded in literature, promoted in advertising, fought over in the courts, and used in so many activities of daily life it boggles the mind.

An evolutionary link has been suggested between the water of the seas that cover a major portion of earth and the water composing 60% of the weight of the adult human body. Salts and nutrients dissolved in the oceans of the world bear a striking similarity by percentage and content to the salts and nutrients contained in the human body.

Water in the human body provides a medium in which oxygen and nutrients dissolve and are used by the body, regulates body temperature through insulation or evaporation, and cushions body parts from injury. Dissolved within the body's water are substances such as potassium and sodium that are known as electrolytes. They are of critical importance in the maintenance of health.

A study of water and electrolytes in the human body is central to the understanding of other body systems. This chapter provides information about normal fluid and electrolyte patterns.

Material about fluid and electrolytes would not be complete without presenting the primary role that the kidneys play in regulating the fine balance of fluids and electrolytes in the human body. Found in Unit VII is a review of the anatomy and physiology of the healthy renal system, renal failures and their causes, replacement therapies, and care of the individual with renal problems.

FLUID COMPARTMENTS
Anatomy

The fluid of the human body is captured in distinct internal spaces referred to as *compartments*. Although the word compartment suggests that the fluid remains stationary within each space, the opposite is true. Fluid movement between compartments is dynamic and constant.

The compartments are separated from each other by thin sheets of tissue known as *membranes*. These membranes have openings (pores) that allow molecules of specific size and molecular weight to pass through while preventing larger, heavier molecules from doing so. This characteristic of the membrane is known as *semipermeability*.

Basically, two fluid compartments are in the human body. The *intracellular* compartment refers to the fluids inside each of the body's cells. It is, by far, the larger compartment, accounting for 40% of an individual's weight.

The remaining fluid is outside the cells in the spaces referred to as the *extracellular* compartment. This compartment is further divided into two subcompartments. The *intravascular* compartment, or blood supply, accounts for 5% of the body's weight. The tissue space, or *interstitial* compartment, is outside both the body cells and blood vessels and contains the remaining 15% of the body weight. Approximate amounts of fluid contained in each compartment are listed in Fig. 29-1, *A*.

The percentage of total body water varies slightly from individual to individual in relationship to age, sex, and body fat content. For instance, a lean adult male will usually have a 60% body water content, whereas an adult female will have closer to 50%. Infants have a body fluid content estimated at 77%; on the opposite end of the age continuum, body fluids decrease and may represent only 46% to 52% of body weight in the elderly.[11] Also, with any increase in body fat, the body fluid percentage decreases because fat does not contain a significant amount of water.

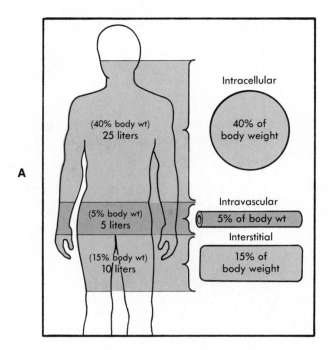
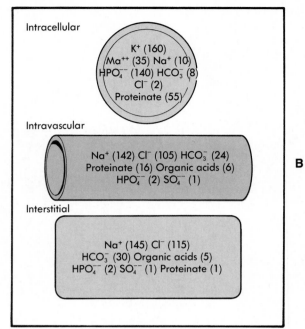

All measurements in MEq/L

Fig. 29-1 **A,** Fluid compartments. **B,** Electrolytes by fluid compartment.

Composition

Any information about body fluids by necessity must involve a description of the substances contained within the fluids. In fact, movement of fluids within the body does not take place without simultaneous movement of these substances.

Electrolytes are elements or compounds that, when dissolved in water, dissociate into parts known as *ions* and give the fluid the ability to conduct an electrical current. The ions carry either a positive (+) or negative (−) charge. Positive ions are known as *cations,* and negative ions are known as *anions.* Electrolytes exist in differing amounts in each of the fluid compartments. The primary electrolytes and other substances of importance are listed by fluid compartment in Fig. 29-1, *B.*

A balance exists between cations and anions and other substances in the compartments. Maintaining this balance is of paramount importance to the normal function of all body systems. For example, the difference between the intravascular and interstitial compartments lies in the amount of proteinate in the vascular compartment.[12] This difference helps maintain a balance between these two compartments. Finally, there are obvious differences in electrolyte compositions between the intracellular and extracellular fluids.

Fluid and Electrolyte Physiology

An overall understanding is needed of both the structures containing or balancing electrolytes and the physiological forces governing movement and balance. Additionally, factors that inhibit or enhance the transfer of fluids and electrolytes are discussed.

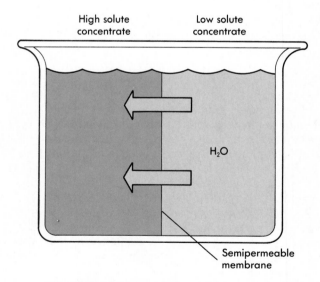

Fig. 29-2 Movement of water by osmosis.

Osmosis. Osmosis is the movement of water through a semipermeable membrane from an area of dilution (greater quantity of water) to an area of concentration. For instance, if distilled water is contained on one side of a semipermeable membrane and a sugar-water solution is on the other, water will travel through the membrane to the sugar-water solution, as illustrated in Fig. 29-2. Osmosis is one of the forces that describes the physiological shift of fluid from one compartment to another. For example, the intravenous infusion of a colloid solution results in an osmotic pull of fluid from the interstitial space into the intravascular space.

Tonicity. *Isotonic, hypotonic,* and *hypertonic* all refer to tonicity, or the *osmolality* of body fluids. Basically, osmolality is defined as the measure of the number of particles in a solution. Measurement of osmolality is in *milliosmoles* and is derived by dividing the milligrams per liter of the substances by their atomic weight. The normal osmolality of body fluids is 280 to 300 mOsm/kg of body weight.[2]

Isotonic means that the number of particles in a solution contained on one side of a membrane or container approximates the number of particles in solution on the other side of the container or membrane. In humans, an isotonic solution is one that has roughly the same tonicity as blood plasma. Therefore cells bathed in an isotonic solution maintain consistency and do not lose fluid to their surroundings (Fig. 29-3, *A*). Care must be exercised to use *isotonic* solutions when their direct contact with the bloodstream is necessary for more than short periods of time.

Hypertonic fluid contains a concentration of particles greater than that inside the cell (Fig. 29-3, *B*). When a hypertonic fluid is infused into the body for a prolonged time, fluid may be drawn out of the cells, causing a withering of the cell called *crenation*. However, if used appropriately, hypertonic solutions such as the osmotic diuretic mannitol can be effective in drawing excess fluid from the cells and interstitial spaces.

Hypotonic solutions contain fewer particles than the solution inside the cell (Fig. 29-3, *C*). As a result, cells suspended in hypotonic fluid swell and burst, a condition known as *hemolysis*. However, if an individual is suffering from dehydration, hypotonic solutions such as 0.45% saline replenish the fluids and some of the lost electrolytes.

Diffusion. Unlike osmosis, the process of diffusion is concerned with the solid particles suspended in the fluid. Diffusion is the movement of particles through a semipermeable membrane from an area of high concentration of particles to an area of low concentration of particles. The particles do not move in an orderly fashion but strike the

membrane randomly and pass through it until equilibration is achieved on either side of the membrane.[11]

For example, urea particles suspended in glomerular filtrate travel through the renal tubules. As water is reabsorbed into the peritubular capillaries, the concentration of urea particles in the tubules rise. A concentration difference exists between the inside of the tubules and the tissue space outside. As a result, urea travels from the tubules into the tissue space and equilibrates the number of particles on either side of the tubular structure.[10]

A force influencing the diffusion of particles across the membrane is known as the *electrical gradient*. Ions carry a positive or negative charge and therefore interact on either side of the membrane by either attracting substances with opposite charges or repelling substances with like charges.[6]

Diffusion also depends on pore size versus molecular size of the particles of a substance. For instance, water molecules are small and diffuse easily, but glucose molecules are larger and pass with difficulty through membrane pores.

Active transport. A concentration difference exists for various electrolytes on either side of the cell membrane. This concentration difference is called a *chemical* or *concentration gradient*. At times there is a need for an electrolyte such as potassium (K^+), which has a low concentration outside the cell, to move inside the cell to an area of high potassium concentration. To move against this chemical gradient (that is, to move from an area of low concentration to an area of high potassium concentration), energy and a substance to carry the potassium are required. The process by which potassium moves against this chemical gradient is called *active transport*. At times sodium also moves by active transport.

Active transport has been likened to a "pump" by which the sodium and potassium are exchanged across the cell membrane and against the concentration gradient. Sodium combines with a carrier substance, a lipoprotein, and travels out of the cell, where it is released. The lipoprotein changes to accept the potassium ion, which is then transported into

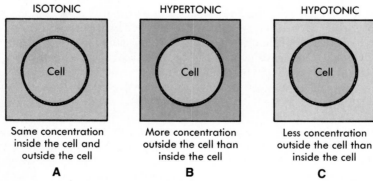

ISOTONIC

Cell

Same concentration inside the cell and outside the cell

A

HYPERTONIC

Cell

More concentration outside the cell than inside the cell

B

HYPOTONIC

Cell

Less concentration outside the cell than inside the cell

C

Fig. 29-3　**A,** Isotonic solution: the extracellular solution concentration is the same as the intracellular concentration. There is no movement of water into or out of the cell. **B,** Hypertonic solution: the extracellular solution concentration is greater than the intracellular concentration. Water moves from the cell into the extracellular compartment. **C,** Hypotonic solution: the extracellular solution concentration is less than the intracellular concentration. Water moves from the extracellular compartment into the cell.

the cell and released. The system continues indefinitely under the influence of adenosine triphosphate (ATP), which provides the energy necessary for the carrier substances to travel.

The active transport mechanism changes the electrical charge on the cell membrane and gives the membrane the "potential" for accepting a message from the nervous system. This process allows contraction of skeletal muscle.

Filtration. Filtration is defined as the movement of fluid and dissolved substances through a semipermeable membrane from an area of high pressure to an area of low pressure[11] (Fig. 29-4). The force of left-ventricular contraction pushes the blood through the circulatory system, causing exertion of pressure by the blood against the vessel walls. This force is known as *hydrostatic pressure.*

The hydrostatic pressure creates the tendency for fluids and dissolved substances to move into the interstitial spaces. If not for other forces counteracting the hydrostatic pressure, fluid would leave the intravascular space until it was depleted. However, whereas hydrostatic pressure creates fluid and electrolyte movement out of the intravascular compartment, the *colloid osmotic pressure* of the plasma tends to hold the fluid and substances in the intravascular space.[16] Colloid osmotic pressure is created by the presence of plasma proteins in the intravascular space.

Movement of water. Forces generated by cardiac contraction, the plasma protein content in the vascular space, and the solute content of both the extracellular fluid (ECF) and intracellular fluid (ICF) result in a constant movement and balance of fluid content throughout the fluid compartments.

For example, fluid movement at the capillary level between the vascular and interstitial spaces is a function of protein content in the plasma (capillary colloid osmotic pressure) and the pressure generated through cardiac contraction, called *capillary hydrostatic pressure.* Similarly, solute and protein content of the tissue space result in generation of interstitial colloid osmotic pressure. Pressure generated through collection and emptying of the lymphatic system creates an interstitial hydrostatic pressure.

An increase in plasma volume results in increased capillary hydrostatic pressure, thereby forcing fluid into the interstitial space and creating edema. Conversely, a reduction in plasma volume causes movement of fluid from the interstitium to the vascular space as a result of the interstitial

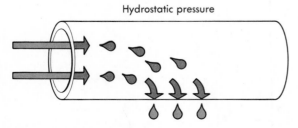

Hydrostatic pressure

Fig. 29-4 Filtration: hydrostatic pressure forces fluid out of the capillary into the interstitial space.

hydrostatic pressure's being greater than the capillary hydrostatic pressure. Also, a loss of plasma proteins in the vascular space lessens the capillary colloid osmotic pressure and results in movement of water to the interstitium.

Movement of fluid between the intracellular space and the extracellular space is primarily a function of the osmolality of the two spaces. For example, hyperosmolality of the ECF, although rare in persons able to obtain oral fluids, will result in movement of fluid from the intracellular space to the extracellular space (cellular dehydration).

Functions of Electrolytes

The specific contributions of the electrolytes to the successful maintenance of overall body functioning are important. Very often, changes in the electrolytes can initiate serious organ dysfunction. Their replacement or reduction is required to restore the necessary equilibrium.

Potassium. Although authorities disagree about which body electrolyte is most essential for normal cellular function, potassium is always ranked among the most important. Without this crucial element, for example, the heart muscle cannot function.

Potassium is the primary *intracellular* electrolyte. For this reason, it is difficult to measure true body stores. However, changes in the intracellular potassium concentration are quickly reflected by the measurement of the extracellular amount. For example, during tissue breakdown potassium leaves the cells; thus the serum potassium level becomes elevated. The normal serum levels of potassium are 3.5 to 5.0 mEq/L.

Diffusion and active transport maintain the very narrow limits of potassium balance. Potassium leaves the cell by diffusion, moving toward the area of lesser concentration outside the cell, but it must be actively transported back into the cell to maintain cellular stability. With this movement, the cell membrane is made ready to accept neural messages, leading to one of the most important of potassium's functions in the body—that of aiding nervous impulse conduction and muscle contraction.

In addition to aiding nervous impulses and muscle contraction, potassium is responsible for enzyme activity that helps produce protein and carbohydrate metabolism for energy production. Also, since it is so abundant in the intracellular fluid, potassium primarily controls the maintenance of intracellular osmolality.

The gastrointestinal (GI) tract and skin excrete small amounts of potassium, but the major controllers of the body's potassium stores are the kidneys. Out of the estimated 50 to 100 mEq/day ingested by an individual, 90% of the potassium will be reabsorbed before arriving at the distal convoluted tubule where the remainder is usually excreted. However, reabsorption and secretion of potassium are influenced by many factors,[14] which are presented in the box on p. 613.

Potassium and sodium are in a constant state of competition within the body, despite the need for both electrolytes and despite their differing functions. The kidneys conserve sodium very carefully, whereas potassium is readily excreted. Potassium wasting may even continue despite the

---

FACTORS AFFECTING REABSORPTION AND SECRETION OF POTASSIUM (K⁺)

Sodium balance: sodium deficit results in increased potassium loss.
Acid-base balance: acidosis results in hydrogen movement into the cell and potassium movement out of it, and the potassium eventually is excreted in the urine.
Use of diuretics (thiazides): their use results in increased distal tubular loss of potassium.
Gastrointestinal (GI) disturbances: disturbances include vomiting and GI suctioning.
Insulin: it promotes potassium's movement back into cells.
Epinephrine: it enhances potassium's reabsorption from the distal tubule.

POTASSIUM

NORMAL SERUM VALUE
3.5-5.0 mEq/L

FUNCTIONS
Promotes transmission of nerve impulses
Maintains intracellular osmolality
Activates several enzymatic reactions
Aids in regulation of acid-base balance
Promotes myocardial, skeletal, and smooth muscle contractility

---

SODIUM

NORMAL SERUM VALUE
135-145 mEq/L

FUNCTIONS
Maintains extracellular osmolality
Maintains the active transport mechanism in conjunction with potassium
Controls body fluids (largely responsible for water movement and retention)
Aids in maintaining neuromuscular activity
Aids in some enzyme activities (helping to create energy)
Influences acid-base balance

---

body's need for potassium, particularly when aldosterone levels are elevated.

A review of the normal values and functions of potassium is in the box above. Potassium is not only important to the human body but is also important in the cells of other plant and animal life.

Sodium. Sodium can easily be called the "great water regulator" because it is primarily responsible for shifts in body water and the amount of water retained or excreted by the kidneys. It is the most abundant extracellular electrolyte. The normal serum value for sodium is 135 to 145 mEq/L.

In addition to water regulation, sodium plays a role in transmission of nerve impulses through the "sodium pump" or active transport mechanism at the cellular level. Sodium also combines with either chloride or bicarbonate to maintain acid-base balance.

The body contains an incredibly complex system of safe-

guards and feedback mechanisms to protect the level of sodium in the ECF. The three organs responsible for regulating sodium balance are the kidneys, the adrenal glands, and the posterior pituitary gland.

Because of the extremely sensitive mechanism for retaining sodium, ingestion of large amounts of sodium is not necessary. In fact, excessive sodium ingestion has for years been implicated in the literature in the development of hypertension and associated disorders. Functions of sodium are listed in the box above.

Calcium. Mention the word *calcium* and the word *bone* immediately comes to mind. Indeed, 99% of the calcium in the body is contained in the bones. Calcium occurs in nature as a very hard crystalline element. It is also the electrolyte of greatest quantity in the human body, with stores estimated at 1200 g. The remaining 1% of the body calcium is contained primarily in the ECF or, specifically, in the bloodstream.

The calcium contained within bone is essentially an inactive form that maintains bone strength and is a ready storehouse for mobilization of calcium to the serum in cases of depletion. The mobilization of calcium is accomplished through the influence of parathyroid hormone (PTH). Since most calcium is contained within bone, it is inactivated for any other purpose. The calcium in the intravascular space is either bound to protein or floats freely in an ionized form, as do sodium and potassium.[15] The protein-bound calcium awaits usage during immediate crisis, whereas the ionized calcium is the active form, which functions in cell membrane stability, blood clotting, and other important functions.

In the ionized form, calcium plays an important role in maintaining the internal integrity of the cell. The amount of ionized calcium in the serum depends on changes in serum pH and on the availability of plasma protein, primarily albumin. Since changes in pH and albumin levels occur with relative frequency, measurement of the serum calcium is often deceptive.

For instance, a change in the serum albumin level will effect the calcium level. As serum albumin levels rise, ionized calcium becomes bound to the newly available protein, thus lowering the ionized calcium. However, since total calcium is measured rather than the ionized fraction, the actual decrease in the ionized calcium may not be accurately reflected.

Conversely, should albumin levels fall, calcium is split free of the protein and creates an actual rise in the ionized calcium level. However, under the influence of the hormone calcitonin, the ionized calcium may be returned to the bone, and the actual availability of the calcium again may not be accurately reflected.

The normal serum calcium level ranges from 8.8 to 10.5 mg/dl. For every increase or decrease in serum albumin of 1 g/dl, a change of 0.8 mg/dl occurs in the total serum calcium.[15] Any serum calcium level should be accompanied by measurement of serum albumin.[15]

Calcium is also responsible for several critically important functions. Myocardial contractility is primarily influenced by calcium. Neuromuscular activity, cell permeability, thickness of cell membrane, coagulation of blood, and hardness of bones and teeth are all dependent on calcium levels. Functions of calcium are reviewed in the box below.

Calcium levels are highly dependent on individual dietary intake and a variety of physiological mechanisms related to absorption. For example, the uptake of calcium is influenced by the level of phosphorus, the amount of vitamin D and its breakdown products, PTH, and the hormone calcitonin.[15] Other factors such as changes in acid-base balance will change calcium levels in the ECF. For example, acidosis ionizes or splits calcium free from albumin, resulting in "ionized" hypercalcemia, whereas alkalosis enhances the binding of calcium to proteins, thereby creating a deficit of ionized calcium.[18]

Magnesium. Magnesium is primarily an intracellular electrolyte; therefore, like potassium, it is measured solely by amounts in serum. Approximately 60% of the body's magnesium is located in bone.[8] Only approximately 1% is actually in the ECF, with the remainder in the ICF. In fact,

---

MAGNESIUM
NORMAL SERUM VALUE 1.5-2.5 mEq/L
FUNCTIONS Aids in neuromuscular transmission Aids in contraction of heart muscle Activates enzymes for cellular metabolism of carbohydrates and proteins Aids in maintaining the active transport mechanism at the cellular level Aids in transmission of hereditary information to offspring

---

other intracellular electrolytes such as calcium and potassium are affected by the level of magnesium present. For example, calcium and magnesium compete for absorption in the GI tract. If the dietary intake is higher in calcium than magnesium, calcium will be preferentially reabsorbed and vice versa.

Magnesium is primarily found in the ICF and helps maintain the correct potassium stores on either side of the cell membrane since magnesium is required for appropriate function of the intracellular "carrier substances" that transport sodium and potassium across the cell membrane. A depletion of magnesium liberates potassium to the ECF and thereby increases renal excretion of potassium, resulting in hypokalemia.[17]

The normal value for magnesium in the serum is 1.3 to 2.1 mEq/L. The most important function of magnesium is in ensuring the transportation of sodium and potassium across the cell membranes. Additionally, magnesium plays roles in transmitting central nervous system (CNS) messages, maintaining neuromuscular activity, and activating enzymes for metabolism of carbohydrates and proteins. A summary of functions and factors affecting magnesium are listed in the box above.

Phosphorus. Phosphorus is often omitted from texts when major electrolytes are considered. However, this intracellular anion plays so many important roles in body function and maintenance that it cannot be ignored.

The normal serum phosphorus level is 2.5 to 4.5 mg%.[15] As with calcium and magnesium, however, the serum values of phosphorus represent a minute portion of actual body stores. Approximately 75% of the phosphorus is found in the bones, and part of the remaining amount is intracellular, thus rendering it difficult to measure. Serum phosphorus levels change frequently and dramatically, particularly in response to ingestion of phosphate-rich foods (milk, red meats, poultry, fish).[3]

The primary function of phosphorus is in the formation of ATP, which is the intracellular energy. The active trans-

---

CALCIUM
NORMAL SERUM VALUE 8.5-10.5 mg/dl or 4.5-5.8 mEq/L
FUNCTIONS Maintains hardness of bone and teeth (crystalline in nature) Contracts skeletal muscle Coagulates blood Maintains cellular permeability Contracts heart muscle

---

PHOSPHORUS

NORMAL SERUM VALUE
2.7-4.5 mg/dl

FUNCTIONS
Aids in structure of cellular membrane
Helps deliver oxygen to the tissues
Is integral part of intracellular energy production (ATP)
Helps maintain bone hardness
Aids in enzyme regulation (ATPase)

CHLORIDE

NORMAL SERUM VALUE
98-108 mEq/L

FUNCTIONS
Maintains body osmolality (in conjunction with sodium)
Aids in body water balance (in conjunction with sodium)
Competes with bicarbonate for recombination with sodium to maintain acid-base balance
Maintains acidity of body fluids (gastric juice)

---

port mechanism cannot function without the energy provided by ATP. Additional functions of phosphorus are as follows: (1) maintenance of cell membrane structure, (2) maintenance of acid-base balance, (3) oxygen delivery to the tissues, (4) cellular immunity, and (5) maintenance of bone strength (see the box above).[4]

Absorption of phosphorus takes place in the GI tract, and excretion, for the most part, occurs in the kidney. At the level of the proximal renal tubule, phosphorus is also reabsorbed when body stores are low. Acid-base balance is, in a minor way, influenced by the availability of phosphorus. Phosphates, available in the renal tubular filtrate, combine with sodium and excess hydrogen ions to form sodium diphosphate (Na_2HPO_4). This complex then dissociates into sodium, which combines with the available bicarbonate and is reabsorbed into the peritubular capillary network. The remaining hydrogen and phosphates are excreted into the urine.[6]

An important reciprocal relationship exists between phosphorus and calcium; high levels of phosphorus will result in low levels of calcium, and, conversely, high levels of calcium will result in low levels of phosphorus. PTH secretion, vitamin D, and the renal tubules are all involved in this complex relationship.

Chloride. Chloride is rarely found in the human body without being in combination with one of the major cations. Therefore changes in serum chloride levels are usually indicative of changes in the other electrolytes or in acid-base balance.

Since chloride combines most frequently with sodium, it plays a major role in maintaining serum osmolality and, subsequently, water balance. Also, since it competes with bicarbonate for combination with sodium, it exerts an effect on acid-base balance. Chloride also combines with hydrogen ions to form the hydrochloric acid present in gastric juice.

Red blood cell oxygenation and the transportation of carbon dioxide depend on adequate chloride levels. The dissociation of carbonic acid inside red blood cells creates hydrogen and bicarbonate ions. The hydrogen usually combines with hemoglobin, and the bicarbonate leaves the cell in exchange for the chloride ions moving into the cell (chloride shift).[6] Therefore carbon dioxide in the form of bicarbonate is liberated to travel to the lungs.

The normal serum chloride level is 98 to 106 mEq/L. It is most often ingested with sodium in the form of salt and, because of this combination with sodium, is reabsorbed or excreted in the renal tubules at the proximal tubular site. Chloride is actively transported out of the tubule into the renal medullary interstitium, again with sodium, to help maintain the high interstitial osmolality and the mechanism for concentrating the urine[10] (see the box above).

Bicarbonate. Rarely does an electrolyte have a solitary purpose in the body. However, bicarbonate, an anion present in extracellular fluid, performs the single, life-sustaining function of maintaining acid-base balance. Although bicarbonate is not solely responsible for acid-base balance, it is the major ECF buffer.

Bicarbonate (HCO_3^-) levels in the body are in balance with carbonic acid (H_2CO_3) levels; the ratio between the two must remain proportional (1 mEq H_2CO_3 : 20 mEq HCO_3^-), or acid-base disturbances result. When the carbonic acid level is elevated, the condition is known as *acidosis*. When the bicarbonate level is high, the condition is known as *alkalosis*. The normal serum level of bicarbonate is 24 to 28 mEq/L, and the normal value for carbonic value for carbonic acid is 1.2 to 1.4 mEq/L[16] (see the box below).

BICARBONATE

NORMAL SERUM VALUE
24-28 mEq/L

FUNCTIONS
Buffers the acidity of body fluids (controls the hydrogen ion concentration and combines with other body salts to maintain acid-base balance)

The amount of bicarbonate available in the ECF is regulated by the kidneys. Reabsorption of bicarbonate occurs primarily from the proximal tubule to the peritubular capillaries. Also, in response to acid-base balance and body requirements, bicarbonate is reconstructed in the distal tubule and reabsorbed into the blood. The kidneys either reabsorb or excrete bicarbonate in response to the number of hydrogen ions present.

Protein. Although proteins are not electrolytes, the role they play in controlling body fluid movement and cell building maintenance cannot be minimized. Proteins are needed for basic cell structure and enzyme formation. When combined with other substances, proteins can also supply energy for body functions.

Protein is a nitrogen compound and is formed from amino acids that are stored in the liver in a process called *anabolism.* The subsequent breakdown of, for example, body tissues, food, and cellular structures is known as *catabolism.* Anabolism and catabolism are usually in dynamic balance within the body.

As previously stated, a secondary function of protein is maintenance of fluid balance, particularly between the intravascular and interstitial compartments. Contained within the intravascular compartment are the *plasma proteins:* albumin, globulin, and fibrinogen. These plasma proteins exert a pull on water molecules and therefore produce a force called *oncotic pressure* or osmotic pressure, that retains fluid within the intravascular compartment. This force is maintained because proteins are large and cannot travel across the membrane unless the permeability of the membrane is changed in some significant way (for example, by burns or infections). The normal total protein is 6.0 to 8.0 g/dl, of which 68% is albumin.[8]

A decrease in serum albumin lessens the oncotic pressure so that the tissue oncotic pressure is greater and pulls fluid from the vascular space into the interstitial space, causing edema. The effects of a low serum albumin level exacerbate when the liver, in need of amino acids for anabolism, breaks down albumin.

With normal kidney function, intact proteins are not filtered through the glomerulus because of their large size. However, in disease states of the kidney, glomerular membrane permeability is altered, and protein molecules pass into the glomerular filtrate and appear in the urine. This appearance of protein in the urine is a cardinal sign of renal compromise and if left unchecked, can result in severely depleted body protein stores.

KIDNEYS AND URINARY TRACT
Anatomy

The human kidneys are physiological marvels in their ability to control and maintain fluid volume and electrolyte concentration precisely. This highly vascular pair of organs receives the entire circulatory volume 20 times per hour and efficiently separates the excesses of fluid, electrolytes, and metabolic by-products to produce urine. Since the kidneys function as primary regulators of fluid and electrolyte balance, a thorough understanding of their structure and function is central to any study of fluid and electrolytes.

Macroscopic structure. The kidneys are "bean-shaped" organs that are approximately 4 inches long, 2 inches wide, and 1 inch thick.[9] The size of one kidney would compare to the size of an adult male's fist. Each kidney weighs 4 to 6 ounces. A slight difference in kidney weight exists in females (closer to 4 ounces) and infants (kidneys are large in proportion to infant's size).

Their location is described as *retroperitoneal,* which means they are located outside and posterior to the abdominal cavity, but lateral and anterior to the lumbar spine. Both are protected by the posterior rib cage, with the right kidney slightly lower than the left as a result of displacement by the liver.[9] This lesser amount of protection often accounts for the majority of traumatic kidney injuries affecting the right kidney.

Atop each kidney on the outer surface lies the adrenal gland. One function of these glands is to produce aldosterone, which allows the kidneys to control sodium and water balance.

An internal view of the kidney (Fig. 29-5) demonstrates the complexity of the filtering and collecting systems. The two distinct divisions of tissue within the kidney are known as the *cortex* and the *medulla.* Lying beneath the fibrous covering of each kidney, the cortical tissue contains the glomeruli and the proximal and distal tubules of the nephrons, which constitute the filtering mechanism of the kidney. The medulla comprises the innermost tissue layer of each kidney and is composed of the loops of Henle and the collecting ducts of the nephrons, which concentrate and collect the urine.

The renal pyramids are triangular divisions within the kidney that extend through both layers of tissue. The base of each pyramid is cortical tissue, and the apex of the pyramid contains collecting ducts, which converge to feed the urine into a canal known as a *calyx.*

As can be seen in Fig. 29-6, leading out of each kidney is a fibromuscular tube, the *ureter,* which is responsible for carrying the filtered and collected urine to the bladder. When entering the bladder, each ureter implants posteriorly under the epithelium.[6]

The bladder is a muscular sac with a capacity of approximately 500 ml. The triple-layered musculature and specialized innervation control urine flow out of the body and prevent back flow.[6] As an extension of the bladder, the urethra, a hollow tube, provides the final conduit for urine to the outside.

The blood flow to the kidney begins with the abdominal aorta, from which the right and left renal arteries stem. Each renal artery further branches into anterior and posterior arteries to provide the blood supply to the entire kidney.[9]

Continuing to decrease in size but increasing in number, the anterior and posterior arteries become the interlobar arteries, which channel between the renal pyramids. The arterial divisions continue through two additional levels until, eventually, the afferent and efferent arterioles which provide circulation to each of the millions of nephrons, are formed.

Microscopic structure. Comprising the kidney tissue are

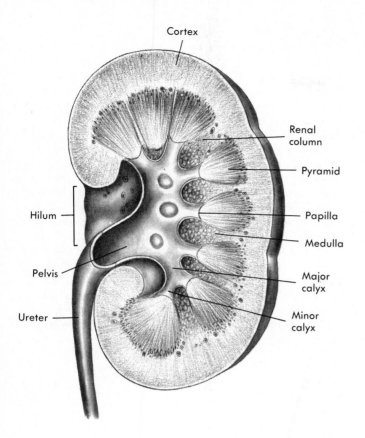

Fig. 29-5 Cross section of the kidney. (From Thompson JM and others: Mosby's manual of clinical nursing, ed 2, St Louis, 1989, The CV Mosby Co.)

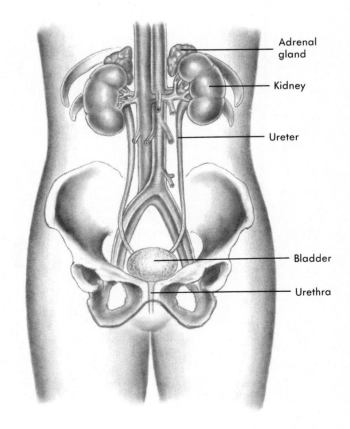

Fig. 29-6 Structures of the urinary system. (From Thompson JM and others: Mosby's manual of clinical nursing, ed 2, St Louis, 1989, The CV Mosby Co.)

approximately 1 to 1.5 million working units known as nephrons. Each nephron consists of the glomerulus, Bowman's capsule, proximal convoluted tubule, loop of Henle, distal convoluted tubule, and collecting duct. Not all of the nephrons function at the same level; some are held in reserve. This means the kidney can continue to function despite the loss of several thousand nephrons.

From the arterial circulation is formed a ball of capillaries known as the glomerulus. The glomerulus forms the beginning of each nephron and is the filtering point for the blood supply. As Fig. 29-7 indicates, the afferent arteriole leads into the glomerulus, and the efferent arteriole leads out of it. There is a distinct difference in the sizes of the afferent and efferent arterioles, with the latter having the smaller lumen size. The size difference is of importance to glomerular filtration in that the larger afferent arteriole allows a greater flow of blood into the glomerulus. The smaller efferent arteriole offers resistance to the outflow of blood, thereby creating the high pressure in the glomerulus that facilitates the filtration of fluid out of the blood, into Bowman's capsule, and subsequently to the tubular network of the nephron.[9]

As the efferent arteriole leaves each kidney, it branches into a mesh of capillaries known as peritubular capillaries. The peritubular capillaries form a meshwork around the tubular structures of each nephron, providing further exchange of fluid, electrolytes, and essential nutrients between the intravascular volume and intratubular filtrate.

The glomerulus is surrounded by the tough, but membranous, tissue known as Bowman's capsule. The space between the capillary walls in the glomerulus and Bowman's capsule holds the initial filtrate from the blood. In other words, fluid, essential nutrients, and wastes are collected in the capsule space and begin to travel through a tubular network that forms the remainder of the nephron.

In the medullary tissue of the kidney, the peritubular capillaries become tiny venules and continue to enlarge until they form the right and left renal veins. This blood flow continues in the same fashion within and through each nephron.

Pathway of renal filtrate. The excess fluid and solutes from the vascular volume filter through the glomerular capillary walls and form *filtrate,* which collects in Bowman's capsule. The filtrate travels through a tortuous section of

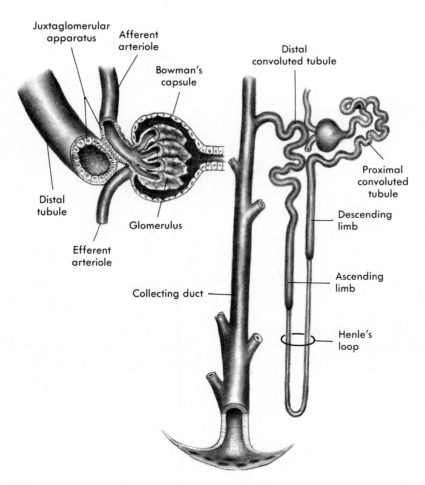

Fig. 29-7   Components of the nephron. (From Thompson JM and others: Mosby's manual of clinical nursing, ed 2, St Louis, 1989, The CV Mosby Co.)

tube known as the *proximal tubule*. The initial exchange of fluid and solutes between the intravascular volume and the intratubular filtrate occurs in this area.

The filtrate continues through a narrower, U-shaped area known as the loop of Henle. While it is contained in this area, concentration or dilution of the filtrate occurs, primarily as the result of gains and losses of sodium, chloride, and water. At various locations along the loop of Henle, permeability to either water, chloride, or sodium ions changes.

For example, the filtrate entering the descending portion of the loop of Henle is isotonic, but it quickly becomes hypertonic as the result of the loss of water to the hyperosmotic medullary interstitium and the reabsorption of sodium from the same area. As the filtrate flows through the ascending portion of the loop, sodium and chloride are lost to the interstitium, with water unable to enter the tubule because of the impermeability to water in this portion of the tubule. Thus as fluid enters the distal tubule, it is hypotonic.

The distal convoluted tubule is the site of potassium excretion, sodium reabsorption, and acid-base balance maintenance in the form of excretion of hydrogen ions and reabsorption of bicarbonate ions. Also, the distal tubule plays a small role in blood pressure regulation as the site for initiation of the renin-angiotensin-aldosterone system.

Specialized cells exist in the wall of the distal tubule at the point where the tubule touches the afferent arteriole. The cells, known as the *macula densa,* sense changes in filtrate flow and sodium concentration. The changes are transmitted to the *juxtaglomerular cells* in the afferent arteriole, and they release substances causing arteriolar constriction or dilation as necessary.[9]

These juxtaglomerular cells release renin, which helps form angiotensin II, a powerful vasoconstrictor. The action of angiotensin II on the efferent arteriole produces a rise in glomerular pressure and increases glomerular filtration.[9]

The macular densa and juxtaglomerular cells form the *juxtaglomerular apparatus,* a specialized area that regulates the renin-angiotensin feedback system (see Chapter 34).

From the distal tubule, the filtrate is pooled in areas known as *collecting ducts.* The collecting ducts allow the loss of water and urea, again resulting in a hypertonic urine. Several collecting ducts join to form the points of the renal pyramids and larger canals known as calyces (calyx—singular form). The calyces become larger still and unite in the renal pelvis, which then forms the ureters. Thus the urine flows from each collecting duct to the calyces and out through the ureters.

Continuing through the urinary tract, the urine is carried by peristalsis (a rhythmic contraction of the muscular ureters) to the bladder. When the bladder's capacity is reached, stimulation is initiated, and the urine flows through the urethra to the outside.

Innervation. The autonomic nervous system supplies the primary innervation to the kidneys and the urinary tract. The kidneys are supplied messages from the lowest splanchnic and inferior splanchnic nerves, which form the renal plexus. The inferior mesenteric plexus, the hypogastric plexus, and the pudic nerve from the sacral region serve the bladder, ureters, and urethra.[1,6]

An example of nervous control in the urinary tract is reflected in the process of micturition, or release of urine. Bladder fullness stimulates stretch receptors in the bladder wall and a portion of the urethra. Signals are sent through nerves in the sacral area and return as parasympathetic messages to contract the detrusor muscle composing most of the bladder. With a full bladder, contractions are usually powerful enough to relax the external sphincter. Sympathetic stimulation returns the external sphincter to contraction after the urine is released. If insufficient urine has collected in the bladder to achieve release, the micturition reflex subsides but repeats regularly, with increasing force, over a period of time.[6]

Additional nervous control exists from the cerebral cortex and brainstem. Control over the micturition reflex, frequency, and external sphincter tone, from the central nervous system, provides conscious control over urinary release.

Functions of the kidneys

Fluid and electrolyte balance depends critically on the continued efficient function of the kidneys. The renal system provides the primary route for reabsorption, excretion, and "fine tuning" of fluid and electrolyte balance and some acid-base balance.

Excretion of nitrogenous wastes. Metabolic processes in the body produce certain waste products that are selectively filtered out of the circulation by the kidneys. Urea, uric acid, and creatinine are the most commonly measured by-products of protein metabolism that the kidneys filter out of circulation.

Clearance is defined as the ability of the kidney to clear certain substances from the plasma.[6] More specifically, clearance represents the volume of plasma that is cleared of a substance during a specific period of time. The unit of measurement representing clearance is milliliters per minute.

Clearance primarily depends on tubular reaction to substances in the glomerular filtrate. For example, the substance may be filtered by the glomerulus and then either reabsorbed or excreted partially or totally.[10] Many factors enhance or reduce clearance of substances through the kidney (see the box, "Factors Affecting Renal Clearance"). Creatinine, a

---

FACTORS AFFECTING RENAL CLEARANCE

Volume depletion
Renal blood flow (hypoperfusion)
Glomerular membrane permeability
Blood pressure (hypertension or hypotension)
Cardiac output (myocardial infarction, pericarditis)
Aging

waste product of muscle metabolism, is produced in standard, predictable amounts by the body, and it is cleared from the blood in predictable amounts; therefore it is used as a standard for gauging the effectiveness of renal activity. The test for creatinine clearance requires that urine be collected for a 24-hour period and be analyzed for volume excreted and amount of creatinine present. At the same time, a blood sample is obtained for analysis of the amount of creatinine present.[5] A mathematical formula is used to calculate the rate of *creatinine clearance* and therefore to predict the adequacy of the kidneys' function. The normal creatinine clearance is roughly proportional to the glomerular filtration rate of 120 to 130 ml/min.

Closely allied with the concept of clearance is that of *glomerular filtration rate* (GFR). The GFR is the volume of plasma cleared of substances through the glomerular membrane per unit of time. The GFR is measured in milliliters per minute, with the normal GFR 125 ml/min.[7]

At least three factors can affect the GFR at any time: (1) glomerular capillary membrane permeability, (2) systemic blood pressure, and (3) the pressure of the blood (effective filtration pressure) entering the afferent arteriole or exiting the efferent arteriole. Any change in these three factors will result in a change in the GFR.[10]

For example, if blood pressure is reduced through vasoconstriction of the afferent arteriole, GFR is significantly reduced. If vasoconstriction of the efferent arteriole occurs, the pressure increases inside the glomerulus and congestion occurs, forcing plasma out into the capsules and thereby reducing the GFR as well.[6]

Regulation of ECF volume. The kidney possesses the unique ability to separate water regulation from electrolyte regulation in the nephron. Water is reabsorbed or excreted to maintain fluid balance. The maintenance of balance is under the control of the *antidiuretic hormone* (ADH), produced by the posterior pituitary gland in the brain.

A multitude of factors control water balance in the body. For example, the conscious intake of fluids provides the source of the fluid, and the kidneys excrete the fluid. In large part body solute content determines this intake and output by stimulating various centers in the brain that regulate the body's water. For example, thirst is controlled by receptors in the vascular system, which sense hypovolemia, or by sensors in the cerebrum, which sense sodium concentration.[13] Thirst, resulting from stimulation of these sensors, results in intake of fluids (if the individual is able). However, water balance is primarily achieved through the suppression or release of ADH and regulation of ECF sodium levels.

ADH release results from signals of the osmoreceptors, baroreceptors, and stretch receptors located in the atria. The receptors send signals to the midbrain where ADH is manufactured and released into the general circulation, eventually resulting in increased fluid reabsorption by the renal tubules. Similarly, stretch receptors in the cardiac muscle sense hypervolemia, resulting in suppression of ADH release.[13]

Regulation of ECF electrolyte concentration. The body controls electrolyte reabsorption in the renal tubules by pro-

viding a mechanism known as the *tubular maximum,* or *threshold*. Basically, the electrolytes and other substances reabsorbed are divided into threshold or nonthreshold substances. The substances and electrolytes useful to the body are reabsorbed in differing amounts to maintain normal plasma levels. For example, sodium, glucose, amino acids, calcium, and phosphorus are almost completely reabsorbed from the tubules.

Although potassium is needed, the amount present in the filtrate usually far exceeds the amount needed; therefore the excess is excreted. In other words, potassium reaches its tubular maximum, and the excess is relinquished. Potassium also retains the distinction of being exchanged for sodium since it occurs in abundance in filtrate.[10]

Nonthreshold substances are usually the waste products such as urea and creatinine that, although not actively reabsorbed, occur in low plasma levels because of passive diffusion into the peritubular network. Primary bulk reabsorption is performed in the proximal tubule, with the distal tubule the site for the fine tuning of, particularly, sodium, potassium, calcium, and phosphates.

Regulation of acid-base balance. The nephron is involved in acid-base regulation by reabsorbing or excreting the various acids and bases. Although the renal mechanism is not as swift in altering acid-base concentrations as that of the lungs, it is meant to regulate the day-to-day balance rather than to cope with the emergencies produced by excesses of either acids or bases.

Bicarbonate, the principal blood buffer, is reabsorbed from the tubules, and hydrogen is secreted into the tubules. Carbonic acid in the renal tubular cells splits and sends hydrogen ions (H^+) to the tubular lumen and bicarbonate ($HCO3$) to the blood. Recombination and further dissociation of carbonic acid in the tubules produces carbon dioxide for perpetuation of the cycle and water for excretion.[3] Hydrogen ions combine with either phosphates or ammonia and are transported into the tubular filtrate and eventually to the urine. Combination with either of these substances will release sodium and bicarbonate for reabsorption into the vascular system through the peritubular capillaries.[3]

REFERENCES

1. Ames SW and Kneisl CR: Essentials of adult health nursing, Menlo Park, Calif, 1988, Addison-Wesley Publishing Co.
2. Ansel J and Elwyn DH: Body composition. In Askanazi J, Starker PM, and Weissman C: Fluid and electrolyte management in critical care, Boston, 1986, Butterworth & Co (Publishers), Inc.
3. Appel GB and Chase HS Jr: Diagnosis and treatment of acid-base disorders. In Askanazi J, Starker PM, and Weissman C: Fluid and electrolyte management in critical care, Boston, 1986, Butterworth & Co (Publisher), Ltd.
4. Baker W: Hypophosphatemia, Am J Nurs 85(9):999, 1985.
5. Fishback FT: A manual of laboratory diagnostic tests, ed 3, Philadelphia, 1988, JB Lippincott Co.
6. Guyton AC: Textbook of medical physiology, ed 7, Philadelphia, 1986, WB Saunders Co.
7. Hyman AI: Renal physiology. In Askanazi J, Starker PM, and Weissman C: Fluid and electrolyte management in critical care, Boston, 1986, Butterworth & Co (Publishers), Ltd.
8. Kavanagh JM: Assessment of the cardiovascular system. In Phipps

WJ, Long BC, and Woods NF: Medical-surgical nursing, St Louis, 1987, The CV Mosby Co.

9. Lancaster LE: Anatomy and physiology of the renal system. In Core curriculum for nephrology nursing, Pitman, New Jersey, 1987, AJ Jannetti, Inc.

10. Lancaster LE: Renal and endocrine regulation of water and electrolyte balance. In Common fluid and electrolyte disorders, Philadelphia, 1987, WB Saunders Co.

11. Metheny NM: Fluid and electrolyte balance—nursing considerations, Philadelphia, 1987, JB Lippincott, Co.

12. Oh MS and Carroll HJ: Regulation of extra and intracellular fluid composition and content. In Arieff AI and Defronzo RA: Fluid electrolyte and acid-base disorders, vol 1, New York, 1985, Churchill Livingstone, Inc.

13. Raymond KH, Reineck HJ, and Stein JH: Sodium metabolism and maintenance of extracellular fluid volume. In Arieff AI and DeFronzo RA: Fluid electrolyte and acid-base disorders, vol 1, New York, 1985, Churchill Livingstone, Inc.

14. Rothkopf MM and Weissman C: Potassium balance. In Askanazi J, Starker PM and Weissman C: Fluid and electrolyte management in critical care, Boston, 1985, Butterworth & Co. (Publishers), Ltd.

15. Shane EJ and Bilezikian JP: Calcium, phosphate and magnesium metabolism. In Askanazi J, Starker PM, and Weissman C: Fluid and electrolyte management in critical care, Boston, 1986, Butterworth & Co (Publishers), Ltd.

16. Soltis B and Cassmeyer VL: Fluid and electrolyte imbalance. In Phipps WJ, Long BC, and Woods NF: Medical-surgical nursing, ed 3, St Louis, 1987, The CV Mosby Co.

17. Thompson JM and others: Clinical nursing, ed 2, St Louis, 1989, The CV Mosby Co.

18. Weisberg LS, Szerlip HM, and Cox M: Disorders of potassium homeostasis in critically ill patients, Crit Care Clin 5(4):835, 1987.

19. Zaloga GP and Chernow B: Hypocalcemia in critical illness, JAMA 256(4):1924, 1986.

30

Renal and Fluids Clinical Assessment

CHAPTER OBJECTIVES

■ *Discuss the rationale involved in developing a consistent, sequential format for performing fluids and renal nursing assessment.*

■ *Perform a thorough nursing assessment of the fluids and renal system on a critically ill patient and interpret the results.*

■ *Identify methods for assessing normal skin turgor.*

■ *Describe the pathophysiological mechanism responsible for the development of edema and ascites and identify the proper method for assessing each one.*

■ *Describe the pathophysiological mechanism responsible for orthostatic hypotension.*

Understanding the anatomical location and physiological workings of the body's fluids and electrolytes is of little or no value if the overt signs and symptoms of problems are not known or understood. The body presents a variety of signs and symptoms that demonstrate fluid and electrolyte disorders. A methodical way of examination presents data that help pinpoint the actual problem. The following section explains the process of taking a fluid and electrolyte history and performing the physical assessment of fluid and electrolyte balance. An outline of this information is presented in the box, "Important Aspects of the Fluid and Electrolyte Assessment."

RENAL AND FLUID HISTORY

A renal and fluid history should begin with a description of the chief complaint, written in the patient's own words. However, it is wise to avoid accepting the patient's estimation of what may have been the cause of the problem. Included in the description of the chief complaint should be its onset, location, and duration and factors that lessen or aggravate the problem.[1] Descriptions of any treatment

sought by the individual, medications taken to alleviate symptoms, or procedures performed to ameliorate the problem are often helpful in delineating the extent of the current complaint.

Of particular concern in gaining a complete renal and fluid history is the patient's past medical history. Similar symptoms, problems, or treatment for complaints in the past may give important clues to current treatment or may aid in establishing the cause of the problem. The patient and his or her family or significant other must provide as much detail as possible about the past history.

The family history may also provide important information to aid in identifying and treating the patient's disorder. For example, the patient may reveal that one or two close family members have always had problems with swelling of the extremities or high blood pressure. These symptoms might lead to questions about any history of kidney problems. A history is investigative and usually progressive in nature, with one question often leading to another.

RENAL AND FLUID ASSESSMENT
Inspection

Renal and fluid assessment begins with looking at neck veins and hand veins. To inspect the patient's neck veins, he or she should be in the supine position, in which normal venous distention is usually noted. If neck veins do not distend with the patient in the supine position, hypovolemia is suspected. After supine inspection, the head of the bed should be elevated to 45 to 90 degrees. If with the bed at 45 degrees the veins remain distended more that 2 cm above the sternal notch, fluid overload may be suspected.[4]

Hand vein inspection is performed simply by observing for venous distention, the expected response, when the hand is held in the dependent position. Venous filling that takes longer than 5 seconds suggests hypovolemia. When the hand is elevated, the distention should disappear within 5 seconds. If distention does not disappear within 5 seconds after the hand is elevated, fluid overload is suspected.

The skin and mucous membranes, when inspected, present readily visible signs of fluid alterations. When a fluid volume *deficit* exists, skin loses elasticity and mucous mem-

---

IMPORTANT ASPECTS OF THE FLUID AND ELECTROLYTE ASSESSMENT

NURSING HISTORY

1. Chief complaint
2. History of present problem
   a. Onset
   b. Duration
   c. Signs/symptoms
   d. Treatments
3. Past history of fluid or renal problems or familial history of fluid or renal problems
4. Dietary likes/dislikes/intake each day
5. Fluid likes/dislikes/intake each day
6. Dentures: if used, oral condition/hygiene
7. Cultural background
8. Educational background

NURSING ASSESSMENT
Fluid status (Deficit/Excess)

1. Skin turgor
2. Mucous membranes
3. Intake and output
4. Presence of edema/ascites
5. Neck and hand vein engorgement
6. Lung sounds—crackles
7. Blood pressure (hypertension or hypotension)
8. Vertigo on rising
9. Blurred vision
10. Diaphoresis
11. Behavioral changes
12. Low grade fever
13. Tachycardia

Electrolyte status

1. Serum osmolality
2. Complete blood count (CBC)
3. Electrolyte levels
4. Electrocardiographic (ECG) tracings (potassium, calcium, magnesium levels)
5. Behavioral changes
6. Chvostek's, Trousseau's signs (calcium levels)
7. Changes in peripheral sensation (numbness, tremors)
8. Muscle strength
9. Gastrointestinal (GI) changes (nausea and vomiting, diarrhea)
10. Therapies that can alter electrolyte status (GI suction, diuretics, antihypertensives, calcium channel blockers)

---

branes become sticky. If a fluid volume *excess* exists, edema is sometimes present, particularly in dependent areas of the body. However, without further assessment the imbalance cannot be positively identified. Other disorders and contributing factors might lead to an inaccurate assumption of a fluid volume disorder. For instance mouth breathing can dry the oral mucous membranes temporarily. A more accurate way to assess the fluid status of the oral cavity is to inspect the mouth, using a tongue blade. Stickiness of this area is more indicative of fluid volume deficit than complaints of a dry mouth.[4]

Assessment of skin turgor provides additional data for identifying fluid-related problems. As the skin over the forearm is picked up and released, the rapidity of its return to its normal position should be observed. Normal elasticity and fluid status allow almost immediate return to shape once the skin is released. However, in fluid volume deficit the skin remains raised and does not return to its normal position for several seconds. Because of the usual loss of skin elasticity in the elderly, this test is not accurate for fluid assessment of this age group. The elderly individual's skin turgor can be assessed in the shoulder area, which retains elasticity.[4]

Changes in skin texture and overall appearance reveal much about fluid status. For example, the patient with renal failure has rough, dry skin and deposits of urate crystals on the skin, called *uremic frost*. These patients frequently have scratch marks because of the pruritis associated with renal failure.

Edema is defined as the presence of excess fluid in the interstitial space. However, the presence of edema does not always indicate true fluid overload; a loss of albumin from the vascular space can cause peripheral edema, yet the patient may be hypovolemic.

Edema is usually assessed by applying fingertip pressure on the skin over a bony prominence such as the ankles, pretibial areas (shins), and the sacrum. If the indentation made by the fingertip does not disappear within 30 seconds, "pitting" edema is present. Pitting edema is indicative of increased interstitial volume and is not in evidence until approximately a 10% weight gain has occurred.[2] It is gauged by a subjective scale of 1 to 4, with +1 indicating only minimal pitting and +4 indicating severe pitting. Edema may also appear in hands and feet, around the eyes, and in the cheeks. Dependent areas such as the sacrum are the most likely to demonstrate edema in patients chronically confined to a wheelchair or bed. Skeletal muscles do not usually reflect changes in fluid status but do reflect changes in electrolyte levels. A skeletal muscle change to weakness or paralysis usually signals a deficit of an electrolyte, particularly of a major cation (potassium and sodium). However, a calcium deficit leads to the opposite extreme—severe cramping and muscle spasm.

Palpation

Although palpation of the kidneys is not directly linked to fluid and electrolye assessments, any subtle changes in kidney function can result in problems with fluids and electrolytes. Palpation of the kidneys is achieved through the bimanual capturing approach. *Capturing* is accomplished

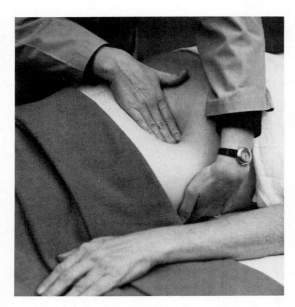

Fig. 30-1 Palpation of the kidney. (From Malasanos L and others: Health assessment, ed 4, St Louis, 1989, The CV Mosby Co.)

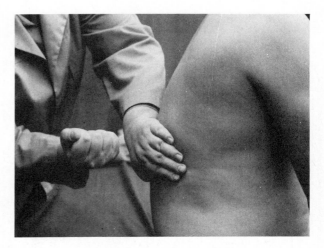

Fig. 30-2 Percussion of the kidney. (From Malasanos L and others: Health assessment, ed 4, St Louis, 1989, The CV Mosby Co.)

by placing one hand posteriorly under the flank of the supine patient with fingers pointing to the midline, while placing the opposite hand just below the rib cage anteriorly. The patient is asked to inhale deeply, while pressure is exerted to bring the hands together (Fig. 30-1). As the patient exhales, the kidney should be felt between the hands. After palpating each kidney in this manner, they should be compared for size and shape. Each should be firm, smooth, and of equal size.[2]

Problems should be suspected if an irregular surface is palpated, a size difference is detected, or the kidney extends significantly lower than the rib cage on either side. However, it should be remembered that the right kidney does extend somewhat lower than the left as a result of its displacement by the liver.

Percussion

Percussion is performed to detect pain in the area of an organ or to determine excess accumulation of air, fluid, or solids in a body cavity. Although percussion of the kidneys per se does not give direct evidence of fluid and electrolyte level abnormalities, it can provide information about kidney location, size, and possible problems that could lead to future fluid and electrolyte level abnormalities.

Percussion of the kidney is performed with the patient in a sidelying or sitting position, with the examiner's hand placed over the costovertebral angle (lower border of the rib cage on the flank) (Fig. 30-2). Striking the back of the hand with the opposite fist will produce a dull thud, which is normal. Pain may be indicative of infection.

Observation and percussion of the abdomen is of value in assessing fluid status also. Percussing the abdomen (using the same procedure as for the kidneys but placing the patient supine) can result in a dull sound (solid bowel contents or fluid) or a hollow sound (gaseous bowel).[1]

Ascites, defined simply as severe fluid distention of the

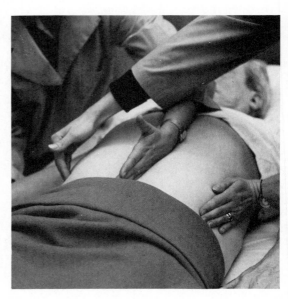

Fig. 30-3 Test for the presence of a fluid wave. (From Malasanos L and others: Health assessment, ed 4, St Louis, 1989, The CV Mosby Co.)

abdominal cavity, is an important observation in determing fluid imbalances. Differentiating ascites from distortion caused by solid bowel contents is done by producing what is called the *fluid wave*. The fluid wave is elicited by exerting pressure to the abdominal midline while one hand is placed on the right or left flank. Tapping the opposite flank produces a wave in the accumulated fluid that can be felt under the hands (Fig. 30-3). Other signs of ascites are a protuberant, rounded abdomen and abdominal striae.

Ascites may or may not represent fluid volume excess. Individuals with a compromised hepatic system may have severe ascites but actually by hypovolemic. The ascites occurs because the increased vascular pressure associated with hepatic dysfunction forces fluid and plasma proteins from the vascular space to the interstitial space and abdominal cavity. On the other hand, individuals suffering from renal failure may be plagued with ascites caused by true volume overload, which forces fluid into the abdomen because of increased capillary hydrostatic pressures.

Auscultation

Although auscultation is perhaps the most difficult area of assessment to master, it provides more accurate information about extracellular fluid (ECF) changes than the areas of assessment previously discussed. Listening for specific sounds in the heart and lungs provides information about the presence or absence of increased fluid in the interstitium or vascular space.

Auscultating the heart calls not only for assessing rate and rhythm, but also for listening for extra sounds such as third and fourth heart sounds. Increased heart rate alone does not offer much data about fluid volume, but combined with a low blood pressure, it may indicate hypovolemia. Often hypertension is accompanied by a third or fourth heart sound, which may indicate the presence of fluid overload. Caution should be exercised, however, in making assumptions about fluid status based on the presence of a murmur, since murmurs may also be present in other cardiac disorders.[1]

Hypertension may be indicative of fluid overload but may also be caused by atherosclerotic or arteriosclerotic vessel changes. Blood pressure readings should be taken at rest with the patient lying, sitting, and standing. A comparison of the three readings should help establish a baseline from which to compare subsequent readings.

A drastic drop in pressure from lying to sitting or from sitting to standing represents an "orthostatic" drop known as orthostatic hypotension. A 20 mm Hg drop in pressure may represent a fluid volume deficit and occurs when the venous circulation is so volume depleted that a sufficient preload is not immediately available after the position change. Orthostatic hypotension produces feelings of weakness or faintness. However, peripheral vascular disease, which often damages the venous circulation of the lower extremities, may be responsible for orthostatic drops in the absence of hypovolemia.

Vascular sounds heard by auscultating major vessels are called *bruits* (Fig. 30-4). A bruit is a blowing or swishing sound, much like cardiac murmurs.[1] Fluid volume excess, coupled with stenosis or any impediment to vascular flow, will produce a loud bruit.

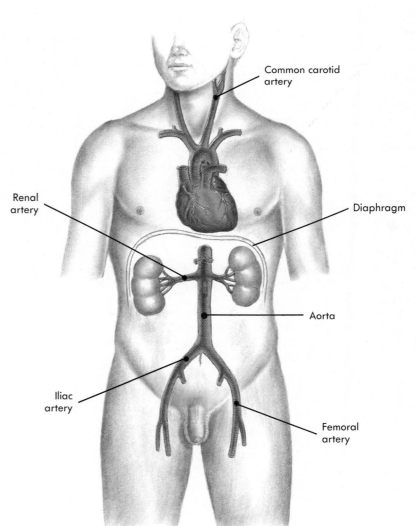

Fig. 30-4 Sites for auscultation of bruits.

Lung assessment is extremely important in gauging fluid status. Dyspnea with any mild exertion or dyspnea at night that prevents sleeping in a supine postion may indicate fluid overload. Shallow, gasping breaths punctuated by periods of apnea may indicate severe acid-base imbalances. Since the lungs are one of the primary controllers of acid-base balance, it is important to identify the types of respiratory changes associated with each condition.

Weight

The single most important assessment of fluid status is the patient's weight. Significant fluctuations in body weight over a 1- to 2-day period are indicative of fluid gains and losses. However, this important sign is often forgotten or ignored when assessing the individual's renal and fluid status.

When possible, the patient should be weighed during admission to the critical care unit. It is important to note whether the current weight differs significantly from the weight 1 to 2 weeks before admission. Thereafter, the patient should be weighed daily for comparison to the previous day. The weight should be obtained at the same time each day, with the patient wearing the same amount of clothing. One liter of fluid equals 1 kg or approximately 2.2 pounds.

The individual's weight is of critical importance to the dialysis nurse caring for a patient with renal failure. The differences in weight from day to day are used in a mathematical formula for calculating the amount of fluid to remove during a dialysis treatment. Therefore setting the appropriate parameters for a safe, comfortable, yet effective hemodialysis treatment depends in large part on obtaining the individual's weight.

Intake and Output

Intake and output can be compared to the patient's weight to evaluate accurately the gain or loss of fluid. Urinary output plus insensible fluid losses (perspiration and water vapor from the lungs) can range widely from 750 to 2400 ml daily. When intake exceeds output, a positive fluid state exists. If disorders such as renal failure perpetuate the positive fluid gain, fluid overload results. Conversely, if output exceeds intake (fever, increased respiration, profuse sweating, vomiting, diarrhea, gastric suction), a negative fluid state exists.

Abnormal output of body fluids not only creates fluid imbalances, but also creates electrolyte and acid-base disturbances. For example, gastrointestinal suction or loss by diarrhea can result in fluid deficit, sodium and potassium

deficits, and metabolic acidosis (from excessive loss of bicarbonate). During a 24-hour period, fever can increase skin and respiratory losses by as much as 75 ml per degree Fahrenheit rise.[4]

In maintaining daily records of intake and output, all gains or losses must be recorded. Having a standard list of the fluid volume held in various containers (for example, milk cartons and juice containers) will ease this process. Discussions about the importance of accurate intake and output with the patient and with his or her family and friends are necessary and can enhance the accuracy of record keeping.

Clinical Observations

Disturbances in fluid and electrolyte levels are often accompanied by signs and symptoms less measurable than those previously mentioned but that are, nonetheless, indicative of serious change.

Changes in mental status such as disorientation are often a result of acidosis. Lethargy, coma, and confusion may result from sodium, calcium, or magnesium excess or deficit. Apprehension may be secondary to sodium deficit or to a shift of fluid from the plasma to the interstitium.[6] Also, individuals with respiratory changes secondary to fluid volume overload are frequently apprehensive.

Finally, apathy and withdrawal often accompany hypovolemic states.[6] Renal failure patients with systemic increases in electrolytes, fluids, and nitrogenous waste products can also exhibit apathy, restlessness, confusion, and withdrawal. It is often difficult to separate the emotional component from the actual physiological mechanism. Nonetheless, the importance of considering a fluid or electrolyte disorder as the cause of a mental or emotional change must be emphasized.

REFERENCES
1. Bates B: A guide to physical examination, ed 3, Philadelphia, 1983, JB Lippincott Co.
2. Grimes J and Burns E: Health assessment in nursing practice, ed 2, Boston, 1987, Jones & Bartlett Publishers, Inc.
3. Malasanos L and others: Health assessment, ed 4, St Louis, 1989, The CV Mosby Co.
4. Metheny NM: Fluid and electrolyte balance—nursing considerations, Philadelphia, 1987, JB Lippincott Co.
5. Poyss AS: Assessment and nursing diagnosis in fluid and electrolyte disorders, Nurs Clin North Am 22(4):773, 1987.
6. Rice V: Problems of water regulation: diabetes insipidus and syndromes of inappropriate anti-diuretic hormone, Crit Care Nurse 32:64, 1983.

CHAPTER

31

Renal and Fluids Laboratory Assessment and Diagnostic Procedures

CHAPTER OBJECTIVES

- *Describe the effect of decreased serum albumin levels on fluid dynamics within the body.*
- *Identify how alterations of both the hemoglobin and the hematocrit levels can signal fluid volume deficit or excess.*
- *Explain why elevations of blood urea nitrogen and creatinine can signal renal dysfunction.*
- *Describe the relationship between serum osmolality and antidiuretic hormone.*

A number of laboratory tests and diagnostic procedures are used to assess renal and fluid status. The most definitive tests are explained in the following narrative.

ASSESSMENT OF BLOOD
Serum Albumin

Serum albumin composes slightly more than 50% of the total plasma protein. It is manufactured in the liver, and its normal blood levels are 3.5 to 5.5 g/dl. Albumin is primarily implicated in the maintenance of colloid osmotic pressure, which functions to hold fluid in the vascular space. The blood vessel walls, because of their impermeability to plasma proteins, prevent albumin from leaving the vascular space. But with third-degree burns (membrane destruction) or nephrotic syndrome (increased glomerular capillary permeability), albumin can escape the vascular space and enter the interstitial space. In this process, the albumin will carry along excess water, thereby creating a fluid shift.

Decreased albumin levels result in a plasma-to-interstitial fluid shift, which creates peripheral edema. A decreased albumin level can occur as a result of protein-calorie malnutrition in which available stores of albumin are depleted, oncotic pressure is decreased, and fluid is shifted from the vascular space to the interstitial space. Liver disease can also cause a fall in albumin levels as the diseased liver fails to synthesize sufficient albumin. Further, severe portal hy-

pertension can force albumin and other plasma proteins into the abdominal cavity, creating ascites.

Increased albumin levels are rare. The body uses a fixed amount of protein for energy and body cell replacement and converts excess protein into stored fat. Most often if all plasma proteins are elevated, fluid volume deficit (hemoconcentration) is suspected.

Hemoglobin and Hematocrit

The hemoglobin (Hgb) and hematocrit (Hct) levels can be indicative of increases or decreases in intravascular fluid volume. Both Hgb and Hct values vary between sexes, with the hemoglobin value in males normally 13.5 to 17.5 g/dl and 12 to 16 g/dl in females. The Hct value ranges from 40% to 54% in males and 37% to 47% in females. Hemoglobin transports oxygen and carbon dioxide; thus it maintains cellular metabolism and acid-base balance.

The Hct expresses the percentage of red blood cells (RBCs) in a volume of whole blood. An increase in the hematocrit often indicates a severe fluid volume deficit, which results in hemoconcentration—hence, the elevated Hct level. Although rare, true disorders of RBC production such as polycythemia can result in an increased Hct level.

Conversely, a decreased Hct level can indicate fluid volume excess because of the dilutional effect of the extra fluid load. However, decreases can also result from anemias, blood loss, liver damage, or hemolytic reactions.[2] The history and bedside assessment will aid in determining whether fluid imbalances and/or disease states are responsible.

Blood Urea Nitrogen and Creatinine

Blood urea nitrogen (BUN) and creatinine are both by-products of protein metabolism. The normal value for BUN is 9 to 20 mg/dl, and the normal value for creatinine is 0.7 to 1.5 mg/dl. The importance of these two serum tests is not with normal levels but with increases or decreases. Both BUN and creatinine levels become elevated when renal function deteriorates.

Creatinine is a by-product of normal cell metabolism and appears in serum in amounts proportional to the body muscle

627

mass. Creatinine is easily excreted by the renal tubules. Tracing the amount of creatinine in the excreted urine and the amount of creatinine in the blood over 24 hours provides accurate information about kidney function.

Creatinine excess occurs most often in individuals with renal failure in whom the diminished renal function impairs creatinine excretion. However, muscle growth disorders such as acromegaly can produce elevations through increased muscle mass. Also, malnutrition can result in transient increases in creatinine levels as the rapid muscle catabolism associated with malnutrition causes "dumping" of increased levels of creatinine into the circulation. Decreased levels of creatinine are rare and are usually associated with muscular dystrophy.[2]

BUN levels are not as accurate an indicator of renal failure as creatinine because BUN levels fluctuate greatly with protein intake, whereas creatinine levels are relatively unaffected by protein intake. Elevations in the BUN level can be correlated with the signs and symptoms of uremia; as the BUN value rises, symptoms of uremia become more pronounced as a result of the irritation this metabolite produces on bodily membranes.

Increased levels of BUN (often called *urea*) also occur with fluid volume deficit (hemoconcentration), infection, excessive protein intake, and renal failure. Decreased levels can result from fluid volume excess, liver failure, or protein malnutrition.[2]

Anion Gap

The anion gap is a calculation of the difference between the measurable cations (sodium and potassium) and the measurable anions (chloride and bicarbonate). The value represents the remaining unmeasurable anions present in the extracellular fluid (for example, phosphates, sulfates, ketones, pyruvate, lactate). The normal value is 10 to 12 mEq/L and should not exceed 14 mEq/L. An increased anion gap level reflects an overproduction and/or poor excretion of acid products.[4]

Renal failure can increase the anion gap value because of retention of acids and altered bicarbonate reabsorption. Diabetic ketoacidosis results in ketone production, which also elevates the level of the anion gap. The measurement of the anion gap is a rapid, effective method for identifying acid-base imbalance, but it cannot be used to pinpoint the actual acid-base disturbance specifically.

Serum Osmolality

The serum osmolality level reflects the concentration or dilution of vascular fluid. The normal serum osmolality level is 275 to 295 mOsm/L.[2] Antidiuretic hormone (ADH) plays an important role in maintaining the serum osmolality level. When the serum osmolality level increases (for example, with insufficient fluid intake), ADH is released from the pituitary gland and stimulates increased water reabsorption, which expands the vascular space and brings the serum osmolality level back to normal. A more concentrated urine also results. The opposite case occurs with a decreased serum osmolality level, which inhibits the production of ADH and results in increased excretion of water through the kidneys, producing a dilute urine and bringing the serum osmolality level back to normal.

Table 31-1 Essential urinalysis tests for diagnosing renal and fluid disorders

Substance	Normal values
Specific gravity	1.003-1.030
Urinary osmolality	300-1200 mOsm/L
Urinary pH	4.5-8.0
Urinary electrolytes	
Sodium	80-180 mEq/24 hr
Potassium	40-80 mEq/24 hr
Chloride	110-20 mEq/24 hr
Calcium	50-300 mEq/24 hr

ASSESSMENT OF URINE

Urinary volume, contents, color, clarity, acidity, alkalinity, and odor provide excellent information about the patient's condition relative to fluids and electrolytes. Specific tests are presented in Table 31-1; several are discussed in greater detail to clarify certain disorders.

Urine pH

Urine pH indicates the acidity or alkalinity of the urine. The normal urinary pH level is 6.0, which is acidic, but it may range from 4.5 to 8.0. As the kidney regulates acid-base balance, far more hydrogen ions are excreted than bicarbonate ions, creating the acidity of the urine. Therefore changes in renal function produce changes in the urinary pH value.

An increase in urinary acidity (decreased level of pH) indicates retention of sodium and acids by the body. Conversely, a decrease in urinary acidity (increased pH or more alkaline level) means the body is retaining bicarbonate. However, urinary pH levels are greatly affected by diet and medications. Certain food groups such as citrus fruits and vegetables lead to an alkaline urine, whereas a diet high in protein can produce an acid urinary pH.

Specific Gravity

Specific gravity measures the density or weight of urine compared to distilled water. The normal urinary specific gravity level is 1.003 to 1.030 as compared to the normal specific gravity level of distilled water at 1.000. Since urine is composed of many solutes and substances suspended in water, its specific gravity level should always be higher than that of water, and it indicates the ability of the kidney to dilute or concentrate the urine.

Decreases in specific gravity values reflect inability of the kidneys to excrete the usual solute load into the urine (less dense with fewer solutes). Increases in specific gravity values (a more concentrated urine) occur with a body fluid volume deficit as the result of fever, vomiting, or diarrhea. An increased specific gravity value can also occur with diabetes or glomerular membrane permeability changes, which allow glucose and protein in the urine, thereby increasing the urine concentrations.[2]

Osmolality

The urinary osmolality value more accurately pinpoints fluid balance than does the serum osmolality value, because the serum osmolality value is actually a reflection of serum sodium concentration and is therefore subject to far more influences than the urinary osmolality value. However, the simultaneous measurement of both the serum and urinary osmolality levels provides a more accurate assessment of fluid status. The normal urinary osmolality level is 300 to 1200 mOsm/kg and depends on reabsorption or excretion of water in the kidney tubules. The urinary osmolality level increases during fluid volume deficit because of the retention of fluid by the body. Conversely, the urinary osmolality level decreases during volume excess because fluid is excreted by the kidneys. In late renal failure, the urinary osmolality value is usually quite low because solutes and fluids are being abnormally retained.[6]

Glucose

Glucose is normally reabsorbed by the renal tubules; therefore urine should be free of glucose. However, the appearance of glucose in the urine may be transient in nature, brought on by ingestion of a heavy carbohydrate load or caused by stress, or resulting from the renal changes accompanying pregnancy.

Consistent appearance of glycosuria occurs during hyperglycemic episodes of diabetes when the renal threshold for glucose is exceeded and the excess glucose is spilled into the urine. However, when renal failure accompanies hyperglycemia, glycosuria cannot be considered indicative of the level of hyperglycemia because of the erratic excretion of glucose by the damaged nephrons.

Protein

Protein, like glucose, is normally absent from the urine because the large protein molecule cannot pass across the normal glomerular capillary membrane. Thus consistent appearance of protein in the urine suggests compromise of the glomerular membrane and possible renal disease.

Transient appearance of protein in the urine can occur as the result of efferent arteriole constriction caused by stress, extreme exercise, or extreme cold. Also, *proteinuria* can occur after ingestion of a high protein meal or can accompany the renal changes associated with pregnancy.

Levels of proteinuria of 0.5 to 4.0 g/day indicate renal compromise, and the amount excreted directly correlates with the severity of the damage.[2]

Electrolytes

Levels of urinary electrolytes are not as frequently measured as are serum electrolytes because of the lesser significance of urinary findings. To measure urinary electrolyte levels, a 24-hour urine sample is required. The electrolyte levels are highly variable, and the electrolytes depend on the kidneys for adequate excretion. Consequently, decreases in urinary electrolyte levels are highly suggestive of renal failure. The urinary sodium level, on the other hand, may increase because of the inability of aldosterone to effect sodium reabsorption in the damaged nephrons.[2]

Urinary Sediment

The presence of epithelial cells and *casts* aids in identifying problems related to the kidneys. Casts are shells or clumps of cellular breakdown or proteinaceous materials that form in the renal tubular system and are washed out in the urinary flow. Although small numbers of epithelial cells normally appear in the urine and an occasional cast may be found, their consistent appearance is abnormal.

The consistent appearance of epithelial cells shed by the nephron may indicate *nephritis*. Casts differ in composition and size, and both characteristics correlate to the severity and type of renal damage. White blood cell casts indicate pyelonephritis and also occur during the exudative stage of acute glomerulonephritis. Red blood cell casts indicate glomerulonephritis, whereas hyaline casts are associated with renal parenchymal disease and glomerular capillary membrane inflammation.

DIAGNOSTIC PROCEDURES
Radiological Assessment

Although laboratory assessment of the patient is used foremost in diagnosing renal and urological problems, radiological assessment confirms or clarifies causes of particular disorders. Radiological assessment ranges from the simple to the sophisticated (Table 31-2) and provides information about abnormal masses, abnormal fluid collection, congenital abnormalities, obstructions, and other disorders of the kidneys and urinary tract.

Kidney, ureters, bladder. A simple flat-plate x-ray film of the kidneys, ureters and bladder (KUB) is often used to detect size, masses, congenital abnormalities, or obstructions.[1] Although the KUB is rarely used in the adult diagnostic workup, especially in the critical care population, it is often used to assess urological or renal conditions in the pediatric population.

Intravenous pyelography. Intravenous pyelography (IVP) offers visualization of the entire urinary tract. A contrast medium is injected parenterally and proceeds through the normal excretory route of the kidneys in which visualization of structural changes, obstructions lesions, or hydronephrosis can be determined. Although a valuable tool, IVP carries with it considerable risk associated with hypersensitivity to the radiological contrast medium. It is important to determine the patient's previous hypersensitivity to the medium and to any iodine-based preparations.

Retrograde radiological tests. Retrograde radiological tests (pyelography, cystourethrography, and cystography) involve instillation of a contrast medium through a catheter into the lower urinary tract to help determine obstructions, bladder anomalies, diverticula, reflux, and the general integrity of the tract.[1,5] Although not used much for renal assessment, these procedures provide much information for prevention of renal disorders secondary to structural or functional changes in the tract. Cystourethrography and cystography are performed with basic urethral catheterization performed during cystoscopy, with insertion of a catheter into the ureter.

Renal arteriogram. Renal arteriography involves injection of a contrast medium into the arterial circulation perfusing the kidneys. This procedure produces radiological

Table 31-2 Renal imaging tests

Tests	Comments
Kidney-ureter-bladder (KUB)	Flat-plate x-ray film of abdomen determines position, size, and structure of kidneys and urinary tract.
	KUB is usually followed by more sophisticated tests.
Intravenous pyelography (IVP)	Intravenous injection of contrast media plus x-ray film allows visualization of internal kidney (parenchyma, calyces, pelves, ureters, bladder).
	Timing of stages can delineate size and shape.
	Obstructions and tumors can be found.
	Drawback can be hypersensitivity to contrast medium.
Retrograde pyelography	Injection of iodine-based contrast medium through ureteral catheter into collection system (calyces, pelves, and ureters) allows visualization of clots, stones, and strictures.
	It may be useful when allergy to IVP dye exists (less chance of hypersensitivity in this test).
Renal angiography	Injection of contrast medium into arterial blood perfusing the kidney allows x-ray visualization of renal blood flow.
	Stenoses, cysts, clots and tumors may be visualized, as may infarctions, traumas, and torn kidneys.
Renal computed tomographic (CT) scan	After administration of a radioisotope, which is absorbed by the kidneys, scintillation photography is performed in several planes.
	Density of the image helps determine tumor, cysts, hemorrhage, calcification adrenal tumors, or necrosis.
	It may be used before or instead of renal biopsy.
Renal ultrasonography	High-frequency sound waves are transmitted to the kidneys and urinary tract and viewed on an oscilloscope. This type of test is usually used to search for fluid accumulation or obstruction.

evidence about the renal vasculature and assists in determining stenoses, hypertensive damage, renal artery diseases, and renal infarctions.[1,5] As with any invasive procedure involving the vessels, this procedure has the risk of bleeding hematoma and thrombus formation.

Renal ultrasonography. Renal ultrasound procedures are used with increasing frequency because they are safe, efficient, noninvasive, and painless. Ultrasonography uses high-frequency sound waves to reverberate off the organs. The echoes are translated into images on a screen. This diagnostic tool allows detection of structural changes, hydronephrosis, cysts, and neoplasms.[5]

Computed tomography and radionuclide imaging. The final radiological tests involve computerized tomographic (CT) scanning and radionuclide imaging of the kidneys. The renal CT scan provides cross-sectional views of the kidneys, which is transferred to images on a viewing screen. Through observation of various areas of density, a determination of vascular defects, masses, filling defects, and renal infarctions can be made.[5] Radionuclide imaging involves special photography of the kidneys after injection of a low-dose radioisotope. This test helps determine the overall structural and functional integrity of renal tissue.

Renal Biopsy

Renal biopsy is the definitive tool for diagnosing disease processes of the kidney. Two methods are used—closed biopsy and open biopsy. In either case, biopsy should be the last resort in diagnostic assessment because of the postprocedural risks of bleeding, hematoma formation, and infection.

Percutaneous needle biopsy (closed method) involves a flank introduction of a cannula (over an obturator) for obtaining a specimen containing both cortical and medullary kidney tissue. Open biopsy is actual surgical visualization of the kidney, at which time a tissue sample is obtained. Specimens are then examined in the laboratory. Biopsy determines the presence of diseases such as glomerulonephritis, amyloidosis, and lupus erythematosus and the cause of renal lesions.

REFERENCES

1. Ames SW and Kneisl CR: Essentials of adult health nursing, Menlo Park, Calif, 1988, Addison-Wesley Publishing Co.
2. Fischbach F: A manual of laboratory diagnostic tests, ed 3, Philadelphia, 1988, JB Lippincott Co.
3. Insel J and Elwyn DH: Body composition. In Askanazi J, Starker PM, and Weissman C, editors: Fluid and electrolyte management in critical care, Boston, 1986, Butterworth and Co (Publishers), Ltd.
4. Narins RG Jr and others: Metabolic acid-base disorders: pathophysiology, classification and treatment. In Arieff AI and DeFronzo RA, editors: Fluid, electrolyte and acid-base disorders, vol 1, New York, 1985, Churchill Livingstone, Inc.
5. Richard C: Assessment of renal structure and function. In Lancaster L: Core curriculum for nephrology nursing, Englewood Cliffs, NJ, 1987, AJ Janetti, Inc.
6. Shorecki KL and Brenner BM: Edema forming states: congestive heart failure, liver disease, and nephrotic syndrome. In Arieff AI and DeFronzo RA, editors: Fluid, electrolyte and acid-base disorders, vol 1, New York, 1985, Churchill Livingstone, Inc.
7. Tilkian SM, Conover MB, and Tilkian AG: Clinical implications of laboratory tests, ed 4, St Louis 1987, The CV Mosby Co.

Renal and Fluids Disorders

CHAPTER OBJECTIVES

- *List signs and symptoms of each of the serum electrolyte disturbances discussed in this chapter.*
- *Identify clinical manifestations of acute and chronic renal failure and of uremic syndrome.*
- *Describe important aspects of the nursing care of a patient with acute renal failure.*
- *Describe important aspects of the nursing care of a patient with chronic renal failure.*

ELECTROLYTE DISTURBANCES
Hypokalemia

Hypokalemia is a potassium deficit of the extracellular fluid (ECF), with a serum potassium level less than 3.5 mEq/L. Potassium deficit occurs as a result of the body's tendency to excrete potassium and is complicated by secondary conditions such as vomiting, gastric suction, and excess aldosterone production and by use of potent diuretics, which further enhance potassium losses.[32]

Potassium in the ECF is constantly in a state of flux. The potassium filtered by the glomerulus is completely absorbed in the proximal tubule, secreted in the distal tubule, and either reabsorbed or secreted in the collecting ducts. Changes in renal tubular function or changes in the adrenal gland secretion of aldosterone (causes potassium excretion) automatically result in potassium level changes (see the box at right).

Clinical assessment of hypokalemia necessitates looking at the serum potassium level, since it is impossible to look at actual total body stores of potassium. The most significant clinical sign related to potassium changes occurs in the electrocardiogram (ECG). Abnormal shifts of potassium in or out of cardiac muscle cells will significantly alter the membrane potentials and subsequently influence conduction. Hypokalemia slows depolarization of the cells and thereby slows conduction velocity of the heart.[8] Hypokalemia has also been implicated in cases of sudden cardiac

death in individuals who have cardiac compromise. See Fig. 13-3, *A* and *B*, for ECG changes associated with hypokalemia.

Individuals suffering from hypokalemia first have symptoms such as anorexia, fatigue, muscle weakness, dizziness, abdominal distention, decreased peristalsis, confusion, and weak irregular pulses.[24]

Treatment of hypokalemia is through oral or parenteral replacement. A diet rich in meats, fruits, and vegetables

---

HYPOKALEMIA

Definition

Deficit of potassium in the ECF

Serum value

Less than 3.5 mEq/L

Causes

Metabolic alkalosis
Decreased potassium intake
Use of diuretics without potassium supplementation
Loss of gastrointestinal (GI) fluids (suction, nausea and vomiting, diarrhea)
Hyperaldosteronism (primary and secondary Cushing's syndrome)

Findings

Muscular weakness
Cardiac irregularities
Abdominal distortion and flatulence
Paresthesia
Decreased reflexes
Anorexia
Dizziness
Confusion
Increased sensitivity to digitalis

---

provides much potassium for the system, and potassium-rich salt substitutes may also be a source of replacement. Parenteral potassium replacement should not exceed 20 mEq/hr or 150 mEq/L/day in adults or 3 mEq/kg in children. Additionally, potassium is *always* diluted for parenteral use.

Potassium levels should be monitored carefully during potassium supplementation. Daily doses can be determined and adjusted according to dietary intake of potassium. Observation of renal function is also necessary to prevent hyperkalemia as a result of potassium retention.[32] Observation of intravenous (IV) sites for extrusion into the tissues is essential, since potassium is very caustic to the tissues.

Hyperkalemia

Hyperkalemia is an excess of potassium in the ECF, with a serum potassium level greater than 5.0 mEq/L. Most cases of hyperkalemia occur secondary to kidney failure. However, decreased aldosterone production, crushing injury, rapid administration of potassium solutions, and administration of potassium-sparing diuretics can result in elevation of serum potassium.[28] Additionally, cell damage resulting from surgery, burns, or myocardial infarction releases potassium into the ECF[28,36] (see the following box).

ECG findings in hyperkalemia are also of value in confirming a diagnosis of hyperkalemia. The appearance of tall,

peaked T waves, a lengthening PR interval, widening QRS complexes, and flattening P waves indicate elevations of potassium[15] (see Figs. 13-1, *A* and *B*, and 13-2). Nausea and vomiting, diarrhea, numbness and tingling, weakness, and bradycardia are also signals to investigate the serum potassium.[24]

Potassium supplementation should be discontinued. Administration of calcium parenterally will temporarily block the effects of hyperkalemia in the heart muscle, but further measures are required to actually decrease serum levels, including sodium bicarbonate injection and the use of a mixture of hypertonic dextrose and insulin, which forces potassium back into the cells. However, eventual excretion of potassium is necessary, particularly in the presence of renal failure. Consequently, cation-exchange resins (for example, sodium polystyrene sulfonate [Kayexalate]) are administered, and hemodialysis should be initiated.[28]

Hyponatremia

Hyponatremia is a deficiency of sodium in the ECF when compared to water. Hyponatremia can be deceptive because in several disorders there is not an actual deficit of sodium but an excess of water in relationship to the sodium. At least three scenarios offer further explanation of the possible alterations in sodium and ECF balance (see the box on p. 633).

The first scenario is hyponatremia associated with an increase in the ECF volume. Commonly known as water intoxication or dilutional hyponatremia, this disturbance is associated with cardiac failure, liver disease, renal failure, and other disorders.[2] A concomitant inability to excrete the excess volume leads to dilution of the existing sodium.

For example, in an individual with renal compromise ingestion of water or infusion of IV solutions beyond the excretion capacity of the kidney results in dilutional hyponatremia. The decrease in glomerular filtration rate (GFR) is implicated as the primary mechanism for this occurrence.

Of particular interest to nursing is the care that must be exercised in monitoring the fluid status of the postoperative patient. Stress, pain, tissue hypoxia, mechanical ventilation, and certain drugs can stimulate the antidiuretic hormone (ADH) to conserve water in excess of desired quantities. Replacement of fluid loss with dextrose in water (D_5W) leads to rapid metabolism of the glucose and can increase water load to the ECF compartment.[24]

Clinical findings include a serum sodium level below 135 mEq/L and a low serum osmolality (<285 mOsm/kg). Symptoms vary from mild to severe but may include fatigue, apprehension, abdominal cramps, nausea and vomiting, headache, and lethargy.[22]

A second picture of hyponatremia is a loss of both sodium and ECF. Implicated in the development of this disturbance are the loss of sodium-rich gastrointestinal (GI) fluids (for example, from nausea and vomiting, diarrhea, GI suction), overuse of potent diuretics, and aldosterone insufficiency.

In the case of GI losses, not only sodium and water are depleted, but potassium is also. With less potassium available for excretion by the distal tubule, the stimulus to release aldosterone is partially lost and sodium is not sufficiently reabsorbed.[2]

HYPERKALEMIA

Definition

Excess potassium in the ECF

Serum value

Greater than 5.0 mEq/L

Causes

Acute or chronic renal failure
Excess intake of potassium
Excess intake through infusions
Burns
Crushing injuries
Potassium-sparing diuretics (spironolactone [Aldactone], triamterene [Dyrenium])
Metabolic acidosis
Transfusions of old blood

Findings

Irritability and restlessness
Anxiety
Nausea and vomiting
Abdominal cramps
Weakness
Numbness and tingling (fingertips and circumoral)
Cardiac irregularities (first tachycardia, then bradycardia)

HYPONATREMIA

WATER INTOXICATION
Definition

Increased ECF volume, with inability to excrete the excess

Serum value

May be less than 125 mEq/L (very mild to severe); serum sodium value of 110-115 mEq/L known to occur

Causes

Excess D_5W solution intravenously
Excess plain water intake
Renal failure

Findings

Disorientation
Muscle twitching
Nausea and vomiting
Abdominal cramps
Headaches
Seizures

TRUE HYPONATREMIA
Definition

Actual deficit of body sodium

Serum value

Less than 135 mEq/L

Causes

Gastric suction
Vomiting
Burns
Use of potent diuretics
Heat exhaustion (excessive sweating)
Loss from wounds and drainage

Use of tap-water enemas
Diarrhea
Adrenal insufficiency

Findings

Apprehension
Dizziness
Postural hypotension
Cold, clammy skin
Decreased skin turgor
Tachycardia
Oliguria

SYNDROME OF INAPPROPRIATE RELEASE OF ADH (SIADH)
Definition

Dilutional state plus sodium loss

Serum value

Less than 120 mEq/L

Causes

Central nervous system (CNS) disorders
Major trauma (stress)
Malignancies (lung, pancreas, thymus)
Certain drugs (oral hypoglycemics, antineoplastics, diuretics, analgesics, bronchodilators)

Findings

Anorexia
Nausea and vomiting
Abdominal cramps
Lethargy and withdrawal
Convulsions
Coma
Urinary osmolality greater than plasma (increased wasting of sodium)

Potent loop diuretics work to disorder the concentrating ability of the loop of Henle and therefore cause increased losses of both sodium and fluid. This hyponatremia is further complicated by a reduction in GFR brought on by the reduced vascular volume.

Treatment for both cases of hyponatremia involves treating the underlying conditions, administering IV sodium chloride solutions, and discontinuing diuretic therapy. Correction of the hyponatremic states with IV saline solutions may prevent the problem of fluid shifts from the ECF to the intracellular fluid (ICF) when sodium is lost.[13]

Finally, hyponatremia can result from the syndrome of inappropriate secretion of ADH (SIADH). Although SIADH is discussed at length in Chapter 41, it must be noted that a rather severe reduction of sodium without ECF loss can occur as a result of this disorder.

The condition results from oversecretion of ADH (va-

sopressin), which permits the continuous reabsorption of water from the renal tubular system. Sodium excretion is high in the urine, whereas large amounts of water are retained under the influence of ADH secretion. Fluid restriction, sodium replacement, mild diuretics, and drugs to control ADH secretion (demeclocycline) represent current treatment for the disorder.[17]

Hypernatremia

Sodium excess of the ECF is extremely dangerous but occurs rarely. Hypernatremia can arise from an actual increase in sodium or from losses of water. However, in all cases of hypernatremia the increase in ECF sodium depletes the cells of fluid and leads to the symptoms commonly associated with this disorder (see the box on p. 634).

Hypernatremia can occur with a loss of both ECF sodium and water, but the water loss far exceeds the amount of

---

HYPERNATREMIA

Definition

Excess sodium in the ECF

Serum value

Greater than 145 mEq/L

Causes

Inability to respond to thirst (decreased fluid intake)
Heatstroke
Diarrhea (excess fluid loss)
Severe insensible loss (ventilation, sweating)
Diabetes insipidus
Excessive administration of sodium solutions (e.g., hypertonic saline, sodium bicarbonate)
Hypertonic tube feedings without water supplement
NOTE: Hypernatremia is usually the result of dehydration of the ECF and subsequent hyperconcentration of the sodium.

Findings

Extreme thirst
Fever
Dry, sticky mucous membranes
Altered mentation
Seizures (later stages)

---

sodium loss. Watery diarrhea or profuse sweating can cause severe hypotonic fluid loss. Moderate-to-severe diarrhea can result in fluid losses of approximately 300 to 3000 ml/day.[33] The fluid loss concentrates the remaining sodium in the ECF, which, in turn, exerts an osmotic pull on the intracellular compartment and depletes the cells of fluid.

True hypernatremia can be caused by administration of high sodium content tube feedings without sufficient water intake and by administration of hypertonic saline solutions for correction of sodium imbalance or administration of sodium bicarbonate during cardiac arrest.[22,27] Plumer[24] even suggests that normal saline solution or D5NS, infused in large quantities, can lead to hypernatremia. This occurrence, however, may be limited to elderly individuals with decreased ability to excrete sodium and water or to postoperative patients with stress-induced renal disturbances.[24]

Finally, hypernatremia can result from only water loss such as occurs with diabetes insipidus. This disorder is classified as either central diabetes insipidus (arising from central nervous system causes) or nephrogenic diabetes insipidus, which results in a loss of the renal response to ADH, causing no reabsorption of water in the collecting ducts. As water is lost, sodium in the ECF rises.[39]

Regardless of the causes of hypernatremia, one particular characteristic remains common—thirst. Thirst is the main defense against hyperconcentration of the fluid compartments. The same osmoreceptors that trigger ADH release are responsible for stimulation of thirst and are stimulated when the serum osmolality rises to 294 mOsm/kg.[34] In patients with diabetes insipidus, an intense thirst is created by the rising serum osmolality, but water is not retained to maintain the fluid compartments. An enormous intake of fluid, however, helps maintain the serum osmolality near normal.

Hypocalcemia

Calcium deficit can be misleading because of the three different ways calcium is held within the body. Ninety-eight to ninety-nine percent of the calcium within the body is bound in bone and is not readily available. The remainder is either protein bound (chelated by phosphate, sulfate, or citrate) or ionized in the bloodstream.[10] Since serum calcium is primarily protein bound, changes in serum protein values will lead to changes in serum calcium values (1 g/dl protein relates to 0.8 mg/dl calcium).[21] Typically, a diagnosis of hypocalcemia means the serum calcium is less than 4.5 mEq/L or 8.5 mg/dl.[38]

Serum calcium stores are replenished primarily through the action of the parathyroid hormone (PTH), which can mobilize calcium from the bone into the vascular space. Absorption of calcium from the intestinal tract, excretion from the kidneys, and constant bone rebuilding help maintain the available store. Disturbances in any of the three areas can result in a deficit or excess of calcium.[9,10]

For instance, a deficit of calcium is possible when renal failure results in poor uptake of calcium in the GI tract, which occurs because the breakdown product of vitamin D, which is metabolized in renal cells, is not available in renal failure; thus, the stimulus to reabsorb calcium from the intestines is lost, and the result is a decrease in serum calcium levels.

The serum calcium level is affected by the inverse relationship that exists between calcium and phosphorus. When phosphorus levels are high, calcium absorption is inhibited; the reverse is also true.[38] Further, serum calcium levels are influenced by the pH of the arterial blood. In acidosis, the lower pH results in the release of more calcium from protein binding, which elevates the ionized calcium. Conversely, an elevated pH results in calcium becoming more highly bound to protein, reducing the ionized calcium.[10] Thus when correcting acidosis, care must be taken to monitor calcium and replace it as needed. Other causes of hypocalcemia may be seen in the box on p. 635.

The person experiencing hypocalcemia may display facial muscle twitching (Chvostek's sign) or carpophalangeal spasm (Trousseau's sign). Cardiac changes are also present with hypocalcemia and are reflected as prolonged QT segments on the ECG and decreased left-ventricular contractility.[10] Both problems result from the decreased availability of calcium to perform its role in cell depolarization and consequent neurotransmission. Treatment for hypocalcemia depends on whether the disorder is acute or chronic. Acute hypocalcemia is treated with IV administration of calcium. An initial bolus of 200 mg is given over 10 minutes, followed by 1 to 2 mg/kg/hour until levels are normal (6 to 12 hours).[38] However, the success of treatment of hypocalcemia often depends on normalizing the levels of other electrolytes. For example, the administration of calcium in the presence of hyperphosphatemia usually results in little success in correcting the original calcium imbalance. If mag-

```
┌─────────────────────────────────────────┐
│              HYPOCALCEMIA               │
├─────────────────────────────────────────┤
```

Definition

Deficit of calcium in the ECF

Serum value

Less than 8.5 mg/dl or 4.5 mEq/L

Causes

Protein malnutrition (decreased albumin causes decreased calcium)
Decreased calcium intake
Burns or infection
Decreased parathyroid function (PTH controls serum calcium availability)
Decreased GI absorption of calcium (diarrhea)
Excessive antacid use (prevents absorption)
Renal failure (decreased vitamin D_3 available to stimulate absorption)

Findings

Irritability
Muscular tetany
Muscle cramps
Decreased cardiac output (decreased contractions)
Bleeding (decreased ability to coagulate)
Fractures

```
┌─────────────────────────────────────────┐
│              HYPERCALCEMIA              │
├─────────────────────────────────────────┤
```

Definition

Excess calcium in the ECF

Serum value

Greater than 10.5 mg/dl or 5.8 mEq/L

Causes

Increased parathyroid activity (increases bone resorption of calcium)
Multiple fractures
Prolonged immobilization
Bone tumors
Other malignancies
Decreased phosphorus (inverse relationship between calcium and phosphate)

Findings

Deep bone pain
Excessive thirst
Anorexia
Lethargy
Weakened muscles

---

nesium levels are low, infusion of calcium only results in its excretion from the kidney in favor of magnesium retention. Drugs that predispose to or prolong hypocalcemia should also be discontinued.[38]

Chronic hypocalcemia such as that associated with renal failure can be treated with oral calcium and vitamin D preparations. Synthetic vitamin D_3 (cholecalciferol) was developed in the late 1970s to increase GI absorption of calcium in these patients.[37] As a preventive measure for individuals with intact renal function, an oral calcium intake of 1 to 1.2 g/day has been recommended. Through the ingestion of milk, vegetables, oral calcium supplements, or bone meal, this level of intake can be achieved.[30]

Hypercalcemia

An excess of calcium in the ECF is known as hypercalcemia. Overstimulation of the parathyroid gland from a tumor, malignancies causing metastatic calcium release, and prolonged immobilization are usually implicated in the development of hypercalcemia. In fact, hypercalcemia is mediated almost exclusively from abnormalities in bone activity rather than absorption and release of calcium into the ECF.[9] The use of diuretics and drugs that stimulate PTH production can worsen existing hypercalcemia.[21]

In patients with hypercalcemia, the serum calcium level is greater than 5.8 mEq/L or 10.5 mg/dl. X-ray examination may demonstrate large areas of bone decalcification.[22] The individual may experience deep bone pain, flaccid muscles,

anorexia, nausea and vomiting, lethargy, confusion, headaches, and even pathological fractures from the demineralization of the bone[9] (see the box above).

Treatment of acute hypercalcemia involves dilution of the calcium using IV fluids and concomitant use of "loop" diuretics (furosemide) to enhance calcium excretion.[9] Thiazide diuretics inhibit excretion of calcium and should not be used in cases of hypercalcemia.[21] Oral phosphorus preparations may be given to increase bone deposition of calcium.[9] However, phosphorus preparations should not be given to those patients with renal failure. Additionally, the diarrhea and/or constipation caused by phosphorus may be undesirable in some individuals. IV phosphate administration is used as a last resort because of the potential for developing soft-tissue calcification from calcium-phosphate precipitates.[21]

In patients with metastatic malignancies causing hypercalcemia, drugs such as plicamycin (Mithracin) or the hormone calcitonin may be used.[9] Plicamycin, a cytotoxic drug, is responsible for slowing bone resorption. However, like many of the antineoplastic drugs, it also risks bone-marrow depression and blood dyscrasias.[9] Calcitonin inhibits PTH activity and thereby slows loss of calcium from the bone.[21]

Hypomagnesemia

Magnesium is involved in enzymatic reaction, cellular permeability, and the maintenance of neuromuscular excitability. Conditions such as malnutrition, chronic alcoholism, prolonged diuresis, and severe diarrhea can lead to magnesium deficits. However, the causes of magnesium deficit

---

HYPOMAGNESEMIA

Definition

Deficit of magnesium in the ECF

Serum value

Less than 1.4 mEq/L

Causes

Malnutrition
Chronic alcoholism (malnutrition)
Diuretics (prolonged use)
Severe diarrhea
Severe dehydration

Findings

Choroid and athetoid muscle activity
Facial tics
Spasticity
Cardiac dysrhythmias

HYPERMAGNESEMIA

Definition

Excess of magnesium in the ECF

Serum value

Greater than 2.5 mEq/L

Causes

Excessive intake of magnesium products (antacids and laxatives)
Renal failure
Severe dehydration if oliguria is present

Findings

CNS depression (especially respiratory)
Lethargy
Coma
Bradycardia

---

are lead by those involving loss from the GI tract[11] (see the box above). The serum magnesium level will be less than 1.4 mEq/L.

Nutritional deficits such as result from administering parenteral nutrition or tube feedings that are magnesium poor can lead to hypomagnesemia. The administration of loop diuretics such as furosemide also can enhance magnesium losses. However, magnesium losses have most commonly been associated with chronic alcoholism, in which losses can stem from diarrhea and vomiting, as well as chronic malnutrition.

The signs and symptoms of hypomagnesemia involve the role magnesium plays in neuromuscular excitability. Severe respiratory muscle depression may occur, rendering the individual in need of mechanical ventilation. Mental apathy and confusion may also be present. Finally, life-threatening dysrhythmias can result from magnesium depletion.[12]

Treatment for hypomagnesemia usually involves IV replacement with magnesium sulfate. However, before treatment is initiated, determination of adequate renal function should be undertaken. Individuals with severe hypomagnesemia may be given 2 g as a 10% solution over 2 minutes, followed by 12 g in 1 L of fluid over 12 hours.[12] Moderate decreases may be treated with 24 to 40 mEq of magnesium sulfate administered parenterally for several days. Oral or nasogastric (NG) supplementation should approach 16 mEq/day.[11]

Hypermagnesemia

The development of excess levels of magnesium in the ECF, although rare, goes hand in hand with chronic renal disease. The renal tubules can no longer excrete magnesium, and dialysis is quite ineffective in removing magnesium.[20] Individuals with renal impairment who chronically take laxatives or antacids containing magnesium will develop hypermagnesemia. Temporary excesses of magnesium can occur as the result of ECF dehydration or its excessive administration for treatment of eclampsia.[22]

The signs and symptoms associated with hypermagnesemia demonstrate profound central nervous system (CNS) involvement. The individual may exhibit muscle weakness, inability to swallow, hyporeflexia, hypotension, and cardiac dysrhythmias[20] (see the box above). The plasma value will typically be greater than 2.5 mEq/L, and the ECG will demonstrate a prolonged PR interval, wide QRS, tall T waves, atrioventricular (A-V) block, and premature ventricular contractions (PVCs).

Treatment for magnesium excess should be vigorous and immediate, with discontinuance of all magnesium-containing drugs, replacement of ECF volume (if secondary to dehydration), and administration of calcium gluconate to counteract the effects of the magnesium.[22] Individuals with severe hypermagnesemia may suffer from respiratory depression secondary to the effect of magnesium on the respiratory centers of the brain. Mechanical ventilation may become necessary to sustain ventilation until the excess is corrected.

Hypophosphatemia

Hypophosphatemia is a deficit of phosphorus in the ECF. Most phosphorus (85%) is held in the bone with calcium, 10% exists in the ECF, and the remainder is in the ICF, where it is responsible for energy formation (ATP), nerve and muscle function, and the acid-base balance of the ECF. Phosphorus shares an inverse relationship with calcium. Losses or gains in either electrolyte cause the kidneys to retain or excrete the other. The serum level indicating hypophosphatemia is less than 3 mg/dl.

HYPOPHOSPHATEMIA

Definition
Deficit of phosphate in the ECF

Serum value
Less than 3.0 mg/dl

Causes
Diabetic ketoacidosis (renal wasting)
Malabsorption disorders
Renal wasting of phosphorus
Prolonged use of IV dextrose infusions
Low-phosphate diets in patients with renal failure
Phosphate-poor total parenteral nutrition solutions

Findings
Hemolytic anemias
Depressed white cell function
Bleeding (decreased platelet aggregation)
Nausea, vomiting, and anorexia
Bone demineralization

Phosphorous loss occurs with conditions such as acute or chronic alcoholism, with excessive administration of electrolyte-poor IV solutions, and with overuse of antacids, which absorb phosphorus in the GI tract. Also implicated in hypophosphatemia are diabetic ketoacidosis and thermal burns[5] (see the box above).

Alcoholism-induced hypophosphatemia is a multifaceted occurrence involving calcium, magnesium, and PTH. An alcoholic's chronically poor nutritional status often results in deficiencies in vitamin D and intestinal irritability. Antacid ingestion to relieve the chronic GI irritability binds significant amounts of phosphate in the intestine. The two-fold assault stimulates PTH for calcium reabsorption, which in turn leads to further excretion of phosphorus in the urine. Also, excessive use of electrolyte-free IV fluids such as D_5W will lead to phosphorus' exiting the cells and its excretion in the urine.

The individual with hypophosphatemia develops bleeding disorders from defective platelets and fragile red blood cell (RBC) membranes. Muscular weakness, paresthesia, and GI distress result from reduced energy and oxygen transport to cells, which phosphorus helps accomplish.[5]

Replacement of phosphorous stores is generally done very slowly because the actual serum level may not reflect a deficit in the intracellular compartment. Oral supplementation is usually achieved through ingestion of skim milk. Fleet's Phospho-Soda can be mixed in water and administered either orally or by NG or feeding tube. Parenteral phosphorus is usually not given unless the serum phosphorus reaches 1.0 mg/dl.[5] Parenteral preparations of phosphorus must be diluted, and care must be taken to monitor levels of phosphorus to prevent precipitation with calcium. Phos-

phate solutions should be administered in quantities no greater than 1 g over 24 hours.[18]

Hyperphosphatemia

Phosphorus excess of the ECF usually occurs in cases of chronic renal failure. The renal tubules no longer excrete phosphorus as before, but uptake continues in the GI tract. Hyperphosphatemia can also result from rapid cell catabolism that releases the cellular phosphorous stores into the ECF. Excessive oral intake of phosphates or intestinal reabsorption of phosphates from enemas can elevate the serum phosphorus. However, elevations seldom become of concern unless phosphate excretion through the kidney is reduced.[18]

The signs and symptoms of hyperphosphatemia (see the box below) closely parallel those of hypocalemia, since these disorders are likely to occur simultaneously. However, muscle tetany and soft-tissue calcifications are usually the more prominent signs of this disorder.[18]

Treatment for hyperphosphatemia may range from simple dietary restriction of phosphorus to ingestion of aluminum antacids, which bind phosphate in the intestine. Adequate hydration and correction of any existing hypocalcemia can enhance the renal excretion of the excess phosphate.[38]

Hypochloremia

Hypochloremia is a deficit of chloride in the ECF. Hypochloremia develops as a result of loss of fluids rich in chloride. These fluids can also be rich in sodium, since chloride combines with sodium. Hypochloremia can be associated with acid-base disorders, particularly metabolic alkalosis, since the retention of bicarbonate, which occurs with metabolic alkalosis, leads to the excretion of chloride

---

HYPERPHOSPHATEMIA

Definition
Excess of phosphate in the ECF

Serum value
Greater than 4.5 mg/dl

Causes
Renal failure
Lactic acidosis
Catabolic stress
Chemotherapy for certain malignancies

Findings
Tachycardia
Nausea
Diarrhea
Abdominal cramps
Muscle weakness
Flaccid paralysis
Increased reflexes

HYPOCHLOREMIA

Definition

Deficit of chloride in the ECF

Serum value

Less than 98 mEq/L

Causes

Loss of gastric contents (vomiting, suction)
Diarrhea (prolonged)
Excessive diuretic use
Excessive sweating
Prolonged use of IV dextrose (dilutes potassium and
    sodium, as well as chloride)
Metabolic alkalosis (more available bicarbonate, so
    chloride excreted)

Findings

Hyperirritability
Tetany or muscular excitability
Slow respirations
Decreased blood pressure (with fluid loss)

---

ions. Other causes of hypochloremia include vomiting, gastric suction, diarrhea, and overuse of potassium-wasting diuretics.[1,22]

In patients with metabolic alkalosis secondary to gastric suctioning, chloride-rich gastric fluids are lost, concentrating the bicarbonate ions in the ECF. Overuse of diuretics leads to potassium wasting, which carries the chloride ions into the urine. The signs and symptoms of hypochloremia primarily result, not from the loss of chloride, but from the loss of potassium and ionized calcium[24] (see the box above).

Treatment for hypochloremia usually involves chloride replacement with a variety of medications such as ammonium chloride tablets or a parenteral solution containing chloride.[24] Treatment of the causative disorder should proceed immediately.

Hyperchloremia

Hyperchloremia is an excess of chloride ions in the ECF. Just as a deficit of chloride is related to acid-base imbalance, so is hyperchloremia. In patients with metabolic acidosis in whom bicarbonate ions are lost excessively, chloride ions are retained. Severe diarrhea, excessive parenteral administration of isotonic saline solution, urinary diversions, and renal failure predispose to bicarbonate (HCO_3^-) loss and concentration of existing chloride stores.[23]

The hyperchloremic individual is initially seen with weakness, lethargy, possible unconsciousness (in later stages), and deep rapid breathing.[24] Serum chloride levels are greater than 108 mEq/L. Treatment for hyperchloremia is based on first treating the underlying cause and correcting the aci-

dosis. Additionally, parenteral administration of sodium bicarbonate can restore bicarbonate stores.[24]

Bicarbonate Deficit

A primary base bicarbonate deficit is referred to as metabolic acidosis. The arterial pH is decreased as a result of loss of bicarbonate. Causes include diarrhea, renal failure, tissue hypoxia, lactic acidosis, diabetic ketoacidosis, malnutrition, and salicylate overdose.[3]

Laboratory findings in patients with bicarbonate deficit include a plasma pH level below 7.35, a urinary pH level below 6, and a plasma bicarbonate level below 22 mEq/L.[24] Signs and symptoms usually include Kussmaul's respirations (deep, fast, rhythmic), weakness, disorientation, coma (in later stages), headache, and anorexia (see the following box).

Bicarbonate deficit occurs in patients with renal failure because the GFR decreases and the available buffers are insufficient to allow acid secretion into the renal tubules. Therefore hydrogen ions are retained in place of bicarbonate, which is lost in the urine.[3] As bicarbonate levels in the ECF drop, potassium exits the cells and floods the ECF, leading to a hyperkalemic state.

Treatment of bicarbonate deficit is achieved by treating the cause and administering oral or parenteral bicarbonate.[24] Replacement of bicarbonate is calculated on the basis of body weight and the desired increment of increase in bicarbonate.[22]

METABOLIC ACIDOSIS

Definition

Bicarbonate deficit of the ECF

Serum value

Bicarbonate level less than 22 mEq/L
Partial pressure of carbon dioxide (Pco_2) normal or less
    than 35 mm Hg to compensate for the low bicarbonate level
pH below 7.35

Causes

Diabetic ketoacidosis
Lactic acidosis
Uremia
Ingestion of acids (e.g., salicylates, alcohol, boric acid)
Starvation
Diarrhea
Some diuretics

Findings

Weakness
Dizziness
Rapid respirations
Coma (later stages)

Bicarbonate Excess

An excess of bicarbonate or excess loss of acid in the ECF is referred to as metabolic alkalosis. Retained bicarbonate is the result of disorders such as loss of acids from vomiting, gastric suction, hyperaldosteronism, or diuretic abuse.[3] Excessive ingestion of medications containing bicarbonate or use of parenteral solutions containing bicarbonate can also predispose the individual to metabolic alkalosis. Potassium levels should also be carefully monitored; metabolic alkalosis causes hydrogen ion release from the cells and a subsequent exchange for potassium, leading to potassium deficit of the ECF.[32]

Metabolic alkalosis can develop from severe fluid and acid losses, causing the retention of bicarbonate, or it can develop from excessive addition of bicarbonate to the body. For instance, the removal of gastric acids through suction depletes the available hydrogen ions and predisposes the patient to an increase in bicarbonate ions.[3]

Clinical observations of bicarbonate excess include a urinary pH level greater than 7, plasma pH level greater than 7.45, and a plasma bicarbonate level greater than 26 mEq/L. Individuals usually experience numbness and tingling of extremities, muscular hypertonicity, slow, shallow respirations with compensatory pauses, bradycardia, and tetany (see the box below).

Treatment of bicarbonate excess primarily involves increasing excretion through the kidney. However, if the patient is taking excessive medications containing bicarbonate, withdrawal of these medications will be necessary. Also, if the cause is a loss in chloride, replacement of the chloride will produce bicarbonate excretion.

Hypoproteinemia

A reduction in protein of the ECF may be rapid or insidious and is a difficult-to-treat malady. Loss of protein can be sudden such as with burns or surgery or very slow and steady such as with renal insufficiency (undetected), malnutrition, bleeding, or liver disease.[24] The serum albumin level is chronically less than 3.8 g (see the box below).

The individual's presenting symptoms may be weakness and fatigue with a flatness of affect. Emotional depression, anorexia, flabbiness of muscles, weight loss, and edema of dependent areas may also be present.[22] Lesions may be unhealed, since insufficient protein is available for wound repair. Traditionally, fluid imbalances related to decreased protein are discussed in relation to albumin, which accounts for 50% to 60% of total protein stores.

The edema associated with hypoproteinemia results from a plasma-to-interstitial fluid shift from a lack of oncotic pressure in the vascular space. For example, in patients with liver disease, insufficient amounts of albumin are produced, thereby lowering oncotic pressure within the vascular system. Portal hypertension increases albumin loss into the interstitium and creates increased edema.

Treatment is difficult because the individual may no longer be able to ingest orally the high amounts of protein needed to replace stores. NG feedings or total parenteral nutrition (TPN) can be used to replace stores, but the course of protein replacement is often lengthy. Human serum albumin can be used to treat hypoalbuminemia. However, albumin must be administered slowly (2 to 3 ml/min) to avoid fluid overload as a result of normalizing oncotic pressure.[24]

METABOLIC ALKALOSIS

Definition

Bicarbonate excess of the ECF

Serum value

Bicarbonate level greater than 26 mEq/L
P_{CO_2} level normal or greater than 45 mm Hg to compensate for the elevated bicarbonate level
pH level greater than 7.45

Causes

Vomiting (with loss of chloride)
Excessive intake of alkalies
Primary aldosteronism (because of loss of potassium)
Diuretic use in patient with congestive heart failure (CHF) (on occasion)

Findings

Hyperexcitability of muscles
Bradycardia
Bradypnea
Numbness and tingling

HYPOALBUMINEMIA

Definition

Deficit of protein in the ECF

Serum value

Less than 3.8 g/dl

Causes

Protein-deficient diet
Burns
Starvation
Surgeries (major, with prolonged recovery phase)
Digestive diseases

Findings

Emotional depression
Muscle wasting
Peripheral edema (fluid shift)
Decreased resistance to infection
Poorly healing wounds

ACID-BASE ABNORMALITIES
Carbonic Acid Deficit in ECF

Carbonic acid deficit in the ECF is usually referred to as *respiratory alkalosis*. The deficit results from any situation causing hyperventilation such as pain, CNS lesions, fever, or assisted ventilation.[25]

The individual who is hyperventilating loses carbon dioxide, which is required to formulate carbonic acid, but retains bicarbonate. The body attempts to compensate for the lost carbon dioxide by allowing excretion of bicarbonate through the kidneys, possibly inducing a deficit of bicarbonate.[19] Also, chloride may be exchanged for bicarbonate at the cellular level, thereby decreasing the available bicarbonate in the ECF.[19]

Besides rapid breathing, the individual may experience tetany (because of the pH and calcium relationship), paresthesia, tingling and numbness (especially around the mouth), blurred vision, diaphoresis, dry mouth, and coma (later stages).[19] Laboratory findings reveal a serum pH level greater than 7.45 and P_{CO_2} level below 35 mm Hg.

Treatment is aimed at reducing the hyperventilation if the cause is known. For instance, sedating the patient may be helpful. Parenteral administration of chloride solutions are helpful in reducing the bicarbonate while the respiratory problem is treated.[3]

Carbonic Acid Excess in ECF

Carbonic acid excess is known commonly as respiratory acidosis. This disorder develops when the lungs fail to rid the body of the appropriate amount of carbon dioxide, resulting in formation of excess carbonic acid from the excess carbon dioxide. Hypoventilatory effort or obstruction to ventilations results in respiratory acidosis. Drugs, anesthetics, CNS damage, neurological disease, or musculoskeletal diseases may be implicated in the development of this disorder. The kidneys compensate for the problem by excreting hydrogen, reabsorbing bicarbonate, and regenerating bicarbonate from the excess carbon dioxide. This process is slow, however (5 days for maximal effect), and other support measures are usually required.[19]

Treatment is aimed at correcting the cause of the hypoventilation or ventilatory distress. Oxygen or mechanical ventilation may be helpful.

RENAL DISTURBANCES
Acute Tubular Necrosis

Description. Acute tubular necrosis refers to damage occurring within the epithelium of the tubular portions of the nephron. Acute tubular necrosis is sometimes used synonymously with acute renal failure but is, in fact, a cause of acute renal failure. Damage to the cellular structures in this area prevents normal concentration of urine, filtration of wastes, and regulation of acid-base, electrolyte, and water balance.[29] A number of disorders can result in ATN, and several contributing factors may work together to bring about tubular damage.[29]

Causes. Common causes of acute tubular necrosis, listed in Table 32-1, are broken into two categories—ischemic and toxic. Ischemic damage occurs irregularly along the

Table 32-1 Causes of acute tubular necrosis

Ischemic	Toxic
Hemorrhage	Rhabdomyolysis
Excessive diuretic use	Gout
Burns	Hypercalcemia
Peritonitis	Gram-negative sepsis
Sepsis	Radiocontrast media
Congestive heart failure	Methanol
Myocardial ischemia	Carbon tetrachloride
Pulmonary emboli	Heavy metals
	Insecticides
	Drugs ("street type" phencyclidine [PCP])
	Aminoglycoside antibiotics
	Analgesics containing phenacetin

tubular membranes, causing areas of tubular cell damage and cast formation. Toxic damage results from nephrotoxins, usually drugs, chemical agents, or bacterial endotoxins, which cause uniform, widespread damage. The renal tubular cells are constantly at risk for damage because of their normally high blood flows, high oxygen requirements, and the constant reabsorption and secretion of metabolites.[4]

Pathophysiology. There are several theories, often discussed and researched, to explain the pathophysiology behind acute tubular necrosis. The *back-leak* theory suggests that tubular injury, whether ischemic or toxic, leads to return of metabolites (for example, creatinine) to the peritubular circulation. This causes decreased urinary production with retention of wastes, water, and electrolytes.[27]

Another theory refers to *tubular obstruction* from interstitial edema or from an accumulation of casts and sloughing tissue creating an obstruction. Filtration ceases when tubular hydrostatic pressure reaches that of glomerular filtration pressure. This decreases the formation of urine because of the nonavailability of filtrate to process.[27]

The *vascular* theories suggest that damage to the tubules is primarily mediated by obstruction in the renal capillary beds. Prolonged ischemia results in afferent arteriolar constriction and a reduction of GFR, which decreases the available filtrate. The exchange between tubules and capillaries is obliterated, and tubular cells fail to receive the necessary blood flow and oxygen to sustain them.[27] *Decreased glomerular membrane permeability* is suggested as a fourth explanation. It restricts filtration but occurs at the cellular level and is independent of blood flow.

Finally, the last theory suggests that *vasoconstriction* reduces renal perfusion and reduces capillary flow in the cortical region of the kidney (site of most of the glomeruli), resulting in acute tubular necrosis.

Assessment and diagnosis. Assessment of acute tubular necrosis usually involves tracking the fluid losses, compartmental fluid shifts, and cardiovascular function and monitoring the patient's general physical condition. Since hypovolemia is the usual precursor of ischemic tubular damage, careful assessment of fluid losses from all potential sources is important. It can be accomplished through accurate intake and output measurements. The patient's weight also is indicative of fluid gains or losses over a 1 to 2 day period. Additional signs such as thirst, decreased skin turgor, and apathy are signs of ECF depletion.[37]

Monitoring blood pressures and hemodynamics is helpful in assessing the fluid changes associated with the progressive course of acute tubular necrosis. Measurement of the abdominal girth for ascites and testing for pitting edema over body prominences and in dependent body areas should be frequent. Finally, cardiac outputs and pulmonary artery pressure (PAP) measurements can indicate a fall in intravascular volume. Cardiac output can decrease with a severe enough initial insult (for example, hemorrhage).

Toxic injury in acute tubular necrosis is frequently caused by bacterial sepsis. Gram-negative organisms produce toxins that have a direct, widespread necrotic effect on the tubular cells. If a hypovolemic state also exists, the toxins are further concentrated in the tubular filtrate, thereby increasing the risk of complicating the injury.[37]

Treatment. Treatment for acute tubular necrosis depends, for the most part, on the phase of the disease. If the patient is oliguric, treatment may include dialysis to remove fluids and toxins, drugs to combat infections and prevent complications, and fluid and dietary regulation with increased nutrients and fluid restrictions to decrease the metabolite load. In the early diuresis phase, output may be stimulated by use of loop diuretics such as furosemide to enhance water excretion.[4]

Nursing care. Because many experts consider acute tubular necrosis as part of acute renal failure, the nursing care would be the same. However, the nurse may actually provide additional preventive care for acute tubular necrosis alone. The nurse is in a unique position to identify individuals at high risk for renal insult, whether in the acute care or public health settings. Patients who have been exposed to toxins associated with acute tubular necrosis should be identified. (See the box at right, "Toxins Associated with Acute Tubular Necrosis.")

The nurse caring for the elderly postoperative patient must be aware that the GFR of the elderly patient may be decreased and that postoperative dehydration can result in hypoperfusion of the kidneys, with subsequent development of ATN. The critical care nurse must be vigilant of hemodynamic parameters (PAP and cardiac output) that provide early information about fluid balance and perfusion of the kidneys. Not only must the nurse be alert for dehydration but for fluid overload as well. Postoperative or trauma patients receiving fluid replacement require as strict attention to output as to intake. Subtle decreases in urinary output may not be observed unless comparisons of intake to output are made on a consistent basis.

Public health nurses and industrial health nurses must recognize those environmental factors that predispose to renal failure in individuals. Since indiscriminate use of some over-the-counter analgesics may predispose to acute tubular necrosis, the public health nurse may provide the link to patient teaching that prevents renal compromise. The industrial health nurse's identification of potential renal toxins

---

Nursing Diagnosis and Management
Acute tubular necrosis and acute renal failure

- Potential Fluid Volume Excess risk factor: renal failure, p. 670.
- Anxiety related to threatened biological, psychological, and/or social integrity, p. 852.
- Potential for Infection risk factors: protein-calorie malnourishment, invasive monitoring devices, pp. 346 and 720.
- Body Image Disturbance related to functional dependence on life-sustaining technology, p. 834.
- Knowledge Deficit: Fluid Restriction, Reportable Symptoms, and Medications related to lack of previous exposure to information, p. 69.
- Sensory-Perceptual Alterations related to sensory overload, sensory deprivation, and sleep pattern disturbance, p. 601.
- Ineffective Individual Coping related to situational crisis and personal vulnerability, p. 850.

TOXINS ASSOCIATED WITH ACUTE TUBULAR NECROSIS

DRUGS
Antibiotics

Cephalosporins
Aminoglycosides
Tetracyclines

Antineoplastics

Methotrexate
Cisplatin

Nonsteroidal antiinflammatory drugs (NSAID)

CHEMICALS

Ethylene glycol

PIGMENTS

Myoglobin (rhabdomyolysis)

CONTRAST MEDIA

---

in the work environment fulfills part of his or her responsibility for preventive health maintenance.

Acute Renal Failure

Description. Acute renal failure can be defined as any rapid decline in GFR with subsequent development of re-

---

CAUSES OF ACUTE RENAL FAILURE

PRERENAL

Hemorrhage
Severe GI losses
Burns
Renal trauma
Volume depletion (actual loss or "third-spacing")
Congestive heart failure, causing decreased renal perfusion
Hypoxia

INTRARENAL

Thrombus
Stenosis
Hypertensive sclerosis
Glomerulonephritis
Pyelonephritis
Acute tubular necrosis
Diabetic sclerosis
Toxic damage

POSTRENAL

Obstructions (stenosis, calculi)
Prostatic disease
Tumors

Table 32-2 Assessment in acute renal failure

Assessment area	Findings
LABORATORY	
Blood	
Hb and Hct	Decreased
Electrolytes	Increased potassium, decreased calcium, decreased sodium
Plasma osmolality	Variable, usually increased
BUN and creatinine	Increased
Urine	
Specific gravity	Decreased (fixed in chronic renal failure)
Urinary sediments	Normal to increased
Osmolality	Decreased
Creatinine clearance	Decreased
Sodium concentration	Decreased
RADIOLOGICAL	
Renal scan	All radiological findings depend on the specific pathology involved
IVP	
Angiographies	
FLUID	
Urinary output	Decreased
Skin turgor	Variable
Edema	Usually present

---

tention of metabolic waste products (azotemia). Acute renal failure is caused by a variety of insults. Mortality rates for it are still very high at approximately 50%, even with advanced critical care and dialysis techniques.[37] GI bleeding, sepsis, and CNS changes are often implicated in deaths related to ARF.[4]

Causes. Causes for acute renal failure are broken into three categories, which are also the categories used to describe causes of chronic renal failure (see the box above). *Prerenal* causes are usually associated with any insult that reduces vascular perfusion to the kidney. *Intrarenal* causes are insults to the kidney tissue such as infections, insults to the nephron such as glomerulonephritis, and scleroses from hypertension and diabetes mellitus. *Postrenal* causes are usually obstructive disorders occurring beyond the kidney in the remainder of the urinary tract. The obstructions cause urine to flow back and swell the kidneys, resulting in a condition known as *hydronephrosis*.

Pathophysiology. Little is known about the exact pathophysiology of acute renal failure. It is suspected that decreased renal perfusion results in renin-angiotensin release, aldosterone release, and vasoconstriction of the blood supply to the nephron. Increased water and sodium uptake further reduces the available filtrate, whereupon renal tubular cells necrose and slough.[27]

Assessment and diagnosis. Assessment for acute renal failure and chronic renal failure are essentially the same. Indeed, acute renal failure may eventually become chronic

renal failure, depending on the extent of damage to the renal tubules.[29] The assessment can be divided into laboratory (blood and urine), radiological, and fluid areas (Table 32-2).

The laboratory assessment always includes a serum test of blood urea nitrogen (BUN) and creatinine levels. BUN is not the sole indicator of ARF and not the most reliable indicator of renal damage because, although it reflects cellular damage, the BUN level is easily changed by protein intake, blood in the GI tract, or cell catabolism. Creatinine, on the other hand, is an accurate reflection of renal damage because it is almost totally excreted by the renal tubules. Elevated levels of creatinine can reflect damage to as much as 50% of the nephrons. However, creatinine may not rise as rapidly as the BUN because creatinine is independent of urinary flow.[27]

The urinalysis can indicate problems with prerenal causes of failure specifically by demonstrating the presence of granular casts or cellular debris. The urinary osmolality level increases (>500 mOsm/L), and the specific gravity level increases (>1.020) as the kidneys conserve water and sodium as a result of decreased perfusion.[29] The urinalysis can also reveal intrarenal causes by demonstrating actual tubular epithelial cells, a decrease in osmolality (from retained solutes), and a high sodium content. Twenty-four hour clearances of BUN and creatinine are typically low.

Table 32-3 Renal imaging tests

Tests	Comments
Kidney-ureter-bladder (KUB)	Flat-plate x-ray film of the abdomen; determines position, size, and structure of the kidneys and urinary tract
	Usually followed by more sophisticated tests
Intravenous pyelography (IVP)	IV injection of contrast media plus x-ray film; allows visualization of the internal kidney (parenchyma, calyces, pelves, ureters, bladder)
	Timing of stages can delineate size and shape
	Obstructions and tumors can be found
	Drawback can be hypersensitivity to the contrast medium
Retrograde pyelography	Injection of iodine-based contrast medium through a urethral catheter into the collection system (calyces, pelves, and ureters); allows visualization of clots, stones, strictures
	May be useful when patient is allergic to IVP dye (less chance of hypersensitivity in this test)
Renal angiography	Injection of contrast medium into the arterial blood source to kidney; allows x-ray visualization of the renal blood flow
	Stenoses, cysts, clots, and tumors may be visualized, as may infarcts, areas of trauma, and torn kidneys
Renal computed tomographic (CT) scan	After patient is given a medium of radioisotope, which the kidneys absorb, scintillation photography is obtained in several planes; density of image helps determine tumors, cysts, hemorrhage, calcification, adrenal tumors, or necrosis
	May be used before or instead of renal biopsy
Renal ultrasonography	Transmission of high-frequency sound waves to kidneys and urinary tract, with imaging on oscilloscope screen
	Used in search for fluid accumulation or obstructions

Most of the electrolytes in the ECF will become increasingly elevated, depending on the cause of damage and length of time the damage has been present. As urinary output decreases, serum electrolytes increase. Typically, elevations of potassium and phosphorus and depression of sodium and calcium occur. Sodium will be depressed in the presence of retention of large amounts of fluids (dilutional effect).[4]

Radiological tests used in diagnosing renal disorders have become increasingly sophisticated and valuable tools. Sonography, tomography, and angiography can help pinpoint the causal mechanism and even help differentiate between acute disease and chronic renal failure (Table 32-3). Radiological contrast media have been implicated, although rarely, in the development or worsening of renal disorders.[31]

Although seldom used today, the kidneys-ureters-bladder (KUB) test can serve as a basic diagnostic tool. This is a flat-plate x-ray film that can reveal kidney enlargement, ureteral blockages, calculi, and masses. Ultrasound, voiding cystourethrograms, and retrograde ureteropyelography visualize the remainder of the urinary tract, as well as the kidneys.[27]

Finally, general assessment of the individual can reveal the effects that renal failure has on other body systems. For instance, hemodynamic monitoring during treatment for prerenal causes is valuable in tracking fluid balance and the need for fluid removal (dialysis) or replacement (IV fluids).[37] The remaining areas of assessment should include a general review of the body systems.

Treatment. Medical interventions for acute renal failure are directed toward three basic goals: (1) correcting the causative mechanism, (2) promoting regeneration of the remaining functional renal capacity, and (3) preventing complications. Medical management is based on the three categories of causes of acute failure. Prerenal failure, involved with perfusion problems and often with fluid losses and shifts, requires two specific methods of management: fluid replacement and stimulation of output with diuretics. Also, the defect causing the initial perfusion problem must be corrected. Care must also be used when using diuretics to avoid creation of secondary electrolyte abnormalities.[4]

Intrarenal failure involves the introduction of increased amounts of water, solutes, and potential toxins into the circulation, so prompt measures are needed to decrease their levels. Hemodialysis is the usual treatment of choice, particularly if volume overload creates pulmonary and cardiac compromise. Severe hyperkalemia almost always necessitates hemodialysis because of the life-threatening cardiac dysrhythmias resulting from hyperkalemia. Dialysis may also be initiated for cases of uremic pericarditis or severe azotemia in which other treatments are contraindicated.[4]

Other forms of dialysis such as continous ambulatory peritoneal dialysis (CAPD) and continuous cycling peritoneal dialysis (CCPD) may be used to attempt correction of the renal failure. Continuous arteriovenous hemofiltration (CAVH) is sometimes used—mainly to remove fluid accumulation but also to reduce the solute load. It is used for patients who cannot tolerate the cardiovascular strain that hemodialysis often produces.[36] A description of hemodialysis, CAPD, CCPD, and CAVH is in Chapter 33.

Drugs, fluid restriction, and dietary control constitute a

large part of the medical treatment for renal failure. Fluid restriction is used to prevent circulatory overload and interstitial edema associated with ARF and is calculated on the basis of daily urinary volumes and insensible losses; thus obtaining daily weights and keeping accurate intake and output records become essential. Patients are usually restricted to 1 L of fluid if urinary output is 500 ml or less and insensible losses range from 500 to 750 ml per day. However, if the patient is nonoliguric, fluid intake may be liberalized on an individual basis, determined by matching the daily fluid outputs.[27]

Electrolyte levels require frequent observation, especially in the initial critical phases of failure. Potassium may quickly reach levels of 6.0 mEq/L and above. Other than through hemodialysis, hyperkalemia can be treated temporarily by IV infusion of insulin and glucose. An infusion of 100 ml of 50% dextrose accompanied by 20 units of regular insulin will force potassium back into the cells.[8] Sodium bicarbonate (40 to 160 mEq) may be infused to promote higher excretion of potassium in the urine.[8] Finally, sodium polystyrene sulfonate (Kayexalate), a cation-exchange resin, is mixed in water and sorbitol and given orally, rectally, or through an NG tube.[6] The resin captures potassium in the bowel, which eliminates it in the feces.

Dilutional hyponatremia, associated with renal failure, can be corrected with fluid restriction. However, if sodium stores are actually depleted, 3% normal saline solution is usually administered intravenously as a replacement.[24] In addition, sodium levels may be raised during dialysis by changing the amount of sodium in the dialysate bath.

Calcium levels are reduced in renal failure, and, as previously described, the reduction is related to multiple factors, among which is hyperphosphatemia. Aluminum hydroxide preparations are administered to bind phosphorus in the bowel and thereby lower its level. Calcium may also be increased by use of calcium supplements, vitamin D preparations, and synthetic calcitriol (Rocaltrol).[38]

The nutritional aspect of renal failure may involve replacement as well as restriction. With the availability of refined products, it has become quite easy to provide total parenteral nutrition (TPN) while the patient is undergoing dialysis. If the patient is anorexic and malnourished, TPN can be provided, and renal formulas are even available.

The renal diet prescription is quite restrictive. Protein, potassium, sodium, and phosphorus are usually limited. For instance, protein restriction may vary from 0.5 to 1.0 g/kg/day to limit azotemia.[29] Carbohydrates are encouraged, primarily to provide needed energy for healing (35 to 45 kcal/kg/day).[16]

Preventing complications in patients with renal failure involves careful monitoring, particularly for indications of infection. Strict asepsis should be used, for example, with dressing changes, use of the vascular access for dialysis treatments, and catheters to prevent bacterial assault on a compromised system. Antibiotic therapy can be used to treat infections but often requires alteration in dose because of reduced clearance through the kidney. Dialysis removes many antibiotics, requiring dosage alteration.[29]

Nursing care. Before initiating nursing care, several points about the patient's current and past history should be explored. If the patient is unable to provide the information, family members may be of invaluable help in developing the plan of care.

Initially, assessment of the urinary output pattern is necessary. Information about the patient's recent urinary pattern should include decreases, increases, pain, frequency, and color to aid the caregiver in planning care for the patient with a renal disorder. Also, it is important to learn if there is a family history of renal disorders.

Careful attention by the nurse to exploring the patient's use of medications (for example, over-the-counter drugs, antibiotics) may provide clues to the cause of the renal failure or to future needs for patient teaching about the use of medications in general. A suspected drug abuse history is also of concern. Any recent medical history or past treatment for the same or related symptoms should be explored, as should an exposure to chemicals or heavy metals in the work place to determine renal damage related to environmental toxins.

Physical assessment should include a check of neurological status, particularly looking for *asterixis*, a "flapping tremor" associated with increased BUN and creatinine levels. By asking the patient to extend the wrist and fingers of the hand, the flapping motion will be present if toxin levels are high. Also, mental status is often depressed, with apathy, lethargy, insomnia, and short-term memory loss present when toxins are at high levels in the serum.[6]

The skin should be checked for bruising, edema, and turgor. Often the skin will be very dry and scaly but may be more so with chronic renal failure than with acute renal failure. Edema is usually present to some extent and can be assessed using the fingerprint method. However, care must be taken to assess edema in hidden areas such as the sacrum, abdomen (abdominal girth), and periorbital areas. Breath sounds should be noted for crackles, indicative of fluid overload.

When listening to heart sounds, a cardinal sign of renal failure is the presence of a cardiac friction rub or a paradoxical pulse, indicative of uremic pericarditis, which develops when toxins irritate the pericardial membrane and cause fluid buildup within the pericardial sac.[6] The patient often will complain of a deep, subscapular pain on the left side. The GI system assessment must include evaluation for nausea and vomiting, hematemesis, and melena because uremic toxins will frequently initiate various ulcerative lesions along the course of the GI tract. Hyperactive, hypoactive, or absent bowel sounds may signal a number of secondary complications such as diarrhea or constipation in the renal patient.[6]

Finally, the musculoskeletal system can provide much information about renal failure. The presence of flaccid muscles may indicate hyperkalemia or tonic contractions caused by hypocalcemia. Also, the patient may exhibit paresthesia and involuntary twitching of the lower legs known as "restless legs," which is commonly caused by *peripheral neuropathy*.[6] The neuropathy is associated with uremic toxins' slowing the nervous response to the limbs and causing "short circuits" of messages to the muscles—thus the involuntary twitching movement.

Meticulous attention to fluid changes, cardiovascular

problems, prevention of infection, and alleviation of symptoms provides more comfort and a better prognosis for the patient in acute renal failure. In addition, providing teaching and emotional support for the patient and family becomes an integral part of the nursing care.

The actual nursing care for the individual with acute renal failure focuses on prevention or control of complications secondary to the disease process. In preventing infection, the nurse must not only frequently monitor for signs of infection but must maintain the patient's pulmonary hygiene, skin integrity, and nutrition. Consideration must be given to limiting invasive procedures and providing strict asepsis when performing dressing changes, catheterizations, or any such invasive procedures. Should the individual be immobile, frequent turning and observation of potential sites for skin breakdown enhance the chances of avoiding infection. If the individual has developed significant anasarca, the use of a circulating air or air-fluid mattress may help prevent skin breakdown.

Frequent assessment of intake and output, particularly the output in response to any administered diuretics, is a necessary part of the nursing care for the patient in renal failure. Daily patient weights correlate with the intake and output to confirm fluid overloads. The nurse should take great care to note the return of urinary output and to seek replacement for the fluids and electrolytes that can be rapidly lost during this phase.

Hyperkalemia, hypocalcemia, hyponatremia, and hyperphosphatemia may all occur during acute renal failure. The nurse must be aware of the signs and symptoms of these electrolyte imbalances and prevent or control their associated side effects. The imbalances with the most potential hazard are hyperkalemia and hypocalcemia, which can result in life-threatening cardiac dysrhythmias. The nurse is involved not only in monitoring signs and symptoms of these imbalances, but in teaching the patient and family ways to avoid imbalances and consequences of the imbalances.

Although the nurse can do little to prevent hyponatremia, nursing care must include frequent assessment for its signs and symptoms. The astute nurse also must remember that as fluid overload worsens in the oliguric patient, dilutional hyponatremia may also develop. Finally, hyperphosphatemia results most often in severe pruritus. Nursing care is subsequently directed at soothing the itching by performing frequent skin care with emollients, discouraging scratching, and administering phosphate-binding medications.

Care in preventing blood loss in the individual with renal failure centers on observation. Irritation of the GI tract from metabolic waste accumulation should be expected, and stools, NG drainage, and emesis should be tested for occult blood.

The nurse must give accurate, uncomplicated information to the patient and family about acute renal failure, including its prognosis, treatment, and possible complications. The nurse should be aware that sleep-rest disorders and emotional upset can occur as complications of acute renal failure and should encourage the patient and family to voice concerns, frustrations, and fears. Searching for ways to allow the patient to control some aspects of the acute care environment or treatment is also essential. However, at times the patient may be disoriented, severely fatigued, or incapable of participating in care.

Chronic Renal Failure

Description. As of 1981, chronic renal failure affected 64,000 individuals in the United States. The cost of caring for these individuals consumed 10% of the Medicare budget.[26] Current health care literature suggests a steady rise in the number of individuals who will face renal failure, either requiring acute or chronic care. Therefore caregivers must be aware of the necessary components of care for these individuals.

Chronic renal failure is defined as *insidious* and *irreversible* damage to the kidneys. Often signs and symptoms develop over a period of years, and the patient will have been treated for a variety of suspected disorders before renal failure is diagnosed. Treatment is usually based on the degree of residual kidney function.

Causes. The causes of chronic renal failure are basically the same as those for acute renal failure. As late as 1983, figures from the Public Health Department revealed at least three main causes of chronic renal failure: (1) glomerulonephritis, (2) diabetes mellitus, and (3) primary hypertensive disease.[26]

Pathophysiology. Glomerulonephritis is initiated in various ways but is characterized as an *immune complex disorder*. Little is known about the initiation of the immune response in glomerulonephritis. However, it is known that certain antigens specific to glomerular tissue are circulated to the glomeruli and, in turn, initiate an inflammatory response in the glomerular basement membrane. The antigens may work to decrease antiglomerular basement antibodies, rendering the glomerulus vulnerable to invasion by infectious agents.[27]

As the glomeruli are damaged and the GFR decreases as a result of sclerosis of the glomerular membrane, protein passes into the tubular filtrate and is eventually excreted in the urine. Sodium and water retention occur, in part because of the body's response in an attempt to alleviate the hypovolemia that results from the protein loss. Interstitial edema develops as a result of decreased protein in the vascular space.[27]

Hypertensive kidney damage can be the sole cause of renal failure or can occur secondary to another disease such as diabetes mellitus. In the hypertensive state, the increased vascular resistance of diseased vessels predisposes to high pressure entering the glomerulus and results in damage to the membrane. Hypertension causes glomerular and tubular problems through malfunction of the renin-angiotensin system. Ischemia and decreased blood volume stimulate the renin-angiotensin system to reabsorb water and sodium from the tubules in an effort to increase volume and thereby the GFR. This creates volume overload, which scleroses the glomeruli by producing a higher vascular pressure. The resulting sclerosis destroys the ability of the glomerular membrane to filter selectively and often reduces available filtrate, leading to eventual necrosis of the tubular structures.[25]

Diabetes mellitus does not directly attack the nephron itself but mediates the damage through thickening arterial walls and eventual thickening of the glomerular basement membrane from the resultant high pressure.[25] Diabetic damage often results not only in renal failure, but in blindness (retinal damage) and cardiac failure because of major blood vessel involvement.

Assessment and diagnosis. The patient assessment for chronic renal failure involves evaluation for many of the same signs and symptoms that occur in patients with acute renal failure (see the box, "Manifestations of Chronic Renal Failure"). However, the progression of chronic renal failure differs from acute renal failure and is characterized by three phases.

The first phase, *diminished renal reserve*, involves the appearance of protein in the urine and elevations of the blood pressure. Mild elevations in BUN and creatinine levels may also be observed. However, for the most part, with fluid and sodium restrictions, the remaining regulatory functions continue within normal limits.[25]

Renal insufficiency, the second phase, is a worsening of kidney function characterized by increases in serum BUN and creatinine levels, mild elevation of the potassium level, impaired concentrating ability, and anemia.

The third phase, *end-stage renal disease*, is often characterized by a set of signs and symptoms known as *uremic syndrome*. At the point end-stage renal disease is reached, the GFR is usually less than 6 ml/min.[7] The signs and symptoms of end-stage renal disease result from the severely elevated BUN, creatinine, potassium, and phosphate levels, as well as the decreased sodium, calcium, Hb, and Hct levels, and fluid retention.[6] (See the box, "Signs and Symptoms of End-Stage Renal Disease.")

Assessment findings of end-stage renal disease clearly reflect uremia. However, not all of the signs and symptoms may be readily noticeable or even present. The insidious nature of chronic renal failure allows time for adaptation to significant changes in the system. For example, a patient may have a serum potassium level of 6.8 mEq/L but not be experiencing muscular lassitude or nausea and vomiting. The tolerance point for the various changes in end-stage renal disease varies widely on an individual basis.

Urinary output is frequently low, and the urine may vary in color from nearly as clear as water to very dark. The patient's weight may elevate by as much as 5 to 10 pounds or more, which will usually correlate with edema of the extremities, dependent areas, and face (periorbital). Blood pressure is usually elevated, but the patient may experience orthostatic drops when standing.[7]

Respiratory sounds may range from clear to crackles and wheezes, depending on the extent of fluid overload and left-ventricular function. The mental status may be depressed, with lethargy, memory loss, and confusion. Neurological checks may reveal asterixis. Headaches often are a complaint and are usually related to blood pressure elevations.[6] Restlessness and insomnia result from uremic toxin irritations in the brain.

The patient will often have a dry mouth and *uremic fetor*, which is a urinelike breath odor. Anorexia, nausea, and vomiting are frequent. Hiccups, burping, diarrhea or constipation, and melena may also be related to renal disease.[6]

The skin is characteristically a pale, greenish-tan color

MANIFESTATIONS OF CHRONIC RENAL FAILURE

CARDIOVASCULAR

Hypervolemia
Hypertension
Dysrhythmias
Congestive heart failure
Pericarditis
Cardiomegaly

PULMONARY

Adventitious lung sounds (crackles)
Dyspnea
Pulmonary edema
Uremic pleuritis

NEUROLOGICAL

Insomnia
Apathy
Confusion
Short-term memory loss
Lethargy
Behavior changes
Peripheral neuropathy
Paraesthesia—asterixis

GASTROINTESTINAL

Nausea and vomiting
Ulcerations
GI bleeding
Uremic fetor
Diarrhea
Constipation

INTEGUMENTARY

Pallor
Pruritus
Color changes (uremic bronzing)
Decreased turgor
Skin fragility

SKELETAL

Joint pain
Joint swelling
Gait changes
Reduced range of motion

HEMATOLOGICAL

Anemia
Platelet defects
Decreased white blood count

SIGNS AND SYMPTOMS OF END-STAGE RENAL DISEASE (UREMIC SYNDROME)

- "Restless legs" and burning sensation of soles of feet
- Apathy
- Confusion
- Stupor
- Flapping tremor of hands (asterixis)
- Insomnia
- Anorexia
- Nausea and vomiting
- Uremic fetor (breath odor)
- Melena
- Dyspnea
- Crackles on auscultation of lungs
- Cardiac dysrhythmias
- Pericardial rub on auscultation
- Additional heart sounds (fluid overload)
- Cardiomegaly
- Edema (dependent areas)
- Poor skin turgor (generalized)
- Pruritis
- Brittle nails and hair
- Anemia (normocytic, normochromic)
- Easy bruising
- Bleeding (gums, nose, GI tract)
- Oliguria or anuria

---

ducing the risk of hypertensive damage to the remaining nephrons.

Normalizing serum electrolytes is often difficult in patients with renal failure. Elevations in potassium may require emergent dialysis or simple alteration in dietary restriction of potassium. Calcium and phosphorous regulation becomes "tricky," depending on the role PTH is playing in maintaining the calcium levels. Phosphorous binders, calcium supplements, and calcium absorption stimulators (calcitriol) are used to normalize calcium and phosphorus. Sodium is usually controlled with a 2-gm sodium (no added salt) dietary restriction.[16]

The anemia of renal failure occurs because of the kidneys' failure to produce the hormone precursor erythropoietin, which acts on bone marrow to stimulate RBC production. Although the exact production points of erythropoietin are unknown, it is suspected that it is produced elsewhere besides the kidney, since minute levels of erythropoietin continue to appear in serum even after bilateral nephrectomy. The decrease in erythropoietin production, blood loss from the dialysis process, and the shortened life span of blood cells caused by uremic toxins result in a normocytic (normal cells), normochromic (sufficient hemoglobin) anemia.[6]

Medications such as androgens, folic acid, and iron preparations are prescribed to increase RBC production and provide a nutritious internal environment for growth and maturation of new RBCs. Folic acid, multivitamins, and ferrous sulfate are often administered to provide nutrition to the RBCs and to enhance their functional abilities. Androgen therapy (fluoxymesterone [Halotestin], nandrolone decanoate [Deca-Durabolin]) is initiated to stimulate RBC production from the bone marrow.[6] However, secondary sex characteristics often result from use of androgens, thereby reducing medication regimen compliance in women.

Transfusions are used as a last resort to provide additional RBCs. They are withheld unless the patient develops Hct less than 20% or has chest pain, dyspnea, or other signs of tissue hypoxia. Multiple transfusions, often required by end-stage renal disease patients, can further depress the bone marrow. Additionally, the risks associated with acquired immunodeficiency syndrome and hepatitis B are of great concern with the administration of frequent blood transfusions. Packed RBCs are given instead of whole blood to reduce the fluid load. The cells are "washed" before administration to patients seeking kidney transplant to prevent the formation of cytotoxic antibodies.[6]

Nursing care. The nursing care for the patient with chronic renal failure is multifaceted. The key to understanding much of the care for this patient is in understanding the following treatments: hemodialysis, peritoneal dialysis, and kidney transplantation. The treatments and their possible associated complications require intense observation and careful management by the nurse.

First, the nurse must be aware of the fluid and electrolyte balances associated with chronic renal failure. Assessment for fluid overload and the signs and symptoms of hyperkalemia remain foremost on the list of nursing care. Daily weights, intake and output measurements, auscultation of the lungs, and assessment of the skin for edema provide a general picture of the fluid status of the patient. The patient's

called *uremic bronze,* caused in part by an inability to excrete certain metabolites and by the pallor of renal failure—associated anemia. The skin is dry, and pruritis is common, usually secondary to the deposition of phosphates.[6]

Often patients report a decrease in libido and demonstrate emotional upsets ranging from discouragement, anxiety, and frustration to depression and withdrawal.[6]

Treatment. Medical and nursing treatment of end-stage renal disease are aimed at preserving as much kidney function as possible, correcting fluid and electrolyte imbalances, correcting problems with the body's organ systems, postponing or eliminating the need for dialysis or transplantation, and providing the patient with the knowledge and support that will enhance the quality of life while coping with the disease.

Correcting fluid and electrolyte problems is of prime concern in treating patients with renal failure. Fluid overload is frequently present, and fluid excess can be removed through hemodialysis or peritoneal dialysis. Fluid and sodium restrictions help control fluid overload. The patient is usually restricted to 1000 to 1500 ml/24 hours of fluid intake, depending on current urinary output.[14] On occasion, patients will experience *nocturnal dehydration,* which can be eliminated by spreading the allotted fluid over the 24-hour period.

Hypertension and congestive heart failure are controlled by providing medications that increase cardiac output and lower blood pressure, allowing less cardiac strain and redevelopment of nausea and vomiting, diarrhea, circumoral and fingertip numbness, and generalized muscle weakness indicates development of hyperkalemia. In addition, an important part of the nurse's care centers on patient teaching about adherence to fluid and dietary restrictions and the consequences of nonadherence.

The nurse frequently collaborates with the physician and dietitian in maintaining the nutritional intake of the patient with chronic renal failure. The nurse can aid the patient in complying with dietary restrictions and in gaining the needed nutrition by obtaining dietary histories from the patient, determining the patient's desires for ethnic choices in the diet, and assessing areas of patient difficulty in compliance with restrictions. In addition, the nurse can reinforce the teaching of the dietician with explanations about the need for adequate nutrition and the consequences of insufficient intake.

The patient with chronic renal failure often copes with pruritis, brittle hair, and skin color changes (pallor, uremic bronzing). The nurse should not only provide skin care but should teach the individual to provide self-care on a consistent basis. Teaching the patient the reasons behind development of skin-care problems may provide the impetus for the patient to adhere to the medication and dietary regimen that helps eliminate the problems. Although little can be done about the hair and skin color changes, encouraging the patient to continue regular beauty salon or barber appointments may, at the very least, help limit changes in his or her body image.

Fatigue and activity intolerance are often voiced as among the most frustrating of complications for the individual with chronic renal failure. Although the usual cause of the fatigue is anemia, fluid overload or secondary cardiac complications can also contribute to the problem. The nurse should monitor Hb and Hct levels for any sudden changes. Patient teaching should include explanations about renal anemia, fluid overload, and cardiac disease and their relationship to fatigue. A discussion with the patient and family about an activity and exercise schedule that allows frequent rest may help alleviate the patient's frustration.

Teaching the patient about the various medicqations prescribed to control chronic renal failure's complications can be a challenging aspect of nursing care. The patient must be taught the reason for taking a medication plus its side effects, the inappropriate combinations of certain agents, and the times at which multiple medications must be taken. Of particular importance is the nurse's care in instructing the patient in the avoidance of overmedication and the use of over-the-counter preparations that might create further complications (for example, kaolin and pectin [Kaopectate], magnesium antacids, and phosphate laxatives).

Finally, as with acute renal failure, focusing attention on the emotional needs of the patient and family coping with chronic renal failure is important. The nurse must be aware that the patient often responds to chronic disease by passing through stages of coping much like those of the grief process. The nursing care involved in providing emotional support should include the following: (1) emphasizing listening to the patient's frustrations, needs, and fears, (2) empha-

---

Nursing Diagnosis and Management
Chronic renal failure

- Potential Fluid Volume Excess risk factor: renal failure, p. 670
- Potential for Infection risk factors: protein-calorie malnourishment, invasive monitoring devices, pp. 346 and 720
- Potential Impaired Skin Integrity risk factors: reduced mobility, poor subcutaneous tissue support (peripheral and sacral edema), uremic pruritis, steroid therapy, p. 725
- Activity Intolerance related to postural hypotension secondary to prolonged immobility, p. 344
- Ineffective Individual Coping related to situational crisis and personal vulnerability, p. 850
- Anxiety related to threatened biological, psychological, and/or social integrity, p. 852
- Body Image Disturbance related to functional dependence on life-sustaining technology, p. 834
- Body Image Disturbance related to actual change in body structure, function, or appearance, p. 833
- Knowledge Deficit: Dialysis Routine, Fluid Restrictions, Medications, Fluid and Dietary Restrictions, Vascular Access Assessment and Care, Reportable Symptoms related to lack of previous exposure to information, p. 69
- Sensory/Perceptual Alterations related to sensory overload, sensory deprivation, and sleep pattern disturbance, p. 601
- Self-Esteem Disturbance related to feelings of guilt over physical deterioration, p. 835
- Altered Role Performance related to physical incapacity to resume usual or valued role, p. 836
- Powerlessness related to health care environment or illness-related regimen, p. 837
- Powerlessness related to physical deterioration despite compliance, p. 838
- Hopelessness related to perceptions of failing or deteriorating physical condition, p. 839
- Altered Health Maintenance related to lack of perceived threat to health, p. 67
- Noncompliance: Self-Care Routine related to lack of resources, p. 68

---

sizing to the patient and family the normalcy of the emotional response to chronic renal failure, (3) providing an avenue for the patient and family to seek professional counseling, (4) suggesting support groups that consider problems of those coping with renal failure, and (5) encouraging the patient and family to take active roles in the treatment process.

REFERENCES

1. Adler S and Fraley DS: Acid-base regulations cellular and whole body. In Arieff AI and DeFronzo RA: Fluid, electrolyte and acid-base disorders, vol 1, New York, 1985, Churchill Livingstone, Inc.
2. Aluis R, Geheb M, and Cox M: Hypo- and hyperosmolar states: diagnostic approaches. In Arieff AI and DeFronzo RA: Fluid, electrolyte and acid-base disorders, vol 1, New York, 1985, Churchill Livingstone, Inc.
3. Appel GB and Stern L: Acute and chronic renal failure. In Askanazi J, Starker PM, and Weissman C: Fluid and electrolyte management in critical care, Boston, 1986, Butterworth & Co (Publishers), Ltd.
5. Baker W: Hypophosphatemia, Am J Nurs 22(4):999, 1985.
6. Carbone V and Bonato J: Nursing implications in the care of the chronic hemodialysis patient in the critical care setting, Heart Lung 14(6): 570, 1985.
7. Chambers JK: Fluid and electrolyte problems in renal and urologic disorders, Nurs Clin North Am 22(4):815, 1987.
8. Commerford PJ and Lloyd EA: Arrhythmias in patients with drug toxicity, electrolyte, and endocrine disturbances, Med Clin North Am 68(5):1051, 1984.
9. Coward DD: Cancer-induced hypercalcemia, Cancer Nurs 9(3):125, 1986.
10. Desai TK, Carlson RW, and Geheb MA: Hypocalcemia and hypophosphatemia in acutely ill patients, Crit Care Clin 5(4):927, 1987.
11. Dickerson RN and Brown RO: Hypomagnesemia in hospitalized patients receiving nutritional support, Heart Lung 14(6):561, 1985.
12. Flink EB: Magnesium deficiency, Hosp Pract 15:116I, 1987.
13. Forse RA: Sodium regulation. In Askanazi J, Starker PM, and Weissman C: Fluid and electrolyte management in critical care, Boston, 1986, Butterworth & Co (Publishers), Ltd.
14. Hoffart N: Nutrition in renal failure, dialysis, and transplantation. In Core curriculum for nephrology nursing, Pitman, New Jersey, 1987, AJ Janetti, Inc.
15. Huerta BJ and Lemberg L: Potassium imbalance in the coronary care unit, Heart Lung 14(2):193, 1985.
16. Hui YH: Essentials of nutrition and diet therapy, Monterey, Calif, 1987, Wadsworth, Inc.
17. Johndrow PD and Thornton S: Syndrome of inappropriate antidiuretic hormone—a growing concern, Focus Crit Care 12(5):29, 1985.
18. Kurokawa K and others: Physiology of phosphorus metabolism and pathophysiology of hypophosphatemia and hyperphosphatemia. In Arieff AI and DeFronzo RA: Fluid, electrolyte and acid-base disorders, vol 1, New York, 1985, Churchill Livingstone, Inc.
19. Laski ME and Kurtzman NA: Acid-base disturbances in pulmonary medicine. In Arieff AI and DeFronzo RA: Fluid, electrolyte and acid-base disorders, vol 1, New York, 1985, Churchill Livingstone, Inc.
20. Lau K: Magnesium metabolism: normal and abnormal. In Arieff AI and DeFronzo RA: Fluid, electrolyte and acid-base disorders, vol 1, New York, 1985, Churchill Livingstone, Inc.
21. Levine MM and Kleeman CR: Hypercalcemia: pathophysiology and treatment, Hosp Pract 22(7):93, 1987.
22. Metheny NM: Fluid and electrolyte balance: nursing considerations, Philadelphia, 1987, JB Lippincott Co.
23. Narins RG and others: Metabolic acid-base disorders: pathophysiology, classification, and treatment. In Arieff AI and DeFronzo RA: Fluid, electrolyte and acid-base disorders, vol 1, New York, 1985, Churchill Livingstone, Inc.
24. Plumer AL and Cosentino F: Principles and practice of intravenous therapy, Boston, 1987, Little, Brown & Co, Inc.
25. Richard CJ: Causes of renal failure, Core curriculum for nephrology nursing, Pitman, New Jersey, 1987, AJ Janetti, Inc.
26. Rubin RJ: Epidemiology of end stage renal disease and implications for public policy, Public Health Rep 99(5):492, 1984.
27. Schrier R: Renal and electrolyte disorders, ed 3, Boston, 1986, Little, Brown & Co, Inc.
28. Schwartz MW: Potassium imbalances, Am J Nurs 87(10):1292, 1987.
29. Sillix DH and McDonald FD: Acute renal failure, Crit Care Clin 5(4):909, 1987.
30. Spencer H and others: Calcium requirements in humans, Clin Orthop 184:270, 1984.
31. Sondheimmer JH and Migdal SD: Toxic nephropathies, Crit Care Clin 5(4):883, 1987.
32. Stanaszek WF and Romankiewicz JA: Current approaches to management of potassium deficiency, Drug Intell Clin Pharm 19:176, 1985.
33. Starker PM and Gump FE: Gastrointestinal disorders. In Askanazi J, Starker PM, and Weissman C: Fluid and electrolyte management in critical care, Boston, 1986, Butterworth & Co (Publishers), Inc.
34. Tonnensen AS: Water balance and control of osmolality. In Askanazi J, Starker PM, and Weissman C: Fluid and electrolyte management in critical care, Boston, 1986, Butterworth & Co, Publishers, Inc.
35. Valladares BK and Lemberg L: Catecholamines, potassium, and beta-blockade, Heart Lung 15(1):105, 1986.
36. Weisberg LS, Szerlip HM, and Cox M: Disorders of potassium homeostasis in critically ill patients, Crit Care Clin 5(4):835, 1987.
37. Whittaker AA: Acute renal dysfunction, Focus Crit Care 12(3):12, 1985.
38. Zaloga GP and Chernow B: Hypocalcemia in critical illness, JAMA 256(4):1924, 1986.
39. Zucker AR and Chernow B: Diabetes insipidus and SIADH, Crit Care Q 6(3):63, 1983.

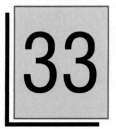

CHAPTER

33

Renal and Fluids Therapeutic Management

CHAPTER OBJECTIVES

- *Identify and describe the various types of vascular access for hemodialysis.*
- *Write a teaching plan for a patient who has recently started hemodialysis.*
- *Explain the differences, including advantages, disadvantages, and nursing care, between peritoneal dialysis, continuous ambulatory peritoneal dialysis, and continuous cycling peritoneal dialysis.*
- *Describe essential aspects of the nursing care for a patient with a renal transplant.*

HEMODIALYSIS

Although other methods of dialysis treatment for chronic renal failure have become more sophisticated, hemodialysis remains the treatment most widely used. As late as 1982, hemodialysis constituted 79% of the total treatments for renal failure in the United States. The wide availability of hemodialysis equipment and the ability to use it rapidly during emergencies predisposes physicians to the selection of hemodialysis as the primary mode of treatment.

Hemodialysis roughly translates as "separating from the blood."[7] As a treatment, hemodialysis literally separates and removes from the blood the excess electrolytes, fluids, and toxins. Although efficient in regulating chemicals, it does not remove all metabolites. Furthermore, electrolytes, toxins, and fluids increase between treatments, requiring performance of dialysis on a regular basis (3 to 4 hours three times per week).

The treatment works by circulating blood outside the body through synthetic tubing to a *dialyzer*, which consists of several membrane pockets (flat-plate type) or tubes (hollow-fiber type) (Fig. 33-1). While the blood flows through the membranes, which are semipermeable, a fluid known as the

dialysate bath bathes the membranes and, through osmosis and diffusion, performs exchanges of fluid, electrolytes, and toxins from the blood to the bath. The blood and bath are shunted in opposite directions (countercurrent flow) through the dialyzer to maintain the osmotic and chemical gradients at their highest.

To remove fluid, a positive hydrostatic pressure is applied to the blood, and a negative hydrostatic pressure is applied to the dialysate bath. The two forces together, called *transmembrane pressure*, pull and squeeze the excess fluid from the blood. The difference between the two values (expressed in mm Hg) represents the transmembrane pressure and results in fluid extraction, known as ultrafiltration, from the vascular space.[6]

Heparin is added to the system just before the blood enters the dialyzer. Without the heparin, the blood would clot since its presence outside the body and its passage through foreign substances initiate the clotting mechanism. Heparin can be administered by bolus injection or intermittent infusion. Administration is determined on the basis of an arbitrary dosage of units per kilogram of weight, followed by monitoring of the response to the particular dose by performing clotting times.[6] Heparin has a very short half-life, so its effects subside within 2 to 4 hours. Also, the effects of heparin are easily reversed through the injection of protamine.

After leaving the dialyzer, the blood continues through synthetic tubing and is returned to the body. Since the systemic blood pressure is not sufficient to propel the blood through this *extracorporeal* (outside the vessels) circuit, a pump is used to provide a consistent flow of blood (200 to 400 ml/minute) through the system. Various monitoring devices prevent blood loss, air embolus, access collapse, or high pressure destruction of the dialyzer or access. The components of a hemodialysis system appear in Fig. 33-2.

The dialyzer, or artificial kidney, is designed as an attempt to mimic the action of the renal tubules. However, since active transport and other physiological mechanisms are not possible with synthetic membranes, the artificial kidney can only provide for partial normalization of the blood. There

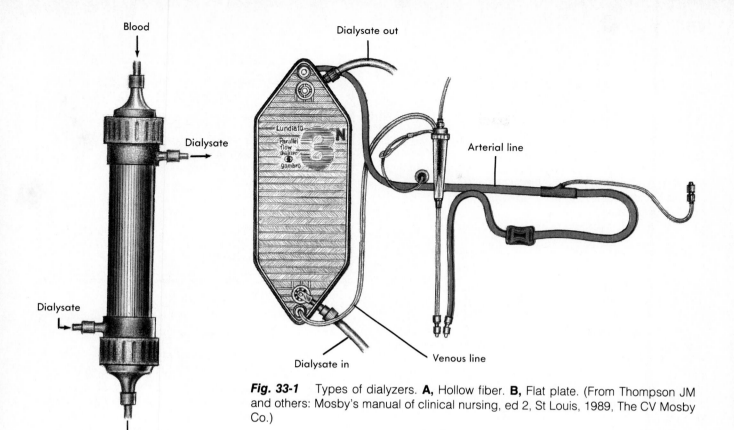

Fig. 33-1 Types of dialyzers. **A,** Hollow fiber. **B,** Flat plate. (From Thompson JM and others: Mosby's manual of clinical nursing, ed 2, St Louis, 1989, The CV Mosby Co.)

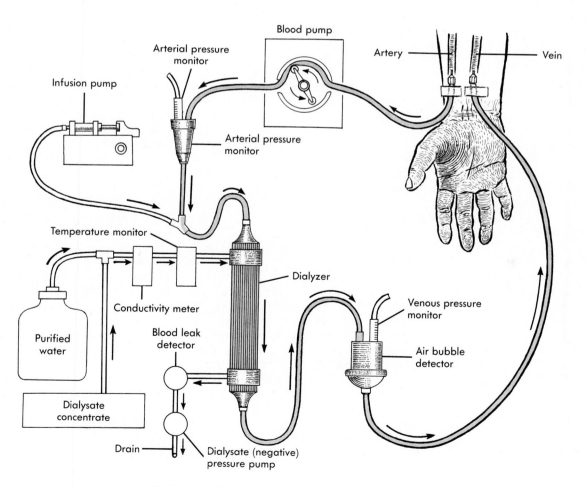

Fig. 33-2 Components of a hemodialysis system.

COMPOSITION OF THE DIALYSATE BATH

Purified water (reverse osmosis process)
Sodium chloride
Potassium chloride
Sodium bicarbonate (used frequently, although sodium acetate may be used as a replacement)
Calcium chloride
Magnesium chloride
Lactic acid

FACTORS AFFECTING THE EFFICIENCY OF DIALYSIS

Composition of dialysate
Temperature of dialysate
Dialyzer configuration (length of flow path)
Membrane's thickness
Membrane's pore size
Flow rate of blood
Flow rate of dialysate
Actual treatment time
Membrane's surface area

---

are two basic types of artificial kidneys—the plate dialyzer and the hollow-fiber dialyzer. Despite the types of artificial kidneys, the process by which they function is the same.

The dialysis process moves blood through either microscopic hollow tubes or thin membranous pockets. The membranes have fixed-sized pores, which allow passage of small molecules (for example, water, glucose, electrolytes) while preventing passage of some large molecules (for example, red blood cells [RBC], white blood cells [WBC], viruses, bacteria).

The dialysate bath is composed of electrolytes, blood buffers, and water in quantities that create a diffusion gradient across the membranes (see the box "Composition of the Dialysate Bath"). For instance, the potassium content may be 2.0 mEq/L in the dialysate to enhance diffusion from the hyperkalemic blood of the renal patient to the dialysate. Calcium absorption is also enhanced by this process. Higher amounts of ionized calcium are placed in the dialysate than are present in the patient's serum. The calcium travels from the dialysate to the patient's vascular space, thereby enhancing calcium stores.

Several factors affect the efficiency of the dialysis treatment. Blood flow rate must be constant and sufficiently fast enough to provide the solute and fluid load that maintain the chemical and osmotic gradient on either side of the membrane. The dialysate flow rate should be 2 to 2½ times that of the blood.[6] The temperature of the dialysate should be comfortable enough (37° C plus or minus 3° C) to maintain blood temperature (98° to 101° F) and to maintain the ability of solutes to diffuse. The dialysate composition should maintain a concentration gradient between the dialysate and the fluid and solute-laden blood. In addition, the direction of flow of the dialysate should be countercurrent, with dialysate flowing in one direction and the blood in the opposite direction. Finally, differences in the pore size, membrane thickness, available membrane surface area, and composition of the membrane can affect the relative efficiency of the dialysis treatment (see box, "Factors Affecting the Efficiency of Dialysis").

Tap water is not safe for use in dialysis; the prevalence of calcium, magnesium, organic and inorganic matter, bacteria, and chloramines in tap water can jeopardize effective dialysis. Therefore purification methods must be undertaken to remove these materials, as well as salts contained in the tap water. Distillation, reverse osmosis purification, and carbon filtering are currently used as methods for obtaining safe water for use in the dialysis treatment.[5]

Vascular Access for Hemodialysis

Hemodialysis can only be performed by obtaining access to the bloodstream. Over many years, various types of accesses such as arteriovenous (A-V) fistulas, A-V shunts, A-V grafts, and femoral and subclavian catheters have been created. The common denominator in most accesses is access to the arterial circulation and return to the venous circulation; femoral and subclavian catheters access the venous circulation only.

It is essential for the nurse to become familiar with each type of access, the potential problems that each can develop, and the nursing interventions each requires. The dialysis patient is often taught that the access is a "lifeline," so care on the part of patient and nurse can prevent complications.

A-V shunt. An A-V shunt is seldom used today as a result of the advent of subclavian and femoral catheters. However, if the temporary catheters cannot be used, access can rapidly be obtained through an A-V shunt. The shunt consists of Teflon vessel tips, Silastic tubing, and a connection joint for creating the circuit between the arterial and venous tubing[9] (Fig. 33-3, *A*). The shunt requires a peripheral artery, usually radial or ulnar, and a peripheral vein such as the cephalic or basilic. A cutdown is performed on each vessel, with the vessel tips inserted and sutured in place. Tubing extends from each vessel tip (outside the body) and is connected, when not being used for dialysis, by a straight connector or a heparin-T device. Blood flows in a U-shaped fashion from artery to vein. Shunts may also be inserted in the thigh or ankle areas. Complications common to A-V shunts are thrombosis, infection, and skin erosion. Nursing care considerations for A-V shunts are listed in Table 33-1.

A-V fistula. The A-V fistula is created by surgically visualizing a peripheral artery and vein, creating an opening in the artery and the vein, and anastomosing the two open areas. Anastomoses may be side-to-side, end-to-side, or end-to-end. The high arterial flow creates swelling of the vein, or a *pseudoaneurysm,* at which point (when healed) a large-bore needle can be inserted to obtain outflow. Inflow is accomplished through a second large-bore needle inserted

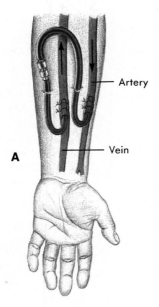

A

Artery

Vein

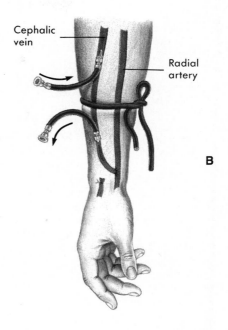

Cephalic
vein

Radial
artery

B

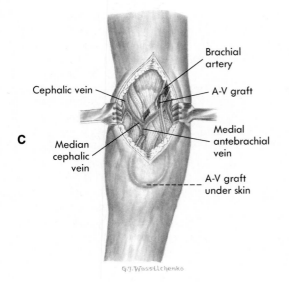

C

Brachial
artery

Cephalic vein

A-V graft

Median
cephalic
vein

Medial
antebrachial
vein

A-V graft
under skin

G.J.Wassilchenko

Fig. 33-3 Circulatory access for hemodialysis. **A,** External (temporary) arteriovenous cannula (shunt). **B,** Internal (permanent) arteriovenous fistula. **C,** Internal (permanent) arteriovenous graft. (**A** and **B** from Thompson JM and others: Mosby's manual of clinical nursing, ed 2, St Louis, 1989, The CV Mosby Co.)

Table 33-1 Care of the A-V shunt

Complications	Nursing Care
Clotting Dislodgment Skin erosion Infection Bleeding	1. Monitor for signs and symptoms of infection. 2. Monitor for signs and symptoms of thrombosis (darkening of blood, separation of serum or cellular compartment blood in tubing, decreased temperature of tubing). 3. Assess insertion site daily for erosion around insertion sites. 4. Use strict aseptic technique during dressing changes at insertion sites. 5. Teach patient to avoid sleeping on or prolonged bending of accessed limb. 6. Keep two shunt clamps attached to patient's clothing or access dressing at all times.

Table 33-2 Care of the A-V fistula

Complications	Nursing care
Thrombosis Infection Pseudoaneurysm Vascular steal syndrome Venous hypertension Carpal tunnel syndrome Inadequate blood flow	1. Teach patient to avoid wearing constrictive clothing on limb containing access. 2. Teach patient to avoid sleeping on or prolonged bending of accessed limb. 3. Use aseptic technique when cannulating access. 4. Avoid repetitious cannulation of one segment of access. 5. Offer comfort measures such as warm compresses or ordered analgesics to lessen pain of vascular steal. 6. Teach patient to develop the blood flow in the fistulas through exercises (squeezing a rubber ball) while applying mild impedance to flow just distal to the access (at least once per day for 10 to 15 minutes).

Table 33-3 Care of the A-V graft

Complications	Nursing care
Bleeding Thrombosis False aneurysm formation Infection Arterial or venous stenosis Vascular steal syndrome	1. Avoid too early cannulation of new access. 2. Teach patient to avoid wearing constrictive clothing on accessed limb. 3. Avoid repeated cannulation of one segment of access. 4. Use aseptic technique when cannulating access. 5. Monitor for changes in arterial or venous pressure while patient is on dialysis. 6. Provide comfort measures to reduce pain of vascular steal (e.g., warm compresses, analgesics as ordered).

into a peripheral vein distal to the fistula (Fig. 33-3, *B*).

Fistulas are the preferred mode of access if the vessels are of quality because of the durability of the individual's own vessels and the relatively few complications in comparison to the other accesses. However, development of sufficient flow to the fistula may require weeks to months. Attempting to obtain flow from the underdeveloped fistulas often causes painful vascular spasm and reduced flow. In addition, internal accesses have the potential for creating arterial insufficiency because of the high arterial blood flow diverted for dialysis purposes. The arterial insufficiency produces a set of symptoms known as *vascular steal syndrome* (pale, cold distal extremity with severe spasmodic pain). Additional complications such as thrombosis, infection (low rate), or venous hypertension can occur with A-V fistulas.[3] The care of the fistula and nursing considerations are listed in Table 33-2.

A-V grafts. Currently, A-V grafts are, by far, the most frequently used access for treating chronic renal failure. Synthetic materials such as Goretex or biological materials such as human umbilical veins provide a wide range of lumen sizes and graft lengths. The graft is a tube formed of the desired material (usually Goretex), which is surgically implanted in the limb. The area is surgically opened, and an artery and vein are located. A tunnel is created (either straight or U-shaped) in the tissue in which the graft is placed. Anastamoses are made with the graft ends connected to the artery and vein. The blood is allowed to flow through the graft, and the surgical area is closed. The graft creates a raised area (looking like a vein) just under the skin and peripheral tissue layers (Figure 33-3, *C*). Two large-bore needles are used for outflow and inflow to the graft. For both grafts and fistulas after needle removal at the end of the hemodialysis treatment, pressure must be applied to stem bleeding. Nursing care for and complications of the A-V graft are listed in Table 33-3.

Subclavian and femoral vein catheters. Sublcavian and femoral vein catheters are used most often in cases of acute renal failure when short-term access is required or when vascular access is nonfunctional in a patient requiring immediate hemodialysis. Both subclavian and femoral catheters can be inserted at the bedside.

Table 33-4 Care of femoral and subclavian catheters

Complications	Nursing care
Hemorrhage Pneumothorax Thrombosis Infection Nerve injury	1. Minimize manipulation of the catheter. 2. Avoid use of catheter for blood sampling, infusions, or monitoring. 3. Obtain a chest x-ray film to ascertain catheter's placement before the first use. 4. Use strict aseptic technique during dressing changes at insertion site. 5. Monitor for signs/symptoms of infection.

The same technique is used for insertion of either the subclavian or femoral vein catheter. A lengthy, large-bore needle is introduced into the vessel, and a guidewire is inserted through the needle hub. The needle is removed, and the catheter is threaded over the guidewire into the vessel. The catheter is sutured to the skin to maintain catheter position, and a sterile dressing is applied.

Femoral catheters may be single lumen, requiring insertion of two catheters into the same vessel, with the outflow catheter placed distal to the inflow catheter.[9] The subclavian catheter, however, usually has two lumens with a central partition running the length of the catheter. The outflow catheter pulls the blood flow through openings that are prox-imal to the inflow openings on the opposite side. This design avoids dialyzing the same blood just returned to the area (recirculation), which can severely reduce dialysis' efficiency.

The nursing considerations and complications for subclavian and femoral catheters are listed in Table 33-4. The subclavian access must *always* be confirmed by chest x-ray film to evaluate the possibility of pneumothorax or hemothorax resulting from catheter insertion. Femoral catheter sites must be carefully observed for any signs of rapidly developing hematomas from femoral artery puncture.[9]

PERITONEAL DIALYSIS

Peritoneal dialysis has existed as a treatment for renal failure approximately 20 years longer than hemodialysis. Because of problems with equipment, technique, and practical, long-term application, peritoneal dialysis was used for cases of acute renal failure only when hemodialysis was not possible. However, in 1978 peritoneal dialysis for chronic renal failure was successfully established.

Peritoneal dialysis involves the introduction of sterile dialyzing fluid through an implanted catheter into the abdominal cavity. The dialysate bathes the peritoneal membrane, which covers the abdominal organs and overlies the capillary beds supporting the organs. By the processes of osmosis, diffusion, and active transport, excess fluid and solutes travel from the peritoneal capillary fluid through the capillary walls, through the peritoneal membrane, and into the dialyzing fluid. After a selected time period, the fluid is drained out of the abdomen by gravity (Fig. 33-4). The process is then repeated.

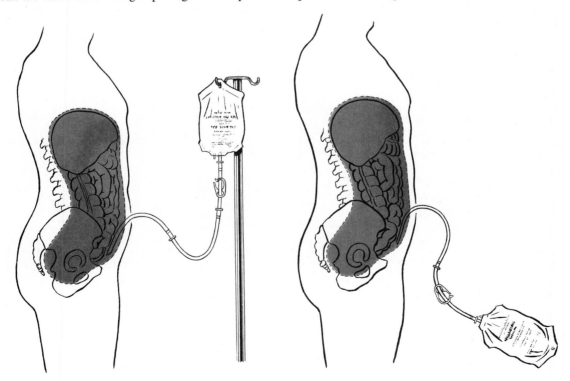

Fig. 33-4 Peritoneal dialysis. (From Thompson JM and others: Mosby's manual of clinical nursing, ed 2, St Louis, 1989, The CV Mosby Co.)

A comparison of the advantages and disadvantages of peritoneal dialysis and hemodialysis appears in Table 33-5. At times peritoneal dialysis becomes a necessity such as when cardiovascular instability or vascular access problems prevent the performance of hemodialysis.

The peritoneal membrane's structure and capillary blood flow to the peritoneum account for the relatively slow nature of peritoneal dialysis. The small capillary pores, the capillary membrane, the interstitium, the mesothelium of the peritoneum, and the fluid film layers in the capillary and the peritoneal cavity provide formidable barriers to fluid and solute passage.[20]

Much about the nature of the membrane is still a mystery, but several factors are implicated in changing the performance of the membrane. For instance, any change in the capillary blood flow changes solute removal but not to a great degree, probably as a result of the relatively poor vasculature of the area in which not all capillaries are perfused at the same time and in which there exists resistance of the capillary membrane to solute transfer.[14]

The volume of dialysate instilled into the abdomen affects the clearance. Research has shown that during acute peritoneal dialysis, 3.5 L/hour will provide a urea clearance of 26 ml/minute.[14] During chronic continuous peritoneal dialysis, 2-L exchanges every 4 hours provide a clearance of 7 ml/minute.[14] The dialysate should be instilled at body temperature for comfort and to provide some vasodilation and increased solute transport in the peritoneum.

The length of time the solution remains in the peritoneal cavity (dwell time) and the solution composition affect the outcome. The dwell time affects the amount of fluid removed from the peritoneal capillaries, although a longer dwell time will not remove proportionately more fluid because of osmotic equilibration across the membranes. The various glucose concentrations of the dialysate provide for different rates of fluid removal. Dialysate compositions and fluid removal characteristics are listed in Tables 33-6 and 33-7.

Table 33-5 Advantages and disadvantages of hemodialysis versus peritoneal dialysis

Advantages	Disadvantages
HEMODIALYSIS	
High efficiency	Safety risks
No protein loss	Requires strict dietary
Fewer metabolic complica-	regimen
tions	Requires anticoagulation
Rapid initiation in emergency	Requires access creation
	Immobility
	Highly technical
	Increased symptoms
PERITONEAL DIALYSIS	
Performed with ease	Low efficiency
Increased mobility	Protein loss
Fewer symptoms	Heavy carbohydrate
No heparin use	loading
Low safety risk	Infection risk

Table 33-6 Composition and characteristics of peritoneal dialysate

Composition	Characteristics
Dextrose—1.5%, 2.5%, or 4.25%	Variable glucose for variable fluid removal
Sodium lactate	Absence of potassium in commercially prepared dialysate because of slow flux of potassium during dwell time
Sodium chloride	
Calcium chloride	
Magnesium chloride	
	Considerable carbohydrate loading for patients because of glucose content
	Variable amounts available for instillation, allowing comfort and tailored regimen for pediatric and adult patients*

*Dialysate is available in sterile containers ranging in size from 250 ml to 3000 ml.

Table 33-7 Peritoneal dialysate solutions and fluid removal characteristics

Standard solution*		Solution type	Fluid removal characteristics	
			Acute PD (1-hr dwell time)	CAPD (4-hr dwell time)
Sodium	132 mEq/L	1.5%	50-100 ml	−40-600 ml
Calcium	3.5 mEq/L	2.5%	100-200 ml	200-300 ml
Magnesium	1.5 mEq/L	4.25%	300-400 ml	150-1100 ml
Chloride	102 mEq/L			
Lactate	35 mEq/L			

Modified from Schoenfeld P: Care of the patient on peritoneal dialysis. In Cogan M and Garavoy M, editors: Introduction to dialysis, New York, 1985, Churchill Livingstone, Inc.
*Available in 1.5, 2.5, 4.25% dextrose concentrations. For continuous ambulatory peritoneal dialysis (CAPD) bags are sterile, prepackaged, and premixed (250 ml to 3L sizes). For acute peritoneal dialysis (PD), sterile bottles of solution are premixed.

CAPD and CCPD

Continuous ambulatory peritoneal dialysis (CAPD) and continuous cycling peritoneal dialysis (CCPD) are variations of peritoneal dialysis that are used as treatments for chronic renal failure. Both are in-home, self-care modes of treatment learned during approximately 2 weeks of training. The patients receive outpatient monitoring on a regular basis.

CAPD involves instilling the contents of a premeasured, sterile bag of solution into the abdomen every 4 hours during the day. The fourth instillation dwells overnight. The empty bag and tubing are continually attached to the catheter and are folded and concealed beneath clothing. Systems allowing disconnection from the catheter have recently been used with excellent results.

CCPD is usually performed at night while the patient sleeps. It uses a mechanical device to which are attached a number of bags of premeasured dialysate. The machine warms the dialysate solution and is programmed to release a given amount of solution periodically through tubing to the dialysis catheter implanted into the patient's peritoneal cavity. From the catheter the same tubing leads to drainage bags. The machine is preset to allow gravity drainage of the previously instilled fluid and gravity filling of fresh, heated fluid. Before the patient arises, the peritoneal cavity is filled, and this last instillation remains throughout the day (long dwell).

The choice between CAPD and CCPD is an individualized decision, incorporating more personal preference and lifestyle factors than actual physiological needs. Both treatments are effective and are rapidly becoming more popular. As of 1985, it was estimated that 10% of the population receiving dialysis rely on CAPD or CCPD.[14]

Catheters. Peritoneal access has changed dramatically over a period of years from the straight, rigid catheters used in acute peritoneal dialysis to the highly sophisticated permanent peritoneal catheters used at present for chronic peritoneal dialysis. All the catheters require surgical implantation; their purpose is delivery to and drainage from the peritoneal cavity. Most catheters have an external segment, a tunnel segment passing through subcutaneous tissue and muscle, a cuff for stabilization at the peritoneal membrane, and an internal segment with numerous holes to quickly deliver and drain dialysate (Fig. 33-5).

Complications. Complications of peritoneal dialysis can be numerous. The complications range from annoying to severe and require careful observation and intervention to control or even prevent further problems. However, with the exception of peritonitis, the complications from peritoneal dialysis are less severe than those associated with hemodialysis. The complications and nursing care related to peritoneal dialysis are listed in Table 33-8.

CONTINUOUS ARTERIOVENOUS HEMOFILTRATION

Continuous arteriovenous hemofiltration was developed in the late 1970s as an alternative to hemodialysis for treatment of certain cases of acute renal failure. It accomplishes the water and solute removal needed in the acutely ill patient while providing the advantage of decreased stress on the cardiovascular system. Additionally, continuous arteriovenous hemofiltration does not require dialysate or the technical equipment necessary for dialysis. It works by using simple convection, and it provides continuous dialysis.[19] Continuous arteriovenous hemofiltration is usually used on patients suffering from acute renal failure and hypervolemia who cannot tolerate the cardiovascular instability associated with hemodialysis.[12]

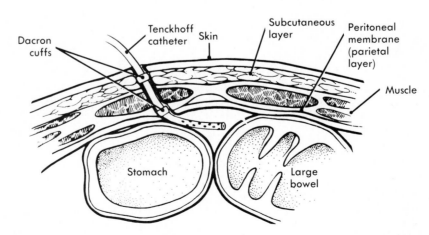

Fig. 33-5 Peritoneal catheter. (From Lewis S and Collier I: Medical-surgical nursing, ed 2, St Louis, 1987, The CV Mosby Co.)

Table 33-8 Complications of peritoneal dialysis

Complications	Nursing care
Peritonitis	Assess for signs and symptoms: cloudy effluent, abdominal pain, rebound tenderness, nausea and vomiting, and fever. Obtain effluent sample for culture. Administer antibiotics as ordered. Teach patient and family signs and symptoms and their prevention.
Exit site infection	Monitor site daily for signs and symptoms of infection: enduration, erythema, purulence, and hyperthermia. Increase daily cleaning of site. Apply topical antibiotics as ordered (this is a controversial practice). Teach patient and family to avoid items such as creams and lotions around exit site.
Catheter tunnel infection	Assess for signs and symptoms of infection: pain along tunnel, enduration for several centimeters away from catheter, erythema leading away from the exit site, and drainage at exit site or as tunnel is "milked" toward exit site. Teach patient and family signs and symptoms of infection. Teach patient and family to avoid pulls or tugs on the catheter or trauma to the exit site. Emphasize the need to maintain cleansing regimen at exit site.
Fluid obstruction	Change position of the patient (i.e., standing, lying, side-lying, knee-chest). Relieve patient's constipation. Irrigate the catheter. Ensure sufficient fluid is in abdomen (sometimes requires a residual reservoir of approximately 50 ml).
Rectal pain	Ensure a sufficient reservoir of fluid. Use slow infusion rate.
Shoulder pain	Ensure that all air is primed from infusion tubing. Attempt draining the effluent with the patient in knee-chest position. Administer mild analgesics as ordered.
Hernias	Monitor for increase in size of or pain in area of hernia. Decrease volume of exchanges as ordered. Dialyze with the patient in the supine position. Use abdominal binder or support for the patient (as long as not binding on catheter exit site). Avoid initiation of peritoneal dialysis until exit site healing has taken place (approximately 1 to 2 weeks if possible).
Fluid overload	Increase use of hypertonic solutions. Decrease by mouth (PO) fluid intake. Shorten dwell times. Weigh patient frequently. Monitor lung sounds and peripheral edema.
Dehydration	Assess patient for decreased skin turgor, muscle cramps, hypotension, tachycardia, and dizziness. Discontinue hypertonic solutions. Increase PO fluid intake. Lengthen dwell times.
Blood-tinged effluent	Monitor for change in effluent color (clear yellow to pink or rusty). Administer heparin, as ordered, to avoid fibrin formation. Obtain patient history about catheter trauma and patient activity before appearance of complication.

At the vascular access (frequently a temporary femoral catheter), tubing is attached, allowing blood flow to the hemofilter (Fig. 33-6). An arterial sampling port and a heparin infusion line are present before the hemofilter is reached. The hemofilter is constructed like the hollow-fiber dialyzer used for hemodialysis except for having a single outflow port for filtrate and no dialysate ports. The blood enters and exits the hemofilter, with the filtrate flowing from the outflow port into the collection device. After exiting the hemofilter, the blood passes through tubing containing the intravenous replacement port and travels back to the vein. The blood is propelled by the systemic blood pressure. A

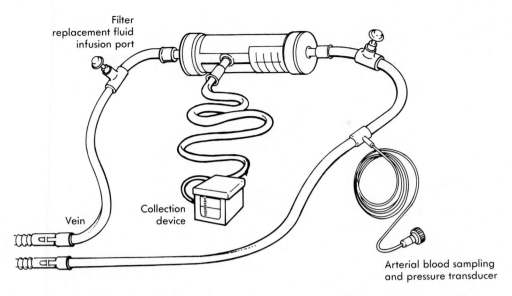

Fig. 33-6 Continuous arteriovenous hemofiltration circuit.

mean arterial pressure of 60 mm Hg is required for continuous arteriovenous hemofiltration to function.[19]

Hemofilters are designed to clear solutes and unbound molecules of 500 to 10,000 daltons. Typical hemodialysis can only clear particles of up to 5000 daltons.[7] Therefore the hemofilter clears many drugs that dialysis cannot remove, along with large amounts of fluids that cannot be removed in as great a quantity through hemodialysis. It has been reported that as much as 14 L of fluid can be removed through the hemofilter in a 24-hour period.[3] Significant fluid removal alone can be accomplished by simply allowing the blood pressure to push the blood continuously through the circuit. A screw clamp applied to the ultrafiltrate port controls the fluid removal.[12]

Ultrafiltration occurs through the combination of the hydrostatic pressure of the blood (blood pressure) and the negative hydrostatic pressure of the outflowing ultrafiltrate. The two pressures are opposed by the oncotic pressure created by the plasma proteins. Ultrafiltration is achieved as long as the oncotic pressure is overcome.

Fluid replacement is based on fluid losses and electrolyte values, with consideration given to achieving the desired reduction in the extracellular fluid volume.[19] Total output minus other intake (such as oral) minus the ordered hourly output equals the hourly replacement amount.[12] Replacement fluids may range from "potassium-free lactated Ringer's solution" to normal saline solution with a variety of additives (for example, calcium chloride, magnesium sulfate, sodium bicarbonate) and D_5W.[19]

Anticoagulation is important, since blood is traveling through an extracorporeal circuit. Commonly, a 20-units/kg dose of heparin is given before initiation of the continuous arteriovenous hemofiltration. Thereafter, 500 units per hour are infused throughout the treatment.[12] Clotting times are frequently determined to monitor anticoagulation.

Nursing care is multifaceted for the patient receiving continuous arteriovenous hemofiltration treatment. Often the nurse is responsible for initiating, monitoring, and discon-

Table 33-9 Nursing care during continuous arteriovenous hemofiltration

Complications	Nursing care
Fluid and electrolyte changes	Observe for changes in central venous pressure or pulmonary capillary wedge pressure. Observe for changes in vital signs. Observe electrocardiogram for changes as result of electrolyte abnormalities. Monitor output values every hour. Control ultrafiltration.
Clotting of hemofilter and circuit	Observe filter and lines once every hour for signs of clotting (dark spots). Monitor blood pressure for decreased flow through filter.
Bleeding	Monitor accelerated clotting time (ACT) no less than once every hour. Adjust heparin dose within specifications to maintain ACT. Observe dressing on vascular access for blood loss. Observe for blood in filtrate (filter leak).
Access dislodgment or infection	Observe access site at least once every 2 to 4 hours. Ensure that clamps are available within easy reach at all times. Observe strict sterile technique when dressing vascular access.

tinuing the treatment, as well as observing for complications such as clotting of the access or extracorporeal unit (hemofilter and lines), fluid and electrolyte imbalances, bleeding, and dislodgment of the access (Table 33-9).

RENAL TRANSPLANTATION

Renal transplantation is another form of treatment for chronic renal failure. Recent developments in the area of immunosuppression have made this treatment a less risky option. However, the posttransplant lifestyle requires ongoing medication and dietary regimens that may burden the individual with lifestyle limitations. Therefore careful pretransplant evaluation and teaching are necessary to provide a greater chance of long-term success. The nurse is instrumental in educating the patient and family, meeting care needs, and monitoring progress of the individual with a renal transplant.

The presurgical preparation involves a thorough medical examination and a psychological and socioeconomic evaluation. The risks of transplantation and the potential complications must be thoroughly discussed with the patient and family. Before the actual surgery, a hemodialysis treatment may be performed to achieve acceptable fluid and electrolyte levels and to keep uremic toxins at low levels.

Immunosuppression

A series of *tissue-matching* tests must be performed to prevent, as much as possible, rejection of the foreign kidney. Even though tissue-matching tests are performed, immunosuppression is still required after surgery. Other tests performed before renal transplant are listed in Table 33-10.

Immunosuppressive therapy includes a number of medications such as corticosteroids (prednisone), purine analogues (azathioprine), antilymphocyte globulin, and cyclosporine, which can be used in combination or supplemented with radiation to effect immunosuppression.

Cyclosporine. Introduced in 1983 and a product of soil fungus, cyclosporine has become the leading immunosuppressant for use in all forms of organ transplantation. Despite its powerful immunosuppression capability, cyclosporine can induce nephrotoxicity, hepatotoxicity, hyperkalemia, and other life-threatening side effects, as well as several less threatening but annoying side effects (Table 33-11). The acute side effects of cyclosporine are usually managed by switching the therapy to azathioprine.[1]

Rejection

Rejection of the transplanted kidney can occur during the actual surgical implantation or months to years later. Rejection has been classified into three types (Table 33-12). Hyperacute rejection is a result of the antigen-antibody response of humoral immunity. Either during surgery or immediately after, the response causes necrosis of the kidney tissue. Crossmatching prevents hyperacute rejection (negative crossmatch required).[1]

Acute rejection occurs weeks to months after the transplantation. Cell-mediated immunity is involved, with the T lymphocytes slowly developing a sensivity to the antigens on the foreign tissue. Necrosis of the kidney tissue occurs,

Table 33-10 Renal tissue-matching tests

Test	Explanation
ABO compatibility	1. Donor and recipient must have same blood type. 2. Compatibility is same as for blood transfusion crossmatching: O, universal donor; AB, universal recipient.
Histocompatibility (antigen matching)	1. Genes determine antigen production and structure. 2. Antigens on the WBCs human leukocyte antigens (HLAs) are of concern in renal transplantation (matches may be achieved between donors and recipients). 3. Identification of the antigens, which occur in pairs—one inherited from each parent, determines the shared antigens between parents, siblings, and children and therefore determines success of crossmatching. 4. Test is performed on venous blood.
Tissue typing, lymphocytotoxicity	1. Lymphocytes are separated and exposed to antisera with known antibodies. 2. Lysis of the lymphocytes indicates that the tissue *will not* match; thus a transplantation will not be successful.
Mixed lymphocyte culture (MLC)	1. Test is performed only in cases of living, related donor transplants (because of lengthy processing time). 2. Lymphocytes of donors and recipients are combined and cultured in a medium. 3. Growth of cells indicates a successful crossmatch. 4. Lysis areas in culture indicate cell death and unsuccessful crossmatch.
WBC crossmatch	1. Identifies antigens between WBCs (process similar to ABO crossmatch).

accompanied by fever and oliguria. The grafted kidney becomes swollen and tender, and the signs of renal failure (oliguria, weight gain, edema, and hypertension) return.[1] Occasionally, aggressive treatment with immunosuppressives and radiation can stop the rejection at a point at which sufficient tissue remains to perform renal function. Diagnosis of acute rejection can be made through monitoring serum creatinine levels, renal scans, ultrasonography, and even kidney biopsy.

Chronic or late rejection is a slow process, occurring over many months to several years. Gradually, function is reduced as tissue becomes sclerosed. The signs of progressive renal failure return (proteinuria, elevated blood urea nitrogen

Table 33-11   Characteristics and side effects of cyclosporine

Characteristics	Side effects
It Interfaces with interleuken release from macrophages. Macrophages can detect the antigen but cannot respond.	Hirsutism
	Gingival hyperplasia
	Tremors
	Headaches
Macrophage production is not affected, so some immune response is intact.	Mild anemia
Hepatotoxicity and nephrotoxicity may result from the toxic levels of the drug.	
Drug has oily consistency (reported by some to have unpleasant taste).	

Modified from Bass M: ANNA J 13(4):196, 1986.

Table 33-12   Types of renal transplant rejection

Type	Characteristics
Hyperacute	1. It occurs promptly after transplant.
	2. Condition is untreatable.
	3. Occurrence is rare if careful pretransplant crossmatching is undertaken.
Acute	1. It occurs 1 to 6 months after transplant.
	2. Signs and symptoms are fever, graft tenderness, hypertension, increased creatinine levels, and decreased urinary output.
	3. Condition may result from surgical complications (e.g., obstruction, thrombus, urological stenosis) or medical complications (e.g., acute tubular necrosis (ATN), hypovolemia, urinary tract infection).
	4. Treatment is undertaken with steroids, antilymphocyte sera, graft irradiation, monoclonal antibodies.
Late	1. Condition occurs 6 months to years after transplant.
	2. It is a slow process, with signs and symptoms of fluid retention, hypertension, and steady rise in blood urea nitrogen and creatinine levels.
	3. It may result from urinary tract infections, vascular complications of the graft, urinary tract obstruction, or a recurrence of the original renal disease.
	4. Treatment usually is aimed at continuing immunosuppressive therapy and measures to support remaining renal function until patient requires dialysis.

and creatinine levels, oliguria, edema, and hypertension). Antirejection therapy is usually ineffective. Causes of late rejection may be related to noncompliance with immunosuppressive therapy, functional vascular damage to the new kidney, or return of the original renal insult (for example, hypertension, diabetes, glomerulonephritis).[1]

Therapy to arrest rejection includes administration of high-dose corticosteroids, which increase neutrophils and decrease T lymphocytes. Antilymphocyte serum has also been used successfully because it binds to T lymphocytes, which, in turn, are subjected to phagocytic activity. Finally, monoclonal antibodies produced through current genetic research have been useful in reducing the T lymphocytes that induce or aid in rejection.[1]

Implantation

The actual surgical implantation of the kidney occurs at the iliac fossa of the recipient (Fig. 33-7). This placement allows ease of attachment to the renal vessels and implantation of the ureter into the bladder. Before the transplant, care is taken to minimize all abnormalities and preexisting disturbances. For example, hypertension is carefully controlled through the use of medications. Gastrointestinal lesions may be treated by drugs or surgical intervention. Prophylactic antibiotic therapy may be initiated. Finally, dialysis is usually performed to remove excess fluid, electrolytes, and waste products to optimize the internal environment.[1]

Donor preparation. Careful preparation and care of the kidney donor must also be performed. The living, related donor must undergo psychological, social, and physical evaluations, and these may prove to be extensive. However, the donor will be placed at no greater surgical risk than the recipient.

Equally careful consideration must be given the cadaver donor and any of his or her family or significant others. Foremost in the mind of the nurse must be the provision of compassionate care to the family. Ensuring that all criteria for donation have been met and obtaining informed consent are other important aspects of nursing care.

Nursing care. Nursing care for the individual considering or actually undergoing renal transplantation ranges from initial explanation of the pros and cons of the surgery to clinical follow-up of compliance to the posttransplant regimen and management of problems. Nursing care of the transplant recipient is outlined in Table 33-13. After reviewing the nursing care for these individuals, it becomes obvious that not only transplant nurses but those providing critical care, general acute care, and home care become involved with patients with renal transplants.

SUMMARY

An overview of the available treatments for chronic renal failure provides the nurse with information with which to guide practice. The challenge to the nurse comes from the rapidity with which technology is altering the treatments described herein. However, the nurse is uniquely able to provide the teaching, intervention, and support that are often omitted in the technological realm.

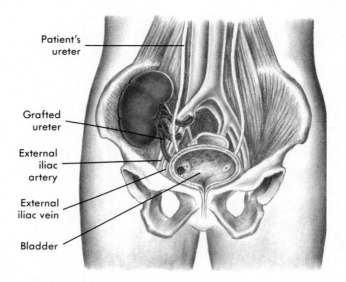

Patient's ureter

Grafted ureter

External iliac artery

External iliac vein

Bladder

Fig. 33-7   Renal transplant. (From Thompson JM and others: Mosby's manual of clinical nursing, ed 2, St Louis, 1989, The CV Mosby Co.)

Table 33-13   Nursing care of the transplant recipient

Nursing Diagnosis	Nursing intervention
Potential for infection	1. Monitor for signs and symptoms of infection.
	2. Use strict aseptic technique with dressing changes, urinary catheters, intravenous infusions.
	3. Monitor immunosuppressant levels for toxicity.
	4. Monitor levels of immunological cell production.
Fluid volume deficit or excess	1. Maintain strict record of intake and output.
	2. Obtain daily weights.
	3. Administer fluids and diruetics as ordered.
	4. Assess for signs of fluid imbalance (dry mucous membranes, decreased skin turgor, dyspnea, edema, headaches, hypertension).
Impaired gas exchange	1. Auscultate lungs frequently.
	2. Provide for pulmonary hygiene (turn, cough, and deep breathe, incentive spirometry).
	3. Monitor for dyspnea.
	4. Obtain arterial blood gas values.
Altered nutrition	1. Assess dietary intake within regimen's restrictions.
	2. Monitor serum electrolytes and glucose levels.
	3. Provide frequent oral hygiene.
	4. Monitor total protein and albumin levels.
Altered tissue perfusion	1. Assess blood pressure and hemodynamic parameters frequently.
	2. Observe for signs of tissue rejection.
	3. Monitor complete blood count as ordered.
	4. Monitor cardiac status for decreased output or dysrhythmias.
Knowledge deficit	Initiate patient education about the following:
	Signs and symptoms of rejection
	Immunosuppressive drugs' actions and side effects
	Dietary restrictions
	Results of noncompliance with regimen

REFERENCES

1. Amend JC and others: Immunosuppression following renal transplantation. In Garovoy MR and Guttmann RD: Renal transplantation, New York, 1986, Churchill Livingstone, Inc.

2. Bass: Common complications of immunosuppression in the renal transplant patient, ANNA J 13(4):196, 1986.

3. Butt MH: Vascular access for chronic hemodialysis. In Nissensen AR and Fine RN: St Louis, 1986, The CV Mosby Co.

4. Carbone V and Bonato J: Nursing implications in the care of the chronic hemodialysis patient in the critical care setting, Heart Lung 14(6):570, 1985.

5. Easterling RE: Water treatment for in-center hemodialysis, including verification of water quality and disinfection. In Nissenson AR and Fine RN: Dialysis therapy, St Louis, 1986, The CV Mosby Co.

6. Gotch FL and Keen M: Dialysis and delivery systems. In Cogan M and Garovoy M, editors: Introduction to dialysis, New York, 1985, Chruchill Livingstone, Inc.

7. Gutch CF and Stoner MH: Review of hemodialysis for nurses and dialysis personnel, ed 4, St Louis, 1983, The CV Mosby Co.

8. Horwood CH and Cook CV: Cyclosporine in transplantation, Heart Lung 14(6):529, 1985.

9. Krupski and others: Access for dialysis. In Cogan M and Garovoy M, editors: Introduction to dialysis, New York, 1985, Churchill Livingstone, Inc.

10. Lancaster LE: Anatomy and physiology for the renal system. In Core curriculum for nephrology nursing, Pitman, NJ, 1987, AJ Janetti, Inc.

11. Lancaster LE: Nursing process and care planning in nephrology nursing. In Core curriculum for nephrology nursing, NJ, 1987, AJ Janetti, Inc.

12. Palmer JC and others: Nursing management of CAVH for acute renal failure, Focus Crit Care 13(5):21, 1986.

13. Ruben RJ: Epidemiology of ESRD and implications for public policy, Public Health Reports 99(5):492, 1984.

14. Schoenfeld P: Care of the patient on peritoneal dialysis. In Cogan M and Garovoy M, editors: Introduction to dialysis, New York, 1985, Chruchill Livingstone, Inc.

15. Thompson JM and others: Mosby's manual of clinical nursing, ed 2, St Louis, 1989, The CV Mosby Co.

16. Tilney NL and Strom TB: Surgical aspects of kidney transplantation. In Garovoy MR and Guttmann RD: Renal transplantation, New York, 1986, Churchill Livingstone, Inc.

17. Ulrick BT and Irwin BC: Renal transplantation. In Core curriculum for nephrology nursing, Pitman, NJ, 1987, AJ Janetti, Inc.

18. Whittaker A: Acute renal dysfunction—assessment of patient at risk, Focus Crit Care 12(3):12, 1985.

19. Winkelman C: Hemofiltration: a new technique in critical care nursing, Heart Lung 14(3):265, 1985.

20. Zappacosta AR and Perras ST: Continuous ambulatory peritoneal dialysis, Philadelphia, 1984, JB Lippincott Co.

34

Renal and Fluids Care Plans

THEORETICAL BASIS AND MANAGEMENT

CHAPTER OBJECTIVES

■ *Discuss the theoretical concepts related to fluid volume deficit.*

■ *Identify and describe nursing interventions that are essential in the treatment of fluid volume deficit.*

■ *Discuss the theoretical concepts related to fluid volume excess.*

■ *Identify and describe nursing interventions that are essential in the treatment of fluid volume excess.*

■ *Discuss factors controlling fluid volume excess and deficit.*

Changes in fluid balance are among the most serious internal threats to human health. The maintenance of this crucial balance results from complex interplay between factors controlling intake and output. Hormonal control from the cerebral cortex and adrenal glands influences both water and sodium reabsorption and excretion. Pressures created by dissolved solutes and the exertion of the cardiovascular system cause movement between compartments and therefore the potential for imbalances.

The kidneys respond to various pressures and hormonal factors by increasing or decreasing the amount of fluid and wastes excreted. Disturbances in any of the intake or output mechanisms result in either an excess or deficit of body fluids.

FACTORS CONTROLLING FLUID VOLUME DEFICIT AND EXCESS
Neurohormonal Control

Antidiuretic hormone (ADH or arginine vasopressin) is secreted by the posterior pituitary gland and functions as the primary controller of extracellular fluid (ECF) volume. Several mechanisms stimulate or inhibit the release of ADH in response to a wide array of stimuli (see the box below). In addition to the usual stimuli, the presence of severe stress, either emotional or physical, is thought to initiate ADH release through the limbic system (surrounding the hypothalamus). However, this mechanism is less well-defined as a source of stimulation than the osmo-receptors in the hypothalamus.[7]

The strongest messages for release of ADH are sent by the osmoreceptors located in the hypothalamus. As serum osmolality rises above 385 mOsm/kg, ADH is released and carried through the circulation to the nephrons in the kidney. There ADH attaches to receptor sites in the loop of Henle, the distal convoluted tubule, and the collecting ducts. The action of ADH at these sites is to increase the permeability of the tubular structures to water. Water can therefore be reabsorbed into the circulatory system at a greater rate, leading to normalization of the serum osmolality and a steep

---

FACTORS STIMULATING RELEASE OF ADH

Hyperosmolality of ECF
Hypovolemia
Increased body temperature
Medications
   Narcotics
   Antineoplastics
   Oral hypoglycemics
   Beta-adrenergic drugs

rise in the urinary osmolality as less water in comparison to solute load is excreted.[7]

ADH can only sustain the effect on the renal tubules to a urinary osmolality of 1200 to 1400 mOsm/L. Therefore a secondary mechanism is required to ensure that appropriate water reabsorption is maintained. That mechanism is thirst, which ensures that fluid will be consciously ingested to prevent water deficit.

Thirst

The thirst center is also located in the hypothalamus and is governed by the same osmoreceptors that stimulate ADH release. Osmoreceptors stimulate the ventromedial nucleus in the hypothalamus and send impulses to the cerebral cortex. The control by the cerebral cortex makes thirst a mechanism that requires conscious effort to satisfy. To individuals who have limited ability to respond such as adults who are comatose or disoriented and infants, thirst may be stimulated in normal fashion but unsatiated; therefore fluid volume deficit may follow.[11]

ADH is easily inhibited by feedback mechanisms as previously discussed. However, the thirst mechanism is less easily inhibited as is evidenced by patients' continued need to ingest fluid in the presence of edematous states such as cardiac and renal failure.[11]

Renin-Angiotensin-Aldosterone System

The inextricable relationship between sodium and water plays a very important role in the influence of the renin-angiotensin-aldosterone system on body water regulation. As diagrammed in Fig. 34-1, a reduction in vascular volume stimulates the release of renin. Renin (in combination with angiotensinogen) splits the substance known as angiotensin

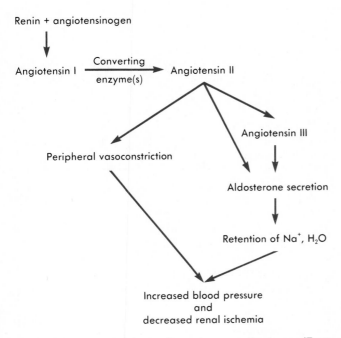

Fig. 34-1 The renin-angiotension mechanism. (From Thompson JM and others: Mosby's manual of clinical nursing, St Louis, 1986, The CV Mosby Co.)

I from the plasma globulins. Angiotensin I, in conjunction with converting enzymes in the lung, forms the powerful vasoconstrictor substance known as angiotensin II.

In turn, Angiotensin II stimulates areas of the adrenal glands to secrete aldosterone (an adrenal mineralocorticoid), which acts on the renal tubules to reabsorb sodium into the circulation. When sodium is retained, water follows. Angiotensin II also constricts the renal vasculature, reducing renal blood flow and available glomerular filtrate, thus sending a signal to the posterior pituitary to release ADH. Frequently, in this way the two systems intertwine, not only to maintain fluid balance but also to maintain electrolyte balance.[3]

Compartmental Fluid Shifts

Deficits and excesses of body fluids occur not through true gains or losses but through shifts between fluid compartments, leaving one compartment with a fluid deficiency and another with fluid overload. Osmotic and hydrostatic pressures influence the movement of fluids between the interstitial and intravascular compartments. A shift may also be the impetus for stimulating, through osmoreceptors or baroreceptors, the aforementioned sodium and fluid control mechanisms.

Colloid osmotic pressure is a pulling force generated by the plasma proteins. Since both the intravascular and interstitial compartments contain plasma proteins, colloid osmotic pressure is generated in both the intravascular and the interstitial space. Plasma colloid osmotic pressure maintains fluid in the intravascular compartment, and tissue colloid osmotic pressure maintains the fluid in the interstitial space. Albumin and, to a lesser extent, globulin generate this pulling force. Any condition that reduces the amount of albumin in the intravascular space (liver disease) or changes the integrity of the membrane containing the proteins in the distinct compartments (burns) will lead to fluid shifts. Although fluid shifts may not be considered true fluid deficits, the somatic responses to a deficit in one ECF compartment and an excess in the other are the same as for true loss of fluid from the body.[12]

Fluid balance depends on the relationship between the hydrostatic pressures in the tissue and vascular spaces and the osmotic pressures in the same spaces.

Hydrostatic pressure is produced through the action of the cardiovascular and lymphatic systems. Capillary hydrostatic pressure is generated by the force of cardiac contraction. Tissue hydrostatic pressure is generated by the drainage of the lymphathic system.[12]

In addition to the differences in pressures, the membranes' permeability to solutes, water, and proteins and the surface area of the capillary endothelium affect water and solute movement.[12]

Renal Fluid Regulation

The dominant forces regulating the renal response to fluid reabsorption and excretion are renal blood flow, glomerular filtration rate, and sodium regulation.[3] Secondary forces mediated by the circulatory system, sympathetic nervous system, and various hormones result in fine-tuning of fluid balance.

For example, inadequate renal blood flow reduces the pressure of the blood traveling into the glomerulus and elicits retention of sodium and water through renin release and the ADH mechanism. However, prolonged reduction in renal blood flow that impairs oxygen delivery produces tubular cell death, which begins to severely limit the ability of the tubules to accomplish excretion and reabsorption.

CAUSES OF FLUID VOLUME DEFICIT
Active Blood Loss

Although many conditions can result in hypovolemia, hemorrhage remains the simplest and most graphic example of alteration in intravascular fluid volume. The rapidity and extent of the blood loss often determine the ability of the body to compensate for the loss. For example, a 10% blood loss decreases cardiac output by 21%, whereas a 20% blood loss decreases cardiac output by 41%, leading to significant impaired tissue perfusion. The ability of compensatory mechanisms to respond to hypovolemia also depends on the rapidity with which fluid is replaced.[10]

The response of the body to hypovolemia is divided into two phases: *compensatory* and *late*. In the compensatory phase, vasoconstriction maintains perfusion to the most vital organs and stimulates renal baroreceptors, resulting in the production of renin, angiotension II, and aldosterone. Stimulation of the sympathetic nervous system results in the release of substances that increase heart rate and cardiac output. Fluid moves from the interstitial spaces into the intravascular space to maintain fluid volume. Hence skin pallor and decreased skin turgor result.

Finally, the decreased hydrostatic pressure in the capillaries decreases available glomerular filtrate and results in the reabsorption of greater amounts of fluid and sodium to replenish the intravascular volume. However, the actions of the compensatory phase cannnot be sustained if fluid replacement is not swift.[10]

The late phase of body response to blood loss results in the signs of shock. This phase primarily results from the failure of the compensatory mechanisms and, therefore, diminished tissue perfusion. Diminished perfusion leaves the cells with reduced substances for ATP (energy) production. Decreased calcium alters the active transport mechanism and thus neurotransmission. In addition, decreased microcirculation leaves toxic metabolic acids such as lactic acid at the cellular level.[10] The subsequent reduction in neurotransmission and in electrolyte balance impairs cardiac output and the balance between the fluid compartments.[10]

Although the initial response to blood loss, as previously noted, is a slight increase in cardiac output, the eventual result of continued loss without replacement is a severely diminished cardiac output. When replacement begins and accurate measurements of fluid status are required, the calculation of cardiac output and measurements of central venous pressure (CVP) and pulmonary capillary wedge pressure (PCWP) are of definite value. Significant blood loss and volume depletion are reflected by CVP less than 6 cm H_2O and PCWP less than 8 mm Hg.[15]

During the late phase of the body's response to hypovolemia when compensatory mechanisms fail, plasma levels of blood urea nitrogen (BUN) and creatinine rise as a result of the decreased oxygen delivery to the renal tubular cells. The ischemia that develops changes the nature of the tubular epithelium and allows "backleak" of waste products into the circulation. The increase in these metabolites also creates hyperosmolality of the serum, again straining the already decompensated mechanisms for fluid reabsorption.[15]

Diarrhea and Wound Drainage

The fluid losses from diarrhea and draining fistulas are usually not the result of water loss alone but of fluid rich in electrolytes. Acute fluid loss through diarrhea may range from 0.5 L to 4 L above daily output.[16] This volume depletion affects not only the ECF but also the intracellular fluid (ICF).[1]

Diarrhea can be divided into three different types: osmotic, secretory, and altered motility. Osmotic diarrhea occurs secondary to the ingestion of solutes that are poorly metabolized and to malabsorption states. Extra fluid and electrolytes are drawn into the stool by the hyperosmolality created by these unprocessed substances.[16] Lactose intolerance, steatorrhea, and ingestion of sorbitol fit this category.[2] Elimination of offending substances or a combination of dietary regulation and proper medication usually resolves this type of diarrhea and thus eliminates the water and solute losses.

Secretory diarrhea stems most prominently from the effects of certain bacterial endotoxins on the intestinal epithelium. However, certain diarrheas of this type have a cause that arises from the influence of hormones on the epithelium. For example, *Staphylococcus aureus* produces a particularly devastating enterotoxin that may permanently scar the intestinal epithelium and reduce the available surface area for fluid absorption. The inflammatory process changes the permeability of the intestinal epithelium and alters fluid and solute exchanges in much the same way as occurs in the renal tubules.[2]

Prostaglandins, along with calcitonin, intestinal peptide, and glucagon, have been implicated in increasing the permeability of the intestinal mucosa. The results of the secretory forms of diarrhea are active water loss, active ion secretion (sodium and chloride), and diminished reabsorption of water and solutes.[2,16]

Diarrhea as the result of altered motility has been observed in patients suffering from diabetic neuropathy. This type of diarrhea, however, so closely resembles the osmotic diarrheas that research has yet to elucidate whether the cause is altered motility or osmotic changes. The loss of fluid and solutes is modest in comparison to secretory diarrhea and tends to be chronic rather than acute.[16]

Sodium loss varies depending on the cause of the diarrhea. However, in most states sodium loss may produce stool sodium levels that approach serum sodium levels. Water loss is so severe, particularly in secretory diarrhea, that ADH production is stimulated. However, because of the sodium loss, the reabsorption of water under the influence of ADH produces a dilutional hyponatremia.

Yet, in osmotic diarrhea the osmotic agents present in the stool cause greater water loss than sodium loss. If the individual fails to ingest sufficient fluid, the result may be ECF hypernatremia.[16]

Ileal fistulas, duodenal stump fistulas, and pancreatic fistuals may drain anywhere from 0.3 to 4 L of extremely sodium-and potassium-rich fluid per day. The results of the fluid and electrolyte losses in these types of wounds are dehydration, metabolic acidosis, hypokalemia, and hyponatremia.[16]

The symptoms of the volume depletion secondary to gastrointestinal (GI) losses depend solely on the amount of diarrheal output versus the amount of fluid replacement. Usually the loss of 2 L of diarrheal fluid will produce tachycardia and hypotension, which indicate compensatory response to the fluid depletion.[9] Also, with any fluid loss a concomitant weight loss can be expected.

Continued losses result in the familiar signs of ECF dehydration: thirst, weakness, decreased skin turgor, increased hematocrit, and increased BUN and creatinine levels, for example. As long as the protective mechanisms are operative and fluid replacement is begun, the kidneys will retain fluid in response to ADH, and aldosterone will be secreted to retain sodium. Yet severe losses reduce the ability of the kidneys to protect the internal environment because of the reduced availability of filtrate.

Burns: Active Plasma Loss

Fluid loss in a patient with a burn injury results from a combination of fluid shift from the intravascular to the interstitial spaces and loss of exudates through the disrupted integument. The primary fluid deficit, however, is intravascular hypovolemia with subsequent interstitial edema, commonly referred to as "third spacing."

Thermal injury disrupts normal capillary permeability and floods the interstitium with plasma proteins. Additionally, the inflammatory process is stimulated, and the lymphathic drainage channels are impaired. Increased osmotic pressure in the interstitial space results from a pull exerted by the plasma proteins that have seeped into the space. The interstitial hydrostatic pressure is also reduced, resulting in congestion of the interstitial space from the inadequate drainage through the lymphathic channels. Blood volume decrease and edema formation are most rapid during the first 8 hours after injury.[14]

Evaporative loss of fluids must also be considered after thermal injury. The loss of the integument removes the barrier that controls evaporative fluid loss. The volume of evaporative loss depends on the extent of the area burned but usually approximates 2 to 3 ml/kg per percent of body surface burned.[6]

Fluid resuscitation during the first 24 hours after injury is directed at maintaining urinary output at 30 to 50 ml/hour. Crystalloid solutions are usually used. A 15% to 20% weight gain is expected during the first 72 hours.[6,14] Later, colloid solutions (plasma or albumin) may be used to restore intravascular volume at 0.3 to 0.5 ml/kg per percent total body surface burned.[14]

Hyponatremia

Most states of hyponatremia are not the result of sodium and water loss but of shifts of water from the ICF to the ECF or of water retention as a result of ADH stimulation. However, vomiting, diarrhea, burns, diuretic therapy, and renal disease may produce hyponatremia through actual sodium and water losses.

Adrenal insufficiency can produce severe water and sodium losses. With decreased production of mineralocorticoids such as aldosterone, sodium is wasted in the urine. The consequence is loss of fluids that accompany the sodium.[5]

Fluid Volume Deficit related to hyponatremia (absolute sodium loss)

DEFINING CHARACTERISTICS

- Central nervous system (CNS) symptoms: headache, lethargy, confusion, muscular weakness
- Postural hypotension
- Tachycardia
- Gastrointestinal (GI) symptoms: nausea, diarrhea, cramping
- Diaphoresis, cold and clammy skin
- Loss of skin turgor and elasticity
- Serum sodium <135 mEq/L
- Urinary specific gravity <1.010
- Elevated red blood cell and plasma protein levels

OUTCOME CRITERIA

- CNS symptoms (e.g., headache, lethargy) are absent.
- Blood pressure and heart rate return to baseline.
- Skin turgor is normal.
- Serum sodium and urinary specific gravity levels are normal.

NURSING INTERVENTIONS *AND RATIONALE*

1. Continue to monitor the assessment parameters listed under "Defining Characteristics."
2. With physician's collaboration, replace fluid and sodium loss with normal saline solution or with hypertonic saline solution (3% or 5%).
3. Provide oral fluids such as juice or bouillon that are high in sodium.
4. Avoid the use of diuretics, especially thiazide and loop diuretics, *because they will further decrease sodium.*
5. If patient is ambulatory, protect from falls until CNS symptoms and/or postural hypotension clears.
6. If performing nasogastric suctioning, irrigate tube with normal saline solution, not water. Additionally, carefully restrict ice chip intake; consider using iced saline solution chips. *Excessive intake of water dilutes serum sodium and can result in water intoxication.*

Fluid Volume Deficit related to active blood loss

DEFINING CHARACTERISTICS

- Cardiac output < 5 L/min
- Cardiac index < 2.5 L/min
- Pulmonary capillary wedge pressure (PCWP), PAD, central venous pressure (CVP) less than normal or less than baseline
- Tachycardia
- Narrowed pulse pressure
- Systolic blood pressure < 100 mm Hg
- Urinary output < 30 ml/hour
- Pale, cool, moist skin
- Apprehensiveness

OUTCOME CRITERIA

- The patient's CO is > 5 L/min and CI is > 2.5 L/min.
- The patient's PCWP, PAD, and CVP are normal or back to baseline level.
- The patient's pulse is normal or back to baseline.
- The patient's systolic blood pressure is > 90.
- The patient's urinary output is > 30 ml/hour.

NURSING INTERVENTIONS *AND RATIONALE*

1. Continue to monitor the assessment parameters listed under "Defining Characteristics." Additionally, a serum lactate level >2 mOsm/L is believed to represent cellular perfusion failure at its earliest stage.
2. Secure airway and administer high flow oxygen.
3. Place patient in supine position with legs elevated *to increase preload.* Consider using low Fowler's position with legs elevated for patient with head injury.
4. For fluid repletion use the 3:1 rule, replacing three parts of fluid for every unit of blood lost.
5. Administer crystalloid solutions using the fluid challenge technique: infuse precise aliquots of fluid (usually 5 to 20 ml/min) over 10-minute periods; monitor cardiac loading pressures serially *to determine successful challenging.* If the PCWP or PAD elevates more than 7 mm Hg above beginning level, the infusion should be stopped. If the PCWP or PAD rises only to 3 mm Hg above baseline or falls, another fluid challenge should be administered.
6. Replete fluids first before considering use of vasopressors, *since vasopressors increase myocardial oxygen consumption out of proportion to the reestablishment of coronary perfusion in the early phases of treatment.*
7. When blood is available or its need is indicated, replace it with fresh packed red cells and fresh frozen plasma *to keep clotting factors intact.*
8. Move or reposition patient minimally *to decrease or limit tissue oxygen demands.*
9. Evaluate patient's anxiety level and intervene through patient education or sedation *to decrease tissue oxygen demands.*
10. Be alert for the possibility of adult respiratory distress syndrome (ARDS) development in the ensuing 72 hours.

Fluid Volume Deficit related to diarrhea, wound drainage

DEFINING CHARACTERISTICS

- Dry mucous membranes and skin
- Weight loss in excess of 10%
- Acute thirst
- Hypotension
- Tachycardia
- Longitudinal wrinkling of the tongue
- Metabolic acidosis
- Serum electrolyte imbalances: hyperchloremia, hypokalemia
- Electrocardiogram (ECG) changes associated with hypokalemia

OUTCOME CRITERIA

- Mucous membranse are moist.
- The patient's weight returns to baseline.
- The patient's blood pressure returns to baseline.
- The patient's heart rate returns to baseline.
- Tongue is moist and nonwrinkled.
- The acid-base balance is normal.
- Serum electrolyte values are normal.

NURSING INTERVENTIONS *AND RATIONALE*

1. Continue to monitor the assessment parameters listed under "Defining Characteristics."
2. With physician's collaboration, replace base and electrolyte losses.
3. With physician's collaboration, replace fluid loss with intravenous isotonic saline solution or dextrose and one-half normal saline solution.
4. Provide oral fluids such as juices that are high in electrolytes.
5. Provide oral potassium replacement according to serum potassium measurements as the metabolic acidosis is corrected.

Fluid Volume Deficit related to active plasma loss and fluid shift into interstitium secondary to burns

DEFINING CHARACTERISTICS

- PCWP, PAD, CVP less than normal or less than baseline
- Tachycardia
- Narrowed pulse pressure
- Systolic blood pressure <100 mm Hg
- Urinary output <30 ml/hour
- Increased hematocrit level

OUTCOME CRITERIA

- The patient's PCWP, PAD, and CVP are normal or back to baseline.
- Systolic blood pressure is >90 mm Hg.
- Urinary output is >30 ml/hour.
- The patient's hematocrit level is normal.

NURSING INTERVENTIONS *AND RATIONALE*

1. Continue to monitor the assessment parameters listed under "Defining Characteristics." Additionally, inspect soft tissues *to determine the presence of edema.*
2. With physician's collaboration, administer intravenous (IV) fluid replacements (usually normal saline solution or lactated Ringer's solution) at a rate sufficient *to maintain urinary output >40 ml/hour.* Colloid solutions are avoided in the initial phases (but can be used later) because of the possibility of increased edema formation *as a result of the increased capillary permeability.*

POTENTIAL VOLUME EXCESS RISK FACTOR: RENAL FAILURE

Whether acute or chronic, renal failure has the potential for ECF excesses of severe proportion. The causes of the renal failure (prerenal, intrarenal, or portrenal) govern the extent of the fluid excess and the permanence of the situation. Prerenal causes stem from the disruption of perfusion to the renal tissues, resulting in temporary or permanent failure of the renal mechanisms. Permanence of the injury usually depends on the length of time of hypoperfusion to the tissue, which may be extremely variable from one individual to another.

Intrarenal causes are the result of direct insult to the kidney tissues by a disease process such as infection or diabetes. Intrarenal insult usually has a prognosis of permanent renal failure; however, this may also vary among individuals.

Postrenal causes result from the blockage of urinary flow from the lower urinary tract, with the flow backing up and congesting the kidney tissues. Removal of the obstruction usually improves the prognosis for swift return of function.

The subsequent fluid and solute handling by the kidney depends on the extent of damage and the area(s) of the nephron damaged. Tubular damage frequently results in inability to concentrate the urine appropriately. Tubular cells can neither excrete solutes and water nor reabsorb the same.[16]

Fluid retention during acute failure results from the function of the compensatory mechanisms governing sodium and water retention. The renin-angiotensin system increases sodium reabsorption and creates peripheral vasoconstriction. ADH is released in response to an increase in plasma sodium, creating decreased output of urine and fluid retention.[13] The increase in ECF, secondary to the decreased urinary output, is reflected as edema when increased intravascular hydrostatic pressure forces fluid into the interstitium.

On the other hand, chronic renal failure produces fluid excess in a slightly different manner. The insult to the kidney produces actual ischemia of the renal tubular cells. Prolonged ischemia produces cell necrosis, with subsequent sloughing of debris, which impedes filtrate flow, thus decreasing urinary production. A decreased glomerular filtration rate (GFR) produces a reduction in creatinine clearance and tubular flow rate. The retention of metabolites such as creatinine produces hyperosmolar ECF and the retention of water. Expansion of the ECF results in increase in the intravascular hydrostatic pressure and edema of the interstitium as discussed previously.[13]

Potential Fluid Volume Excess

RISK FACTOR
- Renal failure

DEFINING CHARACTERISTICS
- Weight gain that occurs during a 24- to 48-hour period
- Dependent pitting edema
- Ascites in severe cases
- Fluid crackles on lung auscultation
- Exertional dyspnea
- Oliguria or anuria
- Hypertension
- Engorged neck veins
- Decrease in urinary osmolality as renal failure progresses

OUTCOME CRITERIA
- Weight returns to baseline.
- Edema or ascites are absent or reduced to baseline.
- Lungs are clear to auscultation.
- Exertional dyspnea is absent.
- Blood pressure returns to baseline.
- Neck veins are flat.

NURSING INTERVENTIONS *AND RATIONALE*
1. Continue to monitor the assessment parameters listed under "Defining Characteristics."
2. Promote skin integrity of edematous areas by frequent repositioning and elevation of areas where possible. Avoid massaging pressure points or reddened areas of skin *because this results in further tissue trauma.*
3. Plan patient care to provide rest periods *to not heighten exertional dyspnea.*
4. Weight patient daily at same time in same clothing, preferably with the same scale.
5. Instruct the patient about the correlation between fluid intake and weight gain, using commonly understood fluid measurments (e.g., ingesting 4 cups [1000 ml] of fluid results in an approximate 2-pound weight gain in the anuric patient.

REFERENCES

1. Aberman A: The ins and outs of fluids and electrolytes, Emerg Med 14:121, 1982.
2. Binder HJ: The pathophysiology of diarrhea, Hosp Pract 19:107, 1984.
3. Hollenberg NK: The kidney in heart failure, Hosp Pract 21:81, 1986.
4. Howard M, Puris VK, and Paidipaty BB: The effects of fluid resuscitation in the critically ill, Heart Lung 13(6):649, 1984.
5. Humes HD: Disorders of water metabolism. In Kokko JP and Tannen RL, editors: Fluids and electrolytes, Philadelphia, 1986, WB Saunders Co.
6. Jacobsen HR: Fluid and electrolyte problems in surgery and trauma. In Kokko JP and Tannen RL, editors: Fluids and electrolytes, Philadelphia, 1986, WB Saunders Co.
7. Johndrow PD and Thornton S: Syndrome of inappropriate ADH-A growing concern, Focus Crit Care 12:29, 1985.
8. Kennedy-Caldwell C: Clinical triads: water metabolism, the NPO patient, and parenteral nutrition, Crit Care Nurse 6:63, 1986.
9. McKeown JW: Disorders of total body sodium. In Kokko JP and Tannen RL, editors: Fluids and electrolytes, Philadelphia, 1986, WB Saunders Co.
10. Myers KA and Hichkey MK: Nursing management of hypovolemic shock, Crit Care Nurs Q 11:57, 1988.
11. Rice V: Problems of water regulation: diabetes insipidus and syndromes of inappropriate ADH, Crit Care Nurse 3:64, 1983.
12. Rice V: Shock management. I. Fluid volume replacement, Crit Care Nurse 4:69, 1984.
13. Richard C: Causes of renal failure. In Core curriculum for nephrology nursing, Pitman, NJ, 1987, AJ Janetti Co.
14. Robertson KE, Cross PJ, and Terry JC: Burn care: the crucial first days, Am J Nurs 85:30, 1985.
15. Urban N: Integrating hemodynamic parameters with clinical decision-making, Crit Care Nurse 6:48, 1986.
16. Whittaker A: Acute renal dysfunction, Focus Crit Care 12:12, 1985.
17. Zucker AR and Chernow B: Diabetes insipidus and syndrome of inappropriate ADH, Crit Care Q 6:63, 1983.

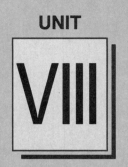
GASTROINTESTINAL ALTERATIONS

CHAPTER

35

Anatomy and Physiology of the Digestive System

CHAPTER OBJECTIVES

- *Identify and briefly describe the physiology of the normal anatomical structures of the gastrointestinal tract.*
- *List and discuss the functions of the gastric secretions and the mediators of gastric juice.*
- *Discuss the formation and function of bile.*
- *List and describe the exocrine functions of the pancreas and discuss how pancreatic secretions promote digestion.*
- *Identify the most important functions of the large intestine, including actions of colonic bacteria.*

The major function of the gastrointestinal (GI) tract is to convert ingested nutrients into simpler forms that can be transported from the tract's lumen to the portal circulation and used in metabolic processes. The digestive system also plays a vital role in detoxification and elimination of bacteria, viruses, chemical toxins, and drugs. Disturbances of the digestive system itself or of the complex hormonal and neural controls that regulate it can severely upset homeostasis and compromise the overall nutritional status of the patient. Furthermore, any circumvention of the normal feeding mechanism (for example, by mechanisms that bypass the oral route such as tube and enteral feeding) can alter digestive processes or contribute to malabsorption.

Thus it is vital for the critical care nurse to have an active knowledge of the normal function of the GI tract to facilitate assessment, diagnosis, and intervention in patients with digestive diseases.

ROLE OF THE BRAIN

Feeding actually begins with the sensation of hunger, the intrinsic desire for food, which is under the control of the feeding center in the lateral nuclei of the hypothalamus. Activation of the feeding center initiates a search for food. The satiety center, which provides the sensation of satis-

faction and fulfillment after a meal and inhibits the feeding center, is located in the ventromedial nuclei of the hypothalamus. Thus the nutritional status of the body is a primary concern of the hypothalamus, which also excites the lower centers and the brainstem in which the mechanics of feeding such as chewing and mastication are controlled.

The selection of specific foods is regulated in higher centers than the hypothalamus, including the amygdala and cortical areas of the limbic system. Appetite is affected by the size of body fat stores, distention of the GI tract, environment, temperature, cultural factors, and experience.

MOUTH, ORAL CAVITY, AND PHARYNX

The mouth and accessory organs, which include the lips, cheeks, gums, tongue, palate, and salivary glands, perform vital functions, including ingestion, mastication, and salivation, in the initial phase of digestion.

Mastication

The mouth is the beginning of the alimentary canal (Fig. 35-1) and is the means for entry of nutrients. The teeth cut, grind, and mix food, transforming it into a form suitable for swallowing and increasing the surface area of food available to salivary secretions. Healthy dentition is vital for this process.

Mucous glands located behind the tip of the tongue and serous glands (Ebner's) located at the back of the tongue aid in the lubrication of food and in its distribution over the taste buds.

Salivation

Salivation has an important role in the first stage of digestion since saliva lubricates the mouth, facilitates the movement of the lips and the tongue during swallowing, and washes away bacteria. Saliva has a pH that ranges from 6.5 to 7.4 and consists of approximately 99% water and 1% mucin and amylase (ptyalin). Saliva also contains a large amount of ions such as potassium and bicarbonate, as well

673

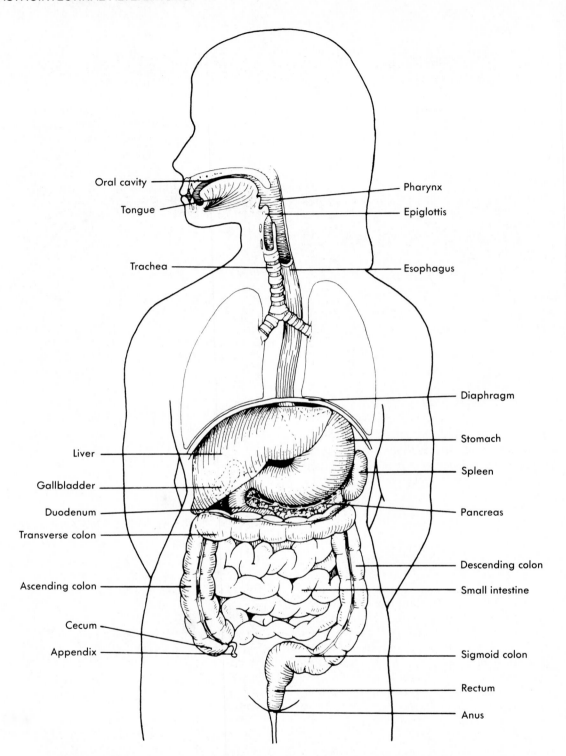

Oral cavity

Tongue

Trachea

Pharynx

Epiglottis

Esophagus

Diaphragm

Stomach

Spleen

Liver

Gallbladder

Duodenum

Transverse colon

Ascending colon

Cecum

Appendix

Pancreas

Descending colon

Small intestine

Sigmoid colon

Rectum

Anus

Fig. 35-1 Anatomy of the gastrointestinal system. (From Broadwell DC and Jackson BS, editors: Principles of ostomy care, St Louis, 1982, The CV Mosby Co.)

as protein antibodies and thiocyanate ions, which are vital in destroying oral bacteria.

Approximately 1000 to 1500 ml of saliva are produced each day by three pairs of salivary glands: the submaxillary glands, the sublingual glands, and the parotid glands. Parotid gland secretions are enzymatic, containing amylase,

which begins the chemical breakdown of large polysaccharides into dextrins and sugars. Only 5% to 10% of starch is digested in the mouth, but amylase continues to break down starch in the stomach for approximately 30 minutes, at which point approximately 40% of the starch is digested.

The mouth and pharynx are also lined with small salivary glands that provide additional lubrication.

Parasympathetic stimulation results in profuse secretions of watery saliva. Sympathetic stimulation causes release of small amounts of saliva with organic constituents from the submaxillary glands. Anticholinergic drugs reduce salivary secretion and a number of GI hormones such as secretin, cholecystokinin, vasoactive intestinal peptide, and gastric inhibitory peptide.

ESOPHAGUS

The esophagus (gullet) is a collapsible tube lacking cartilage. In adults it is 23 to 25 cm (9 to 10 inches) long and 1 to 2 cm (½ to 1 inch) wide. It is the narrowest part of the digestive tube and lies posterior to the trachea and heart with attachments at the hypopharynx and at the cardiac portion of the stomach below the diaphragm (Fig. 35-2). It begins at the level of the C6, C7, and T1 vertebrae and extends vertically through the mediastinum and diaphragm to the level of T11.

The esophagus has two sphincters: the hypopharyngeal, or the upper esophageal, sphincter and the cardiac, or lower esophageal, sphincter. The distal 3 to 5 cm of the esophagus constitute the cardiac sphincter, which, although not grossly discernable, is an area of increased pressure. The stomach forms a 70- to 80-degree angle with the esophagus at this point.

The functions of the esophagus are to accept a bolus of food from the oropharynx, to transport the bolus through the esophageal body by gravity and peristalsis, and to release the bolus into the stomach through the cardiac sphincter. The esophagus also serves as an antireflex barrier and as a vent for increased gastric pressure.

The esophageal phase of deglutition is a visceral response and is reflex in nature. Peristalsis consists of waves of circular contractions and relaxations by which a bolus of food is propelled. A peristaltic wave takes 5 to 10 seconds to reach the stomach from the pharynx. Secondary peristalsis begins in the upper thoracic esophagus and is caused by distention from foods remaining in the esophagus. Body position (standing, recumbent), the acidity of the food bolus, pain, anxiety, and anger can affect transit time. Peristalsis is required for movement of liquids and semisolids in the

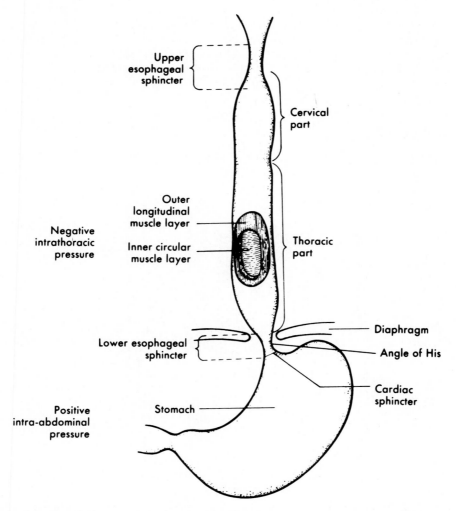

Fig. 35-2   Normal anatomy of the esophagus, with cutaway to show the muscle layers. (From Given BA and Simmons SJ: Gastroenterology in clinical nursing, ed 4, St Louis, 1984, The CV Mosby Co.)

recumbent position. Peristalsis declines with age.

At the cardiac sphincter a pressure of approximately +25 mm Hg is maintained, and it may reach 15 to 20 mm Hg higher than pressure in the fundus. This pressure difference normally prevents reflux of gastric contents and erosion of mucosa from acid-pepsin secretions. In addition, esophageal mucoid secretions provide lubrication and prevent mucosal excoriation caused by food entering proximally or by refluxing gastric contents distally.

ABDOMINAL ORGANS

The abdomen, the largest cavity in the body, consists of the stomach, small and large intestines, liver, pancreas, kidneys, spleen, suprarenal glands, and uterus. The abdominal organs (see Fig. 35-1) are protected by the peritoneum, a serous membrane consisting of mesothelium and connective tissue.

Stomach

The stomach is an elongated pouch approximately 25 to 30 cm (10 to 12 inches) long and 10 to 13 cm (4 to 5 inches) wide at the maximal transverse diameter. It lies obliquely beneath the cardiac sphincter at the esophagogastric junction and above the pyloric sphincter, next to the small intestine. Its anatomical divisions, shown in Fig. 35-3, include the cardia at the proximal end; the fundus, which lies above and to the left of the cardiac sphincter; the body, the central portion; the antrum, an elongated constricted portion; and the pylorus, the distal end connecting the antrum to the duodenum. The greater curvature, which begins at the car-

diac orifice and arches backward and upward around the fundus, is in contact with the transverse colon and the pancreas at the posterior edge. The lesser curvature extends from the cardia to the pylorus. Two sphincters control the rate of food passage: the cardiac at the esophagogastric junction and the pyloric at the gastroduodenal junction.

The shape and size of the stomach vary with body build, position, contents, digestive stage, development of gastric muscles, sex, posture, and condition of adjacent intestine. Its capacity is approximately 1 quart or 1 L of food or liquid. When distended, it may impede the descent of the diaphragm during inhalation.

The stomach wall, like that of the esophagus, has four layers (Fig. 35-4).:

1. The serous coat (tunica serosa), the outermost layer, consists of areolar tissue. It continues as a double fold from the lower edge of the stomach to cover the intestine.
2. The muscular coat (tunica muscularis) has three smooth muscle layers instead of the usual two: (a) an external longitudinal layer; (b) a middle circular layer; and (c) an inner oblique layer, which extends from the fundus to the pyloric antrum.
3. The submucous coat (tunica submucosa) consists of loose areolar connective tissue, blood vessels, lymphatics, elastic fibers, and nerve plexuses.
4. The mucous coat (tunica mucosa), the innermost layer, consists of a muscular layer that is arranged in longitudinal folds, or rugae, that can expand. This layer contains 35 million glands that secrete up to 3000 ml of gastric juice per day.

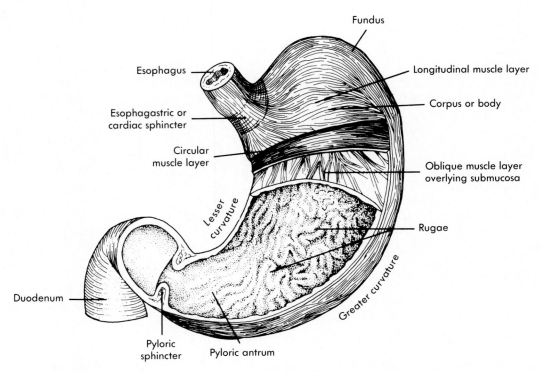

Fig. 35-3 Gross anatomy of the stomach. (From Broadwell DC and Jackson BS, editors: Principles of ostomy care, St Louis, 1982, The CV Mosby Co.)

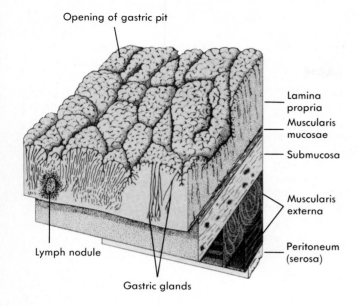

Opening of gastric pit

Lamina propria

Muscularis mucosae

Submucosa

Muscularis externa

Peritoneum (serosa)

Lymph nodule

Gastric glands

Fig. 35-4 Structure of the gastric mucosa. (From Berne RM and Levy MN, editors: Physiology, ed 2, St Louis, 1988, The CV Mosby Co.)

The large blood supply required for the motor and secretory activity of the stomach is provided by the celiac axis. Venous drainage occurs through the portal vein. Numerous lymphatic channels arise in the submucosa and terminate in the thoracic duct.

The stomach receives food and stores it for a period of time, mixes it with gastric secretions, grinds it to a semifluid consistency called chyme, and delivers the chyme to the duodenum in a continuous fashion.

Storage. Food enters the body and fundus of the stomach through the cardiac sphincter and exits through the pylorus. As food enters, the stomach relaxes so there is minimal increase in pressure. This change in muscle tone, mediated by the vagus nerve, is coordinated with the swallowing center. Food may be stored for 30 minutes to 5 hours, depending on its nutrient composition.

Secretion and digestion. The stomach has approximately 35 million glands of various types that secrete 1500 to 3000 ml of gastric juice into the lumen per day, depending on the diet and other stimuli. The major components of gastric juice are hydrochloric acid (HCl), pepsinogen, and mucus. Other components are intrinsic factor, inorganic salts such as potassium, gastric lipase, and protein (gastrin, a hormone produced by the G cells, is secreted into the blood).

Gastric juice has a pH near 1, but when mixed with food, its pH rises to 2 to 3. Peptic activity is optimal at a pH of 3.5. Gastric juice dissolves soluble foods, brings them close to the osmolarity of plasma, and also has bacteriostatic action.

The rate, amount, and type of gastric secretion are tightly controlled. The number of glands in the mucosa and the sensitivity of these glands to stimuli affect secretory activity, but the major stimuli are vagal (acetylcholine) activity, the antral hormone gastrin, and histamine.

Gastric secretion peaks 45 minutes after ingestion of food but never completely stops. By 3 hours after food ingestion, basal secretion is restored.

Motor functions. Motor functions of the stomach include relaxation for storage, peristaltic (mixing) activity, and emptying. Motor functions are regulated by (1) afferent and efferent fibers of the sympathetic and parasympathetic nervous systems, (2) reflexes operating through the celiac and intrinsic plexuses, and (3) gastric hormones.

Storage. At the beginning of a meal, receptive relaxation occurs, mediated by the vagus nerve. The stomach stretches in response to swallowing and gastric pressure and increases to a 1-L volume maximally. Vagotomy decreases the distensibility of the proximal stomach.

Peristaltic activity. The mixing and churning process, which causes semisolid liquid chyme to form, is initiated by neurogenic and hormonal stimuli. Gastric wall distention stimulates mechanoreceptors in the stomach wall. Long reflexes over the vagus nerve and short reflexes through the internal nerve plexuses mediate the resulting augmentation of peristalsis. Contractions propel chyme through the pyloric canal into the small intestine.

Only as much chyme is admitted as can be handled by the small intestine. Chyme having a high fat content is slowed because bile secretion controls its accommodation. Regulation and coordination are provided by duodenal and jejunal enterogastrone. GI hormones gastrin, secretin, cholecystokinin, somatostatin, and gastric inhibitory peptide, (at nonphysiological concentrations) inhibit gastric emptying. Acid chyme is slowed until pancreatic enzymes and mucus neutralize the acidity. In contrast, vasoactive intestinal peptide increases gastric motility and relaxes the pyloric sphincter.

Emptying. The rate of gastric emptying is influenced by the volume, chemical composition, acidity, osmolality, caloric density, and temperature of the chyme. Highly acidic chyme inhibits emptying. Liquids empty before solids, and this emptying occurs faster in the sitting position or when lying on the right side. Hyperosmolar and hypoosmolar solutions slow gastric emptying; fatty acids retard emptying. Unsaturated fatty acids retard emptying more than saturated fatty acids. Temperature extremes (hot or cold) likewise retard emptying. Although the chemical and physical properties of the meal dominate the pace of emptying, other factors are also important. Pain, anxiety, sadness, and hostility inhibit emptying, whereas aggression accelerates emptying.

Narcotic analgesics also inhibit emptying. Anticholinergics can inhibit antral peristalsis and delay emptying but not in conventional doses. Metoclopramide accelerates gastric emptying by facilitating acetylcholine release.

Gastric statis occurs in numerous pathological conditions, including iron deficiency anemia, brain tumor, gastric carcinoma, hepatic coma, hypocalcemia, hypokalemia, irradiation, malnutrition, pancreatic disease, peritonitis, sepsis, uremia, and vagotomy.

Absorption. Epithelial cells of the gastric mucosa are very closely packed and thus serve as a protective barrier, preventing diffusion of hydrogen into the mucosa. Epithelial cells are in a constant state of growth, migration, and desquamation and are shed at a rate of one-half million per minute. Certain lipid-soluble substances can break the mucosal barrier and penetrate the cells, causing their destruction, edema, and bleeding. These substances include alcohol, lysolecithins, regurgitated bile acids, and other aliphatic acids such as acetic, butyric, propionic, salicylic, and acetylsalicylic.

Small Intestine

The small intestine, a coiled, folded tube approximately 7 m (22 to 23 feet) long, extends from the pyloric sphincter to the cecum and fills most of the abdominal cavity. The small intestine has three anatomical divisions:

1. The duodenum, shaped like the letter C, begins at the pyloric sphincter of the stomach. It is 25 cm (10 inches) long and 4 cm (1 to 1½ inches) wide.
2. The jejunum, the middle portion, lies in the left iliac and umbilical regions. It is 250 cm (8 to 9½ feet) long and 4 cm (1 to 1½ inches) wide.
3. The ileum, the terminus, lies in the hypogastric, right iliac, and pelvic regions. It is 375 cm (12 feet) long and 2.5 cm (1 inch) wide.

Although the demarcating line between the jejunum and the ileum is somewhat arbitrary, the ileum is narrower than the jejunum. The ileocecal valve, located at the terminal end of the ileum at the junction of the cecum and colon, controls the flow of small bowel contents into the large intestine and prevents reflux.

The small intestine undergoes extensive growth during the life cycle. At birth, it is 25% of its full length and 13% of its full diameter. The absorptive surface of the infant's small intestine is 950 cm, whereas that of the adult of 7600 cm.

The small intestine has four layers (Fig. 35-5): (1) the outer serosal layer (tunica serosa); (2) the muscular layer (tunica muscularis); (3) the submucous layer (tunica mucosa); and (4) the inner mucous membrane (tunica mucosa).

The mucous and submucous layers are arranged in visible circular folds, which are largest and most numerous in the distal duodenum and proximal jejunum and disappear in the lower ileum. These folds are covered by a second series of folds called villi, which are projections 0.5 to 1.5 mm long that are in constant motion—constricting, lengthening, and shortening. There are 4 to 5 million villi (see Fig. 35-5), which give the intestine a velvety appearance. They are more numerous and larger in the jejunum than in the ileum. Villi contain a network of capillaries and blind lymphatic vessels called lacteals. The villus' core also contains smooth muscle strands and free cells such as lymphocytes, plasma cells, and granular leukocytes. The outer layer of the villus is composed of microvilli. The circular folds of the small intestine, along with the villi and microvilli, increase the digestive-absorptive surface of the small intestine 600 times.

The lymphatic system in the mucosa of the jejunum and ileum includes (1) solitary nodules, which are supplied by one vein and one artery each and their own capillary system, and (2) aggregated, circular-shaped lymph nodes (Peyer's patches), which consist of groups of 20 to 30 nodes and occur only in the ileum.

Extrinsic innervation is provided by both the sympathetic and parasympathetic systems. Sympathetic stimuli (epinephrine and norepinephrine) inhibit motility. Parasympathetic fibers of the vagus nerve (through acetylcholine) increase tone and motility and regulate intestinal reflexes. Resection of the vagus nerve has minimal effect on the small bowel. Intrinsic innervation, which initiates motor functions, is provided by two plexuses (Auerbach's and Meissner's) in the intestinal wall.

Functions. The functions of the small intestine include secretion, digestion, absorption and transport, mixing and peristalsis, and emptying. As chyme enters the duodenum, it encounters secretions derived from the pancreas, liver, gallbladder, and small bowel. Only as much chyme is admitted as can be accommodated by these secretions. Peristalsis and villous movement facilitate the mixing of secretions with chyme. Large molecules of food are thus broken down to smaller ones, and water-insoluble substances are made soluble so that they can be better absorbed. Absorption of nutrients occurs by a variety of mechanisms, depending on the physicochemical properties, the molecular weight, and the osmolality of the nutrient.

Secretion. The small intestine has two major types of glands, Brunner's glands and intestinal glands. Brunner's glands lie in the mucosa of the duodenum and secrete mucous, an alkaline fluid (pH of 9) that neutralizes chyme and protects the mucosa. Intestinal glands are found in pits of the mucosa and are called the crypts of Lieberkühn. These crypts secrete 2 to 3 L per day of yellowish fluid containing enzymes that assist in nutrient digestion.

GI hormones influence the release of secretions from the stomach and other organs emptying into the duodenum. They also regulate small bowel motility, the osmolality of luminal contents, and the duodenal pH (maintained between 7 and 9). There are two families of intestinal hormones: (1) the gastrin type, which includes gastrin and cholecystokinin, and (2) the secretin type, which includes secretin, gastric inhibitory peptide, vasoactive intestinal peptide, and enteroglucagon.

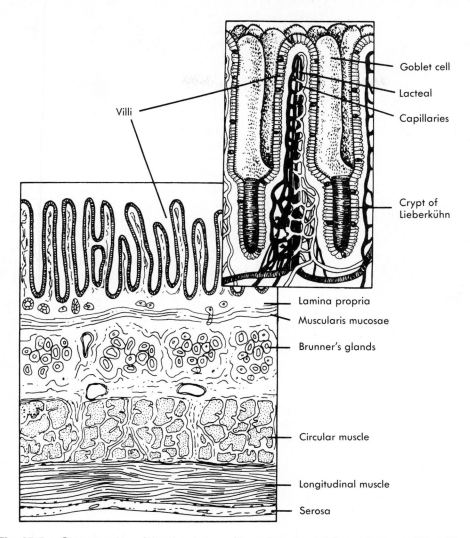

Fig. 35-5 Cross section of the duodenum. (From Broadwell DC and Jackson BS, editors: Principles of ostomy care, St Louis, 1982, The CV Mosby Co.)

Digestion and absorption. The process of digestion, which involves breaking down larger molecules into small ones, is essential for most nutrients absorbed from the small intestine. Optimal conditions for digestion are maintained through pH and osmolality controls within the small intestine. The entry of chyme into the duodenum stimulates the production of secretin, which in turn stimulates the pancreas to secrete a highly alkaline fluid into the duodenum. As chyme enters the duodenum, it is mixed with the combined secretions of the duodenal mucosa and pancreas and bile from the liver and gallbladder.

The small intestine absorbs up to 8 L of fluid per day, passing only a small part of this fluid into the large intestine. Carbohydrates, fats, amino acids, electrolytes, and water constitute the absorbed fluid. Additionally, components of saliva, gastric juice, bile, and intestinal and pancreatic secretions are also absorbed.

Peristalsis in the small intestine is characterized by circular muscular contractions, the purpose of which is to continue the mixing of food and digestive juices. Peristalsis occurs when a portion of the intestinal wall is distended with chyme. This distention initiates contractions along the intestine, giving the small bowel the look of a chain of sausage links. Chyme is chopped 7 to 11 times per minute by these contractions.

Peristalsis within the small intestine is controlled by Auerbach's plexus. Peristaltic waves move chyme 2 to 25 cm (1 to 10 inches) per minute toward the ileocecal valve. Between meals and during fasting and sleeping, an interdigestive sequence of muscle contractions occurs every 90 minutes and proceeds from the antrum to the ileum.

Liver

The liver is the largest internal organ in the body. Weighing 1200 to 1600 g (3 to 4 pounds), it is friable, dark red in color, and of a soft-solid consistency. Located in the right upper abdominal quadrant, it fits snugly against the right interior diaphragm. The liver is surrounded by connective tissue known as Glisson's capsule, which is covered by serosa and contains blood vessels and lymphatics. The peri-

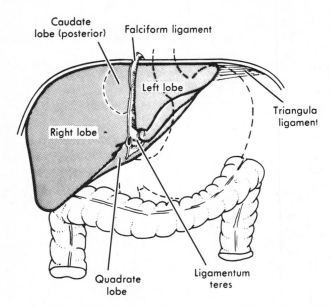

Fig. 35-6 Anatomy of the liver. (From Given BA and Simmons SJ: Gastroenterology in clinical nursing, ed 4, St Louis, 1984, The CV Mosby Co.)

toneum covering the liver forms the falciform ligament, which attaches the liver to the anterior portion of the abdomen between the diaphragm and umbilicus and divides the liver into two main lobes, right and left (Fig. 35-6). The right lobe, which is six times larger than the left, has three sections: the right lobe proper, the caudate lobe, and the quadrate lobe. The left lobe is divided into two sections. Each lobe is divided into numerous lobules.

Circulation. The liver receives one third of the total cardiac output from two major sources: the hepatic artery, which provides oxygenated blood; and the portal vein, which is supplied with nutrient-rich blood from the gut, pancreas, spleen, stomach, and mesentery. The portal vein, which accounts for 75% of the total liver blood flow, branches into sinusoids to transport blood to each lobule. Unlike capillaries, sinusoids lack a definite cell wall but contain a lining of phagocytic (Kupffer's) cells and some nonphagocytic cells of modified epithelium. Sinusoids empty blood into an intralobular vein in the center of the lobule. Intralobular veins empty into larger veins and finally into the hepatic vein, which empties on the posterior surface of the liver and eventually into the vena cava. The hepatic artery also divides and subdivides between the lobules, supplying sinusoids with oxygenated blood before emptying into the hepatic vein.

Lymphatic spaces are between liver cells. Lymph drains into lymphatic vessels surrounding the hepatic vein and bile ducts.

Function. The liver's parenchymal cells (hepatocytes) have a variety of nondigestive functions that are beyond the scope of this text. However, the reader should be aware of the role of the liver in carbohydrate hemostasis, metabolism, and storage. Glycogen, the stored form of glucose, can be synthesized from glucose or from protein, fat, or lactic acid.

Glycogen is broken down to glucose by the liver to maintain normal blood glucose levels. The liver also has a vital role in amino acid metabolism and can synthesize amino acids from metabolites of carbohydrates and fats. The liver synthesizes plasma proteins such as globulins and albumin, important in maintaining the normal osmotic balance of blood, and also synthesizes the clotting factors, fibrogen and prothrombin. The liver deaminates amino acids to produce ketoacids and ammonia, from which urea is formed. In fat metabolism, the liver hydrolyzes triglycerides to glycerol and fatty acids in the process of ketogenesis and synthesizes phospholipids, cholesterol, and lipoproteins. Steroid hormones are conjugated, and polypeptide hormones are inactivated by the liver. Additionally, fat-soluble vitamins, vitamin B_{12}, and the minerals iron and copper are stored by the liver. Finally, detoxification of drugs and toxins and degradation of worn red blood cells occurs in the liver's Kupffer's cells, which belong to the reticuloendothelial system.

Bile. The production of bile makes the liver a vital organ in digestion and absorption. The major components of bile are bile pigments, bile salts, cholesterol, neutral fats, phospholipids, inorganic salts, fatty acids, mucin, conjugated bilirubin, lecithin, and water, with traces of albumin, gamma globulin, urea, nitrogen, and glucose. The principal electrolytes of bile are sodium chloride and bicarbonate, and the major pigment is bilirubin.

Bile functions to emulsify fat globules to facilitate digestion by lipases and to facilitate fat digestion and absorption of fat-soluble vitamins. Bile salts also serve as an excretion route for bilirubin, cholesterol, and various hormones (sex, thyroid, and adrenal). Approximately 80% of bile salts are reabsorbed actively in the distal ileum and are recycled to the liver through the enterohepatic circulation; only 20% are lost in the feces.

Bilirubin, the primary bile pigment, is formed from the heme portion of hemoglobin during the degradation of red blood cells by Kupffer's cells. When released into the bloodstream, billirubin binds to albumin as fat-soluble, unconjugated (indirect) bilirubin. Taken up by liver hepatocytes, indirect bilirubin is conjugated with glucuronic acid to form water-soluble, conjugated (direct) bilirubin, which is then excreted through hepatic ducts into the intestine. In the large intestine, bilirubin is converted to a series of urobilinogen compounds. One of these, stercobilin, gives the stool its color. A very small amount of urobilinogen is reabsorbed into the portal blood and is recycled to the liver. If the amount of bilirubin sent to the liver is in excess, the ability of the liver to conjugate the bilirubin may be taxed; thus free, unconjugated indirect bilirubin will appear in the blood. High levels of indirect (unconjugated) bilirubin in the blood suggest hepatocellular dysfunction, whereas high levels of direct (conjugated) bilirubin suggest biliary tract obstruction.

Bile capillaries, located between liver cells, radiate through the edge of hepatic lobules. After entering interlobular bile ducts, these capillaries become progressively larger until they form the left and right hepatic ducts, which combine to form the hepatic duct. The hepatic duct unites with the cystic duct to form the common bile duct.

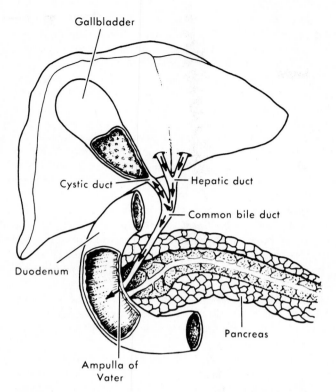

Gallbladder

Cystic duct

Hepatic duct

Common bile duct

Duodenum

Pancreas

Ampulla of Vater

Fig. 35-7 Anatomy of the biliary system. (From Given BA and Simmons SJ: Gastroenterology in clinical nursing, ed 4, St Louis, 1984, The CV Mosby Co.)

Biliary System

The biliary system (Fig. 35-7) consists of the gallbladder and its related ductal system, including the hepatic, cystic, and common bile ducts.

Ductal System. Bile, continuously formed in the liver, is excreted into the hepatic duct, which transports bile to the gallbladder. The hepatic duct then joins the cystic duct, forming the common bile duct, which empties into the duodenum. The common bile duct is surrounded by the sphincter of Oddi, which pierces the wall of the duodenum and controls the flow of bile into the duodenum.

Gallbladder. The gallbladder is a pear-shaped organ 7 to 10 cm (3 to 4 inches) long and 2.5 to 3.5 cm (1 to 1½ inches) wide, lying on the underside of the liver (see Fig. 35-7). It is attached to the liver by connective tissue, peritoneum, and blood vessels.

The main functions of the gallbladder are to collect, concentrate, acidify, and store bile entering it through the cystic duct from the hepatic duct. It can store up to 50 to 60 ml of bile from which approximately 90% of the water is removed so that bile is concentrated approximately 15 to 29 times. Cholesterol and pigment are likewise concentrated. Bile, which is golden or orange-yellow in the liver, becomes dark brown when concentrated in the gallbladder. By altering its shape and volume, the gallbladder regulates pressure within the extrahepatic biliary system. Relaxation of the sphincter of Oddi, which surrounds the common bile duct as it enters the duodenum, is coordinated with gall-

bladder contraction through the regulatory action of cholecystokinin. Psychic factors such as the sight, smell, and taste of food can stimulate gallbladder contraction, whereas fear or excitement decrease contraction. After a meal, the amount of bile entering the duodenum increases as a result of enhanced liver secretion and gallbladder contraction. Intestinal secretion of cholecystokinin and secretin, high levels of bile salts in the blood, and vagal stimulation increase biliary secretion.

Pancreas

The pancreas is a soft, lobulated, fish-shaped gland lying beneath the duodenum and the spleen (see Fig. 35-7). Pinkish-yellow in color, it is 10 to 22 cm (5 to 10 inches) long and 5 cm (1 to 1½ inches) wide. Its anatomical divisions include the head, which lies in the C-shaped curve of the duodenum to which it is attached; the body, the main part of the gland, which extends horizontally across the abdomen and is largely hidden behind the stomach; and the tail, a thin, narrow portion in contact with the spleen.

The main pancreatic duct, the duct of Wirsung, traverses the entire length of the organ. Wirsung's duct empties exocrine secretions into the ampulla of Vater, which is the same lumen draining the common bile duct, at the entrance to the duodenum. (In 40% of the population, the pancreatic duct and common bile duct empty separately into the duodenum. Approximately 15% of the population have an accessory duct, the duct of Santorini, which empties into the duodenum above the ampulla of Vater.)

The internal structural unit of the exocrine pancreas, the lobule, consists of numerous small alveoli lined with secretory cells called tubuloacinar cells (that is, shaped like tiny tubes and grapes). Each acinus has a small duct that empties into lobular ducts. Lobules are joined by connective tissue into lobes, which unite to form the gland. Likewise, the ducts from each lobule empty into the duct of Wirsung.

Exocrine functions. Exocrine functions of the pancreas are limited to digestion. Acinar cells secrete pancreatic juice, which consists of water, sodium bicarbonate, and electrolytes (sodium, potassium) at a highly alkaline pH. Enzymes produced in the pancreas include the following: (1) proteolytic endopeptidases (i.e., trypsin, chymotrypsin, and carboxypeptidase), which are secreted as inactive precursors, and aminopeptidase, which is secreted in the active form, (2) deoxyribonuclease and ribonuclease, (3) amylase, and (4) lipase and cholesterol esterase. Within the secretory cells of the pancreas, a trypsin inhibitor prevents activation of trypsinogen, thus inhibiting autodigestion, the underlying pathology of acute pancreatitis.

Pancreatic exocrine function is regulated by hormonal and neural signals. Hormonal signals are provided primarily by the intestinal hormones secretin and cholecystokinin, which are released from the duodenum and jejunum in response to stimulation by chyme in the intestine. Absorbed by the portal system, these hormones are transported to the pancreas. Secretin causes the pancreas to produce a high volume of fluid rich in water and bicarbonate, whereas cholecystokinin causes it to produce a juice rich in enzymes but low in volume. The two hormones potentiate each other's effects on the pancreas.

Although hormonal controls of the exocrine pancreas are believed only supplemental to vagal regulation, hormonal regulation of the exocrine pancreas is apparently more complex. In addition to secretin, vasoactive intestinal peptide may also mediate an increase in pancreatic fluid and bicarbonate secretion. In contrast to these hormones, which are stimulatory, somatostatin, vasopressin, and calcitonin have inhibitory functions in the exocrine pancreas.

In the duodenum, pancreatic sodium bicarbonate reacts with hydrochloric acid to produce carbonic acid, which is carried to the lungs from which it is excreted as carbon dioxide and sodium chloride.

Parasympathetic stimulation of the pancreas increases exocrine secretions and blood flow to the pancreas. Anticholinergics decrease enzyme production, volume output, and ductal pressure. Alcohol and histamine, by stimulating gastric hydrochloric acid production, indirectly cause an increase in pancreatic secretions. Sympathetic stimulation is inhibitory.

Endocrine functions. Endocrine tissue consists of spherical islets called *islets of Langerhans,* which are embedded within the lobules of acinar tissue throughout the pancreas, especially in the distal body and tail. Endocrine products include insulin (produced in beta cells), glucagon (produced in alpha cells), and gastrin; all of these hormones are secreted directly into the bloodstream. Further discussion of the endocrine functions of the pancreas is in Chapter 39.

Large Intestine (Colon)

The large intestine, or colon, is approximately 150 cm (5 feet) long and extends from the ileocecal valve to the anus. The divisions of the colon are the ascending colon, hepatic flexure, transverse colon, splenic flexure, descending colon, sigmoid colon, rectum, and anal canal. The caliber of the colon decreases as it proceeds distally and averages 1½ to 2 inches in width.

Colonic layers. As with the small intestine, the colon has four layers. Beginning with the outermost layer, they are the serosa, muscular layer, submucosa, and mucosa. The serosa is formed from the visceral peritoneum and covers most of the colon, with the exclusion of the distal rectum. Appendices epiploicae (fat tags) project from the serosa.

The muscular layer contains two smooth muscles: the circular and the longitudinal. These muscles work together to propel fecal matter through the colon and also to "knead" the stool into a compact bolus. The longitudinal muscle consists of three muscular bands (teniae coli) stretching from the cecum to the distal sigmoid colon. These muscular bands create sacculations of haustra, which are important clinical features and are normally apparent on a barium enema radiograph. Haustra aid segmentation so that absorption of fluid from the fecal bolus is achieved. The absence of haustra is associated with severe inflammation of the mucosal layer and may extend into the serosa layer.

The longitudinal muscle and the circular muscle work together to produce two primary types of colonic movement. Segmentation, which is the alternate contraction and relaxation of haustral folds, involves the circular muscle and facilitates (1) the grinding of food masses, and (2) fluid absorption. Peristalsis, the second type of movement, is produced primarily by the longitudinal muscles and propels the fecal bolus forward. Mass peristalsis is a strong, slow contraction in which the distal left colon contracts en masse to move the fecal bolus into the rectum.

The submucosa contains small arteries, veins, and lymphatic vessels and connects the muscular layer to the inner mucosal layer. The innermost layer of the colon is the mucosa, is lined with simple columnar epithelial cells, and contains deep crypts of Lieberkühn (or intestinal glands) that are lined with mucus-producing goblet cells. Mucus is produced to ease the passage of the fecal material and to protect the mucosal surface from trauma. Water and electrolytes are also absorbed through the mucosa.

Rectum. The rectum begins midsacrum, is 12 to 15 cm (5 inches) long, and is quite angulated. These angles, also known as valves of Houston, are important in the defecation process because they tend to slow the passage of fecal material in the rectal vault, thus assisting the continence mechanism.

The rectum is subdivided into three sections: the upper, middle, and lower thirds. These subdivisions allow more precision in describing the location of pathology in the rectum.

The terminal portion of the GI tract, the anal canal, begins at the anorectal junction, ends at the anal verge, and is approximately 3 to 4 cm long. The anal canal is always contracted and is surrounded by strong muscles. Midpoint in the anal canal is an undulating demarcation referred to as the dentate line, or pectinate line. It is near this dentate line that the mucosal epithelium makes the transition from columnar epithelium to squamous epithelium, which resembles true skin.

Sphincters. Two sphincters, the internal and the external, guard the passage of colonic contents along the anal canal. The internal sphincter is an involuntary muscle formed by a circular muscle, and it is always contracted and encircles the dentate line. The external sphincter consists of striated muscles that encircle the entire anal canal. Although both sphincters are maintained at a state of maximal contraction, the external sphincter can be voluntarily relaxed or tightened to control the passage of stool or flatus.

Pelvic floor muscles. The pelvic floor muscles are critical to both bowel and bladder function. Two of these muscles are the puborectalis and the levator ani. These muscles encircle the anal canal and also line the floor of the pelvis. Contraction of these muscles further angulates the rectum to prevent elimination, whereas relaxation allows the passage of stool.

Innervation. The colon has an intrinsic nervous system, which consists of the myenteric plexus (located between muscle layers) and the submucosal, or Auerbach's, plexus (located in the submucosa). These nerves control colonic movement and secretion of mucus, respectively.

Both the sympathetic and parasympathetic branches of the autonomic system innervate the colon. Sympathetic stimulation inhibits colonic activity and relaxes the anal sphincters. Parasympathetic stimulation increases colonic activity and secretion but relaxes the anal sphincter. The sigmoid colon, rectum, and anal canal are richly innervated with parasympathetic fibers to aide in the defecation process.

The mucosa of the distal anal canal is sensitive to pain and touch in contrast to the remainder of the colon, which is sensitive only to stretch.

Functions. The major functions of the colon are as follows:

1. Reabsorption of water, sodium, chloride, glucose, and urea
2. Dehydration of undigested residue
3. Putrefaction of contents by bacteria
4. Movement of the fecal bolus through the colon
5. Elimination of the fecal mass

The colon receives approximately 600 ml to 1000 ml of fluid per day. All but 100 to 150 ml of it will be absorbed in the ascending and transverse colon.

Potassium is secreted into the colonic lumen partially in the potassium-rich mucus secreted by goblet cells. Bicarbonate is secreted by the colon, creating an alkaline fecal matter with a pH of 7.8.

The colon contains billions of anaerobic bacteria that serve the following three functions:

1. To putrefy remaining proteins and indigestible residue
2. To synthesize folic acid, vitamin K, nicotinic acid, riboflavin, and some B vitamins
3. To convert urea salts to ammonium salts and ammonia for absorption into the portal circulation

Common colonic bacteria are *Escherichia coli, Aerobacter aerogenes, Clostridium perfringens,* and *Lactobacillus bifidus.*

Colonic gas is a normal product of swallowed air, diffusion from the blood, and bacterial action. The composition of intestinal gas is oxygen, nitrogen, carbon dioxide, methane, hydrogen, and trace gases. Fecal odor is a consequence of the trace gases.

Feces is expelled from the colon through the defecation process, a complex act involving both autonomic and voluntary efforts. The stimulus for evacuation is distention of the rectum. The box at right lists the normal composition of fecal material.

COMPOSITION OF FECAL MATTER

Bile pigments	Cellulose
Mucus	Epithelial cells
Unabsorbed minerals	5-10 cc sodium
Undigested fats	50-200 ml water
7-10 mEq potassium	pH of 7.8
2 mEq chloride	3 mEq bicarbonate
Meat protein toxins	

Modified from Givens RA and Simmons ST: Gastroenterology in clinical nursing, ed 4, St Louis, 1984, The CV Mosby Co, and Broadwell DC and Jackson BS: Principles of ostomy care, St Louis, 1982, The CV Mosby Co.

REFERENCES

1. Given BA and Simmons SJ: Structure and function of the human gastrointestinal tracts. In Gastroenterology in clinical nursing, ed 4, St Louis, 1984, The CV Mosby Co.
2. Guyton AC: Textbook of physiology, ed 7, Philadelphia, 1986, WB Saunders Co.
3. Heitkemper MM and Morotta SF: Role of diets in modifying gastrointestinal neurotransmitter enzyme activity, Nurs Res 34:19, 1985.
4. Kim MS: Physiologic responses in health and illness: an overview, Ann Rev Nutr Res 5:79, 1987.
5. Moran JR and Greene HL: Digestion and absorption. In Rombeau JL and Caldwell MD, editors: Enteral and tube feeding, clinical nutrition, vol 2, Philadelphia, 1984, WB Saunders Co.
6. Ropka M: Alimentation. In Abels L, editor: Critical care nursing, St Louis, 1986, The CV Mosby Co.
7. Rowlands BJ and Miller TA: The physiology of eating. With particular reference to the role of gastrointestinal hormones in the regulation of digestion. In Rombeau JL and Caldwell JD, editors: Enteral and tube feeding, clinical nutrition, vol 1, Philadelphia, 1984, WB Saunders Co.

36

Gastrointestinal Assessment

CLINICAL AND LABORATORY ASSESSMENT AND DIAGNOSTIC PROCEDURES

CHAPTER OBJECTIVES

- *Discuss the rationale involved in developing a consistent, sequential format for performing a gastrointestinal nursing assessment.*
- *Perform a thorough nursing assessment of the gastrointestinal system on a critically ill patient and interpret the results.*
- *Outline the impact surgery has on a critically ill patient's nutritional status.*
- *Detail the relevant nursing care before, during, and after liver biopsy.*
- *List important diagnostic procedures for detection of large bowel disorders.*

CLINICAL ASSESSMENT
History

An integral part of nursing care is use of information obtained from the patient and/or his or her family during an initial interview. The health history for a critical care unit patient may be obtained by other health care clinicians (for example, a resident or a paramedic) and is very abbreviated because of the rapidly changing status of critically ill patients.

There are two specific considerations in obtaining and using the history and results of the physical examination of the patient with an alteration in the gastrointestinal (GI) system. First, because alterations in nutritional status can be either causative or resultant, an accurate nutritional assessment should be incorporated into the assessment process to provide better patient care. Second, as the population grows increasingly older, the percent of elderly patients admitted to critical care units is increasing, having implications for this area of nursing practice.

Patients with suspected or confirmed GI disorders should have their health history reviewed for the following:
1. Past health history, including any previous surgery (Table 36-1), diseases (Table 36-2), or hospitalizations.
2. Potential nonspecific problems that may affect the GI system—changes in weight, appetite, or activity level.
3. Location and description of symptoms, including the site, pain characteristics, and temporal relationship to events (for example, food intake, time of day).
4. Intake and output (food elimination)—diet (food patterns), nutritional status, bowel characteristics (stool descriptions), use of medication and alcohol.

To help ascertain the nutritional status of a patient, the nurse should review the history, focusing on weight loss, edema, anorexia, vomiting, diarrhea, decreased or unusual food intake, and chronic illness.

Table 36-1   Surgical impact on nutritional status

Organ(s) resected	Nutritional implications
Oropharynx	Tube dependency (loss of gastrointestinal access)
Esophagus	Malabsorption of fat, loss of normal swallowing function, decreased motility, obstruction
Stomach	Dumping syndrome, anemia, delayed emptying, malabsorption
Pancreas	Exocrine and/or endocrine insufficiency
Small bowel	Steatorrhea, bile acid depletion, fat malabsorption, anemia (B_{12} malabsorption), short gut syndrome

Modified from Knox LS: Nurs Clin North Am 18(1):103, 1983.

Table 36-2 Gastrointestinal disorders associated with micronutrient disorders

Disease state or historical feature	Associated deficiency
Pancreatic insufficiency	Vitamins A, D, E, K
Gastrectomy	Vitamins A, D, E, B$_{12}$, folic acid, iron, calcium
Liver disease, alcoholism	Vitamins A, C, D, riboflavin, niacin, thiamine, folic acid, magnesium, zinc
Short bowel syndrome, ileal resection	Vitamin B$_{12}$, folic acid, calcium, magnesium
Blind loop syndrome	Vitamin B$_{12}$
Bile salt depletion, cholestyramine ingestion	Vitamins A, K
Obstructive jaundice	Vitamins A, K
Prolonged antacid therapy, peptic ulcer disease	Thiamine, vitamin C
Miscellaneous disorders:	
Prolonged antibiotic therapy	Vitamin K
Fever	Vitamins A, C, thiamine, riboflavin, folic acid

ASSESSMENT OF THE ORAL CAVITY

INSPECTION

Lips: symmetry, color, edema, surface abnormalities
Tongue: swelling, variation in size or color, coating, ulceration, ability to move
Gums: inflammation, bleeding
Gag reflex: intact
Mouth odors or exudate

PALPATION

Generally performed only during extensive examination of ambulatory patient or if abnormality is detected during inspection

RELATED INFORMATION
Elderly patients (several changes are age-related)

Difficulty in chewing and dysphagia: salivary production slows and thickens; problems can be related to temporomandibular joint degeneration or loose, lost, or worn teeth
Dry mouth, halitosis: salivary production drops and becomes more alkaline
Pale gums: capillary blood supply diminishes
Vermilion border of mouth missing: skin loses elasticity
Yellow papules on oral mucosa: sebaceous glands enlarge (Fordyce's granules)

A compounding problem is the nonspecificity of symptoms as they relate to the GI system; that is, there are systemic manifestations of GI disorders as well as other disorders that have a GI manifestation. The patient's history should be examined for information about multiple drug intake, GI alterations potentially caused by normal aging, and changes in psychosocial parameters that could result in physical problems (for example, lack of money for dentures—dysphagia).

Physical Examination

The clinical assessment helps establish baseline data about the physical dimensions of the patient's situation. In adapting the assessment for the critically ill GI patient, the nurse should do the following:
1. Use the classic four approaches of inspection, palpation, percussion, and auscultation.
2. Modify technique, extent, and frequency of assessment based on the patient's pain level and whether abnormal results are obtained.
3. Use appropriate assessment standards established for elderly persons when reviewing their physical findings.

The assessment should proceed when the patient is as comfortable as possible and is in a supine position; however, the position may need readjustment if it elicits pain. To prevent stimulation of GI activity, the order for the assessment should be changed to inspection, auscultation, percussion, and palpation. Although assessment of the GI system classically begins with inspection of the abdomen, the patient's oral cavity must also be inspected to determine any unusual findings (see the box above).

Percussion and palpation elicit information about deep organs such as the liver, spleen, and pancreas. Because the abdomen is a sensitive area, muscle tension may interfere with assessment. Percussion often helps relax the tense muscles and so is performed before palpation. Percussion, in the absence of any disease, is most helpful in delineating the position and size of the liver and spleen. With percussion, fluid, gaseous distention, and masses in the abdominal region can be detected. Palpation is the technique most useful in detecting abdominal pathological conditions. The box on p. 686 provides a review of the clinical assessment, along with normal and abnormal findings and additional related information.

An examination of the rectal-anal region may be included in a GI assessment. The perianal skin should be inspected for any irritation, lesions, fistulas, or fissures. Hemorrhoids may explain blood noted by the patient with stools but should not be considered the only possible cause. Rectal bleeding requires further evaluation to rule out carcinoma.

The digital rectal examination is commonly used to detect, for example, a polyp, low-lying tumor, or bowel obstruction. Laxity of the sphincter muscle may provide information about fecal incontinence. Hard stool in the rectum may indicate an impaction and explain other symptoms such as constipation, diarrhea, abdominal pain, and/or distention.

CLINICAL ASSESSMENT OF THE ADULT GASTROINTESTINAL SYSTEM

INSPECTION
Procedure

Perform in warm, well-lighted environment with patient in comfortable position with abdomen exposed; view from slightly above and to one side of patient's abdomen.

Observe skin (pigmentation, lesions, striae, scars, dehydration venous pattern), contour, movement (respiratory, symmetry, peristalsis).

Normal findings

Skin: pigmentation varies considerably within normal because of race, ethnic background, occupation exposure; however, abdomen is generally lighter in color than other exposed areas.

Contour: slightly concave or slightly round appearance.

Movement: symmetrical; no visible pulsations or peristaltic waves.

Abnormal findings

Skin: jaundice, skin lesions, tenseness, glistening, stretch marks, scars (keloids), masses.

Contour: distended (asymmetrical/generalized).

Related information

Chart findings, using one of two anatomical maps (four quadrants or nine sections).

Geriatric

Connective tissue changes and lower total body water make determining dehydration through skin assessment difficult.

AUSCULTATION
Procedure

Listen below and to the right of umbilicus for bowel sounds; proceed methodically through all quadrants, lifting and placing diaphragm of stethoscope lightly.

Normal findings

Sounds in small intestine are high pitched and gurgling; colonic sounds are low pitch and have a rumbling quality.

Bowel sounds occur at a rate of 5 to 35/minute.

Abnormal findings

Lack of bowel sounds throughout 5-minute period, extremely soft and widely separated sounds, and increased sounds with characteristically high-pitched, loud rushing sound (peristaltic rush).

Bruits, peritoneal friction rubs, venous hums.

Related information

Normal venous hum is audible at times but is abnormal when heard in periumbilical region and accompanied by a palpable thrill.

Decreased bowel sounds are not significant without added data (for example, nausea, vomiting, digestion).

Geriatric

Pediatric chest piece on stethoscope is useful with emaciated patient.

Aging leads to lessened peristalsis (listen for full 5 minutes) and diminished mucus secretion in esophagus ("popping" sound as food is pushed down dry esophagus).

Laxative intake can cause loud gurgling sounds.

Bell of stethoscope is used to listen to vascular sounds; not uncommon to hear cardiac murmurs over abdominal area.

Because of decreased secretion of digestive enzymes, normal bowel sounds may sound "less combustible."

PERCUSSION
Procedure

Proceed systematically to percuss lightly the entire abdomen, including the liver and spleen.

Normal findings

Stomach: tympanic when empty.

Intestine: tympanic or hyperresonant.

Liver and spleen: dull.

Abnormal findings

Flatness over stomach.

Solid masses and distended bladder: dull sound.

Liver and spleen: dull sounds beyond anatomical borders.

Related information

Geriatric

Upper liver border usually is found in fourth or fifth intercostal space (adults) but in elderly drops to fifth to seventh intercostal space; liver span shrinks to 6 to 12 cm.

Changes in tonal quality in elderly is caused by changes in connective tissue and diminished muscle mass.

PALPATION
Procedure

Perform both light (tender) and deep palpation of each organ and each quadrant of abdomen.

Light: assesses depth of skin and fascia (depth approximately 1 cm).

Deep: assesses beneath rectus abdominis muscle; perform bimanually (4 to 5 cm deep).

Examine any areas in which patient complains of tenderness last.

CLINICAL ASSESSMENT OF THE ADULT GASTROINTESTINAL SYSTEM—cont'd

Normal findings

No areas of tenderness or pain.
No bulges, masses, or hardening.

Abnormal findings

Rebound tenderness, rigidity.
If enlarged, gallbladder (right upper quadrant) palpable as small mass attached to liver.
Spleen palpable only if enlarged.

Related information

Liver sometimes cannot be palpated in healthy adult; how-

ever, in extremely thin but healthy adult, it may be felt at the coastal margin.
Geriatric
Palpation of abdominal organs is easier because of relaxed abdominal musculature.
Loss of muscle tone is apparent, especially in diaphragm and costal margin.
Abdomen is preferred site for palpating skin to assess hydration because of wrinkling and loss of turgor elsewhere.

DIAGNOSTIC PROCEDURES
Liver Biopsy

Liver biopsy is a bedside procedure, usually performed for diagnosis of primary liver disease. Morphological, biochemical, bacteriological, and immunological studies can be performed on the tissue sample. It can also yield information about the progression of the patient's disease and response to therapy. It is performed less frequently for diagnosis of metabolic disease or malignancy or in patients with multisystem organ failure. The procedure requires patient compliance if performed without significant sedation. Generally it involves the following:

1. Anesthetizing the pericapsular tissue
2. Insertion of either a coring or suction needle between the eighth and ninth intercostal space while the patient either breathes lightly or holds his or her breath
3. Withdrawal of the needle with the sample
4. Positioning the patient on his or her right side for several hours (he or she must remain flat for 24 hours after the procedure)

The procedure is brief; however, it is not uncommon for the patient to experience some pain as a result of irritation to the liver tissue. Abdominal or radiating pain from the epigastric area should be reported immediately. Hemorrhage is a rare but serious complication, thus requiring monitoring of vital signs every 30 minutes for 4 hours and every hour for the next 8 hours. Other complications include damage to neighboring organs, bile peritonitis, infection at the needle site, and shock. This procedure is generally not undertaken if the patient is severely debilitated, is unable to cooperate, has bleeding tendencies or sepsis, or if liver dullness cannot be detected. Because of its invasive nature, possible complications, limited total organ assessment ability, and requirement of patient involvement, other techniques (liver scans, endoscopy) have evolved to partially replace the biopsy.

LABORATORY ASSESSMENT

The value of various laboratory procedures used to diagnose and treat diseases of the GI system has often been emphasized. However, no single test provides an overall picture of the various organs' functional state. Also, no single value is predictive by itself. More than 100 laboratory tests have been proposed for the study of the liver and biliary tract alone. For example, in a patient with cirrhosis, prothrombin time, bilirubin, alkaline phosphatase, alanine aminotransferase (ALT), and aspartate aminotransferase (AST) values all elevate, but hemoglobin and hematocrit values drop (secondary to red blood cell destruction and/or GI bleed). In a patient with hepatitis, serum transaminase values rise early then fall as bilirubin rises. Jaundice occurs as the total bilirubin value goes above 2.5 mg/dl. Mild prolongation of prothrombin time and elevation of alkaline phosphatase may occur. With hepatic coma, in addition to those values reflecting the underlying liver disease, a plasma aminogram shows altered amino acid patterns, and serum ammonia levels rise but do not correlate well with level of encephalopathy.

Liver Scans

Liver scans are currently used in assessing a patient's hepatic status. A liver-spleen scan involves intravenous (IV) injection of radioisotopes, the uptake of which is primarily in the liver and spleen with little or no uptake occurring in patients with cirrhosis or splenomegaly secondary to portal hypertension. A liver scan yields information about the size, vascularity, and blood flow of the organs. The scan requires IV injection of radionuclides. These short-lived isotopes concentrate in the bile, allowing visualization of the biliary system and gallbladder, along with emptying into the duodenum; nonvisualization indicates obstruction. The patient is not sedated but must be able to lie flat for 30 to 90 minutes during the scanning. Uptake results can indicate cirrhosis, hepatitis, tumors, abscesses, and cyst.

Endoscopy

Several forms of endoscopy are available for the direct visualization and evaluation of the lower GI tract. The main difference between them is the length of the colon that can be examined.

The proctoscope allows evaluation of only the few centimeters at and above the rectum. The flexible fiberoptic sigmoidoscope can view the anal canal, rectum, and sigmoid colon (up to 60 cm). With this instrument, approximately 60% of the polyps and colorectal cancers are detectable. Lastly, the colonoscope permits direct visualization of the entire colon and often the lower part of the small intestine.

The main value of the various lower GI scopes is their diagnostic potential. However, they also have a therapeutic benefit in that they allow removal of some suspicious lesions (for example, polyps), thus averting surgery.

Invasive tests have risks for the patient. Potential complications include bowel perforation (abdominal pain and distention, rectal bleeding, fever, mucopurulent drainage), hemorrhage, vasovagal stimulation, and oversedation. Fortunately, these complications are rare in the hands of an experienced physician.

Plain and Abdominal X-Ray Studies

Numerous radiological studies are available to investigate large bowel disease further. The most noninvasive are the plain films such as the chest and the abdominal x-ray. Air in the bowel serves as a contrast media to aid in the visualization of the bowel as shown in Fig. 36-1. Gas patterns (the presence of gas inside or outside the bowel lumen and the distribution of gas in dilated and nondilated bowel) are best revealed by plain films. These studies detect bowel obstruction, perforation, foreign bodies, and calcifications.

An erect chest x-ray film or an erect abdominal flat-plate film can demonstrate free gas, suggesting a pneumoperitoneum such as that shown in Fig. 36-2. The supine abdominal x-ray film (abdominal flat plate) also demonstrates the caliber of the bowel, which is an important determination in monitoring megacolon. When a patient is unable to sit or stand for erect films, a left-lateral decubitus radiograph is a good substitute. No special preparation is required for plain films.

Barium Enema

When clearer visualization of the colon is needed, a radiopaque liquid barium suspension is introduced into the colon through the rectum or through a colostomy. A barium enema in indicated when investigating colon cancer, colonic obstruction, diverticular disease, polyps, and inflammatory bowel disease.

Air-Contrast Barium Enema

To enhance the detail of the mucosal surface, air can also be introduced into the colon with the barium. This is called a double-contrast study.

When bowel perforation is suspected, a water-soluble contrast agent such as diatrizoate meglumine (Gastrografin) is the contrast medium used in place of barium. Its use is necessary because barium leakage into the abdominal cavity can cause peritonitis. No preparation is required for this test.

Fistulogram

A fistulogram is performed to visualize a fistulous tract and to identify communicating organs. A water-soluble con-

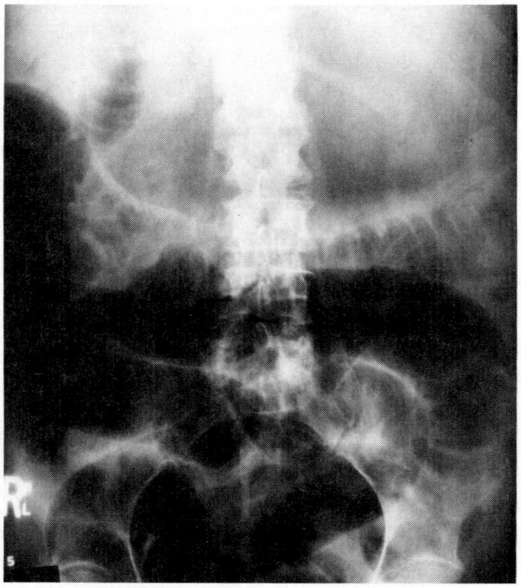

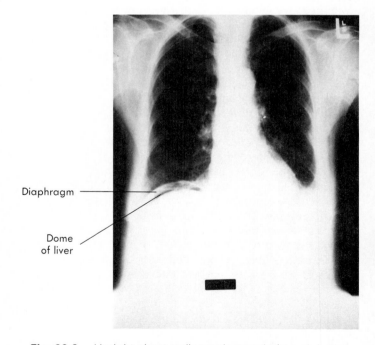

Diaphragm

Dome of liver

Fig. 36-1 Abdominal flat-plate film demonstrates a grossly dilated large bowel *(darker shadows)* and small bowel *(lighter contrast above colon)*. The air in the colon serves as the contrast agent.

Fig. 36-2 Upright chest radiograph reveals free air in the chest as the result of a perforation. Intraperitoneal air is located beneath the right diaphragm *(arrow)* and the dome of the liver *(arrow)*.

trast medium is instilled into the fistula. No special preparation is required for this test.

Ultrasound

Ultrasound is not often used to investigate bowel disorders. When used, the patient usually must have a full bladder.

Computed Tomography

Computed tomography (CT scan) is a radiographic examination that provides cross-sectional images of internal anatomy. It detects mass lesions more than 2 cm in diameter. However, it does not distinguish between benign and malignant tumors, cysts, or abscesses; therefore this type of scan has limited application for colonic disease. It has proven particularly effective in assessing lymph node enlargement and recurrence of colorectal carcinoma.

Magnetic Resonance Imaging

Magnetic resonance imaging (MRI) is a radiological examination that provides multiplanar images of the internal anatomy. This is a relatively new technique based on the emission or absorption of electromagnetic radiation by nuclei when exposed to particular magnetic fields. Since MRI involves use of a powerful magnet, patients with metal implants or cardiac pacemakers cannot undergo this examination.

SURGICAL PROCEDURES

Numerous surgical procedures are used in the treatment of lower GI diseases or conditions. Some of the more common surgical procedures are described in Table 36-3. Surgery may be the primary therapy or may be reserved for the management of complications of a particular disorder.

Stomas

Construction of stomas is often indicated in the management of lower GI problems. A stoma is a surgically created fecal diversion. There is a wide variance in appearance and function. Table 36-4 enumerates the criteria for the evaluation of a stoma.

A stoma can be constructed at almost any point along the alimentary canal. The name of the stoma illustrates the part of the GI tract that has been exteriorized and thus defines the characteristics of the discharge (Table 36-5).

In addition to the type of output, stomas can be defined according to their surgical construction. The surgeon may construct an *end, loop,* or *double-barrel* stoma.

An end, or single-barrel, stoma is created when the proximal part of the bowel is exteriorized through an opening in the abdominal wall. When the stoma is functional, the bowel contents will empty from this opening. The distal part of the bowel can be oversewn and placed back in the peritoneal cavity (as in a Hartmann's pouch) or removed (as in abdominoperineal resection). The removal of the rectum constitutes an irreversible procedure and results in a permanent stoma.

A loop stoma is created when the intact bowel is brought through an abdominal incision and the top of the bowel is opened by cautery. This loop of bowel is secured over some type of external device (such as a rod, bridge, or catheter), or the fascia is sewn together to support the exteriorized bowel. The fascial bridge is preferred, since it requires no special appliance to accommodate the supporting device. However, if an external supporting device is used, it is left in place for 7 to 10 days until the bowel forms adhesions to the abdominal wall. The proximal limb drains stool, whereas the distal limb usually drains mucus. This procedure is not completely diverting since stool can pass from the proximal to the distal bowel.

A double-barrel stoma occurs when the loop stoma is completely divided or when two separate stomas are created. The stomas may or may not be in close proximity to one another. If the stomas are next to each other, they must be incorporated into one pouch. If they are located apart, a drainable pouch would be used over the functional stoma, and a small dressing or closed-end pouch would be used over the distal stoma to contain mucus discharge.

If the patient's distal bowel is not removed and is unobstructed, the patient may continue to pass stool, old blood, and/or mucus through the rectum. The amount of stool passed is dependent on the adequacy of the preoperative bowel preparation and the type of fecal diversion.

Table 36-3 Gastrointestinal surgical procedures

Surgical procedure	Synonymous terms	Description	Fecal diversion	Indications	Nursing concerns
Abdominoperinal resection	APR Miles' procedure	Wide resection of the rectum, surrounding tissues, and lymph nodes is accomplished by an abdominal and perineal approach.	Permanent sigmoid or descending colostomy	Rectal cancer	Patient has both an abdominal and perineal wound. Impotency results in almost every case. Stoma care.
Total proctocolectomy	Panproctocolectomy	Colon and rectum are removed.	Permanent ileostomy	Chronic ulcerative colitis Familial polyposis Crohn's disease	Patient has both an abdominal and perineal wound. Stoma care.
Hartmann's pouch		Distal bowel is closed, and end stoma is created.	Temporary or permanent colostomy, depending on disease	Trauma Incontinence Diverticulitis Rectal cancer (palliative) Obstruction Hirschsprung's disease	Patient may experience long-term mucus discharge from rectal stump. Stoma care.
Subtotal colectomy	Segmental resection	Diseased portion of the colon is removed—may be a one-, two-, or three-staged procedure. One-stage procedure: diseased colon is removed, and bowel is reanastomosed; no stoma is created. Two-stage procedure: diseased colon is removed, and temporary stoma is created; later (usually 6-8 weeks), stoma is taken down. Three-stage procedure: stoma is created to resolve immediate poblem (e.g., obstruction); next, diseased colon is removed; finally, stoma is taken down.	Possibly a temporary colostomy	Diverticulitis Colon cancer Perforation Trauma Crohn's disease Intestinal ischemia Obstruction Intestinal fistulas Chronic ulcerative colitis (not curative) Familial polyposis (not curative)	

Procedure	Description	Indication	Ostomy	Outcomes/Considerations
Ileorectal anastomosis	Colon is removed, and ileum is anastomosed to rectum.	Crohn's disease; Chronic ulcerative colitis (not curative); Familial polyposis (not curative)	Temporary ileostomy if performed in two stages	Patient experiences frequent, liquid stools. Numbers of stools decreases over time as bowel adapts. Perianal skin care is important.
Ileoanal anastomosis	Colon and rectum are removed, and ileum is sutured to the anal canal.	Chronic ulcerative colitis; Familial polyposis; Atonic colon	Temporary ileostomy if performed in two stages	Patient experiences frequent, liquid stools. Number of stools decreases over time as bowel adapts. Perianal skin care is important. Stoma care (temporary).
Continent ileostomy	Colon and rectum are removed; approximately 45 cm of the distal ileum is used to construct internal reservoir and nipple valve.	Chronic ulcerative colitis; Familial polyposis	Permanent continent ileostomy, usually flush with the skin	Postoperatively, stoma is catheterized continuously to avoid overdistention of pouch and tension on the many suture lines. Approximately 14-21 days after surgery, catheter is removed, and patient must intubate stoma to empty the reservoir.
Ileoanal reservoir Restorative proctocolectomy IAR J pouch S pouch Park's pouch Endorectal ileal pouch–anal anastomosis	Procedure is usually performed in two stages. Stage 1: abdominal excision of colon and part of rectum; mucosectomy of rectal stump to dentate line; construction of terminal ileal reservoir; ileostomy. Stage 2: ileostomy takedown.	Chronic ulcerative colitis; Familial polyposis	Temporary ileostomy (usually 6-8 weeks)	Reoperation rate is relatively high. Stoma care. High ileostomy results in large volume output and potential fluid and electrolyte depletion. After Stage 2, patient experiences frequent, liquid stools, transient incontinence, and perianal skin irritation. Conditions improve with pouch adaptation. Long-term results are not known. Stoma care (temporary).
Low anterior resection	Wide resection of upper portion of rectum includes at least a 2-cm distal margin from tumor to anal verge. Procedure includes a hypogastric lymph node dissection in addition to the mesenteric dissection. Splenic flexure may be mobilized.	Rectal cancer (upper one third of rectum)	Possibly a temporary colostomy with a questionable anastomosis	

Table 36-4 Criteria for evaluating a stoma

Characteristic	Ideal	Rationale	Variances
Height	Approximately 2.5 cm	Easier for patient to see and facilitates drainage of effluent	Excessively long stomas may be cosmetically undesirable and difficult to conceal under clothing. Stomas flush with skin may require additional convexity in appliance.
Location of lumen	At apex of stoma	Facilitates drainage of effluent into pouch	If the lumen is at skin level, patient may have problems with leakage and pouch adherence.
Color	Red	Indicates good circulation	Temporary color changes may occur (e.g., anemia, when baby cries) and are normal.
Shape	Round	All presized appliances are round; makes procedure easier for client	If irregularly shaped, patient may need to cut appliances if total skin protection is required.
Location on body	Smooth surface below the beltline	Creases, boney prominences, suture lines, or umbilicus may interfere with pouch adherence Easier to conceal under clothing	

Table 36-5 Characteristic output of gastrointestinal stomas

Type	Amount (ml)	Consistency	pH
Esophagostomy	1000-1500	Saliva	Slightly alkaline
Gastrostomy	2000-2500	Liquid	0.5-1.5
Jejunostomy	1000-3000	Liquid	Slightly acid
Ileostomy	750-1000	Toothpaste	Alkaline
Cecostomy and ascending colostomy	500-750	Toothpaste	Alkaline
Transvere colostomy		Mushy to semiformed	Alkaline
Descending and sigmoid colostomy		Semiformed to formed	Alkaline

REFERENCES

1. Al JAS: Upper abdominal pain: identifying gastrointestinal causes, Consultant 24(12):67, 1984.
2. Bates B: A guide to physical examination, ed 3, Philadelphia, 1983, JB Lippincott Co.
3. Block GJ and Noland JW: The abdomen. In Health assessment for professional nursing: a developmental approach, Norwalk, Conn, 1986, Appleton-Century-Crofts.
4. Carpentino LD: Nursing diagnosis: application to clinical practice, Philadelphia, 1983, JB Lippincott Co.
5. Englert DA: Gastrointestinal system. In Kennedy-Caldwell C and Guenter P, editors: Nutrition support nursing-core curriculum, ed 2, Silver Spring, Md, 1985, American Society for Parenteral and Enteral Nutrition.
6. Field S: Plain films: the acute abdomen, Clin Gastroenterol 13(1):3, 1984.
7. Fischbach F: A manual of laboratory diagnostic tests, ed 2, Philadelphia, 1984, JB Lippincott Co.
8. Greenberger NJ: Gastrointestinal disorders: a pathophysiological approach, ed 2, Chicago, 1981, Year Book Medical Publishers, Inc.
9. Kastrup EK: Drug facts and comparisons, St Louis, 1987, JB Lippincott Co.
10. Lang CE and Shulte CV: Nutritional assessment in critical care—the adult patient. In Lang CE, editor: Nutritional support in critical care, Rockville, Md, 1987, Aspen Publishers.
11. Mansell E and others: Patient assessment: examination of the abdomen, Am J Nurs 74(9):1679, 1974.
12. Meir HB: Ultrasound in gastroenterology, Clin Gastroenterol 13(1):183, 1984.
13. Patras AZ and Brozenec SA: Gastrointestinal assessment: identifying significant problems, AORN J 40(5):726, 1984.
14. Price SA and Wilson LM: Pathophysiology: clinical concepts of disease processes, ed 3, New York, 1986, McGraw-Hill Book Co.
15. Stafford R: Gastrointestinal diagnostic tests, J Enterostom Ther 13(6):242, 1986.
16. Swedberg J, Driggers DA, and Deiss F: Screening for colorectal cancer: the role of the primary care physician, Postgrad Med 79:67, 1986.
17. Thompson JM and others, editors: Mosby's manual of clinical nursing, ed 2, St Louis, 1989, The CV Mosby Co.
18. Varella LD and Kennedy-Caldwell C: Nursing care and specialized nutritional support—the adult patient. In Lang CE, editor: Nutritional support in critical care, Rockville, Md, 1987, Aspen Publishers.
19. Wallach J: Interpretation of diagnostic tests, ed 2, Boston, 1974, Little, Brown & Co.
20. Widmann FK: Clinical interpretation of laboratory tests, ed 9, Philadelphia, 1983, FA Davis Co.

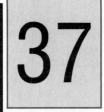

CHAPTER

37

Gastrointestinal Disorders and Therapeutic Management

CHAPTER OBJECTIVES

- *Discuss causes, medical treatment, and nursing care for stress ulcer.*
- *Discuss the high-risk causes, medical treatment, and nursing care of acute gastrointestinal bleeding.*
- *Describe the pathophysiology of acute pancreatitis.*
- *Describe important aspects of the nursing care of patients with acute intestinal obstruction, perforated viscus, and fistula.*

Critical care nurses frequently care for patients with alterations in gastrointestinal (GI) function. The magnitude of health problems related to digestive diseases in the United States is staggering (see the box at top right).

DYSPHAGIA

When a patient experiences difficulty during swallowing or within a few seconds after swallowing, he or she is diagnosed as having dysphagia. When the sensation is described as painful, it is called *odynophagia*. Dysphagia can be caused by a number of physiological and psychological alterations and frequently results from central nervous system damage from a cerebrovascular accident, trauma, or a progressive degenerative disease. In patients with head injury, stroke, motor neuron diseases, and myasthenic disorders, the impairment is usually part of a more widespread disorder. Dysphagia may, however, occur as a fairly isolated problem.

Immediate difficulty swallowing is associated with the thoracic section of the esophagus. Dysphagia can be experienced after intake of either liquids or solids. Assessment and medical diagnosis are based on site of occurrence, type and temperature of food that initiates the symptoms (liquids, semisolids, hot or cold), length of time the symptom has existed, and results from endoscopy, manometry, or a barium x-ray study.

IMPACT OF ALTERATIONS IN GASTROINTESTINAL FUNCTION

Leading cause of hospitalization in the United States
Affects one out of nine Americans daily
Accounts for one out of three major surgeries
Third among causes of economic loss ($50 billion a year)
Second in causes of disability and days lost from work
Fourteen million cases of acute digestive diseases treated annually
As a cause of death:
　Alterations in gastrointestinal function rank third among overall causes (200,000 deaths annually).
　Cirrhosis of liver ranks sixth.
　Thirty percent of all cancer deaths result from cancer in digestive organs.

Modified from Given BA and Simmons SJ: Gastroenterology in clinical nursing, ed 4, St Louis, 1984, The CV Mosby Co.

Nursing Diagnosis and Management
Dysphagia

- Potential for Aspiration risk factor: impaired swallowing, p. 488

CAUSES OF RUPTURE OF THE ESOPHAGUS

TRAUMA

Automobile accidents
Gunshot wounds
Swallowed foreign body
Endoscopy
Traumatic insertion of a stiff tube (e.g., nasogastric tube)
Ingestion of corrosive chemicals

SPONTANEOUS RUPTURE

Severe vomiting

The critical care nurse is most apt to care for dysphagic patients after head injury or spinal cord trauma, for surgical patients who have postoperative cranial nerve injury (for example, after bilateral carotid surgery), for patients with isolated cranial nerve dysfunction in brain-stem strokes (for example, Wallenberg's syndrome), or for patients with bilateral cerebral infarctions that produce spastic paresis of the palatal and pharyngeal muscles ("pseudobulbar palsy").

Some patients with dysphagia are managed by a diet change to semisolid foods. However, critically ill patients with dysphagia who are at risk for aspiration should receive parenteral or enteral nutrition. Enteral nutrition should be initiated after cardiovascular and respiratory stabilization and after the risk of generalized ileus (for example, from spinal injury and trauma) has receded. Tube insertion in the patient with a head injury (especially anterior basal skull fractures) should proceed with great caution because penetration of the intracranial cavity by GI tubes and feeding tubes has been reported.[2] In the patient with cervical spinal injury, nasoenteric tubes must be inserted without moving the neck.

The intraabdominal esophagus is less frequently injured than is the thoracic portion of the esophagus. Blunt or penetrating trauma can occur, however, anywhere along the esophagus (see the box above). Rarely is this area injured alone; thus nursing care is directed toward assessment for concomitant injuries. In spontaneous rupture caused by a Sengstaken-Blakemore tube, for example, the patient should be evaluated for the presence of cyanosis, extreme dyspnea, Hamman's sign (a crushing sound in the precordium), sudden onset of severe pain in the chest or upper abdomen, rigid abdomen, or subcutaneous emphysema.

STRESS ULCER

The term *stress ulcer* (erosive gastritis) covers a spectrum of diseases ranging from superficial mucosal erosions to discrete, mature ulcers. Stress ulcers, which are usually multiple, are located mainly in the fundus of the stomach, although they may involve the entire GI tract. It is the most common cause of upper GI bleeding and the most frequent

pathological process within the stomach. Patients at risk include those in high physiological stress situations such as occur with thermal injury, head trauma, extensive surgery, shock, or acute neurological disease.

Curling's ulcer is the term used for stress ulceration of the stomach and duodenum after burn injury; it occurs in approximately 12% of all patients hospitalized for burns. Punctate hemorrhages and shallow mucosal erosions occur in 90% of patients with burns involving 35% or more of their body surface. Although there are similarities between stress ulcers and Curling's ulcer, their distribution is somewhat different. Curling's ulcer is nearly evenly divided between single and multiple ulcers and between the stomach and duodenum. Another closely related erosion is Cushing's ulcer. Similar in distribution, it is a variety of esophagogastroduodenal lesion that occurs after intracranial operations or trauma. It is unclear if Cushing's ulcer is caused by significant gastric hypersecretion after the insult or if the cause is identical to that of stress ulcers.

Several pathophysiological mechanisms have been suggested as operative in stress ulcer formation (see the box below). The onset can be very rapid (2 to 10 days), and hemorrhage can begin without pain. If hemorrhage goes untreated, mortality can exceed 50%. Patients at risk for development of stress ulcers should be assessed for the presence of hematemesis (red blood or coffee-ground emesis), bloody nasogastric aspirate, and melena (black or dark red stools).

Pharmacological gastric acid neutralization is the accepted treatment for stress ulcers and may even be used prophylactically in high-risk settings. A common regimen includes administering liquid antacids (30 ml every 4 hours) in an attempt to establish and maintain an alkaline gastric environment. At a pH of 5.0, 99.9% of the gastric acid is neutralized, and pepsin activity is essentially nonexistent. Antacids frequently will plug small feeding tubes; therefore a patient may require a 14-French or larger nasogastric tube when antacid administration becomes necessary. Some patients will receive alternating courses of antacids and gastric suctioning. An attempt should be made to keep the pH in the 4.0 to 4.5 range, with additional dosages of antacids

---

CAUSES OF STRESS ULCERS

PRECIPITATING FACTORS

Patient's increased stress level (alteration in equilibrium)
Increased acid level in lumen of stomach (pH <3.5)

COFACTORS

Mucosal ischemia
Hydrogen-ion back diffusion (gastric barrier)
Gram-negative septicemia
Drug intake (e.g., steroids and catecholamines in patients with head trauma)

---

given when the pH falls below 4.0. In addition, courses of cimetidine (Tagamet) or other new hydrochloric acid (H_2) blockers may be used. Although they would seem useful, continuous enteral feedings apparently do not prevent stress ulceration in critically ill patients.[1]

ACUTE GASTROINTESTINAL BLEEDING

Hemorrhage can be a serious symptom or complication of several medical problems (see the box, "Causes of Upper Gastrointestinal Bleeding"). If unrecognized or treated too late, GI hemorrhage can lead to acute GI perforation, peritonitis, sepsis, hypovolemic shock, and ultimately death. In more than one third of patients with GI disease, bleeding will be the initial symptom, and in more than 70% of them, none will have a history of previous bleeding. Generally, gastric surgery patients are not at high risk for postoperative hemorrhage, which, when it does occur, is usually the result of splenic injury or slippage of a suture. Those at highest risk for death from upper GI bleeding are patients who fit any one of the following criteria:

1. More than 60 years of age
2. Disease in three organ systems
3. Required transfusion of five or more units of blood
4. Concomitant lung or liver disease
5. Recent major operation, trauma, or sepsis

Mortality is highest for those patients with bleeding esophageal varices, whereas mortality decreases in those patients with gastric ulcers.

Hematemesis and melena are hallmark manifestations of GI bleeding. Because it is difficult to estimate the amount of blood in emesis or stool, a description of the sample and the patient's clinical picture are the initial sources for a differential medical diagnosis. Laboratory tests help determine the extent of the bleeding by showing a decrease in the hemoglobin, hematocrit, or blood urea nitrogen (BUN) levels or a change in clotting factors. Diagnostic procedures (endoscope) and radiological studies (radionuclide imaging) aid in establishing the site of the bleeding.

Nursing care for GI hemorrhage is similar despite the specific cause. Routine measures include strict bed rest,

---

CAUSES OF UPPER GASTROINTESTINAL BLEEDING*

Peptic ulceration (gastric and duodenal ulcers)—50%-75%

Acute mucosal lesions (gastritis and erosions [stress ulcers])—1%-33%

Unknown—approximately 16%

Esophagogastric varices—approximately 10%

Reflux esophagitis—approximately 2%

Miscellaneous <8%; examples: gastric neoplasms, hepatic trauma, esophagogastric trauma

---
*Reported occurrence ranges.

Nursing Diagnosis and Management
Acute gastrointestinal bleeding

- Fluid Volume Deficit related to active blood loss, p. 668
- Potential for Infection risk factor: invasive monitoring devices, p. 346
- Potential for Aspiration risk factors: gastrointestinal tube, increased intragastric pressure, p. 488
- Anxiety related to threatened biological, psychological, and/or social integrity, p. 852
- Sensory/Perceptual Alterations related to sensory overload, sensory deprivation, and sleep pattern disturbance, p. 601
- Ineffectual Individual Coping related to situational crisis and personal vulnerability, p. 850

---

recording of intake and output, blood transfusions, recording of vital signs at least hourly and in some cases every 15 minutes, and monitoring for further signs of hemorrhage (restlessness, apprehension, increased thirst, and fever). Priorities include the control of bleeding, maintenance of fluid and electrolyte balance, and pharmacological gastric acid neutralization (see "Stress Ulcer"). All patients should be monitored for impending complications of shock, vasovagal responses (especially the elderly), and gastric perforation. In addition to gastric acid neutralization, other treatments include gastric lavage cooling, administration of vasopressin, and surgical repairs such as those procedures used to treat GI hemorrhage (gastroenterostomy, gastroduodenostomy [Billroth I], gastrojejunostomy [Billroth II or subtotal gastrectomy], partial gastric resection, vagotomy, antrectomy, and pyloroplasty).

Gastric perforation constitutes a surgical emergency. When it occurs, the patient will suddenly complain of severe generalized abdominal pain with significant rebound tenderness and rigidity. Other symptoms include fever, tachycardia, dehydration, and ileus. Gastric perforation most often occurs when hemorrhaging results from duodenal ulcer. Mortality is approximately 10% to 20%, with death caused by peritonitis and septicemia. Prompt nursing recognition of the changing status is vital.

ACUTE PANCREATITIS
Description

The pancreas is an organ that has both endocrine and exocrine functions. The chief endocrine disorder is diabetes mellitus, which is discussed further in Chapter 41. Pancreatitis is an inflammation of the pancreas that involves exocrine dysfunction.

Pancreatitis, which may be acute or chronic, is an autodigestive process that results from premature activation of the pancreatic digestive enzymes. These digestive enzymes are normally inactive while housed in the pancreas and become active only in the small intestine. During acute pancreatitis they become active within the pancreas and, in effect, begin the process of digestion before reaching the small intestine. Hence the term *autodigestion* of the pancreas.

Cause and Pathophysiology

Acute pancreatitis is caused chiefly by biliary disease (most commonly gallstones) and by alcoholism. Other causes include reflux of duodenal contents, penetrating duodenal ulcer, surgical trauma (especially of the organs surrounding the pancreas), hyperparathyroidism, vascular disease, and the use of certain drugs (opiates, steroids, thiazide diuretics, sulfonamides, and oral diuretics). Pancreatitis occurs more frequently in women than in men.

Although the common pathogenic mechanism in acute pancreatitis is autodigestion, it is unclear how or why the pancreatic enzymes are activated before reaching the small intestine.

During acute pancreatitis, trypsin, normally inactive in the pancreas, becomes active and triggers the secretion of the proteolytic enzymes, phospholipase A, elastase, and kallikrein. Phospholipase A, in the presence of bile, digests the phospholipids of cell membranes, causing severe pancreatic parenchymal and adipose tissue necrosis. Elastase activation causes dissolution of the elastic fibers of blood vessels and ducts, leading to hemorrhage. Kallikrein activation causes the release of bradykinin and kallidin, resulting in vasodilation and increased vascular permeability. The effects are fluid shifts, hypotension, and pain.

Assessment and Diagnosis

The most prominent symptom of acute pancreatitis is sudden epigastric to midabdominal pain. The pain may vary from mild and tolerable to severe and incapacitating. It is often reported as a "boring" sensation that radiates to the back. Nausea and/or vomiting may accompany the pain. The patient may obtain some comfort by leaning forward or by lying down with knees drawn up. Pancreatic pain is usually steady and lasts 1 to several days. The pathogenesis of this pancreatic pain relates to extravasation of plasma and red blood cells in the area surrounding the pancreas, release of digested protein and lipids of the pancreas, and ductal swelling.

Physical examination may show tachypnea, leukocytosis, hypocalcemia, tachycardia, and/or some degree of shock. The hypocalcemia is thought to result from marked fat necrosis, which results in the release of free fatty acids. They combine with calcium to form calcium soaps. Neuromuscular irritability and tetany may develop. Palpation of the abdomen will reveal tenderness, guarding, and, if peritonitis is present, rigidity. Bowel sounds may or may not be present.

The diagnosis is confirmed by an acute, severely elevated serum amylase level frequently exceeding 250 Somogyi units/dl, and sometimes reaching 400 to 500 Somogyi units (normal is 60 to 180 Somogyi units/dl). Serum lipase levels will also be elevated. Other findings may include hyperglycemia and elevated bilirubin and decreased serum albumin levels.

Complications of acute pancreatitis include development of tetany, diabetes mellitus, pleural effusion, peritonitis, ascites, pancreatic abcess or pseudocyst, secondary infection of the surrounding organs, hypovolemic or septic shock, adult respiratory distress syndrome (ARDS), and disseminated intravascular coagulation (DIC).

Treatment

Treatment includes relief of pain, reduction of pancreatic secretions, and prevention or treatment of complications.

Pain relief is achieved with meperidine rather than opiates since meperidine causes less spasm of the sphincter of Oddi. The patient is placed on nothing-by-mouth (NPO) status, and gastric suction is begun to place the pancreas "at rest" and to eliminate any undue secretion of the digestive enzymes. Total parenteral nutrition will be required for prolonged, severe cases of pancreatitis. Antibiotics are administered to treat secondary infection and/or to prevent pancreatic abcess. Plasma and electrolytes infusion are ordered to treat the fluid shifts.

Nursing Care

Nursing care concerns treating the pain related to acute pancreatitis. Analgesics should be liberally provided, because pancreatic pain can be immobilizing. Because of the pain and the need for high doses of analgesic, the patient's ventilatory pattern should be assessed for depth and rate. Abdominal pain often results in shallow rapid breathing, which can precipitate atelectasis and pneumonia, and high doses of analgesic may further impair the ventilatory pattern. The nursing objective regarding pain control should be achieving pain relief while maintaining ventilations at normal depth and rate. Chest auscultation of breath sounds is essential. Further information on how the breathing pattern affects lung function is found in Chapter 20 in the discussion of atelectasis and in Chapter 22 in the discussion of ineffective breathing pattern.

Measures used to rest the pancreas, the NPO status, and gastric suctioning also assist in pain control. Relaxation techniques may augment analgesia.

Potential or actual fluid volume deficit is another nursing care concern. Assessing central venous pressure (CVP) or pulmonary artery pressures (PAP) yields essential information about fluid volume. Continued monitoring of CVP and PAP is required as intravenous (IV) fluids are infused.

Parenteral nutrition may be required for prolonged cases of pancreatitis in which NPO status must be maintained (usually longer than 5 days). A thorough review of the nursing interventions associated with parenteral nutrition is presented in Chapter 9.

The nurse should be alert for development of complications of pancreatitis. Leukocytosis may signal infection or pancreatic abscess. Pulmonary crackles, previously not found, may mean development of atelectasis, pneumonia, or ARDS.

INTESTINAL ISCHEMIA
Description and Cause

Intestinal ischemia can result from either transient or prolonged insufficient mesenteric vascular supply of the

<table>
<tr><td>

PATHOLOGIES ASSOCIATED WITH INTESTINAL ISCHEMIA

Thrombosis or embolus in splanchnic bed
Cardiopathy or impaired cardiac output
Polyarteritis nodosa
Buerger's disease
Vasculitis secondary to collagen diseases
Strangulation obstruction (e.g., sigmoid volvulus)

</td></tr>
</table>

splanchnic vessels (the celiac axis, the superior mesenteric artery, and the inferior mesenteric artery). Sometimes the progressive increase in collateral circulation compensates for ischemia. See the box above for a list of pathologies commonly associated with intestinal ischemia.

Intestinal ischemia occurs in patients older than 50 years of age who also have a history of arteriosclerosis, cardiac failure, or hemodynamic disorders (for example, multiple myeloma). Ischemic damage can also occur after angioplastic surgery for a ruptured aortic aneurysm or vascular ligations associated with colonic resections.

Assessment and Diagnosis

A confusing array of manifestations accompany intestinal ischemia. There are no specific features and no satisfactory clinical test to confirm the diagnosis. Initially, the patient complains of diffuse or medial abdominal pain. Later,

<table>
<tr><td>

Nursing Diagnosis and Management
Acute pancreatitis

■ Acute Pain related to transmission and perception of noxious stimuli secondary to acute pancreatitis, p. 594

■ Ineffective Breathing Pattern related to abdominal pain, p. 483

■ Fluid Volume Deficit related to wound drainage, p. 669

■ Altered Nutrition: Less than Body Protein-Calorie Requirements related to lack of exogenous nutrients and increased metabolic demand, p. 713

■ Anxiety related to threatened biological, psychological, and/or social integrity, p. 852

■ Sensory/Perceptual Alterations related to sensory overload, sensory deprivation, and sleep pattern disturbance, p. 601

■ Ineffectual Individual Coping related to situational crisis and personal vulnerability, p. 850

</td></tr>
</table>

bloody diarrhea, tenesmus, fever, and hyperleukocytosis can develop. Symptoms are insidious; therefore intestinal ischemia should be suspected in any patient more than 50 years of age who has vague abdominal complaints and a history of heart disease or hemodynamic disorders.

When the sensitive intestinal mucosa becomes hypoxic, mucosal lesions, ulcerations, edema, and hemorrhage develop. The mucosal lesions can heal quickly if the ischemia is brief. However, most of the time the lesions become infected with pathogenic colonic flora. The resulting inflammatory response may conceal the vascular origin and confuse the clinical picture with Crohn's disease or ulcerative colitis. Elevated serum alkaline phosphatase and amylase levels and metabolic acidosis indicate intestinal infarction and evolving gangrenous necrosis.

Radiographic examination of the ischemic colon may reveal "thumbprints" characteristic of mucosal ischemia. Mesenteric arteriography can pinpoint the location of the vascular compromise.

Treatment

Rapid recognition of the disease and rapid treatment are essential. Prognosis is poor because these patients are generally not good surgical candidates because of age and concurrent pathologies such as arteriosclerosis and heart disease. When ischemia is transient, revascularization can be accomplished. Suspected ischemia and necrosis warrant an emergency resection of the involved bowel.

Nursing Care

The nurse should evaluate signs that would indicate intestinal perforation. They might include a change in the pain pattern, increased abdominal girth and rigidity, and a marked deterioration in vital signs. An elevated temperature may indicate an infection secondary to pathogenic colonic flora or perforation.

When diarrhea occurs along with intestinal ischemia, accurate intake and output measurements are necessary. Perianal skin should be evaluated and protection provided to prevent a break in skin integrity.

A nasogastric tube and bowel rest are needed to avoid stress on an already compromised bowel.

ACUTE INTESTINAL OBSTRUCTION
Description and Cause

Acute intestinal obstruction occurs when bowel contents fail to move forward. Functional obstruction, also known as paralytic ileus, results from the absence of peristalsis and frequently occurs with hypokalemia. Mechanical obstruction results from occlusion of the bowel lumen and is most often the result of neoplasms. The box, "Causes of Colonic Obstruction," on the following page lists examples of both types of obstruction.

When the intestinal lumen is obstructed both proximally and distally, a "closed-loop" obstruction exists. A sigmoid volvulus is an example of a closed-loop obstruction because the ileocecal valve resists the backward flow of colonic contents into the ileum. Left-sided obstructions can create enough pressure to perforate the cecum.

CAUSES OF COLONIC OBSTRUCTIONS

FUNCTIONAL OBSTRUCTION
Prolonged intestinal distention
Hypokalemia
Peritonitis
Narcotic use
Intestinal ischemia
Sepsis

MECHANICAL OBSTRUCTION
Contained within lumen

Intussusception
Large gallstones
Meconium
Bezoars
Neoplasms

Extending into bowel wall

Congenital atresia
Congenital stenosis
Inflammatory bowel disease
Diverticulitis
Radiation
Neoplasms

Outside the bowel

Adhesions
Hernias
Neoplasms
Abscesses
Volvulus
Stomal stenosis

Assessment and Diagnosis

Colonic obstructions have minimal forewarning. Typically, patients are initially seen in acute distress, with abdominal distention, obstipation, constipation, cramping abdominal pain, and high-pitched bowel sounds. Emesis is seen only if the ileocecal valve is incompetent or the obstruction prolonged. Hypokalemia may occur when the obstruction is prolonged. Initially, dehydration is unusual and is the result of insufficient intake. When the obstruction is prolonged, dehydration may develop secondary to the movement of fluid and electrolytes into the bowel lumen above the obstruction.

The obstructed bowel lumen accumulates fluid and gas proximal to the point of obstruction. Trapped fluids cause bowel distention, which triggers the secretion of fluid and electrolytes into the lumen and perpetuates the distention. As the distention progresses, the bowel wall edema can ultimately impede venous and arterial supply and cause bowel necrosis and perforation. Once the bowel perforates, peritonitis and sepsis ensue.

A chest x-ray film and serial abdominal flat-plate films taken with the patient standing or sitting and supine will reveal dilated loops of gas-filled bowel. Barium or diatrizoate meglumine (gastrografin) enemas are used to locate the exact site and the degree of obstruction.

Treatment

Medical interventions include replacement of fluids and immediate decompression of the obstruction with nasogastric suction. Use of long GI tubes is contraindicated for colonic obstruction. A sigmoid volvulus can be nonsurgically reduced by inserting a rectal tube during sigmoidoscopy or barium enema, thus relieving the obstruction. Because the volvulus can recur, elective resection at a later date is desirable.

Surgical intervention is required when the obstruction fails to resolve within 24 hours. When the patient is not acutely ill, surgical resection can be a one-stage procedure with reanastomosis of the bowel, therefore eliminating the need for a temporary colostomy. More often a two- or three-stage procedure is used and a temporary colostomy created.

Complications

Bowel necrosis and perforation are potential complications of colonic obstruction, and both can progress to sepsis. Bowel necrosis occurs as a result of impaired circulation associated with volvulus and closed-loop obstruction and with sustained excessive intraluminal pressure. Bowel perforation often results from overdistention of the bowel lumen and is also a sequelae to bowel necrosis. These complications carry a high mortality rate and can be avoided by astute observations and prompt surgical intervention.

Nursing Care

The patient should be observed for signs of bowel obstruction such as abdominal distention, nausea, vomiting, and elevated blood phosphorous or amylase levels. Bowel sounds may be absent or faint and tinkling, depending on the extent of the obstruction. A nasogastric tube should be inserted for decompression. Placement and patency should be checked as needed (prn) to ensure adequate decompression. Outputs greater than 1000 ml/8 hours can occur. Administration of antipyretics will be necessary for treatment of fever. The patient should be monitored for electrolyte imbalance (hyponatremia and hypokalemia) and fluid deficit. Accurate intake and output must be maintained. IV fluids should be administered to prevent dehydration.

PERFORATED VISCUS
Description and Cause

A perforated viscus is a hole in the bowel that results in the spillage of contents into the peritoneal cavity. It is an abdominal crisis that requires an expeditious evaluation, an organized approach, and mature surgical judgment for a successful outcome.

A bowel perforation can be spontaneous, can result from a diagnostic or therapeutic procedure or can be related to trauma (see the box, "Causes of Colorectal Perforations").

The contamination of the peritoneal cavity results in peritonitis, which is an inflammation of the peritoneum caused

---

> ## Nursing Diagnosis and Management
> ### *Acute intestinal obstruction*
>
> - Acute Pain related to transmission and perception of noxious stimuli secondary to acute intestinal obstruction, p. 594
> - Ineffective Breathing Pattern related to abdominal pain, p. 483
> - Decreased Cardiac Output related to decreased preload secondary to fluid volume deficit, p. 337
> - Decreased Cardiac Output related to decreased preload secondary to septicemia, p. 338
> - Potential for Aspiration risk factor: gastrointestinal tube, increased intragastric pressure, decreased GI motility, increased gastric residual, delayed gastric emptying, p. 488
> - Potential Impaired Skin Integrity risk factor: prolonged immobility, p. 725
> - Anxiety related to threatened biological, psychological, and/or social integrity, p. 852
> - Ineffective Individual Coping related to situational crisis and personal vulnerability, p. 850

> ## CAUSES OF COLORECTAL PERFORATIONS
>
> Ruptures (e.g., diverticulum, appendix, pericolic abscess)
> Surgical procedures involving the bowel or contiguous organs
> Diagnostic tests (e.g., endoscopy, barium enema)
> Therapeutic procedures (e.g., polypectomy with endoscopy, insertion of an enema tip, explosions with use of cautery during proctosigmoidoscopy)
> Ingested foreign bodies (e.g., pits, bones)
> Chronic constipation
> Trauma (e.g., gunshot, knife wound)

by bacterial or chemical irritation. The most common bacteria involved are *Escherichia coli*, *Streptococcus*, *Staphylococcus*, *Pneumococcus*, *Pseudomonas aeruginosa*, and *Clostridium perfringens*. Of them, *E. coli* is the most frequent cause, and *Streptococcus* is the most virulent type. Chemical irritation is caused by the enzymes or the pH of the spilled contents.

Assessment and Diagnosis

The hallmarks of a perforated viscus include abdominal pain and "boardlike" rigidity, hypoactive bowel sounds, leukocytosis, and free air in the abdominal cavity. Other symptoms vary with the extent of the peritonitis, its severity, and the type of organism responsible. If left unchecked, the peritonitis will result in sepsis with high fever, dehydration, shock, oliguria, and eventually death.

In addition to a history and abdominal assessment, numerous laboratory tests and flat and upright abdominal x-ray films will be ordered. The films will confirm the presence of free air in the abdomen.

Treatment

Medical interventions are initiated to minimize additional complications. GI decompression is necessary to reduce further contamination of the peritoneum and to decrease the risk of vomiting and aspiration. Nothing is given by mouth to provide bowel rest and eliminate further spillage of GI contents. IV fluids are initiated to correct hypovolemia and electrolyte imbalance, and antibiotics are administered. Oxygen may be useful to decrease intestinal hypoxia and, along with proper patient positioning (head up), to assist oxygenation, which may be impaired because of abdominal distention and pain. Pain control must also be provided.

Surgery is almost always indicated in the treatment of a perforated viscus, and the surgical procedure undertaken is dictated by the primary cause and the patient's overall condition. The aim of surgical intervention is to close the perforation, prevent septicemia, and prevent or drain abscesses. A temporary colostomy may be required to divert intestinal contents away from the perforation and/or infection or to protect a questionable bowel anastomosis.

> ## Nursing Diagnosis and Management
> ### *Perforated viscus*
>
> - Acute Pain related to transmission and perception of noxious stimuli secondary to perforated viscus, p. 594
> - Ineffective Breathing Pattern related to abdominal pain, p. 483
> - Decreased Cardiac Output related to decreased preload secondary to fluid volume deficit, p. 337
> - Decreased Cardiac Output related to decreased preload secondary to septicemia, p. 338
> - Anxiety related to threatened biological, psychological, and/or social integrity, p. 852
> - Potential for Aspiration risk factors: GI tube, decreased GI motility, delayed gastric emptying, increased gastric residual, p. 488
> - Potential for Infection risk factors: invasive monitoring devices, protein-calorie malnourishment, p. 346 and 720
> - Ineffectual individual Coping related to situational crisis and personal vulnerability, p. 850

Nursing Care

Vital signs require assessment every hour. The patient should be checked for signs of peritonitis such as abdominal pain, rigidity, fever, elevated white blood cell (WBC) count, hypotension, tachycardia, and tachypnea. The patient with documented peritonitis should be observed for signs of acute bleeding, including hypotension, tachycardia, tachypnea, decreased urinary output, sudden drop in hemoglobin and hematocrit, warm, dry flushed skin, increased lethargy or drowsiness, restlessness, and changes in sensorium.

Blood cultures and antibiotics may be ordered for febrile episodes.

FISTULA
Description

A fistula is an abnormal communication between two or more structures or spaces. Fistulas are more specifically categorized according to location, involved structures, and volume of output as demonstrated in Table 37-1.

Complications such as fluid and electrolyte imbalance, malnutrition, and sepsis are responsible for the mortality associated with fistulas. High-output fistulas (more than 500 ml per 24 hours) have a poor prognosis because of fluid and electrolyte imbalance. Advances in nutritional support, however, have improved the prognosis.

Cause

Several conditions predispose to fistula formation, including Crohn's disease, trauma, diverticulitis, small bowel obstruction, cancer, ulcerative colitis, and irradiation. Failure of the suture line after an abdominal surgical procedure is the most common cause for fistula formation. Fistulas can develop in irradiated tissue immediately after the therapy or many years later.

Assessment and Diagnosis

An external fistula is usually quite obvious because of the drainage of fluid, feces, or urine through an aperture in the skin. Internal fistulas communicating with the bladder or vagina result in passage of gas, feces, or urine from the urethra or vagina. The patient may also have a fever of unknown origin.

Collection of the effluent and accurate measurements are essential in fistula management. Volume of output and laboratory analysis of the output can aid in identifying the location of the fistula. Table 37-2 lists the electrolyte content of various GI secretions.

The suspicion that a fistula is communicating with the vagina can be validated by placing a tampon into the vagina and instilling methylene blue into the suspected communicating organ. If the packing is unstained when removed in 15 to 20 minutes, a fistula to this particular organ is unlikely. To identify accurately the fistulous tract, the involved organs, and the associated pathologies, radiographic studies using a water-soluble dye should be conducted (for example, fistulogram or diatrizoate meglumine [gastrografin] enema).

Treatment

Medical management requires strict attention to fluid and electrolyte balance, infection control, and nutritional support. Laboratory analysis of the output makes accurate replacement of electrolytes possible.

When fever is persistent, an abscess should be suspected. Vital signs should be taken every 4 hours, and external drainage of the abscess must be established.

Nutritional support is provided either enterally or parenterally. Because oral intake stimulates bowel activity, the patient should be placed on bowel rest when the fistula involves the GI tract. Bowel rest can be achieved with parenteral and specific types of enteral nutrition. In the early treatment phase, parenteral nutrition is preferred. Once the location of the fistula is identified and the patient is stabilized, enteral nutrition may be initiated for colonic fistulas.

To promote wound healing, caloric intake should be 37 to 45 kcal/kg/24 hours, and protein intake should be 1.5 to 1.75 g/kg/24 hours. With intense nutritional support, approximately 50% of the high-volume fistulas will close spontaneously, although doing so may take at least 2 months.

Specific situations can delay or prevent spontaneous fistula closure, thus requiring surgical intervention (see the following box on p. 701). It is best to delay any surgical procedures until the patient is infection free and well nourished. Bowel necrosis or abscess, however, requires immediate surgical attention. Several techniques are used to treat fistulas: diversion, resection, or "patching." The procedure used depends on the location, size, and cause of the fistula and the patient's surgical risks. Irradiation- or neoplastic-induced fistulas rarely heal spontaneously because of the local tissue fibrosis and hypoxia typical of radiation and surgery.

Nursing Care

A patient with a high-output intestinal fistula must be monitored carefully for fluid and electrolyte disturbances. Clinical assessment, including accurate measurement of intake and output, is essential for prompt identification of malabsorption. Dehydration can result in decreased tem-

---

Table 37-1 Nomenclature for fistulas

Category	Terminology	Meaning
Location	Internal	Tract contained within body
	External	Tract exits through skin
Involved structures	Colo-	Colon
	Entero-	Small bowel
	Vesico-	Bladder
	Vaginal	Vagina
	Cutaneous	Skin
	Recto-	Rectum
Volume	High output	More than 500 ml/24 hours
	Low output	Less than 500 ml/24 hours

Modified from Boarini JH, Bryant RA, and Irrgang SJ: Semin Oncol Nurs 2:287, 1986.

Table 37-2 Electrolyte content of gastrointestinal fluid

Fluid	pH	Sodium	Potassium	Chloride	Bicarbonate
Saliva	6.0-7.0	20-80	16-23	24-44	20-60
Gastric juice	1.0-3.5	20-100	4-12	52-124	0
Bile	7.8	120-200	3-12	80-120	30-50
Pancreatic juice	8.0-8.3	120-150	2-7	54-95	70-110
Intestinal juice	7.5-8.9	80-130	11-21	48-116	20-30

Modified from Givens BA and Simmons SA: Gastroenterology in clinical nursing, ed 4, St Louis, 1984, The CV Mosby Co.

FACTORS THAT DELAY OR PREVENT SPONTANEOUS CLOSURE OF FISTULAS

Complete disruption of bowel continuity
Distal obstruction
Foreign bodies in the fistulous tract
Epithelial-lined tract contiguous with the skin
Cancer in the site
Previous irradiation
Crohn's disease
Presence of large abscess

Modified from Irrgang SJ and Bryant RA: J Enterostomal Ther 6(2):211, 1984.

---

perature, increased heart rate, oliguria, and postural hypotension. Hypokalemia can result in a drop in blood pressure, a weak, irregular pulse, electrocardiographic (ECG) changes, and paresthesia, and hyponatremia can result in confusion, apprehension, hypotension, and shock.

Sepsis is a major cause of death in patients with enterocutaneous fistulas. Abscess formation should be suspected in the presence of an elevated temperature and clinical deterioration. Vital signs should be monitored every 2 hours or more frequently. Antipyretics should be administered as ordered.

Management of the effluent and perifistular skin care is discussed in Chapter 38.

PSEUDOMEMBRANOUS ENTEROCOLITIS
Description and Cause

Pseudomembranous enterocolitis is an antibiotic-associated diarrhea in which the bowel mucosa and submucosa become inflamed and necrosis ensues. Because normal bowel flora is altered by antibiotic therapy commonly used in critical care, the environment is conducive for the proliferation of opportunistic microorganisms such as *Clostridium difficile*. As *C. difficile* multiplies, it produces a cytopathic toxin that damages the epithelial cells in the mucosa. A number of antimicrobial agents have been implicated as inciting pseudomembranous enterocolitis, including clindamycin, lincomycin, some cephalosporins, penicillin G, chloramphenicol, tetracycline, and ampicillin.

Assessment and Diagnosis

Patients with pseudomembranous enterocolitis exhibit severe diarrhea, abdominal tenderness, leukocytosis, and fever. Stools are profuse but do not contain blood. The onset of symptoms may begin during antibiotic therapy or may be delayed until after discontinuation of it. As bowel wall necrosis progresses, the patient loses fluid, electrolytes, and albumin. Toxic megacolon, perforation, and peritonitis are potential complications.

Plain abdominal films and colonoscopy will reveal an edematous distended colon, distorted haustra, an erythematous, friable mucosa, yellow-white plaques, and ulcerations. Stool analysis may reveal *C. difficile,* although a negative culture does not absolutely rule out the disease.

Treatment

To prevent the disease from fulminating, antibiotics sensitive to *C. difficile* should be initiated. Colectomy or constructing a diverting ileostomy may be necessary when the symptoms are intractable to medical management or if toxic megacolon develops.

Nursing Care

Profuse diarrhea is a significant problem in the management of these patients. Perianal skin protection is essential. Because the stools are liquid and frequent, the patient may experience fecal incontinence. The nurse should wear gloves and properly dispose of articles soiled with stool. The use of a fecal incontinence pouch is often of value in containing stool and protecting the perianal skin. See Chapter 38.

Vital signs should be monitored frequently to evaluate fluid and electrolyte imbalances secondary to losses. An elevated temperature is common, and administration of antipyretics may be indicated.

Because of the risk of toxic megacolon and perforation, regular abdominal assessments are important. Any increases in abdominal girth or abdominal rigidity should be reported immediately to the physician.

Nursing Diagnosis and Management
Pseudomembranous enterocolitis

Fluid Volume Deficit related to diarrhea, p. 669

THERAPEUTIC MANAGEMENT

Because GI intubation is so common in intensive care patients, it is important for nurses to know the clinical indications and responsibilities inherent in their use. There are four categories of GI tubes based on function: nasogastric suction tubes, long intestinal tubes, therapeutic effect tubes, and feeding tubes (discussed in Chapter 9).

Nasogastric Suction Tubes

Nasogastric suction tubes (Levin, Salem-Sump) remove fluid regurgitated into the stomach, prevent accumulation of swallowed air, may partially decompress the bowel, and reduce the patient's risk for aspiration. The tube is passed through the nose into the nasopharynx and then down through the pharynx into the esophagus and stomach. The length of time the nasogastric tube remains in place depends on its use. Nursing care should prevent the complications common to this therapy, which include the following: ulceration and necrosis of the nares, esophageal reflux, esophagitis, esophageal erosion and stricture, gastric erosion, and dry mouth and parotitis from mouth breathing; interference with ventilation and coughing; and loss of fluid and electrolytes (see the box, "Select Patient Problems Associated with Nasogastric Tubes").

Long Intestinal Tubes

Miller-Abbott, Cantor, Johnston, and Baker tubes are all examples of long intestinal tubes that are placed either preoperatively or intraoperatively. The long length allows removal of contents from the intestine that cannot be accomplished by a nasogastric tube. These tubes can also decompress the small bowel. In addition, they can splint the small bowel intraoperatively or postoperatively. Because progression of the tubes is dependent on bowel peristalsis, their use is contraindicated in patients with paralytic ileus and severe mechanical obstruction. In addition to monitoring for the complications associated with nasogastric tubes, nurses should monitor the patient for gaseous distention of the balloon section, making removal difficult; rupture of the balloon or spillage of mercury into the intestine; overinfla-

---

SELECT PATIENT PROBLEMS ASSOCIATED WITH NASOGASTRIC TUBES

NASOPHARYNGEAL DISCOMFORT

Causes: absence of chewing, which is the normal stimulus to salivary secretions; mouth breathing as a result of the tubes being in place.

Signs/symptoms: sore throat, difficulty with swallowing, hoarseness, thirst, dry mucous membranes.

Plan: lubricate lips, chew sugarless gum, gargle with warm water and a mouthwash solution, use physiological saliva or analgesic and/or anesthetic lozenges for severe discomfort (anesthetic lozenges may decrease swallowing or gag reflexes).

Prevention: symptoms decreased or absent with use of soft, small-bore tubes; use of therapeutic nursing measures.

NASAL EROSIONS AND NECROSIS

Cause: pressure on nasal ala from tube.

Signs/symptoms: erosion of nasal ala.

Plan: tape tube so that no pressure is exerted against nasal ala; apply tincture of benzoin to area in which tape will be applied.

Prevention: use of soft, small-bore tube; tape properly.

ACUTE OTITIS MEDIA

Cause: pressure from the nasoenteric tube at the opening of the eustachian tube, with entry of pathogenic bacteria into the middle ear.

Signs/symptoms: severe, dull, throbbing ear pain, fe-

ver, chills, slight dizziness, nausea, and vomiting; a child may pull on affected ear.

Plan: change nasoenteric tube to other nostril; administer antibiotic therapy if appropriate; perform myringotomy if severe.

Prevention: use of soft, small-bore tubes.

HOARSENESS

Cause: irritation of laryngeal mucous membranes from presence of nasoenteric tube.

Signs/symptoms: hoarseness.

Plan: use soft, small-bore tube, steam or aerosol therapy, warm gargle, anesthetic lozenges.

Prevention: use soft, small-bore tube, adequate hydration, mouth care.

INABILITY TO WITHDRAW THE TUBE

Cause: tube possibly lodged within folds of mucosa or "stuck" to gastric wall.

Signs/symptoms: tube does not respond to gentle pulling motions.

Plan: place the patient in a side-lying position and flush the tube with 20-50 ml of water; then pull back gently on the tube. If unsuccessful, repeat flushing of tube with patient in Trendelenburg position (if not contraindicated). If both measures are unsuccessful, the tube should be cut, allowing evacuation of the lower portion through the rectum.

Modified from Bernard M and Forlaw L: Complications and their prevention. In Rombeau J and Caldwell M, editors: Clinical nutrition, vol 1, Enteral and tube feeding, Philadelphia, 1984, WB Saunders Co.

RESEARCH ABSTRACT

Measures to test placement of nasoenteral feeding tubes

Methany NA, Spies MA, and Eisenberg P: West J Nurs Res 10:367, 1988.

PURPOSE

The purpose of this study was to investigate the reliability of selected techniques to test tube placement and to assess degree of gastric retention.

FRAMEWORK

Many of the practical problems related to enteral nutrient administration remain unsolved, and practice varies widely from institution to institution. Compounding the problem is the recent proliferation in the types of commercially available feeding tubes; they differ in composition, gauge, construction, and methods and sites for insertion. Recent sources report that enteral feeding is emerging as a more cost efficient and physiological mode of nutrition than is total parenteral nutrition. The nursing literature has traditionally recommended that fluid be aspirated from the tube to verify gastric placement and that the degree of gastric retention be measured before introducing more feeding. Both of these measures were developed when only firm, large-bore tubes were in use. Although these measures are often possible with large-bore, firm feeding tubes, some authors report that they are difficult procedures to perform on small-bore pliable tubes, and reports conflict about the usefulness of auscultation of insufflated air to confirm the placement of small-bore feeding tubes. The literature is not specific about how the nurse should confirm that nasoduodenal or nasojejunal feeding tubes are in place. Once the tube is confirmed by radiography as in correct position, one must assume that it has remained in place.

METHODS

This descriptive pilot study was based on data recorded on an instrument designed by the researchers. Seven nursing units that had a large census of tube-fed patients in a large Midwestern hospital were used. All types of nasally placed feeding tubes encountered on the units during the study were included. Night nurses on the identified units were asked to record their responses to questions on the instrument for each nasogastric tube-fed patient they cared for during a 6-month period. They attempted to (1) aspirate at least 5 ml of fluid through a syringe from each tube, (2) auscultate for a gurgling sound over the epigastric region while injecting 10 ml of air through the tube, (3) test the ability of the patient to speak, and (4) measure gastric retention.

RESULTS

Twenty patients with nasogastric tubes and with a total of 128 tube days were studied. Staff nurses also supplied data on 55 patients with nasointestinal tubes with a total of 247 tube days. Simple descriptive statistics were used to analyze the data. Nurses reported being able to aspirate 5 ml of gastric contents in 79% of the patients with traditional large-bore firm nasogastric tubes. Only 45% of the attempts to withdraw fluid from small-bore (8-French) pliable nasogastric tubes were reported as successful. Only 33% of the attempts to aspirate fluid from the small-bore pliable nasointestinal tubes were successful. Of those nurses using traditional large-bore firm tubes, 90% stated that they were able to test adequately for retention as opposed to only 48% of those using the small-bore pliable tubes. Unless the patients were comatose, aphasic, or intubated, all were able to speak. None of the patients had feeding tubes inadvertently placed in the respiratory tract. Air was reportedly heard 18 times when the tube was documented by radiography as located in the stomach. However, air was also heard in the epigastric region when the tip of the tube was documented as elsewhere than in the stomach.

IMPLICATIONS

The data collected during this pilot study indicate that nursing interventions successful in providing safe management to patients with firm large-bore tubes cannot be applied to the care of patients with small-bore flexible feeding tubes. Collapse of some types of flexible tubes reportedly occurs in more than 50% of the attempts to aspirate them. It can also deter nurses from obtaining reliable estimates of the gastric contents and can affect patient safety with a resultant potential for aspiration. Tube placement is also difficult for the newer small-bore tubes. New methods of checking for tube placement must be developed; until they are, protocols that call for periodic x-ray films to determine placement must be used. Bowel sounds should be assessed at regular intervals, and if there is distention or active vomiting, feedings must be withheld.

tion of balloon, leading to intestinal rupture; and reverse intussusception if the tube is removed rapidly.

Therapeutic Effect Tubes

Therapeutic effect tubes most commonly refer to those designed to compress bleeding esophageal and gastric varices. They include the *Sengstaken-Blakemore tube,* and *Linton-Nachlus tube,* the *Edlich tube,* and the *Boyce* modification of the Sengstaken-Blakemore tube. This treatment modality stops acute variceal hemorrhage 85% to 90% of the time. Because the esophagus is totally occluded and rupture of the gastric balloon may result in complete airway obstruction (because of the tube's rising into the nasopharynx), rupture of the esophagus and pulmonary aspiration are major complications that can be fatal.

Because accumulation of secretions in the esophagus is a problem with the Sengstaken-Blakemore tube, a Linton-Nachlus tube may be used instead because it is designed with one gastric balloon and one lumen for aspiration that ends in the stomach and another lumen that ends in the esophagus. In addition, its gastric balloon applies pressure to the intragastric veins because of its larger size; thus esophageal compression is not necessary.

REFERENCES

1. Anderson C and Cerda JJ: Nutritional in GI disease: diets for patients with esophageal and gastric disorders, part 1, Consultant 26(5):25, 1986.
2. Boarini JH, Bryant RB, and Irrgang SJ: Fistula management, Semin Oncol Nurs 2(4):287, 1986.
3. Buschiazzo L and Possanzo C: A 57-year-old man with bleeding esophageal varices, JPEN 12(3):131, 1986.
4. Corman MC: Colon and rectal surgery, Philadelphia, 1984, JB Lippincott Co.
5. Decker SI: The life-threatening consequences of a GI bleed, RN 48(10):18, 1985.
6. Dusek JL: Iced gastric lavage slows bleeding in gastric hemorrhage, Crit Care Nurse 4(4):8, 1984.
7. Eastwood GL: Upper GI bleeding. II. differential diagnosis and management, Hosp Med 23(3):44, 1987.
8. Falconer MW: Falconer's the drug, the nurse, the patient, ed 7, Philadelphia, 1982, WB Saunders Co.
9. Fischer JE: The pathophysiology of enterocutaneous fistulas, World J Surg 7:446, 1983.
10. Fleischer D: Gastrointestinal endoscopy: a look into the future, SGA-J 9(4):171, 1987.
11. Fleischer D: The therapeutic use of lasers in GI disease, SGA-J 7(2):8, 1984.
12. Fuller E: Managing a lower GI bleed, Patient Care 18(6):118, 1984.
13. Gaber A: Endoscopic control of upper gastrointestinal bleeding with bipolar coagulation, SGA-J 7(2):20, 1984.

14. Goldberg SM, Gordon PH, and Nivatvongs S: Injuries to the anus and rectum. In Essentials of anorectal surgery, Philadelphia, 1980, JB Lippincott Co.
15. Guenter P and Slowm B: Hepatic disease: nutritional implications, Nurs Clin North Am 18(1):71, 1983.
16. Hoppe MC, Descalso J, and Kapp SR: Gastrointestinal disease: nutritional implications, Nurs Clin North Am 18(1):47, 1983.
17. Irrgang SJ and Bryant RA: Management of the enterocutaneous fistula, J Enterostom Ther 6(2):211, 1984.
18. Kagan BM: Antimicrobial therapy, ed 3, Philadelphia, 1980, WB Saunders Co.
19. Kurtz RS, Heimann TM, and Aufses AH: The management of intestinal fistulas, Am J Gastroenterol 76:377, 1981.
20. Larson G and others: Upper gastrointestinal bleeding: predictors of outcome, Surgery 100(4):765, 1985.
21. MacFadyen BV, Jr, Dudrick SJ, and Ruberg RL: Management of gastrointestinal fistulas with parenteral hyperalimentation, Surgery 74:100, 1973.
22. Maloney JP: Surgical intervention in the alcoholic patient with portal hypertension, Cleve Clin Q 8(4):63, 1986.
23. Meeroff JC: Algorithm for managing patients with severe GI hemorrhage, Hosp Pract 19(3):186, 1984.
24. Meeroff JC: Management of massive gastrointestinal bleeding, part 2, Hosp Pract 21(5):93, 1986.
25. Padilla GV and others: Subjective distresses of nasogastric tube feeding, JPEN 3:53, 1979.
26. Peppercorn MA: Acute gastrointestinal hemorrhage: pinpointing the source of defining its treatment, Consultant 27(6):61, 1987.
27. Price SA and Wilson LM: Pathophysiology: clinical concepts of disease processes, ed 3, New York, 1986, McGraw-Hill Book Co.
28. Quinless FW: Severe liver dysfunction: client problems and nursing actions, Focus Crit Care 12(1):24, 1985.
29. Rottenberg R: GI bleeding, emergency handbook, Patient Care 20(14):72, 1986.
30. Sabiston DC, editor: Davis-Christopher textbook of surgery: the biological basis of modern surgical practice, Philadelphia, 1977, WB Saunders Co.
31. Saegesser F: II: Acute abdomen from vascular disorders in the elderly, Clin. Gastroenterol 13(1):145, 1984.
32. Smith JL and Graham DY: Variceal hemorrhage: problems of selecting therapy that reduces risk of death, Consultant 23(10):85, 1983.
33. Solomon J, Harrington D, and Gogel HK: When the patient suffers from esophageal bleeding, endoscopic sclerotherapy, RN 50(2):24, 1987.
34. Thomas RJ: The response of patients with fistulas of the gastrointestinal tract to parenteral nutrition, Surg Gynecol Obstet 153:77, 1981.
35. Webb WA: Management of foreign bodies of the upper gastrointestinal tract, SGA-J 9(1):9, 1986.
36. Wetzel DA: Gastrointestinal complications following renal transplantation: nursing implications, J Enterostom Ther 14(1):16, 1987.
37. Winters WA: Coping with the massive GI bleeder: one method—esophga-gastric tamponade, SGA-J 8(2):24, 1985.
38. Yussen PS and LaManna MM: Anatomic localization of acute GI hemorrhage by radionuclide angiography, SGA-J 10(1):12, 1987.

CHAPTER

38

Gastrointestinal Care Plans

THEORETICAL BASIS AND MANAGEMENT

CHAPTER OBJECTIVES

- *Discuss the theoretical concepts related to altered nutrition: less than body requirements.*
- *Identify and describe nursing interventions that are essential in the treatment of altered nutrition: less than body requirements.*
- *Discuss the theoretical concepts related to altered nutrition: more than body requirements.*
- *Identify and describe nursing interventions that are essential in the treatment of altered nutrition: more than body requirements.*
- *Discuss the theoretical concepts related to potential for infection related to compromised nutrition.*
- *Identify and describe nursing interventions that are essential in the treatment of potential for infection related to compromised nutrition.*

ALTERED NUTRITION: LESS THAN BODY REQUIREMENTS
Theoretical Concepts

Nutritional support is an integral part of the comprehensive management of critically ill patients. The rationale for nutritional support is based on an understanding of protein-calorie malnutrition and its relationship to the physiological, hypermetabolic events that accompany critical illness. Cases of starvation and malnutrition have been reported in United States' hospitals since 1955.[56] In 1974 Dr. Charles Butterworth[2] described iatrogenic malnutrition and called attention to the prevalance and cause of protein-calorie malnutrition among hospitalized patients. Common hospital practices that adversely affect the nutritional status of patients were identified and are still the cause of hospital-induced malnutrition today (see the following box).[2]

Since 1984 several publications have documented a 30% to 50% incidence of hospital malnutrition. Bistrian and associates[8,9] documented that 50% of a population of general

---

PRACTICES KNOWN TO ADVERSELY AFFECT THE NUTRITIONAL STATUS OF HOSPITALIZED PATIENTS

1. Failure to order and record height and weight routinely.
2. Maintaining nothing-by-mouth (NPO) status for extended periods, with only glucose and saline solution administered intravenously.
3. Lack of recording patient's calorie counts.
4. Elimination of meals for diagnostic testing.
5. Lack of knowledge about available nutritional products.
6. Lack of knowledge about metabolic response to injury and stress.
7. Failure to assess nutritional status before major surgical procedures.
8. Lack of nutritional intervention after surgical procedures.
9. Lack of nutritional intervention until advanced depletion of lean body mass.
10. Lack of knowledge about nutrition's role in the prevention of infection.
11. Lack of knowledge about the complexities of enteral nutritional support.

Modified from Mosner M and Bader S: Rationale for nutrition support. In Krey SH and Murray RL, editors: Dynamics of nutrition support, Norwalk, Conn, 1986, Appleton-Century-Crofts.

surgical patients in an urban municipal hospital were malnourished, and a later study at the same hospital indicated that 45% of the general medical patients demonstrated symptoms of protein-calorie malnutrition. Weisner and associates[69] prospectively evaluated the nutritional status of medical patients from admission through 2 weeks of hospitalization. The 49% likelihood of malnutrition on admission increased to 69% 2 weeks later. Nutritional status decreased in 75% of those patients who were evaluated as healthy at the time of admission. They demonstrated that this development of malnutrition was hospital related and not just a reflection of nutritional status on admission. Recent studies have focused on critically ill patients, demonstrating a direct relationship between hospital protein-calorie malnutrition and increased mortality and morbidity.[24,26] The causes of hospital malnutrition first noted by Butterworth are still relevant.

The ability to intervene nutritionally when oral intake is not adequate or appropriate was developed in the late 1960s when Dr. Stanley Dudrick demonstrated that long-term, central venous access could be safely maintained and that central venous administration of hypertonic nutrient solutions could result in normal growth and development.[25] Since that time the specialty of nutritional support has grown in prominence among members of all disciplines, focusing attention on the nutritional needs of hospitalized patients.

To assess, administer, and monitor nutritional support therapies, the critical care nurse must have a basic knowledge of both normal and altered nutrient metabolism, nutritional requirements and the body's response to refeeding, and knowledge of currently available methods for parenteral and enteral nutritional intervention.

Nutrient supply. The major macronutrients of the body are carbohydrates, proteins, and fats. For proper metabolic functioning, adequate amounts of vitamins, electrolytes, minerals, and trace elements (micronutrients) also must be supplied. After oral intake all nutrients are broken down by digestion into smaller particles, which are then absorbed by the gastrointestinal (GI) tract. The process by which these nutrients are used at the cellular level is called metabolism. The major purpose of nutrient metabolism is the production of energy and the preservation of protein mass.

Carbohydrates. Of the three macronutrients, carbohydrates provide the preferred source of energy for cellular activity. Through the process of digestion, carbohydrates are broken down into glucose, fructose, and galactose. After absorption from the intestinal tract, fructose and galactose are broken down to glucose. Therefore glucose becomes the final source of used carbohydrates at the cellular level.

The primary function of glucose is to produce the energy needed to maintain cellular functions, including transport of substrates across cellular membranes, secretion of specific hormones, muscular contraction, and the synthesis of new substances. Most of the energy produced from carbohydrate metabolism is used to form adenosine triphosphate (ATP), the principal form of immediately available energy within the cytoplasm and nucleoplasm of all body cells. One gram of carbohydrate will provide 4 kcal of energy.

Glucose metabolism is regulated by the action of two pancreatic hormones, insulin and glucagon. Insulin affects the rate of glucose transport into cells. For example, after a meal has been eaten and there is a rise in blood glucose, insulin is released from the beta cells of the pancreas, causing an increase in glucose transport across cell membranes. Thus blood glucose levels are returned to normal (80 to 100 mg%). Conversely, a fall in the blood glucose level below normal will result in the release of glucagon from the alpha cells of the pancreas. Glucagon causes the conversion of liver glycogen to glucose, thereby raising the blood glucose level to normal, protecting the body against hypoglycemia.

Inside the cell glucose is either stored as glycogen or metabolized for the release of energy. All cells can store glycogen for future use; however, cells of the liver and the muscle have the largest glycogen reserves; which become important sources of glucose during times of metabolic need.

Although excess glucose can be stored as glycogen, only 200 to 300 g of glycogen is stored. These glycogen stores, when converted to glucose, provide only 6 to 12 hours of energy. When the glucose supply is depleted such as during starvation, moderate amounts of glucose can be formed from certain by-products of protein and fat metabolism. This process of manufacturing glucose from nonglucose precursors is called gluconeogenesis, a normal body defense mechanism that preserves the source of energy in time of increased physiological need and limited exogenous supply.[21]

Protein. Protein has important structural and functional activities within the body. It is the structural basis of all lean body mass such as organ mass and skeletal muscle. Proteins are important for visceral (cellular) functions such as initiation of chemical reactions (hormones and enzymes), transportation of other substances (apoproteins), preservation of immune function (antibodies), and maintenance of osmotic pressure (albumin) and blood neutrality (buffers).

Proteins constantly are synthesized, broken down into amino acids, and then resynthesized into new protein. This three-step process is called protein turnover. In very active tissues such as the gut, liver, and kidney, protein turnover occurs every few days. The average turnover time of all body protein has been estimated at 80 days; the rate of turnover is fastest in those proteins such as enzymes and hormones involved in metabolic activities. Therefore, to preserve lean body mass, a constant supply of protein must be assured.

The functional protein compound that is used at the cellular level is the amino acid. Through digestion, complex proteins are broken down into dipeptides and amino acids and are transported to the liver. The liver not only metabolizes the majority of amino acids but also regulates amino acid flow to other cells of the body. Only three amino acids, valine, leucine, and isoleucine, are metabolized outside the liver in skeletal muscle. During times of stress these three amino acids, called branch-chain amino acids, become very important, providing gluconeogenic precursors. One gram of protein provides 4 kcal of energy.

Specific amino acids are *essential;* that is, they cannot be produced by the body. They must be supplied by the diet. Other *nonessential* amino acids can be manufactured by the body under normal circumstances if the *essential* amino acids are in adequate supply (Table 38-1).

Like carbohydrate and fat, amino acid molecules contain

Table 38-1 Amino acids required for synthesis of protein in man

Essential amino acids	Nonessential amino acids	Nonessential amino acids that may be essential under specific circumstances
Leucine	Alanine	Histidine
Isoleucine	Glutamine	Arginine
Valine	Tyrosine	Cysteine
Phenylalanine	Aspartic acid	
Tryptophan	Asparagine	
Methionine	Glutamic acid	
Threonine	Proline	
Lysine	Serine	
	Glycine	

carbon, hydrogen, and oxygen. Amino acids, however, also contain nitrogen in the form of the amine group NH_2. It is the nonamine group that is used to produce glucose in times of need. However, if amino acids are broken down and used for making glucose (that is, gluconeogenesis), proteins are not available for their usual structural and functional activities, resulting in a depletion of both lean body mass (structural protein) and visceral (cellular) proteins, amino acids that are needed for survival. It is, therefore, the sparing of body protein that is the basis for nutritional support of the critically ill.

Fat (lipids). Lipids are also important for the maintenance of body function. They include fatty acids, triglycerides, phospholipids, cholesterol, and cholesterol esters. Aside from their involvement in functions such as the maintenance of cellular membranes and the manufacture of prostaglandins, lipids, primarily in the form of triglycerides, provide a stored source of energy. Triglycerides are more easily stored than glycogen. They are calorically dense molecules, providing more than twice the amount of energy per gram (9 kcal) as protein and carbohydrates.

Dietary lipids, mainly triglycerides, are hydrolyzed in the intestine to form micelles, which are emulsions of chains of fatty acids, monoglycerides, and bile salts. Short-chain fatty acids are passively absorbed through the intestine and are transported to the liver. Long-chain fatty acids are surrounded by specific proteins to form chylomicrons. These chylomicrons are transported out of the intestine through the lymphatic system, finally entering blood circulation through the thoracic duct. A portion of the chylomicrons is taken up by the liver, but the majority are directly transported to other tissues. With the aid of the enzyme lipoprotein lipase, triglyceride-containing chylomicrons are broken down outside the cell and enter the cell as fatty acids and glycerol. Once inside the cell, the fatty acids are oxidized or reformed into triglycerides for storage. Insulin also facilitates the cellular uptake of triglycerides.[21]

During an overnight fast, prolonged starvation, or metabolic stress when glucose supply is low, it is the breakdown of intracellular triglycerides through a process called lipolysis that provides fatty acids for energy production and glycerol for gluconeogenesis. Therefore the use of fatty

acids is directly related to the level of blood glucose.

The fatty acids released from adipose tissue can be used by either the liver or peripheral tissue. In the liver fatty acids are further degraded to ketones (betahydroxybutyrate, acetoacetate, and acetone). In the absence of glucose, fatty acid breakdown and ketone production are increased. Ketone bodies can be directly oxidized by skeletal muscle and used for energy. During prolonged starvation, the brain, which normally uses glucose, can convert to ketones as its primary energy source. This is another body defense mechanism to ensure a supply of energy when exogenous glucose intake is curtailed.

Protein calorie malnutrition. Malnutrition is the lack of necessary nutrients in the body or improper absorption and distribution of them. Although an inadequate supply of both macronutrients and micronutrients can lead to deficiencies and decreased functioning, it is the lack of protein and calories that further debilitates the critically ill patient—thus the use of the term protein-calorie malnutrition. To put it simply, an inadequate exogenous supply of calories for energy results in the breakdown of endogenous protein for gluconeogenesis, severely restricting the availability of protein and amino acids for other peripheral and visceral functions.

Malnutrition can be caused by simple starvation—the inadequate intake of nutrients. It can also be the result of physiological events that increase metabolism beyond the supply of nutrients. In the hospitalized patient the cause of malnutrition usually results from the combined effects of starvation and hypermetabolism.

Metabolic response to starvation and stress. To understand the development of malnutrition in the hospitalized patient, the nurse must understand the metabolic response to starvation and physiological stress.[21,62] Changes in endocrine status and metabolism work together to determine the onset and extent of malnutrition. Nutritional imbalance occurs when the demand for nutrients is greater than the exogenous nutrient supply. The major difference between one who is starved and one who is starved and injured is an increased reliance on endogenous protein breakdown to provide precursors for glucose production to meet increased energy demands. Therefore, although carbohydrate and fat metabolism are also affected, the main concern is with that of protein metabolism and homeostasis.

During the postabsorptive state the normal diet provides exogenous sources of carbohydrate and fat to meet the body's demand for fuel (Fig. 38-1, *A*). Any carbohydrate or fat not immediately used for energy is converted and stored as triglycerides (adipose tissue). Dietary protein enters the amino acid pool and is used to replace protein that has been degraded during routine protein turnover. Ninety-five percent of endogenous protein can be reused if necessary, with the diet providing the remaining 5% for protein synthesis.

During an acute, nonstressed fast the fuel demands of the body must still be met. Some amino acids, instead of being resynthesized into new protein or further broken down and excreted, are shuttled to the liver for gluconeogenesis (Fig. 38-1, *B*). In the liver the amino acid is degraded. The nitrogen-containing amine group is released, is converted to urea, and is transported to the kidney for excretion. The

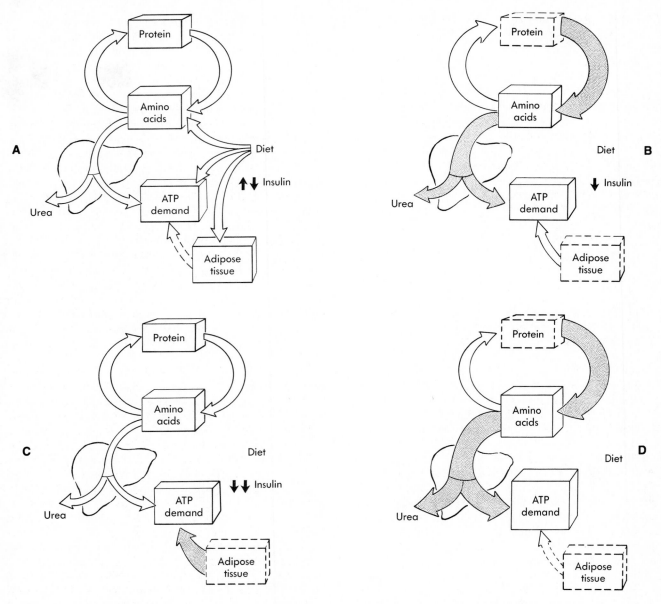

Fig. 38-1 The way substrates are used by the body for energy production changes depending on the supply or lack of supply of exogenous nutrients, as well as on the metabolic milieu (that is, stress/non-stress conditions). When preferred substrates of carbohydrate and fat are unavailable, protein substrates will be used for energy production. *A*, postabsorptive state. *B*, acute fast. *C*, prolonged fast. *D*, stress.

remaining hydrogen, carbon, and oxygen radical (called the carbon skeleton) enters the Kreb's cycle, which eventually produces ATP.

As fasting is prolonged, the metabolic rate decreases, blood levels of insulin fall, and glucagon levels rise. Glucagon promotes the use of glycogen reserves, which are quickly exhausted. Cellular triglycerides (adipose tissue) are therefore mobilized as the primary source of fuel (Fig. 38-1, *C*).

The triglycerides are degraded to fatty acids and glycerol. In the liver the glycerol is used to make glucose, and the fatty acids are further metabolized to ketones, which become the major source of energy. Once circulating levels rise, the

brain is able to use ketones for 70% of its energy. The total body's reliance on glucose as a major energy source is decreased. Protein breakdown and nitrogen excretion also slow as gluconeogenesis from protein precursors decreases. A small amount of protein and amino acids continues to be required for obligatory glucose users. White blood cells, the renal medulla, and 30% of brain function continue to rely on glucose as their preferred source of fuel. However, in general, the events of an acute fast are short lived. In the continued absence of exogenous calories, the body uses degraded triglycerides as its primary energy source. Endogenous protein stores are "spared" from use for gluconeogenesis, and protein homeostasis is partially restored.

Of concern to those caring for critically ill patients is the combination of starvation and the physiological stress resulting from injury, trauma, major surgery, and/or sepsis (Fig. 38-1, *D*). This physiological stress results in profound metabolic alterations that persist from the time of the stressful event until the completion of wound healing and recovery. This metabolic profile of starvation and stress differs greatly from that during unstressed starvation (Table 38-2). The metabolic response to stress, a normal body response, is associated with an increased metabolic rate (hypermetabolism) that necessitates a rise in oxygen consumption and energy expenditure.

Hormonal changes that occur at the initiation of the stressful event begin the hypermetabolic process. Stimulation of the sympathetic nervous system causes the adrenal medulla to release catecholamines (epinephrine and norepinephrine), which in turn stimulate the body's metabolic response to stress. There also occurs an outpouring of adrenocorticotropic hormone (ACTH) and antidiuretic hormone (ADH), as well as glucocorticoids and mineralocorticoids. Insulin resistance caused by the release of glucagon allows nutrient substrates, primarily amino acids, to move from peripheral tissues (for example, skeletal muscle) to the liver for gluconeogenesis.[28]

This hypermetabolic process is an effort by the body to mobilize its supply of circulating nutrient substrates such as glucose and amino acids. Unfortunately, this mobilization occurs at the expense of body tissue and function at a time when the needs for protein synthesis (for example, for wound healing and acute phase proteins) also are high. Hyperglycemia prevails as the effects of insulin and the release of free fatty acids are diminished by the effects of increased catecholamines, glucocorticoids, and glucagon. Again the body becomes reliant on its protein stores to provide substrates for gluconeogenesis because glucose now becomes the major fuel source. Loss of protein results in a negative nitrogen balance and weight loss. The classic response to metabolic stress is the use of protein for fuel.

Nutritional assessment. The primary goal of nutritional assessment is to identify the patient who is at risk for malnutrition because altered nutritional status is associated with adverse clinical outcomes. Although clinical status alone may dictate the need for nutritional intervention, a thorough nutritional assessment consists of collecting and evaluating a variety of clinical and biochemical data (see the box, "Components of Nutritional Assessment"), usually including clinical history and status, physical examination including height and weight, measurement of specific biochemical parameters, and tests of immune function.[36,40] A baseline admission nutritional assessment should be followed by serial assessments throughout the course of hospitalization. Physicians, dietitians, and nurses all have a role in gathering and analyzing pertinent data. The critical care nurse is in a crucial position to identify baseline and ongoing changes in nutritional status since it is the nurse who spends the most time with the patient.

The major components of nutritional assessment reflect alterations in protein homeostasis because significant loss of lean body mass is associated with increased mortality and morbidity. These alterations in protein homeostasis associated with loss of lean body mass result in organic dysfunction and can be clinically observed (see the box, "Signs and Symptoms of Loss of Lean Body Mass"). Although generalized weakness and a lack of endurance reflect the loss of skeletal muscle mass, protein from all body organs is lost. Respiratory function deteriorates as intercostal and diaphragmatic muscles waste, causing progressive deterioration of respiratory effort. A lessened ventilatory response

Table 38-2 Metabolic responses during starvation

	Without stress	With stress
Brief starvation	↓ Metabolic rate Normal body temperature ↓ Blood insulin levels ↑ Blood glucagon levels ↑ Blood free fatty acids levels ↑ Urinary nitrogen excretion	↓ Metabolic rate ↓ Body temperature ↓ Blood insulin levels ↑ Catecholamine, glucagon, cortisol levels ↑ Glucose levels ↑ Blood lactate levels ↑ Plasma free fatty acid levels ↑ Urinary nitrogen excretion
Prolonged starvation	↓ Metabolic rate ↓ Body temperature ↓ Blood insulin levels ↑ Free fatty acid levels ↑ Urinary nitrogen excretion	↑ Metabolic rate → ↓ metabolic rate ↑ Body temperature ↑ Or normal insulin levels ↑ Or normal catecholamine, glucagon, cortisol levels ↑ Or normal blood glucose levels ↑ Blood lactate levels ↑ Free fatty acid levels ↑ Urinary nitrogen excretion

From Forlaw L: Nurs Clin North 18:112, 1983.

COMPONENTS OF NUTRITIONAL ASSESSMENT

HISTORY

- Loss of more than 10% of body weight within previous 6 months.
- Presence of altering factors such as organ failure, sepsis, fever, trauma, burns, use of steroids, antineoplastics, and/or immunosuppressants.
- Inadequate oral intake as a result of NPO status, difficulty with chewing, swallowing, digestion, and/or absorption.
- Long-term negative nutritional effects of chronic disease, chronic dialysis, anorexia, nausea, substance abuse.
- Protracted protein losses such as malabsorption caused by short gut syndromes, dialysis, fistulas, draining wounds, thermal injuries.

PHYSICAL EXAMINATION

Inspection

- Actual weight: less than 90% of ideal or more than 120% of ideal; weight is falsely evaluated because of edema, ascites, organomegaly, tumor bulk, anasarca, amputation.
- Mental status, lethargic, apathetic, listless, irritable, disoriented, obtunded, comatose.
- Hair: fragile, coarse, lackluster, alopecia.
- Eyes: sunken, dull, dry, pale conjunctiva, presence of Bitot's spots, scleral icterus.
- Mouth: mucous membranes possibly dry, pale, red, swollen.
- Lips: dry, cracked, red, swollen, angular stomatitis.
- Tongue: smooth, pale, slick, coated.
- Teeth and gums: swollen, bleeding gums, caries, edentulous, or ill-fitting dentures.
- Gag reflex: decreased or absent.
- Musculoskeletal: evident muscle wasting, thin extremities, flaccid muscles, decreased activity tolerance.
- Skin: dry, scaly, tented, flaky paint dermatosis, edema, draining or unhealed wounds, pressure sores, ecchymoses, subcutaneous fat loss.
- Nails: brittle, thin, flattened, ridged, spoon-shaped.
- Respirations: dyspnea, increased sputum production.
- Abdomen: distention increased girth, ascites.
- Stools: loose or hard-formed; fatty or clay-colored.

Auscultation

- Breath sounds: crackles resulting from protein deficiency–related fluid shifts.
- Bowel sounds: diminished, hyperactive, or absent.

Palpation

- Glands: enlargement of thyroid, parotid.
- Pulses: tachycardia, bradycardia.
- Abdomen: tender on palpation.

DIAGNOSTIC TESTS

Anthropometrics

- Weight for height.
- Tricep skinfold measurement.
- Midarm muscle circumference.

Visceral proteins

- Serum albumin.
- Serum transferrin.
- Thyronin-binding prealbumin.
- Amino acid profile.
- Nitrogen balance studies.
- Blood urea nitrogen.
- Creatinine height index.

Tests of immune function

- Total lymphocyte count.
- Delayed cutaneous hypersensitivity reactions.

Electrolytes and trace minerals

- Serum potassium.
- Serum sodium.
- Serum phosphorus.
- Serum magnesium.
- Serum calcium.
- Serum zinc.

Tests of gastrointestinal (GI) function

- Schilling's test.
- D-xylose test.
- 72-hour stool fat.
- GI series.

---

to hypoxic stimuli results in a potential for increased pneumonia and bronchitis.[45] Renal function deteriorates as decreased urea concentration in the renal medulla results in a loss of the kidney's concentrating ability.[50] Within the GI tract, decreased muscle function leads to decreased motility, malabsorption, and increased transit time.[38] Cardiac muscle, once thought spared during malnutrition, is also diminished. Increased demand for oxygen consumption during hyper-

metabolic states is not met because of decreased stroke volume.[45,53]

The catabolism of body protein is reflected in the renal excretion of urea nitrogen by the kidneys. Twenty-four hour measurements of urinary urea nitrogen are used to measure the degree of hypercatabolism and the response to nutritional support. Nitrogen balance is calculated by subtracting nitrogen excretion from nitrogen (protein) intake. A positive

---

SIGNS AND SYMPTOMS OF LOSS OF LEAN BODY MASS

Decreased muscle mass: skeletal, respiratory, cardiac

Decreased visceral proteins: albumin, prealbumin, transferrin, retinol-binding capacity, negative nitrogen balance

Decreased immune response: lymphocytes, compliment, acute phase proteins, antibodies

Poor wound healing

Poor responses to additional stress, surgery, injury

Organ dysfunction: failure of gut, liver, heart, kidney

---

nitrogen balance exists when intake exceeds output; a negative balance exists when output exceeds intake.

The obese individual can develop malnutrition in spite of an excessive amount of fat and the appearance of being overweight. Intense physiological stress, as previously discussed, can result in protein breakdown. Despite an abundance of fat stores, the obese patient does not convert adipose tissue to triglycerides as a source of energy during critical illness. Malnutrition is frequently not recognized in obese or overweight patients because their size fails to draw attention to their nutritional needs, and excessive body fat may obscure observation of muscle wasting. All critically ill patients, whether underweight or obese, need the same degree of nutritional assessment and aggressive nutritional intervention.

Although many biochemical parameters reflect nutritional status to some degree, visceral proteins are traditional markers. They are hepatic in origin and are particularly sensitive to changes in amino acid supply. Such parameters as serum albumin, transferrin, and more recently prealbumin and retinol-binding capacity have been used as key predictors of protein-calorie malnutrition.[18]

Critically ill patients often do not succumb to their primary disease but to infection and sepsis. Therefore tests of immunocompetence are important. Measurement of total lymphocytes indicates the state of nutrition because of their high metabolic priority. Cell-mediated immunity is an important host defense against infection, reflecting the activity of T cell lymphocytes. Cell-mediated immunity is measured by observing the cutaneous response of delayed hypersensitivity to specific recall antigens placed intradermally. Anergy, a lack of response to intradermal skin testing, is associated with an increased potential for infection.[47]

As endogenous protein is further diminished, wound healing, normally a body priority, also suffers. A lack of protein synthesis at the wound border results in decreased tensile strength, potentiating wound dehiscence. Continued loss of lean body mass will eventually result in increased organ failure and the inability of the body to adapt to additional stressful events. This impaired ability for adaptation restricts survival.

No single parameter of nutritional status can be used in isolation to define the degree of malnutrition. Many of these parameters, reflective as they are of nutritional status, are influenced by nonnutritional physiological events. Clinical status such as fluid overload, the use of agents such as steroids, and the patient's age are but three factors that may result in false-negative or false-positive test results. Thus the importance of referencing biochemical parameters of nutritional status with those of clinical status is key.

Nutritional requirements. Nutritional requirements define the number of nonprotein calories needed to meet energy demands, as well as the grams of protein needed to maintain protein synthesis. Calculation of nutritional requirements is a stepwise process. First, an estimate of basal energy expenditure is calculated. Basal energy expenditure reflects a steady state at which the body is at rest and performing minimal functions needed to maintain life. It is commonly estimated using the Harris-Benedict formula derived in 1912[31] (see the following box). To the basal energy expenditure is added a "stress factor," an estimate of the increase in the energy expenditure required because of physiological stress. Energy requirements for acutely critically ill patients are often in the range of 20 to 35 kcal per kilogram of body weight per day.[16]

In some hospitals the actual energy expenditure is measured using indirect calorimetry. From measurements of actual oxygen consumption and carbon dioxide excretion, calculations of actual energy expenditure can be derived.[67] The energy expenditure calculated from indirect calorimetry measurements compares favorably to calculations derived from the use of the basal energy expenditure formula with stress factors added.

Protein requirements range from 1 to 2.5 g/kg/day for the hospitalized patient. This is higher than the recommended dietary allowance of 0.8 g/kg/day for healthy adults. Increased protein demand can result from the need to repair injured tissue, preserve organ function, restore visceral protein stores, and maintain host defenses. Protein requirements also increase as stress increases; however, the amount of protein that can be used is dependent on hepatic and renal function.[11]

Nutritional requirements for calories and protein also affect micronutrient requirements. The movement of carbohydrate and amino acids into the cell will deplete extracel-

---

HARRIS-BENEDICT FORMULA FOR ESTIMATING BASAL ENERGY EXPENDITURE (BEE)

Men: BEE = 66.47 + 13.7 (kg/ideal weight) + 5 (height in cm) − 0.676 (age)

Women: BEE = 655.1 + 9.56 (kg/ideal weight) + 1.8 (height in cm) − 4.68 (age)

From Harris JA and Benedict FG: A biometric study of basal metabolism in man, Pub No 279, Washington, DC, 1919, Carnegie Institute of Washington.

Table 38-3 Micronutrients

Vitamins	Minerals/trace elements
Vitamin A (retinol)	Calcium
Vitamin B$_1$ (thiamine)	Chromium
Vitamin B$_2$ (riboflavin)	Copper
Vitamin B$_6$ (pyridoxine)	Iodine
Vitamin B$_{12}$ (cobalamine)	Iron
Vitamin C (ascorbic acid)	Magnesium
Vitamin D (calciferol)	Manganese
Vitamin E (α-tocopherol)	Molybdenum
Vitamin K	Phosphorus
Biotin	Selenium
Folic acid (folacin)	Zinc
Niacin (nicotinic acid)	
Pantothenic acid	

lular amounts of these micronutrients (Table 38-3) unless supplementation is provided.[2,54]

Methods of nutritional support. Once nutritional requirements have been estimated, the method of nutritional support must be selected.

The method chosen for nutritional support is dependent on a number of factors, including macronutrient and micronutrient requirements, organ function, GI and intravenous (IV) access, and potential complications that may occur during nutritional support. Complications may be related to access, the metabolic effect of the nutrients on specific organ systems, or infection.

The GI (enteral) route is the route of choice whenever possible. Enteral feeding through nasogastric feeding tubes and gastrostomy and jejunostomy tubes is common. However, in many critically ill patients the gut does not consistently function as a result of trauma, surgical procedures, lack of peristalsis, or intractable diarrhea. Use of the gut may also be contraindicated because of potential pulmonary aspiration of the enteral formula.

The parenteral route allows more constant delivery of nutrients. Because of the hypertoxicity of parenteral nutrient solutions, central venous access must be used for administration to decrease the potential for a chemical phlebitis or severe thrombosis. Peripheral nutritional support is possible, but its use is limited to 5 to 7 days and requires a large fluid load to deliver the number of calories and grams of protein usually needed by a critically ill patient. Because central venous access is at a premium in many patients, the use of multilumen catheters in recent years has allowed the concurrent administration of nutrients with other IV solutions such as IV antibiotics and with hemodynamic monitoring. The use of central venous access can result in a host of mechanical complications, as well as catheter-related infection. The potential for catheter-related complications is well recognized, and strict protocols have been developed to diminish the chance of complications.[51,70]

Standard nutritional support solutions usually are based on the use of glucose as the nonprotein energy source and the use of amino acids to provide protein substrate. To this combination is added the necessary vitamins, minerals, trace elements, and electrolytes. In recent years the availability of IV fat has allowed decreased dependency in the parenteral diet on glucose, especially in those patients in whom hyperglycemia cannot be controlled. A current trend is toward the use of disease- or organ-specific solutions in critical care settings. Current technology allows adjustments in the amounts of carbohydrate, fat, and protein within a specific solution. Specific solutions individualized to take into consideration hepatic, renal, respiratory, and cardiac failure can be formulated. The use of disease-specific solutions also considers potential adverse effects to organ function that might result from the overuse of specific nutrients (see "Altered Nutrition: More than Body Requirements").

ALTERED NUTRITION: MORE THAN BODY REQUIREMENTS
Theoretical Concepts

Alterations in nutrition because of greater than body requirements usually refers to the obese individual. However, the aggressive overuse of nutritional support for critically ill patients has historically been shown to cause undesirable alterations in nutrition. Therefore both situations are discussed in this section.

Obesity. Obesity is a complex medical disorder. For individuals with moderate obesity (130% to 199% of ideal body weight) or morbid obesity (greater than 200% of ideal body weight) a health hazard exists.[37] Obese individuals have a greater incidence of cardiovascular disease, hypertension, renal disease, cholecystitis, diabetes, immobility, infection, pulmonary and ventilatory complications, and thromboembolic disease when compared to individuals who are normal weight for height or who are underweight. Obesity is usually defined as an abnormally high proportion of body fat relative to the amount of lean body mass (protein weight). Obese individuals, both men and women, have increased mortality and morbidity, which can be decreased with weight reduction.[61]

The critically ill obese patient, however, may be protein malnourished. Despite the increased adipose tissue deposits, during critical illness and hypermetabolic states obese patients are not able to use fat stores for energy and are as reliant on endogenous protein sources as are other critically ill patients. The nutritional needs of the obese often are not investigated, because obesity hides skeletal muscle wasting. Critically ill obese patients should receive the same degree of nutritional assessment and support as do other patients since, in most cases, critical illness, with its increased demand for protein and calories, is not the appropriate time during which to begin weight reduction.

The effects of obesity on organ function further complicate treatment. There is an adverse effect on the cardiovascular system. The heart is often enlarged, and cardiac output, stroke volume, and blood volume are increased.[1] Elevated left- and right-ventricular filling pressures and high systemic and pulmonary vascular resistance have been documented.[6] Systemic hypertension is also common. Clinical studies have shown that obese patients who undergo weight reduction have a significant drop in blood pressure, heart

---

Altered Nutrition: Less Than Body Protein–Caloric Requirements related to lack of exogenous nutrients and increased metabolic demand

DEFINING CHARACTERISTICS

- Recent, unplanned weight loss of 10% of body weight within the last 6 months
- Serum albumin <3.5 g/100 ml
- Total lymphocytes <1500 mm^3
- Anergy
- Negative nitrogen balance
- Fatigue; lack of energy and endurance
- Nonhealing wounds
- Daily caloric intake less than estimated nutritional requirements
- Presence of factors known to increase nutritional requirements, e.g., sepsis, trauma, multiorgan failure
- Maintenance of NPO status for >7-10 days
- Long-term use of 5% dextrose intravenously
- Documentation of suboptimal calorie counts
- Drug or nutrient interaction that might decrease oral intake, e.g., chronic use of bronchodilators, laxatives, anticonvulsives, diuretics, antacids, narcotics
- Physical problems with chewing, swallowing, choking, salivation, and presence of altered taste, anorexia, nausea, vomiting, diarrhea, or constipation

OUTCOME CRITERIA

- Patient exhibits stabilization of weight loss or weight gain of ½ pound daily.
- Serum albumin is >3.5 g/dl.
- Total lymphocytes are >1500 mm^3.

- Patient has positive response to cutaneous skin antigen testing.
- Patient is in positive nitrogen balance.
- Wound healing is evident.
- Daily caloric intake equals estimated nutritional requirements.
- Increased ambulation and endurance is evident.

NURSING INTERVENTIONS *AND RATIONALE*

1. Continue to monitor the assessment parameters listed under "Defining Characteristics."
2. Document factors that identify patients at risk for nutritional deficits.
3. Assess patient during physical care for signs of nutritional deficiencies.
4. Measure admission height and weight.
5. Weigh patient daily.
6. Ensure that specimens for biochemical tests of nutritional status are collected properly and on time.
7. Accurately collect blood samples through multilumen catheter.
8. Administer parenteral and enteral solutions as prescribed.
9. Control infusion rate of parenteral and enteral solutions through infusion control devices and check rate every hour.
10. Flush enteral feeding tubes every 4 hours *to maintain patency.*
11. Document oral intake through calorie counts.
12. Perform serial assessments of patient's strength, endurance, conditions of wounds.

---

rate, stroke volume, cardiac output, and oxygen uptake.[37] Since hypertension is so prevalent among obese patients, one would suspect that renal dysfunction would also be more common because hypertension reduces renal blood flow and tubular function.[61]

Of particular concern are the respiratory complications associated with morbid obesity. Morbidly obese patients are particularly susceptible to hypoventilation. They may demonstrate increased ventilatory demand, increased work of breathing, respiratory muscle insufficiency, and hypoxemia. Associated with these findings are increases in total and pulmonary blood volumes and cardiac output.[6] The Pickwickian syndrome, obesity hypoventilation caused by excessive adipose mass around the lungs and diaphragm, can be life-threatening. However, with weight reduction, near normal ventilatory function may be restored.[58]

Obese patients are more prone to wound infections and dehiscence. They are at high risk for wound infections mainly because of the technical difficulties encountered dur-

ing surgical procedures. Their surgical procedures usually take longer and result in more trauma to the abdominal wall and subcutaneous tissues because of vigorous retraction required during abdominal procedures. Another cause of increased wound infection is the excessive amount of poorly vascularized, subcutaneous fatty tissue surrounding the wound, allowing bacteria to thrive. Wound dehiscence is further enhanced because of the technical difficulties in closing the wound and the increased tension on the wound from the subcutaneous adipose tissue.[61]

Recent treatment of morbid obesity has taken two routes. Medically the use of very low carbohydrate diets, fewer than 800 calories per day, has been tried, as has gastric bypass surgery. An excellent review of the medical and surgical treatment of obesity is presented by Hoffer, Palombo, and Bistrian.[37]

Metabolic results from use of nutritional support (more than body requirements). Parenteral and enteral nutritional support alter metabolic events. The overuse of carbohydrate, protein, and fat, in particular, has been associated with well-defined metabolic complications. In recent years, much attention has focused on better methods to define specifically the nutritional requirement of the critically ill patient so that nutritional support does not result in overfeeding. Overfeeding, especially of the macronutrients carbohydrate, protein, and fat, has been associated with organ dysfunction and failure.

Metabolic results from carbohydrate overfeeding

HYPERGLYCEMIA. Hyperglycemia is the most commonly observed metabolic complication related to the use of carbohydrate.[56,60] It is recommended that the blood glucose level be maintained below 150 mg%/dl, a level difficult to achieve in the septic, diabetic, or hypermetabolic critically ill patient. When observed at the initiation of nutritional support therapy, hyperglycemia may be caused by a rapid infusion rate, the inability of the pancreas to increase endogenous insulin production, or the lack of exogenous insulin supplementation. In a patient who previously was glucose tolerant, the sudden presence of hyperglycemia may predict impending infection or sepsis. Hyperglycemia and glycosuria precede the clinical diagnosis of sepsis by 12 to 24 hours. Glycosuria may be observed before a rise in temperature or a rise in the white blood cell count. Patients with renal insufficiency often have a high renal glucose threshold. Certain medications such as steroids may alter the results of urinary glucose testing. In many situations glucose monitoring should be based on blood glucose levels not urinary sugars. Altering the nutritional formula or solution's prescription to include more nonprotein calories as fat may resolve the glucose intolerance and decrease the need for exogenous insulin supplementation.

HYPEROSMOLAR, HYPERGLYCEMIC, NONKETOTIC DEHYDRATION, AND COMA. If hyperglycemia is prolonged and is accompanied by glycosuria and diuresis, the syndrome of hyperosmolar, hyperglycemia, nonketotic dehydration, and coma (HHNC or HHNK) may develop. In more than 40% of cases, this syndrome is fatal.[71] HHNC has been reported during the use of both parenteral and enteral nutrition.[10,41] When a hyperosmolar formula is introduced into the gut's lumen in a haphazard fashion or if the gut's mucosa cannot assimilate the formula quickly, additional water will move into the lumen from the extracellular space in an attempt to neutralize the osmotic effect of the formula. The presence of this additional fluid within the gut's lumen may be accompanied by patient complaints of fullness, nausea, or diarrhea since the movement of water into the gut occurs much faster than the transport of nutrients out of the gut. Infusion of the enteral formula by continuous drip, beginning at dilute concentrations and/or slow hourly rates, will allow gut adaptation. If diarrhea occurs, the concurrent administration of antidiarrheal agents such as tincture of opium or paregoric is beneficial.

Hyperglycemia will occur if enteral nutrient absorption proceeds but, because of a lack of endogenous insulin or a clinically created insulin resistance, glucose uptake by the cells is diminished. At this point in the sequence of events, administration of either glucose-containing enteral formulas or parenteral nutrient solutions will alter metabolism in a similar way, contributing to the development of HHNC.

In the patient with adequate pancreatic beta cell function, hyperglycemia will cause increased endogenous insulin release. However, in patients who have other reasons for glucose intolerance, this additional insulin release will be minimal—sufficient to prevent ketosis but not sufficient to control the hyperglycemia. Hyperglycemia dehydrates the beta cell, also suppressing the production of insulin. Unless exogenous insulin is supplied, the cycle of hyperglycemia, dehydration, and inadequate insulin production and release continues. Regular insulin should be administered to maintain a normal blood glucose level. A continuous insulin infusion may be required in extreme cases, or the nutritional solution may be temporarily discontinued until metabolic problems stabilize. The hyperglycemia, if extreme, should be corrected gradually. If correction of the hyperglycemia occurs too quickly, cerebral edema may develop.[52]

Hyperglycemia leads to glycosuria as the kidney attempts to excrete the increased solute load it has absorbed. Glucose is a very effective osmotic diuretic, even in the presence of adequate ADH. Persistent glycosuria alters the normal osmotic gradient within the renal tubules, causing excretion of large volumes of urine (that is, osmotic diuresis). If renal insufficiency already exists, the ability to concentrate the urine is one of the first functions to diminish; also increasing diuresis, which may lead to clinical signs of dehydration if fluid supplementation is not begun.

Initially during this cycle, the fluid loss is mainly water, but continued diuresis results in a loss of important electrolytes, primarily sodium and potassium. Total body sodium depletion and hypokalemia can result. These electrolyte losses eventually will be accompanied by changes in sensorium as fluid and electrolyte shifts involve the intracellular as well as the extracellular fluid compartments. Treatment is aimed at replacement of sodium and water. At the same time, cautious use of insulin is suggested, because sudden decreases in blood glucose in the presence of total sodium deficits can cause rapid fluid shifts within the central nervous system. These shifts can result in edema, convulsions, coma, and death.[10] Fluid supplementation is important. The use of an isotonic saline solution and electrolyte replacement will repair these deficits, preventing a shift of water back into the intracellular compartment.

HYPERCAPNIA. Excessive production of carbon dioxide has been measured in specific patients who receive nutritional support solutions containing a high concentration of glucose. Hypercapnia has been documented during the administration of both parenteral and enteral nutrition. Much of the early work in this area was done by Askanazi and associates.[5] They demonstrated that the nutritionally depleted patient who is not hypermetabolic and who is fed a large glucose load will respond appropriately by increasing carbon dioxide production, which is accompanied by a minimal increase in oxygen consumption. The hypermetabolic patient also increases his or her carbon dioxide production; however, this increase is accompanied by a large rise (70%) in minute ventilation, which indicates a substantial increase in oxygen consumption.

For those patients with marginal pulmonary function, an increase in carbon dioxide production is of critical concern. For example, the patient with chronic obstructive pulmonary disease who is insensitive to rises in arterial carbon dioxide levels may not be able to ventilate well enough to excrete the additional carbon dioxide. Carbon dioxide retention would result. The increased oxygen consumption and increased carbon dioxide production might precipitate respiratory distress, interfering with the patient's attempts at spontaneous ventilation.[5] Respiratory failure precipitated by high carbohydrate loads during refeeding has been documented.[5] Such a sequence of events would be particularly harmful for the ventilator-dependent patient who is attempting to wean from the ventilator.

It is recommended that the composition of nutritional support solutions for pulmonary compromised or ventilatory-dependent patients be altered to provide 30% to 60% of the nonprotein calories as fat. Fat does not require the same degree of increased oxygen consumption and carbon dioxide production as does the use of glucose.[25]

HEPATIC DYSFUNCTION. Hepatic dysfunction was an early complication associated with parenteral overfeeding or refeeding. Alterations in liver function tests and changes in hepatocyte structure are common. Despite an increasing understanding of metabolism, hepatic dysfunction during nutritional support therapy remains a concern.

Hepatic dysfunction ranges from asymptomatic, transient elevations of liver function test levels to progressive hepatic failure and coma. Physical changes noted within the hepatocytes microscopically include cholestatis, fatty metamorphosis, hepatocellular necrosis, fibrosis, and cirrhosis. Such changes in hepatocyte structure usually are severe only in the neonate or young child. The clinical picture in adults is benign and usually reversible.[43] Elevation of levels in liver function tests occurs in the majority of adult patients who receive total parenteral nutrition (TPN) for more than 2 weeks. In a study of 100 patients, serial comparisons of liver function test results (before TPN and during TPN) demonstrated that serum glutamic-pyruvic transaminase (SGPT) increased to 5.4 times the baseline, serum bilirubin increased to 2.3 times the baseline, and lactate dehydrogenase (LDH) increased to 1.5 times the baseline value.[31] These liver function test elevations lasted from 4 to 10 days.

Patients with preexisting hepatic disease have shown marked progression of liver function changes. Liver biopsies, taken during periods of test result elevations, demonstrate fatty infiltrates of the hepatocytes and increased glycogen stores but no inflammatory or cholestatic changes as are often seen in neonates. At a later date those receiving prolonged TPN may again exhibit liver function test result changes, which often are accompanied by inflammation of the hepatocytes.[18] The cause of these hepatic alterations is unclear. There is a consensus that excessive glucose calories or an inappropriate calorie-to-protein ratio plays a major role.[43] In both animal and human studies, reversible hepatic fatty infiltration has been shown to be related to infusions of high concentrations of glucose. It has been suggested that an upper limit of glucose use exists, especially in the hypermetabolic patient.[15] Delivery of excessive glucose results in the conversion of glucose to intrahepatic fat. The diagnosis of TPN-related hepatic dysfunction is largely by exclusion since biliary disease, sepsis, malignancy, anesthesia, and hepatoxic drugs also cause alterations in hepatic function.

Treatment of hepatic dysfunction during TPN administration has included (1) the provision of adequate but not excessive calories, (2) a decreased reliance on glucose alone as the nonprotein calorie source, (3) the provision of an adequate calorie-to-protein ratio (for example, no higher than 200:1), and (4) the provision of a glucose-free infusion during part of the daily TPN cycle. During this rest period from glucose infusion, the liver is able to clear itself of the accumulated glucose.

Metabolic results from protein overfeeding

AZOTEMIA. Azotemia, a complication related to protein intake, was identified during the early use of nutritional support therapy. In 1968 Gault, Dixon, and Cohen[30] described a tube-feeding syndrome consisting of hypernatremia, azotemia, and dehydration. In those days it was common for the daily protein intake to reach levels greater than 210 g because of the high concentration of protein in blenderized formulas.

Although the cause of this tube-feeding syndrome was the use of high amounts of protein, the sequence of events and potential clinical outcome are similar to those occurring during HHNC. Metabolism of the ingested protein necessitates the production of large amounts of urea by the liver. This urea is sent to the kidneys for excretion, necessitating increased urinary production and excretion for disposal of this increased solute load. In the case of the elderly or those patients with renal dysfunction, the kidney may not be able to adapt to such additional demands.

Patients receiving TPN also may be at risk for azotemia. Amino acid concentrations as high as 11% are used for compounding parenteral nutrition solutions. Clinicians studying the effects of nutritional support on the critically ill have emphasized the need for a lower protein-to-calorie ratio (80:1) as opposed to the traditional 150:1 ratio.[16] High protein intakes in this patient population must be closely monitored since acute renal failure frequently occurs as a part of the primary disease process.

The quantity and quality of amino acids used in various disease states have received increased attention. The first disease-specific study included patients with renal failure.[65] In question was the ability to manufacture nonessential amino acids within the body if only essential amino acids were provided. This was the basis for the "renal failure solutions" used in the past. It is now recognized that both essential and nonessential amino acids are needed exogenously during renal failure and that dialysis should be used, whenever possible, so that the protein needs of the patient can be more easily met without correspondingly increased renal toxicity.[65]

AMINO ACID SERUM IMBALANCE. The ratio of plasma amino acids is of concern and is a potential cause of hepatic encephalopathy. Patients with hepatic dysfunction have decreased ability to metabolize certain amino acids, especially tryptophan and phenylalanine, which must be metabolzied in the liver. Branch-chain amino acids continue to be used (leucine, isoleucine, and valine). They are metabolized only in skeletal muscle. Plasma ratios of aromatic amino acids rise, whereas the ratios of branch-chain amino acids fall.

It is theorized that the aromatic amino acids cross the blood-brain barrier in increased numbers and enter into false neurotransmitter reactions.[32] These false neurotransmitters are thought to be the cause of the central nervous system symptoms of hepatic encephalopathy. Provision of solutions containing an increased percent of branch-chain amino acids have, in some instances, decreased clinical symptoms of hepatic encephalopathy, resulting in less somnolence and lethargy. However, controversy exists about whether or not eventual patient outcome is improved.[32]

Current study of the traumatized and hypermetabolic critically ill patient has lead to further investigation of the role of the branch-chain amino acids. Cerra and associates[16] have demonstrated an improved use of the branch-chain amino acids, especially leucine, in this patient population. However, at this point in time, the relationship of improved metabolism of amino acids to final patient outcome is still a controversial issue.

Metabolic results caused by lipid overfeeding. Despite the demonstrated safety of the currently available fat emulsions, concern over potential complications still exist. However, the overloading syndrome that occurred with the use of the cottonseed oil emulsion available during the 1950s has not been observed with the currently available fat emulsions.

Before hydrolysis, intravenous fat emulsions are taken up by the liver and spleen. Final clearance is through the reticuloendothelial system in Kupffer cells of the liver. Changes in Kupffer cell pigmentation have been observed but apparently are reversible once the fat emulsion has been discontinued.[31]

Infusion of 500 ml of 10% soybean oil emulsion produced a decrease in the pulmonary diffusion capacity of healthy young men, but these changes were no greater than those observed during postprandial lipemia.[34,63] Pulmonary congestion has been attributed specifically to the infusion of the fat emulsion, but similar observations have been reproduced by infusing excessive quantities of normal saline solution.[63]

Observation of alterations in erythropoiesis have been made but are inconsistent and at times contradictory. Hypercoagulability has been reported, but further studies have failed to confirm this observation.[34] Soybean oil apparently does produce a reduction in platelet adhesiveness, lasting several hours after the infusion has been stopped. Prolonged infusion has demonstrated no adverse effect on the platelet count.[63]

Plasma clearance of fat emulsions in critically ill patients has been observed, even in patients with liver dysfunction. This observation has been attributed to the metabolic preference for fat as an energy source during sepsis.[29] However, other researchers question the critically ill patient's ability to use exogenous fat emulsion as an energy source.[16] These reports, although at this time contradictory of each other, should alert one to the need for careful monitoring whenever parenteral fat emulsions are used. Use of the recommended daily dose of 2 to 4 per kilogram should be well tolerated by most patients.[34] Serum triglyceride levels before and during administration should routinely be assessed. Observations of the patient's serum should be made at the time of blood specimen collection, because lipemia can alter other chemistry values (for example, false hyponatremia). Drugs

such as tetracycline have been implicated as causing impaired plasma clearance of triglycerides.

Metabolic monitoring. Many laboratory parameters are monitored during nutritional support therapy. *TPN profiles* or standing laboratory orders are not uncommon during the use of TPN. The need for similar laboratory monitoring during enteral nutrition support has been emphasized. This need has become more apparent as disease-specific nutritional support solutions and formulas have become available (see Table 38-4 for the most frequently ordered laboratory tests). Once a patient's nutritional support prescription has been stabilized, many of these tests may be obtained on an "as needed" basis. Baseline testing, however, is important for adequate observation of trends during the course of therapy.

The nurse has an important role in monitoring patients receiving nutritional support therapy. Ready access to information about the nutritional support prescription, the availability of efficient forms for data documentation and follow-up, and modern equipment such as easy-to-use bed scales, glucometers, and infusion-control devices are required. This attention to detail enhances the nurse's ability to observe and report accurately any changes in the patient's condition that may potentiate or cause metabolic complications related to nutritional support therapy.

Table 38-4 Laboratory monitoring during nutritional support

Test	Frequency (after baseline)
Blood glucose	Daily until stable, then M,W,F
Serum electrolytes (Na$^+$, K$^+$, Cl$^-$, CO$_2$)	Daily until stable, then M,W,F
Creatinine, blood urea nitrogen	Daily or every other day while protein load increasing, then M,W,F
Plasma osmolality	As indicated by electrolyte results
Chemistry profile (total protein, albumin, bilirubin, SGOT, SGPT, LDH, alkaline phosphatase, calcium, phosphorus, magnesium)	At least twice weekly until stable, then once/week
Complete blood count	Weekly
Trace elements	Baseline if losses or need suspected, then as indicated
Triglycerides	M,W,F if fat emulsions used
Folate, B$_{12}$ levels	If supplemented
Hematology studies (Fe, TIBC, ferritin)	Dependent on CBC and laboratory capability
Prothrombin time	Weekly
Urine electrolytes	As indicated
Blood gases	As indicated
Plasma amino acid profile	As indicated
Prealbumin, transferrin	As indicated

From Crocker KS: Metabolic monitoring during nutritional support therapy. In Grant J and Kennedy-Caldwell C, editors: Nutrition support nursing, Philadelphia, 1988, Grune & Stratton, Inc.

Altered Nutrition: Less Than Body Protein-Calorie Requirements related to overfeeding of exogenous nutrients and/or organ dysfunction

DEFINING CHARACTERISTICS

Carbohydrate related
- Blood glucose >150 mg%/dl
- Glycosuria >3+
- Increased urinary output with low specific gravity
- Progressive clinical symptoms: thirst, diuresis, weight loss, clouded sensorium, nausea, headache, poor skin turgor, hypotension, convulsions, coma
- Increased minute ventilation compared to baseline (increased arterial partial pressure of oxygen [PaO_2])
- Increased arterial partial pressure of carbon dioxide ($PaCO_2$) compared to baseline before nutritional support was instituted
- Measured respiratory quotient >1
- >50% of nonprotein calories in nutritional support solution supplied as carbohydrate in a ventilator-dependent patient

Protein related
- Blood urea nitrogen (BUN) greater than baseline
- BUN:creatinine ratio greater than 10:1
- Diuresis or oliguria
- Greater than normal levels of potassium, magnesium, or phosphate, indicative of renal dysfunction

Lipid related
- Lipemia
- Hyponatremia without other cause
- Serum triglyceride level >250 mg/dl
- Decreased platelets without other cause
- Use of fat emulsions at >2-4 mg/kg/hr
- Clinical complaints of nausea, vomiting, headache, altered taste, allergic response

OUTCOME CRITERIA

Carbohydrate related
- Blood glucose is <150 mg%/dl.
- Glycosuria is <2+.
- Fluid balance is evident.
- Clinical symptoms of progressive hyperglycemia are absent.
- $PaCO_2$ level of ventilator-dependent patients is in normal range.
- 30%-50% of nonprotein calories are administered as fat emulsion.
- Measured respiratory quotient is <1.

Protein related
- BUN is within normal limits.
- BUN:creatinine ratio is within normal limits.
- Urinary output is at least 30 ml/hr.
- Serum and urinary levels of potassium, phosphate, and magnesium are normal.

Lipid related
- There is no evidence of lipemia.
- Serum triglycerides <250 mg/dl.
- Serum sodium level >130 mg/dl.
- Platelets are within normal limits for patient.
- Infusion of fat emulsion is in range of 2-4 mg/kg/hr.
- Patient has no clinical complaints.

NURSING INTERVENTIONS *AND RATIONALE*

Carbohydrate related
1. Assess serum glucose level on a daily basis; every 6-hour fingersticks for glucose may be needed.
2. Perform urinary testing for sugar every 6 hours.
3. Maintain infusion control of TPN or enteral infusion nutritional support infusion rates.
4. Maintain accurate intake and output, with tracking of fluid balance.
5. Observe and document clinical signs of progressive hyperglycemia.
6. Supplement with exogenous regular insulin as ordered.
7. Carefully observe and document ventilator-dependent patients' attempts at weaning.
8. Identify patients at risk early (for example, septic, diabetic, hypermetabolic, or elderly patients, renal or pancreatic insufficiencies, use of steroids.)
9. Obtain daily weights.
10. Gradually increase formula's or solution's hourly rates based on documented patient tolerance.

Protein related
1. Monitor serum values of BUN, creatinine, potassium, phosphate, magnesium.
2. Maintain accurate intake and output and measurement of fluid balance.
3. Obtain daily weights.
4. Perform daily assessment of sensorium

Lipid related
1. Monitor laboratory values (triglycerides, platelets).
2. Control infusion of fat emulsion at a rate no greater than 125 ml/hr for 10% solutions and 62 ml/hr for 20% solutions.
3. Observe patient for nausea, vomiting, altered taste, headache, allergic response.

POTENTIAL FOR INFECTION
Theoretical Concepts Related to Nutritional Status

Nutrition and immunocompetence. Infection is a major cause of mortality and morbidity among the critically ill. There is considerable evidence that alterations within the immune system frequently occur during states of malnutrition. Decreased numbers of circulating T lymphocytes and total lymphocytes and decreased response to skin test antigens demonstrate impaired cell-mediated immunity. These defects in immunocompetence have been observed in patients with protein-calorie malnutrition and are related to measurement of parameters of visceral (cellular) protein status.[17] Other abnormalities of the immune system such as depressed levels of complement, reduced amounts of secretory IgA, and nonspecific mechanisms of host defense have also been observed in malnourished animals and humans.[1] Such cumulative adverse effects on the immune system predispose the malnourished critically ill patient to infection.

Several tests of immune function are frequently used as nonspecific indicators of nutritional status, including total lymphocyte count and delayed cutaneous hypersensitivity to skin test antigens. Circulating lymphocytes of importance to infection are T cells, which are very sensitive to malnutrition. A reduction in lymphocyte production, including T lymphocytes, occurs very early during periods of protein-calorie malnutrition. The total lymphocyte count (TLC) is calculated from the white blood count (WBC) and the differential.

$$TLC \; (cells/mm^3) \; = \; WBC \; (cells/mm^3) \; \times \; \frac{\% \; lymphocytes}{100\%}$$

The normal value of circulating lymphocytes is greater than 2000 cells/mm³. Values of 1200 to 2000 cells/mm³ are indicative of mild malnutrition, values of 800 to 1200 cells/mm³ of moderate malnutrition, and values of less than 800 cells/mm³ of moderate malnutrition, and values of less than 800 cells/mm³ of severe malnutrition.[31] Depression of lymphocytes is not specifically related to any one nutritional deficiency and is correlated with other parameters of visceral protein status (for example, albumin, prealbumin).

Several factors other than malnutrition may alter the number of circulating lymphocytes. Surgical patients, in general may have a decreased total lymphocyte count related to the metabolic response to stress and fluctuating albumin levels. A large wound leads to decreased levels of circulating lymphocytes, because lymphocytes migrate to the wound site.[9] Infection and the use of immunosuppressive drugs also may alter lymphocyte values.

The erythematous, indurated skin response to recall antigens has been a standard for studying cell-mediated immunity in malnourished patients. In a classic study, Meakins and associates[47] studied 354 hospitalized patients and found 110 of them had decreased or no reactivity to skin test antigens. Of the 244 patients who did react normally, there was a very low (<4%) rate of sepsis and death (<3%). Of those who were immunodeficient, 50% had septic episodes, and 23% died.

Testing for delayed cutaneous hypersensitivity involves the use of 0.1 cc of a variety of antigens that are injected intradermally in the forearm area. The skin response (erythema and induration) is noted at 24 and 48 hours. If the response is 5 mm or greater, the patient is considered immunocompetent. A failure to respond or a response less than 5 mm after 24 to 48 hours is called anergy and has been well described in patients with protein-calorie malnutrition or decreased visceral proteins. Delayed cutaneous hypersensitivity response is reflective of the patient's previous exposure to the selected antigens, thus the reason for using more than one antigen. Commonly used antigens include purified protein derivative, streptokinase-streptodornase, mumps, *Candida albicans, Trichophyton,* and coccidioidin. Although a traditional marker of nutritional status, there are many problems with antigen testing. Recall response is dependent on prior exposure to the antigen. Contributing factors to false-negative results include age, uremia or liver disease, drug interactions, reader variability, concurrent infections, and anesthesia.[47] Because of these complicating factors, a negative response may be difficult to interpret and directly relate to nutritional status, whereas a positive response does indicate that the patient is immunocompetent.

The precise nutritional deficiencies that result in immune response defects are not known. Patients with protein-calorie malnutrition usually have multiple nutritional deficiencies, any of which, if severe enough, could affect immune system function. Deficiencies of zinc, iron, and selenium have been noted in some immunodeficient patients.[13,22] Immunodeficient states, especially in the children of Third World countries, reverse once the malnutrition has been corrected.[9] Nutritional deficiencies may represent important facilitating factors, permitting the establishment of a principle infective agent in immunodeficient hosts.[7] Despite this nonspecific relationship between immune function and malnutrition, the clinical observation that malnourished patients are more prone to infections and septic episodes is well-known and one reason why aggressive nutritional support should be used in the critically ill patient.[27]

Potential for infection caused by invasive techniques of nutritional support. Administration of nutritional support requires the use of invasive venous catheters and GI feeding tubes. Access devices for nutritional support are usually in place for extended periods of time and thus increase the potential for related infection. Although there is the potential for infection as the result of the contamination of parenteral solutions and enteral formulas, current techniques of compounding them has minimized contamination as a cause of infection.[23,47] Most infections that are specifically related to the use of nutritional support are device related or a result of touch contamination during manipulation of the delivery system and access device.

Device-related infection is the major infectious complication of parenteral nutrition therapy. Infections may be local at the site of insertion or may be systemic, caused by the bacterial seeding of the tip of the device. Most of the research in device-related infection involves central venous catheters.

Colonization of the central venous catheter may occur in several ways. First, the catheter may be contaminated as a result of direct invasion by microorganisms on the skin, at the site of catheter insertion, or along the subcutaneous tract created by the catheter.[48] Second, the catheter may be hematogenously seeded during transient periods of bacteremia or fungemia. A fibrin sheath usually forms around the distal end of most catheters, and it can become colonized by bacterial seeding from distant infection.[51] A third hypothesis recently proposed is that catheters may become infected by intralumen contamination during catheter manipulations.[57,60] This third hypothesis has gained some attention with the increased use of multilumen catheters in the critical care setting.

A variety of risk factors have been associated with catheter-related infection, including susceptibility to infection, the method of catheter insertion, the site of insertion, and the use of the catheter for infusions other than nutritional support. Burn and immunosuppressed patients are at higher risk. Catheters inserted by cutdown are infected more often than those inserted percutaneously. Catheters inserted in the lower extremities, especially the groin, have a higher incidence of infection.

The indwelling central venous catheter has been viewed as a convenient way for administering medications, hemodynamic monitoring, and blood sampling. Use of nutritional support catheters for such multiple purposes may be necessary in patients with limited venous access. Results from studies involving the use of multilumen catheters in which one lumen is dedicated to the nutrition solution are contradictory. Some report an increased incidence of infection, whereas others do not.[22,48]

Prevention of infectious complications of parenteral nutrition therapy depends on strict adherence to principles of infection control and sterile technique (see the box, "Infection Control Guidelines during Nutritional Support").[70] A complete review of catheter care during TPN has been recently published by Murphy and Lipman.[51]

INFECTION CONTROL GUIDELINES DURING NUTRITIONAL SUPPORT

Adhere to nutritional support protocols related to the following:
Solution or formula compounding.
Administration.
Insertion of access devices.
Care of access device.
Evaluation of access device–related infection.
Clinical monitoring.
Maintain quality control during and after solution or formula compounding.
Compound solutions or formulas using sterile or aseptic technique.
Compound parenteral solutions under laminar flow hoods.
Refrigerate all solutions and mixed formulas until used.
Observe 24-hour expiration date.
Complete separate infusion of lipids within 12 hours.
Infuse parenteral dextrose or amino acid solutions using a 0.22 μg filter.
Infuse dextrose, amino acid, or lipid 3:1 solutions using a 1.2 μg filter.

Assist with the insertion and maintenance of central venous catheters by doing the following:
Using sterile attire and drapes during insertion.
Preparing the skin site for 30 seconds with povidone-iodine before catheter insertion.
Suturing catheter in place.
Applying occlusive dressing after insertion.
Evaluating patients with TPN catheters daily for signs of catheter-related infection.
Preparing and redressing catheter insertion site per hospital protocol according to a fixed schedule.
Maintain integrity of administration sets by doing the following:
Changing administration sets every 24-48 hours.
Avoiding unnecessary manipulations of TPN system.
Whenever possible, not using TPN catheters for other influsions.

Potential for Infection

RISK FACTORS

- Malnutrition and immunodeficiencies
- Invasive techniques of nutritional support
- Total lymphocytes: <2000 mm³
- White blood cell count greater than normal
- Anergy
- Temperature >40° C
- Positive blood cultures, with organism same as identified from central venous catheter tip culture
- Clinical signs of sepsis without other cause identified
- Erythema, tenderness, or drainage around skin at site of access device

OUTCOME CRITERIA

- Total lymphocytes are >2000 mm³.
- White blood cell count is within normal limits.
- Positive response to delayed cutaneous hypersensitivity is >5 mm.
- Temperature is normal.
- Blood culture is negative.
- No clinical signs of sepsis are evident.
- Skin integrity surrounding access device is uncompromised.

NURSING INTERVENTIONS *AND RATIONALE*

1. Monitor total lymphocyte counts, WBC, differential.
2. Follow directions for the placement of intradermal skin tests.
3. Monitor vital signs every 4 hours and urinary sugar levels or Accucheks every 6 hours.
4. Perform daily assessment for signs of infection and sepsis.
5. Maintain optimal aseptic environment during access-device insertion.
6. Use aseptic technique during manipulation of nutritional support system.
7. Perform daily inspection of access-device insertion site for erythema, induration, drainage, tenderness, phlebitis.
8. Maintain sterile occlusive dressing over access device according to hospital protocol.
9. Protect access-device site from potential sources of contamination: e.g., ostomies, draining wounds.
10. Refrigerate compounded nutritional support solutions and enteral formulas before use.
11. Maintain a closed sterile nutritional support system using Luer-lock connections.

POTENTIAL IMPAIRED SKIN INTEGRITY
Theoretical Concepts Related to Skin Integrity

All critically ill patients are at risk for impaired skin integrity. Although impaired skin integrity is seldom life-threatening, it can be a site for infection, can delay the patient's progress, and is an avoidable discomfort for the patient. For these reasons, maintenance of skin integrity should be a high priority for the critical care nurse.

Assessment of the patient's integument is essential on admission and is repeated during and after procedures such as dressing changes and repositioning. The critical care nurse must use proper terminology to describe observations so that accurate documentation and evaluation is possible. See the box, "Glossary of Skin Lesions" for a list of common terms used for describing skin lesions.

Insults to skin integrity in the critically ill patient most commonly originate from mechanical forces, chemical drainage, and fungal overgrowth. By recognizing these factors and initiating regular assessment and appropriate measures, the critical care nurse can prevent the development of most of these complications.

Mechanical forces. Several mechanical factors jeopardize skin integrity. Shearing forces are created, for example, when the patient slides in bed. Shear is the movement of a bony prominence over subcutaneous tissue, occluding superficial capillaries and resulting in tissue ischemia or hypoxia with or without necrosis. Typically, ulcers from shear are shallow with uneven edges.

Friction, the rubbing together of two surfaces, is the second type of mechanical factor. It typically occurs with the abrading of elbows against the sheets. Friction can cause superficial tissue damage.

Stripping is the third type of damage to the skin and is the result of removal of the epidermis by mechanical means. Repeated or careless tape application or removal can inadvertently remove epidermal cells. Tape should be applied to the skin without tension, keeping the skin as wrinkle free as possible. When tape is used to secure pressure dressings, formation of blisters along the tape edges is common. These blisters are mistakenly interpreted as an allergic response. Tape should be removed by peeling the adhesive gently from the skin while supporting the skin surface.

Pressure is the most familiar type of mechanical force jeopardizing skin integrity. Capillary closing pressure has been indirectly measured at 11 mm Hg to 32 mm Hg.[42] When pressure that exceeds this range is applied to the skin, capillaries collapse, occluding blood flow. The result is localized tissue ischemia, anoxia, and cellular death.

Three factors determine pressure sore development: the intensity and the duration of pressure and tissue tolerance.[12] Although frequent repositioning does decrease the duration of pressure, it does not affect the intensity of the pressure, and tissue destruction can still result. Pressure ulcers can

LEGAL REVIEW
Skin care in critical care nursing

CASE EXAMPLE: *Ellinghusen v. Flushing Hospital and Medical Center,* 531 N.Y.S.2d 824 (A.D. 2 Dept. 1988).

This lawsuit was brought by Plaintiff Ellinghusen against nurses, their employer (a hospital), and physicians for injuries that Plaintiff sustained during her hospitalization, June 7-17, 1981. The plaintiff was admitted to the hospital through the defendant's emergency room, June 7, 1981. She was in a critical, life-threatening condition, suffering from a strangulated umbilical hernia that had perforated her bowel, causing fecal matter to leak into her abdomen and resulting in peritonitis. She had abdominal surgery performed the following day.

After the operation she was admitted to the critical care unit of the hospital, remaining there for 10 days while her condition stabilized. During that time she was connected to a variety of life-support and monitoring devices, which included a ventilator to assist and control breathing, cardiac monitor, certain venous and arterial monitoring devices, a nasogastric tube to drain her stomach, a sump drain from the incision of the operation, a Foley catheter to her bladder, and various intravenous lines to administer fluids and nourishment.

While she remained in the critical care unit, a sacral decubitus ulcer developed. Nurses' notes of June 13, 1981, first identified the decubitus. Nurses' notes of June 14, 1981, described the decubitus as "an excoriated area of approximately 5 cm by 5 cm in the sacral area." On June 16, 1981, nurses notes' indicated that an air mattress was obtained.

The decubitus became infected and ultimately necessitated corrective plastic surgery and several rehospitalizations for performance of skin grafts and surgical repair. At the time of the injury Plaintiff was 65 years of age, 4 feet 6 inches tall, and weighed 238 pounds.

Plaintiff's expert testified as follows:

1. Nurses' notes did not record that the care needed to prevent decubitus was given;
2. Therefore such care was not given;
3. Fact that patient developed decubitus in itself is indicative that the care required to prevent the decubitus was not given;
4. The hospital regulation entitled, "Skin care Assessment Sheet," requires nurses to record the turning of a patient every 2 hours to prevent decubitus;
5. That this was not done is a breach of a standard of nursing care and led to and was the proximate cause of Plaintiff's injuries; and
6. That nursing staff failed to supply Plaintiff immediately with an air mattress from the inception of her placement in the critical care unit on June 8, 1981, which could have contributed substantially to the prevention of the deterioration of the Plaintiff's condition and materially lessen the possibility of infection caused by fecal contamination.

Plaintiff sought $250,000 in damages and testified about her lifestyle and health before her confinement and her lifestyle and health after the hospital stay on the issue of damages. The issue for the jury was whether the nurses and their employer-hospital breached a standard of nursing care, leading to and causing Plaintiff's injuries. The injury awarded $250,000 to Plaintiff. Although after the trial the judge set aside the verdict, on appeal the higher court held that evidence was sufficient to establish that the hospital (and its nurses) was negligent in its postoperative care of the patient and that such negligence was the proximate cause of the patient's developing a decubitus.

GLOSSARY OF SKIN LESIONS

Denude—loss of epidermis

Epithelization—regeneration of the epidermis across wound surface

Erosion—loss of epidermis

Erythema—redness of skin surface produced by vasodilation

Eschar—hard, black, crusted nonviable tissue

Excoriation—linear scratch marks

Granulation—formation of small capillaries and connective tissue, creating ruddy, red, moist granular surface

Maceration—softening of tissue by soaking in fluid

Necrotic—dead, avascular

Nonviable—dead

Slough—loose, stringy necrotic tissue

Stages—method of categorizing extent of tissue damage:
  Stage 1: erythema
  Stage 2: blister or tissue loss extending into epidermis or dermis
  Stage 3: tissue loss extending into subcutaneous tissue
  Stage 4: tissue loss extending into muscle, bone or tendon

Strip—removal of epidermis by mechanical means; denude

Wound base—bed of wound

Wound margin—rim or border of wound

Modified from Standards of care, dermal wounds: pressure sores, 1987, Irvine, Calif, International Association for Enterostomal Therapy.

SUPPORT SURFACES THAT HELP PREVENT IMPAIRED SKIN INTEGRITY

Pressure-reduction device

Dense, convoluted foam with 3-inch base
Air-filled devices
Gel pads

Pressure-relief beds

Low air loss (e.g., Kin-Air; Flexi-Care)
High air loss (e.g., Clinitron)

POUCH CHANGE PROCEDURE: FISTULA OR STOMA

1. Assemble equipment: pouch with attached skin barrier, material for pattern, skin barrier paste, scissors, closure clip, water, gauze or tissue.
2. Make the pattern.
   a. Lay paper towel or transparent paper over stoma or fistula and trace shape onto paper. Cut out this shape. Pattern should fit snugly around base of protruding stoma and 1/8 inch larger than flush stoma or fistula.
   b. Measuring guides may be used to make pattern.
3. Prepare appliance.
   a. Trace pattern onto pouch.
   b. Cut pouch to size of pattern.
   c. Remove protective backing from pouch and skin barrier.
   d. Set pouch aside.
4. Remove and apply pouch.
   a. Remove pouch, using one hand to push the skin gently away from the adhesive.
   b. Discard pouch and save closure clip.
   c. Control any discharge with gauze or tissue.
   d. Clean skin with water and dry thoroughly.
   e. Apply paste around fistula or stoma. Fill in any uneven skin surfaces with paste. Use a damp finger or tongue blade to apply paste.
   f. Apply new pouch, centering wound site in opening.
   g. Close bottom of pouch with clip.
   NOTE: Empty pouch when one third full.
   Change pouch every 3 days or when leakage occurs.

---

develop both from low pressure applied for long periods of time and from high pressure for short periods of time.[42]

Tissue tolerance refers to the ability of the skin and supporting surfaces to withstand pressure. Several factors have been recognized as decreasing tissue's tolerance for pressure. Restricted or limited mobility and impaired sensorium obscure the patient's perception of pressure. Impaired nutrition weakens tissue tolerance and delays tissue repair. Urinary incontinence macerates epidermal tissues to weaken tissue tolerance to pressure.

Because critically ill patients commonly have many of these variables present, they should all be considered at risk for pressure sore developement. The most vulnerable pressure points for critically ill patients are the heels, sacrum, coccyx, and trochanters. In fact, a pressure ulcer may first manifest as a bruise and then deteriorate into an open skin lesion several days later (for example, after long surgical procedure).

Numerous support surfaces are currently available to redistribute pressure either to reduce pressure or to relieve pressure (see the following box). A critically ill patient with no preexisting pressure ulcer who is stable and is cooperative with repositioning can be placed on a pressure-*reducing* surface. Foam mattress overlays have been used extensively in an attempt to reduce pressure. However, the quality of foam (density, base height) varies widely. The foam with low density and a thin base height provides comfort only. Pressure-*relief* devices are essential for unstable critically ill patients who do not tolerate repositioning. As the patient stabilizes, the pressure-relief device can be replaced with a pressure-reducing device. The selection of the most appropriate, most cost-effective support surface can be confusing. Consultation with an enterostomal therapy (ET) nurse can provide clarity.

Fungal overgrowth. The presence of moisture in conjunction with antibiotic therapy disrupts the skin's normal flora, causing candidiasis, or moniliasis. *Candida albicans* is a resident flora on the skin. However, in a compromised host this opportunistic organism can flourish. Critically ill patients are predisposed to developing candidiasis, because they are often receiving antibiotics and experiencing urinary incontinence, perspiration, or drainage from wound sites.

With candidiasis the skin is macerated and exhibits an erythematous, papular rash that is distributed within an area in which moisture is trapped (for example, dressing sites). Satellite lesions may also be present and are extrafollicular. Subjectively, the patient often comments that the rash itches.

Chemical drainage. Chemical skin irritation is caused by the exposure of the skin to an irritant. Diarrhea, urinary incontinence, fistulas, ostomy output, drainage from a gastrostomy site or drain tube, and harsh solutions (for example, povidone-iodine or acetic acid) applied to wounds can impair skin integrity.

Since stomal function is unpredictable and the effluent caustic, a pouch should be worn at all times by an ostomate. A postoperative pouch should have a solid wafer skin barrier, should be transparent, and should be adjustable by size. Numerous pouches are available. The effectiveness of the pouch is determined by the construction of the stoma, the surrounding skin area, and the characteristics of the discharge. See the box, "Pouch Change Procedure: Fistula or Stoma." An ET nurse can assist in selecting the proper equipment and providing education and follow-up.

Table 38-5 Products used in fistula and ostomy care*

Product	Uses
SOLID WAFER SKIN BARRIER	
Stomahesive (ConvaTec) Premium Barrier (Hollister) Skin Barrier (Bard) Comfeel (Coloplast) Soft Guard XL (United)	Protects skin from output. Wafers vary in degree of flexibility.
SKIN SEALANT	
Skin Prep (United) Skin Gel (Hollister) Protective Barrier Film (Bard) Nu-Gard (NuHope) Shield Skin (Mentor)	Applied to intact skin to protect from latex or acrylic adhesives; also used over powder. Do not apply to eroded skin (contains alcohol).
PETROLEUM-BASED OINTMENT	
Peri-Care (Sween) Moisture Barrier Skin Ointment (Hollister) Uni-Salve (United) Skin Care Moisture Barrier Ointment (Bard) Moisture Barrier Cream (Carrington)	Used with dressings to protect skin from low-volume output or drainage that is not highly caustic; cannot be used when applying a pouch.
SKIN BARRIER PASTE	
Stomahesive paste (ConvaTec) Premium Barrier Paste (Hollister) Comfeel Paste (Coloplast) Karaya Paste (Hollister) Skin Barrier Paste (United)	Used directly around fistula or stoma to increase wearing time; used to fill in creases and to level uneven skin surfaces. Contains alcohol so should not be applied to eroded skin.
SKIN BARRIER POWDER	
Stomahesive Powder (ConvaTec) Karaya powder (many companies)	Used on moist, eroded skin to absorb moisture and to create a dry surface so adhesives can be applied.

*Not intended as an exhaustive list.

The peristomal skin should also be assessed for any abnormalities. The skin around the stoma should look like the skin anywhere else on the abdomen. The presence of any discoloration, prolonged erythema, or lesions is abnormal and must be treated. There are numerous products available to facilitate healing (Table 38-5).

One of the goals for nursing management of fistulas is skin protection (see the box, "Nursing Goals in Fistula Management"). Because fistulous drainage is typically caustic and erodes exposed skin, skin protection is critical. Protec-

---

NURSING GOALS IN FISTULA MANAGEMENT

1. Skin protection
2. Drainage containment
3. Odor control
4. Patient comfort
5. Accurate measurement of effluent
6. Patient mobility
7. Cost containment
8. Nutritional support
9. Psychosocial support

---

tion can be provided by using skin sealants, petrolatum-based ointments, or solid wafer skin barriers (see Table 38-5).

Drainge can be contained by gauze when the output is less than 100 ml per 24 hours and is not odorous. Skin protection must still be provided.

When the fistulous output exceeds 100 ml per 24 hours or contaminates adjacent wounds or incisions, applying a pouch is the management method of choice to achieve containment, skin protection, accurate measurement of output, odor control, patient comfort, and mobility. Deodorants can be used in the pouch to control odor further. Because pouches are changed only every 3 days (or whenever leakage occurs), using a pouch is less costly in equipment and nursing time.

The nurse working in the critical care area is also likely to encounter patients with transient incontinence. These patients are often on medications that alter their level of con-

---

MEDICATIONS THAT MAY CAUSE DIARRHEA*

Antacids containing magnesium hydroxide
Antibiotics
Antihypertensives
Potassium supplements
Ganglionic blocking agents
Laxatives
Alkylating agents

SPECIFIC EXAMPLES

Ampicillin	Neomycin
Cephalosporins	Penicillin
Clindamycin	Propranolol
Colchicine	Quinidine
Guanethidine	Sorbitol
Lactulose	Tetracycline
Lincomycin	

*Partial listing.

sciousness or sensations, thus rendering them unable to respond appropriately to the urge to eliminate. Drugs can also produce undesirable side effects (see the box, "Medications that May Cause Diarrhea"). In addition, the person's mobility and ability to communicate needs may be compromised. In these instances, providing perineal skin protection and containment are important patient care objectives.

Ointments are products with a petrolatum base, and they provide a protective coating for skin that is exposed to an irritant such as stool. Ointments should be applied when the incontinence is first noted and should be applied liberally after gentle cleansing. If fecal incontinence has resulted in perianal skin erosion, the application of a skin barrier powder (for example, Stomahesive) first will allow the ointment to adhere to the moist skin (see Table 38-5).

Pouches have been used successfully to contain stool or urine. For example, a fecal pouch is attached to the perianal skin; the nurse can empty it when it is approximately one third full, or it may be connected to a bedside drainage bag. These pouches usually remain intact for 24 to 48 hours and work best on patients who are not ambulatory. Initiation of the use of these pouches meets with best success when used before diarrhea results in peristomal skin erosion. For a patient experiencing frequent incontinent stools, this method can offer significant time savings for the caregivers and protect the patient's skin from an uncomfortable irritation. The procedure for the application of a perianal pouch is outlined in the box, "Perianal Pouching Procedure."

Using diapers is another method of containment. They are not as effective in containing odor as the pouch but are better suited for patients who are more active or who have occasional incontinence. They can be used in conjunction with ointments if skin integrity is threatened. Although these devices are useful in the management of incontinence, they should not be considered as the treatment of choice.

Another option for managing fecal incontinence is a rectal tube, involving the insertion of a large (18 to 30 Fr) Foley catheter with a 30-cc balloon into the rectum. The inflated balloon usually keeps the catheter in the rectum. The catheter is then connected to a bedside drainage bag.

If stool is profuse or starts to thicken, leakage around the tube can occur. The nurse may need to remove the tube so it can be irrigated and patency maintained. Ointments to protect perirectal skin may be needed.

Even if there is no leakage, many hospital procedures require that the balloon be deflated for a few minutes every 1 to 2 hours to prevent bowel necrosis. Whether there is damage to the rectal mucosa by the presence of the tube is still unclear.

PERIANAL POUCHING PROCEDURE

1. Assemble equipment: pouch, paste, clip, cotton balls, bag for waste.
2. Prepare pouch.
   a. Remove paper backings from skin barrier and tape.
   b. Apply a thick bead of paste around the center opening; set aside.
3. Remove and apply pouch.
   a. Loosen tape and gently push skin away from adhesive.
   b. Discard pouch and save clip (if one is used).
   c. Remove any paste residue, using a dry tissue.
   d. Wash skin with cotton balls and warm water; be sure to remove any greasy residue, using a gentle soap and water. Rinse; dry.
   e. Shave perianal hair if present.
   f. Fold skin barrier of pouch vertically.
      - Position pouch between scrotum or vagina and anus.
      - Roll pouch forward and position barrier above scrotum or vagina then smooth out sides.
      - Encourage pouch seal by pressing gently for 1 minute.
      - Attach clip to open end of pouch or attach spout to straight drainage.

Potential Impaired Skin Integrity

RISK FACTORS

Mechanical factors
- Immobility or reduced mobility
- Malnutrition (hypoalbuminemia)
- Incontinence
- Frequent or repetitive dressing changes
- Impaired cognition or sensorium
- Poor subcutaneous tissue support (e.g., in older patients or those receiving steroids)
- Irradiated skin
- Presence of immobilizing devices

Fungal infections
- Antibiotics
- Moisture (e.g., incontinence, febrile states, damp dressings, pressure-relieving devices that prevent air circulation)
- Compromised host (e.g., diabetes, leukopenia)

Chemical factors
- Ileostomy, colostomy, or fistula
- Drain sites
- Incontinence
- Dressings that use harsh solutions
- Tube feedings
- Medications that can cause diarrhea

DEFINING CHARACTERISTICS

Mechanical factors
- Erythema over bony prominence
- Moist, denuded tissue under adhesives

Fungal infection
- Erythematous papular rash
- Moisture entrapped against skin

Chemical factors
- Erythematous rash surrounding orifice

OUTCOME CRITERIA

Mechanical factors
- No erythema is present over bony prominence.
- Skin under adhesives remains intact.

Fungal infection
- Papular rash does not develop.
- Moisture or drainage is not trapped against skin.

Chemical factors
- Skin around drain sites remains intact.
- No erosion develops around orifice.

NURSING INTERVENTIONS *AND RATIONALE*

1. Continue to monitor the assessment parameters listed under "Defining Characteristics."
2. Mechanical factors.
   a. Prevent shear or friction.
      - Place genuine sheepskin under patient's hips when head elevated. *Sheepskin keeps patient's skin from sticking to sheets.*
      - Allow feet to rest against footboard when head elevated—*prevents sliding.*
      - Provide heel and elbow protectors—*prevent friction against sheets.*
      - Lift patient with lift sheet to reposition—*prevents sliding patient's body against sheets.*
   b. Prevent epidermal stripping.
      - Apply tape without tension—*avoids blistering.*
      - Use porous type—*allows moisture evaporation.*
      - Remove tape by peeling tape away from skin while stabilizing skin—*avoids traumatic removal of epidermis.*
      - Roll gauze or tubular stockinette to secure dressings—*avoids unnecessary use of adhesives on skin.*
      - Apply skin sealants or solid wafer skin barriers under adhesives (see Table 38-5). *Both provide a protective layer over skin for adherence of adhesive, thus serving as a second skin.*
      - Secure wound dressings with Montgomery straps—*provides another means of securing dressing without repeated tape applications so epidermal stripping can be avoided.*
   c. Prevent pressure.
      - Apply pressure-reducing support surface to bed (see box on p. 722)—*redistributes weight.*
      - Reposition patient every 2 hours or more often if bony prominence remains erythematous more than 15 minutes after pressure is relieved. *Frequent repositioning redistributes weight and allows capillary refill. Erythema unresolved within 15 minutes indicates tissue ischemia, which can progress to necrosis if pressure is unrelieved.*

Continued.

Potential Impaired Skin Integrity—cont'd

■ Use pressure-relief support surface if patient is unstable (see box on p. 722). *Pressure-relief device reduces pressure exerted against skin to less than capillary closing pressure so frequent repositioning to relieve pressure is not necessary.*

2. Fungal infections.
   a. Change dressings over drain site as frequently as needed—*keeps dressing from being saturated.*
   b. Apply skin sealant or solid wafer skin barrier under dressings and around drain site (see Table 38-5)—*protects skin from moisture.*
   c. Dust skin folds with cornstarch or lay gauze (unfolded into skin folds—*absorbs moisture.*

3. Chemical factors.
   a. Maintain intact ostomy pouch over fistula and os-

tomy. *Change pouch routinely every 3 days or when leakage develops (see the box on p. 722)—prevents contact of effluent with skin.*

   b. Apply petrolatum-based ointment to perianal skin for treatment of incontinence—*prevents contact of effluent with skin.*
   c. Apply skin sealants or solid wafer skin barrier around drain sites or wounds (see Table 38-5)—*prevents contact of effluent with skin.*
   d. Gently cleanse skin exposed to drainage with cotton balls and water—*prevents mechanical abrasion of jeopardized skin.*
   e. Use rectal pouch for diarrhea (see the box on p. 724)—*protects skin and contains effluent.*
   f. Rule out fecal impaction as source of diarrhea by performing digital examination. *Fecal impaction can function as an obstruction and can stimulate fluid shifts into bowel lumen to create diarrhea.*

REFERENCES

1. Alexander JK and Peterson KL: Cardiovascular effects of weight reduction, Circulation 45:310, 1972.
2. Alpers DH, Clouse RE, and Stenson WF: Manual of nutritional therapeutics, Boston, 1983, Little, Brown & Co.
3. Alterescue W: Theoretical foundations for an approach to fecal incontinence, J Enterostom Ther 13:44, 1986.
4. Boarini J, Bryant R, and Irrgang S: Fistula management, Semin Oncol Nurs 2(4):287, 1986.
5. Askanazi J and others: Respiratory changes induced by large glucose loads of TPN, JAMA 243(14):1444, 1980.
6. Backman L and others: Cardiovascular function in extreme obesity, Acta Med Scand 193:437, 1973.
7. Beach RS and Laura PF: Nutrition and the acquired immunodeficiency syndrome, Ann Intern Med 99:565, 1983.
8. Bistrian BR and others: Prevalence of malnutrition in general medical patients, JAMA 235(15):1567, 1976.
9. Bistrian BR and others: Protein status of general surgical patients, JAMA 230(6):858, 1974.
10. Bivins BA and others: Pathophysiology and management of hyperosmolar, hyperglycemic, nonketotic dehydration, Surg Gynecol Obstet 154(4):534, 1980.
11. Bjornson HS and others: Association between microorganism growth at the catheter insertion site and colonization of venous catheters, J Hosp Infect 2:37, 1981.
12. Braden B and Bergstrom N: A conceptual schema for the study of the etiology of pressure sores, Rehabil Nurs 12:8, 1987.
13. Brinson R: Hypoalbuminemia; diarrhea and the acquired immunodeficiency syndrome, Ann Intern Med 102:413, 1985.
14. Bryant R: Saving the skin from tape injuries, Am J Nurs 58:189, 1988.
15. Burke SF and others: Glucose requirements following burn injury, Ann Surg 190(3):274, 1979.
16. Cerra FB and others: Branched chains stimulate post-operative protein synthesis, Surgery 92(2):192, 1983.
17. Chandra RK: Cell-mediated immunity in nutritional imbalance. Fed Proc 39:3088, 1980.
18. Courtney M and others: Rapidly declining serum albumin values in newly hospitalized patients: prevalence, severity and contributing factors, JPEN 6(2):143, 1982.
19. Crocker KS: Metabolic monitoring during nutritional support therapy. In Grant J and Kennedy-Caldwell C, editors: Nutrition support nursing, Philadelphia, 1988, Grune & Stratton, Inc.
20. Crocker KS: Nutrition support: total parenteral/enteral feeding. In Moorhouse MF, Geissler AC, and Doeneges ME, editors: Critical care plans: guidelines for patient care, Philadelphia, 1987, FA Davis.
21. Crocker KS, Gerber F, and Shearer J: Metabolism of carbohydrate, protein and fat, Nurs Clin North Am 18(1):3, 1983.
22. Crocker KS, Pine RW and Steffee WP: The triple lumen central venous catheter, Nutr Clin Pract 1:90, 1986.
23. Crocker KS and others: Microbial growth in clinically used enteral delivery systems, Am J Infect Control 14(6):250, 1986.
24. Delany R and others: Nutritional support of the acutely ill patient, Heart Lung 12(5):477, 1983.
25. Dudrick SJ and others: Long-term parenteral nutrition with growth, development and positive nitrogen balance, Surgery 64:134, 1968.
26. Echenique MM, Bistrian BR, and Blackburn GL: Theory and techniques of nutritional support in the ICU, Crit Care Med 10(8):546, 1982.
27. Fischer JE Ghory MD: Protein depletion and immunity in the hospitalized patient. In Wright RA and Heymsfield S, editors: Nutritional assessment, Boston, 1984, Blackwell Scientific Publications, Ltd.

28. Forlaw L: The critically ill patient: nutritional implications, Nurs Clin North Am 18(1):111, 1983.

29. Freeman JB Fairfull-Smith RJ: Physiologic approach to peripheral parenteral nutrition. In Fischer J, editor: Surgical nutrition, Boston, 1983, Little, Brown & Co.

30. Gault MH, Dixon ME, Cohen WM: Hypernatremia, azotemia and dehydration due to high protein tube feeding, Ann Intern Med 68(4):778, 1968.

31. Grant JP: Handbook of total parenteral nutrition, Philadelphia, 1980, WB Saunders Co.

32. Grant JP and others: Serum hepatic enzyme and bilirubin elevations during parenteral nutrition, Surg Gynecol Obstet 145(4):573, 1977.

33. Gray RH: Similarities between AIDS and PCM, Am J Public Health 73:1332, 1983.

34. Greene HL, Hazlett D and Demaree R: Relationship between intra-lipid-induced hyperlipemia and pulmonary function, Am J Clin Nutr 29(2):127, 1976.

35. Harris JA and Benedict FG: A biometric study of basal metabolism in man, Pub No 279, Washington, DC, 1919, Carnegie Institute of Washington.

36. Henry M: Fecal incontinence, Nurs Times 79:61, 1983.

37. Hoffer LJ, Palombo J, and Bistrian BR: Theoretical and practical issues in the treatment of obesity. In Rombeau J and Caldwell M, editors: Parenteral nutrition, Philadelphia, 1986, WB Saunders Co.

38. Hoppe MC, Descalso J, and Kapp SR: Gastrointestinal disease: nutritional implications, Nurs Clin North Am 18(1):47, 1983.

39. IAET: Standards of care. Dermal wounds. Pressure sores, Irvine, Calif, 1987, International Association for Enterostomal Therapy.

40. Irrgang S and Bryant R: Management of the enterocutaneous fistula, J Enterostom Ther 11:211, 1984.

41. Kaminski MV: A review of hyperosmolar, hyperglycemic, nonketotic dehydration (HHNK): etiology, pathophysiology and prevention during intravenous hyperalimentation, JPEN 2(5):690, 1978.

42. Kosiak M: Etiology and pathology of ischemic ulcers, Arch Phys Med Rehabil 40:62, 1959.

43. Krevsky B and Levine GM: Hepatic complications of TPN, Nutr Sup Serv 3(5):11, 1983.

44. Krey SH and Murray RL, editors: Dynamics of nutrition support: assessment, implementation, evaluation, Norwalk, Conn, 1986, Appleton-Century-Crofts.

45. McCauley K and Weaver TE: Cardiac and pulmonary diseases: nutritional implications, Nurs Clin North Am 18(1):81, 1983.

46. McLane AM and McShane RE: Bowel elimination, alteration. In Thompson JM and others: Clinical nursing, ed 2, St Louis, 1989, The CV Mosby Co.

47. Meakins JL and others: Delayed hypersensitivity: indicator of acquired failure of host defenses in sepsis and trauma, Ann Surg 186:241, 1977.

48. Miller JJ, Bahman V, and Mathru M: Comparison of the sterility of long term central venous catheterization using single lumen, triple lumen and pulmonary artery catheters, Crit Care Med 12:634, 1984.

49. Morgan J: Nutritional assessment of critically ill patients, Focus Crit Care 11(3):28, 1984.

50. Murphy LM and Cole MJ: Renal disease: nutritional implications, Nurs Clin North Am 18(1):57, 1983.

51. Murphy LM and Lipman TO: Central venous catheter care in parenteral nutrition: a review, JPEN 11(2): 190, 1987.

52. Pesana C: Fluid and electrolytes in the surgical patient, Baltimore, 1977, Williams & Wilkins.

53. Poindexter SM, Dear WE, and Dudrick SJ: Nutrition in congestive heart failure, Nutr Clin Pract 1(2):83, 1986.

54. Recommended daily allowance. In National Research Council: Food and Nutrition Board, ed 9, Washington, DC, 1980, National Academy of Sciences.

55. Reuler JB and Cooney TG: The pressure sore: pathophysiology and principles of management, Ann Intern Med 94:661, 1981.

56. Rhoads JE and Alexander CE: Nutritional problems of surgical patients, Ann NY Acad Sci 63:268, 1955.

57. Ryan JA and others: Catheter complications in total parenteral nutrition: a prospective study of 200 consecutive patients, N Engl J Med 290:757, 1974.

58. Sansky JA and others: Cardiovascular function in extreme obesity, Acta Med Scand 193:437, 1973.

59. Sitges-Serra A, Linares J, and Perez JL: A randomized trial of the effect of tubing changes on hub contamination and catheter sepsis during parenteral nutrition, JPEN 9:322, 1985.

60. Sitges-Serra A and others: Hub colonization as the initial step in an outbreak of catheter related sepsis due to coagulase negative staphylococci during parenteral nutrition, JPEN 8:668, 1985.

61. Strauss RJ and Wise L: Operative risks in the obese patient. In Deitel M, editor: Nutrition in clinical surgery, Baltimore, 1980, Williams & Wilkins.

62. Sttots NA and Friesen L: Understanding starvation in the critically ill patient, Heart Lung 11(5):469, 1982.

63. Tweedle DEF: Metabolic care, London, 1982, Churchill Livingstone, Inc.

64. Twomey P, Ziegler D, and Rombeau J: Utility of skin testing in nutritional assessment: a critical review, JPEN 6:50, 1982.

65. Valgeirdotter K and Munro HN: Protein and amino acid metabolism. In Fischer J, editor: Surgical nutrition, Boston, 1983, Little, Brown & Co.

66. Vanlandingham S and others: Metabolic abnormalities in patients supported with enteral tube feeding, JPEN 5(4):322, 1981.

67. Webb P, Annis JF, and Troutman SJ: Energy balance in man measured by direct and indirect calorimetry, Am J Clin Nutr 33:1287, 1980.

68. Weisier RL, Bacon J, and Butterworth CE: Central venous alimentation: a prospective study of the frequency of metabolic abnormalities among medical and surgical patients, JPEN 6(5):421, 1982.

69. Weisner RL and others: Hospital malnutrition: a prospective evaluation of general medical patients during the course of hospitalization, Am J Clin Nutr 32:418, 1979.

70. Williams WW: Infection control during parenteral nutrition therapy, JPEN 9(6):735, 1985.

71. Witt L: HHNK, Nurs 76(2):66, 1976.

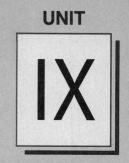
ENDOCRINE ALTERATIONS

39

Endocrine Anatomy and Physiology

CHAPTER OBJECTIVES

- *Identify and briefly describe the physiology of the normal anatomical structures of the endocrine organs discussed in this chapter.*
- *List the target tissues for antidiuretic hormone (ADH), the effect of ADH on the target tissues, and the stimulus for release and inhibition of ADH.*
- *Describe the function of antidiuretic hormone in the maintenance of both serum osmolality and blood volume.*
- *Discuss why the hypothalamus-hypophyseal system is vulnerable with traumatic head injuries.*
- *Describe the function of insulin and glucagon in the maintenance of normal serum glucose.*

Maintaining the dynamic equilibrium of the various cells, tissues, organs, and systems of the human body is a highly complex and specialized process. Two systems regulate these critical relationships: the nervous system and the endocrine system. The nervous system communicates through nerve impulses that control skeletal muscle, smooth muscle tissue, and cardiac muscle tissue.

The endocrine system controls and communicates through the distribution of potent hormones throughout the body (see Fig. 39-1 for a listing of the endocrine glands, hormones, target tissue, and action). When stimulated, the endocrine organ secretes hormones into surrounding body fluids. Once in circulation, these hormones travel to a specific target tissue where they exert a pronounced effect on specialized cells. Receptors found on the cell surfaces or within the cells are equipped with molecules that recognize and bind the hormone to the cell and produce a specific response.

Endocrine hormones may have a direct effect on body functioning (prolactin and the maintenance of milk production for breastfeeding), or the effect may be more generalized (thyroxin and the rate of metabolism in the body). Diseases affecting the endocrine glands usually do not require emergency critical care interventions. However, when an endocrine crises does occur, it often brings with it life-threatening consequences.

Diabetic ketoacidosis (DKA) is an endocrine emergency. It is perhaps the most common endocrine disorder for which the patient is admitted to the critical care unit. Hyperglycemic hyperosmolar nonketotic coma (HHNC) is another endocrine dysfunction involving carbohydrate metabolism. This potentially lethal disorder has a mortality rate greater than 40%[11] and is often seen in the critical care unit as a complication of other serious health problems.

Diabetes insipidus (DI) and syndrome of inappropriate antidiuretic hormone (SIADH) are two pituitary disorders that disrupt the body's regulation of plasma osmotic pressure and circulating blood volume. Each disease is rarely seen alone but rather develops secondary to a precipitating illness.

This unit will focus on these four metabolic disorders.

THE PANCREAS
The Pancreas

The pancreas is generally triangular in shape and is approximately 15 cm (6 inches) long and 4 cm (1.50 to 2 inches) wide. The body of the organ lies horizontally retroperitoneally, with the base end in the C-shaped curvature of the duodenum and the apex extending behind and below the stomach toward the spleen. Specialized exocrine cells within the pancreas secrete digestive enzymes into a 3 mm duct that transverses the pancreas and empties into the duodenum. Fig. 39-2 shows the pancreatic duct, known also as the duct of Wirshung, which forms the passageway for pancreatic juice during intestinal digestion.

The endocrine functions of the pancreas are accomplished by numerous clusters of cells that appear to form tiny islands among the exocrine cells. These islets of Langerhan (named after Paul Langerhan, the German pathologist who identified them in 1869) are composed of four distinct cell types. The cells formerly referred to as alpha, beta, and delta cells are currently called A, B, and D cells (Fig. 39-2). A cells secrete glucagon, B cells secrete insulin, D cells secrete somatostatin. F cells are the most recently identified cells and secrete pancreatic polypeptide hormone.[10]

Glucagon, insulin, somatostatin, and polypeptide hormones are released into the surrounding capillaries to empty into the portal vein where they are distributed to target cells

729

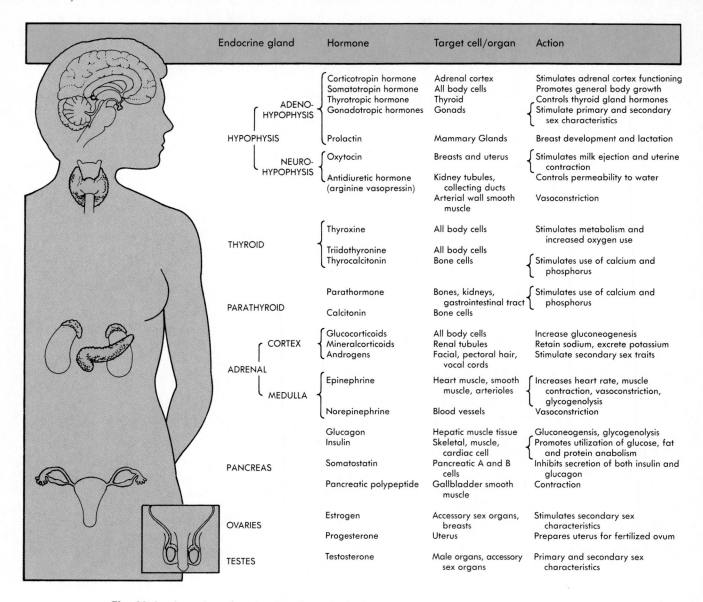

Endocrine gland		Hormone	Target cell/organ	Action
HYPOPHYSIS	ADENO-HYPOPHYSIS	Corticotropin hormone	Adrenal cortex	Stimulates adrenal cortex functioning
		Somatotropin hormone	All body cells	Promotes general body growth
		Thyrotropic hormone	Thyroid	Controls thyroid gland hormones
		Gonadotropic hormones	Gonads	Stimulate primary and secondary sex characteristics
		Prolactin	Mammary Glands	Breast development and lactation
	NEURO-HYPOPHYSIS	Oxytocin	Breasts and uterus	Stimulates milk ejection and uterine contraction
		Antidiuretic hormone (arginine vasopressin)	Kidney tubules, collecting ducts	Controls permeability to water
			Arterial wall smooth muscle	Vasoconstriction
THYROID		Thyroxine	All body cells	Stimulates metabolism and increased oxygen use
		Triidothyronine	All body cells	
		Thyrocalcitonin	Bone cells	Stimulates use of calcium and phosphorus
PARATHYROID		Parathormone	Bones, kidneys, gastrointestinal tract	Stimulates use of calcium and phosphorus
		Calcitonin	Bone cells	
ADRENAL	CORTEX	Glucocorticoids	All body cells	Increase gluconeogenesis
		Mineralcorticoids	Renal tubules	Retain sodium, excrete potassium
		Androgens	Facial, pectoral hair, vocal cords	Stimulate secondary sex traits
	MEDULLA	Epinephrine	Heart muscle, smooth muscle, arterioles	Increases heart rate, muscle contraction, vasoconstriction, glycogenolysis
		Norepinephrine	Blood vessels	Vasoconstriction
PANCREAS		Glucagon	Hepatic muscle tissue	Gluconeogensis, glycogenolysis
		Insulin	Skeletal, muscle, cardiac cell	Promotes utilization of glucose, fat and protein anabolism
		Somatostatin	Pancreatic A and B cells	Inhibits secretion of both insulin and glucagon
		Pancreatic polypeptide	Gallbladder smooth muscle	Contraction
OVARIES		Estrogen	Accessory sex organs, breasts	Stimulates secondary sex characteristics
		Progesterone	Uterus	Prepares uterus for fertilized ovum
TESTES		Testosterone	Male organs, accessory sex organs	Primary and secondary sex characteristics

Fig. 39-1 Location of endocrine glands with hormones, target cell/organ, and hormone action.

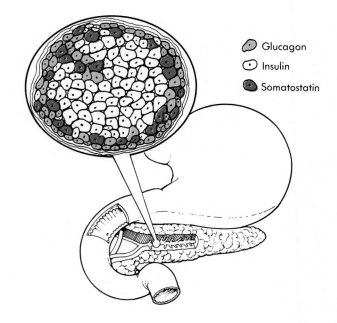

○ Glucagon
○ Insulin
● Somatostatin

Fig. 39-2 Macroscopic and microscopic structure of the pancreas.

Table 39-1 Pancreatic endocrine cells, hormones, stimulant, release factor, target tissue, and response/action

Cell	Hormone	Stimulant	Target tissue	Action
A	Glucagon	↓ Glucose Exercise ↑ Amino acids SNS stimulation	Hepatocyte Myocyte	↑ Glucose in bloodstream ↑ Gluconeogenesis ↑ Glycogenolysis Mobilization fats Mobilization proteins
B	Insulin	Glucose	Skeletal cells Muscle cells Cardiac cells	↓ Blood glucose ↓ Fat mobilization ↑ Fat storage ↓ Protein mobilization ↑ Protein synthesis ↑ Glucogenesis
D	Somatostatin	Hyperglycemia	A cells B cells	↓ Blood glucose ↓ Glycogen secretion ↓ Insulin secretion
F	Pancreatic polypeptide	Acute hypoglycemia	Gallbladder Smooth muscle	↑ Gallbladder contraction ↓ Pancreatic enzyme

Table 39-2 Agents that release or inhibit insulin

Insulin release	Insulin inhibition
Blood glucose level-major stimulant	Low blood sugar
HORMONES	**HORMONES**
Glucagon Corticotropic hormone Thyrotropin Somatotropin Glucocorticoids Secretin Gastrin	Somatostatin Norepinephrine Epinephrine
Vagal stimulation	
DRUGS	**DRUGS**
Beta adrenergic stimulators Sulfonylurea Theophylline Acetylcholine	Beta adrenergic blocking agents Diazoxide Phenytoin Thiazide/sulfonamide diuretics

in the liver. They then go into general circulation to reach other target cells.

Hormones

Insulin. Insulin is a potent anabolic hormone that produces hypoglycemia. It is the only hormone produced in the body that directly lowers glucose levels in the bloodstream.[10] Insulin also augments the transport of potassium into the cells, decreases the mobilization of fats, and stimulates protein synthesis (Table 39-1). The major stimulant for insulin secretion is glucose (Table 39-2). Through the feedback mechanism of plasma glucose, the B cells produce an average of 1 unit of insulin each hour. Insulin levels rise sharply to 6 to 8 units soon after meal ingestion.[18]

Functions of insulin. In the presence of effective insulin, glucose is admitted to the skeletal, cardiac, and adipose cells for use as energy. Excess glucose, in the form of glycogen, is stored in the hepatic and muscle cells for use as fuel at a later time. The movement of glucose from the circulation into the intracellular compartment reduces the presence of glucose in the bloodstream and helps preserve the blood's osmolarity. Simultaneously, glucose is available to the cell as its main energy source.

The central nervous system is freely permeable to glucose and does not rely on insulin for the transport of glucose across the cell membrane. Brain cells store a minimum of glycogen for energy release and are unable to use the end product of gluconeogenesis for energy. Although decreased insulin levels do not damage brain cells, they cannot survive glucose deficiency from hypersecretion of insulin.[2]

Fat metabolism is also affected by adequate, effective insulin levels. In the presence of insulin, fat is stored in connective tissues, thereby reducing fat mobilization and fat catabolism.

Insulin also spares protein from being used as energy and permits protein synthesis. When the cells receive sufficient energy from glucose, amino acids are available for active transport into the cell promoting the conversion of ribonucleic acid (RNA) into new protein.

Abnormal insulin levels. Insufficient or ineffective insulin leads to hyperglycemia and cell deprivation of its energy source. This forces the body to shift from using glucose as fuel to using fat and protein. Fats and protein are catabolized in an attempt to provide a reserve source of glucose through a process called gluconeogenesis. Fats are broken down to fatty acids and glycerol. The glycerol is oxidized as carbohydrate while the fatty acids are converted to ketone bodies. When the ketone bodies accumulate faster than they are metabolized, ketosis results.

Protein is catabolized when the body's stores of carbohydrate and fat are depleted. As part of this process, amino acids are broken down to form ammonia and keto acids. Nitrogen is removed from the amino groups, and the resulting ammonia is detoxified by the liver and removed by the kidneys in the form of urea. Through gluconeogenesis, the ketoacids are converted to glucose.

In a catabolic state, the body is unable to maintain the protein synthesis needed for healthy functioning and blood proteins are used for energy. Without necessary insulin to act on the cell receptor site, blood glucose levels increase. Additionally, the end products of fat and protein catabolism collect in the bloodstream.

Glucagon. Glucagon, synthesized by the A cells, has the opposite effect of insulin. Glucagon counterregulates insulin levels and raises blood sugar levels. It forms glucose from noncarbohydrate sources such as fat and protein through gluconeogenesis. Glucagon is considered a potent gluconeogenic hormone. Glucagon release is stimulated by factors such as a drop in insulin, an increase in blood amino acids, a fall in blood sugar, starvation, exercise, or stimulation of the sympathetic nervous system (Table 39-1). Glucagon is released to protect the body from the hypoglycemia that may result from these conditions.

Initially, glucagon stimulates the release of glycogen stored in the liver and muscle cells to meet short-term energy needs. Through a process called glycogenolysis, the glycogen stored in the liver and muscles is converted back into glucose form to be used by the cells. If the energy needs are long-term, the glucagon stimulates glucose release through a more complex process, gluconeogenesis.[29] In gluconeogenesis, fat and protein nutrients are rapidly broken down into end products that are then changed into glucose.

In the healthy body, a normal blood glucose level is maintained by the insulin-glucagon ratio. When the blood glucose level is high, insulin is released and glucagon inhibited. When blood glucose levels are diminished, glucagon rather than insulin is released (Table 39-3). The insulin/glucagon ratio is considered more important in the overall metabolism of fuel sources than the absolute level of either hormone.[29]

Somatostatin. Somatostatin is a protein hormone that inhibits the release of both insulin and glucagon. Somatostatin is synthesized by the pancreatic D cells, the hypothalamus, gastric mucosa, and elsewhere. The hormone decreases glucagon secretion and in high quantities it decreases insulin release (Table 39-1).

Hyperglycemia stimulates the activity of the D cells. It is theorized that the release of insulin causes somatostatin to keep the beta cells under control. It is also believed that somatostatin allows the gradual influx of glucose into the cell after ingestion of a meal, thus preventing postprandial hyperglycemia.[18]

Pancreatic polypeptide. Pancreatic polypeptide is synthesized by the F cells within the islets of Langerhan. This hormone contracts the smooth muscle tissue of the gallbladder and represses pancreatic enzyme secretion.[29] Pancreatic polypeptide can be stimulated by acute hypoglycemia or by an intake that is high in protein while low in carbo-

Table 39-3 The insulin-glucagon ratio and its effect on carbohydrate, fat, and protein metabolism

Balanced insulin-glucagon	Decreased insulin–increased glucagon
↑ Utilization of glucose by cells	↓ Utilization of glucose by cells
↑ Movement of potassium intracellularly	↓ Movement of potassium intracellularly
↑ Carbohydrate metabolism	↑ Blood glucose
↓ Gluconeogenesis	↑ Gluconeogenesis
↑ Glycogen storage	↓ Glycogen storage
↓ Glycogenolysis	↑ Glycogenolysis
↓ Lipolysis	↑ Lipolysis
↓ Fat mobilization	↑ Fat mobilization
↑ Fat storage	↓ Fat stores
↓ Protein mobilization	↑ Hepatic metabolism fats
↑ Protein synthesis	↑ Ketogenesis
	↑ Mobilization of protein
	↑ Proteolysis
	↑ Lipoprotein

hydrate. Although it currently has no known metabolic function, pancreatic polypeptide is believed to play a role in nutrient homeostasis.[10]

PITUITARY GLAND AND HYPOTHALAMUS

Understanding the structure and function of the pituitary gland is necessary to appreciate the unique relationship that exists between the pituitary and the hypothalamus.

Hypothalamus

The hypothalamus lies superior to the pituitary gland. It is composed of specialized nervous tissue responsible for the integrated functioning of the nervous system and endocrine system, called neuroendocrine control. The hypothalamus weighs approximately 4 gm and forms the walls and lower portion of the third ventricle of the brain. The area composing the floor of the ventricle thickens in the center and elongates. It is from this funnel-shaped portion, called the infundibular stalk (or stem) that the pituitary gland is suspended (see Fig. 39-3). The infundibular stalk contains a very rich vascular supply and a network of communicating neurons that travel from the hypothalamus to the pituitary.[10] The vascular network and neural pathways transport chemical and neural signals and maintain constant communication between the nervous system and the endocrine system.

Pituitary Gland

The pituitary gland, called the hypophysis because it is attached below the hypothalamus, is found recessed in the base of the cranial cavity in a hollow depression of the sphenoid bone called the sella turcica (Greek for Turkish saddle). Secured in such a protected environment, the pituitary is one of the most inaccessible endocrine glands in

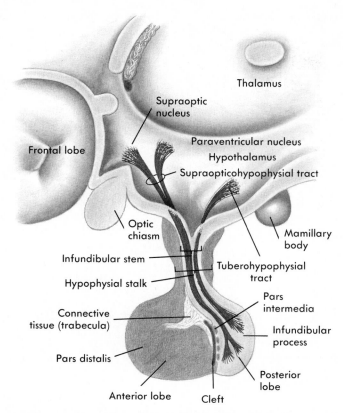

Fig. 39-3 Anatomy of the hypothalamus and the pituitary gland showing the infundibular stem (or stalk) connecting the hypothalamus to the pituitary gland. (From Thompson JM and others: Clinical Nursing, St. Louis, 1986, The CV Mosby Co.

humans. Yet, it is because of this very location that the pituitary gland is susceptible to injury from surgical and accidental trauma of the face and head.

The pituitary gland has been known as the master gland because of the major influence it has over all areas of body functioning. However, it is now known that the pituitary does not act independently. Rather the release and inhibition of its hormones is actually controlled by the hypothalamus. The hypothalamus controls pituitary response by secreting substances known as release-inhibiting factors. These factors then control the release or inhibition of hormones. Virtually every function necessary to maintain the human body in a state of dynamic equilibrium is regulated in this manner.

The hypophysis is composed of three parts (see Fig. 39-3): the anterior lobe, the intermediate lobe, and the posterior lobe, each with its own origin, morphology, and function.[14]

Adenohypophysis

The anterior lobe of the pituitary is the largest portion of the gland. It communicates with the hypothalamus via a vascular network. Several hormones are produced by the glandular tissue of the anterior pituitary, thus it is called the adenohypophysis. Although the exact number of hormones produced here is uncertain,[14] it is undisputed that adrenocorticotropic hormone (ACTH), thyroid-stimulating hormone (TSH), follicle-stimulating hormone (FSH), luteinizing hormone (LH), growth hormone, and prolactin are manufactured here. It is not the purpose of this chapter to discuss these hormones, but information about their target tissue and action is found in Fig. 39-1.

Pars Intermedia

Another lobe of the pituitary, the pars intermedia, is located in the central portion of the pituitary between the anterior and posterior lobes. Although the pars intermedia is present in the fetus, it gradually merges with and becomes indistinct from the posterior lobe in the adult. It is interesting to note that this lobe is larger in some lower vertebrates such as llamas and camels, which are able to withstand long periods of water deprivation.[18] The functions of the pars intermedia are poorly understood, but it is thought to release melanocyte-stimulating hormone (MSH). Melanocyte-stim-

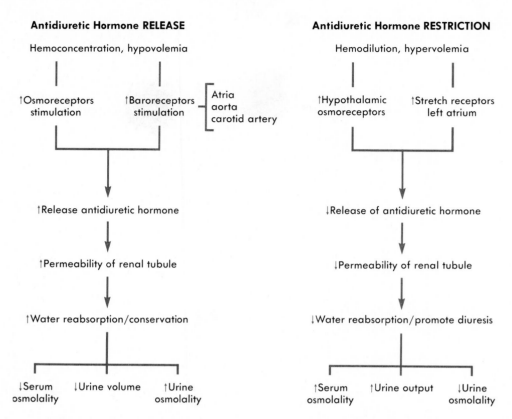

Antidiuretic Hormone RELEASE

Hemoconcentration, hypovolemia

↑Osmoreceptors stimulation   ↑Baroreceptors stimulation   [Atria aorta carotid artery

↑Release antidiuretic hormone

↑Permeability of renal tubule

↑Water reabsorption/conservation

↓Serum osmolality   ↓Urine volume   ↑Urine osmolality

Antidiuretic Hormone RESTRICTION

Hemodilution, hypervolemia

↑Hypothalamic osmoreceptors   ↑Stretch receptors left atrium

↓Release of antidiuretic hormone

↓Permeability of renal tubule

↓Water reabsorption/promote diuresis

↑Serum osmolality   ↑Urine output   ↓Urine osmolality

Fig. 39-4   Physiology of the release and restriction of antidiuretic hormone.

ulating hormone controls color changes of the skin in vertebrates that are able to adjust their skin color for camouflage purposes and blend with the environment.[10]

Neurohypophysis

The posterior lobe of the pituitary is called the neurohypophysis.[14] It retains its continuity with the hypothalamus via neural fibers running through the infundibular stalk. The neurohypophysis does not have glandular properties but functions as an extension of the hypothalamus. It collects, stores, and later releases hormones that are actually produced in the hypothalamus.[10] After hormones are synthesized in the hypothalamus, they are transported to the posterior pituitary until the hypothalamus signals their release. Oxytocin (Pitocin) and arginine vasopressin (antidiuretic hormone) are both manufactured in the hypothalamus and stored in the neurohypophysis.

Hormones

Oxytocin. Oxytocin stimulates smooth muscle contraction of the uterus and causes the myoepithelial cells of the breast to contract and force milk from the alveoli into the secretory ducts. Pathology caused by hypersecretion or hyposecretion of oxytocin has not been identified.[10] Insufficient amounts of oxytocin are known to result in delayed labor and delivery. Exogenous pitocin is used clinically to induce labor, to augment contractions during the first and second stages of labor, and manage postpartum hemorrhage.

Antidiuretic hormone. Antidiuretic hormone (ADH) or arginine vasopressin (AVP) has been identified as the single

most important hormone responsible for regulating fluid balance within the body.[18] ADH has two functions: it constricts smooth muscles within the arterial wall (pharmacological doses may elevate blood pressure), and, most importantly, it maintains the osmolality of the blood in a very narrow range by regulating the permeability of the kidney tubule. In effect, ADH also controls the sodium levels of the extracellular fluid. Plasma osmolality is largely determined by the sodium ion concentration process in the plasma. When sodium levels rise, plasma osmolality increases. ADH is released to stimulate fluid reabsorption at the nephron to maintain water and sodium balance.[9]

In the presence of ADH, permeability of the kidney tubules is increased and water is reabsorbed from the renal filtrate. This decreases water loss from the body and subsequently concentrates and reduces urine volume. Fluid conserved in this manner is returned to the circulating plasma where it dilutes the concentration (osmolality) of plasma (Fig. 39-4). The release of antidiuretic hormone is primarily regulated by the plasma osmotic pressure and the volume of circulating blood. Hemorrhage, sufficient to lower the blood pressure, and emesis, sufficient to reduce fluid volume, will stimulate the release of ADH. Other factors capable of influencing ADH secretion are pain, stress, malignant disease, surgical intervention, alcohol, and drugs [15] (see Table 39-4 for additional factors affecting ADH levels).

Osmoreceptors, believed to be sodium receptors,[9] located in the hypothalamus are sensitive to changes in the circulating plasma osmolality. Stretch receptors located in the

Table 39-4 Factors affecting antidiuretic hormone levels

Antidiuretic hormone stimulation (conserving water by decreasing tubular reabsorption of water)	Antidiuretic hormone restriction (promoting water loss by increasing tubular permeability to water)
Increased serum osmolality	Decreased serum osmolality
Emesis	
Hypovolemia	Hypervolemia
Hemorrhage	Water intoxication
Pain	Cold
	Congenital defect
	CO₂ inhalation
Trauma to hypothalamic-hypophyseal system	Trauma to hypothalamic-hypophyseal system
Accidental	Accidental
Surgical	Surgical
Pathological	Pathological
Stress	
Physical	
Emotional	
Acute infections	
Malignancies	
Nonmalignant pulmonary disorders	
Stimulated pulmonary baroreceptors	
Nocturnal sleep	
Drugs	Drugs
Nicotine	Phenytoin
Barbiturates	Chlorpromazine
Oxytocin	Reserpine
Glucocorticoids	Norepinephrine
Anesthetics	Ethanol
Acetaminophen	Narcotics
Amitriptyline	Lithium
Carbamazeprine	Demeclocycline
Cyclophosphamide	Tolazamide
Chlorpropamide	
K⁺ depleting diuretics	
Vincristine	
Isoproterenol	

left atrium are sensitive to volume changes in the plasma as may be caused by vomiting, diarrhea, or blood loss. ADH is restricted when the blood volume or osmolality is low. Suppression of ADH renders the kidney tubules impermeable to water and causes an increase in the amount of water excreted by the kidneys. This restores the circulating blood volume and normal osmolality (see Fig. 39-4).

Alterations in blood tonicity and circulating blood volume are also controlled by baroreceptors located primarily in the atria, the aorta, and the carotid arteries. Information from these receptors, coupled with change reflected by the osmoreceptors, stimulates the hypothalamus to modify ADH secretion. The result is maintenance of adequate fluid bal-ance within the extracellular and intracellular fluid compartments and normal blood pressure.

The pituitary dysfunctions discussed in Chapter 41 are those brought about by a metabolic derangement of the antidiuretic hormone: hyposecretion resulting in diabetes insipidus (DI) and hypersecretion known as syndrome of inappropriate antidiuretic hormone (SIADH).

REFERENCES

1. Braunwald E and others, editors: Harrison's principles of internal medicine, ed 11, New York, 1987, McGraw-Hill Book Co.
2. Bullock B and Rosendahl P: Pathophysiology, adaptations and alterations in function, ed 2, Glenview, Illinois, 1988, Scott Foresman & Company/Little, Brown College Division.
3. Burch W: Endocrinology, ed 2, Baltimore, 1988, Williams & Wilkins.
4. Butts D: Fluid and electrolyte disorders associated with diabetic ketoacidosis and hyperglycemic hyperosmolar nonketotic coma, Nurs Clin North Am 22(4):827, 1987.
5. Chanson P and others: Ultra-low doses of vasopressin in the management of diabetes insipidus, Crit Care Med 15(1):44, 1987.
6. Fischbach F: A manual of laboratory diagnostic tests, ed 3, Philadelphia, 1988, JB Lippincott Co.
7. Germon K: Fluid and electrolyte problems associated with diabetes insipidus and syndrome of inappropriate antidiuretic hormone, Nurs Clin North Am 22(4):785, 1987.
8. Grindlinger G and Boylan M: Amelioration by indomethacin of lithium-induced polyuria, Crit Care Med 15(5):538, 1987.
9. Guyton A: Textbook of medical physiology, ed 7, Philadelphia, 1986, WB Saunders Co.
10. Hadley M: Endocrinology, ed 2, Englewood Cliffs, NJ, 1988, Prentice-Hall.
11. Harris M and Hamman R, editors: Diabetes in America, Bethesda, Md, 1985, US Department of Health and Human Services, Public Health Service, National Institutes of Health, National Institute of Arthritis, Diabetes and Digestive and Kidney Diseases.
12. Hemmer M and others: Urinary ADH excretion during mechanical ventilation and weaning in man, Anesthesiology 52(5):395, 1980.
13. Henry J, editor: Todd, Sanford, Davidsohn, clinical diagnosis and managment by laboratory methods, ed 17, Philadelphia, 1984, WB Saunders, Co.
14. Hollinshead, W and Rosse C: Textbook of anatomy, ed 4, Philadelphia, 1985, Harper & Row Publishers.
15. Kohler, P, editor: Clinical endocrinology, New York, 1986, John Wiley & Sons.
16. Lubin M and others, editors: Medical management of the surgical patient, Boston, 1988, Butterworths.
17. Marble A and others: Joslin's diabetes mellitus, ed 12, Philadelphia, 1985, Lea & Febiger.
18. Martin C: Endocrine physiology, New York, 1985, Oxford University Press.
19. McEvoy G, McQuarrie G, and DiPietro J, editors: Drug information '87, Bethesda, 1987, American Society of Hospital Pharmacists.
20. Methany N and Snively WD: Nurse's handbook of fluid balance, ed 4, Philadelphia, 1983, JB Lippincott Co.
21. Nerozzi D, Goodwin F, and Costa E, editors: Neuropsychiatric disorders, New York, 1987, Raven Press.
22. Newman R: Bedside blood sugar determinations in the critically ill, Heart Lung 17(6):667, 1988.
23. Nikas D: Critical aspects of head trauma, Crit Care Nurs Q 10(1):19, 1987.
24. Polak J and Bloom S: Endocrine tumours, the pathobiology of regulatory peptide-producing tumours, London, 1985, Churchill Livingstone.
25. Potgieter P: Inappropriate ADH secretion in tetanus, Crit Care Med 11(6):417, 1983.

26. Powers M: Handbook of diabetes nutritional management, Rockville, Md, 1987, Aspen Publishers.

27. Rudy E: Magnetic resonance imaging, new horizon in diagnostic technique, J Neurosurg Nurs 17(6):331, 1985.

28. Schroeder S, Krupp M, and Tierney L: Current medical diagnosis and treatment, 1988, Norwalk, Conn, 1988, Appleton & Lange.

29. Slaunwhite R: Fundamentals of endocrinology, New York, 1988, Marcel Dekker, Inc.

30. Staller A: Systemic effects of severe head trauma, Crit Care Nurs 10(1):58, 1987.

31. Swearingen P, Sommers M, and Miller K: Manual of critical care: applying nursing diagnosis to adult critical illness, St Louis, 1988, the CV Mosby Co.

32. Tepperman J and Tepperman H: Metabolic and endocrine physiology, ed 5, Chicago, 1987, Yearbook Medical Publishers, Inc.

33. Vokes T and Robertson G: Disorders of antidiuretic hormone, Endocrinol Metab Clin North 17(2):281, 1988.

34. Williams C: Lung cancer, Oxford, New York, 1984, Oxford University Press.

Endocrine Assessment

CLINICAL AND LABORATORY ASSESSMENT AND DIAGNOSTIC PROCEDURES

CHAPTER OBJECTIVES

■ *Discuss the rationale involved in developing a consistent, sequential format for performing an endocrine nursing assessment.*

■ *Perform a thorough nursing assessment of the endocrine system on a critically ill patient, interpret the results, and plan nursing interventions that will treat any abnormal findings.*

■ *List the criteria for a health history that would be specific in assessing for diabetic ketoacidosis and hyperglycemic hyperosmolar nonketotic coma.*

■ *Compare and contrast at least three clinical and laboratory manifestations of diabetes insipidus and syndrome of inappropriate antidiuretic hormone.*

■ *List the laboratory tests that will differentiate central diabetes insipidus from nephrogenic diabetes insipidus.*

The majority of the endocrine glands are located deep within the protective encasement of the human body. This protected position safeguards the glands and their link to homeostasis against injury and trauma. Although the placement of the glands provides security for the glandular functions, their inaccessibility prevents the glands from being physically appraised. Most endocrine glands cannot be assessed by palpation, percussion, or auscultation. The thyroid gland and male gonads are unusual in that they are endocrine glands subject to physical examination. The anatomical position of each the thyroid and the testes makes them conducive to palpation. An enlarged thyroid can also be auscultated for a systolic bruit or continuous venous hum.

The endocrine glands that are not assessed by physical inspection can nevertheless be assessed by the clinician who understands the metabolic actions of the hormones involved.

Therefore, since percussion or palpation cannot be used, the nurse monitors the functioning of the target tissue.

Frequently the initial focus of the hormonal disturbance is not on the gland itself but rather on the specific cell receptor or target for the hormonal action. For example, posterior pituitary dysfunction is suspected when the patient has decreased urine output, clinical signs of hypervolemia (bounding pulse, increased blood pressure, elevated pulmonary artery or central venous pressure reading, engorged neck veins), plus serum hyponatremia with hypertonic urine. Understanding that the target cell for antidiuretic hormone is the kidney tubule and reabsorption of urine filtrate is the action of the hormone leads the clinician to suspect a compromise in ADH or posterior pituitary functioning.

Similarly, pancreatic disorders are often recognized by first noting imbalances in the beta cell hormone, insulin, and its systemic effects. The cell receptor site of insulin is found on the adipose and muscle cells. The major action of insulin is to increase the uptake and utilization of glucose by the muscle and fat cells and decrease blood glucose levels. When glucose is utilized for cellular energy, insulin prevents fat and protein from being broken down for fuel. The clinician who understands the metabolic effects of insulin may suspect a dysfunctioning pancreas in a patient who is lethargic and has hot dry skin, oliguria, and a sweet-smelling odor to the breath.

Collecting clues that may signal a dysfunctioning gland poses a challenge to the nurse clinician because target tissues of insulin (adipose and muscle cells) and antidiuretic hormone (kidney tubule) are influenced by numerous other factors. Therefore, the nurse starts with a pertinent data base including history (when available) and precipitating factors. The patient in the critical care unit may not be able to provide an adequate history for the nurse's assessment data base. Changes in level of consciousness and urgent medical/nursing procedures may delay the patient from providing personal perspective of the current problem. This initial phase of the nursing process should not be ignored, however, and sources other than the patient (family, friends, previous medical records) should be used to supply vital information.

CLINICAL ASSESSMENT
Pancreas

Insulin is produced by the pancreas and is responsible for glucose metabolism. The clinical assessment provides information about pancreatic functioning. Assessment of signs and symptoms of abnormal insulin levels identifies the patient response to altered glucose metabolism.

History. A complete health history would include the patient's chief complaint and current health history. Chronic as well as episodic diseases are discussed (acute stress could increase endogenous glucose). Routine treatments such as hyperalimentation, peritoneal dialysis, and hemodialysis are included in the health history because they could be an exogenous source of increased glucose levels.

Also included in the data collection is the patient's past history. Has the patient ever had pancreatic surgery? Was he ever told he had "too much sugar" in his blood or may develop "too much sugar" later in his life? What treatment was prescribed if such a condition existed?

Family history is assessed in respect to present illness. Carbohydrate metabolic imbalance is commonly influenced by hereditary factors.

Included in the medical history are questions pertaining to the patient's use of prescription or over-the-counter medications. Pharmacological drugs may alter pancreatic function by either increasing or decreasing the release of hormones. Drugs may also interfere with hormonal action at the receptor site on the target cell. Epinephrine and phenytoin are two medications that are known to decrease the effect of insulin in the body and increase serum glucose. Glucagon and glucocorticoids increase the breakdown of noncarbohydrate substances into glucose and thereby increase serum glucose levels.

Additionally, information about the immediately preceding health status of the patient is sought. Patients with severe infection or surgical or traumatic injury may develop an inability to balance the body's sudden physiological changes with demands in insulin needs.

The patient or significant other is asked about recent, unexplained changes in weight, thirst, hunger, and urination patterns including frequency and volume during the day and during the night. Review of the patient's activities of daily living and recent changes in activity level gives the clinician information about endurance levels, fatigue, and weakness. This information relates to glucose availability and utilization as fuel. Asking the patient or significant other about vague or obscure changes in behavior or mental status (memory loss, momentary disorientation) may reveal periods of hyperglycemia or hypoglycemia and its effect on the brain tissue.

Physical assessment. Hydration status and skin assessment provide additional information about pancreatic functioning. Normal levels of glucose in the bloodstream contribute to the serum osmolality. The glucose level is a key component in the extracellular and intracellular fluid bal-

ance. This fluid balance is easily identified by the presence of moist, shiny buccal membranes. Skin turgor that is resilient and returns to its original position in less than 3 seconds after being pinched or lifted indicates adequate skin elasticity. (Skin over the forehead and clavicle is the most reliable for testing tissue turgor because it is less affected by aging and thus more easily assessed for changes related to fluid balance.) A well-hydrated patient has skin in the groin and axilla that is slightly moist to touch. A balanced intake and output, absence of thirst, absence of edema, stable weight, and urine specific gravity that falls within the normal range (1.005 to 1.030) all provide the nurse with information indicating the patient's hydration status is adequate for the patient's metabolic demands.

Pituitary Gland

The pituitary gland, recessed in the base of the cranium, is not accessible to physical assessment. Therefore the clinician must be aware of the systemic effects of a normally functioning neurohypophysis to identify pituitary dysfunction.

History. When possible, the patient and/or significant other is asked about the patient's chief complaint and current health history. Does the patient have complaints of headache or fatigue? Is there an active blood loss? (Hypovolemia stimulates the presence of antidiuretic hormone.) Is the patient currently being treated for another endocrine dysfunction that could potentially interfere with the amount of antidiuretic hormone in the body? (Hypothyroidism and adrenal insufficiency stimulate the release of ADH regardless of serum osmolality or volume deficit.[1]) Is there a head injury or neurological disorder that could interfere with the synthesis of ADH in the hypothalamus or its passage down to the posterior pituitary before its release? Equally important is information about pulmonary diseases or malignant diseases—tuberculosis, pneumonia, duodenal carcinoma, and especially oat cell carcinomas. Each is an example of a disease that is capable of causing autonomous production of ADH.

The past history may reveal information about a birth defect involving the infundibular stalk. A family history is assessed in an effort to identify familial tendencies toward ineffective antidiuretic hormone. An inherited disorder involves kidney tubules that are insensitive to the circulating ADH.

A history of the patient's use of medications offers the clinician clues regarding potential ADH imbalance (see Table 39-4 for factors affecting antidiuretic hormone levels). Phenytoin, chlorpromazine, and reserpine, among other drugs, decrease the release of ADH. Barbiturates, anesthetics, vincristine, glucocorticoids, and several other drugs stimulate the release of ADH.

A psychosocial history provides an opportunity to collect data regarding any obsessional neurosis the patient may have experienced. Knowledge of compulsive activities involving insatiable water drinking is useful in determining the cause of antidiuretic hormone imbalance.

The patient and/or significant other is asked about the health status immmediately preceding the acute care episode. Has the patient been complaining of unexplained weight loss? Has there been excessive urination that occurs so frequently that it interferes with the patient's daily living activities and ability to sleep? Has there been an increase in thirst, and if so, is it easily satisfied?

The clinician asks the patient about any changes in mental abilities (increased or decreased fluid levels affected by circulating ADH also affects the serum sodium levels). Sodium imbalance may result from excessive sodium loss in the urine or from a disproportionate amount of extracellular fluid diluting the previously normal sodium level. Alterations in the patient's serum sodium level may first be noticed as a change in the patient's mental status, since difficulty concentrating and confusion may occur. These complaints signal changes in cerebral hydration and serum sodium levels that, unless corrected, will lead to further neurological damage and ultimately death.

Physical assessment. Antidiuretic hormone controls the amount of fluid lost and retained within the body. The nurse uses a hydration assessment to determine the effectiveness of ADH function. A hydration assessment includes skin integrity, skin turgor, and buccal membrane moisture. Blood pressure and pulse are frequently monitored. Decreased blood pressure with an increased pulse is characteristic of hypovolemia, whereas elevated blood pressure and rapid, bounding pulse may indicate hypervolemia. Orthostatic hypotension occurs when there is a decrease in extracellular fluid volume and is identified by a drop in systolic blood pressure of 20 mm Hg and a drop in diastolic blood pressure of 10 mm Hg when the patient changes position from lying to standing.

Daily weight changes coincide with fluid retention and fluid loss. Sudden changes in weight could be a result of a change in fluid balance; 1 L of fluid lost or retained is equal to approximately 2 pounds, 3 ounces of weight gained or lost. To use weight as a true determinant of the body's weight changes, all extraneous variables should be eliminated and the same scale should be used at the same time each day. The patient should also wear similar clothing so as not to affect the reading.

Intake and output is often overlooked as a definitive tool in the critical care unit. It is a simple task which, when performed accurately and conscientiously on *all* routes of fluid intake and loss, provides information about the body's fluid balance. Precise intake and output records are also used as parameters for fluid replacement therapy. Physical characteristics of urine such as concentration, color, and specific gravity are also significant factors in assessing the patient's fluid balance.

The patient's neurological system is frequently evaluated when assessing the pituitary gland. Alterations in serum sodium levels have an adverse effect on brain tissue and disrupt the patient's behavioral patterns as already mentioned. Muscle coordination, deep tendon reflexes, and muscle strength are included in this neurological assessment.

LABORATORY ASSESSMENT
Pancreas

Pertinent laboratory tests for the pancreas measure the amount of insulin produced by the pancreatic B cells and insulin's effectiveness in transporting glucose from the bloodstream into the cell. The test results illustrate insulin's ability to maintain a constant serum glucose level. When insufficient or inefficient insulin is present to permit glucose to be used for fuel, the body is forced to breakdown other noncarbohydrate sources such as fat and protein as alternate energy sources. The rapid, incomplete breakdown of fat and protein leave waste products that affect the body's homeostasis. Tests to determine the osmolality, glucose, and ketone levels identify the residual effects of incomplete glucose uptake and utilization by the cells.

Insulin. When measured by blood test, the normal value of insulin is 5 to 20 μU/ml. The amount of insulin circulating in the bloodstream during a period of fasting is measured by a sensitive radioimmunoassay test. The release of insulin is dependent upon the concentration of blood glucose; when glucose levels rise, insulin levels also rise. Conversely, when serum glucose levels are low, insulin secretion is inhibited. Therefore a fasting blood sample is preferred for evaluation of serum insulin levels.

Glucose. The normal fasting serum or plasma value of glucose when measured by blood test is 70 to 110 mg/dl. The fasting whole blood value is 60 to 100 mg/dl and the nonfasting value is 85 to 125 mg/dl. Circulating blood glucose is derived from three sources: exogenous intake of glucose, release of glycogen stores, and breakdown of noncarbohydrate sources, known as gluconeogenesis. A fasting blood sample is read as a simple, numerical value, but it actually measures many complex, interrelated processes. The glucose reading measures the ability of the pancreatic A cells to balance the release of glucagon with the B cell releases of insulin. Circulating glucose is also dependent on the peripheral uptake of glucose and the functioning of the liver and its role in gluconeogenesis. Consistently elevated glucose levels signal an increase in glucagon production and an insufficient amount of effective insulin. In healthy patients, a fasting serum glucose rarely exceeds 110 mg/dl blood.

Fingerstick glucose test. Fingerstick glucose tests involve a relatively new technique that makes frequent glucose testing rapid, economical, and convenient. This test is commonly used at the bedside for quick, accurate readings that serve as a basis for insulin coverage. The blood test can also be done by the patient as a means of keeping track of daily glucose levels and identifying situations that cause hyperglycemia. It is currently used by patients as a means of obtaining tighter control over glucose levels and keeping the glucose as close to normal as possible with intensive insulin therapy. These test involves a reagent strip and a reflectance meter or a monitor. There are numerous devices available, each with its own specific instructions and guarantee of accuracy. Some strips can be read by comparing the color left by a drop of blood to a color chart. Strips may also be placed into a meter or monitor for an exact reading.

Glycosylated hemoglobin. During the 120-day lifespan of erythrocytes the hemoglobin within each cell binds to the available blood glucose through a process known as glycosylation. In a blood test, 4.0% to 7.0% of hemoglobin is normally glycosylated. The result is Hgb1$_A$, Hgb1$_B$, Hgb1$_C$. Increased levels of circulating glucose cause an increase in glycosylation. Because this process is irreversible, a sample of blood provides information about the average amount of blood glucose that has been present over the previous 3 to 4 months.

This test is not routinely done as a pancreatic screening tool. It is used most frequently for patients diagnosed with diabetes mellitus. It provides information about the degree of hyperglycemia, including the actual increased values over a specific period of time. This test eliminates many variables that could normally affect the accurate interpretation of a glucose test. Fasting state, exercise, stress, and medications do not interfere with this test result. Nor will the test outcome be influenced by patient compliance or changes in a patient's usual habits initiated only to have a fasting blood glucose value read closer to normal than it usually is.

Ketones. In a blood test the normal results are ketones 2 to 4 ml/100 ml blood; acetone 0.3 to 2 mg/100 ml blood. Normally there are no ketones present in the urine so urine tests would be negative. Ketones are byproducts of fat metabolism. Normally, when the body utilizes carbohydrate as its main source of energy, fat metabolism is complete and only a trace of ketones is found in the blood.

In the absence of glucose, fats are burned for energy. Lipolysis (fat breakdown) occurs so rapidly that fat metabolism is incomplete, and ketone bodies (acetone, betahydroxybutyric acid, and acetoacetic acid) collect in the blood (ketonemia) and are excreted in the urine (ketonuria).

Both blood and urine specimens can be tested in the laboratory or with reagent strips. Urine samples can also be tested with specially prepared tablets. Both reagent strips and tables are compared with a color chart.

Ketonemia is observed by a fruity, sweet-smelling odor on the exhaled breath.

Serum osmolality. In blood samples the normal range for serum osmolality is 275 to 297 mOsm/kg. Osmolality is a measurement of the number of particles in a solution and not the size or weight of the particles. This diagnostic test is not a routine screening tool for pancreatic dysfunction. It is commonly used to identify the effects of an imbalance in carbohydrate metabolism and to assess fluid volume status.

An accumulation of ketone bodies and ketoacids results from the rapid, incomplete breakdown of fat and protein. The ketone bodies and ketoacids collect in the plasma as metabolic "debris" and, along with the increasing levels of glucose that cannot enter the cell, drastically increase the number of particles that normally circulate in the plasma. This increase in circulating particles coupled with the fluid loss from osmotic diuresis significantly raises the plasma osmolality.

Pituitary

There is no single diagnostic test that identifies dysfunctioning of the posterior pituitary gland. Diagnosis of pituitary dysfunction is usually made through a combination of laboratory tests combined with the clinical picture of the patient.

The diagnostic tests measure the amount of antidiuretic hormone released into the bloodstream. The tests include both a measurement of the ADH that is produced by the hypothalamus and tests that gauge the subsequent release of ADH by the neurohypophysis.

Serum and urine osmolality tests measure the effectiveness of antidiuretic hormone in maintaining the correct solute concentration for the particular sample of fluid.

Serum antidiuretic hormone. The normal result of blood test for serum antidiuretic hormone is 1 to 5 pg/ml [picogram = $1 \div$ trillion] or <1.5 mg/L). The serum antidiuretic hormone test measures the amount of ADH present in a frozen sample of blood (and/or urine). The direct measurement of ADH is possible by means of a laboratory methodology called radioimmunoassay. This diagnostic procedure provides accurate results and, when available, is used in preference to water load and water deprivation tests (discussed later).

To prepare a patient for this radioimmunoassay testing, all drugs that may alter the release of antidiuretic hormone are withheld for a minimum of 8 hours. Medications that affect ADH levels are morphine sulfate, lithium carbonate, chlorothiazide, carbamazeprine, oxytocin, and certain neoplastic and anesthetic agents (see Table 39-4 for additional drugs). Nicotine, alcohol, both positive and negative pressure ventilation, and emotional stress can also influence the ADH levels and must be considered when interpreting the values.

The test is read by comparing serum antidiuretic hormone levels with the blood and urine osmolality. The presence of increased ADH in the bloodstream compared with a low serum osmolality and elevated urine osmolality confirms the diagnosis of syndrome of inappropriate antidiuretic hormone (SIADH). Reduced levels of serum ADH in a patient with high serum osmolality, hypernatremia, and reduced urine concentration signal central diabetes insipidus.

Urine and blood osmolality. Normal values are serum osmolality 285 to 300 mOsm/L; urine osmolality 300 to 1,000 mOsm/L. Osmolality measurements determine the concentration of dissolved particles in a solution. In a healthy person, a change in the concentration of solutes triggers a chain of events to maintain proper dilution.

Increased serum osmolality will stimulate the release of ADH, which in turn will reduce the amount of water lost at the tubules. Body fluid is thereby retained to dilute the particle concentration in the blood stream. Decreased serum osmolality inhibits the release of ADH, the kidney tubules increase their permeability, and fluid is eliminated from the body in an attempt to regain normal concentration of particles in the bloodstream.

The most accurate results of the body's ability to maintain a fluid balance are obtained when urine and blood samples are collected simultaneously.

Water deprivation test. In the blood and urine test, normal values are urine osmolality >800 mOsm/L; serum osmolality 285 to 300 mOsm/L. The water deprivation test is based on the basic premise that the antidiuretic hormone is released to conserve urinary water when a patient is at risk of becoming dehydrated. This procedure purposely withholds all fluid while laboratory tests determine the body's response to the pending dehydration.

Usually, all fluids are withheld for 24 hours or until a patient has lost up to 5% of his or her body weight.[15] Normally, such a deprivation of fluids would stimulate the release of ADH to conserve urine to maintain serum osmolality. In a balanced state, the serum osmolality would remain constant while the urine osmolality increased.

Patients with reduced levels of ADH are unable to curtail fluid losses through the urine despite increases in blood osmolality. Elevated serum osmolality with a urine osmolality that is either equal to or less than the serum concentration would indicate continued loss of urinary fluid despite hemoconcentration.

The nurse must carefully evaluate the patient's response to this dehydration test to prevent serious fluid imbalances. The patient must be weighed frequently to detect the amount of fluid lost (for every 1 pound, 3 ounces decrease in weight, a quart of body fluid is lost). It is important that variables such as different scales, amount of clothing, and urine level in bladder be eliminated so that the weight recorded will be an accurate reflection of the patient's body mass. Blood pressure is taken every 1 to 2 hours to identify decreased blood volume that could indicate pending vascular collapse. Serum sodium levels are also monitored for a disproportionate rise in sodium compared with the reduced blood volume. Diabetes insipidus is suspected when reduced levels of ADH occur with increased serum osmolality and reduced urine concentration.

Water deprivation test results are usually followed up with a subcutaneous injection of aqueous Pitressin (synthetic antidiuretic hormone). This phase of testing will provide information to differentiate the type of diabetes insipidus. Serial urine samples are collected for 2 hours, and the urine volume and osmolality is measured.

The patient with normal hypophyseal functioning would respond to the exogenous ADH by reabsorbing water at the tubule and raising the urine osmolality slightly less than 5%.[13] In cases of severe central diabetes insipidus, the urine osmolality will rise over 50%. This result indicates that the cell receptor sites on the renal tubules are responsive to Pitressin. Test results in which urine osmolality remains unchanged are suspicious for nephrogenic diabetes insipidus indicating that the target tissue or cell receptor sites are no longer receptive to the ADH.

Water load test. In urine tests normal values are urine osmolality 40 to 1,600 mOsm/L range, 500 to 800 mOsm/L random specimen[20]; urine specific gravity 1.005 to 1.030 range. The water load test is based on the premise that changes in the concentration of particles in the blood stream will affect the release of ADH as the body strives to maintain a homeostatic balance. This test overhydrates the patient and then provides a series of blood and urine tests to monitor the sequence of physiological events leading to a fluid balance.

The patient is given nothing by mouth overnight. He or she is instructed not to smoke (nicotine can stimulate ADH release) and not to take medications that alter ADH levels (see Table 39-4 for additional medications). The patient is asked to drink 20 ml of water per kilogram of body weight within 15 to 30 minutes. Intravenous 5% dextrose in water is given over 8 to 10 minutes if oral fluid cannot be taken.

Serial urine samples are collected for 4 to 5 hours and tested for volume, osmolality, and specific gravity. A serum osmolality is also done at the end of the test and its result is compared with the entire volume of urine collected during the test.

This hypotonic fluid load test would decrease the urine osmolality in a healthy subject. Patients with excessive antidiuretic hormone would have decreased serum osmolality while maintaining either a constant or elevated urine concentration.

This test subjects patients with cardiac or renal dysfunctions to circulatory overload and requires frequent assessment for the signs of cardiac decompensation, such as dyspnea, chest pain, moist breath sounds, jugular vein distension, and elevated central venous pulmonary artery pressures.

Decreasing the patient's serum osmolality with overhydration has a dilutional effect on the serum sodium level resulting in a mild dilutional hyponatremia. Because of this, the patient should be carefully monitored for sodium changes, including gastrointestinal stimulation, cramps, diarrhea, apprehension, and changes in personality.

DIAGNOSTIC PROCEDURES
Pituitary

In addition to the laboratory tests, radiographic examination, computerized tomography, and magnetic resonance imaging are useful in diagnosing hypothalamic-hypophyseal disease. Although these tests may not definitively diagnose diabetes insipidus or syndrome of inappropriate antidiuretic hormone, they are useful in diagnosing the primary causes of these diseases. Cranial bone fractures that injure the hypophyseal stalk and space-occupying masses such as tumors or blood clots that interfere with pituitary circulation are examples of abnormalities identified and studied on diagnostic tests.

Radiologic examination. A basic x-ray examination of the inferior skull views the sella turcica and surrounding bone formation. Bone fractures, or tissue swelling at the base of the brain, apparent on a radiograph, suggests interference with the vascular supply and nerve impulses to the hypothalamo-pituitary system. Dysfunction may occur if the hypophysis, infundibular stalk, or the neurohypophysis is impaired.

Computerized axial tomography. Computerized tomography of the base of the skull (sella turcica) identifies pituitary tumors, blood clots, cysts, nodules, or other tissue masses.

A skull CT scan provides more definitive results than a radiograph and whenever possible is done in preference to a skull radiograph. The 40-minute procedure causes no discomfort to the patient except that it requires the patient to be perfectly still. A radiopaque sodium-iodine solution may be given intravenously to highlight the hypothalamus, infundibular stalk, and pituitary gland. This dye may cause allergic reactions in iodine-sensitive persons, and the patient must be carefully questioned before the start of the test.

Multiple x-ray beams pass through the head from specific angles while detectors record the attenuation (absorption or scattering) of the x-ray beam. The x-rays pass through the head on a various predetermined axis producing images of minute slices or layers of brain tissue. As the x-rays pass through bone, soft tissue, and body fluid, a portion of the beam is absorbed or scattered, depending on the density of the tissue. A computer then calculates the degree of attenuated x-rays over very small areas. The resulting data are then projected on a viewing screen as an image of the head.

The tomogram is interpreted by a radiologist for size and shape of the sella turcica and position of the hypothalamus, infundibular stalk, and pituitary gland. Tissue density changes are noted and a diagnostic impression is made.

Magnetic resonance imaging. Magnetic resonance imaging (MRI) enables the radiologist to visualize internal organs as well as examine the cellular characteristics of specific tissue. MRI uses a magnetic field rather than x-rays to produce images of internal structures of the body. The body part under examination is presented in cross-sectional slices as a high resolution image.

The soft fluid tissue in and immediately surrounding the brain makes the brain especially responsive to MRI scanning. Although the MRI is not a definitive diagnostic test for posterior pituitary hormonal imbalance, its use identifies anatomical disruption of the gland and the surrounding area suggestive or primary causes of DI and SIADH.

REFERENCES

1. Braunwald E and others, editors: Harrison's principles of internal medicine, ed 11, New York, 1987, McGraw-Hill Book Co.
2. Bullock B and Rosendahl P: Pathophysiology, adaptations and alterations in function, ed 2, Glenview, Illinois, 1988, Scott Foresman & Co./Little, Brown College Division.
3. Burch W: Endocrinology ed 2, Baltimore, 1988, Williams & Wilkins.
4. Butts D: Fluid and electrolyte disorders associated with diabetic ketoacidosis and hyperglycemic hyperosmolar nonketotic coma, Nurs Clin North Am 22(4):827, 1987.
5. Chanson P and others: Ultra-low doses of vasopressin in the management of diabetes insipidus, Crit Care Med 15(1):44, 1987.
6. Fischbach F: A manual of laboratory diagnostic tests, ed 3, Philadelphia, 1988, JB Lippincott Co.
7. Germon K: Fluid and electrolyte problems associated with diabetes insipidus and syndrome of inappropriate antidiuretic hormone, Nurs Clin North Am 22(4):785, 1987.
8. Grindlinger G and Boylan M: Amelioration by indomethacin of lithium-induced polyuria, Crit Care Med 15(5):538, 1987.
9. Guyton A: Textbook of medical physiology, ed 7, Philadelphia, 1986, WB Saunders Co.
10. Hadley M: Endocrinology, ed 2, Englewood Cliffs, NJ, 1988, Prentice-Hall.
11. Harris M and Hamman R, editors: Diabetes in America, Bethesda, Md, 1985, US Department of Health and Human Services, Public Health Service, National Institute of Health, National Institute of Arthritis, Diabetes and Digestive and Kidney Diseases.
12. Hemmer M and others: Urinary ADH excretion during mechanical ventilation and weaning in man, Anesthesiology 52(5):395, 1980.
13. Henry J, editor: Todd, Sanford, Davidsohn, clinical diagnosis and management by laboratory methods, ed 17, Philadelphia, 1984, WB Saunders Co.
14. Hollinshead W and Rosse C: Textbook of anatomy, ed 4, Philadelphia, 1985, Harper & Row Publishers.
15. Kohler P, editor: Clinical endocrinology, New York, 1986, John Wiley & Sons.
16. Lubin M and others, editors: Medical management of the surgical patient, Boston, 1988, Butterworths.
17. Marble A and others: Joslin's diabetes mellitus, ed 12, Philadelphia, 1985, Lea & Febiger.
18. Martin C: Endocrine physiology, New York, 1985, Oxford University Press.
19. McEvoy G, McQuarrie G, and DiPietro J, editors: Drug information '87, Bethesda, Md. 1987, American Society of Hospital Pharmacists.
20. Methany N and Snively WD: Nurse's handbook of fluid balance, ed 4, Philadelphia, 1983, JB Lippincott Co.
21. Nerozzi D, Goodwin F, and Costa E, editors: Neuropsychiatric disorders, New York, 1987, Raven Press.
22. Newman R: Bedside blood sugar determinations in the critically ill, Heart Lung 17(6):667, 1988.
23. Nikas, D: Critical aspects of head trauma, Crit Care Nurs Q 10(1):19, 1987.
24. Polak J and Bloom S: Endocrine tumours, the pathobiology of regulatory peptide-producing tumours, London, 1985, Churchill Livingstone.
25. Potgieter P: Inappropriate ADH secretion in tetanus, Crit Care Med 11(6):417, 1983.
26. Powers M: Handbook of diabetes nutritional management, Rockville, Md, 1987 Aspen Publishers, Inc.
27. Rudy E: Magnetic resonance imaging, new horizon in diagnostic technique, J Neurosurg Nurs 17(6):331, 1985.
28. Schroeder S, Krupp M, and Tierney L: Current medical diagnosis and treatment, 1988, Norwalk, Conn, 1988, Appleton & Lange.
29. Slaunwhite R: Fundamentals of endocrinology, New York, 1988, Marcel Dekker, Inc.
30. Staller A: Systemic effects of severe head trauma, Crit Care Nurs Q 10(1):58, 1987.
31. Swearingen P, Sommers M, and Miller K: Manual of critical care: applying nursing diagnosis to adult critical illness, St Louis, 1988, The CV Mosby Co.
32. Tepperman J and Tepperman H: Metabolic and endocrine physiology, ed 5, Chicago, 1987, Yearbook Medical Publishers, Inc.
33. Vokes T and Robertson G: Disorders of antidiuretic hormone, Endocrinol Metab Clin North Am 17(2):281, 1988.
34. Williams C: Lung cancer, Oxford, New York, 1984, Oxford University Press.

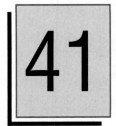

CHAPTER

41

Endocrine Disorders and Therapeutic Management

CHAPTER OBJECTIVES

■ *Define the concepts of plasma hyperosmolality and osmotic diuresis: discuss why and how osmotic diuresis occurs with plasma hyperosmolality.*

■ *Explain the pathophysiology of diabetes ketoacidosis and list at least four signs or symptoms that identify both early and late stages of this disorder.*

■ *List the priorities of nursing care for a patient with early signs or symptoms of diabetic ketoacidosis.*

■ *Identify at least three factors that compose a high risk profile for the patient with hyperglycemic hyperosmolar nonketotic coma.*

■ *List the priorities of nursing care a patient with either diabetes insipidus or syndrome of inappropriate antidiuretic hormone.*

DIABETIC KETOACIDOSIS
Description

Diabetic ketoacidosis (DKA) is a serious complication of diabetes mellitus. It poses a life-threatening situation to the type I, insulin-dependent diabetic patient, although it rarely affects the type II insulin-independent diabetic patient. Diabetic ketoacidosis is a significant community health problem with a major financial impact. Approximately 75,000 hospitalizations for DKA occur annually at a cost of over 120 million dollars. Ten percent of all deaths attributed to diabetes result from DKA.[11] It is estimated, however, that these deaths occur not from the ketoacidotic state alone, but rather from late complications (pneumonia, myocardial infarction, infection) resulting from DKA.[1] Available statistics show that the mortality rate for patients admitted with DKA is 9%, with DKA mortality for females being 50% higher than that for males. The death rate from DKA is three times higher in the nonwhite population than in the white population.[11]

Ketoacidosis may develop over several hours in a person who has had diabetes for a period of time. In an undiagnosed diabetic patient, it may take days to develop and be an abrupt signal of the onset of the disease.

Cause

Ketoacidosis results from an alteration in the insulin-glucagon levels in the body (see the box on p. 744 which lists the possible causes of DKA according to decreased insulin availability and increased presence of glucose in the bloodstream). Changes in diabetic self-management can influence this ratio, as can a decrease in insulin intake, an increase in dietary intake, or a decrease in routine exercise without adequate adjustment in insulin or diet. Lifestyle changes such as growth spurts in the adolescent require an increase in insulin intake. Surgery, infection, and trauma also require an increase in insulin utilization. Although rare, emotional stress can increase glucose levels by releasing epinephrine and/or norepinephrine, which triggers increased glucagon secretion. The person may be continuing a routine insulin dosage that is then inadequate for the rate of glucose entry into the bloodstream from gluconeogenesis and glycogenolysis prompted by the stress hormones.

Recently, diabetic ketoacidosis has been seen in patients who use the new insulin pump devices that aim to provide tighter glucose control. Improper functioning resulting in insulin leakage or pump failure[28] initially causes subtle changes in glucose levels. The patient, believing his or her glucose was aptly controlled by the pump, attributes the physical symptoms to extraneous health problems. Tending to trust the functioning of the pump, the patient delays testing serum glucose and urine ketones while DKA is progressively developing.

Pathophysiology

Insulin is the metabolic key to the transfer of glucose from the bloodstream into the cell where it can be immediately used for energy or stored to be used at a later time. Without the necessary insulin, glucose remains in the blood-

POTENTIAL CAUSES OF DIABETIC KETOACIDOSIS

DECREASED EXOGENOUS INSULIN INTAKE

Lack of knowledge, poor compliance
    Omitting dose
    Insufficient dose to meet glucose requirement
Malfunctioning insulin pump
Pharmacological drugs
    Phenytoin
    Thiazide/sulfonamide diuretics

INCREASED ENDOGENOUS GLUCOSE

Diabetes management changes
    Decreased exercise without decreasing food or in-
        creasing insulin
    Increased dietary intake
Sympathetic nervous system responses
    Stressful events
        Injury
        Surgery
        Infections
            Respiratory tract
            Urinary tract
            Pancreatitis
        Emotional trauma
Increased glucagon
Increased growth hormone
Pharmacological drugs
    Steroid therapy
    Epinephrine/norepinephrine

stream and cells are deprived of their energy source. A complex pathophysiological chain of events follows (Fig. 41-1). The release of glucagon is stimulated when insulin is reduced. Glucagon increases the amount of glucose in the bloodstream by breaking down stored glucose (glycogenolysis) and converting noncarbohydrate molecules into glucose (gluconeogenesis). Blood glucose levels for the patient in diabetic ketoacidosis typically range from 300 to 800 mg/dl blood. The hyperglycemia increases the plasma osmolality, and blood becomes hyperosmolar. Cellular dehydration occurs as the hyperosmolar extracellular fluid draws the more dilute intracellular and interstitial fluid into the vascular space in an attempt to return the plasma osmolality to normal. It is estimated that a serum glucose elevation of approximately 500 mg/dl has the osmotic pull to draw 1 L of intracellular fluid into extracellular compartments.[17]

Excessive urination and glycosuria occur as a result of the osmotic diuresis because the excess glucose cannot be reabsorbed at the renal tubule and "spills" into the urine. The unreabsorbed solute exerts its own osmotic pull in the renal tubules, and less water is returned to circulation via the collecting ducts. As a result, large volumes of water,

along with sodium, potassium, and phosphorus are excreted in the urine.

Polydipsia occurs as the decrease in the circulating blood volume stimulates the osmoreceptors in the hypothalamus and promotes the release of angiotensin II. This initiates a strong thirst sensation intended to curtail the loss of fluids and replenish the circulating blood volume. The fluid volume deficit also stimulates vasoconstriction as a means to preserve blood pressure.

Both the vasoconstriction and the extremely elevated levels of glucose impair the delivery of oxygen to the peripheral cells and impedes the removal of metabolic wastes.

As DKA progresses, gluconeogenesis continues to convert noncarbohydrate molecules into glucose; ketoacidosis occurs as a ketoacid end products accumulate in the blood and rapid, incomplete fatty acid metabolism releases highly acidic substances (acetoacetic acid and B-hydroxybutyric acid) into the bloodstream (ketonemia) and the urine (ketonuria).

The acid ketones dissociate and yield hydrogen ions (H^+) that accumulate and cause a drop in serum pH. Normally, the hydrogen ions react with bicarbonate (HCO_3) to produce carbonic acid (H_2CO_3). Carbonic acid dissociates to form water (H_2O) and carbon dioxide (CO_2), which are eliminated through the kidneys and the lungs, respectively. The patient with gluconeogenesis, however, has ketones accumulating in the bloodstream faster than can be metabolized. The bicarbonate and sodium loss through osmotic diuresis prevents the formation of sodium bicarbonate needed to buffer the increasing carbonic acid. The respiratory rate is altered in an attempt to compensate for the carbonic acid build-up. Breathing becomes deep and rapid (Kussmaul's air hunger) to blow off carbonic acid in the form of CO_2. Acetone is exhaled, giving the breath its characteristic "fruity" odor.

Gluconeogenesis stimulates mobilization of protein and protein catabolism increases. Protein is broken down and converted to glucose in the liver. Continuous, uninterrupted gluconeogenesis would leave no reserve protein available for synthesis and repair of vital body tissues.

Nitrogen accumulates as a protein is metabolized. Urea, added to the bloodstream, increases the osmotic diuresis and accentuates the dehydration. Loss of muscle mass and reduced resistance to infection occur with impaired protein utilization. The combined states of acidosis and osmotic diuresis lead to a loss of phosphorus, further compromising peripheral tissue perfusion. Hypophosphatemia impairs the oxygen function of the hemoglobin by increasing hemoglobin's affinity for oxygen and thereby reducing delivery of oxygen to the cells.[32]

Assessment and Diagnosis

Diabetic ketoacidosis is usually preceded by patient complaints of malaise, headache, polyuria (excessive urination), polydipsia (excessive thirst), and polyphagia (excessive hunger). Nausea, vomiting, extreme fatigue, dehydration, and weight loss follow. Central nervous depression with changes in the level of consciousness can quickly lead to coma.

The patient in DKA may be stuporous or unconscious, depending on the degree of fluid balance disturbance. The

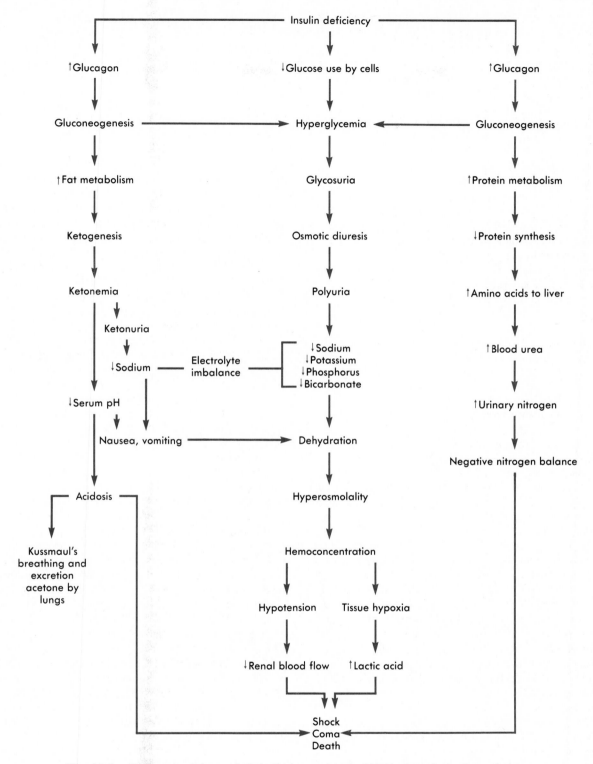

Fig. 41-1 Pathosphysiology of diabetic ketoacidosis (DKA). A carbohydrate derangement affects the metabolism of both protein and fat.

physical examination reveals evidence of dehydration including flushed dry skin, dry buccal membranes, and skin turgor greater than 3 seconds. Frequently "sunken eyeballs," resulting from the lack of fluid in the interstitium of the eyeball, are observed. Tachycardia and hypotension may signal profound fluid losses. Deep respirations (Kussmaul's breathing) become rapid and reveal a "fruity" odor of acetone. Normal or subnormal temperatures exist despite volume depletion. An increased temperature at this point may indicate the presence of infection.[1]

Considering the complexity and potential seriousness of DKA, the diagnosis is straightforward. With a known diabetic patient, a diagnosis of DKA is determined by heavy ketonuria and glycosuria in the presence of hyperglycemia and ketonemia. If the patient is not known to have diabetes, other causes of metabolic acidosis must be differentiated before a course of therapy is begun. Starvation, alcoholism, certain toxic chemicals, lactic acid, and uremia may result in a ketoacidotic state.[1] The treatment plan would vary depending on the cause.

Urine ketones and bedside fingerstick blood sugar determinations provide rapid confirmation of ketoacidosis in the diabetic patient. Laboratory evidence supporting the ketoacidosis includes low arterial blood pH and low plasma bicarbonate.[3]

Dehydration is manifested by an increased serum osmolality, elevated hematocrit, marked leukocytosis (regardless of presence of infection), increased blood urea nitrogen (BUN), and a high urine-specific gravity. Extreme catabolism is seen in severe hypertriglyceridemia, ketonemia, and ketonuria.[26]

Electrolyte imbalances result from the osmotic diuresis and fluid depletion. Vomiting and polyuria cause a decrease in serum sodium and potassium levels. Hyponatremia also occurs from the shift of extracellular sodium to intracellular spaces as the potassium is depleted.

Serum potassium levels vary depending on the phase of ketoacidosis. Potassium levels may be elevated as potassium leaves the intracellular compartment to the extracellular compartment in an exchange for hydrogen ions. Hyperkalemia is quickly reduced as potassium is lost to the body by the vomiting, diarrhea, and osmotic diuresis. Phosphorus levels may also be low, normal, or elevated despite actual serum depletion. Assessment of electrolyte levels must continue throughout the treatment phase as both potassium and phosphorus rapidly reenter the cell when fluid and insulin therapy is provided.

Treatment

Diagnosis of DKA is based on the combined presenting symptoms, patient history, medical history (type I DM), precipitating factors if known, and results of serum glucose and urine ketones. Additional information is obtained from laboratory serum electrolytes, arterial blood gases, urinalysis, and a baseline electrocardiogram. Emergency medical treatment is aimed at reversing the ketoacidosis.

Once diagnosed, diabetic ketoacidosis requires aggressive medical and nursing management to prevent progressive decompensation. Treatment is needed to:

1. Reverse dehydration

2. Restore the insulin-glucagon ratio to:
   Promote cellular use of glucose
   Reduce the counterregulatory hormone, glucagon
   Break the ketotic cycle
3. Treat and prevent circulatory collapse
4. Replenish electrolytes

The diabetic ketoacidotic patient is significantly dehydrated, may have lost 5% to 10% of body weight in fluids, and may have a fluid deficit of 3 to 5 L.[28] There is no consensus among medical practitioners on the use of isotonic or hypotonic solution as a replacement for lost fluid. Initially, normal physiological saline may be given to reverse the vascular deficit, hypotension, and extracellular fluid losses. During the first hour of severe dehydration 1L is infused. The rate, however, is varied depending on urinary output, secondary illnesses, and precipitating factors. To dilute the serum osmolality, infusions of half-strength sodium chloride may follow the initial saline replacement. Since the water deficit exceeds the sodium loss, half-strength sodium chloride can be given at a rate of 300 to 500 ml/hr until the serum osmolality returns to normal and the blood glucose levels decrease.

Once serum glucose is 250 to 300 mg/dl blood, a 5% dextrose solution is infused.[28] Intravenous glucose is necessary to replenish glucose stores, since muscle and liver glycogen reserves may have been depleted during gluconeogenesis. It is also necessary to prevent hypoglycemia, which may result from a relative drop in circulating glucose. Glucose is also given to prevent cerebral edema, which may result when free water is drawn across the blood-brain barrier into brain tissue (the exact mechanism involved in this alteration in the blood-brain barrier is not known[2]). Intravenous glucose is maintained until the patient no longer requires intravenous fluids and is taking liquids by mouth.

Insulin is given simultaneously with intravenous fluids. A reversal of the ketoacidotic metabolic abnormalities gradually occurs as the patient is hydrated and given insulin. The serum glucose level falls as large quantities of glucose are perfused through the kidneys and removed in the urine. The exogenous insulin compliments the fluid therapy and promotes the entry of glucose into the cell (insulin also permits potassium and phosphorous to reenter the cell). Insulin inhibits the release of glucagon and glucose is no longer poured into circulation as a result of gluconeogenesis and glycogenolysis. The ketoacidotic cycle is gradually broken, since ketoacids are no longer produced as a byproduct of incomplete fat metabolism. The serum osmolality is reduced with vigorous fluid replacement coupled with the reduction of glucose, urea, and ketones circulating in the bloodstream. Osmotic diuresis is reversed as the continuous fluids replace fluid losses, and serum glucose levels return to normal.

The traditional use of large doses of insulin has slowly given way to lower, continuous intravenous doses of insulin. A bolus of 0.3 U/kg may be given to saturate the insulin cell receptor sites and compete with any insulin resistance at the cell receptor site. Replacement of low-dose insulin, 0.1 U/kg/hr (approximately 6 to 10 U/Hour), is given intravenously or intramuscularly depending on circulatory perfusion until acidosis is reversed.

Hypokalemia may occur as insulin promotes K^+ return to the cell, and acidosis is reduced. Unless the initial hypokalemia is severe, potassium may not be given for 3 to 4 hours after treatment begins or until the potassium shift stabilizes. Insulin treatment also precipitates hypophosphatemia as serum phosphate returns to the cell. Although the need to administer phosphate is currently debated, its use does seem to improve tissue oxygenation and promote the renal excretion of hydrogen ions.[1]

The replacement of lost bicarbonate is also controversial. While intravenous bicarbonate promotes the rapid acidotic reversal leading to alkalinization, the sudden shift in electrolytes may cause deprivation of oxygen. Tissue hypoxia results from the reduced dissociation of oxygen from hemoglobin of cerebral spinal acidosis. It is generally agreed that bicarbonate is started for critically severe acidotic states (pH <7 and bicarbonate <5 mE/L)[17] and stopped when the pH level reaches 7.2.[28] An indwelling arterial line provides access to hourly sampling of blood gases.

Some comatose patients may require gastric intubation to decompress stomach contents and prevent vomiting and subsequent aspiration. The use of a nasogastric tube also reduces impaired ventilation resulting from abdominal distention.

In addition to vigorous medical treatment the physician investigates the precipitating causes of ketoacidosis. Unless the precipitating factors are known and resolved, DKA will probably recur. After 10 to 12 hours of effective treatment, the patient's hydration and neurological and metabolic status should drastically improve.

Nursing Care

The management of the patient with DKA demands astute assessments, critical thinking, and quick decision-making. Use of the nursing process helps to organize activities and promote reversal of symptoms. Since the nurse will simultaneously monitor several system functions, collect multiple laboratory values, and provide various interventions, an accurately maintained flow sheet is a necessity.

The patient's hydration status is severely compromised in ketoacidosis. Osmotic diuresis and increased insensible loss of fluid from Kussmaul's breathing can result in 10% loss of total body water.[1] Nausea, vomiting, and changes in level of consciousness interfere with the individual's ability to ingest or retain fluids (see the box at right).

Rapid intravenous fluid replacement requires the use of a volumetric pump when possible. Accurate intake and output must be maintained to record the body's use of fluid. Hourly output is used to measure renal functioning. Hourly urine output also provides information that serves as a preventive measure to avoid overhydration or underhydration.

Skin assessment for moisture content provides information about the body's distribution and use of fluid within body tissues. The patient in ketoacidosis has flushed dry skin, dull buccal membranes, parched lips, and ropey saliva. The lips and tongue may adhere to the teeth because of decreased fluids. The conscious patient complains of intense thirst. It may be unwise for the conscious patient to drink large quantities of water if there is a concurrent problem with abdominal distention. Quickly drinking a large volume of fluid may add to the distended abdomen and stimulate

---

HYDRATION ASSESSMENT FOR THE PATIENT IN DKA AND HHNC

HYDRATION STATUS ASSESSMENT INCLUDES:

Hourly intake
Blood pressure changes
   Orthostatic hypotension
   Pulse pressure
   Pulse rate, character, rhythm
Neck vein filling
Skin turgor
Skin moisture
Body weight
Central venous pressure
Pulmonary arterial wedge pressure
Hourly output
Complaints of thirst

---

vomiting. Ice chips may be used as an alternative to quench the patient's thirst, along with reassurance that the intravenous fluids will soon satisfy the need for fluids.

Oral care including lip balm will help keep lips supple and prevent them from cracking. Prepared sponge sticks or moist gauze pads can be used to moisten oral membranes of the unconscious patient. Swabbing the mouth moistens the tissues and displaces the bacteria that collects when saliva and its bacteriostatic action is curtailed by dehydration. The conscious patient removes bacteria and provides oral comfort with frequent tooth brushing and oral rinsing.

Vital signs, especially pulse rate, hemodynamic findings, and blood pressure, are constantly monitored to assess cardiac response to the fluid replacement. Evidence that fluid replacement is effective includes normal central venous pressure (CVP), decreased heart rate, and normal pulmonary artery pressure (PAP). Further evidence of hydration includes a change from the previously weak, thready pulse to a pulse that is strong and full, and a change from a previously low blood pressure to a gradual elevation of systolic blood pressure. Reduced respirations and lowered temperature also signal a return to adequate fluid balance.

Circulatory overload from the rapid fluid volume infusion is a serious complication that can occur in the patient with a compromised cardiovascular and/or renal system. Neck vein engorgement, dyspnea without extertion, elevated CVP and pulmonary artery pressures and moist lung sounds signal circulatory overload. Reduction in the rate and volume of infusion, elevation of head, oxygen and oronasalpharyngeal suctioning as needed may be required to assist the patient to manage the increased intravascular volume.

Urine tests for glucose, ketones, specific gravity, and blood glucose are done every 30 to 60 minutes at the bedside. Serum osmolality is monitored and blood urea nitrogen and creatinine levels are assessed for possible renal impairment related to decreased renal perfusion. Measuring hourly urine is mandatory to assess renal output and adequacy of fluid

Nursing Diagnosis and Management
Diabetic ketoacidosis

- Decreased Cardiac Output related to decreased pre-load secondary to fluid volume deficit, p. 337
- Anxiety related to threat to biological, psychological, and/or social integrity, p. 852
- Knowledge Deficit: Self-Care of Diabetes Mellitus related to lack of previous exposure to information, p. 69
- Knowledge Deficit: Self-Care of Diabetes Mellitus related to cognitive/perceptual learning limitations, p. 70
- Potential Impaired Skin Integrity risk factors: Alterations in tissue perfusion, p. 725
- Body Image Disturbance related to functional dependence on life-sustaining technology, p. 834
- Ineffective Individual Coping related to situational crisis and personal vulnerability, p. 850
- Altered Health Maintenance related to lack of perceived threat to health, p. 67
- Self-Esteem Disturbance related to feelings of guilt over physical deterioration, p. 835
- Powerlessness related to physical deterioration despite compliance, p. 838
- Hopelessness related to perceptions of failing or deteriorating physical condition, p. 839

SIGNS AND SYMPTOMS OF HYPOGLYCEMIA

Restlessness
Apprehension
Irritability
Trembling
Weakness
Diaphoresis
Pallor
Paresthesia
Headache
Hunger
Difficulty thinking
Loss of coordination
Difficulty walking
Difficulty talking
Visual disturbances
  Blurred vision
  Double vision
Tachycardia
Shallow respirations
Hypertension
Changes in level of consciousness
  Seizures
  Coma

SIGNS AND SYMPTOMS OF HYPERGLYCEMIA

Excessive thirst
Excessive urination
Hunger
Weakness
Listlessness
Mental fatigue
Flushed, dry skin
Itching
Headache
Nausea
Vomiting
Abdominal cramps
Dehydration
Wask, rapid pulse
Postural hypotension
Hypotension
Acetone breath odor
Kussmaul's deep breathing
Rapid breathing
Changes in level of consciousness
  Stupor
  Coma

replacement. Catheterizing the alert patient remains a controversy because of the risk of secondary infection.

Insulin is given intravenously to the severely dehydrated patient to ensure absorption when inadequate circulation is present. The insulin dose must be calculated to accommodate the binding that occurs causing insulin to be absorbed by the intravenous container and tubing. It is suggested that 25 U regular human insulin be added to 250 ml of 0.9% saline; 50 ml of this solution is then used to prime the tubing. The prepared solution provides maximum absorption for the container and tubing before starting the infusion.[19] As dehydration and hypotension diminish, insulin is given intramuscularly or subcutaneously. Throughout the insulin therapy, both patient response and laboratory data are assessed for changes relating to glucose levels. Respirations are frequently assessed for changes in rate, depth, and fruity "acetone" odor. When the blood glucose level falls to 250 to 300 mg/100 ml blood a 5% dextrose solution is infused to prevent hypoglycemia. Regular insulin is not stopped as the glucose level reaches a range of 250 to 300 mg, but rather may be decreased. Signs of hypoglycemia such as unexpected behavior changes, diaphoresis, tremors (refer to the box at top right), may occur from a relative drop in glucose. Should hypoglycemia occur, insulin is stopped and the physician notified.

Signs of hyperglycemia such as Kussmaul's breathing, dry skin, fruity acetone breath odor (refer to the box on p.

748), may be related to both physical and emotional stressors that the patient experiences before or during the stay in the critical care unit. Reducing these stressors and their hyperglycemic effects is a worthy challenge for the nurse.

Electrolytes fluctuate throughout the rehydration phase. Standard protocols to administer electrolytes based on laboratory criteria routinely used in the critical care unit may or may not be followed. The nurse must be aware of the obvious and obscure signs indicative of changing electrolyte levels.

Hypokalemia can occur within the first 4 hours of the rehydration-insulin treatment. Continuous cardiac monitoring is required since potassium affects the heart's electrical condition, and hyperkalemia or hypokalemia may lead to cardiac arrest. Hypokalemia is depicted on the cardiac monitor by a prolonged QT interval, a flattened or depressed T wave, and depressed ST segments (see Chapter 13, Figs. 13-3*A* and 13-3*B*). Physical signs of hypokalemia include muscle weakness, decreased gastrointestinal motility (evidenced by abdominal distention or paralytic ileus), hypotension, and a weak pulse. Respiratory arrest can occur as a result of severe hypokalemia.

Hyperkalemia occurs with acidosis or when potassium deficit is treated too aggressively in patients with renal insufficiency. Hyperkalemia is noted on a cardiac monitor by a large, peaked T wave, flattened P wave, and a broad, slurred QRS complex (see Chapter 13, Figs. 13-1*A* and 13-1*B*). Ventricular fibrillation can follow. Additional changes related to increased potassium levels include bradycardia, increased gastrointestinal motility (evidenced by nausea and diarrhea), and oliguria. Neuromuscular signs of hyperkalemia include weakness, impaired muscle activity, and flaccid paralysis.

Serum sodium levels fall as the sodium replaces the potassium that moves out of the cells. Sodium is eliminated from the body as a result of the osmotic diuresis. Additionally, the hyponatremia is compounded by the vomiting and diarrhea that occur during ketoacidosis. Signs of hyponatremia include abdominal cramping, apprehension, postural hypotension, and unexpected behavioral changes.

Sodium chloride is infused as the initial intravenous solution. Maintenance of the saline infusion is dependent on clinical manifestations of sodium imbalance plus serum laboratory values.

Skin care takes on new dimensions for the patient with diabetic ketoacidosis. Dehydration, hypovolemia, and hypophosphatemia interfere with oxygen delivery at the cell site and contribute to inadequate perfusion and tissue breakdown. Patients must be repositioned every hour to relieve capillary pressure and promote adequate perfusion to body tissues. The typical patient with type I diabetes is either normal weight or underweight. Bony prominences must be assessed during position change and circulation promoted with massage. Irritation of skin from shearing force and detergents is to be avoided. Maintenance of skin integrity prevents unwanted portals of entry for microorganisms. Lung sounds are assessed every 8 hours or as needed. Encouraging the conscious patient to cough and deep breathe every hour promotes full ventilation of the lungs and helps prevent pulmonary complications. Strict sterile technique is

used to maintain all intravenous systems. All venipuncture sites are checked every 4 hours for signs of inflammation, phlebitis, or infiltration. Strict surgical asepsis is used for all invasive procedures. Careful sterile technique is used to catheterize the patient if necessary and obtain urine samples for testing. Catheter care is given every 8 hours.

Changes in the patient's neurological status may be insidious. Alterations in level of consciousness, pupil reaction, and motor function may be the result of fluctuating glucose levels and cerebral fluid shifts. Neurological assessments performed every 4 hours or as needed coupled with serum osmolality values serve as an index of the patient's response to the rehydration therapy.

Throughout the treatment, the precipitating causes of the patient's DKA are examined and treated. If the patient is newly diagnosed as having diabetes, teaching about the disease process and self-care is provided. Comprehensive instruction for patients and families involve various health care personnel including the nurse, dietician, and physician. During the instructions, emphasis is placed on reducing the anxiety associated with the critical care unit. However, the patient must appreciate the pathophysiological process of DKA if diabetes is not properly managed.

For previously diagnosed diabetics, the knowledge level and compliance history are important in formulating a teaching plan. Learning objectives include definition of hyperglycemia, its causes, harmful effects, and symptoms. Additional objectives include a definition of ketoacidosis, its causes, symptoms, and harmful consequences. The patient and family are expected to learn the principles of diabetes management during illness. They are also expected to know the warning signs that must be brought to the attention of a health care practitioner. Education of the patient and family or other persons involved in the patient's supportive care is the goal of the teaching process.

HYPERGLYCEMIC HYPEROSMOLAR NONKETOTIC COMA
Description/Cause

Hyperglycemic hyperosmolar nonketotic coma (HHNC) is a frequently lethal complication of diabetes mellitus. The hallmarks of HHNC are extremely high levels of plasma glucose with resulting elevations in hyperosmolality and osmotic diuresis. Inability to replace fluids lost through diuresis or severe diarrhea leads to profound dehydration and changes in level of consciousness. Hyperglycemic, hyperosmolar nonketotic coma has a 40% to 50% mortality rate.[11] The severity of symptoms plus minimal or absent ketosis distinguishes HHNC from DKA (see Table 41-1).

HHNC occurs when the pancreas produces a relatively insufficient amount of insulin for the high levels of glucose that floods the bloodstream (see the box on p. 750, "Potential Causes of HHNC"). The disorder occurs mainly, although not exclusively, in elderly, obese individuals who have underlying conditions requiring medical treatment. The individual may be a patient with type II insulin-dependent diabetes who is treated with diet and hypoglycemic agents. HHNC can also occur in previously undiagnosed and therefore untreated diabetic persons.

Table 41-1 General comparison of DKA and HHNC

	DKA	HHNC
CAUSE	Insufficient exogenous insulin for glucose needs	Insufficient exogenous/endogenous insulin for glucose needs
ONSET	Sudden (hours)	Slow, insidious (days, weeks)
PREDISPOSING FACTORS	Noncompliance to type I DM, illness, surgery, ↓ activity	Elderly with recent acute illness; therapeutic procedures
MORTALITY*	8% to 10%	40 to 50%
POPULATION AFFECTED*	Type I IDDM	Type II IIDM, age >65
SIGNS AND SYMPTOMS	Similarities: dry mouth, polydipsia, polyuria, polyphagia, dehydration, dry skin, hypotension, weakness, mental confusion, tachycardia, changes in level of consciousness	
	Differences: Ketoacidosis, air hunger, acetone breath odor, rapid deep respirations, nausea, vomiting	No ketosis, no breath odor, respirations rapid and shallow, usually mild nausea and vomiting
LABORATORY TESTS		
Serum glucose	300-800 mg/dl	600-2000 mg/dl
Serum ketones	Strongly positive	Normal or mildly elevated
Serum pH	<7.3	Normal
Serum osmolality	<350 mOsm/L	>350 mOsm/L
Serum sodium	Normal or low	Normal or high
Serum potassium	Low, normal, or elevated (total body K$^+$ is depleted)	Low, normal, or high
Serum bicarbonate	<15 mEq/L	Normal
Serum phosphorus	Low, normal, or elevated (may decrease after insulin therapy)	Low, normal, or elevated (may decrease after insulin therapy)
Urine glucose†	3% to 4%	4% or highest concentration
Urine acetone	Strong	Absent or mild

*Harris M and Hamman R, editors: Diabetes in America, Bethesda, Md, 1985, US Department of Health & Human Services, pp. xii-2, xii-10, xii-15.
†Clinitest, 2 drop method.

POTENTIAL CAUSES OF HHNC

Insufficient insulin

Diabetes mellitus
Pancreatic disease
Pancreatectomy
Pharmacological
    Phenytoin
    Thiazide/sulfonamide diuretics

High-calorie enteral feedings
Pharmacological
    Glucocorticoids
    Steroids
    Sympathomimetics
    Thyroid preparations

Increased endogenous glucose

Acute stress
    Extensive burns
    Myocardial infarction
    Infection

Increased exogenous glucose

Hyperalimentation (total parenteral nutrition)
Hemodialysis
Peritoneal dialysis

The extreme hyperglycemia of HHNC can be precipitated by the stress of extensive burns, infection, or other major illness such as myocardial infarction. The syndrome may also be precipitated by iatrogenic procedures that may increase the serum glucose levels and cause an imbalance in the insulin/glucagon ratio. Such procedures include hyperalimentation, high-calorie enteral feedings, hemodialysis, and peritoneal dialysis. Prescription medications that interfere with pancreatic insulin production may precipitate HHNC and include medications such as phenytoin, thiazide diuretics, and diazoxide. Other medications implicated stimulate gluconeogenesis by increasing glucose levels through the metabolism of protein and fats. These medications include the sympathomimetics.

Pathophysiology

The syndrome of hyperglycemic, hyperosmolar nonketotic coma represents a deficit of insulin and an excess of glucagon. Fig. 41-2 schematically presents the pathophysiology. Reduced insulin levels prevent the movement of glucose into the cells, thus allowing glucose to accumulate in the plasma. Glucagon release is triggered by the decreased insulin and hepatic glucose from glycogenolysis is poured into circulation. Glucagon also stimulates the metabolism of fat and protein through gluconeogenesis in an attempt to provide cells with an energy source. Excessive glucose along with the end products of incomplete fat and protein metabolism collect as debris in the bloodstream. As the number of particles increase in the blood, hyperosmolality increases. In an effort to decrease the serum osmolality, fluid is drawn from the intracellular compartment into the vascular bed. Profound intracellular volume depletion occurs if the patient's thrist sensation is absent or decreased, if the patient is unable to respond to thirst, or if fluids are inaccessible.

Hemoconcentration persists despite removal by the kidney of large amounts of glucose through the urine (glycosuria). The glomerular filtration and elimination of glucose by the kidney tubules is not sufficient to reduce serum glucose sufficiently to maintain normal glucose levels. The hyperosmolality and reduced blood volume stimulates the release of antidiuretic hormone to increase tubular reabsorption of water. ADH, however, is powerless in overcoming the osmotic pull exerted by the glucose load. Excessive fluid volume is lost at the kidney tubule with simultaneous loss of potassium, sodium, and phosphate in the urine.

Hypovolemia reduces renal circulation and oliguria develops. Although this conserves water and preserves the blood volume it prevents further glucose loss and hyperosmolality increases.

Ketoacidosis is absent or very mild in HHNC despite the level of free fatty acids resulting from gluconeogenesis. The reasons for lack of ketoacidosis are unclear.[28] It is surmised that the patient may have either a glucagon resistance or sufficient insulin present to prevent the liver from converting fatty acids into ketones.[26]

Failure of the body to regain homeostatic balance further accelerates the life-threatening cycle brought about by hyperglycemia, hyperosmolality, osmotic diuresis, and profound dehydration. In an effort to restore homeostasis, the

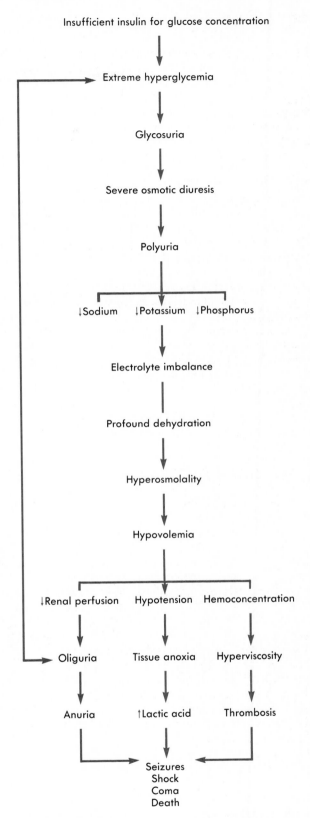

Fig. 41-2 Pathophysiology of hyperglycemic hyperosmolar nonketotic coma (HHNC).

sympathetic nervous system reacts to the body's stress response. Epinephrine, a potent stimulus for gluconeogenesis, is released and additional glucose is added to the bloodstream. Unless the glycemic diuresis cycle is broken with aggressive fluid replacement, the intracellular dehydration affects fluid and oxygen transport to the brain cells. Central nervous system dysfunctioning may result and lead to coma. Hemoconcentration increases the blood viscosity, which may result in clot formation, thromboemboli, and cerebral, cardia and pleural infarcts.[1]

Assessment and Diagnosis

HHNC has a slow, subtle onset. Initially, the symptoms may be nonspecific and may be ignored or attributed to concurrent disease processes in the patient.

History reveals polyuria, polydipsia (depending on patient's thirst sensation), and advancing weakness. Medical attention may not be obtained for these nonspecific, nonacute symptoms until the patient is unable to take sufficient fluids to offset the fluid losses. Progressive dehydration follows and leads to mental confusion, convulsions, and coma.

The physical examination may reveal an obtunded patient with a profound fluid deficit. Signs of severe dehydration include longitudinal wrinkles in the tongue, decreased salivation, and decreased central venous pressure with increases in pulse and respirations (Kussmaul's air hunger is not present).

Serum glucose is strikingly elevated, often double the levels seen in ketoacidosis (reaching 2,000 mg/dl). Serum osmolality, normally 285 to 300 mOsm/L, is greater than 350 mOsm/L, averaging 380 mOsm/L.[17] Elevated hematocrit and depleted potassium and phosphorus levels result from the osmotic diuresis. Serum electrolyte levels vary, depending on the activity and position of the electrolyte when the laboratory test is done.

Serial laboratory tests keep the clinician apprised of the fluctuating serum electrolyte levels and provide the basis for electrolyte replacement. Intracellular potassium is usually depleted as dehydration progresses. However, it quickly reenters the cells when insulin is administered. Phosphate is also carefully monitored and replaced according to insulin activity.

Kidney impairment resulting from the severe reduction in renal circulation is suggested by elevated blood urea nitrogen and creatinine. Metabolic acidosis is usually absent. When acidosis is present, it is usually mild and attributed to other factors. The mild acidosis may be a result of a starvation ketosis, a relative increase in lactic acid circulating in the reduced blood volume, or azotemia caused by impaired renal function.[1]

Treatment

Treatment is necessary to interrupt the glycemic diuresis and to prevent vascular collapse. The underlying cause of HHNC must then be sought. The same basic principles used to treat diabetic ketoacidosis are used for the patient with hyperglycemic hyperosmolar coma: rehydration, electrolyte replacement, restoration of insulin/glucagon ratio, and prevention/treatment of circulatory collapse.

Rapid rehydration is the primary intervention. The fluid deficit may be as much as 25% of the patient's total body water.[17] Current debate exists regarding whether isotonic or hypotonic solutions are more appropriate for treating the severe fluid deficit. Although an isotonic solution would expand the extracellular fluid and treat hypotension, it could compound the serum osmolality and exceed the body's requirement for sodium. A hypotonic solution would reduce the serum osmolality and provide free water for excretion, however, it could result in hypotonic expansion of the cells. The general consensus is to use physiological normal saline (0.9%) for the first 3 L[17] during the first 2 hours of treatment, especially for the patient in circulatory collapse.[1] Half-strength hypotonic saline (0.45%) can subsequently be used to reduce the serum osmolality. The patient may need replacement of 6 to 10 L of fluid in the first 10 hours.[3] Sodium input should not exceed that required to replace the losses. Careful monitoring for sodium and water balance is required to prevent hemolysis as hemoconcentration is reduced.[28] To prevent relative hypoglycemia, the hydrating solution is changed to 5% dextrose in water, in 0.9% saline or in 0.45% saline when the serum glucose levels fall to 250 to 300 mg/dl.

Vigorous fluid therapy alone can reverse hyperosmolar coma.[17] However, intravenous insulin is usually given to facilitate the cellular use of glucose and decrease the serum osmolality more rapidly.[1] Muscle, liver, and adipose cells are usually quite receptive to exogenous insulin levels in the patient with HHNC, and the insulin needs are minimal. Ten to fifteen units of regular insulin is given intravenously as a bolus. Maintenance doses of insulin to control hyperglycemia may range from 0.1 U/kg/hr intravenously until glucose falls to 250 mg[17] to a one time administration of 15 U subcutaneously.[28] Once glucose levels are at 250 mg/dl insulin treatment is usually discontinued. Aggressive treatment of the underlying causes of HHNC (severe infection, therapeutic procedures, medications) are included in the medical treatment to prevent HHNC recurrence.

Diagnostic procedures to identify and plan the treatment of HHNC are the same as those done for diabetic ketoacidosis (see Table 41-1), with differences only in the frequency performed. While arterial blood gases are not repeated as often in HHNC as they are in DKA, the serum osmolality is performed more frequently in HHNC than in ketoacidosis.

Nursing Care

Since hyperglycemic hyperosmolar coma occurs most frequently in the patient with a precipitating stressor or illness, it is not unlikely that the nurse would be the first person to recognize its development. Nursing management of the patient at risk for HHNC involves prompt recognition of changes in the patient's osmolar state. A hydration assessment is outlined in the box on p. 747. The assessment provides beginning signs and symptoms of fluid imbalance signaling dehydration from the increased number of glucose molecules in the bloodstream. Blood values for hematocrit, osmolality, glucose, sodium, and potassium are monitored. Urine values for osmolality and ketones are also followed.

A convenient formula used at the bedside to identify hyperosmolar states using known laboratory values is:

serum osmolality

$$= 2(Na^+ + K^+) + \frac{glucose\ mg/dl}{18} + \frac{BUN\ mg/dl}{2.8}$$

Changes in the patient's personality provide neurological clues to the impact of fluid imbalance on the central nervous system. When unexplained behavior changes are coupled with changing laboratory values and other signs of dehydration, hyperosmolality is to be suspected.

Once hyperglycemia, hyperosmolar nonketotic coma is identified, the nurse plans care to manage the alterations brought about by the fluid deficit, the increase in glucose, and the electrolyte imbalances. Because HHNC occurs most often in the elderly, special care of the elderly is emphasized. Throughout the critical care period, the nurse collects information necessary to identify the precipitating cause of HHNC and educates the patient and family in prevention of its recurrence. Hemodynamic monitoring, including central venous pressure, pulmonary arterial wedge pressure, and pulmonary artery pressure, evaluates the degree of dehydration and the effectiveness of the hydration therapy. Because a preexisting cardiopulmonary or renal problem may exist in the elderly patient, the hemodynamic parameters must be based on the values normal for that patient's age and current medical condition. The nurse is alerted to symptoms of fluid overload while vigorously rehydrating the older patient. Cardiac monitoring for sinus rhythm, central venous pressure, and pulmonary arterial readings continue to provide an evaluation of the patient's fluid tolerance. Symptoms of circulatory overload include elevated CVP and PAP levels, tachycardia, bounding pulse, dyspnea, tachypnea, lung crackles, and engorged neck veins. Decreasing cardiac output is signaled by hypotension and urine output less than 0.05 ml/kg/hr.

Rigorous fluid replacement and low-dose insulin administration are best controlled with electronic volumetric pump devices when possible.

Electrolyte replacement orders are based on the patient response to the treatment plan. Rapid fluctuations of serum potassium and phosphorus further compromises the patient with cardiac or renal problems. Increasing the circulating levels of insulin with therapeutic doses of intravenous insulin will promote the rapid return of potassium and phosphorus into the cell. Potassium imbalances disturb the electrocardiographic tracings (Table 41-2). Continuous cardiac monitoring provides information necessary to maintain or modify electrolyte dosages. Physical changes such as alterations

Table 41-2 Signs and symptoms of hypokalemia and hyperkalemia

Hypokalemia	Hyperkalemia
Generalized muscle weakness	Impaired muscle activity
	Weakness
Fatigue	Muscle pain/cramps
Diminished to absent reflexes	Increased GI motility
Decreased GI motility	Nausea
Anorexia	Diarrhea
Abdominal distention	Intestinal colic
Paralytic ileus	Oliguria
Vomiting	Dizziness
Hypotension	Bradycardia
Decreased stroke volume	Ventricular fibrillation
Dysrhythmias	Irritability
Weak pulse	EKG changes
Respiratory muscle weakness	Flattened P wave
Shallow respirations	Large, peaked T wave
Shortness of breath	Broad, slurred QRS
Apathy	complex
Drowsiness	
Depression	
Irritability	
Tetany	
Coma	
EKG changes	
Prolonged QT interval	
Flattened, depressed T	
wave	
Depressed ST segments	

in gastrointestinal motility and neuromuscular control also signal the effectiveness of electrolyte replacement.

Bedside serum glucose monitoring and urine tests for ketones are done every 30 to 60 minutes to determine effectiveness of treatment.

Alteration in the level of consciousness is directly related to osmotic diuresis and resulting intracellular dehydration. Neurological assessments, including level of consciousness, pupillary response, motor function, and reflexes, are done frequently to monitor the patient's response to treatment. Seizure activity may occur as a result of the hyperosmolar state, which interferes with oxygen delivery to the brain cells. Seizure precautions include nursing actions to protect the patient from injury (padded side rails, bed in low position) and provide an open airway (oral airway, head turned to side without forcibly restraining the patient, suction equipment). Oxygen is administered via nasal cannula. Anticonvulsants, with the exception of phenytoin (interferes with endogenous insulin, see Table 39-2), may be ordered. Documentation of seizures includes onset, duration, and description of seizure activity.

Interference with tissue perfusion by hypovolemia and hypophosphatemia is a serious problem for the severely compromised, dehydrated patient. Fluid replacement, range of motion, frequent positioning, and assessing skin turgor,

---

Nursing Diagnosis and Management
Hyperglycemic hyperosmotic nonketotic coma

▪ Decreased Cardiac Output related to decreased preload secondary to fluid volume deficit, p. 337
▪ Anxiety related to threat to biological, psychological, and/or social integrity, p. 852

color, temperature, and peripheral pulses are used to maintain and monitor skin integrity. Elastic support hose, elastic wraps or antiembolotic stockings may be used in an effort to prevent lower extremity venous stasis.

Combined alertness to the signs and symptoms identifying the underlying cause of the disease is needed to prevent its recurrence. Diabetic teaching plans are necessary if the hyperglycemic coma is the result of untreated diabetes.

DIABETES INSIPIDUS
Description

Diabetes insipidus (DI) occurs when there is an insufficiency or a hypofunctioning of antidiuretic hormone (ADH). Antidiuretic hormone normally stimulates the kidney tubules to reabsorb filtered water when the body needs to increase fluid stores. ADH stimulates the tubules to increase permeability to water when particles in the bloodstream increase in number (rising osmolality) or when blood pressure falls (see Table 39-4 for additional events that restrict ADH). Persons without adequately functioning antidiuretic hormone develop unrestricted serum hyperosmolality. An intense thirst and the passage of excessively large quantities of very dilute urine adds to the characteristics of the disease.

Cause

Diabetes insipidus is categorized into three types according to cause: central diabetes insipidus, nephrogenic diabetes insipidus, and psychogenic diabetes insipidus (see the box at right).

Central diabetes occurs when there is an interruption in the synthesis and release of antidiuretic hormone. It is further divided into primary and secondary categories. Primary DI occurs when structural abnormalities within the hypothalamus, infundibular stalk, and neurohypophysis prevent the release of ADH according to the body's inherent signals. Primary DI may result from an inherited familial disorder or from a neurohypophyseal system that fails to develop at birth. Primary DI may also be "idiopathic" or sporadic and occur without apparent cause.[2]

Secondary diabetes insipidus occurs as a result of trauma to the neurohypophyseal functioning unit. Surgery or irradiation to the pituitary gland, traumatic head injury, tumors (malignant and benign), and infections such as encephalitis, tuberculosis, and meningitis can potentially interfere with the structure and physiology of the unit and compromise the release of ADH.

Nephrogenic diabetes insipidus (NDI) results from the inability of the kidney nephrons to respond to circulating ADH. This may be a result of diseased kidneys and insensitive or inadequate numbers of receptors on the nephron. Drugs can promote NDI by decreasing the responsiveness of the kidney tubules to ADH. Long-term lithium carbonate use is the most common cause of NDI.[8]

Psychogenic diabetes insipidus is a rare form of the disease that occurs with compulsive water drinking. The hypophyseal stalk is functioning adequately in psychogenic DI as are the receptor sites on the kidney nephrons. The cause is believed to be similar to obsessive neurosis as the problem results from the consumption of abnormally large quantities

---

ETIOLOGY OF DIABETES INSIPIDUS

CENTRAL DIABETES INSIPIDUS
Primary

ADH deficiency from hypothalamic-hypophyseal malformation
    Congenital defect
    Idiopathic

Secondary

ADH deficiency from destruction to the hypothalamic-hypophyseal system
    Trauma
    Infection
    Surgery
    Primary neoplasms
    Metastatic malignancies
    Autoimmune response

NEPHROGENIC DIABETES INSIPIDUS

Inability of kidney tubules to respond to circulating antidiuretic hormone
    Decrease or absence of ADH receptors
    Cellular damage to nephron, especially loop of Henle
    Kidney damage, i.e., hydronephrosis, pyelonephritis, polycystic kidney
    Untoward response to drug therapy, i.e., lithium carbonate, demeclocycline

PSYCHOGENIC DIABETES INSIPIDUS

Rare form of water intoxication
    Compulsive water drinking

---

of water.[21] Long-standing psychogenic DI may closely mimic nephrogenic DI, since the kidney tubules decrease responsiveness to ADH as a result of prolonged conditioning to hypotonic urine.

Pathophysiology

ADH is the controlling force in the maintenance of fluid balance. Damage to the hypothalamus, infundibular stalk, or posterior pituitary can lead to a disruption in the normal neuroendocrine communication system, and resulting secretion of ADH (Fig. 41-3 is a diagram of the events postulated to occur with primary diabetes insipidus).

A decreased amount of circulating ADH decreases the kidney tubules' reabsorption of water and leads to excessive water excretion in the urine. As free water is lost from the bloodstream, the serum osmolality rises and elevations in serum sodium stimulate the thirst receptors. Patients who are responsive and able will drink excessive amounts of water to relieve their thirst. This reduces the serum osmolality to a more normal level and prevents dehydration. The disease is debilitating. It interrupts all activities, including sleep, since the patient experiences extreme thirst and con-

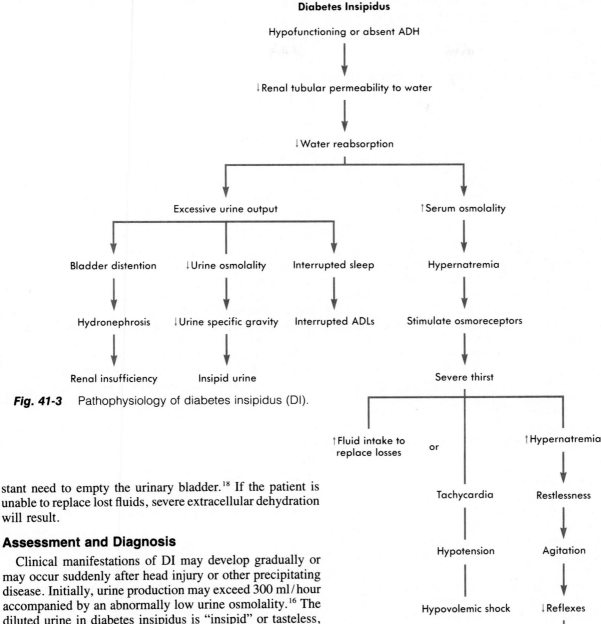

Fig. 41-3 Pathophysiology of diabetes insipidus (DI).

stant need to empty the urinary bladder.[18] If the patient is unable to replace lost fluids, severe extracellular dehydration will result.

Assessment and Diagnosis

Clinical manifestations of DI may develop gradually or may occur suddenly after head injury or other precipitating disease. Initially, urine production may exceed 300 ml/hour accompanied by an abnormally low urine osmolality.[16] The diluted urine in diabetes insipidus is "insipid" or tasteless, as opposed to the sweet honey (mellitus) taste of urine associated with diabetes mellitus. Unless the individual is able to replace the fluid loss, hypernatremia and severe dehydration will result.

Diagnostic tests used to establish the presence of DI evaluate the body's innate ability to balance fluid and electrolytes. Although these tests are early markers for the disease, most are routinely performed and not specific to the endocrine system (Table 41-3). The tests done most frequently include a comparision of serum osmolality, urine osmolality, and serum sodium. In the well-hydrated person, the homeostatic mechanism maintains a 1:3 ratio between serum and urine concentration.[13] The serum osmolality has a narrow range between 285 and 300 mOsm/kg, while urine osmolality can fluctuate between 200 and 800 mOsm with extremes ranging from 300 to 1400 mOsm/L. Severe diabetes insipidus could raise serum osmolality to 330 mOsm/

kg while urine osmolality falls well below normal.[10]

The bedside measurement of urine output identifies polyuria. Urine-specific gravity can be measured more conveniently than urine osmolality because it can be done at the bedside and does not require patient preparation. However, osmolality tests are preferred because they give a more accurate measurement of the renal tubules' reabsorption of water and resulting concentration or dilution of urine.[6]

In the patient with ineffective, absent, or decreased ADH, the urine osmolality is expected to be decreased while the serum osmolality is increased. The degree of serum osmolality is directly related to the degree of urine osmolality. Its measurement can provide data to support the diagnosis

Table 41-3 Laboratory values and intake and output for patients with diabetes insipidus and syndrome of inappropriate antidiuretic hormone

Parameter	Normal	Diabetes insipidus	Syndrome of inappropriate antidiuretic hormone
Serum ADH	1-5 pg/ml	↓ In central DI, may be normal if nephrogenic or psychogenic DI	Elevated
Serum osmolality	285-300 mOsm/L	>300 mOsm/L	<250 mOsm/L
Serum sodium	135-145 mEq/L	>145 mEq/L	<120 mEq/L
Urine osmolality	300-1400 mOsm/L	<300 mOsm/L	Increased
Urine-specific gravity	1.005-1.030	<1.005	>1.030
Urine output	1-1.5 L/24°	30-40 L/24°	Below normal
Fluid intake	1-1.5 L/24°	≥50 L/24°	Unchanged

of diabetes insipidus. For a more accurate reflection of the ADH influence on water balance, the urine sample should be collected and tested simultaneously with the blood sample.

Serum sodium levels mirror the high solute concentration within the bloodstream. Unconscious patients or patients unable to respond to the thirst mechanism accompanying polyuria are at risk of rapidly becoming dehydrated and hypovolemic if diabetes insipidus is not diagnosed and treated. For these patients a gradual rise in serum sodium level signals the fluid imbalance. Some medical clinicians suspect diabetes insipidus in the unconscious patient with hypoosmotic polyuria when the serum sodium level reaches 142 mEq/L before more serious problems with hemoconcentration develop.[5]

Further tests are useful in differentiating DI according to cause. Using a water deprivation or dehydration test, the patient is deprived of fluids for a 24-hour period. During this time, urine and plasma osmolality measurements are taken. Adequate ADH functioning would maintain the plasma osmolality within normal limits while the urine osmolality would increase as high as 800 mOsm/L. Patients with ADH deficiency minimally concentrate the urine following dehydration, while plasma osmolality rises above 300 mOsm/kg and serum sodium >145 mEq/L.

Alternate tests may include quantitative analysis of serum antidiuretic hormone. Absent or decreased levels of serum ADH in the presence of hyperosmolar serum and hypoosmolar urine would indicate primary and secondary ADH deficiency. Normal serum ADH levels (1 to 5 pg/ml or <1.5 mg/L[6]) accompanying clinical manifestations of diabetes insipidus may indicate nephrogenic diabetes insipidus (NDI) in which the kidney tubule is insensitive to ADH. Normal ADH levels with elevated blood osmolality and increased urine output may also suggest pharmacologically induced DI or excessive or compulsive water drinking. The vasopressin concentration level may be measured to differentiate the type of diabetes insipidus present. Exogenous ADH is given parenterally, after which urine and blood osmolality tests are recorded. Water retention and overhydration are risks with this test and it is contraindicated in patients with cardiac dysfunction.

Treatment

Medical intervention is based on the underlying pathology. When possible, treatment involves management of the primary diseased condition that is creating the interference in ADH circulation. Fluid replacement is provided in the initial phase of the treatment to prevent circulatory collapse. Patients who are able are given voluminous amounts of fluid orally to balance output. For those unable to take sufficient fluids orally, hypotonic intravenous solutions are rapidly infused and carefully monitored to restore the hemodynamic balance.

Medications have been used successfully to treat diabetes insipidus (Table 41-4). Patients with primary and secondary DI who are unable to snythesize ADH require exogenous vasopressin replacement therapy.

One form of the hormone available for short-term substitution is aqueous, synthetic Pitressin. It is administered intramuscularly, subcutaneously, or applied topically to the nasal mucosa. Onset of antidiuresis is rapid and lasts up to 8 hours. Chronic DI may be treated with a more potent substitute. Pitressin Tannate is a pituitary extract in oil. The drug is given intramuscularly and never intravenously. The onset of antidiuresis is slow, with the peak activity occurring after 48 hours. The effects of this drug last for several days. Both drugs will constrict smooth muscle and can elevate systemic blood pressure. Water intoxication can also occur if the dose is higher than the therapeutic level.

Another drug for patients with mild forms of DI is a synthetic analogue of vasopressin, desmopressin acetate (DDAVP). It is administered parenterally or via the nasal mucosa (not inhaled). The drug has fewer side effects than other vasopressin preparations. It has minimal effects on the smooth muscle tissue and does not cause hypertension.

Minute dosages of pituitary extract provide greater control of patient's fluid balance with minimal side effects. Recent trial studies have found that ultra low does of pituitrin (bovine posterior pituitary extract of combined oxytocin and vasopressin) have satisfactorily regulated urine output and promoted cardiovascular stability. The dosage is critically measured with a syringe pump to ensure the exact amount of the hormone for the patient's hydration status.[5]

Various drugs have been found that stimulate the pro-

Table 41-4 Medication therapy for the patient with central diabetes insipidus

Trade name	Pituitrin	Pituitrin powder	Pitressin synthetic	Pitressin tannate in Oil	DDAVP	DIAPID nasal spray
Generic name	Posterior Pituitary injection	Posterior Pituitary powder	Vasopression	Vasopressin tannate	Desmopressin acetate	Lypressin
Source	Natural hormone from animals	Natural dried pituitary	Synthetic	Synthetic	Synthetic	Synthetic
Use	Control severe DI	Relief of symptoms from DI	Replacement therapy to correct polyuria, polydipsia	Replacement therapy to correct polyuria, polydipsia	Treatment for temporary polyuria, polydipsia	Treat mild to moderate diabetes insipidus
Route	SC, preferably IM	Absorbed from nasal mucosa	IM, SC, nasally on cotton pledget, spray, or dropper	Deep IM, ONLY	SC, IV, intranasal	Intranasal spray, only
Dose and frequency	5 U to 20 U	Variable	5-10 U, 2-3 times/day, duration 2-8 hours	1.25-5 U every 1-3 days effect last 24°-96° because of slow IM absorption	Parenteral 4 mcg/ml: 0.5 ml to 1 ml/day in 2 divided doses intranasal 0.1 mg/ml = 400 IU/ml 0.1 ml to 0.4 ml/day single or divided doses	1-2 sprays (1 spray = 2 U) into both nostrils 3-4 times/day
Side effects	Increased GI activity: nausea, cramping, flatus, abdominal distention; uterine cramping; facial pallor	Irritation of nasal mucosa limits its use, dyspnea, coughing	Occur most frequently with higher doses related to water intoxication, hypovolemia, hyponatremia; constricts smooth muscle, elevates BP, nausea, vomiting, headache, skin blanching, bronchoconstriction, hypersensitivity		Generally rare, transient headache, nausea, vomiting, cramping; ↑ BP; SC: mild erythema, edema at site; nasal: irritation	Mild and infrequent nasal irritation, congestion, pruritis, rhinorrhea, increased bowel activity
Contraindications	Patient with hypertension, ASHD: CAUTIOUS USE with patients with dysrhythmias, coronary insufficiency, patients receiving barbiturates		Severe coronary artery disease, chronic nephritis, arteriosclerotic heart disease, hypertension; EXTREME CAUTION for patients in whom increased extracellular fluid would be hazardous			

SC = subcutaneous; IM = intramuscular; IV = intravenous.

Continued.

Table 41-4 Medication therapy for the patient with central diabetes insipidus—cont'd

| Nursing interventions | Frequent monitoring of vital signs to observe hemodynamic changes, i.e., ↑ BP, ↑ pulse, change in pulse characteristics, quality | Withhold the drug and notify the MD of symptoms of water intoxication, drowsiness, and confusion; accurate recording of urine output is necessary to indicate drug effectiveness | Warm drug to body temperature, vigorously shake drug to completely disperse medication or incorrect dose and effect may result; only deep gluteus or vastus lateralis, rotate site to avoid lipodystrophy; give 2 glasses of water to patient after each dose to reduce nausea, cramping, and skin blanching | SC: refrigerate drug and inject at 4° C (39.2° F); INTRANASAL: administered in thin, flexible tube; patient instructed to blow end of tube, filled with dose, into own nostril, drug to be deposited deep in nasal cavity; monitor sleep duration and intake and output to determine dose effectiveness | Effects of lypressin therapy impaired in presence of nasal congestion or allergic rhinitis since absorption may be reduced; ask patient about nocturia as dose may be increased to include nighttime dose to ensure uninterrupted sleep; instruct patient to clear nasal passages before dosage |

duction and release of endogenous vasopressin for patients who have ADH present, although in insufficient quantities. These drugs include carbamazepine, an anticonvulsive, clofibrate, a hypolipidemic, and chlorpropamide, an oral hypoglycemic agent.

Nephrogenic diabetes insipidus does not respond to hormonal replacement treatment or to administration of an anticonvulsive or hypolipidemic drug. However, chlorpropamide and tolbutamide have been found to be effective in increasing the responsiveness of the nephron site to circulating antidiuretic hormone. Recent trial studies have shown indomethacin, a nonsteroidal antiinflammatory, is therapeutic in the treatment of lithium-induced polyuria and polydipsia.[8] Certain thiazide diuretics are also used in the treatment of nephrogenic DI. It is not known why diabetes insipidus responds paradoxically to a thiazide diuretic.[18]

Nursing Care

While the basic nursing management of the patient with diabetes insipidus involves a continual, conscientious assessment of the patient's hydration status, diabetes insipidus may be complicated by the primary reason for which the patient was admitted to the critical care unit. Nursing care may then include management of several dysfunctioning systems. Nursing responsibilities for the patient with DI include the following topics (see Table 41-5 for selected outline of nursing care).

Fluid management	Medication administration
Hemodynamic status	Dose effectiveness
Skin care	Side effects
Elimination	Sleep duration
Data collection	Emotional care
Laboratory values	Education
Bedside tests	
Assessment	

Critical assessment and management of the patient's fluid status is the most important concern for the patient with DI. Intake, output measurement, condition of buccal membranes, skin turgor, daily weights, presence of thirst, and temperature form a basic assessment list that becomes paramount for the patient unable to regulate fluid needs and fluid lost. A hypotonic intravenous solution (to reduce the serum hyperosmolality) may be ordered to replace loss[31] plus 50 ml/hr to replace insensible losses.[30] Urine and blood should be simultaneously collected for osmolality studies. Bedside specific gravity analysis gives immediate information regarding variations in kidney tubules' reabsorption of water. If the patient has an indwelling Foley catheter, scrupulous asepsis is required to prevent a nosocomial infection as the closed system is repeatedly entered. Serum sodium and potassium levels are monitored and relayed to the physician as necessary.

Meticulous skin care is necessary to preserve skin integrity and prevent breakdown caused by dehydration. Alterations in elimination are frequently experienced by the patient with DI. Constipation results from fluid loss and, depending on the patient's status, is treated with dietary fiber and/or stool softeners. Diarrhea may accompany the abdominal cramping and intestinal hyperactivity associated with vasopressin drug therapy. Untoward effects are brought

---

Nursing Diagnosis and Management
Diabetes insipidus

- Fluid Volume Deficit related to decreased antidiuretic hormone secretion secondary to diabetes insipidus, p. 766.
- Potential Impaired Skin Integrity risk factor: poor subcutaneous tissue perfusion, p. 725.
- Potential Alterations in Peripheral Tissue Perfusion risk factor: vasopressor therapy (vasopressin), p. 341.
- Anxiety related to threat to biological, psychological, and/or social integrity, p. 852.
- Sensory-Perceptual Alterations related to sensory overload, sensory deprivation, and sleep pattern disturbance, p. 601.

---

to the attention of the physician for dosage modification. Antidiuretic hormone replacement is accomplished with extreme caution in the patient with a history of cardiac disease, since vasopressin tannate may cause hypertension and overhydration. At the first signs of cardiovascular impairment, the drug is discontinued and fluid intake is restricted until urine-specific gravity is less than 1.015 and polyuria resumes.

The patient who is unable to satify sensations of thirst and who is unable to complete any task or self-care activity without the need to urinate is confused and frightened. For patients who are able to verbalize their fears, having someone who is interested and nonjudgmental may help reduce the emotional turmoil. The nurse must recognize the patient's reluctance to engage in any activity because of the polyuria. Having a bedpan or commode constantly in attendance will reduce anxiety for the alert patient.

Educating the patient and the family about the disease process and how it affects thirst, urination, and fluid balance will encourage patients to participate in their care and reduce the feelings of hopelessness. Patients who are discharged with the disease are taught, along with their families, the signs and symptoms of dehydration and overhydration. They are taught to correctly weigh themselves daily and to take urine-specific gravity measurements. Printed information pertaining to drug actions, side effects, dosages, and time table is given to the patient, as well as an outline of parameters that need to be reported to the physician.

SYNDROME OF INAPPROPRIATE ANTIDIURETIC HORMONE
Description/cause

Opposite of diabetes insipidus is the syndrome of inappropriate antidiuretic hormone (SIADH). SIADH occurs when there is an increase in the release of the antidiuretic hormone. The excess antidiuretic hormone secreted in the bloodstream exceeds the amount needed to maintain blood volume and serum osmolality.

Table 41-5 Nursing care outline for the patient with diabetes insipidus

Assessment criteria	Desired outcome	Nursing intervention
HYDRATION		
Intake and output	Intake to equal output, eventual output reduced to 1-2 L/24 hr	Accurate measurement every 1-4 hr; data to be used for fluid replacement; bedpan and commode clean and accessible at all times
Specific gravity	Increase to 1.010-1.030	Bedside test every 4 hr (does not substitute for more accurate laboratory urine osmolality test)
Daily weight	Stable	Same scale, same clothes, same time daily
Skin turgor	<3 seconds	Use clavicle, forehead if decreased subcutaneous tissue caused by aging and weight loss
Buccal membranes	Shiny	
Thirst	Absent	To replace fluids orally, keep ice-cold liquids (patient's preference) accessible at bedside; to replace fluids intravenously, hypotonic solution infused to replace urinary loss plus 50 ml/hr for insensible losses[30]
Blood pressure	Within patient's normal range	
Temperature	Afebrile	
Pulse	60-100/min	
Central venous pressure	Within patient's normal range	
Pulmonary artery wedge pressure	Within patient's normal range	
SKIN		
Skin integrity	Unbroken dry skin; temperature, warm	Preventive measures include: Inspection, especially of bony prominences; palpation; reposition every 1-2 hr and inspect, lubricate skin after bathing to retain moisture; range of motion to all joints; avoid shearing force; bathe perineal area to keep clean and dry after incontinence and/or diarrhea or whenever necessary; special mattress to decrease capillary pressure; mobilize as soon as possible; hydrate according to fluid requirements
ELIMINATION		
Stool consistency, frequency	Resume routine elimination pattern	Hydrate according to fluid requirements; dietary roughage; simulate home routine if possible, i.e., cup hot liquid before toilet use; position to enhance use of abdominal muscles; discuss need for stool softeners with physician
MEDICATION	(see Table 41-4)	
SLEEP		
Sleep pattern	Optimal number of uninterrupted hours of sleep to balance activity	Collaborate with patient to establish urination schedule as needed (every 20 minutes; every 40 minutes); instill confidence in patient by prompt attention to schedule and accessibility of clean bedpan and commode; designate certain time intervals between voiding as uninterrupted time available for sleep; provide darkened, quiet environment conducive to sleep during this time

Table 41-5 Nursing care outline for the patient with diabetes insipidus—cont'd

Assessment criteria	Desired outcome	Nursing intervention
COPING		
Emotional response to illness	Patient verbalization of his or her response/reaction and feelings related to diabetes insipidus	Active listening; supportive enviroment: privacy, determine patient's present coping style, determine positive coping styles used during previous stressors, encourage continued use of appropriate coping mechanisms
EDUCATION		
Knowledge level of diabetes insipidus	Verbalization of at least four major signs and symptoms of dehydration; repetition of physical changes that need to be brought to attention of physician	Teaching strategy most productive for patient and significant other
		Refer to Table 41-4 for critical teaching information regarding use of medications
	Verbalization of long-term measures to treat DI	Obtain identification bracelet and card indicating patient has chronic diabetes insipidus

There are many causes of SIADH, many of which are seen in patients who are critically ill. Causes of SIADH are outlined in the box on p. 762. Central nervous system injury or disease interfering with the normal functioning of the hypothalamo-hypophyseal system may cause SIADH. The most common cause, however, is malignant bronchogenic oat cell carcinoma. This type of malignant cell is capable of synthesizing and releasing antidiuretic hormone. Other carcinomas capable of this autonomous production of ADH involve the pancreas, prostate, duodenum, and thymus. ADH has also been elevated in Hodgkin's disease and leukemia. Ectopic endocrine production of ADH is also identified in certain nonmalignant pulmonary conditions such as tuberculosis and pneumonia. Levels of ADH are also increased by positive pressure ventilators that decrease venous return to the thorax thus stimulating pulmonary baroreceptors to release ADH.[12]

Other causes of SIADH are neurological disorders such as tetanus,[25] meningitis, and Guillain-Barré syndrome. Anesthesia, stress, pain, and drugs such as cyclophosphamide and chlorpropamide have also been implicated.

Pathophysiology

In SIADH, antidiuretic hormone continues to be released into the blood stream despite the feedback mechanism signaling a normal serum osmolality and blood volume (see Fig. 41-4). Hypersecretion of ADH results in hyponatremia and hemodilution.

ADH release increases the kidney tubule reabsorption of water that in turn increases the circulating blood volume. Dilutional hyponatremia occurs as the expanded plasma volume dilutes the previously normal serum levels. The hyponatremia is further aggravated as aldosterone release (normally released to retain sodium at the tubules) is suppressed.[15] Serum hypoosmolality leads to a shift of fluid into the intracellular fluid compartment in an attempt to equalize osmotic pressure. Because there is minimal sodium present in this fluid, edema does not result. Without ADH

and aldosterone, water is retained, urine output is diminished, and further sodium is excreted in the urine. Patients with the syndrome of inappropriate antidiuretic hormone usually excrete a urine that is more concentrated than would be expected for the corresponding concentration of blood.

Assessment and Diagnosis

The patient with SIADH becomes water intoxicated. The clinical manifestations of this condition are related to the excess fluid in the extracellular compartment and the proportionate dilution of the circulating sodium. Although edema is not usually present, there may be slight weight gain from the expanded extracellular fluid volume.

Hyponatremia may initially be asymptomatic. Early signs and symptoms of dilutional hyponatremia include lethargy, anorexia, nausea, and vomiting. As the water and sodium imbalance progresses, neurological signs of hyponatremia predominate. Inability to concentrate, mental confusion, apprehension, and seizures may progress to loss of consciousness and death.

The medical diagnosis is based on various factors. Primary disorders (oat cell carcinoma, CNS disturbance), clinical manifestations, and laboratory tests provide data to substantiate SIADH. Laboratory values provide the clinical hallmarks of SIADH: hyponatremia, serum hypoosmolality, and a urine osmolality grater than would be expected of the hypotonic blood (see Table 41-3 for typical laboratory results for patient with SIADH). The patient with SIADH characteristically displays a serum hypoosmolality less than 250 mOsm/kg with sodium levels less than 120 mEq/L. Urine osmolality that is equal to or exceeds serum osmolality with urinary sodium greater than 20 mEq/L in a patient with normal renal, pituitary thyroid, and adrenal functions indicates the inappropriate excretion of a concentrated urine in the presence of very dilute serum.[20]

To confirm the diagnosis, a water load test is done. After a period of fasting, a dehydrated patient is overhydrated with water. The urine output and serum osmolality are care-

POTENTIAL CAUSES OF SYNDROME OF INAPPROPRIATE ANTIDIURETIC HORMONE

Malignant disease associated with autonomous production of ADH
  Bronchogenic oat cell carcinoma
  Pancreatic adenocarcinoma
  Duodenal, bladder, ureter, prostatic carcinomas
  Lymphosarcoma, Ewing's sarcoma
  Acute leukemia, Hodgkin's disease
  Cerebral neoplasm, thymoma
Central nervous system diseases that interfere with the hypothalamic-hypophyseal system and increase the production and/or release of ADH
  Head injury
  Brain abscess
  Hydrocephalus
  Pituitary adenoma
  Subdural hematoma
  Subarachnoid hemorrhage
  Cerebral atrophy
  Guillain-Barré syndrome
  Tuberculous meningitis
  Purulent meningitis
  Herpes simplex encephalitis
  Acute intermittent porphyria
Neurogenic stimuli capable of increasing ADH
  Decreased glomerular filtration rate
  Physical and/or emotional stressors
    Pain
    Fear
    Trauma
    Surgery
    MI
    Acute infection
    Hypotension
    Hemorrhage
    Hypovolemia

Pulmonary diseases believed to stimulate the baroreceptors and increase ADH
  Pulmonary tuberculosis
  Viral and bacterial pneumonia
  Empyema
  Lung abscess
  Chronic obstructive lung disease
  Status asthmaticus
  Cystic fibrosis
Endocrine disturbances that hormonally influence ADH
  Myxedema
  Hypothyroidism
  Hypopituitarism
  Adrenal insufficiency—Addison's disease
Medications that mimic, increase the release of, or potentiate ADH
  Hypoglycemics
    Insulin
    Tolbutamide
    Chlorpropamide
  Potassium-depleting thiazide diuretics
  Tricyclic antidepressants
    Imipramine
    Amitriptyline
  Phenothiazine
    Fluphenazine
    Thioridazine
  Thioxanthenes
    Thiothixene
    Chlorprothixene
  Chemotherapeutic agents
    Vincristine
    Cyclophosphamide
  Narcotics
  Carbamazepine
  Clofibrate
  Acetaminophen
  Nicotine
  Oxytocin
  Vasopressin
  Anesthetics

fully monitored to discover a decline in serum osmolality resulting from peak moments of overhydration. Patients with SIADH show a decrase in serum osmolality regardless of the fasting state and an inability to secrete dilute urine despite the hydration resulting from the water load.[6]

Treatment

In the critical care unit, SIADH often occurs as a secondary disease. Ideally, recognition and treatment of the primary disease will reduce the production of ADH. If the patient is receiving any of the chemical agents suspected of causing the disease, discontinuing the drug, if possible, may return ADH levels to normal. The medical therapy that is the most successful (along with treatment of the primary disease) is simple reduction of fluid intake[28] to less than 1000 ml/day.[34] Patients with severe hyponatremia <115 mEq/L or those with seizures are infused with 3% to 5% hypertonic saline[33] for rapid but temporary correction of the hemodilution caused by the retention of fluid at the tubules and severe sodium loss. Furosemide is added to further increase the diuresis and prevent risk of pulmonary edema related to the hypertonic saline solution. Hypertonic saline solution is administered very slowly and with extreme caution (0.1 mg/kg/min) until the patient's serum sodium level is increased to 125 mEq/L.[33] Treatment with a hypertonic solution is temporary, as the sodium is continuously re-

Syndrome of Inappropriate Antidiuretic Hormone

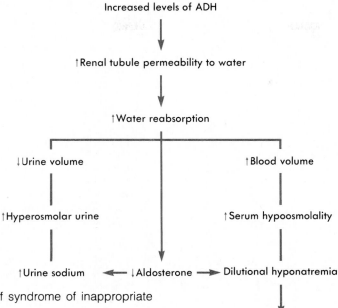

Increased levels of ADH

↓

↑Renal tubule permeability to water

↓

↑Water reabsorption

↓Urine volume　　↑Blood volume

↑Hyperosmolar urine　　↑Serum hypoosmolality

↑Urine sodium　◄──　↓Aldosterone　──►　Dilutional hyponatremia

↓

Anorexia, nausea, vomiting

↓

Irritability

↓

Confusion

↓

Disorientation

↓

Seizures

Fig. 41-4　Pathophysiology of syndrome of inappropriate antidiuretic hormone (SIADH).

moved from the body through the urine.

Narcotic agonists such as oxilorphan and butorphanol reduce the secretion of ADH in many patients with SIADH. However, the drugs do not seem to be effective in patients with SIADH caused by lung malignancies. Patients with lung malignancies are treated with demeclocycline hydrochloride, an antibacterial tetracycline, and lithium carbonate, an alkali metal salt primarily used to alter psychogenic behavior. These drugs inhibit the tubule response to ADH and decrease the water reabsorption at the tubules.[3]

Nursing Care

Thorough, astute nursing assessments are required for care of the patient with SIADH while attempting to correct the fluid and sodium imbalance: the systemic effects of hyponatremia occur rapidly and can be lethal. Evaluation of the patient's neurological status, especially level of consciousness, is done every 1 to 2 hours. Assessment of the patient's hydration status is frequently monitored with serial assessment of urine output, blood and urine sodium, urine-specific gravity, and urine and blood osmolality. Elimination patterns are assessed since constipation may occur when fluids are restricted.

Seizure precautions for the patient with SIADH are provided regardless of the degree of hyponatremia. Serum sodium levels may fluctuate rapidly, and neurological impairment may occur with no apparent warning. The patient's altered neurological response may also be influenced by the acuity of the primary disease, (that is central nervous system infection) and not solely the result of low sodium levels. Seizure precautions include nursing actions to protect the patient from injury (padded side rails, bed in low position when patient is unattended) and to provide an open airway (oral airway, head turned to side without forcibly restraining

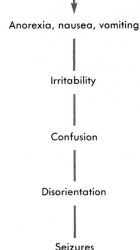

Nursing Diagnosis and Management

Syndrome of inappropriate antidiuretic hormone (SIADH)

▪ Fluid Volume Excess related to increased antidiuretic hormone secretion secondary to SIADH, p. 766

the patient, suction apparatus). Oxygen is administered as needed.

Accurate intake and output is required to calculate fluid replacement for the patient with excessive antidiuretic hormone. All fluids are restricted as ordered, providing only a sufficient intake to equal urine output. Frequent month care may provide comfort during the period of fluid restriction through moistening the buccal membrane. Weights may be taken every 12 hours to gauge fluid retention or loss. Weight gain could signify continual fluid retention, while weight loss could indicate loss of body fluid.

Hemodynamic monitoring, including blood pressure, central venous pressure, and pulmonary arterial wedge pressures, are all expected to be within the normal range for the patient. Elevations in blood pressure or CVP and PAWP could indicate cardiac overload complications from the prescribed hypertonic saline treatment.

Hypertonic saline is infused very cautiously. A volumetric pump is used to deliver 0.1 mg/kg/min[33] or set to deliver a flow rate determined by the serum sodium levels. The saline infusion is usually discontinued when the patient's serum sodium levels reach 125 mEq/L. Hypertonic expansion of the vascular space is a complication of rapid infusion of hypertonic saline that must be avoided. Hypertonic expansion occurs when the hypertonic solution is infused so rapidly that it creates an immediate hyperosmolality of the bloodstream. Fluid is drawn from the more diluted intracellular spaces to the bloodstream in an effort to equalize the concentration of particles. The isomotic conditions or equality of the compartments is not achieved as additional hypertonic solution continues to be rapidly fused. The hypertonic solution is discontinued if signs or symptoms of bounding pulse, increased thirst (to replace depleted cellular fluid), hand vein emptying longer than 5 seconds when the hand is elevated, coupled with increased serum sodium levels, occur.

Signs and symptoms of congestive heart failure and pulmonary edema such as elevated blood pressure, PAWP, CVP are also causes to discontinue the hypertonic saline infusion. Apprehension, abrupt position changes to an upright position to breathe, dyspnea, moist cough, and increased respiratory and pulse rates also indicate the inability of the cardiopulmonary system to accommodate the increased fluid load.

An alteration in bowel elimination resulting in constipation may occur from decreased fluid intake and inactivity. Cathartics or low volume hypertonic enemas may be given to stimulate peristalsis. Tap water or hypotonic enemas should *not* be given as the water in the enema solution may be absorbed through the bowel and potentiate water intoxication.

Rapidly occurring changes in the patient's neurological status may frighten visiting family members. Sensitivity to the family's unspoken fears can be shown by words of empathy and providing time for the patient and family to express their feelings. The nurse should discuss the course of the disease and its affect on water balance with the patient and family. The nurse should also explain the fluid restrictions and the family's role in treating SIADH. Teaching the patient and the family to measure the intake and output will encourage independence and instill a sense of usefulness.

REFERENCES

1. Braundwald E and others, editors: Harrison's principles of internal medicine, ed 11, New York, 1987, McGraw-Hill Book Co.
2. Bullock B and Rosendahl P: Pathophysiology, adaptations and alterations in function, ed 2, Glenview, Illinois, 1988, Scott Foresman & Company/Little, Brown College Division.
3. Burch W: Endocrinology, ed 2, Baltimore, 1988, Williams & Wilkins.
4. Butts D: Fluid and electrolyte disorders associated with diabetic ketoacidosis and hyperglycemic hyperosmolar nonketotic coma, Nurs Clin North Am 22(4):827, 1987.
5. Chanson P and others: Ultra-low doses of vasopressin in the management of diabetes insipidus, Crit Care Med 15(1):44, 1987.
6. Fischbach F: A manual of laboratory diagnostic tests, ed 3, Philadelphia, 1988, J B Lippincott Co.
7. Germon K: Fluid and electrolyte problems associated with diabetes insipidus and syndrome of inappropriate antidiuretic hormone, Nurs Clin North Am 22(4):785, 1987.
8. Grindlinger G and Boylan M: Amerlioration by indomethacin of lithium-induced polyuria, Crit Care Med 15(5):538, 1987.
9. Guyton A: Textbook of medical physiology, ed 7, Philadelphia, 1986, WB Saunders Co.
10. Hadley M: Endocrinology, ed 2, Englewood Cliffs, NJ, 1988, Prentice-Hall.
11. Harris M and Hamman R, editors: Diabetes in America, Bethesda, Md, 1985, US Department of Health and Human Services, Public Health Service, National Institutes of Health, National Institute of Arthritis, Diabetes and Digestive and Kidney Diseases.
12. Hemmer M and others: Urinary ADH excretion during mechanical ventilation and weaning in man, Anesthesiology 52(5):395, 1980.
13. Henry J, editor: Todd, Sanford, Davidsohn, clinical diagnosis and management by laboratory methods, ed 17, Philadelphia, 1984, WB Saunders Co.
14. Hollinshead W and Rosse C: Textbook of anatomy, ed 4, Philadelphia, 1985, Harper & Row, Publishers.
15. Kohler P, editor: Clinical endocrinology, New York, 1986 John Wiley & Sons.
16. Lubin M and others, editors: Medical management of the surgical patient, Boston, 1988, Butterworths.
17. Marble A and others: Joslin's diabetes mellitus, ed 12, Philadelphia, 1985, Lea & Febiger.
18. Martin C: Endocrine physiology, New York, 1985, Oxford University Press.
19. McEvoy G, McQuarrie G, and DiPietro J, editors: Drug information '87, Bethesda, Md, 1987, American Society of Hospital Pharmacists.
20. Methany N and Snively W D: Nurse's handbook of fluid balance, ed 4, Philadelphia, 1983, JB Lippincott Co.
21. Nerozzi D, Goodwin F, and Costa E, editors: Neuropsychiatric disorders, New York, 1987, Raven Press.
22. Newman R: Bedside blood sugar determinations in the critically ill, Heart Lung 17(6):667, 1988.
23. Nikas D: Critical aspects of head trauma, Crit Care Nurs Q 10(1):19, 1987.
24. Polak J and Bloom S: Endocrine tumours, the pathobiology of regulatory peptide-producing tumours, London, 1985, Churchill Livingstone.
25. Potgieter P: Inappropriate ADH secretion in tetanus, Crit Care Med 11(6):417, 1983.
26. Powers M: Handbook of diabetes nutritional management, Rockville, Md, 1987, Aspen Publishers.
27. Rudy E: Magnetic resonance imaging, new horizon in diagnostic technique, J Neurosurg Nurs 17(6):331, 1985.
28. Schroeder S, Krupp M, and Tierney L: Current medical diagnosis and treatment, 1988, Norwalk, Conn, 1988, Appleton & Lange.
29. Slaunwhite R: Fundamentals of endocrinology, New York, 1988, Marcel Dekker, Inc.
30. Staller A: Systemic effects of severe head trauma, Crit Care Nurs Q 10(1):58, 1987.
31. Swearingen P, Sommers M, and Miller K: Manual of critical care: applying nursing diagnosis to adult critical illness, St Louis, 1988, The CV Mosby Co.
32. Tepperman J and Tepperman H: Metabolic and endocrine physiology, ed 5, Chicago, 1987, Yearbook Medical Publishers, Inc.
33. Vokes T and Robertson G: Disorders of antidiuretic hormone, Endocrinol Metab Clin North Am 17(2):281, 1988.
34. Williams C: Lung cancer, Oxford, New York, 1984, Oxford University Press.

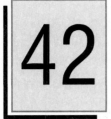

CHAPTER

42

Endocrine Care Plans

THEORETICAL BASIS AND MANAGEMENT

CHAPTER OBJECTIVES

- *Discuss the theoretical concepts related to fluid volume excess resulting from increased secretion of antidiuretic hormone (ADH).*
- *Identify and describe nursing interventions that are essential in the treatment of fluid volume excess related to increased secretion of ADH.*
- *Discuss the theoretical concepts related to fluid volume deficit resulting from decreased secretion of ADH.*
- *Discuss the nursing interventions that are essential in the treatment of fluid volume deficit resulting from decreased secretion of ADH.*

FLUID VOLUME EXCESS
Cause: Increased Secretion of Vasopressin

Antidiuretic hormone (vasopressin) is a powerful, complex polypeptide compound. When released into the circulation by the neurohypophysis (posterior pituitary gland), vasopressin has a widespread effect on the body's regulation of water and electrolyte balance.

ADH activates the receptor cells in the distal tubules and collecting ducts of the nephron. The kidney tubules respond by increasing their permeability to water and by reabsorbing water intended for urinary output. ADH also activates the receptor cells located in the smooth muscles of the arterial wall to cause constriction of the vessel lumen. Injecting large, nonphysiological doses of ADH into the body could potentially cause the blood pressure to rise.

Hyperosmolality (increased concentration of dissolved particles within the blood) and hypovolemia (diminished circulating blood volume) are two conditions that cause the body to release ADH. Hypotension is another causative factor stimulating vasopressin release. Several disease con-

ditions such as oat cell carcinoma can result in the abnormal increase in metabolism and/or release of ADH.[6]

Normally osmoreceptors in the hypothalamus and baroreceptors in the aortic arch and in the major veins signal the release of vasopressin from the posterior pituitary gland.[3] ADH is then circulated to its primary target cells in the nephron. The nephron stimulates the tubules to conserve water. The reabsorption of water dilutes the plasma and decreases serum osmolality. The quantity of urinary output is diminished, and the urine's concentration is increased.

The syndrome of inappropriate secretion of antidiuretic hormone (SIADH) suggests increased amounts of circulating ADH unrelated to physiological needs. Profound fluid and electrolyte disturbances result from the unsolicited, continuous release of the hormone into the bloodstream. Rather than providing a water balance within the body, excessive ADH stimulates the kidney tubules to retain fluid, regardless of need. Furthermore, excessive ADH alters the extracellular fluid's sodium balance, reducing the sodium concentration to critically low levels.[3]

Defining Characteristics

The reabsorbed fluid at the kidney tubule dilutes the blood and lowers the plasma osmolality. The increased fluid has a dilutional effect on the circulating sodium levels, and dilutional hyponatremia develops. The decrease in serum sodium levels is progressive throughout the course of SIADH.

The urine has an increased osmolality from the reduction in water excretion. Urinary concentration is also increased by the continuous loss of sodium into the urine. It is believed that despite the hyponatremia, the increased release of ADH promotes sodium loss through the kidneys. It is likely that the dilute serum enters the cells in an attempt to balance the intracellular serum sodium concentration. This intracellular transport suppresses the release of aldosterone, which would normally conserve the sodium ion at the renal tubule, and sodium loss in the urine continues.[2] Left un-

Fluid Volume Excess related to increased secretion of ADH

DEFINING CHARACTERISTICS

- Weight gain *without edema*
- Hyponatremia (dilutional)
- Decreased urinary output
- Urinary osmolality above normal, exceeding plasma osmolality
- Urinary specific gravity >1.030
- Evidence of water intoxication:
  - Fatigue
  - Headache
  - Abdominal cramps
  - Altered level of consciousness
  - Diarrhea
  - Seizures

OUTCOME CRITERIA

- Weight returns to baseline.
- Serum sodium is 135-145 mEq/L.
- Urinary output is >30 ml/hr.
- Urinary osmolality is 300-1400 mOsm/L.
- Urinary specific gravity is 1.005-1.030.
- Patient has no evidence of water intoxication.

NURSING INTERVENTIONS *AND RATIONALE*

1. Continue to monitor the assessment parameters listed under "Defining Characteristics." Additionally, monitor patient closely for evidence of cardiac decompensation caused by excessive preload, i.e., elevated pulmonary artery diastolic pressure (PADP) or pulmonary capillary wedge pressure (PCWP), tachycardia, lung congestion.
2. Anticipate administration of demeclocycline, lithium carbonate, furosemide, and/or narcotic agonists.
3. With physician's collaboration, administer intravenous hypertonic sodium chloride *to temporarily correct hyponatremia.*
4. Weigh patient daily at same time in same clothing, preferably with same scale.
5. Maintain fluid restriction.
6. Monitor hydration status.
7. Initiate seizure precautions, *since severe sodium deficit can result in seizures.*

---

treated, serum hyponatremia results in neurological changes that could ultimately lead to loss of consciousness and death.

FLUID VOLUME DEFICIT
Cause: Decreased Secretion of ADH

ADH is the hormone directly responsible for maintaining fluid balance within the body.[5] The body releases ADH in an effort to maintain blood tonicity and circulating blood volume. When released into the bloodstream, ADH has a twofold effect. One effect is to promote reabsorption of fluid at the distal convoluted tubule and the collecting ducts of the kidneys. The other effect is to stimulate the vascular walls to constrict.

When ADH is absent, inefficient, or secreted in insufficient amounts, the kidney tubules prevent the reabsorption of urinary substrate, and an excessive amount of water is lost to the body. This pathological condition is known as diabetes insipidus.

Defining Characteristics

Polyuria develops as the kidneys fail to reabsorb tubular fluid and to concentrate the urine. Almost pure water is excreted, and the body is depleted of the fluid necessary for hydration. Urinary osmolality and specific gravity decrease.

As excessive fluid is eliminated, the serum osmolality rises, leaving an excessive sodium concentration (hypernatremia) in the vascular space.

In a healthy body capable of balancing fluid losses, the rising serum osmolality triggers synthesis and release of ADH, which activates the kidney tubules to decrease their permeability, and water is conserved. This action would return fluid to the vascular space, thereby diluting or decreasing the osmolality. Consequently, the concentration of electrolytes, especially sodium, returns to a balanced state. In the individual with the pathological condition of decreased ADH secretion, however, this negative feedback system is interrupted, and ADH is either not released or is ineffective.

As the extracellular dehydration ensues, hypotension and hypovolemic shock can occur. The thirst mechanism is stimulated. Extreme polydipsia develops as the individual attempts to replace lost fluids.[5] The dramatic cycle of polydipsia and polyuria interferes with the individual's ability to work, eat, or sleep. Unless the lost fluids are replaced, severe hypernatremia, decreased cerebral perfusion, and dehydration disrupt the individual's neurological system. Seizures and loss of consciousness may lead to death.

Fluid Volume Deficit related to decreased secretion of ADH

DEFINING CHARACTERISTICS

- Polyuria (15 L per day)
- Serum sodium 145 mEq/L (particularly in patients who are not drinking to replace losses)
- Intense thirst
- Polydipsia (alert patients)
- Urinary specific gravity <1.005
- Urinary osmolality <300 mOsm/L
- Plasma osmolality >300 mOsm/L

OUTCOME CRITERIA

- Urinary volume, specific gravity, and osmolality are normal.
- Thirst is reduced.
- Plasma osmolality and serum sodium level are normal.

NURSING INTERVENTIONS *AND RATIONALE*

1. Continue to monitor the assessment parameters listed under "Defining Characteristics." Additionally, monitor for signs of critical volume deficits, i.e., hypotension, fall in pulmonary artery pressures, tachycardia.

2. With physician's collaboration, administer intravenous electrolyte replacement solutions, *because critical electrolyte loss occurs along with water loss.* Replace losses milliliter for milliliter plus 50 ml/hr for insensible losses. Avoid replacement of losses with intravenous dextrose solutions *because of the risk of water intoxication.*

3. If he or she is alert, allow the patient to satisfy partially his or her replacement needs by drinking according to thirst. Caution should be observed regarding the patient's excessive ingestion of water (typically, the patient will crave iced water) *because of the risk of water intoxication.*

4. With physician's collaboration, administer vasopressin intravenously, intramuscularly, or per the nasal route.

5. For patients after hypophysectomy, teach the administration of vasopressin and its reportable side and toxic effects, the monitoring of intake and output measurement, and the documentation of daily weights.

REFERENCES

1. Barton R: Diabetes insipidus and obsessional neurosis. In Nerozzi D, Goodwin F, and Costa F, editors: Neuropsychiatric disorders, New York, 1987, Raven Press.
2. Ganong W: Review of medical physiology, ed 12, Los Altos, Calif, 1985, Lange Medical Publications.
3. Guyton A: Textbook of medical physiology, ed 7, Philadelphia, 1986, WB Saunders Co.
4. Hadley M: Endocrinology, ed 2, Englewood Cliffs, NJ, 1988, Prentice-Hall, Inc.
5. Martin C: Endocrine physiology, Oxford, NY, 1985, Oxford University Press.
6. Williams C: Lung cancer, Oxford, NY, 1984, Oxford University Press.

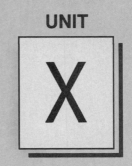

UNIT

X

MULTISYSTEM ALTERATIONS

CHAPTER

43

Burns

CHAPTER OBJECTIVES

- *Differentiate full-thickness and partial-thickness burn injuries using the recommended classification criteria.*
- *List the American Burn Association's criteria for determining burn injuries that should be referred to a regional burn center.*
- *Describe emergency management of chemical, electrical, and tar and asphalt burns.*
- *Develop nursing diagnoses and management approaches for the burn injury patient in the resuscitation, acute, and rehabilitation phases.*
- *Identify medical and nursing management approaches to burn wound closure.*
- *State common stressors in the specialty practice of burn nursing.*

The care of burn patients requires all the knowledge and skills discussed in this textbook. Burn patients have dramatic physiological alterations that are multisystem in scope, as well as psychosocial alterations that challenge the expertise of a comprehensive burn team. This *burn team* comprises nurses, physicians, psychologists, physical therapists, occupational therapists, recreational therapists, nutritionists, social workers, family, and spiritual support staff.

Approximately 2 million persons sustain burn injuries each year. Of them, approximately 100,000 are hospitalized, and 10,000 burn victims die each year.[3] Those who survive can expect to be in rehabilitation seven times longer than their stay in the hospital and they sometimes require years of psychological intervention. The purpose of this chapter is to promote an understanding of the complexities of the burn patient and motivate the creative application of the nursing process in burn care.

CAUSE AND PATHOPHYSIOLOGY OF BURNS

Burns can be thermal, chemical, electrical, or from hot tar and asphalt. The most commonly thought of burns are thermal burns caused by steam, scalds, contact, and fire injuries. Chemical burns are caused by acids such as sulfuric or nitric, alkalies such as caustic soda and anhydrous ammonia, and organic compounds. Generally, alkali burns are more serious than acid burns because alkalies penetrate deeper and burn longer. The concentration of the chemical agent and the duration of exposure are the key factors determining the extent and depth of damage.

Electrical burns can be caused by low-voltage (alternating) current or high-voltage (alternating or direct) current. Electrical burns are most often associated with industrial injuries, do-it-yourself home electricians, inappropriate use of small electrical appliances around or in water, and toddlers placing conductive material in outlets. Too frequently these incidents are fatal.

Tar and asphalt burns are serious and rather common injuries. Approximately 70% of these burns occur on the hands and the remaining 30% on other extremities.

Classification of Burn Injuries

The severity of the burn is determined by several factors, including the burn's depth, size, and location, the patient's age and medical history, and cause of the burn.

Burns are classified by their depth and size. Traditionally, the terms first-, second-, or third-degree were used to discuss burns; however, these terms are not descriptive of the burn surface. Currently, the classification of the burn (partial thickness or full thickness) is based on the surface appearance of the wound. There are two types of partial-thickness burns: superficial and deep. *Superficial partial-thickness burns* (first degree) involve only the first two or three of the five layers of the epidermis. From the surface inward the five layers are stratum corneum, stratum lucidum, stratum granulosum, stratum spinosum, and stratum basale. Superficial partial-thickness wounds appear red and moist and result in local pain. Common examples of these burn injuries are sunburns and minor steam burns experienced while

769

cooking. Generally, these wounds heal in 2 to 7 days and do not require medical intervention.

A *deep partial-thickness burn* is deeper, involving the entire epidermal layer and part of the dermis. The dermis is composed of two layers: the papillary layer next to the stratum basale and the reticular layer. The dermal layer contains the sweat and sebaceous glands, sensory motor nerves, capillaries, and hair follicles. The predominant fiber in the dermis is collagen. Mast cells in the connective tissue perform the functions of secretion, phagocytosis, and production of fibroblasts. In the burn-injured patient, the mast cells release histamine.

These burns are often the result of very severe sunburns, contact with hot liquids, or flash burns from gasoline flames. Usually more painful than deeper burns, which destroy nerve endings in the skin, a deep partial-thickness burn will appear red or mottled, and the epidermis will be blistered or broken, with subcutaneous edema and weeping. It will be sensitive to circulating air movement.

The severity of this type of injury is considered *minor* if less than 15% of the body surface is involved; *moderate* if it involves 15% to 30% of the body surface; and *critical* if the burn is complicated by respiratory tract injury and other system involvement and if it involves more than 30% of the body surface. Partial-thickness injuries can become full-thickness injuries if they become infected, if blood supply is diminished, or there is further trauma to the site.

Depending on their size and depth, these wounds spontaneously heal within 3 to 35 days as the epidermal elements germinate and migrate until the epidermal surface is restored. Left untreated and depending on the size, these wounds can heal with unstable epithelium, late hypertrophic scarring, and marked contracture formation.

Full-thickness burns (third degree) involve all the layers of the skin and the subcutaneous tissue. The subcutaneous tissue is composed of adipose tissue, includes the hair follicles and sweat glands, and is poorly vascularized. A full-thickness burn appears pale white or charred, red or brown, and leathery. At first a full-thickness burn may appear like a partial-thickness burn. The surface of the burn may be dry, and if the skin is broken, fat may be exposed. Full-thickness burns are painless and insensitive to pin pricks. The area involved may be very edematous.

The severity of this type of injury is considered minor if it involves less than 2% of body surface area (BSA); it is considered moderate if the burns involve 2% to 10% of BSA and do not involve face, hands, genitals, feet, or circumferential burns. This injury is critical if it is complicated by respiratory tract injury, fractures, or other major system involvement or if it involves the face, hands, and feet or more than 10% of the BSA.

Extremely small wounds, less than a 4-cm area, may be allowed to heal by granulation. However, more severe wounds generally need some type of graft to achieve wound closure. The primary goal of wound healing is to restore the protective mechanism of the integumentary system. Extensive full-thickness wounds leave the patient extremely susceptible to infections, fluid and electrolyte imbalances, alterations in temperature regulation, and metabolic alterations.

BURN REFERRAL

Burn injuries that are partial-thickness injuries of less than 15% of total BSA in adults or 10% in children or full-thickness burns of less than 2% can be treated in local emergency rooms or outpatient burn settings. They must be followed on an outpatient basis until the risk of infection has been eliminated and wound healing is well under way.

The following burn injuries can be treated in a community hospital that has appropriate facilities and personnel to implement complex wound healing procedures: ones that are not complicated; partial-thickness injuries of 15% to 25% total BSA in adults and 10% to 20% in children; and full-thickness injuries of less than 10%.

According to the American Burn Association (ABA), the following types of burn injuries should be referred to burn centers:

- Full-thickness burn covering more than 10% of the BSA
- Partial-thickness burn exceeding 20% of the BSA and full-thickness burn exceeding 10% of the BSA in the adult
- Burns involving the face, hands, feet, perianal or genital area, or joints
- Circumferential burns of an extremity or chest wall
- Burns involving the genitalia
- Chemical burns
- Electrical burns
- Inhalation burns
- Burns complicated with other major injuries

ESTIMATION OF BURN AREA

Several different methods can be used to estimate the size of the burn area. One method is known as the "Rule of Nines." In this method the adult body is divided into surface areas of 9%. Each of the following areas is considered to compose 9% of the body—the head, each arm, each anterior leg, and each posterior leg; the anterior surface and the posterior surface of the trunk are each considered 18%, and the perineum is counted as 1%, making a total of 100%.

In infants and very small children the head and the anterior and the posterior surfaces of the trunk are each 18%, each arm is 9%, each leg is 14%, and the perineum is 1%. This is the most commonly used method of estimating burn area sizes.

Berkow's method is also used to estimate burn size for infants and children, because it accounts for the proportionate growth. (This method requires special charts provided by the National Burn Institute, which are not always available in local hospitals but may be in a designated burn center.)

The Lund and Browder method (Fig. 43-1) is the most accepted method for determining the percentage of burn. It has been highly recommended for use with children less than 10 years of age for some time because it corrects for smaller surface areas of the lower extremities. Currently, it is also used for adult burn victims because it provides additional accuracy in adults.

Small areas of burns can be calculated using the principle that the palmar surface of the victim's hand represents 1% of the total BSA.

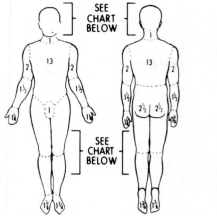

AGE:_____
SEX:_____
WEIGHT:_____
HEIGHT:_____

COLOR CODE
RED - Full
BLUE - Partial
GREEN - Available donor sites

AREA	Inf.	1-4	5-9	10-14	15	Adult	Part.	Full	Total	Donor areas
HEAD	19	17	13	11	9	7				
NECK	2	2	2	2	2	2				
ANT. TRUNK	13	13	13	13	13	13				
POST. TRUNK	13	13	13	13	13	13				
R. BUTTOCK	2½	2½	2½	2½	2½	2½				
L. BUTTOCK	2½	2½	2½	2½	2½	2½				
GENITALIA	1	1	1	1	1	1				
R.U. ARM	4	4	4	4	4	4				
L.U. ARM	4	4	4	4	4	4				
R.L. ARM	3	3	3	3	3	3				
L.L. ARM	3	3	3	3	3	3				
R. HAND	2½	2½	2½	2½	2½	2½				
L. HAND	2½	2½	2½	2½	2½	2½				
R. THIGH	5½	6½	8	8½	9	9½				
L. THIGH	5½	6½	8	8½	9	9½				
R. LEG	5	5	5½	6	6½	7				
L. LEG	5	5	5½	6	6½	7				
R. FOOT	3½	3½	3½	3½	3½	3½				
L. FOOT	3½	3½	3½	3½	3½	3½				
						TOTAL				

Fig. 43-1 Lund and Browder burn estimate diagram. (From Jacoby FG: Nursing care of the patient with burns, St Louis, 1976, The CV Mosby Co.)

Tar and Asphalt Burns

After a tar or asphalt injury, the removal of tar and asphalt is best accomplished with the use of Medisol.* This product is the most efficient in removing tar without damaging the underlying burn wound. Mineral oil, petroleum ointments, lard, margarine, or antibiotic ointments may also be used to remove tar. The tar should not be peeled off because of potential damage to the hair and skin incorporated in the tar (Fig. 43-3).

There no longer is controversy about the need for immediate or aggressive removal of tar or asphalt. No documentation exists that infection or complication is less likely with early removal of tar or asphalt. According to Hill, Achauer, and Martinez,[4] there is no real advantage to early tar removal, and nothing is gained by aggressively removing the material other than a great deal of patient discomfort. It is believed there is much better patient acceptance to delayed removal. Daily wound care, consisting of debridement of loose skin and tar, followed by application of an antibiotic-containing emollient, is preferable.

SPECIAL CONSIDERATIONS IN THE MANAGEMENT OF NONTHERMAL BURNS
Chemical Burns

In the past, irrigating acid, alkali, and organic compound burns with neutralizing solutions was recommended to limit the extent and depth of chemical burns. However, neutralizing agents may produce reactions that are exothermic, thereby increasing the extent and depth of the burn. It is also possible that the neutralizing agent is not known im-

*Orange-Sol, Inc.

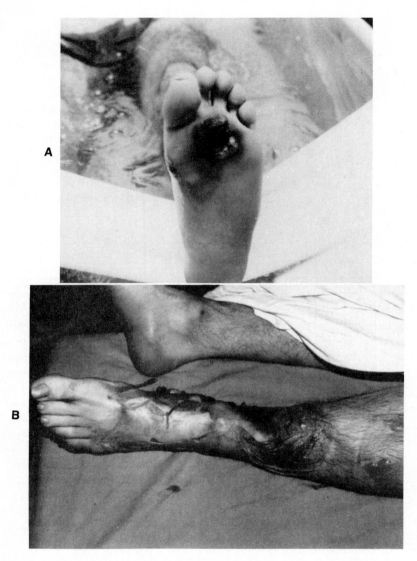

Fig. 43-2 **A,** Exit site of electrical burn on sole of foot. **B,** Same leg several days later, illustrating extension of tissue damage after the injury.

mediately or is not available. Therefore the use of large amounts of water to flush the area is recommended. Alkali burns of the eyes require continuous irrigation for many hours after the injury.

Electrical Burns

In electrical burns the type and voltage of the circuit, resistance, pathway of transmission through the body, and duration of contact should be taken into consideration in determining the amount of damage sustained. Frequently in these situations the rescuer also may become a victim because he or she may become part of the electrical circuit. The rescuer must disconnect the electrical source to break the circuit or must know how not to become part of the circuit. Using appropriate insulated equipment that diverts the circuit elsewhere is essential. Extreme caution should be used in the rescue of victims.

Electricity always travels toward the ground. It travels

most quickly through the circulatory system, then through nerves, muscles, the integumentary system, and finally bone. Electrical burns frequently are much more serious than their surface appearance. As the electrical current passes through the body, it damages the inner tissues, leaving little evidence of a burn on the skin surface (Fig. 43-2, *A* and *B*).

The electrical burn process can result in a profound alteration in acid-base balance and the production of myoglobinuria, which poses a serious threat to the renal system. Myoglobin is a normal constituent of muscle; with extensive muscle destruction it is released into the circulatory system and is filtered by the kidney. It can be very toxic and can lead to intrinsic renal failure.

The immediate management of an electrical burn includes placement of a large-bore intravenous (IV) line and a Foley catheter to monitor kidney function. In the presence of red urine, one must assume that myoglobinuria and acidosis are

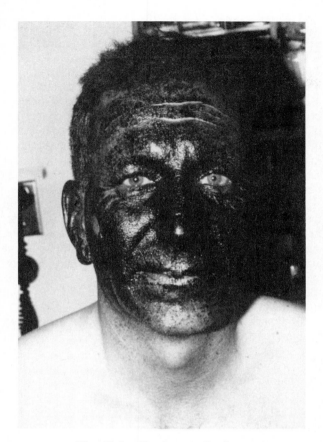

Fig. 43-3   Tar burn to the face.

admitted to an appropriate medical facility and prepared for care of the burn injury. Preadmission guidelines and extensive education may be provided by the regional burn center to the outlying emergency medical system, emergency facilities, and hospitals.

As with any major trauma victim, the first hour is crucial, but the first 24 to 36 hours are also vitally important in burn patient management. This time interval has a major impact on the survival and ultimate rehabilitation of the patient. Preadmission or prereferral of major burn patients is vital to this end. Each burn unit should have a protocol that includes immediate measures to save life and to estimate the injury and criteria for transfer to the burn center closest to the location of injury and capable of appropriate care for the injury. This protocol should be developed by the burn unit team and disseminated to local and regional emergency rooms and the emergency medical transfer systems. It is ideal if the nurses and physicians from the burn unit visit these sites to present workshops and seminars.

Arresting the burn process is vital. Clothing must be removed as quickly as possible to stop the continued burning of flammable fabric and the burning process caused from fabric and materials that smolder and melt (for example, polyester fabric) (Fig. 43-4). Quick and appropriate action can reduce the size and depth of the burn, thus reducing complications and improving the rate and length of recovery. Additionally, complete evaluation of the patient requires removal of all clothing, including jewelry and footwear.

Immediate measures to save the life of the burn patient includes management of the airway. The burn patient may present few, if any, signs of airway distress. However, ther-

present. Sodium bicarbonate may be administered (only when the acidosis has been documented) to bring the pH into normal range. IV mannitol may also be administered until the qualitative myoglobinuria has disappeared.

THE CONTINUUM OF BURN MANAGEMENT

Management of the burn patient can be divided into three phases: resuscitation, acute, and rehabilitation. Each phase is unique and has its own set of actual and potential problems.

The resuscitation phase is the period from immediately after injury to the onset of spontaneous diuresis, the hallmark that demonstrates the capillaries have regained their integrity. This period generally lasts 2 to 7 days.

The major focus of the acute phase that follows is wound healing and closure and the prevention of infection and other complications. The rehabilitation phase overlaps the acute phase and may continue for up to 2 years after the burn injury. The rehabilitation phase focuses on support for adequate wound healing and prevention of scarring and contractures.

Burn Management Before Hospitalization

The resuscitation phase begins immediately after the burn insult has occurred; therefore the nurse is concerned with how the patient is managed at the scene until he or she is

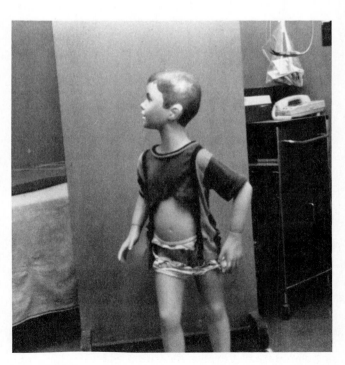

Fig. 43-4   Flammable fabric causing extension of the burn process.

mal injury to the airway should be anticipated if there are facial burns, singed eyebrows and nasal hair, carbon deposits in the oropharynx, or carbonaceous sputum or if the history suggests confinement in the burning environment. Any of these findings indicate acute inhalation injury and require immediate and definitive care. The use of immediate intubation and respiratory support should be considered before tracheal edema occurs. Performing intubation before the onset of edema may decrease the difficulty of the intubation and prevent the necessity of tracheostomy or cricothyroidotomy.

A patient with a burn involving more than 15% of the BSA will need support for the circulating blood volume. Initially, two large-bore (14-gauge) peripheral catheters or one femoral IV catheter should be inserted. Placement of central venous catheters (cephalic, juglar, or subclavian) may be necessary, but not immediately. Acceptable practice is to insert IV catheters initially through the burn wound; however, this procedure is being done less frequently. If possible, it is best to establish lines outside the burn injury area.

A burn patient with a total BSA involvement of 70% might require 18 L or more of fluid in the first 24 hours. Generally, it is easier to establish the IV lines and begin administering the required fluids during the first hour after injury before the interstitial fluid shifts occur.

Use of narcotics, analgesics, and sedatives should be carefully considered before their administration. The severely burned individual with full-thickness burns may be experiencing more anxiety than actual pain. Use of IV diazepam (Valium) may be considered to reduce anxiety; however the respiratory depression produced is not reversed by naloxone (Narcan). Morphine titrated intravenously is probably the better choice for decreasing discomfort and anxiety. It is important to remember that the severely burned patient's absorption from muscular tissue is impaired. Therefore narcotics, analgesics, and sedatives should be administered only by the IV route.

Obtaining a history of the nature of the injury is extremely valuable in managing the burn patient. Water heat, propane gas, grain elevator, and other types of explosions frequently throw the patient some distance and may result in internal injuries and fractures. It is valuable to know the specific chemicals involved if the burns are chemical in nature. It also helps to know what was burned and inhaled and how long the patient was exposed to super-heated air.

The history should include the typical survey of allergies, illnesses (including diabetes, hypertension, and cardiac or renal disease), current drug therapy, and drug or alcohol abuse. The status of tetanus immunization should be ascertained. Unless a booster immunization has been given with the last 5 years, the patient should receive 0.5 ml tetanus toxoid subcutaneously. The unimmunized patient should receive 250 units of human immunoglobin intramuscularly.[3,13]

Wound care before the transfer to the burn unit is limited. Partial-thickness burns result in pain when air passes over the burn surface. Covering the patient with clean linen will relieve some of the pain by dissipating the air current and will minimize external contamination of the wounds. Blis-

ters should not be broken, and antiseptic preparation should not be applied to the burn surface because its removal, which is necessary before the application of antibacterial agents, would cause the patient considerable discomfort.

Application of or immersion in iced water should not be used for any burn. Cold packs or ice should never be used because of possible further tissue damage and conversion of the thermal injury to a frost bite injury. The application of ice or cold packs may intensify shock, possibly resulting in ventricular fibrillation. Cool water may be applied to the face for comfort but should be avoided on the hands or feet because of the potential for altering microcirculation.

The personnel involved in transporting the patient from the site of injury to the hospital must be able to provide, maintain, and manage an airway; establish baseline vital signs; stop the burning process by removing all burning or smoldering clothing; avoid contamination of the wounds by using clean linen; establish an IV line and administer the required fluids; and deliver oxygen because of the potential for carbon monoxide poisoning.

If the burn victim must be transported from the primary hospital to a burn center, several considerations are necessary. The responsibility of the transfer is with the accepting physician. The physician must consider the amount of time required for transfer, which will in turn influence other decisions (for example, the need to intubate, the amount of fluid to transport, the oxygen delivery system needed, and the extent of supplies to carry.

Maintenance of the core temperature can be a problem with long transport times. Hypothermia can be managed with layers of dressing and blankets, but the transportation team must be aware of this possibility if the cabin is air-conditioned or the environmental temperature is low. An organized, adequately planned, well-instituted plan for primary and secondary transportation minimizes the complication and morbidity that can occur and ensures the potential for an optimal outcome.[3]

Comprehensive Burn Management

Oxygenation alterations. Forty to fifty years ago, burn shock accounted for most burn deaths, followed in more recent years by burn wound sepsis. Currently, inhalation injuries have emerged as the most frequent cause of death in burn patients. Three separate oxygenation complications are associated with smoke inhalation during the resuscitation phase: *carbon monoxide poisoning, upper airway obstruction,* and *chemical pneumonitis.* Early diagnosis of inhalation injuries is vital to minimize complications and improve the mortality rate.

When assessing a patient for inhalation injury, the following items should be included: physical assessment, arterial blood gas analysis, carboxyhemoglobin levels, chest radiography, flexible fiberoptic bronchoscopy, xenon-133 lung scan, and pulmonary function tests.[2]

Impaired gas exchange. The most common burn complication is carbon monoxide poisoning. Inhalation of carbon monoxide, a by-product of the incomplete combustion of carbon, results in its bonding to available hemoglobin, producing carboxyhemoglobin (HbCO), which effectively decreases oxygen saturation of hemoglobin. Carbon monoxide has an affinity for hemoglobin 220 times that of oxygen.

Symptoms associated with carbon monoxide poisoning include headache, dizziness, nausea, vomiting, dyspnea, and confusion. In severe cases carbon monoxide poisoning may lead to myocardial ischemia and central nervous system complications caused by lowered oxygen tension and the already compromised circulatory system. The shortage of oxygen at the tissue level is worsened by a leftward shift of the oxyhemoglobin dissociation curve, reflecting a heightened affinity of carbon monoxide for the hemoglobin molecule. Early signs of carbon monoxide poisoning may include cherry-red skin and membranes, tachycardia, tachypnea, confusion, and light-headedness. As the level of carbon monoxide rises, the patient will demonstrate a decreased level of responsiveness, which may progress to unconsciousness and respiratory failure.

The treatment of choice is high-flow oxygen administered at 100% through a face mask with a rebreathing mask or through an endotracheal intubation. The half-life of carbon monoxide in the body is 4 hours on room air (21% oxygen), 2 hours on 40% oxygen, and 60 to 80 minutes on 100% oxygen. The half-life of carbon monoxide is 30 minutes in a hyperbaric oxygen chamber at three times atmospheric pressure. Currently, the use of hyperbaric oxygen is not recommended for the majority of burn patients.

Chemical pneumonitis is caused by inhalation of the by-products of combustion such as substances present in burning cotton, aldehydes, oxides of sulphur, and nitrogen. Burning polyvinylchloride yields at least 75 potentially toxic compounds, including hydrochloric acid and carbon monoxide. Within 2 to 3 days after a burn, patients with chemical pneumonitis frequently develop adult respiratory distress syndrome (ARDS), with the chief manifestation hypoxemia refractory to oxygen therapy. Early signs include increased pH, decreased partial pressure of carbon dioxide (Pco_2), and increased respiratory rate. Ventilatory support with the use of positive end-expiratory pressure (PEEP) is the treatment of choice. See Chapter 20 for a discussion of ARDS.

Ineffective airway clearance. Laryngeal swelling and upper airway obstruction generally occur 4 to 6 hours after the burn injury. Endotracheal intubation should be accomplished early, because this simple procedure can become extremely difficult in the presence of laryngeal edema. However, there is generally time to intervene after obtaining the patient's history and transporting the patient to the primary hospital. Edema may continue to develop for 72 hours after the burn incident. An oral airway may adequately maintain airway patency. If the patient is not initially intubated, he or she should be carefully assessed during this critical period.

Predicting an upper airway obstruction is based on consideration of the following variables: extent of injury to the face and neck, the presence of blisters on or redness of the posterior pharynx, signs of burned nasal hair, increased carboxyhemoglobin levels, increased rate and decreased depth of breathing, hoarseness (which indicates a significant decrease in the diameter of the airway), increased amount of sputum, and the circumstances of the burn event (that is, whether it occurred in a closed space and/or if it involved

superheated gases [steam]). Only steam has a heat-carrying capacity many times that of dry air and is capable of overwhelming the extremely efficient heat-dissipating capabilities of the upper airway.

Extubation of these patients should occur only if they can meet extubation criteria: awake level of conciousness, intact cough and gag reflexes, inspiratory effort greater than -25; vital capacity of 10 cc/kg; and decreased volume and tenacity of the sputum.[2]

Laryngeal spasm is another complication that, although not frequently seen, should be addressed. It is generally brought on by airway irritation secondary to inhalation of noxious agents.

Ineffective breathing pattern. Circumferential full-thickness burns to the chest wall can lead to restriction of chest wall expansion and decreased compliance. Decreased compliance requires higher ventilatory pressures to oxygenate the patient. In the nonintubated patient, the signs and symptoms may include rapid, shallow respirations; poor chest wall excursion; and severe agitation.

Escharotomies should immediately be performed to increase compliance, leading to improved ventilation. Eschartomies are incisions made to relax the pressure and tension of the edema that is being exerted against the venous and arterial systems and, in this case, the chest wall. Only the dead eschar is incised. These incisions are generally made down the lateral sides of the chest. The wound spreads spontaneously as the edema continues to form. Electrocautery or a scalpel can be used to perform the escharotomies.

Fluid volume deficit.* Burn injuries result in the loss of fluid and electrolytes, leading to hypovolemic shock, commonly referred to as "burn shock" in this population of patients. The burn injury causes damage to the capillary bed and other tissue, increasing the capillary permeability. As capillary permeability increases, the capillaries leak fluid into the interstitial spaces. This rapid shift of plasma from the vascular compartment into the interstitial area and/or to the surface of the burn is the primary cause of hypovolemia in the burn patient. If the water vapor barrier, the stratum corneum, has been extensively damaged, a great deal of fluid can be vaporized from the burn surface.

Tissue damage after the burn insult is complicated by the physiological effects of the burn. Coagulation factors are affected, protein is denatured, and cellular content is ionized. These factors, coupled with the dilation of capillaries and small vessels, lead to increased capillary permeability and fluid shifts. The lymphatic system, which would normally carry away the increased interstitial fluid, may be damaged or be overloaded and unable to function to its normal capacity.

In addition to the protein and electrolyte shift, there is an increased insensible water loss. In the healthy adult this loss is estimated at 35 to 50 ml per hour. The burn patient's insensible loss may be as much as 300 to 3,000 ml. This increase may be related to temperature elevation, tracheostomy, and the size of the burn.

---

*See also "Fluid Volume Deficit related to active plasma loss and fluid shift into interstitium secondary to burns," p. 669.

Table 43-1 Formulas for fluid replacement resuscitation

Formulas	First 24 hours			Second 24 hours		
	Electrolyte	Colloid	Glucose in water	Electrolyte	Colloid	Glucose in water
ABA Consensus	Lactated Ringer's solution, 2-4 ml/kg/% BSA to maintain urinary output at 30-50 ml/hour					
Brooke	Lactated Ringer's solution, 1.5 ml/kg/% burn	0.5 ml/kg/% burn	2000 ml	One half to three quarters of first 24-hour requirement	One half to three quarters of first 24-hour requirement 20%-60% of calculated plasma volume	2000 ml
Parkland	Lactated Ringer's solution, 4 ml/kg/% burn					
Hypertonic sodium solution	Volume to maintain urinary output at 30 ml/hour (fluid contains 250 mEq sodium/L)			One third of salt solution orally, up to 3500 ml limit		

Modified from Hudak C, Gallo B, and Lohr T: Critical care nursing: a holistic approach, ed 4, Philadelphia, 1986, JB Lippincott Co.

Burn shock is proportional to the extent and depth of injury. The loss of plasma begins almost immediately after the injury and reaches its peak within the first 48 hours. Fluid volume deficit must be addressed during the first 24 to 36 hours of the resuscitation phase.

Several formulas are used to guide fluid resuscitation, each with its advantages and disadvantages (Table 43-1). They differ primarily in terms of administration, volume, and sodium content. The Consensus Formula of the ABA is lactated Ringer's solution at 2 to 4 ml/kg body weight/%BSA burned. The first half is given during the first 8 hours after the burn and the second half during the next 16 hours. The goal is to maintain a urinary output of 30 to 50 ml/hour. Ringer's lactate is the crystalloid solution of choice because of its physiological similarity to the composition of extracellular fluid. In addition, it is an excellent volume expander because of its large molecules. Whichever fluid resuscitation formula is used, it is only a guideline. The actual amount of fluid given to any patient should be based on that individual's response.

Desired clinical responses to fluid resuscitation include a urinary output of 30 to 50 ml/hour, pulse rate below 120, blood pressure in normal to high ranges, central venous pressure less than 12 cm H_2O or a pulmonary capillary wedge pressure below 18 torr, clear lung sounds, clear sensorium, and the absence of intestinal events such as nausea and paralytic ileus. Heart rate, blood pressure, and central venous pressure values are not always accurate or reliable predictors of successful fluid resuscitation.

Potassium and sodium are the two electrolytes of concern during the resuscitation period, and they should be carefully monitored until the wounds are healed. *Hyperkalemia* can occur during the resuscitation phase because of the release of potassium from damaged cells, metabolic acidosis, and/or impaired renal function secondary to hemoglobinuria, myoglobinuria, or decreased renal perfusion and the patient should be assessed for its signs and symptoms. Treatment should include correction of acidosis. However, during the resuscitation phase it is not recommended to use cation-exchange resins or IV insulin and hypertonic dextrose to transport potassium back into the cell.

Hypokalemia can also occur during the resuscitation phase because of the massive loss of fluids and electrolytes through the burn wounds or because of hemodilution. During the acute phase it may be related to hemodilution, inadequate replacement, loss associated with diuresis, diarrhea, vomiting, nasogastric drainage, long hydrotherapy sessions, and/or the shift of potassium from the intravascular space to the cell after the acidosis has been corrected. Nursing interventions include treating nausea and vomiting, limiting hydrotherapy sessions, preventing fluid volume excess, and monitoring potassium replacement.

Hyponatremia is not uncommon during the resuscitation phase because of the loss of sodium through the burn wound, the shift into interstitial space, vomiting, nasogastric drainage, diarrhea, and/or the use of hypotonic salt solutions during the early phase of resuscitation. During this phase it may be necessary to monitor the serum sodium every 2 to 4 hours. Hyponatremia may also occur during the acute phase because of hemodilution, loss through the wound, lengthy hydrotherapy sessions, and excessive diuresis resulting from the fluid shift back into the intravascular space. Interventions should be followed for treating nausea and vomiting, hydrotherapy sessions should be limited, and consideration should be given to the replacement of sodium intravenously. During diuresis, which occurs during the acute phase, restricting free water intake is usually the only required intervention to increase the serum sodium.

Potential for infection.* Preventing infection in the burn patient is a true challenge and involves complex decision making. There are pros and cons to both invasive and non-invasive physiological monitoring. Monitoring of a major burn victim is multisystem and complex in nature.

Invasive monitoring. Before deciding to use invasive techniques, careful consideration should be given to the potential risk factors and to how the data collected will actually influence the course of treatment. Invasive monitoring should certainly be considered if treatment seems ineffective or if there are complicating factors such as severe respiratory involvement, major life-threatening injuries, head injuries, pneumothorax, or preexisting medical conditions such as chronic obstructive pulmonary disease (COPD), congestive heart failure, and renal failure.[12]

During the past 10 years invasive cardiovascular monitoring has become commonplace. This procedure includes direct measurement of central venous pressure, pulmonary artery pressure, arterial pressure, core temperature, cardiac output, systemic vascular resistance, and pulmonary vascular resistance.

The use of *arterial lines* is considered if knowing serial and frequent arterial blood gas values is required for respiratory management or if vasoactive drugs are being titrated. *Central venous catheters* are often required for fluid resuscitation in the early stages to deliver the massive amount of fluids required. The physician placing these catheters should consider where the burns are located and the purpose of the catheter. It is preferable not to insert these catheters through burns. It may be appropriate to use a multilumen catheter that can be used for fluid resuscitation and maintanence, antibiotic therapy, and vasoactive drugs. The risks involved include the increased chance of infection, potential for pneumothorax, and difficulty with the procedure if the patient is hypovolemic.

Pulmonary artery catheters should be placed only when necessary for optimal care. They may be absolutely essential to the survival of the septic patient despite the risks involved. Pulmonary artery catheters can provide data about pulmonary artery wedge pressure, cardiac output, systemic and pulmonary vascular resistance, core temperature, and oxygen saturation, all of which are discussed at length in other chapters.

These catheters require meticulous care. Strict guidelines should be established and monitored. It is highly recommended that these catheters be changed over a guidewire every 3 days and the site rotated every 6 days. All catheters should be inserted under sterile conditions, and the dressings should be changed under the same conditions.

Laboratory assessment. Laboratory assessment is another important aspect of burn care. Because of the invasive nature of drawing blood, it should be done only if absolutely indicated. Consideration should be given to the age of the patient, the size of the burn, the time since injury, and any underlying disease process.

---

*See also "Potential for Infection risk factors: invasive monitoring devices, p. 346, and "Universal Precautions," Appendix E.

White blood cell (WBC) counts are usually followed as a sign of sepsis. However, it is not unusual for the WBC count to fall below 5000/mm^3 within the 48 hours after injury. It may drop even lower—1500 to 2000 mm^3—with the use of silver sulfadiazine. If the WBC count stays in this range for more than 12 hours, the use of a different topical agent is recommended. The WBC count will generally become normal again. At this point the use of silver sulfadiazine can be tested again by applying it to a small area. If the WBC count does not drop again within 12 hours, its use can be continued. In practice discontinuation of silver sulfadiazine is not common but should be considered if the WBC count continues to fall.[11]

Infection control practices. There has been considerable discussion in recent years about the type of isolation precautions to use with burn patients. Studies[5,7] suggest that handwashing and the use of gowns, gloves, and masks alone are effective in controlling contamination and infection in the adult patient with burns. Significant contributors to infection are autocontamination from exogenous sources. Cross-contamination by direct contact is the most significant source of infection and subsequent cause of sepsis.[11]

Handwashing cannot be overemphasized. Hands should be washed and gloves changed when moving from area to area on the same patient. For example, after changing the chest dressing, which may be contaminated with sputum from the tracheostomy, hands should be washed and gloves changed before moving to the legs. Gowns, gloves, and masks should be changed and hands washed before caring for a different patient.

Whichever precautions are used, it is vital that everyone coming in contact with the patient (including the family and visitors) be knowledgable about the standard for infection control and that it be strictly followed by all. Precautions should have sound rationale and must not increase the work load or the frustration of the burn team. Otherwise, compliance and consistent application of the standard will not occur, increasing the risk of infection and sepsis for the burn patient.

Altered renal tissue perfusion. Urinalysis to determine the myoglobin level should be performed early in burn care. Myoglobinuria can be detected grossly by a dark, port wine color of the urine. Myoglobin is extremely toxic to the kidneys and can cause massive tubular destruction. It is best treated with rapid fluid administration and forced diuresis with mannitol, an osmotic diuretic. The goal is an hourly urinary output that is at least double the general recommendations to flush the tubules. All other diuretics should be avoided because they will deplete the already compromised intravascular volume.

Maintaining and monitoring the renal system is vital in burn patient management. Impairment of the renal system may be related to hemoglobinuria, myoglobinuria, and hypoperfusion related to hypovolemia. Urinary output should be monitored every hour for the first 48 to 72 hours, and specific gravity values should be used to determine adequacy of hydration status and renal competency. Urinary glucose is monitored, as are urinary sodium, creatinine, and blood urea nitrogen (BUN). Use of a Foley catheter is appropriate for the first 48 to 72 hours. Because of the tremendous risk of infection related to indwelling catheters, they should be discontinued as soon as possible. Leaving the catheter in place may be necessary if perineal burns are involved. Oliguria is usually related to inadequate fluid resuscitation but may be associated with acute renal failure. An adequate urinary output is generally considered 0.5 to 1 ml/kg for the adult. Other signs of renal failure include increasing creatinine, blood urea nitrogen (BUN), phosphorus, and potassium levels; weight gain; edema; elevated blood pressure; lethargy; and confusion.

The presence of glucose in the urine will cause osmotic diuresis, which does not necessarily reflect the patient's volume status and may, in fact, suggest the need for additional fluid to make up for the compensatory mechanism.

Altered cerebral tissue perfusion. Assessment of the patient's neurological status should also be performed frequently during the first few days. Changes in the neurological status of the patient may be related to an associated head injury that occurred with the burn, hypoperfusion related to hypovolemia, hypoxemia associated with inadequate ventilation, carbon monoxide poisoning, and/or electrolyte imbalances. Patients with electrical burns or major thermal burns may have peripheral neurological injuries, but they may not become evident for several days after the injury. The neurological assessment should include using the *Glasgow Coma Scale,* detailed elsewhere in this text. It is not unusual for the patient to be agitated, restless, and extremely anxious during the emergent phase of burn injury as a result of hypovolemia or the patient's fear of death. However, the possibility of neurological involvement should not be overlooked.

Altered peripheral tissue perfusion. Altered peripheral tissue perfusion results from third spacing of fluid during the emergent phase, which restricts blood flow to extremities. As hypovolemia ensues, vasoconstriction increases and can be potentiated by the loss of body temperature. Peripheral tissue perfusion should be monitored carefully in all burn patients. The patient's blood pressure, pulse, and respirations should be monitored as previously discussed. Unburned areas should be carefully assessed for warmth, color, and peripheral pulses. Capillary refill time should be less than 3 seconds. Any signs or symptoms of diminished systemic tissue perfusion should be reported immediately.

Nursing actions should be taken to minimize any compromise of peripheral circulation. Fluid resuscitation must be maintained and monitored to enhance peripheral circulation. Care should be taken not to position the patient in a way that compromises blood flow such as crossing legs, pillows under knees, or dependent positioning. If possible, limbs should be elevated to decrease the peripheral edema by enhancing venous return.

Monitoring the peripheral circulation is vital in the burn patient with circumferential full-thickness burns of the extremities. The resulting edema may severely compromise the venous system and then the arterial system. Neurovascular integrity of extremities with circumferential burns should be assessed every hour for the first 24 to 48 hours using the "six P's": *pulselessness, pallor, pain, paresthesia, paralysis,* and *poikilothermia.* The use of a Doppler flowmeter may be necessary. Loss of pulses may be a late sign.

If any other changes are noted, the physician should be notified immediately. Numbness and paresthesias can occur in 30 minutes. Irreversible nerve ischemia resulting in a loss of function may begin after 12 to 24 hours.[12]

A most unfortunate scenario results when the patient's reports of ischemic pain and paresthesias in a circumferentially burned extremity go unheeded and neurovascular compromise is allowed to persist. Sensory nerve fibers become damaged, and altered sensations cease, which may be misinterpreted as improvement in neurovascular status. Permanent disability and quite possibly loss of limb are eventual outcomes.

Extremities should be elevated and put through passive range-of-motion exercises to reduce edema. This, however, may not be sufficient intervention to improve circulation. Performing an escharotomy, which is an incision into the full thickness of the eschar, allowing the underlying tissue to expand, may become necessary. In deeper wounds it may be necessary to do a fasciotomy, which involves incision of the fascia. These procedures can be performed at the bedside using either a scalpel or electrocautery (Fig. 43-5). Because these are full-thickness wounds, no local anesthesia is required. There may, however, be localized bleeding.

Altered gastrointestinal tissue perfusion. Paralytic ileus is a common gastrointestinal (GI) complication during resuscitation or when the patient becomes septic. The abdomen and the bowel sounds should be assessed every 2 hours during the initial phase and every 4 hours thereafter. If there are signs and symptoms of a paralytic ileus, all oral intake should be withheld and a nasogastric tube inserted, using low to medium suction.

A paralytic ileus can be related to hypokalemia, the sympathetic response to severe trauma, and/or decreased tissue perfusion related to hypovolemia. The patient may develop a stress ulcer (Curling's) as a result of decreased tissue perfusion to the GI tract, a change in the quantity or quality of mucus (which has a pH of 1), and/or an increase in gastric acid secretion resulting from the stress response. Gastric acid should be maintained above pH 5 through the administration of antacids, cimetidine, or ranitidine to prevent the development of these ulcers. The patient should be carefully monitored for GI bleeding. All stools and gastric content should be tested for occult blood. The patient should be assessed for epigastric discomfort or fullness, decreased blood pressure, or increased pulse.

Impaired tissue integrity. Management of the burn wound is the top priority after the resuscitation phase. Expedient closure of the wounds will decrease the potential for multiple complications such as fluid and electrolyte imbalances, loss of proteins and nitrogen, and infection.

Eschar is the nonviable tissue that forms after the burn injury. This tissue has no blood supply. Therefore polymorphonuclear leukocytes, antibodies, and systemic antibodies cannot reach these areas. Eschar provides an excellent medium for bacterial growth; thus it is vital that the burn wounds be cleared and debrided on a daily basis to remove this eschar.

The use of tangential excision of the wounds is becoming more popular currently in light of better techniques for administration of anesthetics and better critical care support.

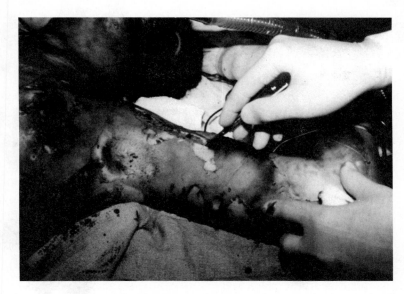

Fig. 43-5   Performance of fasciotomy on the upper arm to release tension from burn wound and to improve peripheral perfusion. An escharotomy, which was performed to improve chest expansion that was restricted by a circumferential full-thickness burn wound to the chest, can be seen in the midaxillary line of the patient's chest.

This surgical debridement technique may begin as early as 3 to 5 days after the burn insult when the patient is hemodynamically stable. It involves excision of full-thickness tissue down to freely bleeding and viable tissue. The area that has been excised is immediately grafted with temporary biological or synthetic dressings. This procedure is not without risk because the blood loss can be significant (up to 200 ml per percent of burn tissue removed. Therefore the procedures may be staged. Use of this method may require many surgical procedures spaced several days apart. Generally, the wound can be covered and grafted much sooner by using this method, thereby decreasing the potential for wound infections or sepsis.

Several other methods of debridement are commonly used. Washing and friction can remove much debris. Hydrotherapy facilitates the removal of debris and eschar. Daily immersion of the wound in a tub of plain water or dilute povidone-iodine solution should not begin until the patient is hemodynamically stable. Generally, this therapy is performed once or twice daily and should last no longer than 20 or 30 minutes per session. The patient's vital signs should be carefully monitored during this time, especially body temperature and blood pressure. Mechanical debriding with scissors and forceps can be done during these treatments.

Total immersion is not as popular as it once was. Currently, spray tables and specially designed upright and chair showers are being used. The force of the spray assists in debridement. The areas not being sprayed can be covered. The procedure can be accomplished in less time, decreasing the potential loss of electrolytes and potential reduction in core temperature. Patients report experiencing less discomfort with this method.

After debridement, burn wounds are managed in one of three methods. The *open method* is to leave the burn open with only a topical agent applied. Advantages to this method are (1) the wound can be easily assessed, (2) there are no dressings that would limit range of motion, and (3) the risk of diminishing circulation is decreased. However, there are several disadvantages to the open method, including the need for strict isolation techniques. Additionally, patients experience more discomfort with this method because of exposure of the wound to air currents and environmental temperatures.

The *semiopen method* consists of covering the wound with topical antimicrobial agents and then applying a thin layer of gauze and netting material to keep the antimicrobial agent in place. This method, combined with hydrotherapy once or twice a day, enhances wound debridement and the development of granulation tissue and makes grafting of the wound possible sooner.

The *closed method* of management generally consists of the application of gauze impregnated with topical antimicrobials, followed by a bulkier gauze kept in place by a pressure dressing. Disadvantages of this method include the amount of nursing time required to change these dressings, the inability to assess the wound directly, and the increased risk of impaired peripheral circulation.

Blister management. Blister management is a controversial area of burn care. Each of its three approaches is acceptable and is an option that each burn team should consider: (1) leave the blister intact and allow the underlying wound to heal in the sterile fluid environment, (2) evacuate the blister fluid and allow the overlying skin to cover the underlying wound, and (3) debride the blister. To use the first two options, the blister must be sterile with no evidence of contamination or infection. If this is not the case, the blister is debrided.

Burn wound closure. The primary goal of burn wound

There are many methods for achieving this goal. When the burn injury covers a large BSA and there are inadequate amounts of uninjured skin to cover the affected areas, temporary skin substitutes may be used.

A nationwide survey was done by Nowicki and Springer[15] to identify and report on the skin substitutes used in burn centers throughout the United States. Skin substitutes that they identified were pigskin, allograft, biosynthetic skin substitute, elastomeric polyurethane, Xeroform, and scarlet red. These materials temporarily restore the protective barrier that the skin provides naturally.

Skin substitutes may be biological or synthetic. Biological substitutes include cadaver skin, animal skin, or tissue derivatives such as collagen. Synthetic skin substitutes are man-made and include elastomeric polyurethane, biosynthetic skin substitute, and Xeroform.

Skin barrier substitutes must possess several properties to accomplish their desired effect as a temporary wound covering to protect the granulating tissue and/or to preserve a clean, viable wound surface for future autografting. The most important property of these materials is adherence so that the skin substitute can simulate the function of the skin. Adherence must be uniform to prevent fluid accumulation beneath its surface, which could lead to bacterial proliferation.

Ideal properties of skin substitutes include the following[15]:
- Adherence
- Minimal discomfort or pain
- Easy application and removal
- Intact bacterial barrier
- Shelf storage capability
- Inexpensive in relation to alternatives
- Nonantigenic
- Similar to normal skin in transport of water vapor
- Nontoxic
- Elastic
- Hemostatic
- Decreased protein and electrolyte loss
- Enhanced natural healing processes

For application of skin substitutes, the wound must be clean and ideally have a bacterial count of less than 10^{-5} organisms per gram of tissue. The burn wound must be free from eschar, and hemostasis must be present. Both eschar and blood provide an excellent medium for bacterial proliferation, and the presence of blood may interfere with adherence. The surfaces should be cleaned and rinsed with saline solution, and the skin substitutes should be applied according to established procedures, using sterile techniques.[11]

BIOLOGICAL SKIN SUBSTITUTES

Allograft. Allograft, or homograft, is a graft transferred from one individual to another of the same species to provide temporary coverage. Fresh human cadaver skin is considered by many as the ideal biological skin substitute barrier. It has been commonly used as the standard for comparison for other skin substitutes. It possesses all the physical qualities of those previously mentioned as ideal. However, the disadvantages include its antigenicity, lack of accessibility, difficulties with storage and quality control, expense of procurement, and possibility of disease transmission from the donor. The microbiological cleanliness of the cadaver skin is of extreme concern because of the burn patient's debilitated immunological condition.

Allografts are generally available only in centers in which the rigorous processing procedure can be achieved. These centers usually have skin and tissue bank facilities. Procurement of the allograft is much the same as for any other donated organ. However, the public is not nearly as well educated about this organ as it is about eyes, kidneys, and hearts.

As part of a burn team, educating the public and members of the medical team about the importance of allografts is vital. Nurses need to know the advantages and disadvantages of allografts, how the procedure is done, how the donor's appearance will be affected, and how to approach a family in crisis to request this important organ donation. Often it is fear of the unknown that stops people from requesting such a donation.

Allografts are harvested during the first 4 hours after death. They are generally taken from the abdomen, thighs, and back. Partial-thickness grafts are obtained, leaving the graft sites looking as if they were sunburned. These areas generally do not interfere with the presentation or appearance of the body at the funeral.

Allografts are used to cover full-thickness burn wounds temporarily before autografting. They may also be used to enhance the healing of partial-thickness burns. When the allograft is applied to the wound, it becomes vascularized and "takes" to the recipient site. The graft can remain in place for approximately 3 to 5 weeks before the host rejects it as a foreign body. This rejection phenomenon is delayed in the burned patient because of the patient's existing immunosuppressed state.

The allografts are applied to clean wounds after daily cleaning or in the operating room. Allografts should be handled and applied very carefully. They should be placed with the shiny surface down and should be wrinkle free. They should not overlap each other or lap over infected areas or uninjured areas. The grafts can be dressed with fine mesh gauze and soaked with saline solution and are usually not changed for 24 hours (Figs. 43-6 and 43-7).

Xenograft. Xenograft, or heterograft, is a graft transferred between two different species to provide temporary wound coverage. The most common and widely accepted xenograft is pigskin (porcine). Pigskin is available in frozen and shelf forms, with each type having a much longer storage life than allografts. Depending on how the pigskin has been prepared, it can have a shelf life of 1 month to 1 year. The pigskin is packaged in a variety of ways and in variable sizes. It can be treated with silver sulfadiazine and can be meshed or nonmeshed.

Pigskin can be used for temporary coverage of full- and partial-thickness wounds, burn wounds, and donor sites. It meets many of the ideal skin substitute properties mentioned previously. However, it does have two disadvantages: it is antigenic, and it has the potential for digestion by the wound collagenase, possibly leading to infection.

Pigskin is applied in the same manner as allografts (Fig. 43-8). If the pigskin is frozen, it is thawed in a warm saline solution bath. If it has been treated with silver sulfadiazine,

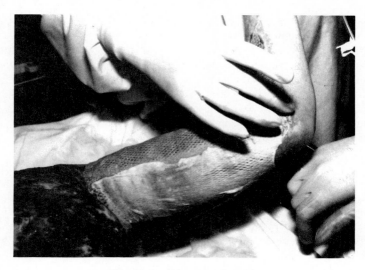

Fig. 43-6   Human allograft.

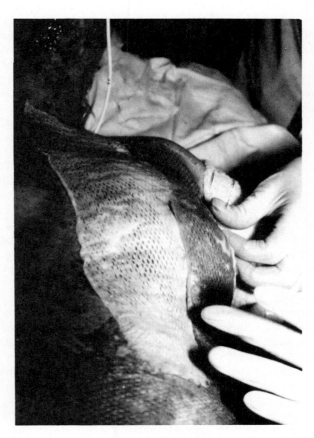

Fig. 43-7   Human allograft.

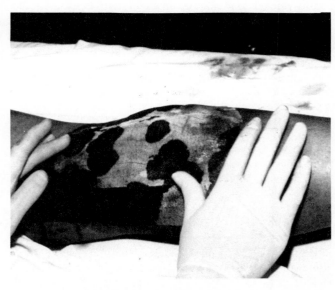

Fig. 43-8   Xenograft (pigskin).

management is closing the wound during the acute phase. it is thawed in water. The pigskin is placed on the wound with the dermal side down (the dermal side faces the center of the roll) and may be distinguished by its tendency to curl toward the dermal surface when held up at one end. Shelf-stored pigskin may be applied with either side to the wound. Once the pigskin is in place, it may be dressed with anti-bacterial-impregnated dressings or other forms of dressings. Pigskin is usually removed in 3 to 4 days. If sloughing or purulent drainage occurs, the xenograft should be removed.[15]

SYNTHETIC SKIN SUBSTITUTES

Biosynthetic skin substitute. The use of biosynthetic skin substitute has gained popularity throughout the United States during the last 5 to 10 years. It is composed of a nylon and Silastic membrane combined with a collagen derivative. It also can be used on several types of wounds, including partial- and full-thickness burns and wounds, granulating wounds, and donor sites and over split-thickness grafts (Fig. 43-9).

Biosynthetic skin has many of the properties of an ideal skin substitute. It has two advantages that other skin substitutes do not share. Biosynthetic skin has elasticity in all directions and conforms well to surfaces that are difficult to dress such as breast, joints, and axilla. Also, because of its porosity, it allows the passage of some topical antibiotics such as silver sulfadiazine to penetrate its membrane, reducing the bacterial count of the burn wound.

Biosynthetic skin may be applied after daily cleaning at the bedside or in the operating room. It is applied with the dull or nylon mesh side facing the wound. It can be held in place with sutures, staples, steri-strips, or stent. If fluid accumulates under the biosynthetic skin, it may be slit and the fluid expressed. If a large amount of fluid accumulates, the biosynthetic skin should be removed and replaced. Biosynthetic skin initially adheres to the wound fibrin, which binds to the collagen and nylon backing of the material.

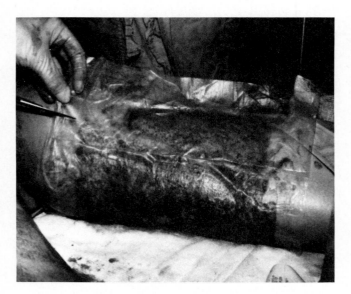

Fig. 43-9 Biosynthetic skin substitute.

Later the cells migrate into the nylon mesh and further bind to the wound.

Elastomeric polyurethane. Elastomeric polyurethane film is primarily used in the coverage of donor sites, but some practitioners report using it over some partial-thickness burn wounds. Like biosynthetic skin, elastomeric polyurethane possesses many of the properties of an ideal skin substitute. Its major disadvantages include limited water permeability and lack of adherence to the wound itself. Fluid accumulation between the film and wound creates a potential environment for maceration and infection. When fluid collects, it often leaks and decreases the adherence of the dressing. The fluid can be removed with a needle and syringe; however, the needle puncture must be patched with a small piece of elastomeric polyurethane film.

Elastomeric polyurethane film has as adhesive side that is designed to adhere to normal skin adjacent to the wound. It generally takes two persons to apply large pieces of elastomeric polyurethane film because of its tendency to wrinkle and stick to itself. The dressing may be further secured with an elastic wrap or netting material. Donor sites generally head within 1 or 2 weeks using this type of dressing.

Scarlett red and Xeroform. Scarlet red and Xeroform are considered dressings rather than skin substitutes. However, they possess many of the desired properties of a skin substitute and are used as such by many burn centers in the United States.

Scarlet red is a fine mesh gauze impregnated with a blend of lanolin, olive oil, and petroleum and is primarily used over the donor sites. It possesses many of the ideal skin substitute properties; however, it has several serious disadvantages. It causes red stains on clothing and linen and can cause discomfort related to the way the material dries, hardens, stretches, and pulls underlying skin.

Xeroform is a fine mesh gauze that contains 3% bismuth tribromophenate in a petrolatum blend. It, too, is generally used on donor sites. Xeroform has no major disadvantages and possesses many of the ideal properties. Application is easy, and it does not have the disadvantages of scarlet red.

As the donor site heals, the edges of the scarlet red and Xeroform loosen and may be trimmed. These dressings should not be removed forcibly, because this would interfere with the reepithelialization process.

Research in the area of skin substitutes may significantly change the approach to wound care in the very near future. Green and colleagues[15] are investigating the development of cultured autologous human epithelium. Burke, Yannas, and associates are developing the "artificial skin."[15]

Autograft. Autograft is a skin graft transferred from one location to another on the same individual to provide permanent coverage of the wound. Autografts are the only grafts that provide permanent coverage. Preferred sites for obtaining these grafts are thighs, back, and abdomen. However, grafts can be harvested from almost anywhere. Grafts that are placed on the face, neck, lower arms, and hands are generally sheet grafts. Grafts that are meshed can cover more area but may not produce the cosmetic appearance desired and therefore are usually placed on areas generally covered by clothing.

Autografting is usually performed in the operating room.

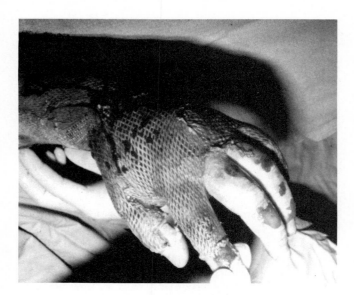

Fig. 43-10 Autograft.

The grafts can be sutured or stapled into place and can be left open to air or dressed with occlusive dressings. These dressings usually remain intact for 48 hours (Fig. 43-10). Great care should be taken not to disturb the graft. Care of the donor site is as equally important, because it represents a wound similar to that of a partial-thickness injury. One of the synthetic dressings mentioned previously can be used in its care. Healing of donor site generally occurs in less than 2 weeks.

Topical antibiotic therapy. Burn injuries destroy the function of the skin's protective mechanism, including that of the sebaceous glands. Sebaceous glands normally secrete sebum, which contains fatty acids, including oleic acid. In addition to lubricating the skin, sebum is believed to help destroy some microorganisms such as streptococci and some strains of staphylococci. In addition, serum is lost from damaged capillaries, providing a rich nutritional medium for bacterial colonization. Topical antibiotics are used to control this colonization.

Effective antibacterial agents should control colonization so that wound biopsies reflect fewer than 10^{-4} microorganisms per gram of tissue. More microorganisms than this make control of wound sepsis with topical antibiotics questionable. Consideration must then be given to parenteral therapy.

Topical antibiotics selected should meet the following criteria: side effects should be minimal, resistant strains should not develop with use, application should be easy and rapid, and use should be relatively economical. Currently, the most commonly used topical antibiotics are silver sulfadiazine (Silvadene), silver nitrate-sulfadiazine, and mafenide acetate (Sulfamylon).

Silver sulfadiazine has bactericidal action again many gram-negative and gram-positive bacteria. It does not penetrate as readily as mafenide acetate. However, its application is much more comfortable for the patient. Caution should be used with any patient with altered renal function.

BUN and creatinine values should be monitored closely. Electrolyte imbalances generally do not occur with the use of silver sulfadiazine; however, toxic symptoms may occur with prolonged use and include nausea, vomiting, granulocytopenia, oliguria, anuria, jaundice, and skin rashes. If the patient has a glucose 6-phosphate dehydrogenase deficiency, hemolytic anemia can occur.

Mafenide acetate penetrates through burn eschar and is bacteriostatic against many gram-negative and gram-positive organisms. Its application is generally uncomfortable for the patient. However, some of the newer spray applications are much better tolerated. Metabolic acidosis that results from use of mafenide acetate is not uncommon. The patient should be monitored closely for hyperventilation.

Research is being conducted to determine the effectiveness of parenteral antibiotics used as topical agents. Antibiotics being studied are aminoglycosides, cephalosporins, penicillin, colistin (Coly-Mycin), and amphotericin B (Fungizone). In one study[11] application of these antibiotics was done with wet dressing, spray, or immersion. Toxicity from topical solutions of parenteral antibiotics did not occur in this study. Peaks and/or troughs of the aminoglycosides did not approach the low therapeutic ranges of the drugs. It is believed that much of the bolus of the topical antibiotic solution is sequestered in the burn wound eschar and an indeterminate amount is evaporated. The strength and amount of the solution required to control microorganisms within the acceptable range apparently are small enough for this to be an economically sound approach.[11]

Closed burn wound care. Two to six weeks after wound closure, there is frequently a problem with the formation of tiny water blisters. These blisters usually open and heal without incident in 3 to 5 days. These areas should be kept clean with mild soap and should be covered with a bland ointment.

Recently healed partial-thickness wounds are very dry. For 6 to 8 weeks, a mild lanolin skin cream should be applied every 4 hours to these areas to lubricate the skin until natural lubrication occurs. Pruritus is common in the maturing burn wound. Patients can be relieved of this discomfort by the administration of antipruritics such as diphenhydramine hydrocholoride or hydroxyzine and by the use of moisturizing creams.

Another concern with burn wound healing is the prevention or reduction of hypertropic scarring. Its prevention or reduction depends on the timely application of uniform pressure. Hypertrophic scarring can be controlled with the use of tubular support bandages applied within 5 to 7 days after the graft. Bandages are available in a variety of sizes and have the advantage of applying pressure to selected body areas while allowing the remaining burned area to heal sufficiently. They are also readily available for immediate use while waiting for the commercially prepared elastic pressure garment for long-term use, which can take up to 3 or 4 weeks for manufacture.

Tubular support bandages apply a tension in the medium range of 10 to 20 mm Hg. Tensions lower than this do not exert adequate pressure to control scarring, and higher tensions tend to cause edema in the distal parts of the extremities and may be too abrasive to newly grafted skin. Tension

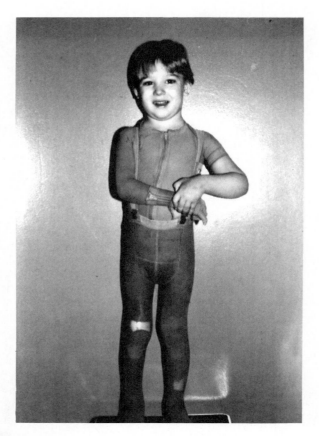

Fig. 43-11 Custom-made elastic pressure garment.

can be elevated if needed by placing silicone foam under the tubular support bandages over areas such as the axilla and knees.[6]

Custom-made elastic pressure garments are generally worn for 6 months to 1 year after grafting. It is important to assess the patient for pressure points during this time as weight is gained and as children grow (Fig. 43-11). It is also necessary to assess the garment for elasticity; with many washings over time this property may be decreased.

Adjunct therapy in burn wound healing. For patients with extensive posterior burns or large graft sites and those immobilized for long periods of time, providing adjunct support should be considered. Support may be the use of fluidized air therapy or controlled air suspension. Each has its advantages and disadvantages.[16]

To allow better wound healing, it is useful to reduce skin pressure as much as possible, because skin pressure is significantly less than capillary pressure. Fluidized air therapy reduces this pressure, reduces shearing force, and reduces moisture to the posterior surface through flotation and the circulation of dry air. Because of these advantages, conversion of wounds from partial thickness to full thickness is reduced, wound infections are reduced, healing time is improved, and patient comfort is enhanced.[20]

There are, however, three areas of concern that must be addressed if fluidized air therapy is used. The most significant complication is dehydration, which is related to the evaporation as the dry air circulates around the patient. Evaporation can increase insensible fluid loss by twice the normal amount. In the burn patient there is already a significant loss of fluid related to the loss of skin integrity. This complication must be carefully considered when using this therapy and appropriate steps taken to maintain the patient's fluid and electrolyte balance. This risk factor can be reduced by the use of a latex sheet, which decreases the dry air circulating around intact body surface areas. Contractures of the shoulders can also occur. This is usually an anterior rotation that can be avoided by using a foam wedge under the shoulders several times a day. The use of the foam will decrease the advantages of the therapy, so it should not be used for several hours at a time. The last concern with this therapy is that patients occasionally become confused and disoriented when they are suspended in this "weightless" state. This concern can generally be compensated by stopping or freezing the flotation of the bed.

One of the significant issues involved in burn care and wound management is development of an explicit protocol and adequate education of the staff. Constant review of outcomes within the burn unit is mandatory. What works well in one unit may not in another for a multitude of reasons.

Acute pain.* Pain is an individualized and subjective phenomenon. It is comprised of both physiological and psychological aspects. Pain after burn injury is significant. Physiological changes associated with pain include the damage or exposure of the nerve endings within a partial-thickness burn, donor sites, range of motion of the affected limbs, tightening scar tissue, and/or extensive and frequent treatments in tubs and debridement. Other pain-producing interventions include arterial punctures, chest physical therapy, injections, and use of nasogastric tubes, suction, and pressure garments. Loss of control, forced dependence, loneliness, and separation from home and family can all contribute to anxiety, which heightens the patient's perception of the pain. The patient's fears abound in thoughts of disfigurement, loss of love, function, and job.

The psychological experience or subjective component may be related to past experiences, anxiety, and altered coping mechanisms. Attention to the psychological component of the patient's pain may lead to very useful strategies in decreasing his or her perceived pain. If possible, how the patient usually responds to pain and interventions, if any, he has used in the past that have been successful in relieving pain should be determined.

Patients with partial-thickness burns experience a great deal of discomfort. The slightest air current to the surface of the burn may stimulate pain. Covering wounds with topical agents, dressings, and linen will significantly decrease the pain.

Use of narcotics in burn patients is an area of controversy. Pharmacokinetics of drugs such as aminoglycosides, digitalis, phenytoin, and meperidine are altered in the burn patient. Perry and Inturrisis[17] studied the pharmacokinetics of morphine in eight patients with burns less than 40% of

---

*See also "Acute Pain related to transmission and perception of noxious stimuli," p. 594.

BSA and at least 2 weeks old. Their findings in this limited sample showed that burn patients could eliminate morphine normally and could receive effective pain relief when plasma concentration was sufficient. However, the effects on the respiratory system, fear of iatrogenic addiction, the pharmacokinetics of patients immediately after burn injury, and the influence of the size of the burn are causes of concern.

Narcotics and other sedatives should be administered intravenously. Intramuscular injections should not be used until the patient is hemodynamically stable and has adequate tissue perfusion.

Nonpharmacological techniques such as imagery, hypnosis, distraction, and methods adapted from some of the popular childbirth techniques can be very effective in reducing anxiety and the pain experience. Giving the patient some control of his or her management can also reduce the anxiety and the pain experience. The perception of pain is often increased in the patient who is anxious and lacks control of the situation. A study[18] was done to determine if interrupted debridement would decrease the pain experienced during daily tub treatments. Patients could suspend debridement for 15 seconds each minute. It was predicted that this increased sense of control would decrease anxiety and thereby diminish the pain experience. It was found that having a choice in the method of debridement did make a difference in the patient's pain experience. It was also found that during continuous debridement, nurses were not conscious of the patient's continuous pain; during continuous debridement procedures there was no correlation between the patient's and nurses' ratings of distress and pain. During the interrupted procedures there were high positive correlations between nurses and patients. In the continuous procedures nurses consistently underestimated the pain, anxiety, and distress of the patient, perhaps because of their intense concentration on the physical task at hand. Nurses involved in the interrupted procedures, however, were much more aware of patients' pain and their reaction.[18]

Altered nutrition: less than body requirements.* The basic metabolic rate of a burn patient may be elevated 40% to 100% above the normal rate, depending on the amount of BSA involved. The metabolic rate is influenced by the amount of protein and albumin lost through the wounds, the catabolic response associated with stress and other associated injuries, fluid loss, fever, infection, immobility, sex, and the height and weight of the patient before the injury.[19]

The goal in nutritional management of the burn patient is to provide adequate calories to prevent starvation and to enhance wound healing. To achieve this goal nutritional support is imperative, and the reduction of energy demand is also vital. Every effort should be made to reduce the release of catecholamines which increase metabolic rate. Release of catecholamine stores is stimulated by pain, fear, anxiety, and cold. Appropriate interventions for each of these stimuli should be performed.

The use of enteral and oral routes is preferred in the management of burn patients. Caloric requirements should

be calculated based on the size of the burn; the age, height, and weight of the patient; and the stress factors. Protein and caloric requirements of each patient are highly individualized and should be assessed on a daily basis. The daily protein requirement for the burn patient will be elevated in light of a negative nitrogen balance. The daily protein requirement may increase to two to four times the normal 0.8 g/kg of body weight. Carbohydrates and fat are used for energy and to spare proteins required for wound healing. Daily caloric intake can be 2 to 20 times higher than normal.

Vitamins and minerals are generally given in doses higher than normal. Serum iron, zinc, calcium, phosphate, and potassium values should all be monitored and supplements given as indicated.

Impaired physical mobility. Tremendous advances have been made in the physical care of the burn patient over the last 10 to 15 years. The survival rate of patients with full-thickness burns greater than 40% of total BSA has increased significantly. Currently, survival of patients with burns greater than 90% is not unusual. As patients with larger and deeper burns survive, the challenge to maintain their optimal mobility and cosmetic appearance has increased.

It is imperative that rehabilitation needs are addressed early in burn care. Nursing prescriptions for range-of-motion exercises, positioning, splinting, ambulation, and activities of daily living are initiated within the first 48 hours of hospitalization.

Contractures may develop after a burn injury because of a variety of factors: the extent, depth, location, and configuration of the burn; the position of comfort the patient most frequently assumes; the relative underlying muscle strength; and the patient's motivation and compliance. Positioning the affected body parts in *antideformity positions* is vital. Frequent change of position is also important and may need to be done as frequently as every hour. Burn patients are at greater risk for developing pressure sores than the general hospital population, in addition to possibly converting their partial-thickness burns to full-thickness burns.

Splints can be used to prevent and/or correct contractures or to immobilize joints after grafting (Fig. 43-12). If splints are used, they should be checked daily for proper fit and effectiveness. Splints used to immobilize body parts after grafting should be left on at all times except to assess the graft site for pressure points every shift. Splints to correct severe contractures may be off for 2 hours per shift to allow burn care and range-of-motion exercises. Mild contractures may be in splints for 4 hours and off for 4 hours to promote exercise and mobility.[14]

Active exercise should be encouraged and is preferred, although active-assisted or gentle-passive exercise may also be an important part of the rehabilitation program. Active exercise maintains muscle mass, aids in restoring protein structures within the muscle tissue, aids in venous and lymphatic return, and reduces the risk of pulmonary embolus and deep vein thrombosis. Patient tolerance should be carefully evaluated. The number of repetitions should be proportional to the degree of anticipated contracture and the patient's tolerance.

Anticipation of the patient's pain should also be carefully considered. Before range-of-motion exercises and activities

---

*See also Unit III, "Nutritional Alterations," Chapters 9 and 10.

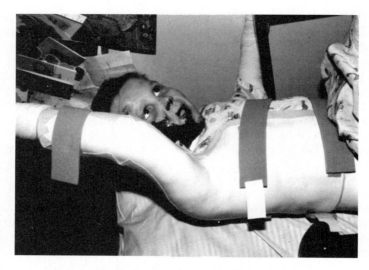

Fig. 43-12   Splinting in the antideformity position.

of daily living are performed, the need for pain medication should be assessed.

Self-concept alterations*

Body image disturbance. Patients experience changes in self-perception after their burn injuries because of changes in physical appearance, alterations in mobility, and sensory losses. The experience will vary with each individual. A patient with a 10% BSA burn on his or her back that will be covered with clothing most of the time may have an extremely difficult time accepting this new body image. This reaction may seem disproportionate when compared to a patient with a 95% BSA burn who appears to adapt well to his or her new image. It is vital that each patient be considered individually. Patients with cosmetic changes to their face, neck, and hands may have a more difficult time adjusting to their new image than others, but this should not be taken as a generalization. Each patient should be encouraged to verbalize his or her feelings about the burns and their appearance. The burn team should be acutely aware of the nonverbal cues of the patient's reactions.

The burn team should assist the patient to adjust to the new image by first helping him or her cope with the effect of the burns. The staff members should demonstrate acceptance of the patient's experience and appearance. They may demonstrate this through empathetic listening, therapeutic touch, and frequent visits and may encourage the significant others to do the same. The patient should not be forced to use a mirror until ready, at which time the staff should be available to provide support and encouragement. Cosmetic alterations should be discussed with the patient and alternatives suggested. Interventions might include plastic surgery, new makeup techniques, a new hairstyle, and/or different styles of clothing.

Within the burn unit the patients should be encouraged to make contact with one another to help test and reestablish their new images. Once they are comfortable in this setting, they should begin to interact with others outside the unit by taking small progressive steps, using situations in which they would be exposed to only one or two nonburn patients at first, and by progressively involving themselves with more people in a variety of circumstances. Ideally, the patient should be accompanied by a staff member through each step.

Powerlessness. Powerlessness is frequently experienced by patients in the hospital environment. This experience can be compounded for the burn patient. Patients frequently believe they have lost control over their situation. They may become so discouraged or despondent that they may believe that nothing they do will influence their eventual outcome.

Powerlessness can be expressed in a variety of ways. Patients may verbally express their feelings of having no control over their care or their eventual outcome, or they may be apathetic and passive. They may become totally dependent on the burn team. It can not be stressed enough how vital it is to include the patient in establishing goals, planning his or her care, and evaluating the outcomes. The burn team must establish the problem list, priorities, and the outcome criteria. But these must be carefully and thoroughly explained to the patient, and when possible, the patient's input should be incorporated. Every effort should be made to allow the patient personal expression and some control of the environment, treatments, and therapies.

Altered role performance. It is not unusual for burn patients to experience either a perceived or actual disturbance in role performance. This alteration is interrelated with the patient's self-esteem, body image, and personal identity. The patient and significant others should be allowed to discuss perceptions of their roles before the burn injury and how they believe these roles have changed or may need to change. It is important to have some knowledge of their past history in terms of role performance; however, this may take some time to establish. As many of the patient's preinjury roles as possible (for example, major income producer, planner, caretaker, money manager, father, son, student, employee, employer) should be identified.

Continued involvement in all of the identified roles should

*See also Chapter 47, "Self-Concept Alterations."

be encouraged. If the patient was always the decision maker within the family, he or she still needs to be included. Patients can be devastated if they feel they have lost their role or roles within the family. The burn team must be aware of how these perceived or actual changes can influence the patients' eventual recovery. Any misconceptions about limitations, physical activity, sexual functioning, returning to work, and role function should be clarified as soon as possible. Patients must be helped to recognize how their roles may need modification, to plan for lifestyle changes, and to realistically prioritize changes that might be necessary.

The burn team should not lose sight of the fact that the patient's significant others are included in this process. They must also be assisted with their new roles, for example, if they must become the caretaker or the income producer of the family. Conflicts in roles can cause great turmoil for the patient which may slow recovery and decrease potential full recovery.

Outpatient burn care. Outpatient burn care should be considered for minor burns. It is cost effective and removes the potential for a wound infection from endemic, drug-resistant microorganisms within the hospital environment. The hospital environment also changes many of the self-care routines such as diet, family contact, hygiene, and coping mechanisms. However, patients considered for outpatient burn care should be well screened. Nursing evaluation of the patient and/or family includes consideration of motivation, willingness to participate in care, ability to understand and perform the necessary procedures, potential aversions to wound care or dressing changes, and reliability of transportation. Medical considerations include hemodynamic stabilization, nutritional status, fluid and electrolyte balance, adequate pain control, and ruling out any complications.

It is possible to overtreat burn wounds, leading to complications such as localized infections and delayed wound healing. However, in general, small burns should be washed daily with a mild soap and water, and a bland ointment and/or synthetic antimicrobial agent can be applied and held in place with dressings. Initially, these wounds should be followed daily and then on a weekly basis until the wound matures. Generally, if epithelialization (maturing) of these wounds has not occurred in 2 to 3 weeks, use of primary excision and grafting should be considered.

Partial-thickness injuries should be followed until the epithelialization has occurred to check for evidence of hypertrophic scarring. If hypertrophic scarring occurs, compression dressings should be fitted and worn until the wound becomes quiescent, requiring 12 to 18 months.

Stressors of Burn Nursing

Burn units are fascinating environments in which to work. They offer the fast-paced, high-tech atmosphere of any critical care setting, the complexity of advanced nursing management, and the dynamics of an interdisciplinary, collaborative model of practice. All of these elements combined, however, contribute to a potentially stressful work environment for the nurse.

The physical environment can be a difficult one in which to work for a variety of reasons. The amount of equipment necessary to maintain the patient can be overwhelming and can limit the work space dramatically. The temperature of the room is generally kept at approximately 85° F and can get much warmer, depending on the amount of equipment in the room. Odors vary and can be very unpleasant. Noise levels within a unit are also distressing. These variables exact a physical toll on the nursing staff.

Additionally, there are patient care complexities unique to burn nursing. The daily tub treatments and dressing changes are extremely stressful for both the nurse and the patient. The nursing management of patient's pain is a complex issue in burn care and is one that contributes significantly to the stress of burn nurses. The psychodynamics associated with the patient's burn injury experience are just that—*dynamic*—and require constant, high-level nursing assessment and intervention.

The decision to specialize in burn nursing is a meaningful one, an important one; this decision, however, must also be an informed one. For an excellent discussion of the nature of stress in critical care nursing and specific stress management strategies, see Chapter 50. Self-care and care of other nurses are just as important as the care of the patient and his or her significant other.

SUMMARY

The burn patient presents a unique set of challenges to the team of professionals specialized in his or her care. The burn team is not only concerned with the care of the burn victim but also with the prevention of burn casualties. Successful patient outcomes depend on the knowledge and commitment of the members of the burn team.

The Advanced Burn Life Support Course (ABLSC), endorsed by the American Burn Association, was designed by physicians and nurses across the United States. The National Advisory Committee for the ABLSC is composed of individuals who are experts in burn care and burn research. The course is designed to teach improved burn resuscitation to rural and metropolitan caregivers. Additional details about the course may be obtained by writing to Nebraska Burn Institute, 4600 Valley Road, Lincoln, NE, 68510.

REFERENCES

1. Demling RH and Tortella B: The effect of lipid infusion on pulmonary function in burn patients with inhalation injury, J Burn Care Rehabil 6(3):222, 1985.
2. Desai MH: Inhalation injuries in burn victims, Crit Care Q 7:1, 1984.
3. Gillespie RW: Preadmission/prereferral treatment of patients with major burns, Kansas City, Mo, 1980, Marion Laboratories, Inc.
4. Hill ME, Achauer BM, and Martinez S: Tar and asphalt burns, J Burn Care Rehabil 5:271, 1984.
5. Jacoby F: Care of the massive burn wound, Crit Care 7:44, 1984.
6. Judge JC, May R, and Declement FA: Control of hypertrophic scarring in burn patients using tubular support bandages, J Burn Care Rehabil 5:221, 1984.
7. Kealey CP and others: Cytomegalovirus infection in burn patients, J Burn Care Rehabil 8(6):543, 1987.
8. Kibbee E: Burn pain management, Crit Care Q 7:54, 1984.
9. Klein DG and O'Malley P: Interventions for persons with burns. In Phipps WJ, Long BC, and Woods NF, editors: Medical-surgical nursing: concepts and clinical practice, ed 3, St Louis, 1987, The CV Mosby Co.

10. Kravitz M and others: Thermal injury in the elderly: incidence and cause, J Burn Care Rehabil 8:487, 1985.

11. Mangus DJ and others: Quantitative evaluation and laboratory studies of topical antibiotic therapy in burns, J Burn Care Rehabil 6:39, 1985.

12. Moore S and Marvin JA: Monitoring the burn patient. In Boseick JA, editor: The art and science of burn care, Rockville, Mass: 1987, Aspen Publication.

13. Moylan JA: First aid and transportation burn patients. In Boseick JA, editor: The art and science of burn care, Rockville, Mass, 1987, Aspen Publication.

14. Nadel E and Kozerefski PM: Rehabilitation of the critically ill burn patient, Crit Care Q 7:19, 1984.

15. Nowicki CR and Springer CK: Temporary skin substitutes for burn patients: a nursing perspective, J Burn Care Rehabil 9:209, 1988.

16. Peltier GL, Poppe SR, and Twomey JA: Controlled air suspension: an advantage in burn care, J Burn Care Rehabil 8:558, 1987.

17. Perry S and Inturrisis CE: Analgesia and morphine disposition in burn patients, J Burn Care Rehabil 4:276, 1988.

18. Powers PS and others: Interrupted debridement, J Burn Care Rehabil 5:398, 1985.

19. Schane J, Goede M, and Silverstein P: Comparison of energy expenditure measurement techniques in severely burned patients, J Burn Care Rehabil 8:366, 1987.

20. Scheulen JJ and Munster AM: Clinitron air-fluidized support: an adjunct to burn care, J Burn Care Rehabil 4:271, 1983.

21. Weinsier RL and others: Cost containment: a contribution of aggressive nutritional support in burn patients, J Burn Care Rehabil 6:436, 1985.

CHAPTER

44

Trauma

CHAPTER OBJECTIVES

- Compare and contrast the current methodologies of trauma patient classification systems.
- Plan a systematic approach to the physical assessment of and intervention for trauma patients, using primary and secondary surveys.
- Describe LeFort's classification of facial fractures.
- Discuss common abdominal injuries.
- Differentiate between immediately life-threatening thoracic injuries and potential life-threatening thoracic injuries.

Death and taxes are the two most frequently stated inevitabilities of life; trauma qualifies as a legitimate third.[25] In fact, each person in the United States has a 1 in 70 chance of being hospitalized for traumatic injury this year.[25] Trauma, or unintentional injury, is a major health problem throughout the world. In the United States it is the fourth leading cause of death surpassed only by heart disease, cancer, and stroke.[4] Trauma is the leading killer of individuals ages 1 through 44; and for individuals ages 5 through 44, it kills more people than all other causes combined.[4] The average age of death is 77 for individuals with heart disease, 68 for cancer, and 27 for trauma. Trauma accounts for more lost years of productive life than cancer, heart disease, and stroke combined.

Despite these staggering figures, limited public awareness has been directed toward this disease. By definition, a disease is a *destructive force* or *an alteration in the function of a specific organ or being.* There is a common belief that trauma, or *accidents,* are not preventable and are unpredictable and result from chance or bad luck.[17] In fact, many injuries are preventable and are not random events. There has been an overwhelming association between alcohol use or substance abuse and traumatic injury. Likewise, ignorance of safety devices such as restraints and helmets and poor observance of highway speed limits have resulted in dramatic increases in traumatic injury.

Society has also failed to recognize trauma as a legitimate disease. In 1984 traumatic injury costs totaled close to $100 billion in the United States,[16] which equals approximately $9 million per hour. The number of life years lost in 1984 was 4,100,000 and 1,700,000 for trauma and heart disease respectively; yet allocated research dollars were $112,000,000 for trauma and $998,000,000 for heart disease.[8] Civilian interest in trauma has only developed recently. Sustained educational programs that call for prevention and improved methods of care are still unheard of for trauma, unlike the other major diseases. Samuel Johnson's observation[25] that "Man needs more often to be reminded than informed" is a harsh reality of today's society. With heightened awareness and further research efforts, this disease can be controlled like other disease processes such as tuberculosis and smallpox.

HISTORY

George Santayana[21] once said, "Those who cannot remember the past are condemned to repeat it." As far back as 3000 BC, injury was a major health problem. The Egyptians, having performed lithotomies and extraction of cataracts and foreign objects, are basically regarded as the first trauma surgeons, despite the fact that the surgical knife was never mentioned.[9] During the time of Hippocrates, growth in knowledge and experience in the field of trauma continued. Wound management consisted of healing through secondary intention. Wounded soldiers were carried to barracks or ships to receive medical care as is vividly described by Homer in *The Iliad.* This concept of removing the injured from the scene for treatment would be expanded in the nineteenth century when Dominque Jean Larrey, a surgeon in Napolean's army, developed the precursor to the *air ambulance,* or *ambulance volante,* the horse-drawn carriage.[23] Wounded soldiers were removed from the battlefield by these carriages and were transported to safety for definitive care.[10]

Trauma care in the twentieth century advanced through the work of George Crile,[9] who was involved in the study of hemorrhagic shock. He is credited with revolutionizing intravenous (IV) fluid therapy by administering seawater for the treatment of hypovolemic shock. Meanwhile, use of a systematized approach to trauma care was beginning in the military.

A correlation between time of injury to receipt of definitive therapy can be recognized in Homer's *The Iliad,* in which the mortality rate was as high as 77%, partially because of the prolonged delay in intervention. During World War I the time lapse between injury and surgery averaged 12 to 18 hours, with a mortality rate of 8.5%. This time lapse was decreased by 33% in World War II, and the decrease was reflected by a 5.8% mortality rate. Over the 10-year period of the United States involvement in Vietnam, the time from injury to definitive care was reduced to a mere 65 minutes, reducing mortality to 1.7%. This "golden hour of trauma" remains a standard for acute resuscitation. The 60-minute time frame incorporates activation of the emergency medical system, stabilization and transportation in the prehospital setting, and rapid resuscitation on arrival in the emergency department. Thus getting the *right patient* to the *right facility* at the *right time* is essential in combating impairments in circulation and respiration.

RESUSCITATION PRIORITIES

Johann Goethe once remarked, "An ox cart is as useless as a rocketship if you do not know where to go." The patient suffering multiple injuries requires an aggressive, predetermined approach to treatment. Using the head-to-toe assessment approach that was handed down from the Egyptians ensures that the immediately life-threatening injuries will be readily evaluated. The American College of Surgeons (ACS) has developed programs such as the Advanced Trauma Life Support Course (ATLS) to address the need for rapid assessment. A similar nursing model, the Trauma Nurse Core Course (TNCC), has recently been introduced by the Emergency Nurses Association (ENA). Other programs include the Basic Trauma Life Support Course (BTLS) and the Prehospital Trauma Life Support Course (PHTLS). All of these programs emphasize the need for a systematized approach to the assessment and resuscitation of the multiple trauma patient.

Fortunately, only 10% to 20% of all injuries are classified as immediately or potentially life-threatening injuries.[7] Using the assessment techniques taught in the trauma programs, the practitioner can rapidly assess for the presence of these injuries, using the primary survey, secondary survey, and resuscitation and management.

PRIMARY SURVEY

The primary survey includes the following hallmarks of assessment: the *ABCs*—A, Airway; B, Breathing; C, Circulation *and* Cervical spine immobilization; plus *D* and *E*—D, Disability (minineurological examination); E, Exposure (removal of clothes).

Airway

During this primary survey airway patency and mode of oxygen delivery are evaluated. The most common airway obstruction is caused by the tongue, followed in descending order by blood, teeth, vomitus, and foreign objects. A simple chin thrust may be all that is necessary to open the airway. This is performed by grasping the patient's lower jaw and moving the mandible in a forward motion. All patients must receive supplemental oxygen during the initial examination. It can be delivered through a variety of methods, including nasal, orotracheal, or nasotracheal routes or the cricothyroidotomy, or "surgical airway." If there is loss of consciousness, intubation should strongly be considered for airway maintenance. Patients who have suffered massive facial injuries or fractures of the facial bones and who require airway protection should undergo cricothyroidotomy. Time should not be spent attempting orotracheal or nasotracheal intubation because it will probably be unsuccessful as a result of the amount of bloody secretions in the oropharynx.[1] Likewise, the conscious patient or the patient with suspected or proven midface or basilar skull fracture should *not* have nasotracheal intubation attempted. Because of possible disruption of the cribriform plate, *any* nasally placed tube can penetrate the intracranial contents.[1]

Breathing

Examination of the respiratory component uses the *look, listen,* and *feel* method. Respiratory rate and quality should be recorded and continually assessed. Supplemental oxygenation should be used in all trauma patients, since aerobic metabolism is dependent on saturation of hemoglobin with oxygen. "Supersaturation" with supplemental oxygen may be necessary for the patient with hemorrhage.

Circulation

During the primary survey the systemic blood pressure can be rapidly evaluated by using the *80-70-60* method. If a radial pulse is palpable, the minimal systolic pressure is 80 mm Hg. A systolic pressure of 70 mm Hg should be present with a carotid pulse and a systolic pressure of 60 mm Hg with a femoral pulse.[18] Capillary refill should be determined, as should skin temperature and pulse quality.[18] Capillary refill time greater than 3 seconds indicates that the capillary beds are not receiving adequate circulation.

Cardiac monitoring should also be initiated to detect rhythm disturbances. Common cardiac dysrhythmias in the trauma population include sinus tachycardia, premature ventricular contractions (PVCs), atrial fibrillation, ventricular fibrillation, ventricular tachycardia, asystole, bundle branch blocks, and ST segment changes. Placement of large-bore catheters (14 to 16 gauge) should be used for IV access. Primary peripheral access should be at a level above the diaphragm (upper extremities). Central venous access should be used as a secondary site in most instances. Restoration of volume can be accomplished through administration of crystalloid (lactated Ringer's solution or 0.9% saline solution), colloid (plasma or albumin), and/or blood products. Using the pneumatic antishock garment should be considered. It encompasses the two lower-extremity and the abdominal sections; inflation of these compartments is thought to shunt blood from the periphery to enhance perfusion of the brain, heart, and kidneys.

Disability

After the ABCs have been assessed, a brief neurological assessment should be performed. It is designed as a brief assessment of level of consciousness (LOC) only. During the secondary survey a more detailed assessment is emphasized; during the primary survey, time is essential. By using the AVPU pneumonic, which was devised by the American College of Surgeons,[1] confusing terminology can be avoided:

A, Alert
V, Verbal
P, Pain
U, Unresponsive

Each of these letters can be used to describe the patient's level of consciousness. Spontaneous eye opening and appropriate response to questioning would classify the patient as alert. Eye opening to verbal stimuli only would classify him in the verbal category, thus indicating a decrease in the patient's mental status. Assessment of pain can be obtained in a variety of humane methods. Pinprick to all extremities and sternal rubbing can elicit response to light pain, whereas compression of the nailbed with the side of a pocket penlight can be used to assess deep pain. Spinal cord injury could provide a falsely depressed Glasgow Coma Scale (GCS) in the unconscious patient with a minor closed head injury. Alterations in mental status can also result from hypovolemia, hypoxia, hypoglycemia, or ethanol and/or illegal substance abuse.

Once venous access and laboratory specimens are obtained, 50% dextrose, thiamine, and naloxone can be administered to reverse metabolic causes of depressed mental status. When preparing the site for venous access, isopropyl alcohol preparations interfere with the serum ethanol results. A povidone-iodine solution is recommended to prevent this occurrence. Of major concern in all patients with depressed mental status is airway protection. It should be continually assessed in all patients with changes in mental status.

Exposure

All clothing should be removed from the trauma patient as quickly as possible, and all body surfaces should be inspected for the presence of injury. Glass particles and metal fragments can remain in the clothing and cause secondary injury to the clinician and patient. Once the clothes have been cut down the center of both legs and arms, the patient can be logrolled (while cervical spine immobilization is maintained through in-line cervical traction), and his or her undersurface can be inspected and the clothing and all jewelry removed. The patient's dignity should always be protected.

SECONDARY SURVEY

A more detailed head-to-toe assessment is performed after the primary survey. An in-depth explanation of this begins on p. 800. During the secondary survey adjuncts such as 12-lead electrocardiography (ECG), cervical spine, thoracic, and pelvic radiographs, arterial blood gas determination, contrast-enhanced radiography, and diagnostic peritoneal lavage can be used. The history is one of the most important aspects of the secondary survey. The prehospital providers (paramedics, emergency medical technicians [EMTs], first responders) can usually provide most of the vital information pertaining to the accident. Unfortunately, this resource is not frequently used, and prehospital providers are sometimes allowed to leave the emergency department before complete information has been obtained. To use valuable time better, it is suggested that a member of the trauma team (nurse, physician, or both) should meet the transporting vessel and help "unload" the patient. While this is being performed, a thorough description of the accident scene can be obtained. The first question that should be answered relates to the mechanism of injury—is it *blunt* or *penetrating?* If a penetrating mechanism is responsible for the injury, the following issues should be addressed:

- Weapon used (handgun, shotgun, rifle, knife)
- Caliber of weapon (if known and applicable)
- Number of shots fired (if applicable)
- Sex of assailant (if known)
- Position of victim and assailant when injury occurred

If the injury mechanism is blunt, the following should be addressed:

- Length of fall (greater than or equal to 15 feet)
- Temperature extremes (hot or cold)
- Motor vehicle accident (MVA) extrication time
- Passenger compartment intrusion (in MVA)
- Ejection
- Location in automobile (passenger, driver; frontseat, backseat)
- Restraint status (lapbelt, shoulder harness, lapbelt-shoulder harness combination, unrestrained)
- Speed of involved automobile(s)
- Occupants (number of and morbidity status)
- Amount of external damage
- Amount of internal damage
- Speed of automobile if pedestrian accident

History

The AMPLE mnemonic, developed by Freeark and Baker of the Cook County Hospital in Chicago, is a quick, dependable method of obtaining the patient's history[6a]:

A, Allergies
M, Medications (current)
P, Past illness and surgeries
L, Last meal/Loss of Consciousness
E, Events preceding the accident

Allergies. Of immediate concern are allergies to antibiotics, analgesics, shellfish (iodine), and horse serum (vaccinations).

Medications. Information about over-the-counter (OTC) medications, "recreational" drugs ("street" drugs, ethanol), prescription medications, their route of administration, and their length of use should be ascertained. Use of prophylaxis against withdrawal of appropriate agents should be considered.

Past medical history. Information about previous surgeries, injuries, and relevant medical illnesses (for example, myocardial infarction, hypertension, blood dyscrasias) should be obtained, as should information about complications from illness, surgery, or anesthesia.

Last meal. Information about the time, quality, and type of ingested food or beverage should be obtained if possible, especially if the patient will undergo emergency surgery.

Events. Obtaining all information about the time immediately preceding the accident is necessary to prevent overlooking an injury. If a detailed history is obtained, occult injury should not go undetected.

LABORATORY AND RADIOLOGICAL TESTS
Laboratory Studies

McSwain[14] states that there are three reasons for obtaining laboratory studies in the acute trauma patient:

1. Diagnosis of the patient's injury to influence how that injury will be managed.
2. Management of the patient during the postoperative phase.
3. Screening purposes only.

Treatment should not be delayed for the sole purpose of obtaining specimens for laboratory analysis. For medicolegal purposes, serum ethanol and toxicology screening cannot not be randomly performed without patient consent. In some institutions, serum ethanol screening is performed on all trauma admissions; to prevent "selection bias" and its possible legal implications, ethanol levels must be determined on *all* admissions. In settings in which determination of serum ethanol levels cannot be rapidly obtained, the formula described by Unkle, Clements, and Ross[24] ($-1.055 + 0.00365 \times$ Serum *osmolality = Ethanol*) can be used to predict accurate ethanol levels.

Routine toxicological screening has not been shown clinically useful in the acute setting, nor is its use cost-efficient for *every* patient. When assessing the patient's behavior and mental status, it is unwise to assume that aberrant behavior is the result of a positive ethanol or toxicological report. Patients *should* and *must* be considered to have clinical pathology until proven otherwise.

The multiple trauma patient should have the following laboratory studies performed:

1. Complete blood count (CBC) with differential
2. Serum electrolyte profile to include sodium, potassium, chloride, carbon dioxide, glucose, urea nitrogen, and creatinine
3. Platelet count
4. Coagulation parameters (prothrombin time, partial thromboplastin time)
5. Type and screen (ABO compatibility)
6. Urinalysis with microscopic examination
7. Serum amylase
8. Serum osmolality
9. Serum ethanol
10. Liver function study (serum glutamic-pyruvic transaminase [SGPT])

Radiographic Studies

Radiological examination of the trauma patient is a tertiary concern, following the subjective response and ob-

jective physical assessment. Only after these two phases have been completed can other diagnostic tools be used. In all patients with traumatic injury, one should automatically assume that the cervical spine is injured until proven otherwise. For the cervical spine to be considered "cleared," or without anatomical injury, it should be evaluated from the following three radiological views: (1) cross-table lateral; (2) opened-mouth odontoid; and (3) anterior-posterior (A-P).

All seven vertebral bodies should be visualized, including the entire body of the first thoracic vertebra. If this cannot be successfully achieved, the patient should remain in a cervical collar (Philadelphia collar) until computerized tomographic (CT) views can be obtained. Flexion-extension views may be required to rule out ligamentous injury to the cervical spine. It is important to remember that unstable injury can be present *without* cervical tenderness.

The next series of films that should be obtained are either the supine pelvis or the upright chest view. Points can be made for choosing either first, since they both detect life-threatening injury. If pelvic fracture is suspected and the patient is hemodynamically stable, it has been suggested that the pelvis view be chosen first. Unstable bony fragments can worsen or initiate arterial and venous hemorrhage. The upright chest film should be the first view taken of the chest. Mediastinal widening greater than 8 cm indicates great vessel injury and can be appropriately demonstrated in this view. Should a supine chest view be chosen, a false-positive mediastinal widening will be seen in the majority of cases.

After the above-mentioned views have been obtained, the following studies may be performed: contrast enhanced CT, arteriography or angiography, IV pyelography, retrograde cystogram, or plain film examination of extremities or other injury sites.

PATIENT CLASSIFICATION

Numerous clinical methods for patient classification are in existence today. For purposes of this chapter, the tools that are pertinent to the trauma population are discussed. The described methodology has many implications in the acute setting: triage of patients, standardization of injury, and prediction of morbidity and mortality. The reader is encouraged to refer to the references for a more extensive review of these tools.

Anatomical Injury Scale (AIS)

Both the Anatomical Injury Scale (AIS)[16] and its spinoff, the Injury Severity Score (ISS),[17] have been recognized as indicators of the magnitude of traumatic injury and as predictors of mortality. The AIS divides the body into six anatomical regions: head/neck, face, thorax, abdomen, extremities, and external (integumentary). Injuries are classified on a sliding scale, with 1 a minor injury and 5 a critical injury with survival uncertain. The anatomical regions with the three highest scores are then squared. The sum is considered the ISS. For example, a patient with a fractured femur, a concussion, and a unilateral pneumothorax would have the following AIS pattern: extremity (AIS = 3), head (AIS = 2), and thorax (AIS = 3). This would equate to an ISS of $(3 \times 3 = 9) + (2 \times 2 = 4) + (3 \times 3 = 9) = 22$. An injury that is classified as *non-survivable* is assigned an AIS = 6, with an automatic score of 75. Civil and Schwab have devised an easy-to-use sheet that can be maintained and updated at the patient's bedside (Tables 44-1 and 44-2).

Trauma Score

The Trauma Score devised by Champion and associates[6] (Table 44-3) is a physiological method of categorizing the multiple trauma patient. It incorporates the Glasgow Coma Scale (GCS), as well as the variables of respiration and circulation. The ranges of the Trauma Score are from a high of 16 and to low of 1. The probability of survival (Table 44-4) can be estimated using the Trauma Score. Other tools

Text continued on p. 800.

Table 44-1   Sample sheet demonstrating use of AIS and Injury Severity Score—Blunt Injury

	1 Minor	2 Moderate	3 Severe: not life-threatening	4 Severe: life-threatening	5 Critical: survival uncertain
Head/neck	Headache/dizziness secondary to head trauma Cervical spine strain with no fracture or dislocation	Amnesia from accident Lethargic/stuporous/obtunded; can be roused by verbal stimuli Unconsciousness <1 hr Simple vault fracture Thyroid contusion Brachial plexus injury Dislocation or fracture spinous or transverse process of C-spine Minor compression fracture (≤20%) C-spine	Unconsciousness 1-6 hrs Unconsciousness <1 hr with neurological deficit Fracture base of skull Comminuted compound or depresed vault fracture Cerebral contusion/subarachnoid hemorrhage Intimal tear/thrombosis carotid A Contusion larynx, pharynx Cervical cord contusion Dislocation or fracture of laminar body, pedicle, or facet of C-spine Compression fracture >1 vertebra or >20% anterior height	Unconsciousness 1-6 hrs with neuro deficit Unconsciousness 6-24 hrs Appropriate response only to painful stimuli Fractured skull with depression >2 cm, torn dura or tissue loss Intracranial hematoma ≤100 cc Incomplete cervical cord lesion Laryngeal crush Intimal tear/thrombosis carotid A with neuro deficit	Unconsciousness with inappropriate movement Unconscious >24 hrs Brainstem injury Intracranial hematoma >100 cc Complete cervical cord lesion C4 or below
Face	Corneal abrasion Sup. tongue laceration Nasal or mandibular ramus* fracture Tooth fracture/avulsion or dislocation	Zygoma, orbit*, body* or subcondylar mandible* fracture LeFort I fracture Scleral/corneal laceration	Optic nerve laceration LeFort II fracture	LeFort III fracture	

*Add AIS 1 to these fractures if open, displaced, or comminuted
†*Add AIS 1 if associated with hemothorax, pneumothorax, or hemopneumomedeastinum*
‡*Add AIS-1 if involving face, hand or genitalia.*
Modified from Civil ID and Schwab CW: J Trauma 28:87, 1988.

Continued.

Table 44-1 Sample sheet demonstrating use of AIS and Injury Severity Score—Blunt Injury—cont'd

		1 Minor	2 Moderate	3 Severe: not life-threatening	4 Severe: life-threatening	5 Critical: survival uncertain
Thorax		Rib fracture† Thoracic spine strain Rib cage contusion Sternal contusion	2-3 rib fractures† Sternum fracture Dislocation or fracture spinous or transverse process T-spine Minor compression fracture (≤20%) T-spine	Lung contusion/lac. ≤ lobe Unilateral h' or p'thorax Diaphragm rupture ≥4 rib fractures† Intimal tear/minor lac/ thrombosis subclavian or innominate A Inhalation burn, minor Dislocation or fracture of laminar body, pedicle, or facet of T-spine Compression fracture >1 vertebra or more than 20% height Cord contusion with transient neurological signs	Multilobar lung contusion or laceration H'p'mediastinum Bilat h'p'thorax Flail chest Myocardial contusion Tension p'thorax Hemothorax >1000 cc Tracheal fracture Intimal aortic tear Major lac subclavian or innominate A Incomplete cord syndrome	Major aortic laceration Cardiac laceration Ruptured bronchus/ trachea Flail chest/inhal burn requiring mechanical support Laryngotrach separation Multilobar lung laceration with tension p'thorax, h'p'mediastinum, or >1000 cc hemothorax Cord laceration or complete cord lesion
Abdomen		Abrasion/contusion, superficial lac scrotum, vagina, vulva, perineum Lumbar spine strain Hematuria	Contusion/sup. laceration stomach, mesentery, SB bladder, ureter, urethra Minor contusion/lacerations kidney, liver, spleen, pancreas Contusion duodenum/colon Dislocation or fracture spinous or transverse process L-spine Minor compression fracture (≤20%) L-spine Nerve root injury	Sup. lac. duodenum/ colon/rectum Perforation SB/mesentery/bladder ureter/ urethra Major contusion/or minor lac. with major vessel invol, or h'periton >1000 cc of kidney/ liver/spleen/panc Minor iliac A or V laceration Retroperitoneal hematoma Dislocation or fracture of laminar body, facet, or pedicle of L-spine Compression fracture >1 vertebra or >20% anterior height Cord contus. with trans neuro signs	Perforation stomach duodenum/ colon/rectum Perforation with tissue loss stomach/bladder SB/ ureter/urethra Major liver laceration Major iliac A or V lac Incomplete cord syndrome Placental abruption	Major lac with tissue loss or gross contamination of duodenum/colon/rectum Complex rupture liver, spleen/kidney/pancreas Complete cord lesion

Table 44-1 Sample sheet demonstrating use of AIS and Injury Severity Score—Blunt Injury—cont'd

	1 Minor	2 Moderate	3 Severe: not life-threatening	4 Severe: life-threatening	5 Critical: survival uncertain
Extremities	Contusion elbow, shoulder, wrist, ankle Fracture/dislocation finger, toe Sprain A-C joint, shoulder, elbow, finger, wrist, hip, ankle, toe	Fracture humerus,* radius,* ulna,* fibula, tibia,* clavicle, scapula, carpals, metacarpals, calcaneus, tarsals, metatarsals, pubic rami, or simple pelvic fracture Dislocation elbow, hand, shoulder, A-C joint Major muscle/tendon lac Intimal tear/minor lac axillary, brachial, popliteal A; axillary, femoral, popliteal V	Comminuted pelvic fracture Fractured femur Dislocation wrist/ankle/knee/hip Below-knee or upper-extremity amputation Ruptured knee ligaments Sciatic nerve laceration Intimal tear/minor lac, femoral A Major lac. ± thrombosis axillary or popliteal A; axillary, popliteal or femoral V	Pelvic crush fracture Traumatic above knee amputation/crush injury Major laceration femoral or brachial artery	Open pelvic crush fracture
External	Abrasions/contusions ≤25 cm on face/hand ≤50 cm on body Superficial lacs ≤5 cm on face/hand ≤10 cm on body 1° burn up to 100% 2° burn/degloving injury <10% total body	Abrasions/contusions >25 cm on face or hand >50 cm on body Laceration >5 cm on face or hand >10 cm on body 2° burn 10%-19% total body‡ 3° burn/degloving injury‡ <20% total body	2° or 3° burn or degloving injury‡ 20%-29% of total body	2° or 3° burn or‡ degloving injury 30%-39% total body	2° or 3° burn or degloving injury 40%-89% total body

AIS = 6	MAXIMAL INJURY AUTOMATICALLY ASSIGNED ISS = 75
HEAD/NECK	Crush fracture, crush/laceration brainstem Decapitation Cord crush/laceration or total transection with or without fracture C3 or above
THORAX	Total severance aorta Chest massively crushed
ABDOMEN	Torso transection
EXTERNAL	2° or 3° burn or degloving injury ≥90% TBS

AIS '85

INJURY SEVERITY SCORE (ISS)		
ISS BODY REGION	**AIS SCORE**	**SQUARED**
HEAD/NECK	_____	_____
FACE	_____	_____
THORAX	_____	_____
ABD/PELVIC CONTENTS	_____	_____
EXTREMITIES/ PELVIC GIRDLE	_____	_____
EXTERNAL	_____	_____
ISS (sum of squares of 3 most severe only)		_____

Table 44-2 Sample sheet demonstrating use of AIS and Injury Severity Score—Penetrating Injury

	1 Minor	2 Moderate	3 Severe: not life-threatening	4 Severe: life-threatening	5 Critical: survival uncertain
Head/neck	PI = PENETRATING INJURY	PI to neck with no organ involvement	Complex PI to neck with tissue loss/organ involvement Minor lac carotid/vertebral A; internal jugular V Transection ± segmental loss jugular V Thyroid laceration Superficial lac larynx/pharynx Cord contusion with transient neurological signs	Minor lac carotid/vertebral A with neurological deficit Transection carotid/vertebral A; int jugular V Segmental loss int jugular vein Perforation larynx/pharynx Cord contusion with incomplete cord syndrome	PI with entrance and exit wounds PI of cerebrum/cerebellum Segmental loss carotid/vertebral A Complex laceration larynx/pharynx Cord laceration Complete cord lesion
Face	PI with no tissue loss	PI with superficial tissue loss Corneal/scleral lac	PI with major tissue loss		
Thorax	PI with no violation of pleural cavity	Thoracic duct laceration Pleural laceration	Complex PI but no violation of the pleural cavity Sup lac innominate/pulmonary/subclavian, and other named smaller veins Sup lac trachea/bronchus/esophagus Lung laceration ≤ lobe Unilateral h' or p'thorax Diaphragmatic laceration Cord contusion with transient neurological signs	Sup aortic laceration Major lac innominate/pulmonary/subclavian and other named smaller art; vena cava/brachiocephalic pulmonary/subclavian and other named smaller veins Transection/tissue loss other named smaller veins Perforation trachea/bronchus esophagus Multilobar lung laceration H'p'mediastinum Bilateral h'p'thorax Tension p'thorax H'thorax >1000 cc Cardiac tamponade Cord contusion with incomplete cord syndrome	Major aortic laceration Transection/segmental loss vena cava/pulmonary/brachiocephalic V and other named smaller arteries Lac trachea/bronchus/esophagus with tissue loss Multilobar lung lac with tension p'thorax/>1000 cc Myocardium/valve laceration Cord laceration Complete cord lesion

Modified from Civil ID and Schwab CW: 28:87, 1988.

Table 44-2   Sample sheet demonstrating use of AIS and Injury Severity Score—Penetrating Injury—cont'd

	1 Minor	2 Moderate	3 Severe: not life-threatening	4 Severe: life-threatening	5 Critical: survival uncertain
Abdomen	PI with no peritoneal penetration	PI with superficial tissue loss but no peritoneal penetration Sup lac stomach/SB/mesentery/bladder/ureter/kidney/liver/spleen/pancreas Laceration through peritoneum	PI with significant tissue loss but no peritoneal penetration Sup lac vena cava/iliac and other named smaller arteries and veins Sup lac duodenum/colon/rectum Full-thickness laceration SB/mesentery/bladder/ureter Major lac or minor lac with major vessel injury/>1000 cc h'peritoneum; kidney/liver/spleen/pancreas Cord contusion with transient neurological signs	Minor aortic laceration Major lac vena cava/iliac A and V and other named smaller arteries and veins Transection/segmental loss iliac and other named smaller veins Full thickness lac stomach/colon/duodenum/rectum Tissue loss/gross contamination stomach/SB/mesentery bladder/ureter Cord contusion with incomplete cord syndrome	Major aortic laceration Transection/segmental loss vena cava/iliac and other named smaller arteries Tissue loss/gross contamination duodenum/colon/rectum Tissue loss kidney/liver spleen pancreas Cord laceration
Extremities	Sup lac brachial and other named veins	Simple PI with no internal structure involvement Sup lac axillary/brachial/popliteal A; axillary/femoral/popliteal V Major lac ± segmental loss brachial vein and other named smaller arteries and veins Lac median/radial/ulnar/femoral/tibial/peroneal N Major tendon/muscle lac	Complex PI with internal structure involvement Sup laceration femoral A Major lac axillary/popliteal A; axillary/femoral/popliteal V Segmental loss axillary/femoral popliteal V Sciatic nerve laceration >1 nerve lac in same extremity Multiple tendon/muscle lacerations in same extremity	Major lac brachial/femoral artery Segmental loss brachial/axillary/popliteal artery	Segmental loss femoral A
External	Superficial laceration ≤5 cm on face or hand ≤10 cm on body PI with no tissue loss	Laceration >5 cm on face or hand >10 cm on body PI with superficial tissue loss			

Continued.

Table 44-2 Sample sheet demonstrating use of AIS and Injury Severity Score—Penetrating Injury—cont'd

		INJURY SEVERITY SCORE (ISS)		
AIS = 6	MAXIMAL INJURY AUTOMATICALLY ASSIGNED ISS = 75	**ISS BODY REGION**	**AIS SCORE**	**SQUARED**
		HEAD/NECK	_____	_____
HEAD/NECK	Brainstem laceration	FACE	_____	_____
THORAX	Aortic transection	THORAX	_____	_____
	Segmental loss aorta/innominate pulmonary/subclavian arteries	ABD/PELVIC CONTENTS	_____	_____
	Complex myocardial laceration	EXTREMITIES/ PELVIC GIRDLE	_____	_____
ABDOMEN	Aortic transection/segmental loss	EXTERNAL	_____	_____
	AIS '85	ISS (sum of squares of 3 most severe only)		_____

Modified from Civil ID and Schwab CW: J Trauma 28:87, 1988.

Table 44-3 Trauma score

Category	Value	Points
A. Respiratory rate	10-24	4
	25-35	3
	>35	2
	<10	1
	0	0
B. Respiratory effort	Normal	1
	Shallow or absent	0
C. Systolic blood pressure	90	4
	70-90	3
	50-69	2
	<50	1
	0	0
D. Capillary refill	Normal	2
	Delayed	1
	None	0
E. Glasgow Coma Scale (GCS)		
1. Eye opening	Spontaneous	4
	To voice	3
	To pain	2
	None	1
2. Verbal response	Oriented	5
	Confused	4
	Inappropriate words	3
	Incomprehensible words	2
	None	1
3. Motor response	Obeys commands	6
	Purposeful movement (pain)	5
	Withdraw (pain)	4
	Flexion (pain)	3
	Extension (pain)	2
	None	1

Total GCS points	Score
14-15	5
11-13	4
8-10	3
5-7	2
3-4	1
TOTAL GCS POINTS _____	TRAUMA SCORE _____
(1 + 2 + 3)	(TOTAL POINTS = A + B + C + D + E)

Modified from Champion HR and others: Crit Care Med 9:672, 1981.

Table 44-4 Probability of survival (Ps) for Trauma Score values

Trauma Score	Ps (%)		
1	2.3	9	61.7
2	6.1	10	66.7
3	6.2	11	75.2
4	14.3	12	80.4
5	21.6	13	90.7
6	31.7	14	95.0
7	38.3	15	97.6
8	52.2	16	99.1

From Champion NR and others: Major trauma outcome study and quality assurance, 64th annual meeting, American College of Surgeons, Committee on Trauma, Ft. Lauderdale, Fla, May 14, 1986.

such as the Trauma Index[12a] have proven less accurate as predictors of injury severity and are used infrequently.

CLINICAL ASSESSMENT

A systematic, head-to-toe approach should be the cornerstone of physical assessment of the multiple trauma patient. Only the most common and severe injuries are discussed in this chapter.

Cranium

Cranial injury is caused in many ways: direct impact, the stationary head striking a relatively stationary object, or a moving object striking a relatively stationary cranium (Fig. 44-1). These mechanisms are referred to as deceleration and acceleration. Likewise, cranial injury can result from indirect forces, for example, a force transmitted through the spinal canal, such as occurs with certain types of falls. Furthermore, cranial injury can be classified as closed (without violation of the cranium and usually the result of blunt injury) or open (violation or fracture of the cranium by either blunt or penetrating mechanisms).

Physical assessment of the cranium should include a visual inspection for bony defects, lacerations, and foreign objects. Scalp lacerations in and of themselves are serious injuries and can result in hypovolemic shock and death. The presence of "raccoon eyes" (periorbital ecchymosis) should be noted and is indicative of basilar skull fracture. Battle's sign, or bruising in the mastoid region, is also indicative of skull fracture.

Head

Concussion. Concussion is usually the result of a low-velocity, blunt injury. Amnesia for the event, brief loss of consciousness, and headache are commonly observed. Recovery is usually brief and without lasting sequelae. Headaches may persist and cognitive function remain impaired for 6 months or longer.

Contusion. Like cerebral concussion, contusion is usually the result of blunt injury. In cerebral contusion there is disruption of the microvascular supply, causing a bruise-like appearance on the brain. Contusions can be minimal or diffuse and are frequently referred to as coup (same side as impact) and/or contrecoup (opposite side of impact). Short to prolonged episodes of mental status depression can occur, as can residual neurological, psychological, and personality defects. Treatment of contusion depends on the degree of injury and can range from symptomatic interventions to assisted hyperventilation to ensure hypocapnia. After lowering the partial pressure of carbon dioxide (PCO_2), a decrease in cerebral edema and intracranial pressure should follow.

Epidural hemorrhage. Epidural hemorrhage is bleeding between the cranium and the dura. It is usually the result of an arterial injury (middle meningeal artery) from a linear skull fracture, although it can be venous in nature. Since the locus is usually arterial, an epidural hemorrhage is considered a rapidly expanding lesion that can depress mental status function, thus requiring prompt surgical intervention. Typically, with this injury the patient will have a period of unconsciousness, followed by a lucid interval and then another period of unconsciousness. Neurological impairment (ipsilateral pupil dilation and contralateral hemiparesis, vomiting, seizures, headaches, and paralysis) can be observed. Loss of consciousness apparently is a significant prognosticator of functional outcome. Hence it is imperative that the prehospital providers be questioned about the patient's neurological state on all admissions so that rapid intervention can be implemented.

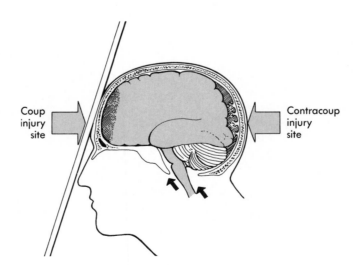

Fig. 44-1 Coup or contrecoup injury. Sudden cessation of forward motion of the skull does not stop the forward motion of the brain. Thus the leading side of the brain can be contused against the skull (coup injury), and the opposite side of the brain can be contused during the succeeding backward motion (contrecoup injury). Both injuries can result in cerebral hemorrhage.

Subdural hemorrhage. Subdural hemorrhage is bleeding between the dural and arachnoid layers of the brain and is usually venous in nature. It can be classified according to the time from the onset of symptoms: acute (24 to 72 hours), subacute (72 hours to 14 days), or chronic. As with cerebral contusion, ipsilateral pupillary dilation and contralateral hemiparesis occur. The mortality rate frequently corresponds inversely to the appearance of symptoms (high mortality rate with acute subdural hemorrhage versus approximately a 10% mortality rate with chronic subdural hemorrhage). Mortality rate is primarily associated with length and level of consciousness on admission. Surgical intervention is required to relieve the mass effect of the bleed.

Intracerebral or brain stem injuries. Intracerebral or brainstem injuries can result from contusion or from direct injury (either blunt or penetrating mechanisms) and can be either venous or arterial in nature. Markedly decreased mental status and neurological function (contralateral hemiparesis and ipsilateral pupil dilation) are usually observed. Level of consciousness on admission has a direct effect on mortality; the mortality rate approaches 50% with an unconscious patient. Secondary brainstem injury can result from increased intracranial pressure (ICP) and herniation. Treatment consists of optimizing cerebral perfusion through ventilatory support, osmotic diuresis, and positioning to facilitate cerebral venous drainage.

Goals of care. The primary goals in caring for the head-injured patient are maintaining adequate oxygenation and implementing measures to decrease intracranial pressure and edema. The arterial partial pressure of oxygen (Pao_2) should be at least 90 mm Hg and the $Paco_2$ should be maintained at 25 to 30 mm Hg to decrease ICP. Cerebral perfusion pressure (CPP = ICP − MAP [mean arterial pressure]) should be kept at 60 to 100 mm Hg. Measures to achieve this effect include endotracheal intubation and mechanical ventilation instituted in patients with depressed levels of consciousness (GCS <12) to maintain airway patency.

Face

Ophthalmological and otoscopic examination should be included in every physical examination. Pupillary reaction and extraocular movement should also be assessed in detail, and a repeat Glasgow Coma Score and a full cranial nerve assessment should be performed. The facial bones should be visually inspected and palpated for defects such as those in LeFort's classification of facial fractures (Table 44-5).

LeFort I fracture. LeFort I, or Guérin's, fractures are horizontal fractures of the maxilla and are the most common of LeFort's classifications.

LeFort II fracture. A LeFort II fracture is an extension of a LeFort I fracture into the orbit, ethmoid, and nasal bones. The cribriform plate is commonly involved, and a cerebrospinal fluid (CSF) leak can be observed. The nasal and auditory canals should be examined for the presence of discharge. The "ring test" should be performed to determine if the discharge is CSF: the fluid is placed on a paper towel and allowed to set; if, when the fluid dries, a double ring is formed, the fluid is considered CSF. The fluid will also have an elevated glucose level.

LeFort III fracture. In LeFort III fracture, there is independent movement of the cranial and facial bones (craniofacial separation). CSF leaks frequently occur with these fractures, as does airway obstruction. Oral intubation should not be attempted, because it is frequently unsuccessful. Airway control should be used through surgical intervention (cricothyroidostomy).

The oropharynx and mouth should be inspected for foreign bodies, loose or weakened teeth, malocclusion, and glossal injury. The neck is examined first for obvious external injury. As previously mentioned, the victim of traumatic injury is assumed to have a bony abnormality of the cervical spine, along with the potential for spinal cord damage, until proven otherwise. The cervical vertebrae should be palpated for changes in the curvature or a "step-off" (change in vertebral continuity). Tenderness and spasm also

Table 44-5 LeFort's classification of facial fractures

Fracture	Clinical presentation	Surgical approach
LeFort I (transverse)	Pain in upper jaw, numb upper teeth, midfacial edema, ecchymosis, epistaxis, malocclusion, mobile maxillary dentition	Disimpaction, fixation with skull cap, or internal fixation to pyriform margin
LeFort II (pyramidal)	Pain in midface; numb upper lip, lower lid, and lateral nasal area; midfacial edema; ecchymosis; epistaxis; malocclusion; mobile midface; nasal flattening; anesthesia in infraorbital nerve territory	Disimpaction, fixation with suspension to solid structure above fracture
LeFort III (craniofacial dysjunction)	Pain in face, airway obstruction, "donkey-face" deformity, malocclusion, mobile face, marked facial edema and ecchymosis, epistaxis, cerebral spinal fluid, rhinorrhea.	Fixation and cranial suspension to wire fixation at frontal bones; direct wiring through brow incisions, nasoorbital incisions

Modified from Trunkey DD and Lewis FR: Current therapy of trauma, vol 2, Philadelphia, 1986, Brian C Decker, Publisher.

warrant further examination. The patient with penetrating injury to the neck requies surgical exploration in most cases.

Goals of care. Soft-tissue injuries of the face caused by either blunt or penetrating mechanisms always present a challenge to the practitioner. Aggressive airway management should be instituted. Cervical spine injury should also be suspected in the patient with facial trauma. Placement of tubes (nasogastric, nasotracheal) into the nasal orifice should be discouraged, since violation of the cribriform plate could result in its cranial placement. Likewise, orotracheal intubation should not be considered in the patient with massive facial injuries, since successful attempts are a rarity. Airway management should be instituted through placement of the surgical airway or cricothyroidostomy. Surgical intervention is required for all of these facial fractures. Prevention of infection and addressing the alterations in body image should also be of concern with these patients.

Thorax

The Edwin Smith Papyrus, written between 3000 and 1600 BC, documents 48 cases of traumatic injury, of which one was a penetrating injury to the sternum.[9] Most open wounds to the chest were mortal in those times, a fact that remained unchanged through the nineteenth century. As recently as the Franco-Prussian War, (late 1870s), mortality rates from chest wounds were greater than 55%. Dramatic advances were made during both the Korean and Vietnam Wars; however, traumatic injury to the thorax currently results in a 25% mortality rate because of the organ systems involved.[12] When the indirect effects of thoracic injury are factored into place, an additional 25% mortality can be included.[12] The average length of stay for a patient with thoracic injury requiring hospital admission, observation, and tube thoracostomy (chest tubes) is 3 days. If the patient requires thoracotomy, the length of stay is almost quadrupled. These injuries can be equally devastating *without* thoracotomy, as is seen in the patient with a flail chest. The majority of these patients may never return to work or will have a disability that prevents their returning to their previous occupation.

Thoracic injuries can be classified using the system established by the American College of Surgeons (ACS).[1] *Immediately life-threatening* thoracic injuries include pericardial tamponade, massive hemothorax, tension pneumothorax, open pneumothorax (sucking chest wound), and flail chest. *Potentially life-threatening* thoracic injuries include pulmonary contusion, aortic disruption, diaphragmatic hernia, tracheobronchial disruption, myocardial contusion.

Injury to the thorax occurs as a result of either blunt, penetrating, or blast mechanisms. Blunt injury accounts for the majority of thoracic injuries and predominantly occurs secondary to motor vehicle accidents. Sudden deceleration of the human body commonly results in parenchymal injury to the lung. In addition, shearing of vessels from fixed structures such as with the aorta's tearing from the ligamentum arteriosum (Fig. 44-2), and/or compression of intrathoracic structures can occur (Fig. 44-3). Secondary intrathoracic or intraabdominal injury can occur from rib or sternal fractures.

Penetrating injury can result from use of a variety of

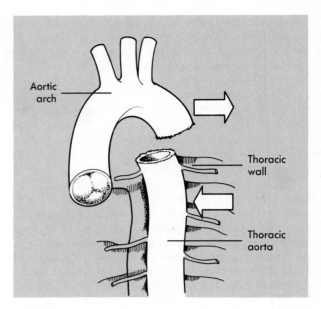

Fig. 44-2 Laceration of the aortic arch can result when the upper portion of the arch is thrust forward during acute deceleration because it is free to move while the lower portion of the arch remains stationary because it is fixed to the posterior thoracic wall.

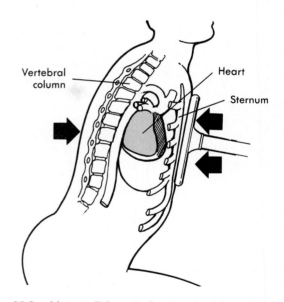

Fig. 44-3 Myocardial contusions and rupture can result when, during sudden impact, the heart is compressed between the sternum and the veterbral column.

weapons, including handguns, shotguns, rifles, and knives. Weapons are commonly classified by velocity—either low, medium, or high. Examples of these weapons are listed below.

1. *Low velocity* (less than 1000 feet/second): handguns, knives, spears, and arrows.
2. *Medium velocity* (1000 to 2000 feet/second): civilian weaponry (.357 Magnum, .44 Magnum).
3. *High velocity:* (>2200 feet/second): military weaponry (Russian AK-47, M-16, M-14).

Finally, indirect forces such as the blast mechanism can result in thoracic injury that frequently involves the pulmonary parenchyma, resulting, for example, in pulmonary contusion and adult respiratory distress syndrome (ARDS). When assessing the trauma patient, the clinician's knowledge about the causative mechanism will assist him or her in the classification, diagnosis, and treatment of thoracic injury.

Specific Thoracic Injuries

Pericardial tamponade. The pericardial sac is a fixed, fibrous structure, normally containing approximately 20 to 30 ml of serous fluid. When myocardial trauma and injury occur, it is imperative that the possibility of cardiac tamponade be addressed. As bleeding into the pericardial sac occurs, the sac fills to a point and then can no longer expand. As the bleeding continues, the pressure of the blood in the pericardial sac compresses the heart. Attempts to correct this deficiency by increasing the heart rate and contractility are often effective but temporary since the bleeding within the pericardial sac will further depress ventricular filling. Eventually, the right atrial pressure increases, enlarging the pressure gradient between the right atrium and right ventricle and is termed *pulsus paradoxus*. The clinical signs of pericardial tamponade are listed below.

Signs	*Description*
Pulsus paradoxus	Drop in systolic blood pressure of more than 10 mm Hg during inspiration
Muffled heart sounds	Result from increased pericardial fluid
Neck vein distention	Reflects increase in right atrial pressure, usually in excess of 15 mm Hg
Narrowed pulse pressure	Difference between systolic and diastolic pressure readings (normally 40 mm Hg; will be less than 30 mm Hg in pericardial tamponade)

The combination of muffled or distant heart sounds, neck vein distention, and narrowed pulse pressure is commonly referred to as *Beck's triad*. Not every patient with pericardial tamponade will exhibit these findings, which may be present in various combinations. The treatment of pericardial tamponade consists of relieving the congestion through either pericardiocentesis or creation of a pericardial window.

Massive hemothorax. Massive hemothorax indicates intrapleural blood volumes exceeding 1500 ml and is usually a result of penetrating injury. Percussion of the chest will elicit dullness along with a decrease in audible breath sounds on the side of injury. Hypotension, respiratory distress, and tracheal shift to the opposite side of injury occur, with great vessel or parenchymal lung injury usually responsible. Insertion of large-bore IV lines and placement of large-bore chest tubes should be initiated in the emergency department before surgical intervention.

Tension pneumothorax. Tension pneumothorax results when atmospheric air enters the pleural space during inhalation and does not escape during exhalation. The consequence is a buildup of volume and pressure in the pleural space. When this buildup is not relieved, a mediastinal shift is inevitable. Percussion of the thorax will produce a hyperresonant sound. Hypotension, alterations in breathing patterns, and tracheal deviation away from the pneumothorax or site of injury are the common symptoms.

Treatment of tension pneumothorax consists of decompression of the pleural space, which can be accomplished by inserting a large-bore needle (18 gauge) into the second or third intercostal space at the midclavicular line. A hissing sound should be heard as the tension pneumothorax is converted to a simple pneumothorax. A chest tube should then be placed, and surgical intervention should be considered, depending on the primary cause.

Open pneumothorax. Open pneumothorax ("sucking chest wound") is created when there is a communication between the atmosphere and the intrapleural space. A tension pneumothorax allows air to enter during inhalation and *not* during exhalation; the open pneumothorax allows free air passage during both inhalation and exhalation. Air preferentially moves through any opening that is approximately two thirds the diameter of the trachea (1.8 cm). With an open pneumothorax, air moves through the defect in the chest wall during inhalation, thus bypassing the trachea. Unless this situation is rapidly corrected, the patient will succumb to tissue hypoxia. Treatment consists of placing a nonocclusive dressing that is taped on three sides of the wound. It will prevent air's entering during inhalation yet will allow air to escape during exhalation. Should the patient develop respiratory distress, the dressing should be "burped" to express any accumulation of air. A large-bore chest tube should also be placed distal to the site to allow for lung reexpansion.

Flail chest. Flail chest is usually the result of blunt trauma and commonly occurs in the unrestrained occupant of a motor vehicle whose chest becomes crushed under extreme force. The average 70-kg occupant involved in a motor vehicle accident at 40 to 50 miles per hour produces approximately 25,000 pounds of pressure per square inch on contact with the interior of the vehicle. The majority of this energy is imparted to the thorax. Rib and/or sternal fractures usually occur. The thoracic cage is considered a "ring" structure. When subjected to external forces, structures such as rings will break in more than one place; on careful examination, a contralateral break is usually apparent (this can be demonstrated by attempting to break a hard, rounded pretzel between the thumb and third finger). When two or more ribs are injured in two or more places, a flail, or "free-floating," segment occurs, and underlying great vessel, myocardial, or pulmonary injury can result. This free-floating segment moves inward during inhalation and outward during exhalation (paradoxical breathing), leading to hypoxemia, tissue hypoxia, and respiratory failure. Negative and positive intrathoracic pressures are altered, and the resulting pain causes a decrease in tidal volume. A mediastinal shift toward the uninjured side results in a decrease in preload, thus decreasing cardiac output.

Treatment is centered on stabilizing the flail segment (usually with ventilatory support), allowing adequate exchange of oxygen and carbon dioxide and pain relief. External support of the flail segment with sterile towel clips around the flail segment are currently seldom used. Maintaining the Pao_2 greater than 60 mm Hg on room air, the respiratory rate at 12 to 24 breaths per minute, and a tidal volume of at least 10 ml per kilogram of body weight ensures aerobic tissue metabolism. If the patient develops respiratory distress or has either preexisting cardiac or pulmonary disease or acute head or orthopedic injuries, controlled ventilation should be instituted. It would also allow internal splinting through the use of positive end-expiratory pressure (PEEP) and intermittent mandatory ventilation (IMV) modalities. Pain control can be achieved through various routes such as IV, epidural, or intercostal analgesia and/or transcutaneous electrical nerve stimulation (TENS). Since an underlying injury such as pulmonary contusion may be present, fluid administration should be conservative. Diagnostic studies to detect either myocardial or great vessel trauma should be implemented.

Pulmonary contusion. Pulmonary contusion, a bruising of pulmonary parenchyma, is the most common sequela of thoracic trauma. It can be seen with or without a flail chest. Children rarely present with a flail chest because of the flexibility of their rib cage. Treatment of pulmonary contusion is based on the same goal as that of flail chest— ensuring adequate oxygenation. Since intraalveolar and interstitial edema occur, lower airway obstruction can result. Use of IV fluid therapy should be minimized, except in the presence of hypovolemic shock, to prevent noncardiogenic pulmonary edema. Adequate oxygenation can be achieved either through assisted or spontaneous respiratory mechanisms. The parameters for nonintubation include:

- PaO_2 >60 mm Hg on 0.50 fraction of inspired oxygen (FIO_2)
- Respiratory rate of <24 and >12
- Spontaneous tidal volume of >5 ml/kg of body weight
- Voluntary vital capacity of >10 ml/kg of body weight

Although pulmonary contusion differs from ARDS in that contusion occurs within minutes of the injury, the latter is a commonly associated sequela.

Aortic disruption. Injuries to the aorta can occur through either a blunt or a penetrating mechanism and predominantly result from motor vehicle accidents. Unfortunately, 80% to 90% of patients with aortic injury will not reach the hospital with signs of life.

The ascending aorta is a fairly mobile structure, and the descending aorta is fixed, resulting in the shearing effects commonly seen with acute deceleration (see Fig. 44-2). Common sites for aortic disruption are the ligamentum arteriosum, the innominate artery fork, the diaphragm, and the area superior to the aortic valve annulus.

Aortic disruption can manifest the following signs:

- Anterior or posterior thoracic pain
- Hoarseness or stridor
- Dysphagia
- Upper-extremity hypertension
- Lower-extremity hypotension
- Paraplegia
- Hypovolemic shock

Radiographic evidence on an upright anterior-posterior view includes the following:

- Widening of the superior mediastinum
- Loss of the aortic knob
- Pleural capping (left apical hematoma)
- Tracheal deviation to the right

- Esophageal deviation to the right
- Depression of left mainstem bronchus
- Elevation of the right mainstem bronchus

Aortic injury should be highly suspected if the following are present:

- Thoracic spine fracture
- Multiple left rib fractures
- Scapular fractures
- Sternal fractures
- Fracture of rib 1, 2, or 3

The diagnosis of aortic injury is confirmed by aortography; once it is confirmed, surgical intervention is mandated.

Diaphragmatic injury. The diaphragm is a large muscular band that serves as an anatomical separation between the thoracic and abdominal cavities and facilitates ventilation. Anatomically, the diaphragm rises to the fourth intercostal space (level of fourth rib on the right, fifth on the left). Blunt or penetrating injury can result in herniation of the diaphragm. If the injury results from blunt trauma, the patient will relate a history of rapid deceleration, most commonly occurring when an unrestrained driver of an automobile crashes against a steering wheel or when a backseat passenger, restrained by a lapbelt apparatus (without shoulder harness), decelerates against the belt. Direct injury to the abdomen (crush injuries, falls) can also result in herniation.

The first record of a diaphragmatic injury is attributed to Sennertus in 1541, and the injury occurred after a penetrating chest wound.[20] Diaphragmatic injuries from penetrating trauma are usually the result of gunshot or stab wounds. The majority of diaphragmatic injuries occur on the left side (85%) because the liver protects the diaphragm on the right. Penetrating mechanisms usually produce small rents in the diaphragm, whereas blunt injury causes larger, linear tears.

The diagnosis of diaphragmatic injury is rarely obvious. This injury should be highly suspected in patients with penetrating injuries to the anterior thoracoabdominal regions and with deceleration injuries. It should also be suspected in patients with lower rib fracture and hemothorax or lower lobe pulmonary contusion. Radiographic evaluation may reveal gastric contents in the thorax (for example, a nasogastric tube may be visualized, or the hemidiaphragm may be elevated). The patient may complain of sharp shoulder pain and increasing respiratory distress. Laparotomy is indicated for all patients, regardless of the mechanism. If the herniation is discovered during thoracotomy for penetrating thoracic injury, intraabdominal involvement should be expected and a laparotomy anticipated. Use of the pneumatic antishock garment is not recommended for hypotensive patients with diaphragmatic injury because it may enlarge the tear, forcing abdominal contents into the thoracic cavity and further impeding respiration and circulation.

Tracheobronchial injury. Seuvre,[20] in 1873, reported the first case of traumatic bronchial rupture. Sanger[19] performed the first successful suture of a bronchial laceration in 1945, and Beskin[5] repaired a complete rupture of the trachea in 1957. As a result of anatomical position, both the esophagus and trachea can be injured by blunt or penetrating mechanisms. Sudden increases in intrathoracic pressure against a closed glottis, massive blows to the chest (for example, in rapid deceleration), and direct injury are common causes of tracheobronchial injury.

Pain is usually present and is accompanied by severe respiratory distress and upper airway obstruction. Subcutaneous emphysema, pneumothorax, associated rib fractures, hoarseness, dysphagia, stridor, and hemorrhage may occur. Radiographic signs include pneumomediastinum, pneumothorax, free intraperitoneal air, retroesophageal air, and peribronchial air. Contrast radiography and flexible endoscopy are most commonly used for confirmation of the diagnosis. Decompression of the thorax through a chest tube and direct repair through thoracotomy are indicated.

Goals of care. Nursing care of the patient with intrathoracic injuries centers on maintenance of the process of ventilation (ensuring, when possible, adequate exchange of carbon dioxide and oxygen) and circulation. Providing adequate analgesia is essential for the patient with flail chest. Constant reassessment for "missed injuries" is essential regardless of the body system involved.

Abdomen

Intraabdominal injury can occur with either blunt or penetrating mechanisms. The majority of blunt abdominal injuries results from motor vehicle accidents. Numerous landmarks have been proposed for separating the intraabdominal and intrathoracic regions. Since thoracic and abdominal injuries frequently coincide, examination should focus on the entire thoracoabdominal region.

When determining the mechanisms of blunt injury, especially in victims of motor vehicle accidents, occupant location and restraint status are two of the most important areas to be probed. In the front-seat passenger, hepatic injury should be suspected when the point of impact is on the same side as the passenger. Likewise, a driver should be assessed for injury to the spleen in an impact on the driver's side. Use of the lapbelt, without shoulder harness, is associated with distal thoracic and proximal lumbar spine fractures (T12 to L2). In penetrating mechanisms, determining the size, shape, and configuration of the object, as well as the position of the assailant and victim, adds valuable information to the assessment.

Assessment. Unlike most instances, determining injury to a specific abdominal organ is a secondary goal that falls behind determining the need for surgical intervention. Using the components of an accurate history and physical examination, surgical need can be determined. The first component of the examination is the visual appearance. Entrance and exit wounds from penetrating objects or bruising from blunt injury should be investigated. In victims of motor vehicle accidents the area of bruising usually documents the anatomical area that absorbed the force.

The presence of bowel sounds should be documented and compared with results at a later examination. Should bowel sounds be present on admission and disappear on later physical examination, peritoneal irritation should be suspected. One of the hallmarks of the abdominal examination is the presence of pain. The examiner should keep in mind that "guarding" and abdominal pain do not occur until peritoneal irritation is present. Rebound tenderness is also a sensitive

predictor of peritoneal irritation. Additional methods for detecting peritoneal irritation (through external transmission of force) include shaking the bed, percussion of the heel while the knee is locked, "pelvic rocking" of the iliac crests, and asking the patient to cough.[15]

Laboratory analysis. Results from laboratory analysis in the patient with acute abdominal injury can be nonspecific. Leukocytosis in the early stage is usually the result of either splenic or hepatic injury. Infection will also cause elevation of the white blood count (WBC); however, this elevation does not occur for at least 4 hours after injury. Hemoglobin and hematocrit results may not reflect actual values as a result of hemoconcentration.

Radiographic studies. Radiographic examination of the abdomen includes the supine plain film, upright chest film, and retrograde cystogram. If invasive radiography is being used to document extraabdominal injury (for example, aortic injury), an intravenous pyelogram (IVP) can be obtained during arteriography to assess for genitourinary injury. The chest film is useful in detecting diaphragmatic injury, whereas the abdominal film is primarily used to detect the missile tracks of penetrating trauma. It is important to localize all bullets before surgical intervention. Missiles that enter one body region may terminate in another.

Computerized tomography and peritoneal lavage. Additional means of abdominal assessment are computerized tomography (CT) and diagnostic peritoneal lavage. The reported sensitivity or specificity and accuracy of both of these methods are similar. Diagnostic peritoneal lavage is of limited use because it is not organ specific and cannot discriminate retroperitoneal blood from peritoneal injury in pelvic fracture. Likewise, CT is of limited use because performing it requires a hemodynamically stable patient. Therefore, diagnostic peritoneal lavage is indicated for patients with questionable intraabdominal pathology who exhibit hemodynamic instability or those patients in whom CT cannot be performed for physical reasons.

The diagnostic peritoneal lavage is performed through an incision through the skin to the peritoneum. A small catheter is placed through a small opening into the peritoneum. Use of bladder decompression through urethral catheterization and gastric decompression through a nasogastric or orogastric tube is imperative to prevent secondary trauma. If gross blood is visualized on entering the peritoneal cavity, the procedure is aborted, and the patient is immediately transported to the surgical suite. If gross blood is not initially encountered, rapid infusion of either 1 L of lactated Ringer's solution or physiological solution of sodium (0.9% normal saline solution) is indicated (in the pediatric patient 10 ml of fluid per kilogram of body weight is infused). The IV bag is then placed in a dependent position and allowed to drain. The inability to read newspaper print through the bag is considered a positive result. This crude but accurate method detects the subtle cloudiness of blood or other contaminant in the diagnostic peritoneal fluid. Likewise, a WBC >500 high power frequency (hpf), red blood count (RBC) >100,000/hpf, or the presence of bile, bacteria, or gastric contents is criteria for further exploration.

Spleen. The spleen remains the organ most commonly injured by blunt trauma and is second only to the liver as a source of life-threatening hemorrhage. Traditionally, splenic injury resulted in splenectomy, although currently the emphasis is shifting to splenorraphy when possible. The incidence of postsplenectomy sepsis is approximately 3%, with a mortality rate that approaches 50%. Therefore, as long as the spleen is not pulverized, attempts at repair should be made. Contraindications for repair include the presence in a patient of prolonged, severe hypotension or of a major associated injury, either intraabdominal or extraabdominal. Such a patient should not have prolonged attempts at splenic repair. Pneumococcal vaccination (Pneumovax) should be instituted after splenectomy.

Physical examination of the patient manifesting splenic injury reveals diffuse abdominal tenderness for peritoneal irritation. Kehr's sign (pain in the left shoulder) is also indicative of splenic injury. Complicating the assessment are adjacent injuries such as multiple rib fractures or posterior penetrating injuries that can easily be missed. Diagnosis of splenic injury is accomplished either through peritoneal lavage or CT.

Liver. The liver is the second most commonly injured organ in blunt trauma and the primary organ injured with penetrating mechanisms. Hemoperitoneum and severe hypotension commonly occur in the presence of hepatic injury. Detection of this injury, as in all intraabdominal pathology, is accomplished through the combination of physical assessment and the use of diagnostic peritoneal lavage or CT. Once the diagnosis of hepatic injury has been established, surgical therapy can usually correct the defect in the majority of cases. In massive injuries, resection of devitalized tissue is mandated. Occasionally, ligation of one of the hepatic arteries or veins is necessary to control the hemorrhage. Postoperative care is directed toward volume replacement, correction of coagulation defects, and nutritional enhancement.

Duodenum, small bowel, and colon. Injuries to the duodenum, small bowel, and colon are usually the result of penetrating mechanisms. The patient who sustains hollow viscus injury from blunt trauma presents a diagnostic dilemma and requires careful abdominal assessment. The combination of physical examination, laboratory studies (amylase, CBC), and peritoneal lavage or abdominal CT should prevent these injuries' going undetected. Resection and direct repair are routine surgical interventions.

Pelvic Fractures

Like the thoracic cage, the pelvis is considered a ring structure. Thus, since a ring will typically break not only on the side of injury but also on its contralateral side, the patient with pelvic injury should be examined for opposing breaks. Areas with injuries associated with pelvic fractures include the abdominal viscera, perineum, retroperitoneum, and the lower extremity. The mortality rate from pelvic fractures ranges from less than 10% in patients with a simple, isolated, closed fracture to approximately 50% in patients with an open pelvic fracture. Classic signs of pelvic fracture include perineal ecchymosis (testicular or labial), pain on palpation or "rocking" of the iliac crests, and obvious deformity. Diagnostic tests include plain film examination of the pelvis, CT angiography (for diagnosis of iliac

vessel injury and to control hemorrhage), and cystourethrography (to detect for genitourinary injury). Major pelvic fractures should be ruled out before obtaining an upright chest film in the hemodynamically stable patient, since worsening of the stability of the fracture and increasing vascular injury can occur.

A major complicaiton of pelvic fractures is hemorrhage. Treatment usually involves a combination of the use of a pneumatic antishock garment, fluid and blood component replacement, vessel embolizaiton, and surgical reduction of the fracture(s). Although surgical intervention is usually necessary, some minor fractures are treated with bed rest. Application of an external fixation device allows early mobilization of the patient and assists in the prevention of deep vein thrombophlebitis and pulmonary complications.

Femoral Fractures

The patient with a femoral fracture will initially have pain in the extremity although he or she may not necesarily have an obvious deformity. Obtaining a careful history about the mechanism of injury should alert the clinician to this possibility. Depending on the severity of injury, surgical intervention may be required. Like pelvic fractures, fractures of the femur are associated with major hemorrhagic complications. Other complications of femoral fracture include avascular necrosis of the femoral head, malunion, rejection of fixation devices, and refracture.

SUMMARY

The care of the multiple trauma patient is based on lessons learned not only from the American military experience, but the experiences of the Egyptians and Romans many years ago. On June 21, 1876, 4 days before the Battle of Little Big Horn, James DeWolf, physician to General Custer, made the following observation: "I think it is very clear that we shall not see an Indian this summer."[18a] This serves to demonstrate that a decision based solely on one observation can prove to be detrimental. Such is the case when caring for patients with traumatic injury. These patients demand constant reassessment of their injuries, as well as the possible detection of "missed" injuries. An organized, aggressive approach is essential to achieving a favorable outcome in these patients.

REFERENCES

1. Advanced Trauma Life Support Text, Chicago, 1984, American College of Surgeons.
2. American Association for Automotive Medicine: The abbreviated injury scale (AIS), Morton Grove, Ill, 1985, The Association.
3. Baker SP and O'Neill B: The injury severity score: an update, J Trauma 16:882, 1976.
4. Baker SP, O'Neill B and Karpf RS: The injury fact book, Lexington, Mass, 1984, DC Heath & Co.
5. Beskin CA: Rupture separation of the cervical trachea following a closed chest injury, J Thorac Surg 34:392, 1957.
6. Champion HR and others: Trauma score, Crit Care Med 9:672, 1981.
6A. Collicott PE: Initial assessment of the trauma patient. In Mattox KL, Moore EE, and Feliciano DV, editors: Trauma, Norwalk, Conn, 1988, Appleton & Lange.

7. Committee on Trauma of the American College of Surgeons: Hospital and prehospital care of the injured patient, Am Coll Surg Bull 68:10, 1983.

8. Committee on Trauma Research, Commission of Life Sciences, National Research Council, and the Institute of Medicine: Injury in America: a continuing public health problem, Washington, DC, 1985, National Academy Press.

9. Davis JH: History of trauma. In Matox KL, Moore EE, and Feliciano, DV, editors: Trauma, Norwalk, Conn, 1988, Appleton & Lange.

10. Hau T: The surgical practice of Dominique Jean Larrey, Surg Gynecol Obstet 154:89, 1982.

11. Hunter J: A treatise on the blood, inflammation, and gunshot wounds, Birmingham, England, 1982, LB Adams.

12. Jones KW: Thoracic trauma, Surg Clin North Am 60:957, 1980.

12A. Kirkpatrick JR and Youmans RL: Trauma index: an aide in the evaluation of injury victims, J Trauma 11:711, 1971.

13. Madding GF, Lawrence KD, and Kennedy DA: Forward surgery of the severely injured, Second Aux Surg Group 1:307, 1942.

14. McSwain NE: Patient assessment and initial management. In McSwain NE and Kerstein MD, editors: Evaluation and management of trauma, Norwalk, Conn, 1987, Appleton-Century-Crofts.

15. McSwain NE: Abdominal trauma. In McSwain NE and Kerstein MD, editors: Evaluation and management of trauma, Norwalk, Conn, 1987, Appleton-Century-Crofts.

16. National Safety Council: Accident facts, Chicago, 1985, The Council.

17. O'Neill B: Biomechanics of trauma, Norwalk, Conn, 1984, Appleton & Lange.

18. Prehospital Trauma Life Support Text, Educational Training, Akron, Ohio, 1986, Emergency Training.

18A. Rich NM: Missile injuries, Am J Surgery 139:414, 1980.

19. Sanger PW: Evacuation hospital experience with war wounds and injuries of the chest, Ann Surg 122:147, 1945.

20. Seuvre M: Crushing injury from wheel of omnibus: rupture of the right bronchus, Bull Soc Anat (Paris) 48:680, 1873.

21. Trunkey DD: Reflections of our origins. In Najarian JS and Delaney JP, editors: Trauma and critical care surgery, Chicago, 1987, Year Book Medical Publishers, Inc.

22. Trunkey DD: Torso trauma: an overview. In Trunkey DD and Lewis FR, editors: Current therapy of trauma, Philadelphia, 1986, Brian C Decker, Publisher.

23. Trunkey DD: Trauma, Sci Am 249:28, 1983.

24. Unkle DW, Clements CP, and Ross SE: Osmolality as a predictor of intoxication in the trauma patient: usefulness in clinical practice, unpublished manuscript. Proceedings from the Second Annual Nursing Symposium: Management of Multiple Trauma and Burns, Cleveland, Ohio, May 19-20, 1988.

25. Walt AJ: Trauma. In Mattox KL, Moore EE, and Feliciano DV, editors: Trauma, Norwalk, Conn, 1988, Appleton & Lange.

CHAPTER

45

Anaphylaxis

CHAPTER OBJECTIVES

- *Describe the basic mechanism for initiation of the immune response for both anaphylactic and anaphylactoid reactions.*
- *List and explain the triad of physiological effects that occur in patients with anaphylaxis.*
- *List at least two causative agents of anaphylaxis from each of the following categories: medications, food, chemicals, and animal stings or bites.*
- *Describe distributive shock, using anaphylactic shock as an example.*
- *Identify three nursing diagnoses and interventions relevant to the care of the patient experiencing anaphylaxis.*

Millions of Americans have a history of systemic or localized reactions to a variety of substances such as penicillin or bee stings. Each year an estimated 50 deaths result from bee-sting anaphylaxis. Allergic reactions to insect stings occur in approximately 0.4% of the population each year.[16,20] The realization that most anaphylaxis-related deaths occur within the *first 30 minutes* after exposure to the foreign antigen stresses the need for prompt intervention.

DESCRIPTION

Anaphylaxis is a potentially life-threatening allergic reaction. It is described as a hypersensitivity reaction to an invading substance *(antigen)* that causes release of powerful vasoactive substances such as histamine and bradykinin into the bloodstream. The somatic responses to the vasoactive substance release include bronchospasm, generalized edema, hypotension, urticaria, and hives (Fig. 45-1).

Allergic reactions are categorized into four types, because their pathogenesis cannot be attributed to one mechanism (Table 45-1). Of greatest importance for this discussion is type I, also known as an anaphylactic reaction. As defined by Gell, Coombs, and Lachman,[10] *true anaphylactic reactions* (type I) occur only when immunoglobulin E (IgE)

reacts with an antigen in a *previously sensitized person.* IgE is a type of antibody that is produced in response to a specific antigen; it remains inactive until rechallenged by that same antigen.

In contrast, *anaphylactoid reactions* (types II to IV), when triggered, produce allergic reactions through nonimmunologically (nonIgE) mediated mechanisms. Anaphylactoid reactions are produced in persons *not previously sensitized* and can occur with the first exposure to an antigen such as radiopaque dye or medication.

Vasoactive substances will, however, be liberated (with similar clinical results) in both cases. Patients with either anaphylactic or anaphylactoid reactions can manifest all of the life-threatening signs of anaphylactic shock.[17] The terms anaphylaxis and hypersensitivity reaction are used interchangeably in this chapter.

CAUSE

Almost any substance can cause a hypersensitivity reaction. Such a substance, also known as antigen, is usually introduced by injection or by ingestion and is less commonly introduced through the skin or the respiratory tract. The most common offenders are listed in the box on p. 810.

Many medications, including opiates, dextran, muscle relaxants, antibiotics, thiamine, and iodinated radiocontrast media, can cause a hypersensitivity reaction.[16] Patients become sensitive to penicillin more than to any other antibiotic. It is estimated that three of every 2000 patients without known sensitivity will develop some allergic symptoms while taking penicillin. One fatality occurs for every 100,000 persons taking penicillin.[2,16,24]

The most commonly used radiocontrast medium is a hyperosmolarity thiiodinatobenzoate such as diatrizoate or metrizoate.[13] Approximately 1.7% of patients undergoing radiocontrast procedures develop anaphylactoid symptoms. It is estimated that one fatality occurs for every 50,000 intravenous pyelograms (IVPs).[2] Recently, low osmolarity radiocontrast media (for example, iopamidol) have been developed that produce fewer side effects and that have been shown, in vitro, to produce less basophilic histamine release. It is hoped that these low osmolarity agents will

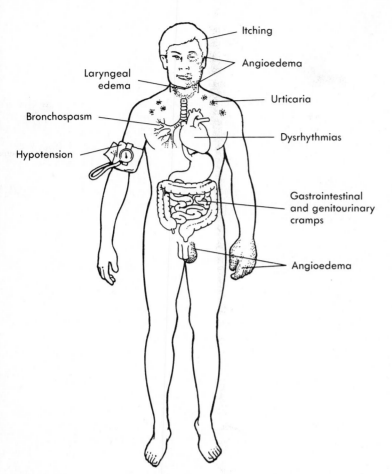

Itching

Angioedema

Laryngeal edema

Urticaria

Bronchospasm

Dysrhythmias

Hypotension

Gastrointestinal and genitourinary cramps

Angioedema

Fig. 45-1 Clinical manifestations of anaphylaxis. Laryngeal edema, bronchospasm, and hypotension are the major contributors to patient morbidity and mortality. (From Price S and Wilson L: Pathophysiology: clinical concepts of disease processes, ed 3, St Louis, 1986, The CV Mosby Co.)

decrease the incidence of anaphylactoid reactions.

Virtually every food has been known to cause a hypersensitivity reaction. The incidence of food allergies in children ranges from 0.3% to 7.5%.[16] Anaphylaxis generally occurs in the sensitized person within minutes of ingestion of the offending food.

Many clinical reactions to insect stings and food have been considered strictly immunologically mediated (IgE), requiring presensitization to the offending substance. However, literature describing allergic reactions to these substances on the patient's first exposure suggest that a non–IgE-mediated cause may account for the immediate hypersensitivity and anaphylaxis.[16,18,27,35]

PATHOPHYSIOLOGY

The mast cell and the basophil are the primary effector cells for anaphylaxis. Mast cells are found in the connective tissue of all organs, particularly in small blood vessels. Basophils (a form of white blood cell) circulate in the bloodstream. Both type I (IgE) anaphylactic reactions and types

Table 45-1 Classification of allergic reactions by Gell and associates

Type	Synonyms	Antibody	Complement	Effector cells	Chemical mechanism	Examples
I	Anaphylactic Immediate hypersensitivity	IgE	Not involved	Mast cells Basophils	Antigen or allergen binds to IgE on the surface of mast cells and basophils with release of mast-cell products.	Anaphylaxis Cutaneous wheal and flare Extrinsic asthma
II	Cytotoxic	IgG IgM	Fixed and activated	Polymorphonuclear cells	IgG or IgM binds to allergen on cell membranes; complement system is activated with cellular destruction.	Transfusion reactions Hemolytic anemia Rh disease
III	Immune complex	IgG IgM	Fixed and activated	Polymorphonuclear cells	IgG or IgM binds to allergen in the fluid phase and deposits in small blood vessels; complement system is activated with cellular destruction.	Serum sickness Glomerulonephritis Arthus reactions
IV	Delayed hypersensitivity Cell-mediated immunity	Not involved	Not involved	Thymus-derived lymphocytes	Sensitized cells bind to allergen and release, on activation, effectors known as lymphokines.	Contact dermatitis Tuberculin immunity

Modifed from Levy JH and others: Spine 11(3):283, 1986.

CAUSES OF ANAPHYLAXIS

ANIMAL STINGS AND BITES

Order Hymenoptera: honeybees, yellow jackets, New and Old World hornets, wasps
Jellyfish
Stingrays
Ants

MEDICATIONS

Antibiotics, particularly penicillin
Aspirin
Local anesthetics, e.g., lidocaine (Xylocaine)
Opiates, e.g., morphine, codeine
Tetanus antitoxin and other serums
Blood and blood products
Insulin (obtained from animals)
Radiological iodinated contrast media
Chymopapain

FOODS

Peanuts
Chocolate
Eggs
Seafood and shellfish
Strawberries
Milk

CHEMICALS

Hand lotion
Soaps
Perfume

OTHER

Exercise
Hemodialysis filtration membrane

II to IV anaphylactoid reactions act on mast cells and basophils to produce an allergic reaction.

Powerful vasoactive substances, including histamine, leukotrienes, kinins, eosinophil chemotactic factor (ECF-A), and prostaglandins, are produced inside mast cells and basophils. All of these substances are released when the mast cells or basophils swell and rupture *(degranulate)* during the anaphylactic and anaphylactoid reaction.

When released into the bloodstream, *histamine* causes vasodilation, increased capillary permeability, bronchoconstriction, coronary vasoconstriction, and cutaneous reactions (wheals, flares). Increased capillary permeability and vasodilation are largely responsible for the hypotension occurring during anaphylaxis. Fluid movement out of capillaries accounts for the characteristic edema of the face, body, and airway, as well as the pulmonary edema found in anaphylaxis. Upper-airway edema with obstruction and bronchoconstriction contributes significantly to the mortality in patients with hypersensitivity reactions. Histamine also con-

stricts the smooth muscle in the intestinal wall, bladder, and uterus, resulting in cramping, vomiting, abdominal pain, diarrhea, incontinence, and vaginal bleeding.

The *leukotrienes* (including slow-reacting substance of anaphylaxis [SRS-A]) are more than 1000 times as potent as histamine in constricting the small airways of the bronchial tree and are potent coronary vasoconstrictors. Coronary vasoconstriction causes severe depression of myocardial contractility. *Prostaglandins* act on bronchial smooth muscle and affect mucus gland activity and the viscosity of mucus secretions. In patients with allergic reactions, prostaglandins produce inflammation, excessive mucus secretion, bronchoconstriction, peripheral vasodilation, and increased capillary permeability. Leukotrienes, prostaglandins, and chemical mediators join to stimulate nerve endings, causing itching and pain. *Bradykinin* and the other *kinins* also increase capillary permeability, cause vasodilation, and contract smooth muscles.

(ECF-A) promotes chemotaxis of eosinophils, thus facilitating the movement of eosinophils into the area. During allergic reactions, *eosinophils* phagocytize the antigen-antibody complex and other inflammatory debris and release enzymes that inhibit vasoactive mediators such as histamine and SRS-A.[14-17]

Although all of the aforementioned antigenic responses are meant to protect the body, frequently they result in serious organ dysfunction, which occurs because both the antigenic agent and the normal tissue surrounding the agent become involved in the allergic process. Further, many of the most serious responses to anaphylactic and anaphylactoid reactions are systemic in nature (increased capillary permeability, vasodilation, bronchoconstriction) and produce life-threatening consequences if not controlled. One of the most serious consequences of an anaphylactic reaction is anaphylactic shock.

Distributive (Low-Resistance) Shock

In a healthy person adequate perfusion is achieved through the blood volume, the heart pump mechanism, and the normal tone maintained in the vascular bed. During shock one or more of these elements are severely compromised, resulting in decreased perfusion. Inadequate tissue perfusion is the common denominator of all states of shock, regardless of the cause.

Anaphylactic shock is a form of *distributive (low-resistance) shock*. With distributive shock, vascular tone is lost because of the presence of vasodilators (anaphylactic or septic shock) or the loss of autonomic nervous innervation (spinal or neurogenic shock). The end result of distributive shock is profound vasodilation of the circulatory system and a decrease in systemic vascular resistance. Profound vasodilation increases the size of the vascular bed, producing decreased venous return to the right side of the heart, decreased stroke volume and cardiac output, and decreased blood pressure.

During anaphylactic shock, the three principal elements responsible for adequate perfusion (size of vascular bed, blood volume, and the pump mechanism) are all impaired. As in all forms of distributive shock, anaphylaxis results in maldistribution of the blood volume in the peripheral circulation. Vasoactive substances such as histamine and kinins produce vasodilation and poor vascular tone, particularly in the terminal arterioles. Histamine and other substances also increase capillary permeability, causing fluid shifts from the intravascular to the interstitial space. Although the total blood volume does not change, the large amount of fluid pooled in the interstitial space is not available to maintain cardiac output, creating a *relative hypovolemia*. Decreased cardiac output and hypotension follow. Lastly, the cardiovascular system is compromised by depressed myocardial contractility and coronary artery vasoconstriction produced by release of leukotrienes from degranulated mast cells and basophils.

ASSESSMENT AND DIAGNOSIS

Localized allergic reactions, anaphylaxis, and anaphylactic shock are products of the same mechanisms. The severity of each clinical situation is appraised on a *continuum* from localized signs, to systemic allergic reactions, to life-threatening conditions of anaphylactic shock. Each patient may manifest signs of each phase on this continuum or may progress or deteriorate during the course of the episode. It is the challenge of the clinician to monitor the patient closely for changes in status and to adjust treatment accordingly.

The patient in *less severe anaphylaxis* will exhibit slight hypotension from vasodilation and increased capillary permeability. Smooth-muscle contraction in the bronchial tree produces wheezing, hoarseness, dyspnea, and chest tightness. The patient may feel that his or her "throat is closing" because of the laryngeal edema. Additionally, the patient may have the classic symptoms of an allergic reaction: generalized pruritus (itching), urticaria (hives, wheals), angioedema (nontraumatic swelling, particularly perioral, periorbital, and in the areas of contact to the antigen), gastrointestinal (GI) upset, anxiety, and restlessness.

Patients with signs of allergic reactions or less severe anaphylaxis can deteriorate in a matter of minutes. Signs of *severe anaphylaxis* include *profound hypotension, decreased level of consciousness (LOC), and respiratory distress with severe stridor and cyanosis*. As vital organs become hypoxic, cardiac dysrhythmias and seizures may occur. Death may result from airway obstruction and/or cardiovascular collapse.[16]

TREATMENT

Treatment is directed toward preservation of tissue oxygenation and normalization of blood pressure. For systemic allergic reactions and anaphylaxis, *epinephrine* (adrenaline) is the cornerstone of treatment and should be administered as quickly as possible. Its actions on peripheral vasculature and on histamine-releasing mast cells and basophils make epinephrine's role essential. Every effort must be made to administer the medication by intravenous (IV), endotracheal, or subcutaneous routes. Performing *airway management* with positive pressure and endotracheal intubation is also essential to maintain airway patency and adequate alveolar ventilation. Other modalities include the use of medical antishock trousers (MAST), diphenhydramine (Bena-

dryl), corticosteroids, fluid resuscitation, and vasopressor drugs (dopamine). The offending substance also must be removed or discontinued as soon as possible.[22,23]

Epinephrine

Epinephrine is an endogenous catecholamine with both alpha- and beta-adrenergic activity. Its functions counter the life-threatening triad of anaphylaxis: vasodilation, increased capillary permeability, and bronchospasm. Epinephrine stimulates alpha$_2$ receptors in blood vessels and the surrounding vascular beds to produce *peripheral vasoconstriction* that elevates the blood pressure. Additionally, the beta-adrenergic properties of epinephrine will prevent progression of anaphylaxis by increasing intracellular cyclic AMP, which inhibits the release of histamine and other vasoactive substances from mast cells and basophils.[22] Epinephrine's beta-agonist properties enhance inotropic and chronotropic cardiac activity while promoting bronchial smooth muscle relaxation.[15,28]

Epinephrine can be administered in many ways: subcutaneously, intravenously, endotracheally, or intraosseously.[1,5,19] Intracardiac injections are not performed because of the frequency of complications such as laceration of coronary arteries and pneumothorax.

The standard adult subcutaneous dose is 0.2 to 0.5 mg of a 1:1000 solution. Children can receive 0.01 mg/kg (0.01 ml/kg of 1:1000 solution) to a maximum of 0.5 mg. In both adults and children injections may be repeated every 10 to 15 minutes until the desired effect is achieved (increased blood pressure, decreased laryngeal edema) or until significant side effects of epinephrine administration (for example, tachycardia with chest pain) occur. This route is reserved for systemic allergic reactions and less severe anaphylaxis because medications given into subcutaneous tissue in the presence of increased capillary permeability and edema are poorly absorbed into the central circulation. Additionally, once resuscitation is successful and peripheral perfusion restored, medications sequestered in subcutaneous tissue can enter the bloodstream at a time when their effects are no longer needed and can result in mild to severe side effects.

The IV and endotracheal (ET) dosages are the same[9]: (1) adults—0.1 to 0.5 mg of a *1:10,000* solution, which may be repeated in 10-minute intervals (not to exceed 0.5 mg in 10 minutes, and (2) pediatric dose (<12 years)—0.01 mg/kg or 0.1 ml/kg (where 0.1 mg = 1 ml).

Epinephrine administered by the IV or ET route is reserved for patients in severe anaphylaxis with signs and symptoms of poor perfusion, including severe hypotension. (blood pressure <70-80 mm Hg systolic), with decreased LOC and cyanosis.[32] Medications administered endotracheally must be diluted to a total of 10 ml for adults and to 0.1 ml/kg for children to effect adequate distribution in the bronchial tree. When epinephrine is given IV, the IV line must be flushed before sodium bicarbonate and other alkalotic preparations are administered to prevent precipitation of the drugs within the line.

IV epinephrine has some significant side effects: supraventricular tachycardia, ventricular irritability, hypertension, palpitations, nervousness, chest pain, GI upset, tremulousness, and anxiety.[28] However, because of epinephrine's ability to reverse life-threatening anaphylaxis, it must be given, regardless of the patient's age or state of health. In the person with a history of cardiac disease or in the geriatric patient, the dosage can be modified or reduced to prevent additional side effects and complications of treatment.

After resuscitation the patient will probably be given a subcutaneous injection of a long-acting preparation of epinephrine such as *Sus-Phrine* to prevent recurrence of the reaction. Sus-Phrine has all the alpha and beta properties of epinephrine, as well as its side effects and complications. It comes in an aqueous suspension at a dilution of 1:200 and is administered by subcutaneous injection, with an onset of action of 15 minutes and a maximal duration of 8 hours. Sus-Phrine is usually not given more frequently than every 6 hours and is *never given IV,* since the medication is suspended in peanut oil.[28]

Airway Management

Airway management is best effected by endotracheal intubation in the semiconscious or unconscious patient. Achieving this can be difficult because of the large amount of laryngeal edema often associated with anaphylaxis. Until intubation can be performed, 100% oxygen by mask must be instituted. If the patient is apneic or bradypneic, the clinician must assist ventilation with positive pressure by a bag-valve-mask device or by another oxygen delivery system.

The severity of the allergic reaction and its effect on ventilation are best determined by the clincial condition, that is, by the presence of cyanosis, air hunger, stridor, diminished lung sounds or wheezes, and resistance to positive pressure ventilation and by the extent of angioedema in or around the mouth and throat. Obtaining arterial blood gas values is essential in determining the efficiency of ventilation and the extent of acid-base imbalance and hypoxemia. Sodium bicarbonate dosages should be adjusted accordingly. However, waiting for arterial blood gas results should not delay the initial treatment of anaphylaxis with administration of epinephrine, airway management, and MAST trousers.

Medical Antishock trousers

The medical antishock trousers (MAST; also called military antishock trousers) and the pneumatic antishock garment (PASG) are effective against hypotension created by vasodilation and increased capillary permeability, the two major pathological features of anaphylaxis. The MAST suit exerts a squeezing effect, external counterpressure, which is theoretically capable of sustaining capillary integrity for the tissue surrounded by the device. By increasing the intracapillary pressure and decreasing the radius of the blood vessel, the external counterpressure counters the leakage of fluid and increases impedance to flow in the lower extremities. Arterial blood pressure and cardiac output are quickly restored.[3] It is no longer accepted that the MAST suit improves cardiac output by forcing blood from the lower extremities into the central circulation (autotransfusion).[11]

Clinicians often encounter certain dilemmas in anaphylaxis; for instance, peripheral IV lines can be difficult to insert because of massive edema in the extremities. In this case IV fluids and medications cannot be administered for correction of severe hypotension, but MAST suit can be applied to engorge the superficial veins of the upper extremities, significantly aiding in venous cannulation.[12,23,37]

Alternatively, when an IV is in place, the clinician may face the dilemma that there is little response to treatment. It has been conclusively shown that application of the MAST suit can preserve blood pressure and cerebral perfusion *despite clinically profound vasodilation.*[12,23,37] In one retrospective study of 1200 cases in which the MAST suit was used in a variety of shock situations, the greatest response was noted when the MAST suit was applied to anaphylactic shock patients.[37] The application of the suit resulted in an increase in mean systolic blood pressure, a decrease in pulse rate, and an overall increase in survival rates.

The MAST suit has been used extensively in patients with hypovolemia occurring secondary to trauma. It has also been used in patients with numerous low-flow states, including cardiogenic shock, drug overdose, diabetic ketoacidosis, ruptured aortic aneurysms, ruptured ectopic pregnancies, postpartum hemorrhage, and pulseless idioventricular rhythm.[23] Additionally, prehospital personnel have used the device to tamponade bleeding sites and to splint long-bone fractures in the lower extremities.

Critical care nurses must be well versed in the indications and application of use of the MAST suit. A complete set should be accessible to the staff at all times. The only strict contraindication to its use is the presence of cardiogenic pulmonary edema secondary to left-ventricular dysfunction. Since application of the MAST suit will increase systemic vascular resistance and afterload, it may further impair left-ventricular emptying and exacerbate the pulmonary edema. Caution should be exercised with those patients experiencing shortness of breath or vomiting. In these patients, the pressure exerted by the inflation of the abdominal compartment of the MAST suit may complicate the patient's symptoms; the inflation pressure in the abdominal compartment can be adjusted to relieve shortness of breath or vomiting.

Other Treatment Modalities

Fluid resuscitation. Having IV access is critical for medication administration and fluid therapy. Isotonic fluids such as lactated Ringer's or saline solution are given to preserve intravascular volume compromised by vasodilation and extravasation of fluid into the interstitial spaces. Once resuscitation is effective, the patient should be evaluated for possible fluid volume overload.

Other medications. Other medications administered to patients with systemic allergic reactions and anaphylaxis include aminophylline, diphenhydramine, corticosteroids, and vasopressors. *Aminophylline* is administered to produce bronchodilation when epinephrine has not significantly improved the patient's ventilatory status.[36] In the hypoxic patient, the cardiac-stimulating properties of aminophylline can produce dysrhythmias; therefore careful monitoring for these side effects is required.[28,32]

Diphenhydramine (Benadryl) is an antihistamine used to prevent a further antigen-antibody reaction. It cannot reverse the reaction once started; epinephrine counters the reaction once in progress. Large doses of *corticosteroids* such as hydrocortisone and dexamethasone inhibit the enzymes and white blood cells responsible for the allergic response in anaphylaxis and thus may ease bronchoconstriction and cardiac dysfunction.[17] However, the efficacy of corticosteroid use in the treatment of anaphylaxis remains in debate since there is a 6- to 10-hour latent period before this medication becomes pharmacologically effective, even if given intravenously.[17,36] When the patient does not respond to epinephrine or other treatments, *vasopressors* (for example, dopamine) are used to counter the profound hypotension and to restore cerebral perfusion. Dopamine is given in high enough doses (20 to 40 μg/kg/minute) to produce vasoconstriction in peripheral tissues.

NURSING CARE

Nursing care of the patient with an acute hypersensitivity reaction is aimed at assessment of the respiratory and cardiovascular status, support of respiratory and cardiovascular functions, identification and removal of the offending antigen or allergen, and education and referral of the patient to prevent further life-threatening events.

The nurse assesses the patient for signs and symptoms of a hypersensitivity reaction to establish a baseline and to monitor the patient's status on the continuum between localized, systemic, or severe anaphylactic reactions. Priority should be given to the respiratory and cardiovascular status (Table 45-2).

Ineffective Airway Clearance

Upper airway or laryngeal edema may be seen as stridor, cyanosis, perioral edema, swollen tongue, facial swelling, or a subjective feeling of air hunger or panic. Bronchial or lower airway narrowing is manifested by wheezing (audible with or without a stethoscope), tachypnea, intercostal or supraclavicular retractions, and/or diminished lung sounds (indicating severe bronchoconstriction). If the patient's breathing is being assisted with positive pressure (for example, Ambu bag or mechanical ventilation), bronchoconstriction may be manifested by an increased resistance to airflow during inhalation when compressing the positive-pressure device. The patient's LOC is a sensitive indicator of the adequacy of his or her cellular oxygenation, with a decreased LOC implying cerebral hypoxia. Arterial blood gas values, when available, are very helpful in monitoring oxygenation and acid-base status.

Maintaining proper airway management is essential in the critically ill patient. The airway must be kept patent, either through proper positioning and/or insertion of an endotracheal tube or oral or nasal airway. When ventilatory failure is present, an endotracheal tube is the airway of choice since it will maintain airway patency despite upper airway edema. However, it cannot ensure ventilation past severely bronchoconstricted airways. Placement of any airway may be difficult or impossible because of upper airway edema and may actually make the swelling worse. Early and careful placement of airways is strongly advised when progression of symptoms seems likely. Suctioning of the airway may be necessary because of increased mucus production associated with allergic reactions. The nurse should administer 100% oxygen by mask or by positive pressure device if the patient is apneic, bradypneic, or hypoventilating.

Decreased Cardiac Output Related to Widespread Vasodilation and Third Spacing

Although blood pressure is the most commonly practiced assessment of cardiovascular status, significant angioedema implies profound third-spacing, with extravasation of volume and relative hypovolemia. Monitoring of extremity edema (often full body), abdominal girth, and angioedema is helpful in determining the availability of body fluid.

Fluid shifts can be dramatic in patients with anaphylaxis. When treatment of anaphylaxis is successful, the excess extravascular fluid should move into the vascular space as evidenced by increased urinary output and increased blood pressure.

Additional swelling, despite treatment, implies unresponsiveness to treatment modalities, overaggressiveness with fluid resuscitation, or organ dysfunction (heart, kidney). Pulmonary artery catheter monitoring can be helpful in identifying, assessing, and treating these problems. Assessment then requires scrupulous attention to all organ systems and frequent monitoring of vital signs (blood pressure, pulse, and respirations), LOC, lung sounds, respiratory effort, heart sounds (S_3), intake and output, and arterial blood gas values. Signs and symptoms of hypersensitivity should be monitored and documented. Dysrhythmias on the electrocardiogram (ECG) may indicate hypoxemia (from a number of causes) or adverse responses to therapy (epinephrine, aminophylline).

A large-bore IV catheter must be inserted to provide a delivery route for medication and fluid resuscitation. In the patient with full-body swelling, hypovolemia, and hypotension in whom peripheral vessels are not visualized, application of the MAST suit will increase peripheral vascular resistance and blood pressure, promoting engorgement of peripheral vessels to facilitate cannulation. Fluid resuscitation is titrated to achieve a desired blood pressure (systolic = 100). Lung sounds must be monitored frequently for indications of fluid overload, often heralded by auscultation of "crackles" (rales), particularly in the posterior bases and dependent areas of the lung fields. The patient should be continuously monitored with an ECG for dysrhythmias. Cardiac resuscitation equipment and medications must be

Table 45-2 Assessment of anaphylaxis

Sign/symptom	Cause
Hypotension	Vasodilation and increased capillary permeability
Stridor	Laryngeal edema
Bronchospasm	Bronchoconstriction
Angioedema	Increased capillary permeability
Itching	Leukotrienes, prostaglandins
Dysrhythmias	Hypoxemia, coronary vasoconstriction

available at all times. If necessary, cardiopulmonary resuscitation (CPR) and advanced cardiac life support (ACLS) may be required.

The critical care nurse should monitor the patient to determine further recurrence of the allergic reaction or signs of deterioration of a previously stable condition. Sequential assessment and documentation of the patient's response to therapy is essential. The nurse must never leave the patient unattended.

Knowledge Deficit: Prevention of Anaphylaxis

The critical care nurse can play an important role in identifying knowledge deficits that may account for recurrence of severe allergic reactions. Education of the patient and family while he or she is in the critical care unit may be the first important step in safeguarding the allergic patient from further morbidity or mortality.

Avoidance of insects and known allergens, possession of emergency medication, and desensitization or venom immunotherapy are the cornerstones of prophylaxis.[20] Skin testing should be performed to identify the causative agent(s) so they can be avoided. When outdoors, the venom-sensitive patient should wear protective clothing and avoid activities that promote contact with insects (cooking or eating food, visiting the environs of insects). Venom-allergic patients should be taught how to extract the stinger and apply a constrictive band (see the following box).

All patients should wear a *Medic Alert bracelet,** indicating their specific allergies and medical history. Patients

---

*Medic Alert Foundation International, Turlock, CA 95381-1009 (1-800-ID-ALERT).

FIRST AID FOR ENVENOMATION

If an allergic reaction has been precipitated by a bite, sting, or other form of injection on an extremity, remove all rings and bracelets from the affected extremity so they will not hamper distal circulation in the event of swelling.

The patient or a bystander should apply a *constrictive band* to impede further absorption of the toxin. A soft rubber tubing or Penrose drain can be used to wrap around the extremity. After checking for the presence of a distal pulse, the band is applied 1 inch proximal to the site. The nurse should tuck one end of the band under itself as if applying a band to draw a blood sample—but looser. Two fingers should easily fit under the band. *(This is not a tourniquet; blood flow must be maintained.)* Reassess the pulse. If swelling in the extremity increases, the constrictive band may need reapplication.

If the stinger is still in place, gently *scrape* the object out of the skin. *Do not grab the stinger* since to do so would further inoculate the patient with venom.

---

who are allergic to shellfish may also have a cross-sensitivity to radiopaque dyes. Before performing all radiographic dye studies, the nurse should question the patient about shellfish allergies and any possible reactions during previous radiocontrast studies. Aspirin and nonsteroidal antiinflammatory agents are common sources of allergic reactions.[33] Patients with known allergies to these medications should be advised to identify the ingredients in all over-the-counter preparations.

Individuals with histories of anaphylaxis should be instructed about and should carry an *anaphylactic kit,* which contains injectable epinephrine, oral antihistamines, and a constrictive band. At the least, injectable epinephrine should be on hand at all times. These emergency self-care kits are meant for use as prompt treatment before the patient is transported to a medical facility; they are not to substitute for definitive medical care. Their use can mean the difference between an uncomfortable experience and possible fatality. In one allergy medical practice, more than 40% of the patients admitted to not having epinephrine available at all times, despite patient education with reinforcement.[20] This anecdotal data underscores the importance of continuous education with these at-risk patients.

Epinephrine is available for self-administration in two delivery systems. The *Ana-Kit* (Miles Laboratories) contains a syringe with the needle preloaded with 0.6 ml of 1:1000 epinephrine and with a plunger lock to prevent administering more than 0.3 ml per dose. With the Ana-Kit, it is possible to administer fractional doses. The physician who prescribes this kit must give detailed instructions on how to use the device and must be confident that the patient will actually be able to carry out the injection procedure. For the patient unwilling or unable to perform the self-injection, the *EpiPen* or *EpiPen Junior* (Center Laboratories) may be more practical (Fig. 45-2). The EpiPen contains a spring-loaded automatic injector that delivers 0.3 ml of 1:1000 epinephrine (0.15 ml in Junior version). Using graduated doses is not possible with the EpiPen. The medication is injected when the device is triggered by applying pressure to it on the thigh.[20]

Despite the existence of *immunotherapy* (desensitization) for many specific allergies, a large population of susceptible individuals remains unprotected. Immunotherapy is almost 100% effective in preventing hypersensitivity reaction from known allergens.[2,36] People at risk for severe allergic reactions or anaphylaxis should be advised to seek this preventive treatment. Based on skin test results, immunotherapy is instituted at the appropriate dose, which is incrementally increased until the maintenance dose is achieved. This therapy is continued indefinitely. Premature discontinuation of immunotherapy may result in a substantial risk of anaphylaxis if the patient is exposed to the offending allergen.

In the future *vaccines* against specific allergens may be available; they are currently being developed. New medications are also being marketed to relieve the distress of allergies. *Ketotifen (Zaditen)* is an oral antiallergic, antiasthmatic drug that has been shown effective in the prevention of systemic reactions to food allergies.[21]

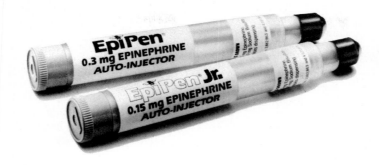

Fig. 45-2 EpiPen and EpiPen Junior. (Courtesy Center Laboratories, Port Washington, New York.)

SUMMARY

Anaphylactic and anaphylactoid reactions are immediate hypersensitivity reactions to a foreign substance, with a release of histamine and other vasoactive chemicals. Anaphylaxis is the most acute, life-threatening expression of these allergic reactions, producing the triad of bronchoconstriction, vasodilation, and an increase in capillary permeability.

Ventilation is severely compromised by upper airway edema and narrowing of the bronchi. Hypotension is produced by the combination of vasodilation and increased capillary permeability. Fluid and proteins shift from the vascular to the interstitial space (third-spacing), creating a relative hypovolemia. Insufficient volume to maintain vascular integrity and cardiac output produces shock. Changes in the capillaries also produce the full-body edema characteristic of anaphylaxis. The chemical mediators of anaphylaxis produce the cutaneous signs of wheals (urticaria), pruritus (itching), and pain.

If the patient is left untreated, death results from asphyxiation secondary to edema of the upper airway, with total airway obstruction, hypoxemia secondary to bronchospasm, vascular collapse from vasodilatation, and/or cardiac dysfunction.[36]

According to one source, respiratory complications will claim the majority of the patients (70%) who die from anaphylactic reactions, whereas 24% will succumb to cardiovascular problems.[16]

The critical care nurse plays an essential role in the prevention, identification, and treatment of this life-threatening disorder. Knowledgable assessment and prompt action can spell the difference between life and death for the patient in anaphylaxis.

REFERENCES

1. American Heart Association: Textbook of advanced cardiac life support, Dallas, 1987, The Association.
2. Anderson J and Adkinson F: Allergic reactions to drugs and biologic agents, JAMA 258(20):2891, 1987.
3. Bickell WH and Dice WH: Military anti-shock trousers in a patient with adrenergic-resistant anaphylaxis, Ann Emerg Med 13:189, 1984.
4. Bourg P, Sherer C, and Rosen P: Standardized nursing care plans for emergency patients, St Louis, 1986, The CV Mosby Co.
5. Cahill SB and Balskus M: Intervention in emergency nursing: the first 60 minutes, Rockville, MD, 1986, Aspen Publishers, Inc.
6. Cohan R, Dunnick N, and Bashore T: Treatment of reactions to radiographic contrast material, AJR 151(2):263, 1988.
7. Costa AJ: Anaphylactic shock. Guidelines for immediate diagnosis and treatment, Postgrad Med 83(4):368, 1988.
8. Dickerson M: Anaphylaxis and anaphylactic shock, Crit Care Nurs Q 11:68, 1988.
9. Fincke M and Lanros N: Emergency nursing: a comprehensive review, Rockville, Md, 1986, Aspen Publishers, Inc.
10. Gell PG, Coombs RR, and Lachman PJ, editors: Clinical aspects of immunology, ed 3, Oxford, 1975, Blackwell Scientific Publications, Ltd.
11. Goldsmith SR: Comparative hemodynamic effects of antishock suit and volume expansion in normal human beings, Ann Emerg Med 12:348, 1983.
12. Granata AV, Halickman J, and Borak J: Utility of the antishock trousers (MAST) in anaphylactic shock—a case study, J Emerg Med 2(5):349, 1985.
13. Greenberger PA: Contrast media reactions, J Allergy Clin Immunol 74:600, 1984.
14. Griffin J: Hematology and immunology: concepts for nursing, Norwalk, Conn, Appelton-Century-Crafts, 1986.
15. Guyton A: Textbook of medical physiology, ed 7, Philadelphia, 1986, WB Saunders Co.
16. Keahey TM, Yancey K, and Lawley T: Immediate hypersensitivity, J Am Acad Dermatol 17:826, 1987.
17. Levy JH, Roizen M, and Morris J: Anaphylactic and anaphylactoid reactions. A review, Spine 11(3):282, 1986.

18. Lockey RF and others: Fatalities from immunotherapy (IT) and skin testing (ST), J Allergy Clin Immunol 79(4):660, 1987.

19. Manley L, Haley K, and Dick M: Intraosseous infusion: rapid vascular access for critically ill or injured infants and children; J Emerg Nurs 14:63, 1988.

20. McLean DC: Insect sting allergy, Primary Care 14(3):513, 1987.

21. Molkhow P and Dupont C: Ketotifen in prevention and therapy of food allergy, Ann Allergy 59:187, 1987.

22. Netzel MC: Anaphylaxis: clinical presentation, immunologic mechanisms, and treatment, J Emerg Med 4(3):227, 1986.

23. Oertel T and Loehr MM: Bee-sting anaphylaxis: the use of the medical anti-shock trousers, Ann Emerg Med 13(6):459, 1984.

24. O'Leary MR and Smith MS: Penicillin anaphylaxis, Am J Emerg Med 4(3):241, 1986.

25. Orlowski JP: An animal model for anaphylactic shock (letter), Ann Emerg Med 15(8):979, 1986.

26. Price SA and Wilson LM: Pathophysiology: clinical concepts of disease processes, New York, 1987, McGraw-Hill Book Co.

27. Reisman R and Osur S: Allergic reactions following first insect sting exposure, Ann Allergy 59(6):429, 1987.

28. Rodman M and Others: Pharmacology and drug therapy in nursing, ed 3, Philadelphia, 1985, JB Lippincott Co.

29. Sheehy SB and Barber J: Emergency nursing: principles and practice, ed 2, St Louis, 1985, The CV Mosby Co.

30. Sheffer AL: Anaphylaxis, J Allergy Clin Immunol 81:1048, 1988.

31. Stephens GW, Bernard D, and Idelson B: Anaphylaxis: an unusual complication of hemodialysis, Clin Nephrol 24(2):99, 1985.

32. Stoelting R: Pharmacology and physiology in anesthetic practice, Philadelphia, 1987, JB Lippincott Co.

33. Szczeklik A: Adverse reactions to aspirin and nonsteroidal anti-inflammatory drugs, Ann Allergy 59:113, 1987.

34. Toogood JH: Risk of anaphylaxis in patients receiving beta-blocker drugs, J Allergy Clin Immunol 81:1, 1988.

35. Trevino RJ: Food allergies and hypersensitivities, Ear Nose Throat J 67:42, 1988.

36. Valentine MD and Lichtenstein LM: Anaphylaxis and stinging insect hypersensitivity, JAMA 258(20):2881, 1987.

37. Wayne MA: Clinical evaluation of the antishock trouser: retrospective analysis of 5 years of experience, Ann Emerg Med 12:342, 1983.

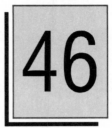

Disseminated Intravascular Coagulation

CHAPTER OBJECTIVES

- *List at least four disorders from both coagulation pathways (intrinsic and extrinsic) that can precipitate acute disseminated intravascular coagulation (DIC).*
- *Describe the most common clinical presentation of acute DIC and its cause.*
- *List important laboratory findings that are highly suggestive of DIC.*
- *Outline the medical management of DIC, including the purpose and actions of heparin, antithrombin III, epsilonaminocaproic acid (EACA), whole blood, platelets, fresh frozen plasma, and cryoprecipitate.*
- *Discuss three nursing diagnoses and their interventions that are related to the treatment of DIC.*
- *Explain the nursing actions specific to "bleeding precautions."*

Disseminated intravascular coagulation (DIC) is a hemorrhagic disorder produced by the effects of both *thrombotic* (clot formation) and *fibrinolytic* (clot digestion) processes. As the name implies, DIC causes microvascular clotting in organ systems throughout the body, but, paradoxically, its lethality stems from the profound bleeding resulting from the depletion (consumption) of clotting substances (Fig. 46-1). Since both clot formation and clot digestion consume clotting factors, the most dramatic manifestation of DIC is the *acute generalized hemorrhage* secondary to the inability of blood to coagulate. The thrombotic processes of DIC can also result in infarction of major organs. The severity of DIC depends on the magnitude of the underlying disease that precipitates this syndrome of intravascular coagulation. Mortality increases with the patient's age, the extent of his or her clinical manifestations, and the severity of abnormal laboratory results.[10]

DIC can be either *acute* or *chronic*. Additionally, both acute and chronic clinical forms can be designated *subclinical*. Subclinical DIC implies lack of significant clinical symptomatology; the presumptive diagnosis is based on abnormal laboratory findings.

Acute DIC, which can develop rapidly in critically ill patients, is the most serious of the acquired coagulation disorders. Mortality in acute DIC is high—estimated at 50% to 70%. Acute DIC occurs in approximately 1 in every 1000 hospital admissions, although this estimate is probably low.[11,12] In one study elderly patients with infections were most at risk for developing acute DIC.[17]

Chronic DIC is characterized by episodic changes in coagulation in the chronically ill patient. Malignancy is the most common cause, especially mucin-producing adenocarcinomas of the prostate and pancreas, solid tumors of the lung, colon, and stomach, and metastatic disease.[2,12] Chronic DIC is also associated with connective tissue diseases, renal disease, liver disease, metabolic disease, collagen vascular disease, lymphoma, and myeloma.[2,12] Unlike those with acute DIC, patients with chronic DIC manifest thrombotic complications such as thrombophlebitis, nonbacterial thrombotic endocarditis, and pulmonary embolism. Exacerbation of hemorrhage may also occur. Longterm therapy is usually required, with careful monitoring of clotting studies.

CAUSE

All forms of DIC occur secondary to some underlying disease or disorder. Scores of clinical disorders cause DIC, with infection (sepsis) the most common (see the box on p. 819). Every type of infection (for example, bacterial, viral, or chlamydial) has been implicated in the pathogenesis of DIC. Unfortunately, the mortality rate for patients with DIC associated with severe infections is 80%.[2] DIC is frequently encountered in patients with obstetrical emergencies, major trauma, and "low-flow states," that is, conditions such as cardiopulmonary arrest and shock characterized by inadequate perfusion of the major organs. Abruptio placentae is the most common obstetrical cause of DIC and accounts for a significant number of maternal deaths secondary to hemorrhage.[2] Acute and chronic forms of DIC occur with many forms of cancer. DIC is particularly prevalent among patients with acute promyelocytic leukemia; 80% to 90% of

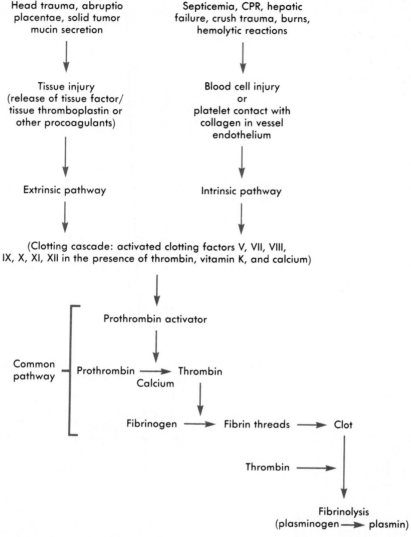

Fig. 46-1 Normal coagulation. (Modified from Guyton A: Textbook of medical physiology, ed 6, Philadephia, 1981, WB Saunders Co.)

all these patients will develop DIC.[10] (See the review by Carr[2] for a more extensive list of DIC causes.)

The mechanisms initiating coagulation, and thereby DIC, are as varied as the underlying disorders. In some disorders the coagulation process is started through red blood cell (RBC) damage or platelet contact with collagen in the endothelial lining of blood vessels.[5] In other cases disorders that cause or result from tissue injury stimulate the release of *procoagulants* (substances that promote coagulation), including *tissue factor* (tissue thromboplastin).

Gram-negative septicemia can initiate both coagulation and fibrinolysis through activation of the Hageman factor (factor XII) in the intrinsic pathway.[10] One hypothesis suggests that the endotoxins of infection roughen and expose the endothelial lining of blood vessels and initiate clotting.[5] Low-flow states and vasculitis also damage the vessel endothelium, with release of tissue thromboplastin. Crush trauma, burns, aortic aneurysms, hyperthermia or hypothermia, giant hemangiomas, and radiographic procedures can cause severe, local endothelial injury, with activation

of the intrinsic coagulation pathway.[12] Antigen-antibody complexes produced during anaphylactic reactions can also result in endothelial damage.

Although RBCs contain only small amounts of thromboplastin, significant RBC hemolysis secondary to multiple transfusions or transfusion incompatibility can release sufficient amounts of thromboplastin to initiate DIC. In addition, certain snake venoms contain enzymes that activate prothrombin or activate platelets and initiate thrombosis in organ microvasculature.[15]

PATHOPHYSIOLOGY
Cycle of Thrombosis and Hemorrhage

In the healthy person there is a balance between (1) clot formation (thrombosis), which is needed to minimize blood loss and to repair blood vessels, and (2) clot lysis (fibrinolysis), which maintains the patency of blood vessels. In a patient with DIC this balance is upset; *DIC is an exaggeration of the normal coagulation process.* The normal

CAUSES OF DIC

INFECTIONS

> Bacterial
> > Gram-negative sepsis *(Neisseria, Klebsiella, Pseudomonas aeruginosa, Escherichia coli)*
> > Gram-positive septicemia (Staphylococcus, Streptococcus)
>
> Fungal (aspergillosis)
> Mycobacterial (tuberculosis)
> Protozoal (malaria)
> Rickettsial (Rocky Mountain spotted fever)
> Viral (chicken pox, measles, herpes simplex, influenza)

MALIGNANCIES

> Carcinoma (breast, colon, lung, stomach, pancreas, prostate, ovary)
> Leukemia (acute promyelocytic, acute and chronic myelocytic)
> Other (pheochromocytoma, polycythemia vera)

TRAUMA

> Burns
> Multiple injury
> Head injury
> Snakebite
> Fat embolism

SURGERY

> Extracorporeal circulation
> Transurethral prostatectomy

OBSTETRICAL DISORDERS

> Abruptio placentae
> Missed abortion
> Amniotic fluid embolism
> Septic abortion
> Dead fetus syndrome
> Toxemia of pregnancy
> Eclampsia
> Hydatidiform mole

IMMUNOLOGICAL DISORDERS

> Incompatible transfusion reactions
> Anaphylaxis
> Systemic lupus erythematosis

HEMATOLOGICAL DISORDERS

> Sickle cell crisis
> Use of prothrombin concentrate in patient with liver disease

OTHERS

> Pulmonary embolism
> Intravenous pyelogram
> Diabetic ketoacidosis
> Postcardiac arrest
> Aortic aneurysm
> Hyperthermia or hypothermia

Modifed from Carr M: J Emerg Med 5(4):312, 1987.

processes of thrombosis and fibrinolysis are magnified to life-threatening proportions corresponding to the severity of the precipitating disorder (Fig. 46-2).

Since DIC results from increased thrombin activity, the disorders precipitating DIC produce a systemic hypercoagulation state—thrombosis is no longer localized but is generalized *(disseminated)*. Thrombosis does not act as a protective mechanism but causes microvascular changes in major organ systems, with the possibility of organ ischemia and infarction. Thus the *initial component* of DIC is thrombosis of major vessels. The severity of the thrombosis is dependent on the intensity of the precipitating disorder.

Although no organ system is spared, organs with larger blood flow are more likely affected.[2] The skin, lungs, and kidneys are the organs most commonly involved and damaged during DIC (Table 46-1). Rapidly developing hemorrhages of the skin (purpura fulminans), cyanosis of the hands and feet (acral cyanosis), mottled or cool extremities, and gangrene may result from thrombosis. Depending on the site of the vessel occlusion, the patient may also develop signs and symptoms of thrombophlebitis, pulmonary embolism, cerebral vascular accident, gastrointestinal (GI) bleed or obstruction, or renal failure. The thrombosis continues to extend within vessels if the precipitating disorder is not removed or corrected or if lysis is not accomplished. Ischemia or infarction of organ(s) can contribute to the patient's death.

The *second component* of DIC is hemorrhage. Lysis of clots (fibrinolysis) is naturally activated by coagulation (specifically by thrombin). In a patient with DIC the intensity of the thrombosis activates a similar intensity of lysis. Unlike what occurs in normal situations, the thrombosis in DIC is so generalized and of so great a magnitude that lysis cannot keep pace to maintain the patency of vessels.

Although the lysis is not sufficient to meet the great demand, the consequences of lysis produce the classic, life-threatening hemorrhage of DIC. As fibrin and fibrinogen are digested by plasminogen during lysis, fibrin-split products are formed and exert a powerful anticoagulant effect. Their presence is a *very* characteristic feature of DIC, although fibrin-split products can appear in other disorders.

Additionally, DIC is termed a *consumption coagulopathy.*

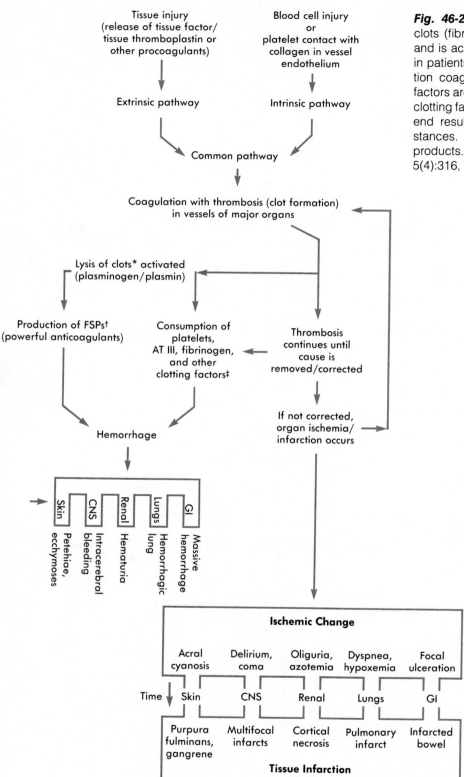

Fig. 46-2 Pathophysiology of DIC. Lysis of clots (fibrinolysis) is a natural consequence of and is activated by coagulation. It is intensified in patients with DIC. DIC is termed a consumption coagulopathy. During thrombosis clotting factors are used to form clots. During fibrinolysis clotting factors are destroyed inside the clot. The end result is a depletion of coagulation substances. *FSP,* Fibrin-split or fibrin-degradation products. (Modified from Carr M: J Emerg Med 5(4):316, 1987.

Table 46-1 Organ damaged by DIC

Usually involved	Often involved	Occasionally involved
Skin	Heart	Testes
Kidneys	Liver	Lymph nodes
Lungs	Brain	Bladder
	GI tract	Pituitary gland
	Pancreas	

From Carr M: J Emer Med 5(4):316, 1987.

The enzymes of fibrinolysis break down the clotting factors within the thrombosis and platelets, fibrinogen, and thrombin are consumed in large quantities. Additionally, the ongoing coagulation also consumes these same substances. The end result is a depletion of coagulation substances. Thrombocytopenia (low platelet count), hypofibrinogenemia, and the presence of fibrin-split products are typical laboratory abnormalities occurring in patients with DIC. The lack of clotting substances and the presence of powerful anticoagulants (fibrin-split products) produce a generalized hemorrhagic state. Ironically, this frequently fatal bleeding phenomenon is triggered by an underlying thrombotic process, and a vicious cycle of thrombosis and hemorrhage is established. The pathological consequences of fibrinolysis with hemorrhage will continue until the precipitating cause is removed or corrected and the thrombotic process is terminated.

ASSESSMENT AND DIAGNOSIS

Since the pathological sequelae of DIC are generalized and no organ is spared, assessment of each organ system must be accomplished. Particular attention should be paid to pathological manifestations in the skin, since the vasculature of the skin is frequently involved in DIC and pathological signs and symptoms are readily apparent. Although hemorrhagic signs and symptoms are the most dramatic, the critical care nurse should also note evidence of thrombotic-ischemic changes. Laboratory findings also play an important role in the diagnosis and treatment of DIC.

Thrombotic Signs and Symptoms

Skin involvement produces the most apparent signs and symptoms. Occlusion of capillaries and small vessels can produce red, indurated areas along the vessel walls or diffuse skin infarction (purpura fulminans).[10,15] Signs of acral cyanosis (generalized diaphoresis, with mottled, cool fingers and toes) may be present. With occlusion of terminal arterioles, necrosis of the fingers and toes, nose, and genitalia may occur. Signs of distal occlusion may also include cool, pale extremities; mottling; cyanosis; or edema.

Involvement of the renal vasculature can result in *renal failure*. The nurse must monitor urinary output (reporting oliguria of less than 30 ml/hour) and assess for gross or occult hematuria. Increased serum potassium, creatinine, or

blood urea nitrogen (BUN) levels may indicate renal insufficiency and should be considered suggestive of DIC in a susceptible patient.

Cerebral infarcts or embolization can produce focal neurological deficits such as hemiplegia or loss of vision or nonspecific changes, including an altered level of consciousness, confusion, headache, seizures, or coma. Alterations in neurological function may indicate intracerebral infarction or hemorrhage.

Bowel infarction manifests signs of acute intraabdominal pathology, including melena, hematemesis, abdominal distention, and absent or hyperactive bowel sounds.

Deep vein thrombosis can result in *thrombophlebitis*. Thrombophlebitis of the deep venous network of the lower extremities may be manifested as muscle pain and tenderness, fever and chills, venous distention, and Homan's sign (pain in calf with dorsiflexion of foot). *Pulmonary embolism* is a potentially life-threatening complication of thrombophlebitis and/or DIC. The patient may experience dyspnea, anxiety, sharp, stabbing chest pain, or hemoptysis.

Hemorrhagic Signs and Symptoms

The generalized bleeding characteristic of DIC can be *spontaneous* and cause hemorrhage into body cavities and skin surfaces. The *classic presentation* of DIC is oozing or bleeding from invasive-line insertion sites or from body orifices. Petechiae, purpura, or ecchymosis may be apparent. On examination the patient may exhibit gingival, nasal, or scleral hemorrhages.

Bleeding from body orifices such as the rectum, vagina, urethra, nose (epistaxis), and ears, as well from the lung and GI tract, occurs frequently. Signs of bleeding can take many forms; melena, hematemesis, or hemoptysis indicate hemorrhage in the GI tract and lungs. The nurse should test all voidings, stool, and other body discharge for the presence of blood.

Hemorrhage in a patient with DIC can occur into all body cavities, including the peritoneal space, the retroperitoneal space, the cranium, and the thorax. Occult bleeding can be detected by vital sign and orthostatic changes associated with decreased blood volume such as decreasing blood pressure, narrowing pulse pressure, rapid and thready pulse, postural hypotension, syncope when erect or dangling, pallor, and altered level of consciousness. Besides classic signs of fluid volume deficit and blood loss, the nurse should assess for subtle changes such as lethargy and weakness.

Laboratory Findings

There are no generally accepted diagnostic criteria for DIC, nor is there a laboratory test that is pathognomonic for DIC. Strong indicators of DIC include thrombocytopenia (low platelet count), prolonged prothrombin time (PT), hypofibrinogenemia, and elevated levels of fibrin-split products (in the patient *without* underlying liver disease) (Table 46-2). A low platelet count occurs in nearly all DIC patients. The PT is prolonged in more than 90% of patients with DIC. The hallmark of DIC, an elevated fibrin-split/fibrin-degradation product level, strongly suggests DIC and is also found in more than 90% of DIC patients. Normal or sus-

Table 46-2 Clotting studies in patients with DIC

Laboratory test	Abnormality	Reason
Prothrombin time	>15 seconds	Elevated fibrin-split products and decreased plasma clotting factor levels
Platelet count	<150,00	Platelet consumption
Fibrinogen	<160 mg/dl	Consumption by clotting cascade and destruction by plasmin
Fibrin-split Products	> One-eighth dilution	Fibrinogen destructon by plasmin
Antithrombin III	Decreased	Massive complex formation with active coagulation substances

picious laboratory results must be viewed in the context of the clinical presentation.

TREATMENT

The four aspects of the medical treatment of DIC—(1) treatment of the underlying illness (the precipitating factor), (2) the control of hemorrhage, (3) the termination of the thrombotic process, and (4) the treatment of complications—address the major elements that constitute the disorder (Fig. 46-3). First and foremost, the clinician must treat the underlying illness. In patients with septicemia and malignancies, use of antibiotics and chemotherapeutic agents is required.[9] The control of hemorrhage is accomplished in three ways: (1) through reconstitution of the patient's blood with RBCs and clotting factors, (2) through interruption of coagulation by blocking the action of thrombin through antithrombotic therapy, and (3) through termination of fibrinolysis with epsilon aminocaproic acid (AMICAR) in extreme cases. The use of heparin and antithrombin III prevents further thrombosis and breaks the thrombosis-fibrinolysis cycle.[10] The life-threatening complications of DIC must be addressed, including hypotension, acidosis, and hypoxemia. Since acute renal failure may often develop during DIC, hemodialysis may be necessary.

Blood Component Therapy

RBCs may be lost through frank or occult hemorrhage or through hemolytic processes, depending on the cause of the DIC. Large quantities of clotting substances (including antithrombin III and platelets) are consumed in the microvascular clots in major organs and from the breakdown of clots during fibrinolysis.

RBC transfusions and replacement of blood clotting factors may be performed. If the platelet count falls below 30,000/mm³ (or if hemorrhage is ongoing), administration of *platelets* is indicated. *Fresh frozen plasma* contains all clotting factors (V, VIII, XIII, and antithrombin III) and is also used for volume expansion.[10] Each unit of fresh frozen plasma will raise each clotting factor by approximately 5%. Appropriate laboratory tests should be monitored to determine further requirements for RBCs, platelets, and other clotting substances.[12]

Treatment of severe hypofibrinogenemia (<50 mg/dl) is the administration of *cryoprecipitate,* a concentrated source of fibrinogen and factor VIII from fresh frozen plasma. Each unit contains approximately 200 mg of fibrinogen, increasing the levels of fibrinogen and factor VIII by 2%.[10,12]

Antithrombotic and Antifibrinolytic Therapies

Anticoagulants can be given to terminate the coagulation (thrombotic) process. *Heparin* produces an anticoagulant effect by potentiating the action of *antithrombin III,* which is a naturally occurring inhibitor of clotting proteins. With the formation of a heparin-antithrombin III complex, the speed of inactivation of clotting enzymes significantly increases. This complex has been shown to produce a 2000-time increase in the degradation of thrombin.[13]

Heparin. The activity of heparin is affected by several factors. Antithrombin III must be present in sufficient amounts for heparin to work properly. It is recommended that heparin not be administered if the serum antithrombin III level is less than 80% because decreased production of antithrombin III as a result of liver failure or dysfunction retards the effectiveness of heparin. Heparin dosages should be adjusted according to the partial thromboplastin time (PTT), hepatic, and renal studies.

In the presence of intense bleeding, use of heparin therapy for DIC remains controversial. There have been no prospective randomized controlled studies to demonstrate the efficacy of using heparin in patients with DIC. Heparin is indicated, however, when there are clinical signs of thrombosis and when heparin therapy is administered concurrently with blood component therapy. General clinical indications for its use include deteriorating renal or neurological function and, under certain conditions, life-threatening bleeding unresponsive to blood product support.[7] Heparin apparently is an accepted treatment when DIC has been precipitated by amniotic fluid embolism, severe incompatible blood transfusion reactions, retained nonsurviving fetus, venous thrombosis, septic abortion, septicemia, acute promyelocytic leukemia, or heat stroke.[2,12]

Heparin is the treatment of choice in patients with chronic DIC; it is initially administered by intravenous (IV) infusion, then by subcutaneous injections for long-term maintenance. Heparin is most commonly used in these patients to treat venous thrombosis or overt skin infarction. Low-dose heparin may be given prophylactically to prevent thrombosis. Long-term heparin therapy may be necessary since use of coumarin derivatives (for example, warfarin [Coumadin] or Dicumarol) shows little effectiveness. As in patients with acute DIC, hemorrhage in patients with chronic DIC is first treated with blood products, and heparin is added if bleeding continues.[15]

Antithrombin III. Antithrombin III is a naturally occurring inhibitor of the active clotting process that binds with throm-

Therapy

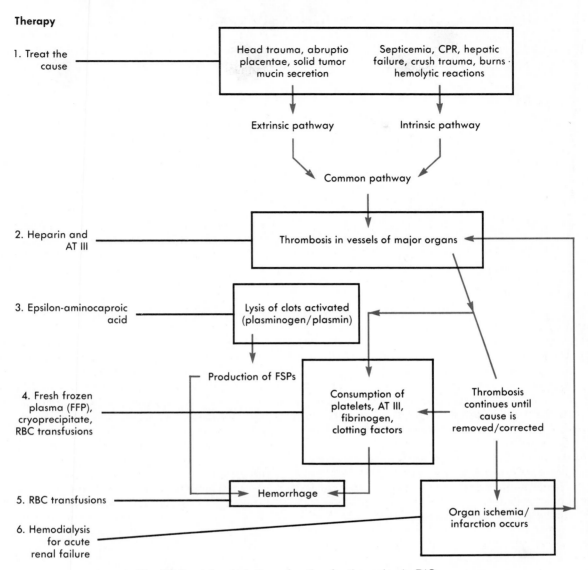

Fig. 46-3 Intended sites of action for therapies in DIC.

bin and other clotting factors to form an inactive complex. It helps produce the natural balance in the body between thrombosis and fibrinolysis. It can be administered alone or in conjunction with heparin. In patients with DIC increased amounts of antithrombin III are consumed, chiefly in individuals with thrombotic vascular occlusions. Critically ill patients with septicemia commonly have antithrombin III levels 50% of normal; if the levels return to normal, chances for survival increase. A principal reason for the unabated thrombotic process of DIC is the low antithrombin III levels since there is less inhibition of the active substances of coagulation. Administration of antithrombin III shortens the course of the disorder and decreases the complications of DIC.[13]

An average dose of 1 unit per kilogram will raise antithrombin III activity by 1%. In severe cases in which the level is below 50%, the antithrombin III level should be monitored every 4 hours, and antithrombin III should be administered to obtain a level of 100%. No undesirable side effects, including incompatibility reactions, have been reported with use of antithrombin III, and there have been no reported cases of hepatitis acquired from its use.[13]

Aminocaproic acid. In approximately 5% of DIC cases, bleeding cannot be controlled with heparin. In this life-threatening situation aminocaproic acid can be given to interrupt the fibrinolytic process through inhibition of plasmin. Aminocaproic acid is a potent inhibitor of plasminogen activators and, to a lesser degree, it inhibits fibrinolysin. It must be given only in the presence of DIC and not for other causes of fibrinolysis. There must also be reasonable certainty that the thrombotic process has already been controlled by heparin or other measures. The greatest complication—and the greatest barrier—to using aminocaproic acid is the potential for large-vessel thrombosis. Aminocaproic acid has also produced endocardial hemorrhage in laboratory animals, and it should be used with caution in patients with cardiac dysrhythmias. Cardiac, renal, and electrolyte studies should be followed closely during its use.[1,10]

NURSING CARE

The nursing management of a patient with DIC is directed at the prevention and/or recognition of hemorrhagic or thrombotic complications. It ranges from continuous assessment of the course of the disorder to intensive treatment maneuvers during acute hemorrhagic episodes. Prompt attention to any sign of hemorrhage or thrombosis may spell the difference in patient morbidity and mortality.

The nursing diagnoses and interventions for the patient with DIC can be grouped into four categories: fluid volume deficit: hemorrhage, altered tissue perfusion, potential for venous thrombosis, and anxiety.

Fluid Volume Deficit: Hemorrhage

For the patient with DIC, the nurse should institute *bleeding precautions,* which are intended to prevent blood loss. These precautions act to minimize tissue and vascular trauma, which, even in mild form, can precipitate bleeding.[4] Gentle technique is used during personal care and during turning, because exerting even normal force during these activities can produce subcutaneous bleeding. Obtaining blood pressure measurements by auscultation should be done as infrequently as possible since pressure on subcutaneous tissue can cause bleeding, with bruising or hematoma formation. Using invasive hemodynamic monitoring is preferable, although complications of line placement can result in significant hemorrhage. The use of intramuscular (IM) injections is avoided since the bolus of medication can rupture capillary walls from a pressure effect. If IM injections are required, the nurse should use the smallest needle gauge possible, inject the medication slowly, and monitor the site of injection for bleeding. Oral, IV, and subcutaneous injections (with small-gauge needles) are the preferable routes of medication administration.[10]

Other bleeding precautions include avoiding the use of rectal temperatures, vaginal or rectal suppositories, enemas, and digital examinations of the rectum and vagina. Only paper tape should be used to secure tubes, invasive lines, and indwelling catheters since silk, plastic, and adhesive tape can cause tissue trauma and bleeding when removed.[14] Shaving a patient must be performed gently with an electric razor, never a straight blade. Use of aspirin, all aspirin-containing products, and many nonsteroidal antiinflammatory drugs (NSAIDs) is strictly contraindicated since they decrease platelet aggregation and promote bleeding.

Every effort must be taken to avoid trauma to mucous membranes and to the skin. Performing frequent mouth care is necessary, since ischemia is common in the mouth. Gentle use of foam swabs for oral care, using a mild solution of saline, peroxide, or baking soda is preferable to the use of toothbrushes. Mouthwash solutions containing alcohol act as irritants and should be avoided.[10] Other oral and GI irritants include dental flossing, highly spiced or high rough-

age foods, harsh laxatives, and ill-fitting dentures.[4] Constipation or hemorrhoids can cause rectal irritation or straining at the stool; thus the use of stool softeners and increased fluid intake should be instituted.

Dry or cracking skin can become a site for bleeding or oozing. The nurse must keep the skin moist and intact through frequent application of lubricants to skin and lips, maintenance of adequate humidity in patient care areas, and prevention of patient injury.[4,12]

Potential for Altered Tissue Perfusion: Cerebral, Cardiopulmonary, Renal, Gastrointestinal, Peripheral

The potential for arterial thrombotic embolization to any major organ system is ever present in patients with DIC. The critical care nurse's contribution to the management of this problem consists of surveillance as detailed in the section, "Assessment and Diagnosis." Surveillance is meant to detect changes in organ function at the earliest possible moment; the problem is then referred to the physician for appropriate medical intervention.

Anxiety

The patient and significant others undergo a great deal of stress when coping with DIC and its life-threatening complications. Frequent opportunities for the patient and significant others to ask questions and voice concerns promote emotional well-being. All treatments and procedures should be explained to and understood by the patient. Some significant others benefit by assisting in patient care. The patient should be kept advised of his or her health status, progress, and plans for treatment. Since it has been hypothesized that stress increases fibrinolytic activity, nursing measures that help alleviate the patient's anxiety and provide emotional support take on special importance.[4]

REFERENCES

1. American Medical Association Department of Drugs, Division of Drugs and Technology: Drug evaluations, ed 6, Chicago, 1986, The Association.
2. Carr M: Disseminated intravascular coagulation: pathogenesis, diagnosis, and therapy, J Emerg Med 5(4):311, 1987.
3. Dangel R: Injury: potential for, related to disseminated intravascular coagulation (DIC). In McNally J, Stair J, and Somerville E, editors: Guidelines for cancer nursing practice, Orlando, Fla, 1985, Grune & Stratton, Inc.
4. Griffin J: Hematology and immunology, concepts for nursing, Norwalk, Conn, 1986, Appleton-Century-Crofts.
5. Guyton A: Textbook of medical physiology, ed 6, Philadelphia, 1981, WB Saunders Co.
6. Johanson BC and others: Standards for critical care, ed 3, St Louis, 1988, The CV Mosby Co.
7. Ockelford P: Heparin 1986: indications and effective use, Drugs 31:81, 1986.
8. Pesola G and Carlon G: Pulmonary embolus-induced disseminated intravascular coagulation, Crit Care Med 15(10):983, 1987.
9. Price S and Wilson L: Pathophysiology: clinical concepts of disease processes, ed 3, New York, 1986, McGraw-Hill Book Co.
10. Rooney A and Haviley C: Nursing management of disseminated intravascular coagulation, Oncol Nurs Forum 12:15, 1985.

11. Sheehy S and Barber J: Emergency nursing: principles and practices, ed 2, St Louis, 1985, The CV Mosby Co.

12. Siegrist C and Jones J: Disseminated intravascular coagulopathy and nursing implications, Semin Oncol Nurs 1(4):237, 1985.

13. Vinazzer H: Clinical use of antithrombin III concentrate, Vox Sang 53(4):193, 1987.

14. Weber B, Speer M, and Swartz D: Irritation and stripping effects of adhesive tapes on skin layers of coronary artery bypass graft patients, Heart Lung 16(5):567, 1987.

15. Weitz J: Disseminated intravascular coagulation. In Brain MC and Carbone PP, editors: Current therapy in hematology-oncology, Toronto, 1988, Brian C Decker, Publisher.

16. Zbilut J: Disseminated intravascular coagulation, J Emerg Nurs 7(5):213, 1981.

17. Zbilut J: Incidence of disseminated intravascular coagulation in patients admitted through the emergency department: a 5 year retrospective study, Heart Lung 9(5):833, 1980.

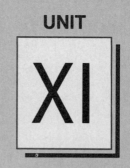

UNIT

XI

PSYCHOSOCIAL ALTERATIONS IN CRITICAL CARE

Self-Concept Alterations

CHAPTER OBJECTIVES

- Describe the theoretical bases of self-concept and its related nursing diagnoses: body image disturbance, self-esteem disturbance, altered role performance, powerlessness, and hopelessness.
- Identify defining characteristics and causes of the above nursing diagnoses.
- Identify situations that increase the risk of disturbances of self-concept.
- Point out assessment strategies of use with patients experiencing a disturbance in self-concept.
- Given a situation in which a patient experiences a self-concept alteration, match relevant interventions with expected outcomes.

The human self-concept comprises attitudes about oneself; perceptions of personal abilities, body image, and identity; and a general sense of worth. Included in this chapter are discussions of the nursing diagnoses of disturbances in self-concept, that is, body image disturbance, self-esteem disturbance, altered role performance, powerlessness, and hopelessness. The nursing diagnosis personal identity disturbance, included as a subcomponent of the human self-concept by the North American Nursing Diagnosis Association (NANDA), is omitted because it is not yet sufficiently developed for useful application to clinical practice. The four subcomponents of the human self-concept appear in Fig. 47-1.

This chapter focuses on the theoretical basis for each diagnosis. Each nursing diagnosis is defined and then discussed in terms of defining characteristics, expected outcomes, and interventions. The problems common to critical care nursing are the major concerns.

SELF-CONCEPT

Over the years many writers in the behavioral sciences have been interested in the self-concept, its development,

and its importance to the individual.[9,38,44,45] In Rogers' writings on client-centered psychotherapy,[38] he focused on the client's self-concept as currently organized and functioning. He believed that there were elements of the self that the person could not face or clearly perceive; therefore he defined self-concept as an organized body of perceptions that were admissible to awareness. Included were perceptions of one's characteristics, abilities, relationships with others and the environment, values, goals, and ideals.

Sullivan[44,45] first used the concepts of *significant others* and *reflected appraisals* in his interpersonal theory of psychiatry. He believed the self is developed from social interaction, especially in dynamic patterns of interaction with significant people, especially the mother. Based on interactions that provide reward and punishment, the individual develops a self-concept that reflects the appraisals of others.

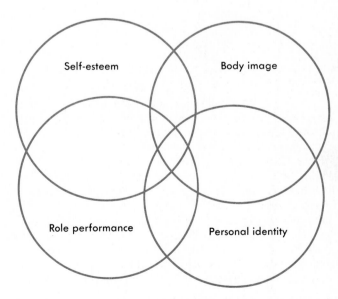

Fig. 47-1 Four subcomponents of the human self-concept (NANDA).

827

Perception is the focus of the theory of self-concept of Combs and Snygg.[9] The part that one regards as *I* or *me* (the beliefs about oneself and one's abilities) determines what one thinks and how one behaves. Although self-concept controls perceptions and eventual behavior, these perceptions and behaviors also affect the self-concept in a cyclic process. Some of the perceptions of self are basic or central and are highly resistant to change. Others are less important and more readily subject to change. Self-perceptions become more clear as the individual matures. These perceptions exist in a framework that is the individual's own private conception of himself or herself. Combs and Snygg named this construction the *phenomenal self,* which encompasses the central, vital concepts of the person. The phenomenal self is set in a *perceptual field,* which includes all the perceptions about the person plus the things outside the person.

Self-concept is a construct that is useful for understanding individuals and their behavior. Although it is relatively stable, it can be modified. It influences how one reacts to and manages problems in daily life. Self-concept is a major concern for nurses who care for patients because nursing interventions that do not consider the individual in his or her wholeness, including the self-concept, will probably be ineffective.

DISTURBANCES IN SELF-CONCEPT

Three major subcomponents of the self-concept are discussed in this chapter: body image, self-esteem, and role performance. Alterations may involve any or all of these interrelated components. Pertinent to all these diagnoses are the following key factors that affect an individual's self-concept[14]:

1. Previous perception of appraisals about self from significant others.
2. Previous experience with developmental and situational crises and how they were managed.
3. Past experiences with success and failure and current expectations of self.
4. Positive and negative feelings of self-worth from interpersonal experiences.
5. Level of physiological functioning.

Causes of Disturbances of Self-Concept

Causative factors related to self-concept disruptions may be categorized as biophysical, cognitive-perceptual, psychosocial, and cultural or spiritual. Major causative factors include (1) cognitive-perceptual difficulties, that is, knowing deficit, altered thought processes, and sensory-perceptual alterations, (2) biochemical changes in the body, (3) inability to adjust to and integrate body changes, (4) repeated negative interpersonal experiences, (5) absence of significant role models, (6) inability to learn new behaviors in response to transitional states, (7) poor identity development, (8) loss of control related to health care environment and illness-related regimen, (9) prolonged activity restriction, and (10) deteriorating physical health.[25]

Assessment of the Self-Concept

The self-concept is what one believes about oneself; the self-report is what one is willing to share about oneself.

When assessing the self-concept of the critically ill patient, Lee's phases of response to illness or injury[21] are useful. She identified four phases: impact, retreat, acknowledgment, and reconstruction. Patients in critical care units are primarily in the first two phases. During phase one, impact, signs of despair, discouragement, passive acceptance, anger, and hostility may be present. Shock, anxiety, numbness, strangeness, and unreality may be the immediate responses. During the retreat phase the patient may try to avoid reality; denial is common. Patients are not ready to look at the meaning or implications of the situation. They may repress or suppress reality and then, when this is no longer possible, become intensely angry. The patient is usually transferred to an intermediate unit before the acknowledgment phase occurs. This phase is marked by the conflicting emotions associated with recognition of the changes or losses that have or will occur. In the final phase, there is an attempt at a new approach to life.

The disturbances of self-concept are examined individually in this chapter. It must be remembered, however, that although each subcomponent has unique characteristics, some characteristics are shared with several or all the other subcomponents.

BODY IMAGE DISTURBANCE

Body image is the mental picture an individual has of his or her body and its physical functioning at any given time. It is based on past and present perceptions and includes one's attitudes and feelings about one's body. The body image develops over time from internal-sensation postural changes, contact with people and objects in the environment, emotional experiences, and fantasies.[41] Although the body image is a stable part of the self-concept, it changes over time; it is influenced by cognitive growth and physical changes in the body. Fisher[16] suggested that body experiences can be dampened or minimized, or they can be magnified to the point where they are the center of attention. He also described the *body boundary,* the demarcation between the self and the environment and the pattern of body awareness. The latter refers to the variation in attention given to different parts of the body; more attention is given to the parts that have symbolic significance or that are currently being threatened.

A change in the body's appearance, structure, and/or function necessitates a change in the body image. Such changes may be caused by disease, trauma, or surgery. The cause of body image disturbance may be biophysical, cognitive-perceptual, psychosocial, cultural, or spiritual. Body image disturbances arise when the person fails to perceive or adapt to the changed body. Such disturbances are manifested by verbal or nonverbal response to the actual or perceived change in appearance, structure, or function. A patient admitted to a surgical intensive care unit after a traumatic amputation may awake to find his or her leg missing with no prior knowledge of the loss. Reliving the accident and receiving explanations about the need for the amputation are priorities for such a patient. The critical care nurse must begin the process of helping the patient live with this alteration. Interventions by the nurse and others on the health team focus on helping the person manage the physical changes and the changes in the psychosocial areas affected. Helping the person recognize, accept, and live with the resultant change requires recognition that self-esteem and role performance may also be affected.

Body image has received considerable attention in the nursing literature.[2,5-8,25,32,34] This body of knowledge forms the basis for interventions with patients experiencing the losses associated with altered body image. Body image may also be altered by the need to incorporate a prosthetic device or a donated body part.[33]

The meaning of the alteration (appearance, structure, or function) varies with the individual. What is lost? What value is placed on it? What did the body part or function enable the person to enjoy or accomplish? What disability results? The values of the culture are important; wholeness, independence, and attractiveness are important in society today. The person's ability to cope, the responses from others significant to him or her, and the help available to him or her and the family are important factors in the outcome of body image disturbances.

SELF-ESTEEM DISTURBANCE

Self-esteem develops as a part of self-concept through the reflected appraisals of significant others. The way in which such information is interpreted is probably more important than the content. Self-esteem is only partly related to material, economic, or social conditions. The need for self-esteem is a part of the hierarchy of human needs postulated by Maslow.[23] Having high self-esteem helps one deal with the environment and face more easily the maturational and situational crises of life. A low self-regard impairs one's ability to adapt. Overall, the goal is to maintain a high positive regard for oneself in the midst of ever-changing views of oneself. This goal, when met, contributes to the quality of life of the individual. Persons with a well-developed self-esteem are at less risk for disturbances of self-esteem than those with poorly developed self-esteem.

Disturbances in self-esteem arise when a person experiences a decrease in self-worth, self-respect, and self-approval or self-confidence. Causative factors of the decrease include repeated negative interactions with significant others, as well as cognitive-perceptual difficulties. Low self-esteem may be manifested by (1) inability to accept positive reinforcement, (2) lack of follow-through, (3) nonparticipation in therapy, (4) not taking responsibility for self-care (self-neglect), (5) self-destructive behavior, and (6) lack of eye contact.

Self-esteem is an important concept for nurses and other health professionals. It has been studied frequently in a variety of contexts.* Nurses have a significant impact on patients who are experiencing illness. When the illness is critical, a patient's self-esteem level may be imperiled. Perhaps the patient caused the accident that injured him or her and others, including family members. Perhaps he or she was under the influence of alcohol or drugs. Perhaps he or she will be subject to arrest if he or she survives. Perhaps he or she will lose his or her job or be unable to return to

his or her previous occupation. The nurse who expresses negative reactions to a patient, either openly or covertly, will reinforce a patient's low self-esteem. An aloof, insensitive, or superficial relationship with a patient who has acquired immunodeficiency syndrome (AIDS), for example, can cause the patient to feel rejected, humiliated, and stigmatized.[47]

Antonucci and Jackson[1] pointed out that, although a link between self-esteem and mental illness has been confirmed, the link with physical health is not clear. Self-esteem level may be an outcome, a predisposing factor, or an insulating factor in situations involving physical health. In their study of self-esteem and physical health, self-esteem was lower as the severity of the health problem increased, as the perception of ill health increased, and as the degree of disability increased. The study stresses the need for awareness that patients with health problems probably have a lowered self-esteem that may negatively affect behavior during illness.

The antecedents of self-esteem were the focus of Coopersmith's book.[10] He identified four major factors that contribute to the development of self-esteem:

1. The amount of acceptance and concern from significant persons in one's life.
2. The successes in one's past and one's status and position in the world.
3. The values and aspirations to which one commits oneself.
4. The manner in which one responds to devaluing experiences.

Of special importance to the development of high self-esteem were three conditions: (1) total or near-total acceptance of the child by the family, (2) clearly defined limits that are reasonable, rational, and enforced, and (3) respect and allowance for individual actions within the defined limits.

Basic self-esteem as described by Crouch and Straub[12] is that which is established early in life and, once firmly established, is relatively unchanging. They also described a functional level of self-esteem that varies from day to day according to ongoing evaluations of interactions. Such self-esteem may be more or less than the basic self-esteem. The functional level can be changed in response to interventions of the person himself or herself, the family, co-workers, or health professionals. Functional self-esteem may be increased through individually oriented, short-term approaches that attempt to improve the person's view of his or her worth.

Self-esteem throughout the life span was discussed by Stanwyck.[43] He found that overall self-esteem was relatively stable and was based on critical elements of experience, including significant others, social role expectations, psychosocial developmental crises, and the communication and coping patterns of the family. In adulthood self-esteem is affected by intimate relationships, progress in social relationships, and career development. One's self-esteem needs the esteem of others. Experiences may confirm or modify self-esteem. Both failures and successful experiences are important. Such information may be ignored or disqualified as useful evidence. Hence the focus on perception of reflected appraisals is important.

In old age, a person faces loss of autonomy that may lower self-esteem. Changes in the expectations of others for

*References 1, 10, 11, 13, 18, 26, 27, 35, 40, 43.

one's behavior and capacity may occur. Losses related to health alterations and sensory impairment related to aging, dependency, retirement, and deaths of friends and family may affect self-esteem. If nurses are impatient with performance deficits, the patient may feel inadequate and guilty. If patients are treated as children, they may believe themselves burdens and react with resentment. Failure to include them in decision making may cause them to feel useless and rejected. On the other hand, people with a strong sense of self-worth are likely to be adjusted, happy, and competent.

Defensive self-esteem attempts to defend against the person's perception of a gap between his or her real self and his or her ideal self. High self-esteem is associated with a low need for social approval, comfort with intimacy and self-disclosure, and the ability to acknowledge personal failures. Rubin[40] discussed the loss of self-esteem that accompanies the loss of control of functioning in relation to time and place. This loss is associated with a decrease in self-esteem. A sense of shame accompanies this private judgment of failure.

A person's level of self-esteem is an important factor in the response to a critical illness, and behavior during illness may be negatively affected by lowered self-esteem. The patient with severe burns may interpret the avoidance behavior of nurses and family who are appalled by the appearance of the patient and the odor in his or her room as a devaluation of himself or herself. He or she may refuse to cooperate with the treatment regimen and may judge himself or herself a failure and be unable to see a future in which he or she will return to a productive life. Anticipatory interventions that assist the staff and family in their care of the patient would help to avoid such a situation.

ALTERED ROLE PERFORMANCE

Interactions with others that create and modify roles are an important part of the self-concept. The roles one chooses reflects one's beliefs and feelings. Persons have primary, secondary, and tertiary roles. Primary roles are those associated with gender, age, and developmental stage. Secondary roles are those of daughter, sister, and so forth. Tertiary roles are those assumed by choice such as scout leader or churchgoer. Illness, when it occurs, disrupts secondary and tertiary roles.

Role performance alterations are those problems that arise when a person experiences difficulties in making life transitions. Causative factors include lack of significant role models, inability to learn new roles because of life transitions, and cognitive-perceptual difficulties. Altered role performance may be manifested by (1) change in self-perception of role, (2) denial of role, (3) change in others' perception of role, (4) conflict in roles, (5) change in physical capacity to resume role, (6) lack of knowledge of role, and (7) change in usual patterns of responsibility.

Meleis[28,29] has examined role theory from a nursing perspective and pointed out that nursing deals with people who are experiencing transitions, that is, a change in role status. They may be completing a transition or about to begin one. Such transitions involve loss and addition to role relationships and may involve developmental, situational, or health status–related events. Each of the types of transition can have implications for nursing. Examples include the teen-aged girl who becomes pregnant (developmental), a young adult whose father dies (situational), and an older adult who experiences an acute onset of illness (health-illness event). All these transitions require changes in roles of the persons and families involved. The individuals concerned must incorporate new knowledge, alter behaviors, and change their self-concepts.

Role transitions occur in patients with critical illness. Role change in the transition from wellness or chronic illness to acute illness is a concern for the critical care nurse because role transitions mean changes in role relationships, expectations, or abilities and can be major concerns for the critically ill patient.

The rapid and potentially drastic changes that accompany critical illness may seriously interfere with role performance. The male patient after a myocardial infarction wonders about his role as husband, breadwinner, and careerist. The psychosocial needs of the patient in such a situation depend on age, gender, occupation, family roles, previous experience with illness, suddenness of onset, extent of illness, and prognosis. Nurses are frequently involved with situations that include alterations in role performance in individuals and families.

The patient may be unable to meet the demands of such changes and thus experience role insufficiency.[28] The use of role supplementation is an approach nurses can use in such a situation. As described by Meleis,[28] this intervention involves both preventive and therapeutic efforts. Using communication and interaction with patient and family, information or experience is conveyed that increases the awareness of the new roles and interrelationships necessary because of the role transition. For example, role insufficiency may be displayed in behaviors that reflect fear of moving from the critical care unit to the intermediate care unit. A variety of nursing activities can anticipate and facilitate this transition.

POWERLESSNESS

The concept of powerlessness may be defined as the perceived inability to influence or control an outcome. Powerlessness as a nursing diagnosis is defined as the perception of the individual that one's own action will not significantly affect an outcome. Powerlessness is a perceived lack of control over a current situation or immediate happening. Unrelieved powerlessness may result in hopelessness, which is discussed in the next section.

The causes of powerlessness include factors in the health care environment, interpersonal interactions, illness-related regimen, and a lifestyle of helplessness. A severe level of powerlessness may be manifested by (1) verbal expressions of having no control or influence over the situation, (2) verbal expressions of having no control or influence over the outcome, (3) verbal expressions of having no control over self-care, (4) depression over physical deterioration that occurs despite the patient's compliance with regimens, and (5) apathy. Moderate levels of powerlessness may be reflected by nonparticipation in care or decision making when opportunities are provided; expressions of dissatisfaction and frustration over inability to perform previous tasks and/or activities; not monitoring progress; expression of doubt about role performance; reluctance to express true feelings, fearing alienation from caregivers; passivity; inability to seek information about care; dependence on others that may result in irritability, resentment, anger, and guilt; and no defense of self-care practices when challenged. Low powerlessness may be reflected in passivity.

Both actual and perceived control over present or impending events are important.

An alert patient with widely spread metastatic carcinoma of the breast was admitted to the medical intensive care unit for treatment of septic shock. She was Japanese and had been married for many years to a US serviceman. After a conference with the physician, the husband gave permission for a "do not resuscitate" order. The nurses caring for her soon found that the patient was expecting to get better and to go home. A conference involving her and her husband and the staff clarified the situation. Treatments for her cancer would continue, but heroic measures would not be used. Every effort to get her ready to go home again would be made.

In this situation, there were cultural expectations that the husband would make all decisions. However, every effort should be made to permit the patient the right to make decisions about care to the extent he or she desires.

Most people expect to have the power to participate in making decisions that affect them. Feelings of powerlessness are avoided if possible. When patients feel their choices are limited, they may act against their own best interests.[19] Given enough frustration, any exercise of control—even one with negative outcomes (such as signing out of the hospital against medical advice [AMA])—can become attractive.

Individuals vary in the amount of control they prefer.[37] A patient may feel power, but he or she may or may not desire it. Important variables in this regard are the illness; values, traits, attitudes, and past experiences; the hospital setting; and social displacement. Personality, age, religion, occupation, income, residence, and race may all be pertinent factors. Apparently there is an increase in variability in the amount of control preferred as people age. Rodin[37] pointed out that giving a person more control than desired may result in negative outcomes: stress, worry, self-blame. The critical care unit routines may oppose or preclude any control by the patient. The person to whom control is important should be helped to continue to control as many areas of life as possible. On the other hand, a patient must be given the opportunity to choose not to control.

One explanation or this variable interest in control is the concept of *locus of control*. This idea of expectancy of control developed by Rotter[39] has been particularly helpful in explaining the variability of responses of people to similar situations. The locus of control is a personality characteristic, a relatively stable tendency to perceive events and outcomes as within or outside one's control regardless of the situation.

The Internal-External Locus of Control Scale developed by Rotter is useful in assessing this personality trait. A person with an internal locus of control tends to believe that events are under one's personal control. A person with an external locus of control, however, tends to believe that events are related to chance, fate, or powerful others. Situations exist in which the person with an internal locus of control has made serial lifestyle changes based on medical advice and then has experienced a major illness, typically a myocardial infarction. This experience forces him or her to believe that his or her own actions will not (because they have not) significantly affect the outcome. Repeated or significant experiences with illness may reinforce belief in an external locus of control for people who originally possessed an internal locus of control. Nursing interventions that support the power or influence the individual does wield help prevent an all-encompassing sense of powerlessness.

Another aspect of powerlessness is *learned helplessness*. Seligman[42] suggested that repeated experiences with uncontrollable events result in diminished motivation, lessened ability to perceive success, and increased emotionality. Interventions suggested to prevent or reverse learned helplessness include opportunities to exert control.

In the critical care unit, threats to a patient's control include the unusual signs and symptoms of his or her illness and inadequate knowledge about the situation.[36] The disease process and the personal, psychological, and social situation interact to affect the patient's perception of control or lack of control. If control is defined as the ability to determine the use of time, space, and resources, admission to a critical care unit strips away control to varying extents. Patients no longer can decide about physical care, socializing, or privacy. They are under the close scrutiny of the nurses and physicians and have decreased physical strength.

On admission persons lose their independent status. They become patients. Use of clothes and other personal belongings is usually restricted in a critical care unit. Patients cannot decide who enters the room, who provides personal care, or who intrudes with painful treatments. The hospital rules usually are not open to modification. Patients may feel anxious because they are separated from a familiar environment, have restrictions on visitors, and must depend on others for their care. They may fear death or permanent loss of function and may feel guilty if they have contributed to the cause of their illness or injury. They may resent the invasion of their privacy.

By virtue of their experiences of critical illness and care, people may lose sight of areas of influence they retain over themselves because so much control is taken from them. Nursing emphasizes this intact influence and control and thus helps to preserve it.

The extent of powerlessness is determined by the situation. Critically ill patients generally have experienced a rapid onset of illness without time to acquire the illness role. A sense of powerlessness in such situations is not unexpected. Poor interactions with the health care providers may make the situation worse. Patients may react aggressively, may try bargaining, or may refuse to comply with diagnostic and treatment regimens.

To assist further in understanding powerlessness, a brief examination of the bases of power is useful. French and Raven[17] identified five bases: *reward, coercive, legitimate, referent, and expert*. The perceived ability to reward or punish, an acknowledged right to influence, possession of personal characteristics with which another person identifies, and possession of special knowledge may be attributed to a person and thus enable this person to control or influence others.

In the critical care unit legitimate and expert power are usually most important. On admission the patient agrees to the rules and regulations of the setting (legitimate) and accepts the directives of the nurses and physicians (expert). In reality, patients may not be in the hospital voluntarily and may believe they are being coerced. They may fear retaliation if they refuse to agree to tests or to follow treatment regimens.

Miller[30,31] has written extensively about powerlessness in the chronically ill patient. Her ideas are useful in thinking about the acutely ill patient. Many patients in the critical care unit are chronically ill or will become so as a result of the event that precipitated the admission to the unit. Miller developed a powerlessness assessment tool to be used with chronically ill patients.[31] Control factors that increase or decrease a patient's control were categorized as (1) behavioral—responses available to influence or modify the situation, (2) cognitive—the interpretation of the situation, and (3) decisional—the choice of alternative.

Powerlessness in acutely ill persons is related to (1) the uncertainty of the outcome, (2) the strange, threatening, overwhelming experience in the critical care unit, including diagnostic and treatment events, and (3) the lack of knowledge about the situation. The nurse has a primary role in preventing and alleviating the perception of personal powerlessness in the patient and family.

HOPELESSNESS

Hopelessness is a subjective state in which an individual sees limited or no alternatives or personal choices available and is unable to mobilize energy on his or her own behalf. To help clarify this nursing diagnosis, a definition of hope is included—a feeling that what is wanted will happen, that desire is accompanied by anticipation or expectation.[46] Most people agree that an element of hope must be maintained no matter how hopeless things appear. Hope is a force that helps one survive. It is an attitude toward the future, and it occupies a key position between the present and future. The absence of hope is a serious situation.

Causative factors related to hopelessness include (1) prolonged activity restriction, creating isolation, (2) a failing or deteriorating physiological condition, (3) long-term stress, (4) abandonment, and (5) a lost belief in transcendent values or God.

Hopelessness is defined in terms of negative expectations concerning oneself and one's future life.[3] Motivation is lost; a decision is made not to want anything, to give up, and not to try to get something. The future seems dark, vague, and uncertain.

Hope often arises in the presence of crisis. The idea of giving up is vigorously resisted. The help of others in the situation supports the patient's belief. Hope wards off despair, mental anguish, disorganization, helplessness, and hopelessness.

A female patient with cancer who is receiving chemotherapy develops pneumonia and is placed on neutropenia precautions in the medical intensive care unit. She may believe she has no chance of recovery, since she feels isolated from staff and family and believes that her body will not fight the infection successfully because the drugs for the cancer have lowered her ability to combat infection. She may despair, become desperate, and despondent. What causes these feelings in critically ill patients? Why do they feel helpless? Their bodies have lost control. No longer do their physiological mechanisms adapt to changes. They need external help.

Hopelessness can take control and immobilize the patient. The sense of impossibility can block attempts to change the situation. A system of negative expectancies about oneself and the future may result in a sense of overwhelming defeat. The hopeful person can imagine a future and that the storm will pass. The hopeless one gives up.

Jones[20] pointed out that one tends to find what one expects in interactions with others. Processing information is selective. Expectancies cause an individual to act in ways that elicit behaviors that can be interpreted as confirming those expectancies, even when such expectancies are mistaken. This response is the behavioral confirmation of an expectancy, the self-fulfilling prophecy. This idea is important in instances of hopelessness. Staff members may feel helpless when patients do not respond to their care; they may label patients as hopeless. Patients recognize this attitude and react to confirm this expectancy by giving up. Engel[15] identified the "giving up–given up" syndrome and included hopelessness as one component. Other components included a depreciated self-image; lack of gratification from roles and role relationships; interference with continuity of the past, present, and future; and reawakened painful memories. The acutely ill individual is highly susceptible to such a situation. Persons may give up hope, believing that they have been given up by others—a self-fulfilling prophecy.

Illness influences hopelessness by threatening internal resources (one's ability to cope) and external resources (one's perceptions of who can help). A patient's autonomy, self-esteem, independence, strength, and integrity may be at risk.

The critically ill patient is a multiproblem patient. Nurses and physicians are tempted to focus on the crisis and overlook the patient in his or her totality. The critical care unit is noisy and frightening; it increases the patient's sense of vulnerability and the fear of death. The patient's degree of hopelessness is related to the perception and duration of his or her powerlessness. Thus feelings of hopelessness are not uncommon in critical care units. Therefore it is important to foster a realistic sense of hope. Science has progressed and can accomplish many things. Even if long-term survival is not likely, patients can be helped to plan to live the remaining life to the fullest. The critical care nurse must try to feel hopeful and identify some aspect of the situation in which hope is warranted, no matter how grave the situation, and must try to channel feelings toward some positive outcome.

Body Image Disturbance related to actual change in body structure, function, or appearance

Definition: Problem that arises when a person fails to perceive or adapt to a change in the body's appearance, structure, or function.

DEFINING CHARACTERISTICS

- Actual change in appearance, structure, or function
- Avoidance of looking at body part
- Avoidance of touching body part
- Hiding or overexposing body part (intentional or unintentional)
- Trauma to nonfunctioning part
- Change in ability to estimate spatial relationship of body to environment
- Verbalization of the following:
  Fear of rejection or reaction by others
  Negative feelings about body
  Preoccupation with change or loss
  Refusal to participate in or accept responsibility for self-care of altered body part
- Personalization of part or loss with a name
  Depersonalization of part or loss by use of impersonal pronouns
  Refusal to verify actual change

OUTCOME CRITERIA

- Patient verbalizes the specific meaning of the change to him or her.
- Patient requests appropriate information about self-care.
- Patient completes personal hygiene and grooming daily with or without help.
- Patient interacts freely with family or other visitors.
- Patient participates in the discussions and conferences related to planning his or her medical and nursing care in the critical care unit and transfer from the unit.
- Patient talks with trained visitors (support group representatives) about his or her loss at least twice.

NURSING INTERVENTIONS *AND RATIONALE*

1. Continue to monitor the assessment parameters listed under "Defining Characteristics." Additionally, assess patient's mental, physical, and emotional state; recognize assets, strengths, response to illness, position in Lee's phases (see p. 828), coping mechanisms, past experience with stress, support systems, and coping mechanisms.
2. Appraise the response of family and significant others. *Body image is derived from the "reflected appraisals" of family and significant others.*
3. Determine the patient's goals and readiness for learning.
4. Provide the necessary information to help the patient and family adapt to the change. Clarify misconceptions about future limitations.
5. Permit and encourage the patient to express the significance of the loss or change; note nonverbal behavioral responses.
6. Allow and encourage the patient's expression of anxiety. *Anxiety is the most predominant emotional response to a body image disturbance.*
7. Recognize and accept the use of denial as an adaptive defense mechanism when used early and temporarily.
8. Recognize maladaptive denial as that which interferes with the patient's progress and/or alienates support systems. Use confrontation.
9. Provide an opportunity for the patient to discuss sexual concerns (see Chapter 49).
10. Touch the affected body part *to provide patient with sensory information about altered body structure and/or function.*
11. Encourage and provide movement of altered body part *to establish kinesthetic feedback. This enables the person to know his or her body as it now exists.*
12. Prepare the patient to look at the body part. Call the body part by its anatomical name (e.g., stump, stoma, limb) as opposed to "it" or "she." *The use of impersonal pronouns increases a sense of fantasy and depersonalization of the body part.*
13. Allow the patient to experience excellence in some aspect of physical functioning—walking, turning, deep breathing, healing, self-care—and point out progress and accomplishment. *This helps to balance the patient's sense of dysfunction with function.*
14. Avoid false reassurance. Acknowledge the difficulty of incorporating the altered body part or function into one's body image. *This evidences the nurse's sensitivity and promotes trust.*
15. Talk with the patient about his or her life, generativity and accomplishments. *Patients with disturbances in body image frequently see themselves in a distortedly "narrow" sense. Encouraging a wider focus of themselves and their life reduces this distortion.*
16. Help the patient explore realistic alternatives.
17. Recognize that incorporating a body change into one's body image takes time. Avoid setting unrealistic expectations and *thereby inadvertently reinforcing a low self-esteem.*
18. Suggest the use of additional resources such as trained visitors who have mastered situations similar to those of the patient. Refer patient to a psychiatric liaison nurse or psychiatrist if needed.

Body Image Disturbance related to functional dependence on life-sustaining technology (ventilator, dialysis, IABP, halo traction)

DEFINING CHARACTERISTICS

- Actual change in function requiring permanent or temporary replacement
- Refusal to verify actual loss
- Verbalization of the following: feelings of helplessness, hopelessness, powerlessness, fear of failure to wean from technology

OUTCOME CRITERIA

- Patient verifies actual change in function.
- Patient does not refuse or fight technological intervention.
- Patient verbalizes acceptance of expected change in lifestyle.

NURSING INTERVENTIONS *AND RATIONALE*

1. Continue to monitor the assessment parameters listed under "Defining Characteristics." Additionally, assess patient's response to the technological intervention.
2. Assess responses of family and significant others. *Body image is derived from the "reflected appraisals" of family and significant others.*
3. Provide information needed by patient and family.
4. Promote trust, security, comfort, and privacy.
5. Recognize anxiety. Allow and encourage its expression. *Anxiety is the most predominant emotion accompanying body image alterations.*
6. Assist patient to recognize his or her own functioning and performance in the face of technology. For example, assist the patient to distinguish spontaneous breaths from mechanically delivered breaths. *This activity will assist in weaning the patient from the ventilator when feasible. To establish realistic, accurate body boundaries, a patient needs help to separate himself or herself from the technology that is supporting his or her functioning. Any participation or function on the part of the patient during periods of dependency is helpful in preventing and/or resolving an alteration in body image.*
7. Plan for discontinuation of the treatment, e.g., weaning from ventilator. Explain procedure that will be followed, and be present during its initiation.
8. Plan for transfer from the critical care environment.
9. Document care, ensuring an up-to-date care plan is available for all involved caregivers.

Self-Esteem Disturbance related to feelings of guilt about physical deterioration

Definition: Problem that arises when a person experiences a decrease in self-worth, self-respect, self-approval, or self-confidence.

DEFINING CHARACTERISTICS

- Inability to accept positive reinforcement
- Lack of follow-through
- Nonparticipation in therapy
- Not taking responsibility for self-care (self-neglect)
- Self-destructive behavior
- Lack of eye contact

OUTCOME CRITERIA

- Patient verbalizes feelings of self-worth.
- Patient maintains positive relationships with significant others.
- Patient manifests active interest in appearance by completing personal grooming daily.

NURSING INTERVENTIONS *AND RATIONALE*

1. Continue to monitor the assessment parameters listed under "Defining Characteristics." Additionally, assess the meaning of health-related situation. How does the patient feel about himself or herself, the diagnosis, and the treatment? How does the present fit into the larger context of his or her life?
2. Assess the patient's emotional level, interpersonal relationships, and feelings about himself or herself. Recognize the patient's uniqueness (how the hair is worn, preference for name used).
3. Help the patient discover and verbalize feelings and understand the crisis by listening and providing information.
4. Assist the patient to identify strengths and positive qualities that increase the sense of self-worth. Focus on past experiences of accomplishment and competency. Help patient with positive self-reinforcement. Reinforce the obvious love and affection of family and significant others.
5. Assess coping techniques that have been helpful in the past. Help the patient decide how to handle negative or incongruent feedback about the situation.
6. Encourage visits from family and significant others. Facilitate interactions and ensure privacy. Help family members entering critical care unit by explaining what they will see. Increase visitors' comfort with equipment; offer chairs and other courtesies.
7. Encourage the patient to pursue interest in individual or social activities, even though difficult in the critical care unit.
8. Reflect caring, concern, empathy, respect, and unconditional acceptance in nurse-patient relationships.
9. Remember that for the patient the nurse is a significant other who provides important appraisals of the patient and who can facilitate the change process.
10. Help the family support the patient's self-esteem.
11. Provide for continuity of nurse assignment to assure consistent contacts that can *facilitate support of the patient's self-esteem.*

Altered Role Performance related to physical incapacity to resume usual or valued role

Definition: Problem that arises when a person experiences difficulty making life transitions.

DEFINING CHARACTERISTICS

- Lack of acknowledgement of role change
- Change in usual patterns of responsibility
- Change in self-perception of role
- Denial of role
- Change in other's perception of role
- Conflict in roles

OUTCOME CRITERIA

- Patient verbalizes a beginning plan to alter lifestyle to meet restrictions imposed by physical incapacity.
- Patient verbalizes plans to adjust personal and family goals rather than to abandon them.
- Patient expresses willingness to interact with significant others.

NURSING INTERVENTIONS *AND RATIONALE*

1. Continue to monitor the assessment parameters listed under "Defining Characteristics." Additionally, identify the primary, secondary, and tertiary roles of the patient. Assess the patient's developmental stage and whether there are maturational and situational crises in addition to the health-related event. *Illness disrupts role performance and makes life transitions difficult.*

2. Assess past experiences with role change, the degree of attachment to the role, and the ability or capacity to modify the role.

3. Assess the patient's perception of the role change or role loss, the responses of others, and the likelihood of a new role performance consistent with role expectations.

4. Explore with the patient the expected role change; permit patient to express his or her fears and concerns. Recognize role(s) that will continue.

5. Help the patient establish realistic goals and expectations.

6. Reinforce and support positive behaviors with verbal praise. Help the patient face any conflicts.

7. Teach the new skill(s) needed. Convey information and experience necessary to patient and family. Provide environmental supports that permit mastery of new skills (equipment and time for practice). Be sure expectatons are clear. Reward mastery behavior.

8. Use role supplementation strategies (role clarifying, role-taking, role-modeling, role-rehearsal, and reference group interaction).

Powerlessness related to health care environment or illness-related regimen

Definition: The perception of an individual that one's own action will not sufficiently affect an outcome. Powerlessness is a perceived lack of control over a current situation or immediate happening.

DEFINING CHARACTERISTICS

Severe
- Verbal expressions of having no control or influence over situation
- Verbal expressions of having no control or influence over outcome
- Verbal expressions of having no control over self-care
- Depression over physical deterioration that occurs despite patient's compliance with regimens
- Apathy

Moderate
- Nonparticipation in care or decision making when opportunities are provided
- Expressions of dissatisfaction and frustration about inability to perform previous tasks and/or activities
- Lack of progress monitoring
- Expressions of doubt about role performance
- Reluctance to express true feelings, fearing alienation from caregivers
- Passivity
- Inability to seek information about care
- Dependence on others that may result in irritability, resentment, anger, and guilt
- No defense of self-care practices when challenged

Low
- Passivity

OUTCOME CRITERIA

- Patient verbalizes increased control over situation by wanting to do things his or her way.
- Patient actively participates in planning care.
- Patient requests needed information.
- Patient chooses to participate in self-care activities.
- Patient monitors progress.

NURSING INTERVENTIONS *AND RATIONALE*

1. Continue to monitor the assessment parameters listed under "Defining Characteristics." Additionally, assess the patient's feelings and perception of the reasons for lack of power and sense of helplessness.
2. Determine as far as possible the patient's usual response to limited control situations. Determine through ongoing assessment the patient's usual locus of control; i.e., believes influence over his or her life is exerted by luck, fate, powerful persons (external locus of control) or influence is exerted through personal choices, self-effort, self-determination (internal locus of control).
3. Support patient's physical control of the environment by involving him or her in care activities; knock before entering room if appropriate; ask permission before moving personal belongings. Inform the patient that, although an activity may not be to his or her liking, it is necessary. *This gives the patient permission to express dissatisfaction with the environment and regimen.*
4. Personalize the patient's care using his or her preferred name. *This supports the patient's psychological control.*
5. Provide the therapeutic rationale for all the patient is asked to do for himself or herself and for all that is being done for and with him or her. Reinforce the physician's explanations; clarify misconceptions about the illness situation and treatment plans. *This supports the patient's cognitive control.*
6. Include patient in care planning by encouraging participation and allowing choices wherever possible, e.g., timing of personal care activities and deciding when pain medicines are needed. Point out situations in which no choices exist.
7. Provide opportunities for the patient to exert influence over himself or herself and his or her body, thereby affecting an outcome. For example, share with the patient the nurse's assessment of his or her breath sounds and explain that they can be improved by self-initiated deep breathing exercises. *Feedback that the patient has been successful in helping clear his or her lungs reinforces the influence he or she does retain.*
8. Encourage family to permit patient to do as much independently as possible *to foster perceptions of personal power.*
9. Assist the patient to establish realistic short- and long-term goals. *Setting unrealistic or unattainable goals inadvertently reinforces the patient's perception of powerlessness.*
10. Document care to provide for continuity *so the patient can maintain appropriate control over the environment.*
11. Assist the patient to regain strength and activity tolerance as appropriate, *thus increasing a sense of control and self-reliance.*
12. Increase the sensitivity of the health team members and significant others to the patient's sense of powerlessness. Use power over the patient carefully. Use the words "must," "should," and "have to" with caution *because they communicate coercive power and imply that the objects of "musts" and "shoulds" are of benefit to the nurse vs. the patient.*
13. Plan with the patient for transfer from the critical care unit to the intermediate unit and eventually to home.

Powerlessness related to physical deterioration despite compliance

DEFINING CHARACTERISTICS

- Verbal expressions of having no control over the situation
- Verbal expressions of having no control or influence over outcome
- Despondency over physical deterioration
- Nonparticipation in care or decision making when opportunities are provided
- Dependence on others that may result in irritability, resentment, and anger
- Apathy

OUTCOME CRITERIA

- Patient verbalizes a sense of control.
- Patient verbalizes an increased ability to cope with the stress of illness.
- Patient demonstrates commitment to option(s) selected.
- Patient recognizes that efforts to delay the progression of the disease are worth his or her effort.

NURSING INTERVENTIONS *AND RATIONALE*

1. Continue to monitor the assessment parameters listed under "Defining Characteristics." Additionally, assess the patient's feelings and perceptions of the reasons for lack of power and a sense of hopelessness.
2. Determine through ongoing assessment the patient's usual locus of control; i.e., believes influence over his or her life is exerted by luck, fate, powerful persons (external locus of control) or influence is exerted through personal choices, self-effort, self-determination (internal locus of control).
3. Redefine the situation to change the patient's thought process about hospitalization to modify inappropriate beliefs and expectations.
4. Actively involve the patient in care and decision making.
5. Provide choices; make clear the realistic options available.
6. Assist the patient to exercise physical control when possible. Provide information that patient's efforts have had desired effects. For example, suggest that the patient can reduce his or her heart rate and even dysrhythmias by performing relaxation techniques. Then provide feedback that heart rate and ectopy have decreased when true.
7. Communicate desirable, positive behaviors by subtly providing examples.
8. Focus on attainable goals *so to not inadvertently reinforce perceptions of person's powerlessness*
9. Make explicit the positive appraisal of patient's personal resources and expectations for a successful outcome.

Hopelessness related to failing or deteriorating physical condition

Definition: A subjective state in which an individual sees limited or no alternatives or personal choices available and is unable to mobilize energy on own behalf.

DEFINING CHARACTERISTICS

Major
- Passivity
- Decreased verbalization
- Decreased affect
- Verbal cues (despondent content, "I can't," sighing)

Minor
- Lack of initiative
- Decreased response to stimuli
- Decreased affect
- Verbal cues (hopeless content, "I can't," sighing)
- Turning away from speaker
- Closing eyes
- Shrugging in response to speaker
- Decreased appetite
- Increased sleep
- Lack of involvement in care or passive allowance of care

OUTCOME CRITERIA

- Patient looks at speaker.
- Patient verbalizes, "I will try" (hopeful content).
- Patient initiates conversation with staff, family.
- Patient requests involvement in self-care activities.
- Patient's conversation reflects affect (hope, anger, disagreement, anticipation).

NURSING INTERVENTIONS *AND RATIONALE*

1. Continue to monitor the assessment parameters listed under "Defining Characteristics." Additionally, assess the patient's total health situation realistically. Do not offer false reassurance. What is the patient's perception of treatment and the environment?

2. Assist the patient to look for alternatives. Help patient establish realistic short-term and long-term goals.

3. Offer help and assist the patient as needed, *thus conserving the patient's energy for things the patient wants to do.*

4. Encourage and help the patient to have something for which to plan. Help him or her imagine a future, even a short-term one. Support the possibilities.

5. Offer information before events occur. Facilitate control and predictability of events when possible.

6. Be careful not to create a hopeless environment. Convey hopefulness despite being helpless to alter the outcome.

7. Support the patient's sense of security and inner strengths. Enhance his or her feelings of being understood. Support what the patient finds in the situation as grounds for hope. Do not renounce hope prematurely.

8. Facilitate close personal contacts between patient and nurse, as well as between patient and family and significant others. Help them to feel involved.

9. Inspire hope. Consider the patient's religious and cultural background. *Faith and hope in God are strengthening for some patients and families.*

10. Recognize the influences of others such as family, clergy, and friends.

11. Communicate an attitude of quiet confidence, genuine interest, and mutual trust. *This does much to support the patient's hope.*

12. Help the family members not to "give up." *Their struggle, as well as that of the nurse, is important. The family can regain and sustain hope from the nurse's example.*

REFERENCES

1. Antonucci TC and Jackson JS: Physical health and self-esteem, Fam Commun Health 6(4):1, 1983.
2. Baxley KO and others: Alopecia: effect on cancer patient's body image, Cancer Nurs 7(6):499, 1984.
3. Beck AT and others: The measurement of pessimism: the hopelessness scale, J Couns Clin Psychol 42(6):861, 1974.
4. Bonham PA and Cheney AM: Concept of self: a framework for nursing assessment. In Chinn P, editor: Advances in nursing theory development, Rockville, Md, 1983, Aspen Systems Corp.
5. Brown MS: Distortions in body image in illness and disease, New York, 1977, John Wiley & Sons, Inc.
6. Brown MS: Normal development of body image, New York, 1977, John Wiley & Sons, Inc.
7. Brundage DJ and Broadwell DC: Altered body image. In Phipps WJ, Long BC, and Woods NF, editors: Medical-surgical nursing: clinical concepts and practice, ed 3, St Louis, 1987, The CV Mosby Co.
8. Champion VL, Austin JK, and Tzeng O: Assessment of relationships between self-concept and body image using multivariate techniques, Issues Mental Health Nurs 4(4):299, 1982.
9. Combs AW and Snygg D: Individual behavior: a perceptual approach to behavior, New York, 1959, Harper & Row, Publisher.
10. Coopersmith S: The antecedents of self-esteem, San Francisco, 1967, WH Freeman & Co.
11. Cormack D: Geriatric nursing: a conceptual approach, Oxford, 1985, Blackwell Scientific Publications, Ltd.
12. Crouch MA and Straub V: Enhancement of self-esteem in adults, Fam Commun Health 6(4):65, 1983.
13. Driever MJ: Problems of low self-esteem. In Roy C, Sr, editor: Introduction to nursing: an adaptation model, Englewood Cliffs, NJ, 1976, Prentice-Hall, Inc.
14. Driever MJ: Theory of self-concept. In Roy C, Sr, editor: Introduction to nursing: an adaptation model, Englewood Cliffs, NJ, 1976, Prentice-Hall, Inc.
15. Engel GL: A life setting conducive to illness: the giving up–given up syndrome, Ann Intern Med 69:293, 1968.
16. Fisher S: Body experience in fantasy and behavior, New York, 1970, Appleton-Century-Crofts.
17. French JRP, Jr and Raven BH: Bases of social power. In Cartwright D, editor: Studies in social power, Ann Arbor, Mich, 1959, University of Michigan Press.
18. Hirst SP and Metcalf BJ: Promoting self-esteem, J Gerontol Nurs 10(2):72, 1984.
19. Janis IL and Rodin J: Attribution, control, and decision-making: social psychology and health care. In Stone GC and Adler NC, editors: Health psychology—a handbook, San Francisco, 1979, Jossey-Bass, Inc, Publishers.
20. Jones EE: Interpreting interpersonal behavior: the effects of expectancies, Science 234:41, 1986.
21. Lee JM: Emotional reactions to trauma, Nurs Clin North Am 5(4):577, 1970.
22. Martinez C: Nursing assessment based on Roy adaptation model. II. Self-concept. In Roy C, Sr, editor: An introduction to nursing: an adaptation model, Englewood Cliffs, NJ, 1976, Prentice-Hall, Inc.
23. Maslow AH: Motivation and personality, New York, 1954, Harper & Row, Publisher.
24. McCloskey JC: How to make the most of body image theory in nursing practice, Nurs 76 6(5):68, 1976.
25. McFarland GK and McCann J: Self-perception–self-concept. In Thompson JM and others, editors: Mosby's manual of clinical nursing, ed 2, St Louis, 1989, The CV Mosby Co.
26. Meisenhelder JB: Self-esteem: a closer look at clinical interventions, Int J Nurs Stud 22(2):127, 1985.
27. Meisenhelder JB: Self-esteem in women: the influence of employment and perception of husband's appraisals, Image: J Nurs Schol 18(1):8, 1986.
28. Meleis AI: Role insufficiency and role supplementation: a conceptual framework, Nurs Res 24(4):264, 1975.
29. Meleis AI: The evolving nursing scholarliness. In Chinn PL, editor: Advances in nursing theory development, Rockville, Md, 1983, Aspen Systems Corp.
30. Miller JF: Coping with chronic illness: overcoming powerlessness, Philadelphia, 1983, FA Davis Co.
31. Miller JF: Development and validation of a diagnostic label: powerlessness. In Kim MJ, McFarland GK, and McLane AM, editors: Classification of nursing diagnoses: proceedings of the fifth national conference, St Louis, 1984, The CV Mosby Co.
32. Murray RLE: Symposium on the concept of body image, Nurs Clin North Am 7(4):593, 1972.
33. Muslin HL: On acquiring a kidney, Am J Psychiatry 127:1185, 1971.
34. Norris CM: The professional nurse and body image. In Carlson C and Blackwell B, editors: Behavioral concepts and nursing intervention, ed 2, Philadelphia, 1978, JB Lippincott Co.
35. Norris J and Kunes-Connell M: Self-esteem disturbance, Nurs Clin North Am 20(4):745, 1985.
36. Roberts SL: Behavioral concepts and the critically ill patient, ed 2, Norwalk, Conn, 1986, Appleton-Century-Crofts.
37. Rodin J: Aging and health: effects of the sense of control, Science 233:1271, 1986.
38. Rogers CR: Client-centered therapy: its current practice, implications, and theory, Boston, 1951, Houghton-Mifflin Co.
39. Rotter JB: Generalized expectancies for internal versus external control of reinforcement, Psychol Monogr 80(1):1, 1966.
40. Rubin R: Body image and self-esteem, Nurs Outlook 16:20, 1968.
41. Salkin J: Body ego technique, Springfield, Ill, 1973, Charles C Thomas, Publisher.
42. Seligman ME: Helplessness: on depression, development and death, San Francisco, 1975, WH Freeman & Co.
43. Stanwyck DJ: Self-esteem through the life span, Fam Commun Health 6(4):11, 1983.
44. Sullivan HS: Conceptions of modern psychiatry, Washington, DC, 1946, William A White Psychiatric Foundation.
45. Sullivan HS: The interpersonal theory of psychiatry, New York, 1953, WW Norton & Co, Inc.
46. Webster's new world dictionary of the American language, Cleveland, 1966, The World Publishing Co.
47. Wolff PH and Colletti MA: AIDS: getting past the diagnosis and on to discharge planning, Crit Care Nurs 6(4):76, 1986.

Coping Alterations

CHAPTER OBJECTIVES

- *Discuss the following coping strategies as they relate to the critically ill patient: stress inoculation training, cognitive therapy, relaxation techniques, biofeedback, and psychotherapy.*
- *List and discuss factors that enhance coping.*
- *Discuss the importance of social support for the critically ill patient.*
- *Describe the needs and coping mechanisms of families of critically ill patients.*
- *Discuss interventions and nursing management for patients with coping alterations.*

helping relationship with the patient. The purpose of this chapter is to provide a brief overview of theories related to stress and coping as relevant to the critical care patient. Specific stressors are identified that have implications for the critical care nurse. Finally, nursing care plans for the patient experiencing coping alterations are presented.

THE CRITICAL CARE EXPERIENCE

Wong,[47] a psychiatrist, wrote of his personal experience as a patient in an intensive care unit. He described "losing connection" with the world and having no sense of time or sleep. He was immobile, experienced pain, and was attached to a ventilator, urinary catheter, gastric tube, intravenous (IV) lines, and chest tubes. A growing awareness of the tubes and lines entering his body helped him to get in touch with his sense of self. He realized his loss of control over

Patients in critical care units receive intensive and highly technical treatments for multiple health problems under the supervision of many health professionals. Nursing care enhances the effects of treatment modalities through specific interventions such as monitoring the patient's progress during treatments and administering specific treatments in collaboration with the physician and other health care providers. Most importantly, the nurse supports patients as they cope with the complexities of illness and the critical care environment. The ability of the nurse to support the coping resources of patients is related to an understanding and acceptance of the behavior exhibited by patients. Patients may rely on a nasogastric tube for nourishment, may be connected to numerous invasive lines, or may be dependent on oxygen and mechanical ventilation to sustain life. A nurse may efficiently and accurately monitor the equipment, vital signs, and subtle physiological changes in conditions while, at the same time, ignoring the critical question not asked but implied by the patient: "Am I all right?"

Understanding and acceptance of the patient's behavior will be enhanced through knowledge and a conscious willingness on the part of the nurse to work at maintaining a

---

COMMON COPING STRATEGIES

1. Seek information; get guidance.
2. Share concern; find consolation.
3. Laugh it off; change emotional tone.
4. Forget it happened (suppression).
5. Keep busy; distract yourself.
6. Confront the issue; act accordingly.
7. Redefine the problem; take a more optimistic view.
8. Resign yourself; make the best of what cannot be changed.
9. Do something, anything, perhaps exceeding good judgment.
10. Review alternatives; examine consequences.
11. Get away from it all; find an escape.
12. Conform, comply; do what is expected or advised.
13. Blame or shame someone or something such as a spouse, the job.
14. Ventilate; feel emotional release.
15. Deny as much as possible.

himself and his world. He used humor and denial and became alert to indications of improvement of his body functions as each mechanical support was removed. Then, in a state of hypomania (excessive emotion, elation, and motor activity) he discussed his work and made plans to return to the job in 2 weeks. He was suprised at the pain he experienced during his first meal. He fought to be rational but experienced hallucinations.

People cope with the critical care experience in many ways, and a complete listing of strategies would be impossible. Weisman[45] identified 15 common coping strategies, which are found in the box on p. 841. The nurse supports the patient as he questions his experience, that is, what he feels, hears, sees; as he wonders what his caregivers and significant others think of him; as he expresses his needs and wants against what he can realistically expect of himself or others; and as he learns new skills and adapts old ones. The nurse is essential to the patient's overall understanding and acceptance of the critical care experience.

COPING THEORIES

The reactions of patients to the critical care unit are varied as are the theories that explain feelings, thoughts, and behaviors of persons in such situations. Eisendrath[7] used Erikson's developmental theory to explain the psychosocial repression of individuals in the critical care unit, and Roberts[39] applied Piaget's theory of cognitive development to the egocentric behavior of the critically ill adult.

Other writers have focused on the emotional responses experienced by patients. Shine[40] described cardiac patients' reactions in terms of anxiety, that is, its manifestations, its undesirable physiological effects, and its frequent sources. Thomas[44] described the loneliness of the individual, and Quinless[38] wrote of the helplessness, powerlessness, hopelessness, and anxiety experienced in the critical care unit. Behavior has also been described as a manifestation of a psychiatric disorder, that is, the psychopathology of trauma patients,[41] and the "overload depression" of patients in the critical care unit.[5]

Coping as a concept offering interpretation of feeling, thought, and experience resulting in behavior after a stress-producing situation is presented in this chapter to offer further understanding of the patient and his behavior. Coping has been defined as "efforts to master conditions of harm, threat, or challenge when a routine or automatic response is not readily available."[32] Four models describing the process involved in coping, response to illness, cognitive appraisal, emotional processing, and conflict theory of decision making, are presented to assist the nurse in choosing interventions that are realistic and effective.

Response-to-Illness Model

Leventhal and Nerenz[28] described coping in terms of the self-regulating process that occurs when an individual adapts to illness. It is seen as a feedback system with processing loops that make interventions possible at any point in the process.

Input stage. During the input stage, or interpretation process, the individual registers and integrates the stimulus into

LEGAL REVIEW
Coping alterations in critical care patients

CASE EXAMPLE: *Cowan v. Doering,* 522 A.2d 444 (1987)

Two critical care unit nurses were found negligent in this case for failing to properly monitor a patient's condition and for failure to take appropriate precautionary steps to prevent the patient from attempting to commit suicide.

The plaintiff in this case was a registered nurse who became extremely depressed over severe marital problems and a romantic attachment to a physician where she worked. On two occasions she swallowed a large quantity of pentobarbital (Nembutal) in an attempt to commit suicide. Both attempts resulted in hospitalization and admission to an intensive care unit. During the first hospitalization plaintiff never became violent, but she attempted to disconnect the intravenous tubes and remove herself from chest and wrist restraints. Her physician requested a psychiatric consultation. During the second hospitalization plaintiff was again restrained. In addition, plaintiff was connected to a cardiac monitor, which had a screen at the central nurses' station. If the patient were to disengage herself from this device, the screen would show a straight line and an alarm would sound. Although plaintiff initially appeared extremely lethargic, she subsequently became agitated and attempted to remove the restraints and disconnect the intravenous tubing. Although aware of these developments, the doctor did not order a suicide watch. One evening the plaintiff's lover appeared in her room, ordered the critical care unit nurse to leave, and closed the door. The nurse went into another area to assist another patient and later heard the plaintiff's door close again. She returned to the plaintiff's room and found her bed empty, saw the open window, and heard moaning from outside. Plaintiff was found lying on the ground two stories below.

The jury awarded $600,000 to the plaintiff and apportioned fault among the doctors (85%) and nurses (15%). The nurses' portion of the award was $90,000.

his perceptual system. Pain, hot, cold, strong lights, nausea, loud noises, someone saying, "That is intravenous fluid," are examples of sensations experienced in the critical care unit. Strong emotions such as fear or anxiety increase the impact of the stimulus on the system.

Further processing of the stimuli occurs after the sensory registration. Different features of the experience arouse memories, and the attention is directed toward a particularly meaningful aspect of the memory. Then other associated memories are activated to the point that information may reach consciousness. Interpretation of the stimulus or body sensation is related to the individual's schemata, or framework, for understanding what is occurring. Examples of this process are as follows: the sensation, that is, "Crushing"; specific aspects of it, that is, "Chest"; the label given to the sensation, that is, "Heart attack"; the prognosis, that is, "Impending death"; the cause, that is, "My arteries are clogged"; and the temporal features, that is, "It will be better in a few minutes."

Other aspects of the schemata are the perceptual and conceptual memories. Perceptual memories are what an individual heard, saw, or felt during a certain experience. The interpretations that an individual makes, based on mostly perceptual memory, are associated with automatic responses. The conceptual memories are abstract and verbal representations of an experience that result in interpretations and a conscious determination of action.

Coping stage. The individual plans and generates actions during the coping stage. These actions are directly related to the interpretation of the illness. Plans are made for objective features of the illness such as the symptoms, how to seek help, treatments, length of time required for recovery, causes of illness, changes in lifestyle, and prognosis. Problem-solving strategies are used, and the individual deals with the emotional reactions. A threat to life, loss of body part, or loss of control frequently takes procedence over objective problem-solving actions.

Leventhal and Nerenz[28] support the importance of setting goals or temporal sequencing in smaller steps. In other words, an individual needs to know when his goals are more emotional (to tolerate the fear and helplessness) in contrast to more problem solving (to find ways to sleep despite the light and noise). Problem solving may be postponed until emotional reactions are managed. It is difficult to delay satisfaction or to endure pain, but some individuals are able to do so when they have a long-range view of the illness and its treatment. More frequently, the emotional features are so overwhelming that problem solving activities such as decision making are advised against. Problem-solving goals and activities can be achieved later when emotions are less intense.

The person in the critical care unit experiences a threat to the self (powerlessness). He must depend less on self and rely more on others for assistance, and emotional resources are taxed during a critical illness. How a person generates actions or the coping responses is not precisely known. A major resource is behavior that was used in the past, and knowledge and skill gained from past experiences are helpful. At times, previous experiences may be disruptive. For example, a person takes a pill for a headache, and it is relieved; Then he takes a pill for hypertension, but he cannot feel the effects. Nevertheless, the person must learn to take the pill daily, despite his feeling of wellness—a conscious intervention.

Monitoring stage. The third stage is the monitoring, or appraisal, stage. The outcomes of the coping responses are judged as ineffective or effective in relation to the goals and criteria set by the individual. Goals may be too concrete, confused, idealistic, or poorly related to time; thus an individual may conclude that his responses are not appropriate. The appraisal process is also related to emotional or objective feedback. Awareness of affect is a cue for the individual that the coping responses are controlled by the

automatic emotional process. The emotions signal a need for help to change the situation. The problem-solving behavior may become less effective because emotional information is incorrect, leading to misinterpretation and inappropriate actions.

The regulatory system repeats the processes of interpretation, coping, and monitoring as the individual responds to stressful events. Signs of an unstable regulatory system would include inconsistent, uneven, purposeless, and haphazard behavior, expressions of increased threat, distressed appearance, and verbalizations of general unhappiness.

Implications for practice. Leventhal and Nerenz[28] suggested further implications of the model for practice. First, the entire regulatory system must be considered: the interpretation of the illness or stress, the coping skills, and the appraisal criteria. Patients may be assisted by beginning with data to alter outcome appraisals. An analysis of the stressor and the patient's representation of it may reveal inconsistencies and areas for active intervention. The emotion experienced by the patient must be identified, and it is assigned a supposed cause or expectation. The explanation related to the emotion generates automatic coping responses, for example, fight, flight, hide. The explanations offered by staff are sometimes inappropriate in stress situations because of physiological changes occurring in the individual that cause an emotional reaction in the individual. The emotional reaction of the individual may also be unnoticed and result in inappropriate or insufficient staff interventions.

To change the objective and affective representations, alteration of schemata, both concrete and abstract, is required. The concrete perceptual memories seem to serve as an organized focus of responses, for example, fear of injections. To reduce these fears, verbal persuasion is not effective. Gathering information about the object itself and about one's ability to approach and deal with the emotion generated and having a rehearsal for approaching the object are important. For altering the automatic responses to situations, biofeedback training may be useful.

Inherent in the model is the setting of goals and time lines to promote self-regulation. Achievement of appropriate goals is assured, failures are less frequent, and self-regulation and coping effectiveness are enhanced. Sharing the model of self-regulation with the patient can promote his or her own appraisal of his efforts, make failure a less negative experience, and make swings between stability and instability less stressful.

Cognitive Appraisal Theory

Lazarus and colleagues[9-11,23,25-27] have developed a dynamic multivariate multiprocess of stress and coping. Cognitive appraisal and coping are mediating processes between the person-environment encounters and the immediate and long-term outcomes.

Cognitive appraisal is the process that the individual uses to evaluate his or her encounters with the environment. If the environment is considered endangering, impairing, diminishing, or overwhelming to his or her resources and well-being, stress is interpreted. *Primary appraisal* refers to the evaluation of what is at stake—is there benefit or harm to his or her values, self-esteem, goals, or commitments? The *secondary appraisal* identifies actions to take, or the coping options. Together, these appraisals determine whether the interaction or encounter with the environment is threatening, with a chance of harm or loss, or challenging, with a chance of benefit or mastery.

Coping refers to "the person's cognitive and behavioral efforts to manage (reduce, minimize, master, or tolerate) the internal and external demands of the person-environment transaction that is appraised as taxing or exceeding the person's resources."[10] This definition focuses on the coping process: what the person thinks and does, what comes first, second, and so on. Its concerns are with the situational context of the demand—what the demand is itself, the resources available, the constraints, and the time involvement. Coping is not considered good or bad, effective or ineffective, successful or unsuccessful, reality oriented or defensive. The coping efforts are significant in and of themselves.

Coping generally encompasses two functions: (1) regulation of emotions (emotion-focused coping) and (2) alteration in the person-environment encounter (problem-focused coping). The idea that emotion-focused coping strategies are pathological, ineffective, or maladaptive is questionable. Lazarus[24] posited that emotion-focused coping is harmful when it impairs important actions and is helpful when it reduces threats. Precise definition and assessment of emotion-focused coping strategies in context are necessary to specify appropriate outcomes.

The mediations of the person's appraisal and coping strategies have immediate and long-term effects. Changes of affect, physiology, and quality of encounters are the immediate effects identified by the theory. Long-term effects are important considerations because, although a person-environment problem may be temporarily resolved, the person may be in conflict with his goal or value, not be able to meet social or role expectations, or may exhibit behaviors that create additional problems.

Emotional Processing Model

Foa and Kozak[8] outlined a framework for the study of emotional processing that focuses on fear as a structure in the memory of individuals. The fear structure in the memory consists of the stimulus that produces fear and the responses, that is, physiological activity, subjective report, and overt behavior. A program to escape or avoid danger is thus constructed and placed in memory.

A stimulus presents information to the memory where it is encoded. Memory is searched, and if the information matches the fear structure, the fear response is activated, for example, the heart rate is increased. The person states that he or she is experiencing fear, and avoidance or escape behaviors are noted. As the stimulus continues, the physiological response decreases and a plateau is reached. Habituation occurs, or, in other words, the body becomes accustomed to the stimulus. The information that there is a decrease in the physiological response affects the memory structure, the behavior responses, and the meanings assigned to the experience. Corrective information can be integrated into the system at this point. With less potential harm perceived and less fear experienced, the need to escape is also lessened.

Foa and Kozak[8] proposed two strategies for fear reduction. The first is activation of the memory structure by providing fear-relevant information, for example, the threatening situation, the responses, or the meanings. Ways to access a fear memory include confrontation with actual situations, written or verbal descriptions, pictures, role playing, poems, and movies. In systematic desensitization the fear stimulus is first presented to a person as he or she is using relaxation techniques. The intensity of the fear stimulus is gradually increased; thus the relationship between the stimulus and response is diminished. Another technique, flooding, produces changes by continuous presentation of the fear stimulus, which eventually results in no fear reaction.

The following is an example of the application of these two strategies in the critical care unit. Before the procedure a patient who has a fear of blood's being drawn is taught deep breathing exercises as a way to relax. While in a relaxed state, the patient listens as the nurse tells him or her that the technician will be there at 7AM. Relaxation exercises continue, and feelings of intense fear abate. The patient is asked to describe the blood-drawing procedure. Seeing no signs of increasing fear in the patient, the nurses describes the event more vividly. The presentation of the procedure by the nurse in more and more realistic terms as the patient remains relaxed occurs repeatedly until the patient demonstrates a marked reduction in the fear response or no fear. Flooding occurs as a result of the patient's being in the critical care unit surrounded (or flooded) by new and strange, sometimes painful, stimuli 24 hours a day. It is an experience that happens to the patient by virtue of being exposed again and again to the critical care environment. The result is that the patient's fear is eventually obliterated.

Conflict Theory Model of Decision Making

The conflict theory model of decision making proposed by Janis and Mann[16,18] examines the decision and coping patterns associated with responses to threats such as life-threatening illnesses. Five patterns were identified: uncomplicated inertia, defensive avoidance, unconflicted change, hypervigilance, and vigilance.

Uncomplicated inertia. Uncomplicated inertia, or immobilization and inactivity, is related to misjudgment that stems from ignorance about the threat at hand, for example, illness, treatment, or procedure. This pattern can easily be changed by providing correct information about the threat and associated actions.

Defensive avoidance. A person who demonstrates defensive avoidance is either placing responsibility for decision making on another, procrastinating in making a decision or action, rationalizing a choice that is the least harmful, or ignoring threatening symptoms. Correction can occur as the person experiences hope about a positive outcome from the information and receives reassurances from the staff. For example, the patient questions that his or her doctor knows what to do in his or her case; the nurse encourages the patient to decide for himself or herself and assures patient that he or she has the ability to do so.

Unconflicted change. Unconflicted change is displayed when a person consents to do anything and everything the health care providers say and does not show any sign that he or she is worried, does not understand, or does not know what to do. When information is provided, the patient is selectively inattentive and afterwards is angry, feels he or she has been misled, and is not cooperative.

Providing too much knowledge about what will occur and developing overconfidence lead to the "work of worrying." During this time, the patient experiences anticipatory fear, rehearses what will occur, reassures himself or herself, and develops expectations for self and others. If this work of worrying cannot be done because of a pattern of suppressing the anticipatory fear, because the event was totally unexpected or accidental, because warnings were not given, or because reassurances were over-encouraging, then the individual cannot work through his or her emotional state.

Hypervigilance. Individuals may experience a near panic state when faced with danger, and they subsequently manifest hypervigilance coping patterns. During these periods full or complete information is not sought, and decisions to act are made impulsively. The person is emotionally excited and cognitively restricted, has a short memory span, oversimplifies or ignores complicating factors, and often repeats words and phrases over and over.

Janis[16] asserted that hypervigilance coping patterns were frequently used by critical care patients. Patients who have experienced "near misses" (for example, had a cardiac arrest), observed activities in the unit with other critical patients, or have a worsening condition have an increased probability of having a hypervigilance pattern. Lack of time to find a way to escape the danger and perceived impending loss or death predispose the patient to its use.

The environment itself also adds to the probability of hypervigilance because of environmental factors such as invasive and monitoring lines and equipment that restrict movement. Physical symptoms may include pain, nausea, dizziness, hypothermia or hyperthermia, and altered mental status caused by analgesics. Sensory deprivation or overload is another condition that may lead to hypervigilance. Examples in critical care are the continuous noise of machines and alarms, bright lights, repetitive questions, multiple caregivers and staff, and frequent procedures and treatments. The timing of the stress event (for example, frequent around-the-clock disturbances) also leads to hypervigilance.

Use of an alternative coping pattern is encouraged by giving the patient meaningful explanations of what has happened and what will be occurring in the future. The patient needs encouragement and reassurance that he or she has the ability to cope and that support is available to him or her. In addition, actions can be taken to reduce hospital and critical care restrictions and to approximate normal daily activity.

Vigilance. The vigilance pattern is characterized by examining the situation for appropriate goals, carefully gathering information, assimilating information, examining possible consequences of actions, and planning action strategies. By using this pattern, the person has three basic beliefs: (1) the decision he is making involves risk, (2) the solution can be potentially satisfying, and (3) sufficient time will be available before a choice is made. For example, when faced with a decision about consenting to a coronary angiogram,

the patient knows that there is risk involved, that he or she can gain the satisfaction of knowing whether he or she has coronary disease, and (in the case of a nonemergent elective procedure) that he or she will have time to consider the decision.

COPING INTERVENTIONS

Moos and Schaefer[33] described five major tasks that form the basis for treatment of patients in stressful situations: (1) establishing personal meaning for the crisis, (2) confronting the demands and reality of the crisis, (3) maintaining relationships with family and helpers, (4) managing emotions aroused by the crisis, and (5) sustaining a positive self-image. These goals can be achieved by the patients through the use of processes such as self-regulation, cognitive appraisal, coping with the emotional arousal, and decision making.

Stress Inoculation Training

Stress inoculation training was developed by Meichenbaum in 1977, has evolved into a treatment for impending stress, and is particularly effective for developing coping skills.[29,30] The first of three phases of stress inoculation training is conceptualization, during which the focus is on developing a collaborative relationship with the stressor, achieving an understanding of the stressor and its consequence, and reinterpreting reactions to the stressor. The second phase is one of skills acquisition, in which rehearsal with new skills is practiced and explored for usefulness to the person in stressful situations. Specifically, skills of relaxation, cognitive restructuring, and inoculation to failure, problem solving, and self-instructional training are taught. The final phase is one of application and follow-through, in which training is extended to the future with a focus on relapse prevention.

Cognitive Therapy

Cognitive therapy consists of a therapist assisting the patient to describe thoughts, feelings, and interpretation of events. The patient is encouraged to explore associations among the various thoughts, gather more information as necessary, and to validate interpretations of his or her thoughts and feelings. During this process both negative and positive thoughts are brought to the patient's awareness, and incorrect interpretations are identified. Overall, self-inquiry and correct validation of information are promoted.

Relaxation Techniques

Techniques of relaxation produce a decrease in pulse, breathing rate, blood pressure, anxiety, and pain. Benson[4] offered four components necessary for the relaxation response to occur: quiet environment, passive attitude, mental capability, and a comfortable position. Benson's technique involves maintaining a comfortable position with eyes closed in a quiet place, relaxing all of the muscles, beginning with the toes and moving to the head, becoming aware of breathing and focusing on it, and maintaining this state of relaxation for 10 to 20 minutes.

RESEARCH ABSTRACT

Effect of the family visit on the patient's mental status

Bay BJ and others: Focus Crit Care 15:10, 1988.

PURPOSE

The purpose of this study was threefold: (1) to determine the relationship between a family member's visit and the mental status of the critical care unit patient, (2) to determine the degree of family closeness and the mental status of the critical care unit patient, and (3) to determine the relationship between the family member's level of anxiety and the mental status of the patient after the visit.

FRAMEWORK

Literature reporting the interaction between the family and the critically ill patient has been conflicting. Some studies have viewed the family as an additional stressor and the nurses as patient centered. However, the importance of the supportive, nurturant role of the family is evidenced in critical care philosophy and in studies that show the positive effect family social support has on its members during stress. The stress of the patient is compounded by the complex critical care unit environment and routine. Behavioral manifestations of anxiety, changes in cognition, visual and auditory hallucinations, restlessness, illusions, and feelings of prosecution can be experienced by the patient when he or she is deprived of meaningful experiences. Because the family members have communication networks and intimacy functions that are already established, they could intervene in reducing the mental changes in their loved one during visiting. Crisis situations may impair the family's ability to help the ill family member. Anxiety may be transferred to the patient and have negative effects on his mental status.

METHODS

This exploratory study included a convenience sample of 74 patients and their families in three different general medical-surgical critical care units. Subjects were in the unit for a minimum of 24 hours, and, when appropriate, surgery had been performed at least 24 hours earlier. A revision of Adams Mental Status Examination (MSE) was used to assess the critical care unit patient's mental status. The Family Closeness Tool was used to assess family characteristics of mutuality-isolation and clear-unclear communication. The Spielberger State-Trait Anxiety Inventory was used to measure anxiety of the patient. Data on anxiety, demographic variables, and family closeness were collected before the visit. The MSE was administered to the patient before the visit, the family was allowed a 15-minute visit, then the MSE was administered to the patient a second time.

RESULTS

The average length of stay in the critical care unit was 4.45 days, and the mean patient age was 55 years. Thirty percent of the patients received antianxiety drugs within 24 hours of data collection, and more than half of the population received 4.46 narcotic doses in the same time period. Most family members had lived with the patient for more than 9 years. Age and the surgical status of the patient, i.e., younger age and those having undergone surgical procedures, were the only two variables that showed significant relationships with improved mental status after family visits. Using analysis of variance, a relationship was demonstrated between closeness and mental status. Family members who saw themselves as having moderate amounts of mutuality with the patient had the most positive effect on the patient's mental status. No significant relationships were found between state and trait anxiety and mental status change score.

IMPLICATIONS

Nurses can assess the patient's mental status before and after a visit to determine how the visit affects the patient's thoughts. Data collection about the family's closeness and communication practices would also be useful. A more specific instrument that focuses on assessing specific areas of mental status needs development. After specific abnormal behaviors are identified, various nursing interventions can be introduced and their effects noted. Critical care nurses need to be continuously aware of the family's dynamics and state of crisis. Holistic care includes the patient-family system, and it will be enhanced if nurses can gain insight into the precrisis system and how the illness has affected the family unit.

Biofeedback

Biofeedback is closely associated with relaxation techniques and is used to monitor the responses of the body as the individual attempts to exert control over these responses. Miller[31] offered examples of the use of feedback response and relaxation techniques in critical care. After administration of pain medication, the patient is instructed in the use of relaxation techniques. The change from focusing on the pain to focusing on the breathing pattern and chest movement is a diversion that helps to reduce pain. Information is given to the patient about changes in the heart rate that occur as the result of his or her efforts. By using these techniques, the patient can learn to relax, monitor the state of tension, and divert his or her thoughts as a way to reduce pain and manage stress.

Wilson-Barnett[46] reviewed 43 studies on intervention to reduce stress responses over a 20-year period. Information, particularly sensory information, was found significantly to reduce anxiety and promote recovery. Positive reappraisal regarding selected concerns was more effective in reducing stress than general information about the stressors. Moss[34] reported providing patient and family preoperative instruction is an effective method for decreasing fear and anxiety.

Psychotherapy

Brief psychotherapy, which focuses primarily on processing the painful event with a qualified psychotherapist, is another approach to the treatment of stress. Bellak, Leopold, and Siegel[3] described an exploration with patients of the meaning of surgery, anesthesia, possibility of death, and secondary gains of the surgery. Owen and Harrision[35] also used brief psychotherapy to examine stress and fears of patients who had experienced cardiac arrest. Psychodynamic considerations after heart surgery might include reducing hostility, widening sources of pleasure, stressing the value of relaxation, or developing less competitive and perfectionistic attitudes.[14]

Crisis intervention, conceptualized by Aguilera and Messick,[1] is a form of brief psychotherapy. During this process an assessment is made of the person's perception of the precipitating event, what support systems are available, and what coping mechanisms might be helpful. Based on this assessment, an action plan is developed. Interventions are related to the skill of the therapist and involvement and capabilities of the patient. Interventions may include assisting the patient with an intellectual understanding of the crisis, exploring feelings, helping him to identify coping mechanisms, and assisting him to reestablish social support.

Slaby and Glicksman[42] specified 40 principal factors related to adaptation to life-threatening illnesses such as cancer, heart disease, and near-fatal trauma. Those factors specifically related to enhancing coping are listed in the following box.

COPING AND SOCIAL SUPPORT
Stress-Buffering Model

The Stress-Buffering Model, developed by Thoits,[43] integrates coping strategies and social supports. Sources of stress are identified as threats to survival or loss of self-regard (emotional) or as reactions to the situation (situational). The major modes of changing the stressors are behavioral and cognitive.

Social support is conceptualized as a method of coping with stress in which the individual receives assistance in varying forms from other individuals. The form of support is not simply reassuring words but rather is derived from actions to help others deal with emotional and situational aspects of the stress. Helpers are identified as those who have faced similar situations or who have had similar reactions and who can provide empathetic understanding. Functions of empathetic understanding include validation of the experience and acceptance of one's feelings. The helper can accurately identify aspects of the situation and specific feelings that form the basis of the stress reaction.

FACTORS ENHANCING COPING

PATIENT

Patient and family's knowledge of the illness and treatment

Awareness of the relationship of past experiences and conflicts to anger being experienced with current stress

Use of age-appropriate adaptive mechanisms

Obtaining care from person of one's own choosing

Acknowledging psychological pain and seeking relief

Receiving support from someone else who has the illness

Identifying stages of adaptation, i.e., denial, anger, acceptance

Tolerating dependence on others for care and assistance

Finding strength and meaning in the experience

HEALTH CARE PROFESSIONALS

Giving truthful information to the patient as changes in illness and treatment occur

Demonstrating a positive, rational view of the illness, treatment, and prognosis

Providing ways for the patient to express self-control and autonomous decision making

Emphasizing the strengths and capabilities of the patient

Recognizing that denial is an adaptive phase during illness

Collaborating with the patient and family on care and treatments

Allowing time—particularly time to mourn loss of body function or capabilities

---

A summary of the Stress-Buffering Model is found in Table 48-1.

Families and Social Support

The family is part of the patient's primary social support system and, as such, demands the attention and concern of the critical care nurse. Pearlmutter and colleagues[37] described the needs of families of critical care patients at various stages. Families should be immediately reassured that the reactions they are experiencing do not imply incompetence but are felt by others in similar situations. They should be given explanations of policies and procedures and should be told that there will always be qualified staff to care for their loved ones. Further contacts are necessary to demonstrate respect and acceptance for the family's reactions such as hostility, sadness, and withdrawal; to listen to complaints and problems without invoking fear of reprisal; and to assist in the grief process. Finally, the family needs assistance during the transition from the critical care unit to

Table 48-1 Stress-Buffering Model

Sources of stress	Modes of altering response		Modes of assistance	
	Behavioral	**Cognitive**	**Behavioral**	**Cognitive**
Situation	Avoidance Withdrawal Distancing Altering threatening features to produce pleasure Constructing plans	Reinterpretation of situation as less threatening Deliberate distraction from stressors Devaluing Comparison with others having more problems	Removing distressed person from situation Advising how to change situation	Assistance in reinterpreting the situation Assistance in reinforcing the less-threatening aspects by repetition and selective intervention Distraction Diversion
Emotions	Acting on physiological sensations with stimulants or depressants, e.g., exercise, relaxation techniques	Biofeedback training Manipulation of expressive gestures through play-acting more appropriate feelings Reinterpretation of emotional state by relabeling with less-negative or socially appropriate phrase	Offering drink or other item Suggesting food and sleep to deal with emotional state	Assistance in focusing on internal state that is more comforting Coaching in biofeedback, meditation, desensitization Responding to appropriate expressive gestures Relabeling situation, using a less-threatening label or reinforcing the individual's new label

a step-down or general medical-surgical unit. During this time separation, loss of support, development of new relationships, and adjustment to a new environment and staff serve as new stressors to families.

Family coping mechanisms. Nine coping mechanisms of families of critically ill patients were identified by King and Gregor[21,22]: (1) turning to others for support, (2) remaining close to loved one, (3) review of events, (4) information seeking, (5) intellectualization, (6) rehearsal of potential future situations, (7) minimizing the situations, (8) repetition, and (9) hope. Nursing interventions to assist the family may consist of developing a helping relationship, listening, providing information, fostering hope, providing realistic expectations and goals, and assisting in an evaluation of previously used coping strategies.

Gaglione[13] identified behaviors of families of patients in the coronary care unit. Shock and disbelief were early responses, followed by anxiety, the need to be useful, the need to know that the patient is receiving the good care, and the need for emotional support. Informational, physical, and spiritual needs were only minimally mentioned.

COPING ASSESSMENT

Assessment involves the judgment of the nurse regarding the stress-coping patterns of the patient in the critical care unit. Several points must be considered when assessing the coping pattern of patients. The situational context of the critical care setting is in itself threatening. The various treatment procedures have profound physiological and psycho-

---

COPING ASSESSMENT QUESTIONS

CURRENT SITUATION

1. What is the nature of the threat, i.e., is it threatening to life, goals, values, or self-esteem, or to the ability to manage or cope?
2. What is the meaning of the event in terms of the past, present, and future?
3. What abilities, skills, and resources are available to meet the threat?
4. Is there an available support system?

COPING BEHAVIORS

1. What is the nature and range of emotion-focused behaviors?
2. What is the nature and range of cognitive-focused behaviors?
3. What are the effects of the current situation on self-esteem?
4. What are the effects of the coping behaviors on relationships with others?
5. Are there conflicts between values, beliefs, and needs?
6. How may the coping behavior affect the desired outcome?

logical effects on the patient. The numerous brief encounters with a variety of professionals and limited contact with significant others add to the stressful experiences. The emotional reactions and cognitive understanding accompanied by multiple coping behaviors are human responses to severe illness and major treatment procedures. An emotion is a behavior in itself and may not be effective as a coping mechanism. Suggested assessment questions are delineated in the box on p. 848.

RESEARCH ABSTRACT

Need satisfaction levels of family members of critical care patients and accuracy of nurses' perceptions

Lynn-McHale DJ and Bellinger A: Heart Lung 17(4):447, 1988.

PURPOSE

The purpose of this investigation was to gather information about the level of need satisfaction as perceived by family members and the extent to which nurses are able to identify accurately those areas of relatively high and low family member satisfaction.

FRAMEWORK

Incorporating family members into the patient's plan of care can have a significant impact on a patient's ability to cope during the stay in a critical care unit. When a patient is admitted to a critical care unit, both the patient and the family members must be viewed as experiencing major life crises. Therefore the likely contributions by these family members in terms of the patient's recovery will be influenced by the extent to which they are able to deal with their own crisis state. Crisis theory, in which family functioning is threatened or disrupted, formed the basis for this study. The family members' perception fo the crisis event and available support systems and their past and present coping mechanisms will affect their ability to assist the family to return to equilibrium or the precrisis state. The critical care nurse is in an ideal position to identify and coordinate interventions to deal with the stressors of family members, and the literature reflects this centrality of locus. For nurses to assist family members more effectively during crises, it is important that they be able to identify accurately those needs perceived by family members as unsatisfied.

METHODS

Fifty-two family members of 52 patients in critical care units of two large general hospitals in a metropolitan area formed the first study group. Family members were at least 18 years of age and had visited the patient in the critical care unit. The patient they had visited had to have been in the unit for 24 to 72 hours. Ninety-two critical care nurses in the two hospitals from which the family-member sample unit sample was drawn constituted the second sample group. Individuals in the registered nurse sample had to have been working in critical care a minimum of 1 year. Data were collected using a questionnaire consisting of 46 statements of needs that relatives of critically ill patients may have.

RESULTS

The mean age of family members was 48.5 years, and 73% were women. The mean age of the critical care nurses was 29.6 years, and 56% had their baccalaureate degree in nursing. Family members reported being more satisfied than dissatisfied for 43 of the 46 needs. They were relatively well satisfied with those needs that pertained to personal support systems, visitation, and information. They were less satisfied with those that related to psychological aspects, the environment, and institutional support services. Critical care nurses were moderately accurate at identifying the extent to which family members perceive their needs as being met. However, numerous items were identified for which marked disagreement was found. Those needs identified by families as the five most important were (1) to receive support from friends, (2) to see the patient frequently, (3) to feel that the hospital personnel care about the patient, (4) to feel that there is hope, and (5) to feel accepted by the hospital staff.

IMPLICATIONS

Whether unmet needs are accurately or inaccurately identified, they constitute a prescription for nursing interventions and deserve consideration in the care plan. The importance that each family member attaches to each need also must be taken into consideration. Family needs can be identified by using a family assessment form, which can be incorporated into the initial admission patient assessment. Data obtained should reflect family roles, relationships, strengths, weaknesses, and overall family functioning. A standard of care may be developed by the critical care unit staff for families who have potential for ineffective coping related to admission of their family member to the critical care unit. Subsequent investigations might include instrument development to assess specific needs and studies to identify the needs that patients and their families viewed as important but unmet.

Ineffective Individual Coping related to situational crisis and personal vulnerability

Definition: Ineffective coping is the impairment of a person's adaptive behaviors and problem-solving abilities for meeting life's demands and roles.

DEFINING CHARACTERISTICS

■ Verbalization of inability to cope. *Sample statements:* "I can't take this anymore." "I don't know how to deal with this."
■ Ineffective problem solving (problem lumping). *Example:* "I have to eliminate salt from my diet; they tell me I can no longer mow the lawn; this hospitalization is costing a mint; what about my kids' future? who's going to change the oil in the car? this is an incredible amount of time away from work."
■ Ineffective use of coping mechanisms.
    Projection: blames others for illness or pain.
    Displacement: directs anger and/or aggression toward family. *Examples:* "Get out of here; leave me alone." Curses, shouts, or demands attention; strikes out or throws objects.
    Denial of severity of illness and need for treatment
■ Noncompliance. *Examples:* activity restriction; refusal to allow treatment or to take medications (see Chapter 49, "Sexuality Alterations," for interventions with patients using adaptive denial vs. patients using maladaptive denial or no denial).
■ Suicidal thoughts (verbalizes desire to end life).
■ Self-directed aggression. *Examples:* disconnects or attempts to disconnect life-sustaining equipment; deliberately tries to harm self.
■ Failure to progress from dependent to more independent state (refusal or resistance to care for self).

OUTCOME CRITERIA

■ Patient verbalizes beginning ability to cope with illness, pain, and hospitalization. *Sample statements:* "I'm trying to do the best I can." "I want to help myself get better."
■ Patient demonstrates effective problem solving (lists and prioritizes problems from most to least urgent).
■ Patient uses effective behavioral strategies to manage the stress of illness and care.
■ Patient demonstrates interest or involvement in illness or environment. *Examples*—patient does the following:
    Requests medications when anticipating pain.
    Questions course of treatment, progress, and prognosis.

Asks for clarification of environmental stimuli and events.
Seeks out supportive individuals in his environment.
Uses coping mechanisms and strategies more effectively to manage situational crisis.
Demonstrates significant reduction in impulsive, angry, or aggressive outbursts (projection, shouting, cursing) directed toward family.
Verbalizes futuristic plans, with cessation of self-directed aggressive acts and suicidal thoughts.
Willingly complies with treatment regimen.
Begins to participate in self-care.

NURSING INTERVENTIONS *AND RATIONALE*

1. Continue to monitor the assessment parameters listed under "Defining Characteristics."
2. Actively listen and respond to patient's verbal and behavioral expressions. *Active listening signifies unconditional respect and acceptance for the patient as a worthwhile individual. It builds trust and rapport, guides the nurse toward problem areas, encourages the patient to express concerns, and promotes compliance.*
3. Offer effective coping strategies to help the patient better tolerate the stressors related to his illness and care. Give him or her permission to vent feelings in a safe setting. *Sample statements:* "I don't blame you for feeling angry and frustrated." "Others who are ill like you have expressed similar feelings." "I will listen to anything you want to share with me." "We don't have to talk; I'd like to sit here with you." "It's perfectly OK to cry." *Individuals who are provided with opportunities to express their feelings will be better able to release pent-up emotions and derive a greater sense of relief and comfort. Thus they are less likely to resort to overly impulsive, aggressive acts, which may harm self or others.*
4. Inform the family of the patient's need to displace anger occasionally but that you will be working with the patient to help him or her release his or her feelings in a more constructive, effective way. *Family members who are well-informed are better equipped to cope with their loved one's emotional anguish and outbursts. They are less likely to waste energy on feel-*

Ineffective Individual Coping related to situational crisis and personal vulnerability— cont'd

ings of guilt, fear, anger, or despair and can use their strength to help the patient in more constructive ways. The knowledge that their loved one is being cared for emotionally as well as physically will offer family members a greater sense of comfort and understanding. They will feel nurtured and respected by the nurse's attempt to include them in the process.

5. With the patient, list and number problems from most to least urgent. Assist him or her in finding immediate solutions for most urgent problems; postpone those which can wait; delegate some to family members; and help him or her acknowledge problems that are beyond his control. *Listing and numbering problems in an organized fashion help break them down into more manageable "pieces" so that the patient is better able to identify solutions for those that are solvable and to suppress those that are less relevant or not amenable to interventions.*

6. Identify individuals in the patient's environment who best help him or her to cope, as well as those who do not. Validate your observations with the patient. *Sample statements:* "I notice you seemed more relaxed during your daughter's visit." "After the clergy left, you were able to sleep a bit longer than usual; would you like to see him more often?" "Your grandson was a bit upset today; I'll be glad to talk to him if you like." *Supportive persons can invoke a calming effect on the patient's physiological and psychological states. Conversely, well-meaning but nonsupportive individuals can have a deleterious effect on the patient's ability to cope and must be carefully screened and counseled by the nurse.*

7. Teach the patient effective cognitive strategies to help him or her better manage the stress of critical illness and care. Help him or her construct pleasant thoughts, situations, or images that can simultaneously inhibit unpleasant realities. *Examples:* a day at the beach, a walk in the park, drinking a glass of wine, or being with a loved one. *Pleasant thoughts or images constructed during critical illness and care tend to inhibit or reduce the intensity of the unpleasant, stressful effects of the experience.*

8. Assist the patient in using coping mechanisms more effectively so he or she can better manage his or her situational crisis:

   Suppression of problems beyond his or her control.

   Compensation for illness and its effects; focusing on his or her strengths, interests, family, and spiritual beliefs.

   Adaptive displacement of anger, fear, or frustration through healthy, verbal expressions to staff.

   Effective use of coping mechanisms helps to assuage the patient's painful feelings in a safe setting. Thus the patient is strengthened and need not resort to the use of more ineffective defenses to rid itself of anxiety.

9. Initiate a suicidal assessment if the patient verbalizes the desire to die, states that life is not worth living, or exhibits self-directed aggression. *Sample statement:* "We know this is a bad time for you. You're saying repeatedly that you want to die. Are you planning to harm yourself?" If the response is yes, remain with the patient, alert staff members, and provide for psychiatric consultation as soon as possible. Continue to express concern to the patient and protect him or her from harm. *Suicidal thoughts as a result of ineffective coping or exhaustion of coping devices are not an uncommon occurrence in critically ill patients. If the mood state is distressing enough, a patient may seek relief by attempting a self-destructive act. Although the patient may not imminently have the energy to succeed in his or her attempt, voicing specific plans signifies a depressed mood state and a depletion of coping strategies. Thus immediate intervention is needed since the attempt may be successful when the patient's energy is restored.*

10. Encourage the patient to participate in self-care activities and treatment regimen in accordance with his or her level of progress. Offer praise for his or her efforts toward self-care. *Patients who take an active role in their own treatment and progress are less apt to feel like helpless or powerless victims. This greater sense of control over their illness and environment will guide them more swiftly toward becoming as independent as possible.*

Anxiety related to threat to biological, psychological, and/or social integrity

Definition: A vague, uneasy feeling, the source of which is often nonspecific or unknown to the individual.

DEFINING CHARACTERISTICS
Subjective
- Verbalizes increased muscle tension.
- Expresses frequent sensation of tingling in hands and feet.
- Relates continuous feeling of apprehension.
- Expresses preoccupation with a sense of impending doom.
- States has difficulty falling asleep.
- Repeatedly expresses concerns about changes in health status and outcome of illness.

Objective
- Psychomotor agitation (fidgeting, jitteriness, restlessness).
- Tightened, wrinkled brow.
- Strained (worried) facial expression.
- Hypervigilance (scans environment).
- Startles easily.
- Distractibility.
- Sweaty palms.
- Fragmented sleep patterns.
- Tachycardia.
- Tachypnea.

OUTCOME CRITERIA
- Patient effectively uses learned relaxation strategies.
- Patient demonstrates significant decrease in psychomotor agitation.
- Patient verbalizes reduction in tingling sensations in hands and feet.
- Patient is able to focus on the tasks at hand.
- Patient expresses positive, futuristic plans to family and staff.
- Patient's heart rate and rhythm remain within limits commensurate with physiological status.

NURSING INTERVENTIONS *AND RATIONALE*
1. Continue to monitor the assessment parameters listed under "Defining Characteristics."
2. Instruct the patient in the following simple, effective relaxation strategies:
   - If not contraindicated cardiovascularly, tense and relax all muscles progressively from toes to head.
   - Perform slow, deep breathing exercises.
   - Focus on a single object or person in the environment.
   - Listen to soothing music or relaxation tapes with eyes closed.

Progressive toe-to-head relaxation releases the muscular tension that may be a stress-related effect resulting from the threat or change in the patient's health status and outcome of illness. Deep breathing exercises provide slow, rhythmic, controlled breathing patterns that relax the patient and distract him or her from the effects of his or her illness and hospitalization. Focusing on a single object or person helps the patient dismiss the myriad of disorienting stimuli from his or her visual-perceptual field, which can have a dizzying, distorted effect. A clear sensorium allows him or her to feel more in control of his or her environment. (See "Sensory-Perceptual Alterations," p. 601.) Music or words expressed in soft, low tones tend to produce soothing, relaxing effects that counteract or inhibit escalating anxiety and provide respites from the patient's situational crisis. Closed eyes eliminate distracting, visual stimuli and promote a more restful environment.

3. Perform Therapeutic Touch. (See Appendix D.)
4. Actively listen to and accept the patient's concerns regarding the threats from his or her illness, outcome, and hospitalization. *Active listening and unconditional acceptance validate the patient as a worthwhile individual and assure him or her that his or her concerns, no matter how great, will be addressed. Knowledge that he or she has an avenue for ventilation will assuage anxiety.*
5. Help the patient distinguish between realistic concerns and exaggerated fears through clear, simple explanations. *Sample statements:* "Your lab results show that you're doing OK right now." "The shortness of breath you're experiencing is not unusual." "The pain you described is expected and this medication will relieve it." *A patient who is informed about his or her progress and is reassured about expected symptoms and management of care will be better equipped to maintain a more realistic perspective of his or her illness and its outcome. Thus anxiety emanating from imagined or exaggerated fears will likely be assuaged or averted.*
6. Provide simple clarification of environmental events and stimuli that are not related to the patient's illness and care. *Sample statements:* "That loud noise is coming from a machine that is helping another patient." "The visitor behind the curtain is crying because she's had an upsetting day." "That gurney is here to bring another patient to x-ray." *Clarification of events and*

*From Bigus KM: West J Nurs Res 3:150, 1981.

Anxiety related to threat to biological, psychological, and/or social integrity—cont'd

stimuli that are unrelated to the patient helps to disengage him or her from the extant anxiety-provoking situations surrounding him or her, thus avoiding further anxiety and apprehension.

7. Assist the patient in focusing on building on prior coping strategies to deal with the effects of his or her illness and care. *Sample statements:* "What methods have helped you get through difficult times in the past?" "How can we help you use those methods now?" (See Ineffective Individual Coping care plan for interventions that assist patients to use coping strategies effectively.) *Use of previously successful coping strategies in conjunction with newly learned techniques arms the patient with an arsenal of weapons against anxiety, providing him or her with greater control over his or her situational crisis and decreased feelings of doom and despair.*

8. Give the patient permission to deny or suppress the effects of his or her illness and hospitalization with which he or she cannot cope or control. *Sample statements:* "It's perfectly OK to ignore things you can't handle right now." "How can we help ease your mind during this time?" "What are some things or tasks that may help distract you?" *Adaptive denial can be helpful in reducing feelings of anxiety in patients with life-threatening illness. Bigus* reports that in studies of two groups of patients with myocardial infarction, the group that used adaptive denial demonstrated significantly fewer symptoms of state anxiety than those patients who failed to use it. (See Chapter 49, "Sexuality Alterations," for interventions with patients using adaptive denial vs. patients using maladaptive denial or no denial.)*

REFERENCES

1. Aguilera DG and Messick JM: Crisis intervention: theory and methodology, St Louis, ed 5, 1986, The CV Mosby Co.
2. Barrier D and others: Practice: a family assessment tool for family medicine. In Christie-Seely J, editor: Working with the family in primary care: a systems approach to health and illness, New York, 1984, Praeger.
3. Bellak L, Leopold R, and Siegel H: Handbook of intensive, brief and emergency psychotherapy, Larchmont, NY, 1984, CPJ, Inc.
4. Benson H: The relaxation response. In Monat A and Lazarus RS, editors: Stress and coping: an anthology, ed 2, New York, 1985, Columbia University Press.
5. Bronheim HE and others: Depression in the intensive care unit, Crit Care Med 13:985, 1985.
6. Carpenito L: Nursing diagnoses: application to clinical practice, Philadelphia, 1987, JB Lippincott Co.
7. Eisendrath SJ: Psychological concepts in the care of intensive care unit patients, Int J Psychosomat 31:8, 1984.
8. Foa EB and Kozak MJ: Emotional processing of fear: exposure to corrective information, Psychol Bull 99:20, 1986.
9. Folkman S and Lazarus RS: Stress process and depressive symptomatology, J Abnorm Psychol 95:107, 1986.
10. Folkman S and others: Appraisal, coping, health status, and psychological symptoms, J Pers Soc Psychol 50:571, 1986.
11. Folkman S and others: Dynamics of a stressful encounter: cognitive appraisal coping and encounter outcomes, J Pers Soc Psychol 50:992, 1986.
12. Frenn M, Fehring R, and Kartes S: Reducing the stress of cardiac catheterization by teaching relaxation, Dimens Crit Care Nurs 5:108, 1986.
13. Gaglione KM: Assessing and intervening with families of CCU patients, Nurs Clin North Am 19:427, 1984.
14. Heller S and Kornfeld D: Psychiatric aspects of cardiac surgery, Adv Psychosom Med 15:124, 1986.
15. Janis IL: Adaptive personality changes. In Monat A and Lazarus RS, editors: Stress and coping: an anthology, ed 2, New York, 1985, Columbia University Press.
16. Janis IL: Coping patterns among patients with life-threatening diseases. In Speilberger CD and Sarason I, editors: Stress and anxiety: a source book of theory and research, New York, 1986, Hemisphere Publishers.
17. Janis IL: Stress inoculation in health care: theory and research. In Monat A and Lazarus RS, editors: Stress and coping: an anthology, ed 2, New York, 1985, Columbia University Press.
18. Janis IL and Mann L: Decision-making: a psychological analysis of conflict, choice and commitment, New York, 1977, Free Press.
19. Johnson SJ: Ten ways to help the family of a critically ill patient, Nursing 86 16:50, 1986.
20. Kim MJ, McFarland GK, and McLane AM: Pocket guide to nursing diagnoses, ed 3, St Louis, 1989, The CV Mosby Co.
21. King KB: Psychological aspects of critical care, Heart Lung 14:579, 1985.
22. King SL and Gregor FM: Stress and coping in families of the critically ill, Crit. Care Nurs 5:48, 1985.
23. Lazarus RS: Psychological stress and the coping process, New York, 1966, McGraw-Hill Book Co.
24. Lazarus RS: The costs and benefits of denial. In Monat A and Lazarus RS, editors: Stress and coping: an anthology, ed 2, New York, 1985, Columbia University Press.
25. Lazarus RS and Folkman S: Coping and adaptation. In Gentry WD, editor: The handbook of behavioral medicine, New York, 1984, Guilford.
26. Lazarus RS and Folkman S: Stress, appraisal and coping, New York, 1984, Springer-Verlag New York, Inc.
27. Lazarus RS and others: Stress and adaptational outcomes: the problem of confounded measures, Am Psychol 40:770, 1985.
28. Leventhal H and Nerenz DR: A model for stress research with some implications for the control of stress disorder. In Meichenbaum D and Jaremko ME, editors: Stress reduction and prevention, New York, 1983, Plenum Publishing Corp.
29. Meichenbaum D: Stress inoculation training, New York, 1985, Pergamon Press.

30. Meichenbaum D and Novaco R: Stress inoculation: a preventive approach. In Speilberger CD and Sarason I, editors: Stress and anxiety: a source book of theory and research, New York, 1986, Hemisphere Publishers.

31. Miller BK: Teaching biofeedback techniques in critical care, Dimens Crit Care Nurs 4:314, 1985.

32. Monat A and Lazarus RS: Stress and coping: some current issues and controversies. In Monat A and Lazarus RS, editors: Stress and coping: an anthology, ed 2, New York, 1985, Columbia University Press.

33. Moos RH and Schaefer JA: Life transitions and crises. In Moos RH and Schaefer JA, editors: Coping with life crises: an integrated approach, New York, 1986, Plenum Publishing Corp.

34. Moss RC: Overcoming fear: a review of research on patient, family instruction, AORN J 43:1107, 1986.

35 Owen PM and Harrison JW: Brief psychotherapy after survival from cardiac arrest, Heart Lung 14:18, 1985.

36. Panzarine S: Coping: conceptual and methodological issues, Adv Nurs Sci 7:49, 1985.

37. Pearlmutter DR and others: Models of family centered care in one acute care institution, Nurs Clin North Am 19:173, 1984.

38. Quinless F: Assessing the client with acute cardiovascular dysfunction, Top Clin Nurs 8:45, 1986.

39. Roberts SL: Piaget's theory reapplied to the critically ill, Adv Nurs Sci 2:61, 1980.

40. Shine KI: Anxiety in patients with heart disease, Psychosomatics 25:27, 1984.

41. Silverman JJ and others: Surgical staff recognition of psychopathology in trauma patients, J Trauma 25:544, 1985.

42. Slaby AE and Glicksman AS: Adapting to life-threatening illness, New York, 1985, Praeger Publishers.

43. Thoits PA: Social support as coping assistance, J Consult Clin Psychol 54:416, 1986.

44. Thomas SA: Reducing loneliness in critical care, Dimens Crit Care Nurs 5:68, 1986.

45. Weisman AD: The coping capacity: on the nature of being mortal, New York, 1984, Human Sciences Press.

46. Wilson-Barnett J: Interventions to alleviate patients' stress: a review, J Psychosom Res 28:63, 1984.

47. Wong N: Psychological aspects of physical illness, Bull Menninger Clin 48:273, 1984.

Sexuality Alterations

- *Formulate nursing diagnoses for a patient whose sexual activity is compromised because of cardiovascular or chronic lung disease.*
- *Conduct a nursing interview that assesses the sexual concerns of patients with cardiovascular or chronic lung disease.*
- *Contrast the symptoms and causes of anginal pain, the pain of myocardial infarction, and chest wall pain.*
- *List appropriate patient responses and treatment strategies for the three types of chest pains that may occur during sexual activity.*
- *Describe nursing management of cardiac patients who demonstrate adaptive and maladaptive denial related to sexual concerns.*
- *Assist patients in correlating expended sexual energy with comparable MET equivalents.*
- *Inform patients and partners about alternate positions recommended for safe sexual activity.*
- *Facilitate opportunities for patients and partners to experience physical contact as a precursor to healthy sexual expression.*

Sexuality is a unique, highly individual expression and experience of the self as a sexual, erotic being. It is a holistic experience in that it encompasses both the mind and the body and a part of the character of a person also termed the personality.

To express oneself in a sexual way means to define who one is and what one feels in the most basic sense on one hand and yet in the most deep, profound sense on the other. Sexuality does not solely reflect the technique and mastery of sexual intercourse but is part of a being's relationship to and with all other beings throughout one's lifetime.

Sexuality may therefore be expressed in the most simple ways such as in the solitary activities of studying or walking in the park and also in the more physical demonstrations such as kissing, embracing, and sexual intercourse. Whichever way sexuality is expressed, most authorities agree that rapport and communication are two vital aspects of the sexual experience.

SEXUAL EXPRESSION

Sexual expression at its best is more than just attainment of coitus and orgasm. It also encompasses love, warmth, sharing, and touching between people and an emotional union of hearts and minds, all of which transcend purely physical pleasure. It is the culmination and coming together within the individual of biological, psychological, and cultural influences that result in sex-role behavior or sexual expression of self (Fig. 49-1).[7]

Sensuality, although a necessary component of sexual fulfillment, does not in itself reflect sexual activity. It refers to the pleasure one derives through the senses such as touch, smell, sight, and sound, which enhance the total sexual experience.

Sexual health is defined as "the integration of the somatic, emotional, intellectual and social aspects of a sexual being, in ways that are positively enriching and that enhance personality, communication and love."[31]

Sexual function is limited by very few inevitable, physiological truths—men normally impregnate women, and women are normally able to ovulate, menstruate, lactate, and gestate. All other differences, including aggressive behavior and even sex roles, have not been found specifically related to either man or woman.[10]

Most authorities concur that in today's society there is a wide range of accepted behaviors leading to sexual gratification. Sex without love or marriage has long been practiced, and although double standards exist, small vociferous groups claiming moral and religious propriety have failed to quell the sexual revolution.

A larger portion of society may frown on extramarital sex, or what is loosely defined as promiscuity, but unless one is engaged in illegal sexual practices such as prostitution or incest, sexual behavior is considered an individual decision. Legalized abortion and inexpensive, accessible birth

Call Mrs. Jones

at 555-4396

my wife of 46 years

and ask her to bring —

(1) Long box of kleenex.

(2) Three ink pens like this.

(3) Razors.

(4) One tube of Preparation H.

(5) Tell her I love her and that we'll think of each other on our 46th wedding anniversary, June 23rd

Bob

Fig. 49-1 Handwritten note from patient.

control methods have enhanced freedom of sexual expression.

Oral and anal sexual practices, bisexuality, homosexuality, and promiscuity are currently being more closely scrutinized as the result of information about the life-threatening, sexually transmitted disease acquired immunodeficiency syndrome (AIDS).

SEXUAL DYSFUNCTION

Masters and Johnson[15] originally introduced the term sexual dysfunction in 1970. It was originally interpreted to mean "sexual problem" or "sexual disorder." More recently (1979), Masters and Johnson, along with their associates,[12] first discussed sexual apathy and sexual aversion, calling these conditions "nondysfunction," or problems stemming from a "lack of desire or arousal," differentiating them from organic dysfunctions related to the sex organs themselves. It was thus clarified that sexual dysfunctions, according to Masters and Johnson[12], are "those sex problems that appear as difficulties on the physical level, such as problems with orgasms, erections or penetration." These physical symptoms are absent from or play only a small part in the bulk of sex problems.[11,16]

It is beyond the scope of this chapter to do justice to the works of leading authorities in the field of human sexuality. The literature is vast, interesting, and in some areas contradictory. For further information about things such as sexual anatomy and physiology, the phases of the human sexual response cycle, organic and nonorganic impotence, and intensive counseling related to sexual expression, refer to the works of experts such as Masters and Johnson, Robert Kolodny, Helen Singer Kaplan, and Bernard Apfelbaum.

This chapter uses the term sexual dysfunction as defined by the North American Nursing Diagnosis Association (NANDA)[4]: The state in which an individual experiences or is at risk of experiencing a change in sexual health or sexual function that is viewed as unrewarding or inadequate.

This chapter emphasizes common problems related to physiological and psychological stressors that threaten the sexual function of the male and female cardiac patient, with some attention given to the patient with chronic lung disease. The role of sexual partners is included throughout the discussion. Patients with sexual dysfunction related to neurological deficits are not discussed in this chapter, since the major portion of sexual assessment and intervention for that group of patients is better addressed during the rehabilitation phase versus critical care.

ASSESSMENT OF SEXUAL ACTIVITY INTOLERANCE

Most sources agree that critical care nurses should seize the earliest opportunity to teach patients and their partners about myocardial infarction and how to recognize and manage the different types of chest pain and control the symptoms of fatigue, dyspnea, and rapid heart rate during times such as sexual activity. Since chest pain is the most frightening symptom, the nurse needs to begin by teaching patients the specific language that describes the characteristics of the various types of chest pain. In this way he or she can help patients differentiate chest wall pain from anginal pain and anginal pain from the pain of myocardial infarction. The nurse can then assist patients and partners in connecting each type of pain with its probable cause, symptoms, duration, and mode of prevention and treatment. She or he can instruct patients how to monitor changes in breathing and heart rates and to determine if they are within normal parameters in relation to the amount of energy expended. The nurse can alert patients to be aware of thoughts that may invoke anxious feelings that can contribute to the physical symptoms and then demonstrate strategies to reduce anxiety. "Thoughts that attempt to fight chest pain are more likely to increase anxiety than are those that go beyond the immediate pain experience and focus on the idea that the pain will quickly pass."[24]

The nurse needs to inform patients and partners that some or all of these symptoms may occur during sex, partly because the work load of the damaged cardiac muscle increases to provide the oxygen needed to satisfy the body's demands for energy. Also, anxiety could arouse the nervous system into provoking or sustaining the physical symptoms.[22,24]

Angina pectoris is the chest pain associated with myocardial ischemia. Patients with ischemia have an imbalance of regional myocardial perfusion in relation to the demand for myocardial oxygenation. This transient imbalance is precipitated by conditions that increase the heart rate such as exercise, anger, anxiety, or postural changes. The location of the pain may be substernal or extrathoracic (neck, jaw, shoulder, arm) and may include variable degrees of discomfort. Patients who experience anginal pain during sexual activity may benefit from the prophylactic use of nitroglycerin, the use of long-acting nitrate preparations, or the use of beta-blocking agents such as propranolol. Some types of anginal pain may be experienced as indigestion or a toothache. Since anginal pain is precipitated by activities and exercise, it is relieved within minutes by rest or the use of nitroglycerin.

Myocardial infarction (MI) involves cellular damage and death of a portion of the cardiac muscle as a result of prolonged ischemia of more than 30 to 45 minutes. Permanent cessation of contractile function occurs in the necrotic or infarcted area. The degree of ventricular dysfunction depends on the size, location, collateral circulation, compensatory mechanisms, and function of the uninvolved myocardium. The patient suffering from myocardial infarction typically experiences severe, prolonged chest pain, frequently associated with sweating, nausea, vomiting, and a feeling of impending doom. If symptoms of chest pain, chest tightness, or severe shortness of breath persist, sexual activities must cease, and the physician must be notified immediately. Hospitalized patients should be instructed that this type of pain can always be treated with narcotic-analgesics.[22]

Chest wall pain is caused by a "tightening" of the chest wall muscles, which generally results from poor posture and is exacerbated by anxiety. "Hunching" of the back during sexual intercourse can strain the chest wall muscles and produce dyspnea. Patients should be taught to decrease anxiety by focusing on the idea that the pain will pass versus attempting to fight the pain. Dyspnea can be controlled by straightening the back and performing slow, deep-breathing exercises. Patients can learn to associate anxiety-producing thoughts such as fear of recurrent myocardial infarction and/or death with the occurrence of chest wall pain and recognize that such thoughts exacerbate otherwise normal symptoms of activity intolerance. Once patients successfully master relaxing the chest wall muscles, the cessation of pain will afford them confidence and control during sexual activity and will help them better distinguish between the three types of chest pain.[24]

PSYCHOLOGICAL FACTORS AFFECTING SEXUAL FUNCTION

Many authorities agree with the substantial evidence that recovery from myocardial infarction can be viewed from a psychological as well as biological perspective.

The meaning one ascribes to one's heart in human terms encompasses a multitude of emotions and feelings such as love, courage, sympathy, affection and survival itself. The heart and its attributes are romanticized throughout literature, music and the art world, to the extent that the very thought of it failing is to reduce it to the mere organ that it is and to bring one face to face with mortality.[24]

According to several outcome studies researched by Mayou, Foster, and Williamson[17] and Wishnie, Hackett, and Cassem,[31] approximately 50% of postmyocardial infarct patients continue to suffer from fear, anxiety, and depression, as well as low energy and fatigue, as long as 1 year after the heart attack. Between 20% and 30% of individuals suffer from a morbid fear of returning to normal functions and activities, including sexual activity. Adverse effects from severe anxiety and heightened somatic concern during the early phase of recovery have been associated with dysrhythmias, chest pain, and death. Patients who experience sexual problems as a result of drug therapy and who complain of chest pain, even with mild exertion, are in the minority.[11,24]

During interviews with spouses and partners of myocardial infarct patients, varying degrees of anxiety, depression, and sexual dissatisfaction were expressed. Both British and American studies[24,30] revealed that wives coped by overprotecting their husbands (for example, attempting to restrict husband's activities in general). Some resentment was also identified and was attributed to the wives' perceived loss of emotional support from their ill husbands. It probably contributed to the ensuing marital discord, although clear causality was not established.

Several authorities document the following psychological fears[11]:

1. Sudden death will occur from exertion.
2. Sexual activity will impose physical difficuilties in sexual function.
3. Heart attack is a "warning" that the aging process reflects a deterioration of sexual capacity.
4. Excitement and orgasm will cause another heart attack.

A study[19] was designed to demonstrate the influence of a brief marriage enrichment relationship skills training program (ME-RSTP) on marital satisfaction and quality of life in couples in the recovery phase of cardiovascular disease. It was established that adequate adaptation to life-threatening and lifestyle-threatening illness required that couples draw on previous relationship skills and coping styles honed from many years of marriage and past experience with stressful situations. It was concluded that only couples whose relationship skills and coping styles were inadequate to meet the demands of adapting to physical illness would truly benefit from such a program. Sexual counseling, no matter how well-intentioned, is not for everyone.

Couples who find in each other "a confidant—one with whom a person can have a close intimate relationship— . . . will be better able to sustain intimacy and satisfy the emotional needs of the relationship, in illness, as they did in health."[4]

Assessment of Sexual Concerns

Myocardial infarct patients who are at high risk for sexual dysfunction because of psychological concerns may be identified early in the critical care unit. For the critical care nurse, eliciting the patient's adaptive or maladaptive responses to myocardial infarct points the way to distinct interventions that may help him or her vent feelings and overcome loss of sexual function and fear of death (see the box below).

INTERACTIVE STRATEGIES

1. Provide privacy for patient and partner. This illustrates respect and consideration.
2. Demonstrate how they can comfort, touch, and hold each other. Explain the equipment so that they are not intimidated by it.
3. Begin slowly, with less personal topics, to build trust and rapport. Discuss topics such as diet, medications, and breathing treatments.
4. Bring in topics such as activities and discuss restrictions that this illness may impose on them (e.g., housework, gardening, playing golf).
5. Ask patient if he or she has any concerns about how these restrictions may affect sexual relations as well. If it is expressed that sex has not played a big part in the lives of the patient and partner for years but that they are still close in many ways, there is no need to pursue the subject. Simply move on to other areas. If a sexually active lifestyle is revealed, proceed to step 6.
6. Determine if the patient feels that the disease has affected, or may affect, his or her sexual activity and to what extent.
7. Ask whether he or she would like to continue sexual relations but is concerned or anxious about the shortness of breath that accompanies the sex act.[6]

One study by Sulman and Verhaeghe[28] revealed there are two distinct groups of patients in need of sexual counseling.

Group I patients demonstrate grieving behaviors such as poor appetites, saddened affects, and passive resistance to treatment and exercise regimen. These patients can develop growing anxiety or depression as a result of exaggerated concern about the effect of the illness on their sexual integrity and self-esteem and may require psychiatric consultation.

Group II patients demonstrate angry, "bullying" behaviors such as being uncooperative and noncompliant to treatment in a belligerent manner. These patients may deny the extent of their illness by continuing to smoke and work while in the hospital and threatening to resume sexual relations at a dangerous pace on discharge. They generally exhibit difficulty in absorbing important information about their illness and frequently verbalize their eagerness for discharge with impatience and frustration.

The researchers identified a third group of patients who comply with treatment in spite of their anxiety and depression. Unlike the patients who clearly display their need for intervention, these patients demonstrate more subtle symptoms, which may be deceptive. They are generally perceived as "good patients," since they make benign requests for encouragement and readily acknowledge apprehension and sadness. Often, their compliance is credited to their expressed feelings, so staff members fail to recognize their growing anxiety and depression. This group of patients requires preventive intervention such as positively acknowledging their participation in treatment regimens. Their consequent sense of mastery reinforces ego strength and promotes adaptive denial.

This same study stipulates that, occasionally, male myocardial infarction patients will verbalize sexually explicit comments interspersed with humor, jokes and "adolescent" type behaviors directed at the staff or visitors. This is considered a "normal" means by which some patients cope with the fear of sexual dysfunction and threat of death. The denial is considered adaptive as long as they *comply* with the treatment and exercise program. In dealing with this personality type, the nurse is advised to ignore the content of the conversation and "go along with the intent" in a light exchange of banter, as long as it allows the patient to cope in a healthy manner.

EXERCISE PHYSIOLOGY AND PATIENT EDUCATION

Experts suggest that during the acute phase of hospitalization (first 3 to 4 days) the critical care nurse should inform the patient and partner that walking, running, sex, and other activities will be possible and can be regained gradually through participation in a progressive cardiac rehabilitation program. Eighty percent of postcoronary patients can resume sexual relations 2 to 4 weeks after discharge (4 to 8 weeks after MI), as long as there is no history of complications (50% are uncomplicated) and if exercise can be tolerated to the extent of raising the heart rate to approximately 110 to 120 beats per minute (bpm) without precipitating angina or severe shortness of breath. Exercise tol-

erance can be ascertained by formal testing such as the use of a calibrated bicycle ergometer or a submaximal treadmill test.[9,19]

Although sexual intercourse is one of the most physically demanding exercises, conjugal sexual activity in middle-aged males (and females) with uncomplicated cardiac pathology invokes only modest physiological exertion with maximal cardiac stress lasting only 10 to 15 seconds. Sexual activity, including coitus and orgasm, can be compared in terms of oxygen consumption and work load of the heart to activities equal in energy expenditure. Activity progression is based on METs, a term used to describe the energy expenditure for many activities. A MET is a metabolic equivalent that can be assigned to activities regardless of a person's weight. One MET represents the energy expenditure of a person at rest and equals approximately 3.5 ml of oxygen per kilogram of body weight per minute.[1]

Most patients will need to perform three to four MET-level activities when they return home, and hospitals gear exercise programs toward that goal. Some of the activities that are considered comparable in oxygen consumption and energy expenditure to sexual activity, including coitus and orgasm, are as follows[1]:

1. Climbing two flights of stairs (20 steps in 10 seconds) without difficulty (this task is considered by experts to be the most standard test).
2. Taking a brisk walk (3 to 4 METS equal 4.8 km or 2½ mph).
3. Performing ordinary tasks in many occupations and recreations such as pushing a light power mower or pulling a light golf bag cart (Table 49-1).

The nurse can also teach the patient to assess his or her own readiness to return to sexual intercourse by checking the pulse rate during comparable activities. When it rises to 110 to 120 beats/min without causing shortness of breath, chest pain, or fatigue, sexual activity can be resumed. This generally occurs 4 to 6 weeks after discharge when the patient is still under the care and scrutiny of the physician.[21] One author[25] says 6 to 8 weeks but defers to physician's final assessment for decision.

Authorities[18,21,25] cite four danger signals that may indicate that sexual intercourse is causing physiological problems because of increased work load of the heart beyond the patient's endurance and should be ceased and a physician notified immediately: (1) dyspnea or increased heart rate that lasts longer than 5 minutes after intercourse, (2) extreme fatigue the day after intercourse, (3) insomnia after intercourse, and (4) chest pain during intercourse that is unrelieved by vasodilators, cessation, rest, and/or use of relaxation and breathing techniques.

Sexual activities such as hugging, kissing, and embracing should begin in the critical care unit to prepare for the more strenuous activity of sexual intercourse and to provide a more natural transition to sex for the patient and partner. Continuation of intimacy in illness also maintains healthy sensual relations between couples, which promotes overall wellness. Some patients may find it reassuring to attempt masturbation (3 to 4 METs) before intercourse for these same reasons.[14]

Patients also need information about the medications that

Table 49-1 Approximate metabolic cost of activities

	Occupational	Recreational
1½-2 METs* 4-7 ml O$_2$/min/kg 2-2½ kcal/min (70-kg person)	Desk work Auto driving† Typing Electric calculating machine operation	Standing Walking (strolling 1.6 km or 1 mile/hr) Flying,† motorcycling† Playing cards† Sewing, knitting
2-3 METs 7-11 ml O$_2$/min/kg 2½-4 kcal/min (70-kg person)	Auto repair Radio, television repair Janitorial work Typing, manual Bartending	Level walking (3.2 km or 2 miles/hr) Level bicycling (8.0 km or 5 miles/hr) Riding lawn mower Billiards, bowling Skier,† shuffleboard Woodworking (light) Powerboat driving† Golf (power cart) Canoeing (4 km or 2½ miles/hr) Horseback riding (walk) Playing piano and many musical instruments
3-4 METs 11-14 ml O$_2$/min/kg 4-5 kcal/min (70-kg person)	Brick laying, plastering Wheelbarrow (45.4 kg or 100-lb load) Machine assembly Trailer-truck in traffic Welding (moderate load) Cleaning windows	Walking (4.8 km or 3 miles/hr) Cycling (9.7 km or 6 miles/hr) Horseshoe pitching Volleyball (6-person, noncompetitive) Golf (pulling bag cart) Archery Sailing (handling small boat) Fly-fishing (standing with waders) Horseback (sitting to trot) Badminton (social doubles) Pushing light power mower Energetic musician
4-5 METs 14-18 ml O$_2$/min/kg 5-6 kcal/min (70-kg person)	Painting, masonry Paperhanging Light carpentry	Walking (5.6 km or 3½ miles/hr) Cycling 12.9 km or 8 miles/hr) Table tennis Golf (carrying clubs) Dancing (foxtrot) Badminton (singles) Tennis (doubles) Raking leaves Hoeing Many calisthenics
5-6 METs 18-21 ml O$_2$/min/kg 6-7 kcal/min (70-kg person)	Digging garden Shoveling light earth	Walking (6.4 km or 4 miles/hr) Cycling (16.1 km or 10 miles/hr) Canoeing (6.4 km or 4 miles/hr) Horseback ("posting" to trot) Stream fishing (walking in light current in waders) Ice or roller skating (14.5 km or 9 miles/hr)
6-7 METs 21-25 ml O$_2$/min/kg	Shoveling for 10 min (4.5 kg or 10 lb)	Walking (8.0 km or 5 miles/hr) Cycling (17.7 km or 11 miles/hr)

Modified from Fox SM, Naughton JP, and Gorman PA: Mod Concs Cardiovas Dis 41:6, 1972.
NOTE: Includes resting metabolic needs.
*MET is the energy expenditure at rest, equivalent to approximately 3.5 ml O$_2$/kg body weight/minute.
†A major excessive metabolic increase may occur because of excitement, anxiety, or impatience during some of these activities, and a physician must assess his or her patient's psychological reactivity.

Table 49-1 Approximate metabolic cost of activities—cont'd

	Occupational	Recreational
7-8 kcal/min (70-kg person)		Badminton (competitive)
		Tennis (singles)
		Splitting wood
		Snow shoveling
		Hand lawn mowing
		Folk (square) dancing
		Light downhill skiing
		Ski touring (4.0 km or 2½ miles/hr) (loose snow)
		Water skiing
7-8 METs	Digging ditches	Jogging (8.0 km or 5 miles/hr)
25-28 ml O$_2$/min/kg	Carrying 36.3 kg or 80 lb	Cycling (19.3 km or 12 miles/hr)
8-10 kcal/min (70-kg person)	Sawing hardwood	Horseback riding (galllop)
		Vigorous downhill skiing
		Basketball
		Mountain climbing
		Ice hockey
		Canoeing (8.0 km or 5 miles/hr)
		Touch football
		Paddleball
8-9 METs	Shoveling for 10 min (6.4 kg or 14 lb)	Running (8.9 km or 5½ miles/hr)
28-32 ml O$_2$/min/kg		Cycling (20.9 km or 13 miles/hr)
10-11 kcal/min (70-kg person)		Ski touring (6.4 km or 4 miles/hr) (loose snow)
		Squash racquets (social)
		Handball (social)
		Fencing
		Basketball (vigorous)
10+ METs	Shoveling for 10 min (7.3 kg or 16 lb)	Running:
32+ ml O$_2$/min/kg		6 mph = 10 METs
11+ kcal/min (70-kg person)		7 mph = 11½ METs
		8 mph = 13½ METs
		9 mph = 15 METs
		10 mph = 17 METs
		Ski touring (8+ km or 5+ miles/hr) (loose snow)
		Handball (competitive)
		Squash (competitive)

act to decrease cardiac work load, because they may be prescribed by the physician for use before intercourse to prevent chest pain.[2,18]

It is also important for nurses to inform patients about medications that can alter or interfere with sexual function and performance. Sometimes simply adjusting the dose of some drugs can ameliorate the problem.

A commonly shared perception has been that during the sex act the partner with the heart disease should assume the dependent or "patient-on-bottom" position. However, experts[19] have reported no significant difference in either heart rate or blood pressure when healthy men were studied while they engaged in sexual intercourse in either position. Peak heart rates were 114 beats/min for the "male-on-top" position, with a peak, mean blood pressure of 163/81 mm Hg. Findings during the "male-on-bottom" position were a peak heart rate of 117 beats/min and a blood pressure of 161/77 mm Hg.

Experts agree that patients with coronary artery disease who can perform a comparable level of activity without symptoms can safely resume sexual activity as long as they *avoid* sex in the following situations:

- After a heavy meal—food and/or drink disrupts circulatory efficiency and diverts blood flow from the heart and great vessels to the gut.[8]
- For at least 3 hours after alcohol ingestion—alcohol, even in small amounts, decreases cardiac index and stroke index in patients with heart disease[17]; avoid heavy drinking.[8]
- Positions requiring isometric exertion—they are more apt to increase the heart rate or precipitate dysrhythmias.[18,27]
- Anal intercourse—this could cause vagal stimulation and bradycardia.
- Extreme room temperatures—extreme hot or cold can add stress on the heart.

- When fatigued or during an emotional outburst—rest is beneficial before intercourse; and work load on the heart is increased during extreme tiredness, and there is increased stress on the heart during a highly emotional state.[17]

Most authorities agree that patients should avoid sex with unfamiliar partners because it is assumed that a greater level of excitement occurs, which may act as a stressor on the heart. However, no current scientific information supports this belief.[11]

Sex and Sudden Death

In a frequently cited study done in Japan,[29] 34 of 5559 cases of sudden endogenous death (0.6%) occurred during coitus. Eighteen of the 34 deaths were thought of cardiac origin, and 27 of them occurred during or after extramarital sex.

It may be, however, that alcohol use or other unknown variables affected the outcome of this study, since there are no reliable data to indicate the actual magnitude of the risk involved.[12]

PATIENT WITH SEVERE HEART DISEASE

Physical activity in general does not tend to induce ventricular tachycardia in patients whose conditions are well-controlled; but for the patients with severe heart disease, possible heart failure is a problem, and symptoms of angina, fatigue, and dyspnea must be considered warning signals. For these patients it is difficult to allay the fear of an impending episode of ventricular tachycardia and possible death.[5]

Experts suggest more investigation into the effect of sexual intercourse in provoking episodes of ventricular tachycardia. Since reliable data do not exist for this category of patient, guarantee of safe sexual experience cannot be made.[17]

The importance of the nurse's role as a caring, concerned communicator cannot be stressed enough. For patients who express difficulty in maintaining satisfying love relationships because of the realistic possibility of future abstinence, the nurse should remind them that intimate relationships can be sustained by less vigorous demonstrations such as hand holding, caressing each other, and possibly conjugal masturbation; the latter activity requires the physician's approval and is dependent on the patient's cultural beliefs, preferences, and activity tolerance.[24]

Loss of physical capacity is frequently perceived as a severe threat to self-esteem and concepts of masculinity or femininity (body image). Without appropriate counseling, the patient may well transfer these negative feelings to other areas of life such as work, recreation, and the parenting role. The nurse should be aware of the possiblity of the patient's developing overwhelming anxiety or depression and should seek psychiatric consultation if necessary.[25]

PATIENT WITH CHRONIC LUNG DISEASE

Another commonly seen group of patients who may have sexual dysfunction as a result of activity intolerance and shortness of breath are patients with chronic lung disease, for example, chronic obstructive pulmonary disease (COPD), cancer of the lung, or bronchiectasis. Because of the advanced age of some of these patients, the nurse should review the medical history carefully for other possible causes of sexual dysfunction unrelated to the respiratory problem such as excessive alcohol intake, renal disease, hypertension, diabetes mellitus, or use of medications. The history may uncover long-standing sexual problems that existed before the chronic respiratory illness. Such variables would alter the focus of the approach to sexual counseling.[6]

Anxiety caused by the shortness of breath is the most common complaint of patients with respiratory disease. The fear is so great that all physical activity, including sex, is avoided, often resulting in a decreased desire for sex and subsequent feelings of worthlessness and isolation. The desire for intimacy and close contact is also diminished because of the coughing, sputum production, and foul mouth odor that accompany respiratory disease.[13]

Nurses can reduce their own anxiety by increasing their knowledge about respiratory disease and sexuality and by recognizing the importance of sexual expression regardless of age, illness, disability, and course of treatment.

SUMMARY

Knowledge based on the long-term findings of experts in the field of cardiac pathology and exercise physiology and their effects on the work load of the heart during sexual activity, including intercourse and orgasm, can provide the critical care nurse with two major tools: (1) the scientific data base which affords accurate and inclusive information to the patient and his or her partner about sexual function and activity tolerance of the heart; and (2) the impetus to promote nursing research in the critical areas of cardiopulmonary physiology and human sexuality.

Sexual Dysfunction related to activity intolerance secondary to myocardial infarction

Definition: The state in which an individual experiences a change in sexual function that is viewed as unsatisfying, unrewarding, or inadequate.

DEFINING CHARACTERISTICS

- Verbalized reluctance to resume preillness levels of sexual activity because of decrease in energy and increase in fatigue (EXAMPLE STATEMENT: "I won't be the same in bed after this setback. I just don't have the stamina.")
- Chest pain, dyspnea, and increased heart rate during routine hospital activities, which patient assumes will occur during sexual activity (EXAMPLE STATEMENTS: "I get chest pain and out of breath just by moving around in my room and my heart speeds up when I exert myself. How is this going to affect my sex life?" "How will I know when I'm in danger of having another heart attack during sexual activity?")

OUTCOME CRITERIA

- Patient lists activities that are comparable in METs to energy expenditure and oxygen consumption during sexual activity, including orgasm. (see Table 49-1).
- Patient states with accuracy the specific vocabulary that describes and contrasts the three types of chest pain (chest wall, anginal, and infarct), their individual symptoms, conditions that provoke them, and actions taken for relief.
- Patient demonstrates correct monitoring of pulse rate while performing activities comparable, according to METs, in energy expenditure to sexual intercourse.
- Patient states which medications may alter or decrease sexual desire or performance.
- Patient verbalizes understanding of activities and situations to avoid before and during sexual intercourse.
- Patient describes symptoms related to sexual activity and orgasm that are considered life-threatening and must be reported immediately to a physician.
- Patient participates in progressive cardiac rehabilitation program.
- Patient and partner express they have achieved a mutually gratifying preillness level of sexual function as measured by patient's increased energy and decreased fatigue, dyspnea, heart rate, and chest pain 6 weeks after myocardial infarction.

NURSING INTERVENTIONS *AND RATIONALE*

1. Continue to monitor the assessment parameters listed under "Defining Characteristics." (See box entitled "Sample Interview Guidelines.")
2. Review METs (Table 49-1) with the patient and partner and explain which activities are comparable to sexual activity in energy expenditure and oxygen consumption (3-4 METs) such as climbing two flights of stairs in 10 seconds, walking briskly (2½ miles in 1 hour), pushing light power mower, or pulling light golf-bag.
3. Demonstrate monitoring of heart rate to be practiced by patient during activities that are equivalent to energy expenditure during intercourse and explain that coitus can be performed safely when heart rate is maintained within 110 to 120 beats/min without precipitating angina or severe shortness of breath.
4. Teach the patient the specific vocabulary that describes each type of chest pain, and ask him or her to associate each type of pain with its symptoms, provocation, and actions for relief such as the following:
   - *Chest wall pain. Symptoms:* tightness in chest muscles, sore to touch, shortness of breath. *Caused by* "hunching" of back, which strains chest muscles and/or anxiety. *Actions:* straighten back; relax chest muscles; take slow, deep breaths; and focus on idea that pain will go away. If not relieved within 5 minutes, notify physician.
   - *Anginal pain. Symptoms:* jaw pain or substernal pain that may radiate to left arm and/or shoulder; may be felt as indigestion or toothache. Caused by increased stress (exercise, anger, extremes of hot or cold temperatures). *Actions:* prevent by taking vasodilator before sex; should be relieved in minutes by use of vasodilator (nitroglycerin), cessation of sex, and rest. If pain persists or worsens, notify physician immediately.
   - *Infarct pain. Symptoms:* severe, persistent, "crushing" chest pain may be accompanied by sweating, severe shortness of breath, and feeling of impending doom. *Caused by* inability of narrowed coronary arteries to meet oxygen needs of heart muscle. *Actions:* notify physician and alert emergency facility immediately to obtain relief with narcotic-analgesics and oxygen.
5. Inform the couple that studies indicate the "patient-on-bottom" position during sex uses nearly as much energy as "patient-on-top" position but that isometric exercises (tightening of muscles, including heart) may increase heart rate more than safe parameters and should be avoided.
6. Construct a list of the patient's medications that may alter or decrease libido, performance, and/or sexual activity, and explain that the physician's adjusting the dose of some drugs may correct the problem.
7. Reassure the couple that safe sexual activity is possible, provided that situtations that dangerously increase the work load of the heart are avoided before sexual activity. Such activities include ingesting a large meal, consuming alcohol either excessively or 3 hours before sexual activity, fatigue, and emotional outburst.

Continued.

Sexual Dysfunction related to activity intolerance secondary to myocardial infarction—cont'd

8. Instruct the couple to avoid the following situations during sexual activity, and state the reasons why they should be avoided: anal intercourse, isometrics or "tightening" of muscles, extreme hot or cold temperatures, and sexual intercourse with a new partner.

9. Inform couple that if the following symptoms occur as a result of sexual activity, the physician should be notified immediately, *since it is a signal that the heart's work load is greater than its capacity to meet the body's energy demands:* shortness of breath that persists more than 5 minutes after orgasm, increased heart rate or palpitations that persist more than 5 minutes after orgasm, extreme fatigue the day after intercourse, insomnia the day after intercourse and chest pain during or after intercourse that is unrelieved by measures listed in interventions for chest wall pain and anginal pain (may indicate infarct pain).

10. Teach patient that, while in the hospital, his or her exercise tolerance during sex will be ascertained by formal testing such as monitoring heart rate during treadmill tests, the use of calibrated bicycle ergometer, and before and after walking briskly down the hospital corridor.

11. Reassure patient and partner that compliance with treatment regimen and participation in rehabilitation program will reduce work load of the heart and promote mutually satisying sexual activity, with increased energy and decreased fatigue, chest pain, and shortness of breath, within 4 to 6 weeks after myocardial infarction.

SAMPLE INTERVIEW GUIDELINES

LESS PERSONAL [TO BUILD TRUST AND RAPPORT]

Reflect observed behaviors: "Mr. Jones, you've been very quiet for the last 2 days and not eating very much. You hardly spoke to your wife today."

Voice concerns: "The staff and I are concerned that you don't seem interested in your treatment program. How can we help you?"

Sit in silence: "I'd like to sit here with you for a few moments." (Patient may choose to vent feelings or cry, in which case gently touching the patient's hand or arm is appropriate.)

Elicit feelings (open-ended approach):

"Tell me, what is it about your illness that troubles you the most?"

Offer information: "I have some information about your heart condition that will help you understand that there are some activities you will still be able to do, but they must begin now while you're in the hospital."

Praise accomplishments: "Mr. Jones, you are doing very well with your exercise program. If you continue, you'll be able to play golf again in about 6 weeks."

PERSONAL

Refocusing (open-ended approach): "Mr. Jones, you said that you've been married for 25 years. Tell me about your relationship. What kind of activities do you enjoy together?"

Open (direct approach): "Has this illness been associated with any problems in sexual relations?"

Offering reassurance (effective in connecting patient with others and alleviating fear and embarrassment and isolation): "Other patients have expressed some concerns about their sexual relations after an illness such as yours. Do you have any such concerns?"

Confrontive: "I'd like to clear up some concerns you have about your ability to experience healthy sexual relations in the future."

Positive closure: "It sounds as though you and your partner enjoy a close, intimate relationship. Hugging and kissing while in the hospital are healthy expressions of love. With your continued work toward recovery, you should enjoy healthy, satisfying sexual relations in 6 to 8 weeks."

Altered Sexuality Patterns related to fear of death during coitus secondary to myocardial infarction

Definition: The state in which an individual experiences concern about his or her sexuality.

DEFINING CHARACTERISTICS

■ Patient and partner demonstrate behaviors indicating sexual intercourse is a threat to patient's cardiac integrity and life function (EXAMPLE STATEMENTS *[patient]*: "I guess I'll have to take life easy from now on." "My [sexual partner] and I will have to be satisfied with holding hands" [affect anxious, voice tremulous].)

■ Partner demonstrates overprotective attitude toward patient, which invokes a shared sense of anxiety (sense of impending doom); partner verbalizes that patient "won't have to lift a finger from now on" (facial expression strained)

■ Patient demonstrates grieving behaviors, indicating diminished sense of self-worth related to threat to sexual performance and perceived body image change, including the following:
  a. Saddened affect (stares into space with bland facial expression)
  b. Lack of interest in food, treatment, and exercise program
  c. Apathy toward sexual information offered by nurses
  d. Resistance to sexual partner's intimate attempts such as kissing and hugging

■ Patient exhibits behaviors indicative of *maladaptive denial* (unconscious defense mechanism used to decrease anxiety and protect the ego against a painful, unacceptable reality—in this case fear of death and threat to sexual integrity) such as the following:
  a. Lack of cooperation with staff (uses loud, "bullying" tones)
  b. Nonparticipation in treatment and exercise program
  c. Refusal to pace activities (states intentions to " . . . work, drink, smoke, and have sex as usual")
  d. Strong rejection of information about sexuality.

OUTCOME CRITERIA

■ Patient demonstrates positive attitude with decreased anxiety (steady voice tone, calm body movement, eye contact when discussing illness, recovery, and sexual potential).

■ Patient rejects overprotective behaviors of partner (feeds and grooms self). This defuses partner's anxiety and builds mutual confidence in future sex roles.

■ Patient does the following:
  1. Exhibits brightened affect (animated facial expression and expressive voice tone) and indicates interest in life and a positive self-esteem.
  2. Actively participates in treatment and exercise program and reflects acceptance of body image change and potential for sexual participation.

3. Accepts sexual information offered by nurses about METs and repeats it accurately in a calm manner.
4. Responds to intimate advances of sexual partner and indicates decreased fear of resuming sexual activity on discharge.

■ Patient does the following:
  1. Refrains from using "bullying" behaviors (angry, demanding voice tone), and displays calm, cooperative attitude toward staff and sexual partner.
  2. Requests information about how safely to pace activities such as work, drink, cigarette smoking, and sex and repeats information accurately.

Long-term outcome (after discharge)

■ Patient and partner will verbalize transition to mutually satisfying preillness sexual function without fear of recurrent myocardial infarction or fear of death within 4-6 weeks (measured by increase in desire and frequency of the sex act and absence of feeling of impending doom during sex).

NURSING INTERVENTIONS *AND RATIONALE*

1. Continue to monitor the assessment parameters listed under "Defining Characteristics."
2. Clarify any misconceptions about myocardial infarction, contrasting realistic concerns with irrational fears about future sexual function and performance (Refer to "Sexual Dysfunction related to activity intolerance secondary to myocardial infarction" for specific information about cardiac work load during sexual activity.)
3. Inform the patient and partner early in the rehabilitation program that activity and independence are crucial to the patient's emotional and physical recovery in which sexual function plays a role. The ability to feed oneself is one indication of such progress.
4. Do the following:
   ■ Use therapeutic communication skills to elicit feelings of fear and anxiety about the effect of sexual intercourse on the function of the heart muscle and the life of the patient.
   ■ Encourage and provide privacy for intimate behaviors between patient and partner and for masturbation if feasible.
   ■ Provide clear, concise information about rationale for medical protocol and provide role-modeling of calm, controlled, adult behavior. *Knowledge provides power, which builds self-esteem and decreases anxiety. Use of adult behavior influences patient to respond in like manner.*
   ■ Praise the patient generously for participation in cardiac rehabilitation program, for pacing activities of daily living, for displays of intimacy, and for calm, controlled, adult behavior.

Altered Sexuality Patterns related to fear of death during coitus secondary to myocardial infarction—cont'd

- Discuss resumption of sexual activity in nonthreatening, matter-of-fact manner, beginning with discussion of the least personal activities such as gardening to the most personal areas. See box entitled "Sample Interview Guidelines." (EXAMPLE STATEMENT: "I'd like to discuss how you can safely incorporate activities, including sexual activity, back into your life.")

Interventions for long-term outcome
1. Refer patient to cardiac rehabilitation support group on discharge for help with continued sexual participation and enrichment.
2. Consult psychiatrist or sex therapist if patient demonstrates progressively depressed mood and affect related to sexual fear and anxiety that are unrelieved by nursing interventions.

Sexual Dysfunction related to activity intolerance secondary to chronic lung disease

DEFINING CHARACTERISTICS

- Patient and partner express the need to avoid or experience decreased frequency in sexual activities because of patient's dyspnea on exertion during all activities. (EXAMPLE STATEMENT: "It's too hard to breathe during any kind of exertion, so sex is probably out of the question.")
- Patient verbalizes anxiety or fear about life-threatening respiratory distress and increased heart rate during sexual activity. (EXAMPLE STATEMENT: "Sex is just not worth the risk to my life. I need to conserve my energy to survive.")
- Patient expresses feelings that increased mucus production, which is exacerbated by activities, including sex, may be repulsive to partner. (EXAMPLE STATEMENT: "My breath smells horrible with all this sputum, and it's worse during activities. How can anyone come close to me?")
- Patient avoids or rejects efforts by partner to kiss or embrace in the critical care unit.

OUTCOME CRITERIA

- Patient demonstrates intimate behaviors with partner and masturbates, if feasible, while in critical care unit (affords patient the opportunity to monitor return of pulse and respiratory rate to normal after orgasm).
- Patient expresses willingness to engage in sexual intercourse after taking appropriate rest periods to conserve energy, decrease mucus production, and reduce dyspnea.
- Patient verbalizes desire to try alternative, energy-saving positions during sexual intercourse.

- Patient lists appropriate medications or treatments for use before sexual activity.
- Patient states knowledge of effects of drug therapy, alcohol consumption, and heavy meals on sexual activity.

Long-term outcomes (after discharge)
- Patient monitors pulse and respiratory rates before, during, and after sexual activity to note return of rates to normal after coitus.
- Patient and partner expresses they have mutually gratifying sexual activity and patient has increased energy, decreased mucus production, and minimal episodes of dyspnea.
- Patient and partner enroll in pulmonary rehabilitation program.

NURSING INTERVENTIONS *AND RATIONALE*

1. Continue to monitor the assessment parameters listed under "Defining Characteristics."
2. The nurse will inform the patient about the following:
   - Sexual intercourse will increase the pulse and respiratory rates, but they will normally return to baseline very quickly. (Demonstrate how to monitor pulse rate.)
   - Sexual intercourse with orgasm uses approximately the same amount of energy as climbing two flights of stairs in 10 seconds, walking briskly (2 ½ miles in 1 hour), pushing tight power, or pulling light golf bag. (See Table 49-1.)

Continued.

Sexual Dysfunction related to activity intolerance secondary to chronic lung disease—cont'd

- The "patient-on-top" position, although shown in most studies to require nearly the same amount of energy expenditure as the "patient-on-bottom" position, should be avoided by the respiratory patient *because it may tend to produce more dyspnea. On the other hand, the "patient-on-bottom" position could lead to compression of the chest, which may also lead to shortness of breath.* Thus, the following alternative positions should be tried:

  Side-to-side, rear, or front entry (by male) except for the hypoxemic individual *who may not be able to tolerate having head and upper chest in a flat position.* In this situation, *upright position augments ventilation and perfusion and improves oxygenation status.*[3]

  Patient in chair with feet on floor and partner (female) astride.

  Masturbation and oral-genital sex (if feasible). Remember that age, religion, cultural beliefs, and desire should be considered before suggesting these alternatives. Although oral-genital sex may be difficult because of the dyspnea, cough, and sputum production, it is up to the patient to determine how bothersome this is compared to the pleasure of sexual fulfillment. Some authorities believe that masturbation can begin in the critical care unit, depending on the couple's inclination and the condition of the patient. They believe that *patients who masturbate while in the critical care unit set the stage for a smoother transition toward resumption of "normal" or "near-normal" sexual function after discharge as their conditions allow.*

  - *Holding, touching, and caressing are acceptable behaviors in the critical care unit. Also, whenever couples express anxiety about having sex when at home, they should be advised to relax, "cuddle up," and enjoy a glass of wine together at home.*

- *Inhaled bronchodilators can be used by patients with asthma before, during, and after sex to decrease anxiety and shortness of breath.*
- Taking medications 30 to 60 minutes before sexual activity *may decrease dyspnea.*
- Use of steroids and theophylline have no effect on sexual functioning. (In some instances, adjusting the dose with physician's advice may increase libido and potency.)
- If oxygen is used at home, increase the liter flow by 1 L/min during intercourse with the recommendation of the physician.
- Intercourse should be avoided after a heavy meal. *A full stomach can restrict ventilatory movement because of the raised diaphragm.*
- Excessive alcohol consumption decreases sexual function.
- Sexual intercourse is best initiated after a rest period such as in the morning hours, but if there is excessive sputum production at that time, it may be better to plan sexual activities for the afternoon after a nap.
- The use of a waterbed is recommended by some[7] who believe that *there is decreased demand for energy during sexual intercourse because of the rhythm of the bed.*
- Attending a pulmonary rehabilitation program to learn about the techniques that aid breathing and conserve energy and about exercises that can increase activity tolerance during sex is crucial after discharge.[6]

REFERENCES

1. American College of Sports Medicine: Guidelines for graded exercise testing and exercise prescription, ed 2, Philadelphia, 1980, Lea and Febiger.
2. Baggs J: Nursing diagnosis: potential sexual dysfunction after myocardial infarction, Dimens Crit Care Nurs 5(3):178, 1986.
3. Campbell ML: Sexual dysfunction in the COPD patient, Dimens Crit Care Nurs 6(2):70, 1987.
4. Carpenito LJ: Nursing diagnosis: application to clinical practice, ed 3, Philadelphia, 1989, JB Lippincott Co.
5. Cassels C, Eckstein A, and Fortinash K: Retirement: aspects, response, and nursing implications, J Gerontol Nurs 7(6):335, 1981.
6. Cohelo A and others: Treadmill testing in patients with recurrent sustained ventricular tachycardia, Circulation 64:IV, 1981.
7. Cooper D: Sexual counseling of the patient with chronic lung disease, Focus Crit Care 13(3):18, 1986.
8. Ebersole P and Hess P: Toward healthy aging, human needs, and nursing response, ed 3, St Louis, 1989, CV Mosby Co.
9. Gould L and others: Cardiac effects of a cocktail, JAMA 218:1799, 1971.
10. Hellerstein HK and Friedman EH: Sexual activity and the postcoronary patient, Arch Intern Med 125:987, 1970.
11. Johnson BS: Psychiatric mental health nursing, adaptation and growth, Philadelphia, 1986, JB Lippincott Co.
12. Kolodny RC and others: Textbook of human sexuality for nurses, Boston, 1979, Little, Brown & Co.
13. Krajicek MJ: Developmental disability and human sexuality, Nurs Clin North Am 17:173, 1982.
14. Kravetz H: Sexual counseling for the patient with chronic lung disease, Sexual Medicine Today, 17(3):377, 1981.
15. Masters WH and Johnson VE: Human sexual inadequacy, Boston, 1970, Little, Brown & Co.
16. Masters WM and Johnson VE: Human sexual response, Boston, 1966, Little, Brown & Co.
17. Mayou R, Foster A, and Williamson B: Psychosocial adjustment in patients 1 year after myocardial infarction, J Psychosom Res, 22:447, 1978.
18. McCauley K and others: Learning to live with controlled ventricular tachycardia: utilizing the Johnson Model, Heart Lung 13(6):633, 1984.
19. Moore K, Folk-Lightly M, and Nolen MJ: The joy of sex after a heart attack, Nurs 77 7(6):52, 1977.
20. Nemec ED, Mansfield L, and Kenneley J: Heart rate and blood pressure responses during sexual activity in normal males, Am Heart J 92:274, 1976.
21. O'Shea MD: An evaluation of a marriage enrichment and relationship skills training program (ME-RSTP) for couples coping with heart disease, doctoral dissertation, Atlanta, 1984, Georgia State University.
22. Phipps WJ, Long BC, and Woods ND: Medical surgical nursing, ed 3, St Louis, 1987, The CV Mosby Co.
23. Price SA and Wilson LM: Pathophysiology, ed 3, New York, 1986, McGraw-Hill Book Co.
24. Puksta NS: All about sex . . . after a coronary, Am J Nurs 77:602, 1977.
25. Runions J: A program for psychological and social enhancement during rehabilitation after myocardial infarction, Heart Lung 14(2):117, 1985.
26. Scalzi C, Burke L, and Greenland S: Evaluation of an inpatient educational program for coronary patients, Heart Lung 9:46, 1980.
27. Stein RA: The effect of exercise training on heart rate during coitus in the post-myocardial infarction patient, Circulation 55:738, 1977.
28. Sulman JY, Verhaeghe N: Myocardial infarction patients in the acute care hospital: a conceptual framework for social work intervention, Soc Work Health Care 11:1, 1986.
29. Ueno M: The so-called coition death, Jpn J Legal Med 17:333, 1952.
30. Watts RJ: Dimensions of sexual health, Am J Nurs 79:1572, 1979.
31. Wishnie MA, Hackett TP, and Cassem N: Psychological hazards of convalescence following myocardial infarction, JAMA 215:1291, 1971.
32. World Health Organization: Education and treatment in human sexuality: the training of health professionals, Tech Rep 572, Geneva, 1975, The Organization.
33. Zalar MK: Role preparation for nurses in home sexual functioning, Nurs Clin North Am 17(3):152, 1982.

STRESS IN THE CRITICAL CARE UNIT

50

Stress and Critical Care Nursing

Vital signs, pulmonary pressures, cardiac rhythms, intakes, outputs, level of consciousness, blood gas values, cardiac outputs, wound healing, nutrition, and other physiological parameters; anger, depression, grief, anxiety, disorientation, family dynamics, desire to live, ethical dilemmas, communication, and additional psychosocial indicators; infusion pumps, central lines, ventilators, chest tubes, mouth care, turning, feeding, and bathing—these are all but a glimmer of the myriad features composing the work environment of a critical care nurse. What response is generated by thoughts of this critical care world? Do they evoke energy, opportunity, and a sense of challenge, or do they elicit exhaustion, danger, and a feeling of threat? In either case, the reaction can be described by the term *stress*.

Cannon pioneered the study of stress in the early 1900s.[74,75] Since then, various individuals have continued to develop the stress concept to include Selye's physiological orientation, Pearlin's sociological view, and Lazarus' psychological perspective. Stress as a concern in the workplace first received attention in the mid1950s.[46] Occupational stress continues to be a pressing concern because of its potentially averse effect on health.[11,49,69,93]

Nursing represents an occupation in which stress has been scrutinized. Menzies[77] was one of the first individuals to address the stress experienced by nurses, and a multitude of additional reports have followed.[18,48,51,71] As Marshall[71] commented, "The nurse's role is . . . implicitly and chiefly one of handling stress." The physical labor, the human suffering, the work hours, the staffing, and the interpersonal relationships have all been mentioned repeatedly as sources of stress in nursing.

Not only are there stressors inherent in nursing, but stress is exacerbated when traditional beliefs, norms, and structures are realigned.[96] Therefore the prevalence of high technology, high patient acuity, and the transition to prospective payment are creating additional turbulence in the health care environment.[79,80,101] These changes have the potential to escalate the stress experienced by nurses.

The purpose of this chapter is to consider the issue of stress in nursing—particularly critical care nursing. The discussion covers six topics: (1) a brief overview of stress, (2) special challenges of critical care nursing, (3) potential sources of stress in critical care, (4) signs of stress, (5) effects of stress, and (6) stress management.

AN OVERVIEW OF STRESS
Definition

Stress is commonly discussed and commonly experienced, but what is stress? Despite its pervasive, persistent, and popular use, the precise nature of stress remains elusive. The term has generated much confusion and controversy. Some individuals have even suggested that the usefulness of stress as a concept is doubtful.[57,58,76,102] For example, if stress is defined as a particular physiological response, psychological differences among individuals can affect the meaning of a situation to the extent that even physiological reactions are altered.[17,27]

Pearlin[90] concurs that stress is complicated but offers an optimistic alternative: rather than discard the concept because of its problems, it would be useful to continue dealing with its complexity. However, ambiguity and the lack of consensus regarding its meaning complicate using the term stress. Fortunately, models such as the person-environment

(P-E) fit framework afford a way to integrate the complexities of work stress so that they can be discussed more meaningfully.

The person-environment fit model. The P-E fit model is a framework that considers relationships between job stress and health.[32,41] According to the P-E model, occupational stress is experienced when there are discrepancies between perceived environmental demands and individual abilities.[41] This definition is congruent with that proposed by Lazarus and Folkman[64] who state that stress is "a particular relationship between the person and the environment that is appraised by the person as taxing or exceeding his or her resources and endangering his or her well-being." Stress can therefore be minimized by balancing the abilities and needs of the person with the supplies and demands of the environment.

It is apparent that demands and abilities are influenced, in part, by subjective evaluation that affects an individual's awareness and understanding. This subjective element is known as perception; perception gives meaning to events. Perception not only determines the presence or absence of stress but also whether stress is viewed as a challenging, positive force or a negative threat. The person ponders, "am I in trouble or being benefited . . . and in what way."[64]

Although stress has a negative connotation, it is not inherently deleterious. Stress has the potential for positive outcomes. In fact, Selye[99] emphasized that the complete freedom from stress is death; it is not so much what happens to people but the way they interpret it. However, perception and interpretation do give meaning to events. It is not possible to specify which circumstances will engender stress because what might be distressing and bothersome for one individual could be satisfying and challenging for another. Additionally, perception contributes to the ever-changing nature of stress, establishing stress as a process, not an event.[57,58,64,92]

Coping. Another aspect of stress involves coping or how the individual evaluates what can be done about the event. Stress and coping are clearly interrelated; both are dynamic processes. The purpose of coping is to help an individual manage demands that are perceived as stressful.[64] This may be accomplished by modifying the situation, modifying the meaning of the situation, or managing symptoms provoked by the situation.[91] The way a person copes is partially determined by the individual's resources. Therefore coping evolves from personal characteristics such as health, energy, and positive beliefs or from constituents of the environment such as social support.

Coping differs between the genders. Johnson and Johnson[54] found that men used more denial than women in coping with the stress of parenthood. It is therefore possible that stress experienced by working women from occurrences external to the work milieu might transfer into the work setting. Furthermore, Pearlin and Schooler[91] found that coping strategies differ between men and women; men were more likely to use effective coping modes such as maintaining optimism and a positive outlook and possessing a sense of mastery over events. In addition, they found that coping for both genders was more useful in attenuating problems related to marriage and children and least effective in thwarting stress engendered by work. These issues are extremely cogent to a female-dominant profession such as nursing. If socialization limits women's repertoire of coping skills and nonwork stress is carried into the work setting, the stresses in the workplace might be perceived more harshly.

Related Concepts

Additional confusion in the stress nomenclature arises from the lack of precision in using various terms that are similar to but different from stress. Strain and burnout represent the problem. In the occupational literature stress and strain are typically separated, with stress preceding strain. For example, stress may arise from role conflict or role ambiguity. Role-related stress could contribute to strain, which might be manifested as job dissatisfaction.[11,18,32,69]

Burnout, like strain, is a consequence of stress. It is a more extreme condition, however, because burnout is the final stage of coping with negative conditions. Burnout is a psychological response to the chronic stress experienced by professionals employed in human service occupations,[29,33,72,100] and it is characterized by emotional exhaustion, depersonalization, and loss of personal motivation.[14,73]

This overview is only a sketchy beginning of a detailed portrait of stress. Nevertheless, it does help to convey that stress is indeed complicated. Making definitive statements about stress is both dangerous and difficult because, as French and Caplan[31] convey, what may be psychological poison for some people may be less toxic for others and vice versa. With these cautions in mind, it is possible to turn more specifically to stress in critical care units.

SPECIAL CHALLENGES OF CRITICAL CARE
Historical Perspective

The advent of recovery rooms in the 1940s marked the actual origin of critical care.[19,25] However, coronary care units, which are more prototypical of contemporary critical care settings, did not evolve until 1962.[45] Since the 1960s, an ongoing interest in critical care has led to an impressive number of studies, many of which indicated the critical care environment to be filled with stress.[1,4,50]

In addition to noting the valuable knowledge gained from early studies of stress in critical care, it is equally important to address their limitations. The most evident limitation is the emphasis on critical care irrespective of other patient care areas. As early as 1960, Menzies[77] stated, "Nurses experience a great deal of stress in their work. This may seem so obvious as hardly to merit comment. For nurses confront suffering and death as few other people do." Nevertheless, the implicit message in many early studies was that critical care was more stressful than other hospital-based nursing settings.[12,13,44,110] Perhaps this belief evolved from a study in which critical care and noncritical care nurses were compared.[35] The findings suggested that critical care nurses were more inclined to experience negative affective states, thereby perpetuating the belief that critical care nursing was more stressful. However, this disproportionately small number of noncritical care nurses in the sample may have skewed the comparison. The caution appropriate to such a limitation was not transmitted along with the results. Nevertheless, in using a comparison group, this study made an important contribution to knowledge about stress in the critical care milieu.

Contemporary View

Despite a lapse of 10 years, the idea of comparing critical care nurses to those in other patient areas surfaced again. Perhaps there never really was a difference in the stress experienced by critical care and noncritical care nurses. Perhaps the current health care environment, typified by escalating patient acuity and accelerating technological advances, has obliterated whatever differences there were at one time. In either case, more recent studies indicate that stress is an occupational problem in the nursing profession regardless of specialty.[60,67,109]

Nonetheless, as patient care becomes more complicated in all health care arenas, it only stands to follow that the critical care population represents the sickest of the sick. Advances in medical knowledge enable people to live longer despite aging and chronic illness. In addition, it is currently possible to treat patients with problems that were previously untreatable. All of these changes have an impact on nursing and nurses. Critical care nurses, therefore, are exposed to the most acutely ill patients and the most sophisticated, state-of-the-art technology. Consequently, even though stress is common in all facets of nursing, it becomes important to consider stress as it relates to critical care nurses.

POTENTIAL SOURCES OF STRESS IN CRITICAL CARE
Major Origins of Critical Care Stress

Several hallmark studies, summarized in two review articles,[10,104] have identified the major sources of stress in the critical care setting, which can be organized into five general categories: (1) the environment, (2) the work load, (3) patient acuity, (4) interpersonal relationships, and (5) responsibility for life and death decisions. Examples of conditions representing each of these categories are in Table 50-1.

The complexity of stress, however, makes it impossible to predict with certainty whether potential sources of stress will in fact generate stress. The following discussion briefly addresses how perception, personality, life's spheres, and chronic versus acute stress complicate identifying origins of stress in critical care.

Complexity of Stress in Critical Care

Perception. The importance of perception in the stress process is underscored by reemphasizing that the same situation can evoke different responses among individuals. In the critical care setting this means that the same activities identified as threatening by some staff members are stimulating for others.[4,6,83,87] The positive aspects of stress, however, are often overlooked because of the predominantly negative connotation. Furthermore, the positive side of stress highlights the difficulty that can arise when trying to moderate stress—it would seem unwise to remove or reduce sources of satisfaction. As expressed by one critical care nurse, "cardiac arrest and the amount of rapid decisions that

Table 50-1 Sources of stress in critical care

Category	Examples
Environment	Equipment
	Complexity
	Malfunction
	Nonavailability
	Physical features
	Inadequate storage
	Inadequate work space
	Inaccessible supplies
	Too much noise
	Too few windows
Work load	Patient
	Patient:staff ratio
	Patient acuity
	Frequent, repetitive routine
	Nonpatient
	Documentation
	Family interactions
	Staff competence and mix
Severity of illness	Emergencies
	Death and dying
	Requisite knowledge: physiological, psychosocial, pharmacological, technological
	Requisite repertoire of skills
Interpersonal relations and communication	Interactions with the following:
	Unit staff
	Other nursing units
	Hospital departments
	Other health care professionals
	Nurse managers
	Hospital administrators
	Families
	Patients
Decision making	Responsibility for decisions
	Conflicting opinions
	Adequacy of knowledge and information
	Accountability for effects of decisions
	Ethical dilemmas
	Fear of making mistakes

must be made are what I would call positive stressors—without these, my job wouldn't be exciting, challenging, and interesting."[83]

The dynamics of perception are further exemplified in a series of remarks originating from one of the early accounts of stress experienced by coronary care nurses.[13] A well-known cardiologist responded to the article by commenting in part, "It seems to me that coronary care is one of the less stressful and more restful atmospheres in which a nurse can work."[70] However, a registered nurse took issue with the cardiologist's remarks and stated, "Every coronary-care unit is different in terms of its demands" and "Awaiting the unexpected can be more anxiety provoking than active physical engagement."[2] This situation is not a case of who is right and who is wrong. Rather it clearly portrays how perception affects one's interpretation of stress. Nevertheless, there are sufficient sources of stress that are perceived only in a negative sense. It is these stressors that warrant modification.

Personality traits. Additional complexity is added to understanding critical care stress when considering the influence of personality. Why are some people seemingly tolerant of stress, whereas others are more vulnerable to its effects? Many personality variables have been identified as relevant to the stress process, including hardiness, locus of control, and Type A and B behaviors.[58,61,71,92] The effect of personality on the stress experienced by the critical care nurse has only recently been explored.

Hardiness, a three-faceted trait comprising challenge, commitment, and control, is purported to enhance tolerance for stress. Characteristics of the hardy personality have been found among both critical care and noncritical care nurses,[59,68] with less burnout experienced by nurses with high hardiness scores. Nurses with higher internal locus of control—a belief that the individual can influence life events to some degree—had fewer deleterious responses to stress.[30,62,86] Nurses with both Type A and Type B behaviors experienced stress, although the sources of stress differed.[51]

Life's spheres. A third complexity in determining sources of stress arises because it is not possible to compartmentalize the many components of one's work and nonwork life. As a result, stress may be experienced in the work environment because of the work itself, or it may be that the stress is actually provoked by occurrences external to the work environment.[42,89,93]

The interrelatedness of life's spheres is particularly salient for nursing, a profession that is predominantly composed of women. The movement of women out of the home and into the work world has been cited as a chief source of female role strain, or the dissonance experienced when expectations and demands of different roles conflict with one another.[89,94] However, the stress imposed by combining work, marriage, and family, for example, cannot be attributed solely to work.[43,56,66,108]

Consequently, it may be very difficult to isolate work stress. Although staffing constraints may be an obvious source of stress, it could be that dealing with a sick child, unpredictable child care, or an unsupportive spouse are the more potent provocations of stress, the effects of which may be experienced at work. In fact, it was determined that the most stressful situation for a group of 79 critical care nurses was dealing with a personal crisis while working.[87] Similarly, in a study of head nurses from a variety of clinical settings, it was apparent that stress from both work and nonwork sources had undesirable effects on the head nurses' mental health.[53]

Chronic versus acute stress. A final consideration demonstrating the complex process of stress is the influence of two different sources of stress. At one end of the continuum are the sudden, recent, acute events. It is possible to state rather precisely when these events occurred. Examples include motor vehicle accidents, death, divorce, policy changes, the arrival of new physicians, and starting a new job. Acute stressors are bothersome, not simply because they generally provoke change, but because they are often viewed as undesirable or uncontrollable.[42,64,89,92]

On the other end of the continuum are the less apparent, daily occurrences that are chronic sources of stress. Lazarus and Folkman[64] refer to them as daily hassles. These ongoing, enduring, wearing conditions are often taken for granted. Although they do not leave the same immediate impression as many acute stressors, the chronic stressors are nonetheless stressful.[42,64,89,92] Chronic stressors can arise from all segments of life such as family discord, conflict among one's roles, life-cycle changes, the medical hierarchy, inadequate staffing, and shift work. It is also possible that enduring features of acute stressors move them into the chronic end of the continuum. Feelings engendered by loss encountered because of death or divorce, for example, may linger for a considerable time. Teasing apart these intricacies of the stress process compounds the complexity of occupational stress in general and critical care stress in particular.

SIGNS OF STRESS

Despite its complexities, stress does occur, and when it does, it evokes many signs and symptoms. However, the indicators of stress are somewhat nonspecific insofar as they could accompany several conditions. Actually, Selye[98] referred to stress as a nonspecific response of the person to demands that are either pleasant or noxious; regardless of the demand or response, the body makes compensatory adjustments to maintain a harmonic balance.

Probably all people have experienced the pounding heart, sweaty palms, and knotted stomach that frequently accompany stressful events. Many of these responses arise from the neuroendocrine effects of preparing to deal with stress and attempting to sustain one's equilibrium. The box on p. 111 represents a composite of physical, mental, and behavioral manifestations of stress. Although these indicators might be associated with a variety of conditions, they could be signs of stress. The nonspecificity of these manifestations also further conveys the vagueness that is inherent to the entity known as stress.[11,40,65,97]

EFFECTS OF STRESS

Although stressors in the critical care setting have been identified, a reasonable next question might be, "So what?" That is not meant to sound glib but to demonstrate further that the presence of stress is not automatically detrimental. What are the sequelae of stress? To reiterate a point made at the beginning of this chapter, occupational stress, specifically stress in nursing, is a concern because of the serious health problems it generates.[11,49,69,93] Both individual and organizational health suffers from the deleterious effects of stress. Employers have been held legally accountable for stress-related mental injuries,[9,78] and lowered work quality, increased absenteeism, and increased turnover are additional sequelae of work stress.[63]

Physical problems induced by work stress must be considered too. This issue is often overlooked by those who have underscored that the demands of stress may be viewed

INDICATORS OF STRESS

PHYSICAL MANIFESTATIONS

Cardiovascular

Tachycardia
Increased blood pressure
Chest pain
Palpitations
Cold hands and feet

Neurological

Headache
Hyperreflexia
Trembling; excessive energy
Insomnia
Lethargy

Pulmonary

Tachypnea
Cough

Endocrine

Increased metabolic rate
Increased appetite
Anorexia

Gastrointestinal

Decreased peristalsis
Intestinal cramping
Indigestion
Diarrhea
Nausea

Genitourinary

Urinary urgency
Sensation of full bladder
Urinary frequency

Integumentary

Cool, pale skin
Blushing
Increased perspiration
Rashes

Musculoskeletal

Back pain
Joint pain

Other

Dry mouth, eyes
Dysphagia

PSYCHOLOGICAL MANIFESTATIONS

Anger
Frustration
Depression
Apathy
Fear
Hostility
Denial
Other defensive responses

BEHAVIORAL MANIFESTATIONS

Complaining
Crying
Panicking
Quarreling
Withdrawal
Disorientation
Indecisiveness
Helplessness
Irritability
Reduced productivity
Reduced quality of performance
Forgetfulness
Inattention to detail
Preoccupation with other things
Inability to concentrate
Reduced creativity
Increased use of drugs, alcohol, tobacco
Increased absenteeism and illness
Lethargy
Accident proneness
Disinterest
Blaming others
Increased errors
Inefficiency
Speech changes

as either challenge or threat. Regardless of how stress is perceived, irrespective of whether a nurse views events in the critical care setting as positive or negative, the biological sequelae are the same. Neuroendocrine responses evoke the same physiological reactions which, over time, may give rise to disease.[38] It is therefore not surprising that Pelletier[93] warns, "Caution: Work May Be Hazardous To Your Health."

Another relevant issue involves a curious paradox: although the goal of health care providers is to enhance the health of others, their own health may be at risk.[52] Although the preceding statements have an intuitive appeal, some of the outcomes of critical care stress are more speculative than factual at present. It is therefore helpful to examine the research-based evidence regarding the effects of stress on critical care nurses.

Individual Effects

Cleland's early investigations of stress in nursing[15,16] are unique in that they considered stress in relation to select effects. In one report, the expected curvilinear relationship between nurses' performance and stress was demonstrated,[15] and in another an inverse relationship was found between the quality of nurses' thinking and stress.[16] Most research concerning stress in nursing, however, has been limited to identifying stressors.[82] It is only recently that critical care stress has been considered in relation to outcome variables. Some of the information is conflictive, and all of it is preliminary, but the findings are nonetheless compelling. For example, most of the stressors identified by a large group of critical care nurses were *not* related to two outcome measures—job satisfaction and psychological distress.[83]

No pathology was found in two small groups of critical care nurses whose psychological health was examined.[28,30] However, in a group comprising 180 critical care nurses, 87% of the participants' psychological symptom scores exceeded normal, with 10% of them reaching levels comparable to psychiatric outpatients.[83] The findings from this latter study suggests that stress does have an undesirable effect. Although additional evidence is needed to elucidate clearly the effect of stress on mental health, it is important to pursue this problem.

Another outcome that is important to individuals is job satisfaction. It is often suggested that stress contributes to job *dis*satisfaction. However, the empirical evidence is weak. In the previously mentioned study of 180 critical care nurses, only 3 of 16 stressful situations were related to low job satisfaction.[83] Further, personality traits, characteristics that vary greatly among individuals, have been noted to alter job satisfaction.[62]

Burnout is also a possible outcome of stress. Here, too, the relationship is complicated, but an association between job stress and burnout has been found among critical care nurses.[21,59] A preliminary profile of the burnout-prone critical care nurse is beginning to emerge. Symptoms of burnout are often found in male nurses, younger nurses, and nurses educated at the baccalaureate level and higher.[5,59] Nurses who are inclined to burnout were also found to be less experienced in nursing and to have less effective coping skills.[106] This profile emphasizes that specifying sequelae of stress is complicated by many factors. Although it is probable that a similar profile could be developed for organizational features that enhance and reduce the development of burnout, no such studies have yet been published.

A gap in knowledge exists regarding the effects of stress on nurses in that the physiological effects of stress and physical illnesses have not been studied. Nevertheless, stress has been related to many disorders such as headache, hypertension, coronary artery disease, asthma, gastric and duodenal ulcers, diabetes, arthritis, allergies, cancer, mental disorders.[22,23,47,98] It would be valuable to know how or if the stress of nursing contributes to the development of any of these maladies.

Organizational Effects

An index of organizational health might be determined by considering stress-related issues such as absenteeism, turnover, or the quality of work. These factors are reflections of individual responses to stress; however, these indicators may also affect the productivity and the financial status of the organization. For example, the organization experiences the impact of individual stress in that stress-induced illnesses contribute to escalating costs of medical benefits. Organizational expenditures related to work stess have been estimated at $75 billion annually.[111]

Despite the obvious importance of these organizational effects of stress, they have been studied only limitedly in nursing. Turnover has received the most attention. Stress has been implicated as one of the contributors to turnover.[1,3,112,114] Turnover involves the cost of recruiting, orienting, and socializing replacements.[8] The cost of attracting and hiring nurses for a 450-bed hospital has been estimated at $62,000, with an additional $20,000 in expenditures annually to replace nurses who leave. The current nursing shortage has further emphasized how turnover can adversely affect organizational health.

These findings alone would seem to provide ample stimuli to motivate organizations to seriously attempt to reduce stress. Additional organizational outcomes related to stress are more hunches at this point than evidence established by careful study. However, the speculations seem credible and would therefore benefit from more formal investigation. Examples of these ideas include that stress interferes with patient care, thereby affecting quality of care, and stress lowers staff morale. In a labor-intensive occupation such as nursing, the impact of stress for individuals and organizations cannot be overlooked.

STRESS MANAGEMENT

The most obvious way to manage stress is to intervene in the process. However, that is not as simple as it seems. After considering the innumerable sources of stress and the influence of perception, it is unclear what specific interventions would ameliorate certain of the undesirable conditions. For example, there are not ready answers to questions such as what is adequate staffing, where can both space and money be obtained to renovate the environment, and exactly how can interpersonal relationships be made more satisfactory?

House[49] offers a valuable insight by noting that work organizations may believe their responsibility is only to help individuals learn how to deal with stress. This approach is necessary but not sufficient. It is not totally clear how effective the use of individual stress remedies are. In addition, attending only to the individual detracts from examing the organization. Although restructuring work environments to reduce stress is a difficult task, it may ultimately be the only tenable approach to dealing with work stress.

To date, however, the methods of stress reduction that have dominated nursing are those that focus on helping the individual cope. Coping, to reiterate, is an individual response used to reduce internal tension; it protects against stress and it represents individual attempts to reestablish a harmonic balance. One of the first steps in coping with stress is to trace its origin. Because of the interrelationship among life's spheres, sources of stress originating from the non-

RESEARCH ABSTRACT
Noise-induced stress as a predictor of burnout in critical care nurses

Topf M and Dillon E: Heart Lung 17(5):567, 1988.

PURPOSE

The purpose of this investigation was to assess the degree and sources of noise-induced stress in critical care nurses who have long-term exposure to unpredictable noise and uncontrollable noise. A second purpose was to evaluate whether noise-induced stress was linked with burnout in critical care nurses.

FRAMEWORK

Noise-induced stress has been defined as any sound that is physically arousing and subjectively annoying. Consistent with stress theory, unpredictable and uncontrollable noise is perceived as more stressful, compared with continuous noise that is under a person's control. Burnout has been defined as a syndrome of emotional exhaustion, depersonalization, and decreased personal accomplishment. It is the result of the chronic stress of work. Empirical evidence has demonstrated a potential link between noise-induced stress and burnout. Several of the effects of stress on human performance have been associated with noise-induced stress. It was therefore hypothesized that a greater degree of noise-induced stress would be associated with a greater degree of burnout in critical care nurses. Furthermore, nurses who were more sensitive to noise were expected to have greater noise-induced stress and consequently greater burnout than less-sensitive nurses.

METHODS

A convenience sample of 100 nursing employees from two large university-affililated hospitals on the West Coast volunteered for the survey. Participants were from cardiac, medical-surgical, urology, neonatal, and pediatric critical care units. Six instruments were administered to measure the dependent variables. The Life Experience Survey was used to measure life events' stress in nurses. The Nursing Stress Scale measured other occupational stress (other than noise induced). Weinstein's Noise Sensitivity Scale was used to determine the nurses' sensitivity to noise. A modified version of the Disturbance Due to Hospital Noise Scale was used to assess stress caused by hospital sounds. The Maslach Burnout Inventory (MBI) and 20 items from Jones' Staff Burnout Scale for Health Professionals (SBS-HP) were used to measure burnout. Nurses were instructed to fill out the questionnaires at home and return them in 3 days.

RESULTS

The top four types of noises ranked as stress for nurses from both hospitals were continuous beeping of patient monitoring devices, alarms on equipment, telephones, and excessive traffic on the unit. Analysis of combined hospital results for demographic variables showed nonsignificant relationships with study variables with the exception of shift. Eight-hour shift nurses were more distressed by noise, and nurses who rotated shifts underwent more emotional exhaustion. Noise-induced occupational stress was positively related to burnout as measured by the SBS-HP ($r = 0.369$, $p, < 0.001$) and the emotional exhaustion subscale of the MBI ($r = 0.300$, $p, < 0.01$). Hierarchal multiple regressions confirmed these results once variance in burnout linked with life stressors and other occupational stressors were considered. Furthermore, an interaction term, noise-induced stress X intrinsic sensitivity to noise in the person, did not account for significant variance in burnout once independent variance linked with noise-induced stress was identified. That is, nurses with intrinsic sensitivity to noise were no more at risk for burnout linked with noise-induced stress than were less-sensitive nurses.

IMPLICATIONS

The results provided support for the contention that noise-induced stress is positively related to burnout in critical care nurses. The noise level in the critical care units studied may have been great enough to distress nurses, regardless of the degree of their intrinsic sensitivity to noise. The present positive descriptive findings provide support for designing experimental studies involving modification of the critical care noise environment. Noise-induced stress and burnout could be evaluated in nurses before and after acoustical modifications in the structure of units and equipment. Noisy equipment or staff conferences might be housed in a soundproof room, and consideration should be given to modifying the ringing of telephones. Innovative alternatives might be designed to replace alarms and beeping monitors at the bedside. Straightforward interventions could include signs that redirect foot traffic on the unit or that enhance awareness of noises easily reduced by staff.

STRATEGIES TO MANAGE WORK STRESS

INDIVIDUAL STRATEGIES

Recognize the presence of stress or feelings of disequilibrium
Enhance clinical knowledge and skills
Manage time and set priorities
Improve all facets of communication
Assess one's assets and abilities
Evaluate one's attitudes, values, beliefs, and expectations
Reconsider expectations of self and work
Reframe the meaning of situations
Assert one's needs
Break out of the "stressed-out" mold
Adopt self-care measures
    Exercise
    Proper diet
    Imagery, meditation, relaxation
    Recreation
    Vacation

ORGANIZATIONAL STRATEGIES

Recognize stress and its undesirable effects
Support educational endeavors
Develop leadership styles that reduce stress
Offer group-based experiences
    Facilitated staff meetings
    Support groups
    Liaison psychiatric involvement
Create a stress-resistant environment
    Promote high social support
    Structure or restructure the physical features
    Assess effects of shift changes and scheduling
    Introduce a shared-governance model

---

work setting must be contemplated along with work factors. By pinpointing the problem—is it child care or critical care—it is possible to mobilize coping resources that are best suited to manage the particular difficulty. This discussion, however, focuses on those individual and organizational coping strategies, as summarized in the box above, relevant to stressors intrinsic to the work setting.

Individual Strategies

Individual coping strategies are those techniques arising from self-awareness and a sense of responsibility for self. Several reports have suggested that the most crucial step in the coping process is recognizing that stress is present and that either one's equilibrium is endangered or that the imbalance has already occurred.[42,87,97,105] Only after stress is recognized can decisions be made about which specific tactics might enhance coping. The armamentarium of individual coping strategies is extensive, and the approaches may be used either separately or in various combinations. As Sutterley[107] underscores, however, although approaches to

stress management are eagerly sought, the efficacy of most approaches remains to be established.

Clinical knowledge and skills can be expanded to enhance one's sense of competence in the critical care setting. Techniques for judiciously managing time and setting priorities may enhance one's sense of control and accomplishment. Stress might also be reduced by learning better communication skills such as expressing one's needs and concerns, truly listening to and hearing what is being said, and recognizing the divisiveness and destructiveness of ineffective communication tactics.

There is also a large collection of self-care measures such as exercise and proper diet that might be tried.[42,85,97] Taking a personal asset inventory may also help to embellish personal coping skills.[88,97] Although limitations are often sources of frustration, identifying one's strengths helps to accentuate the positive. This process enables the individual to cultivate strengths and potentials rather than succumb to a false sense of complete ineptitude.

Another coping technique involves recognizing how individual attitudes, values, beliefs and expectations affect the stress experience. It is possible that job stress is largely the product of unfulfilled expectations. In the past work was primarily viewed as a source of income; today work is also expected to contribute to personal fulfillment, thereby posing women with the challenge of filling multiple roles simultaneously. These issues are cogent for nurses, who are predominantly females. The doors of opportunity have been opened to new sources of gratification and satisfaction. The opportunities also bring with them a spectrum of complexities and challenges for the "super" person of the late twentieth century who tries to juggle a variety of demands not encountered by previous generations.[53]

Expectations may also affect the sense that the "grass is greener" elsewhere. Things may seem better at another institution—or is that an illusion created by wishful thinking? By reframing situations, reconsidering expectations, and reevaluating the real significance of events, some of the self-induced stress dynamics can be diminished. Harris[40] phrases it well by stating, "Is . . . dropping a bedpan really a major life threat?" Whether an event is viewed as a major catastrophe or as somewhat humorous, human error does alter the stressfulness of the occurrence.[97]

A final comment about individual coping has to do with the voguish, stylish reputation that stress has developed. Being "stressed out" is almost an expectation of current life. Perhaps part of coping with stress is to realize it is all right *not* to be stressed; it is acceptable to feel relaxed and contented. Because it has become customary to complain about stress, it may even be stressful to be free from the clutches of stress. Perhaps one of the best ways to break the cycle of stress is to express more vocally the good sensations, the happy thoughts, and the pleasantries that are not as stylish as stress.

Organizational Strategies

Along with individual coping efforts, a variety of organization-based approaches are available to attenuate stress. For example, not only is education an important individual intervention, but it is also a viable organizational strategy as well. Education includes programs to enhance a staff member's knowledge about both critical care and stress. This education might be offered as in-service workshops, university-based courses with tuition assistance from the health care agency, or continuing education seminars and symposia.[81,95,113]

An assortment of group activities aimed at facilitating stress management might also be generated and sustained by organizations. Well-managed staff meetings, support groups, and exchanges with liaison psychiatric personnel have the potential to diminish stress.[7,30,34,103] If group approaches to stress reduction are to be effective, at least one facilitator skilled in the dynamics of group interactions must help with the group. In addition, although group approaches to stress management can be very helpful, they also require commitment from participants to keep the group viable over a sufficient period of time to allow the group process to reach its full potential.[103]

Another organizational tool for managing stress would be to sustain a climate that fosters social support—interactions that have the potential to both diminish stress and enhance health. Many definitions of social support exist, but the essence of it is based in positive relationships that leave the participants feeling cared for, esteemed, and respected.[49] Supportive relationships are not always pleasant or free from conflict. However, even when disagreement prevails, the persons continue to feel valued.[52] Such dynamics require maturity and insight from both the recipient and the giver of support.[85] In the work environment supervisors and co-workers are obvious sources of social support. For nurses social support has demonstrated efficacy in reducing burnout[20,21] and lowering symptoms of psychological distress.[46,84]

Leadership characteristics are also relevant organizational features that may ameliorate stress. Leadership has two components—consideration or concern for group members and structure or emphasis on task completion. In a study of neonatal critical care nurses, it was determined that staff members who perceived head nurses as considerate leaders experienced less burnout and more job satisfaction.[26] Others have also cited the importance of the head nurse in attenuating stress.[34,36,39] The responsibilities and possibilities for administrators to modify the effects of stress are apparent from the investigations of both social support and leadership.

Restructuring the critical care environment is a costly alternative to managing stress, but it may be a necessary consideration. For example, Norbeck[83] found that, more than any other stressors, features of the physical environment such as inaccessible supplies and inoperable equipment contributed to psychological distress and job dissatisfaction. Gorny[37] also underscored that critical care nurses are predisposed to sensory disequilibrium because of the excessive sensory stimuli present in the critical care environment. Such information must be heeded by those responsible for planning and constructing new critical care settings. This information must also be considered by individuals renovating and remodeling existing facilities.

For institutions in which environmental changes are not anticipated, it is imperative that environmental stressors be acknowledged as more than sources of an insignificant expression of disgruntlement or idle complaining. Rather,

it would be wise to contemplate at what point the cost of replacing staff, either because of turnover or illness, exceeds the expense of altering the environment to reduce sources of stress from the physical plant itself.

A very important point must be considered in regard to managing stress with the aforementioned techniques—both individual and organizational. With a few exceptions, intervention strategies have been neither extensively nor carefully evaluated.[81,95] Although many of the suggestions are extremely appealing, their effectiveness in reducing work stress is not really known. Consequently, it is important to be cautious in regard to which interventions are implemented. To overcome this deficit in knowledge, regardless of which plan is tried, it is essential that the program be evaluated.

Program evaluation must not only consider overall effectiveness but also the duration of effectiveness. Perhaps retraining or reexposure should occur at critical points after the intervention if it is an activity that is not ongoing. More apparently is known about the effects of interventions that are within the purview of the organization. Although it is important to study these tactics for managing stress, it is equally necessary to carefully evaluate the individual modes of managing stress. For example, at what point does an exercise program become a source of stress rather than a way to cope? The cost of a fitness club membership, dislike for the activities, or time conflicts in using the facilities could all serve to negate the intended benefits of exercise. None of the strategies for managing stress is a panacea; nor are the strategies replacements for more directly modifying the actual sources of stress.

SUMMARY

Stress is a complex entity that evokes responses and problems that are equally complicated. It is therefore not surprising that managing stress is also intricate and elusive. However, stress is a common aspect of life, of nursing, and of critical care. Developing an understanding of stress is one way to begin to deal with this pervasive process. Occupational sources of stress have been placed in the spotlight because of their potentially deleterious effects on health. Nursing represents a very stressful profession. The stresses originate not only from the work and the work environment but also from nonwork problems such as how to manage career, home, and family.

The past has made an impressive contribution to identifying sources of stress in nursing, particularly critical care nursing. It is a task for the future to build on that foundation by delineating more precisely the effects of stress and how to intervene in the stress process. It is the responsibility of the present to use the information that does exist to establish a more harmonious equilibrium for critical care nursing.

REFERENCES

1. Anderson CA and Basteyns M: Stress and the critical care nurse reaffirmed, J Nurs Adm 11(1):31, 1981.
2. Babbini LJ: Letter to the editors regarding Cassem and Hackett: Stress on the nurse and therapist in the intensive-care unit and the coronary-care unit, Heart Lung 5:328, 1976.
3. Bailey JT: Stress and stress management: an overview, J Nurs Educ 19(6):5, 1980.

4. Bailey JT, Steffen SM, and Grout JW: The stress audit: identifying the stressors of ICU nursing, J Nurs Educ 19(6):15, 1980.
5. Bartz C and Maloney JP: Burnout among intensive care nurses, Res Nurs Health 9:147, 1986.
6. Bilodeau CB: The nurse and her reactions to critical-care nursing, Heart Lung 2:358, 1973.
7. Bohannan-Reed K, Dugan D, and Huck B: Staying human under stress: stress reduction and emotional support in the critical care setting, Crit Care Nurse 3(3):26, 1983.
8. Brief AP: Turnover among hospital nurses: a suggested model, J Nurs Adm 6(8):55, 1976.
9. Brodsky CM: Long-term work stress, Psychosomatics 25:361, 1984.
10. Caldwell T and Weiner MF: Stresses and coping in ICU nursing. I. A review, Gen Hosp Psychiatry 3:119, 1981.
11. Caplan RD and others: Job demands and worker health. Main effects and occupational differences, Washington, DC, 1975, NIOSH Government Printing Office.
12. Cassem NH and Hackett TP: Sources of tension for the CCU nurse, Am J Nurs 72:1426, 1972.
13. Cassem NH and Hackett TP: Stress on the nurse and therapist in the intensive-care unit and the coronary-care unit, Heart Lung 4:252, 1975.
14. Cherniss C: Staff burnout. Job stress in the human services, Beverly Hills, Cal, 1980, Sage Publications.
15. Cleland VS: The effect of stress on performance, Nurs Res 14:292, 1965.
16. Cleland VS: Effects of stress on thinking, Am J Nurs 67:108, 1967.
17. Cohen F and others: Panel report on psychosocial assets and modifiers of stress. In Elliott GR and Eisdorfer C, editors: Stress and human health. Analysis and implications of research, New York, 1982, Springer Publishing Co.
18. Colligan MJ, Smith MJ, and Hurrell J: Occupational incidence rates of mental health disorders, J Human Stress 3(3):34, 1977.
19. Conboy CF: A recovery room, Am J Nurs 47:686, 1947.
20. Constable JF and Russell DW: The effect of social support and the work environment upon burnout among nurses, J Human Stress 12(1):20, 1986.
21. Cronin-Stubbs D and Rooks CA: The stress, social support, and burnout of critical care nurses: the results of research, Heart Lung 14:31, 1985.
22. Dembrowski TM and others: Moving beyond Type A, Advances 1(1):16, 1984.
23. Dimsdale JE and Herd JA: Variability of plasma lipids in response to emotional arousal, Psychosom Med 44:413, 1982.
24. Donovan L: The shortage, RN 43(6):21, 1980.
25. Dunn FE and Shupp MG: The recovery room. A wartime economy, Am J Nurs 43:279, 1943.
26. Duxbury ML and others: Head nurse leadership style with staff nurse burnout and job satisfaction in neonatal intensive care units, Nurs Res 33:97, 1984.
27. Elliott GR and Eisdorfer C: Conceptual issues in stress research. In Elliott GR and Eisdorfer C, editors: Stress and human health. Analysis and implications of research, New York, 1982, Springer Publishing Co.
28. Esteban A, Ballesteros P, and Caballero J: Psychological evaluation of intensive care nurses, Crit Care Med 11:616, 1983.
29. Farber BA: Introduction: a critical perspective on burnout. In Farber BA, editor: Stress and burnout in the human service professions, New York, 1983, Pergamon Press.
30. Fawzy FI and others: Preventing nursing burnout: a challenge for liaison psychiatry, Gen Hosp Psychiatry 5:141, 1983.
31. French JRP and Caplan RD: Organizational stress and individual strain. In Marrow AJ, editor: The failure of success, New York, 1972, AMACOM.
32. French JRP, Rodgers W, and Cobb S: Adjustment as person-environ-ment fit. In Coelho GV, Hamburg DA, and Adams JE, editors: Coping and adaptation, New York, 1974, Basic Books.
33. Freudenberger HJ: Burnout: contemporary issues, trends, and concerns. In Farber BA, editor: Stress and burnout in the human service professions, New York, 1983, Pergamon Press.
34. Gardner D, Parzen ZD, and Stewart N: The nurse's dilemma: mediating stress in critical care units, Heart Lung 9:103, 1980.
35. Gentry WD, Foster SB, and Froehling S: Psychologic response to situational stress in intensive and nonintensive nursing, Heart Lung 1:793, 1972.
36. Gil R and Sumner M: Establishing a leadership style that shows you do care, Nurs Success Today 2(4):32, 1985.
37. Gorny DA: Maintenance of sensory equilibrium for the critical care nurse, Top Clin Nurs 6(4):44, 1985.
38. Grout JW, Steffen SM, and Bailey JT: The stresses and the satisfiers of the intensive care unit: a survey, Crit Care Q 3(4):35, 1981.
39. Guy ML: Leadership style and approaches in critical care nursing, Crit Care Q 5(1):17, 1982.
40. Harris JS: Stressors and stress in critical care, Crit Care Nurse 4(1):84, 1984.
41. Harrison RV: Person-environment fit and job stress. In Cooper CL and Payne R, editors: Stress at work, New York, 1978, John Wiley & Sons, Inc.
42. Hartl DE: Stress management and the nurse, Adv Nurs Sci 1(4):91, 1979.
43. Haw MA: Women, work and stress: a review and agenda for the future, J Health Soc Behav 23:132, 1982.
44. Hay D and Oken D: The psychological stresses of intensive care unit nursing, Psychosom Med 34:109, 1972.
45. Hilberman M: The evolution of intensive care units, Crit Care Med 3(4):159, 1975.
46. Hirsch BJ and Rapkin BD: Social networks and adult social identities: profiles and correlates of support and rejection, Am J Community Psychol 14:395, 1986.
47. Holroyd KA, Appel MA, and Andrasik F: A cognitive-behavioral approach to psychophysiological disorders. In Meichenbaum D and Jaremko JE, editors: Stress reduction and prevention, New York, 1983, Plenum Press.
48. Holsclaw PA: Nursing in high emotional risk areas, Nurs Forum 4(4):36, 1965.
49. House JS: Work stress and social support, Reading, Mass, 1981, Addison-Wesley Publishing Co.
50. Huckabay LMD and Jagla B: Nurses' stress factors in the intensive care unit, J Nurs Adm 9(2):21, 1979.
51. Ivancevich JM and Matteson MT: Nurses and stress: time to examine the potential problem, Superv Nurs 11(6):17, 1980.
52. Jennings BM: Social support: a way to a climate of caring, Nurs Adm Q 11(4):63, 1987.
53. Jennings BM: Stress, social support, and locus of control: effects on head nurses' mental health, doctoral dissertation, San Francisco, Cal, 1987, University of California.
54. Johnson CL and Johnson FA: Attitudes toward parenting in dual-career families, Am J Psychiatry 134:391, 1977.
55. Kahn RL and others: Organizational stress: studies in role conflict and ambiguity, New York, 1964, John Wiley & Sons, Inc.
56. Kandel DB, Davies M, and Raveis VH: The stressfulness of daily social roles for women: marital, occupational and household roles, J Health Soc Behav 26:64, 1985.
57. Karamus W: Working conditions and health: social epidemiology, patterns of stress and change, Soc Sci Med 19:359, 1984.
58. Kasl SV: Epidemiological contributions to the study of work stress. In Cooper CL and Payne R, editors: Stress at work, New York, 1978, John Wiley & Sons, Inc.
59. Keane A, DuCette J, and Adler DC: Stress in ICU and non-ICU nurses, Nurs Res 34:231, 1985.

60. Kelly JG and Cross DG: Stress, coping behaviors, and recommendations for intensive care and medical surgical ward registered nurses, Res Nurs Health 8:321, 1985.

61. Kobasa S: Stressful life events, personality, and health: an inquiry into hardiness, J Pers Soc Psychol 37:1, 1979.

62. Kosmoski KA and Calkin JD: Critical care nurses' intent to stay in their positions, Res Nurs Health 9:3, 1986.

63. Lawler EE: Can the quality of work life be legislated? The Personnel Administrator 21:17, 1986.

64. Lazarus RS and Folkman S: Stress, appraisal, and coping, New York, 1984, Springer Publishing Co.

65. Lindsey AM and Carrieri V: Stress response. In Carrieri V, Lindsey AM, and West C, editors: Pathophysiological phenomena in nursing: human responses to illness, Philadelphia, 1986, WB Saunders Co.

66. Long J and Porter KL: Multiple roles of midlife women. A case for new directions in theory, research, and policy. In Baruch G and Brooks-Gunn J, editors: Women in midlife, New York, 1984, Plenum Press.

67. Maloney JP: Job stress and its consequences on a group of intensive care and nonintensive care nurses, Adv Nurs Sci 4(2):31, 1982.

68. Maloney JP and Bartz C: Stress-tolerant people: intensive care nurses compared with non-intensive care nurses, Heart Lung 12:389, 1983.

69. Margolis BL, Kroes WH, and Quinn RP: Job stress: an unlisted occupational hazard, J Occup Med 16:659, 1974.

70. Marriott HJL: Letter to the editors regarding Cassem and Hackett: Stress on the nurse and therapist in the intensive-care unit and the coronary-care unit, Heart Lung 4:802, 1975.

71. Marshall J: Stress amongst nurses. In Cooper CL and Marshall J, editors: White collar and professional stress, New York, 1980, John Wiley & Sons, Inc.

72. Maslach C: Burned-out, Hum Behav 5(9):16, 1976.

73. Maslach C: Understanding burnout: definitional issues in analyzing a complex phenomenon. In Paine WS, editor: Job stress and burnout, Beverly Hills, Cal, 1982, Sage Publications.

74. Mason JW: A historical view of the stress field, part I, J Human Stress 1(1):6, 1975.

75. Mason, JW: A historical view of the stress field, part II, J Human Stress 1(2):22, 1975.

76. McLean A: Occupational "stress"—misnomer. In McLean A, editor: Occupational stress, Springfield, Ill, 1974, Charles C Thomas, Publisher.

77. Menzies IEP: Nurses under stress, Int Nurs Rev 7:9, 1960.

78. Minnehan RF and Paine WS: Bottom lines. Assessing the economic and legal consequences of burnout. In Paine WS, editor: Job stress and burnout, Beverly Hills, Cal, 1982, Sage Publications.

79. Naisbitt J and Elkins J: The hospital and megatrends, Hosp Forum 26(3):9, 1983.

80. Naisbitt J and Elkins J: II. The hospital and megatrends, Hosp Forum 26(4):52, 1983.

81. Newlin B: Stress reduction for the critical care nurse: a stress education program, Occup Health Nurs 32:315, 1984.

82. Norbeck JS: Coping with stress in critical care nursing: research findings, Focus Crit Care 12(5):36, 1985.

83. Norbeck JS: Perceived job stress, job satisfaction, and psychological symptoms in critical care nursing, Res Nurs Health 8:253, 1985.

84. Norbeck JS: Types and sources of social support for managing job stress in critical care nursing, Nurs Res 34:225, 1985.

85. Noroian EL and Yasko J: Care for the critical care-giver. Strategies for the prevention of burnout, Dimens Crit Care Nurs 1:97, 1982.

86. Numerof RE and Abrams MN: Sources of stress among nurses: an empirical investigation, J Human Stress 10(2):88, 1984.

87. Oskins SL: Identification of situational stressors and coping methods by intensive care nurses, Heart Lung 8:953, 1979.

88. Otto HA: The human potentialities of nurses and patients, Nurs Outlook 13(8):32, 1965.

89. Pearlin LI: Role strains and personal stress. In Kaplan HB, editor: Psychological stress. Trends in theory and research, New York, 1983, Academic Press.

90. Pearlin LI: The social contexts of stress. In Goldberger L and Breznitz S, editors: Handbook of stress. Theoretical and clinical aspects, New York, 1982, The Free Press.

91. Pearlin LI and Schooler C: The structure of coping, J Health Soc Behav 19:2, 1978.

92. Pearlin LI and others: The stress process, J Health Soc Behav 22:337, 1981.

93. Pelletier K: Healthy people in unhealthy places, New York, 1984, Delacorte Press.

94. Perun PJ and Bielby DD: Towards a model of female occupational behavior: a human development approach, Psychol Women Q 6:234, 1981.

95. Randolph GL, Price JL, and Collins JR: The effects of burnout prevention training on burnout symptoms in nurses, J Contin Educ Nurs 17(2):43, 1986.

96. Schwab JJ: Stress: a psychosocial view, J Ky Med Assoc 82:115, 1984.

97. Scully R: Stress: in the nurse, Am J Nurs 80:912, 1980.

98. Selye H: Stress and a holistic view of health for the nursing profession. In Claus KE and Bailey JT, editors: Living with stress and promoting well-being. A handbook for nurses, St. Louis, 1980, The CV Mosby Co.

99. Selye H: The stress of life, ed 2, New York, 1976, McGraw-Hill Book Co.

100. Seuntjens AD: Burnout in nursing—what it is and how to prevent it, Nurs Adm Q 7(1):12, 1982.

101. Shaffer FA, editor: DRGs: changes and challenges, New York, 1984, National League for Nursing.

102 Sharit J and Salvendy G: Occupational stress: review and reappraisal, Hum Factors 24(2):129, 1982.

103. Simon NM and Whiteley S: Psychiatric consultation with MICU nurses: the consultation conference as a working group, Heart Lung 6:497, 1977.

104. Stehle JL: Critical care nursing stress: the findings revisited, Nurs Res 30:182, 1981.

105. Stillman SM and Strasser BL: Helping critical care nurses with work-related stress, J Nurs Adm 10(1):28, 1980.

106. Stone GL and Others: Identification of stress and coping skills within a critical care setting, West J Nurs Res 6:201, 1984.

107. Sutterley DC: Stress management: grazing the clinical turf, Holistic Nurs Pract 1(1):36, 1986.

108. Verbrugge LM: Role burdens and physical health of women and men, Women Health 11(1):47, 1986.

109. Vincent P and Coleman WF: Comparison of major stressors perceived by ICU and non-ICU nurses, Crit Care Nurse 6(1):64, 1986.

110. Vreeland R and Ellis GL: Stresses on the nurse in the intensive-care unit, JAMA 208:332, 1969.

111. Wallis C: Stress: can we cope? Time, p 48, June 6, 1983.

112. Wandelt MA, Pierce PM, and Widdowson RR: Why nurses leave nursing and what can be done about it, Am J Nurs 81:72, 1981.

113. Warren JJ: Developing a stress-management program, Dimens Crit Care Nurs 1:307, 1982.

114. Wolf GA: Nursing turnover: some causes and solutions, Nurs Outlook 29:233, 1981.

APPENDIXES

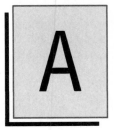

North American Nursing Diagnosis Association's (NANDA) Taxonomy I Revised*

In 1973 a group of nurses met in St. Louis and organized the First National Conference for the Classification of Nursing Diagnoses. They began the formal effort to identify, develop, and classify nursing diagnoses. Seven conferences have been held since that time with the last, the Eighth, being held in 1988.

Following the first conference, Gebbie (1974) identified four steps necessary for the development of a classification system; they are useful today. The first step in developing a classification is to identify all those things which nurses locate or diagnose in patients. The second step is to reach some agreement about consistent nomenclature that can be used to describe the domain of nursing as identified in step one. The third step in the classification process is the grouping of identified diagnoses (the labels) into classes and subclasses so that patterns and relationships among them can emerge. The final step in the process is the substitution of numbers or equivalent abbreviations for terminology so that data related to the various diagnoses can be manipulated more readily by hand or computer.

The first conferences were invitational. Participants were placed into groups and asked to generate diagnoses related to a specific functional system. They relied on their recall of patient situations to generate the signs and symptoms. Diagnoses were accepted by a majority vote of the participants. In 1982 the conferences were opened to the nursing community at large. The process for generating and accepting diagnoses moved through several stages incorporating submission and review by clinical experts. Acceptance, which was initially by conference participants, now requires positive vote of the membership of NANDA. No formal action was taken on new diagnoses at the 1982 and 1984 conferences while the diagnostic review process was being evaluated. However, since that time, the Guidelines for Submission and review of new diagnoses have been developed.

*This is largely the work of the North American Nursing Diagnosis Association.

After much dialogue, the participants at the First Conference could not agree on a scheme to classify the newly developed diagnoses, and so the decision was made to list the diagnoses alphabetically. Though the list was expanded over years, the alphabetic system was not changed until 1986 when the NANDA Taxonomy I was endorsed for development and testing.

The structural basis for the taxonomy was derived from the work of a group of nurse theorists during the third, fourth, and fifth conferences, chaired by Sr. Callista Roy. The nurse teorist group was asked to develop a conceptual framework for the classification of nursing diagnoses. Using an inductive methodology, they studied the alphabetic list of nursing diagnoses and generated several broad patterns that grouped the individual diagnoses. Their final work proposed the nine patterns of unitary man as the conceptual framework for the diagnostic classification system (Fifth Proceedings, Roy, p. 31, 1984). During this process, different theoretical levels of abstraction were identified among the diagnoses. Depending on the specificity of the diagnoses, some were very abstract and general whereas others were specific and concrete.

At the Fifth Conference, a taxonomy special interest group chaired by Phyllis Kritek was charged with the task of generating an initial taxonomy for the nursing diagnoses labels. The group focused on the existing list of diagnoses and the theorists' patterns of unitary man. The labels were separated into four levels of abstraction, Level I subsuming Levels II, III, and IV; Level II subsuming Levels III and IV, etc., with Level 1 being the most abstract and Level IV being the least abstract. During this time, members observed that Level IV diagnoses were the most useful for the practicing nurse. In the final analysis the Level I categories were identified as alterations in human responses and were categorized under the nine patterns of unitary man. This was the stage of taxonomy development at the end of the Fifth Conference.

On acceptance of the NANDA Bylaws and election of officers, the Taxonomy Committee began its work of formalizing and modifying the work that had gone before. The term *Human Response Patterns* was introduced to replace the less familiar term of *Patterns of Unitary Man*. This change was based on the advice of reviewers who critiqued the proposed taxonomy between the sixth and seventh conferences. The nine patterns constitute Level I concepts, the most abstract level, and provide the organizing framework for the taxonomy. Conference participants accepted this change without debate. The purposes of a taxonomy are to provide a vocabulary for classifying phenomena in a discipline, provide new ways of looking at the discipline, and play a part in concept derivation. The taxonomy provides a beginning classification scheme that can be used to categorize and classify nursing diagnostic labels. It is not meant for use as a theoretical framework or as an assessment framework in the strict sense of those constructs. After much discussion and work, the taxonomy was presented to the membership at the seventh conference which endorsed Taxonomy I for development and testing.

The following are rules of classification and guidelines used by the Taxonomy Committee:

1. There is no inherent order, that is, one pattern is not considered better than another, in the numbering of the nine patterns. The first pattern developed in the taxonomy was numbered one. It so happened that it was *Exchanging,* but it could have been any of the other patterns. This system of numbering was retained for the inclusion of each new diagnosis.
2. The level of abstraction (general to specific, abstract to concrete) determines the level of placement within the taxonomy. Supporting literature from the submitter, the opinion of experts, and nursing literature assist in determining placement.
3. The diagnosis is classified by considering the definition of the pattern and the definition of the diagnosis. They must be consistent.
4. The placement of the diagnosis is conceptually consistent with current theoretical views within nursing.
5. Categories in brackets were developed by the committee to clarify why certain diagnoses were placed at a specific level or in a specific pattern and from a collaborative effort with the American Nurses' Association. It is hoped that these categories will be researched and submitted as diagnoses or that new diagnoses will be submitted to replace them. This practice was only instituted to clarify the thinking of the committee so that nurses using the taxonomy could understand the placement of diagnoses.
6. The numbering system was developed to facilitate computerization of the taxonomy. At this point in the development of nursing diagnoses, one digit at each level was determined to be sufficient. In the future this may need to be changed.

This has been a brief history of the development of Taxonomy I and its subsequent revisions. It is hoped that it assists the nurse in using the taxonomy more knowledgeably and efficiently.

Concomitantly, NANDA is working to further develop the taxonomy and the coding of nursing diagnoses for the possible inclusion in the World Health Organization International Classification of Diseases. The first version of Taxonomy II will be presented at the 1990 NANDA conference.

DEFINITIONS FOR TAXONOMY I REVISED*

Classification: systematic arrangement in groups or categories according to established criteria; an arrangement of phenomena into groups based on their relationships

Defining characteristics: clinical criteria that represents the presence of the diagnostic category

Actual
1. Major defining characteristics: present 80% to 100% of time if researched, 100% of time if not researched
2. Minor defining characteristics: present 50% to 79% of time if researched or less than 100% of time if not researched

Potential
1. Risk factors

Level of abstraction: the concreteness or abstractness of a concept
1. Very abstract concepts are theoretical and cannot be directly measurable, defined by concrete concepts, inclusive of concrete concepts, disassociated from any specific instance, or independent of time and space; very abstract concepts have more general descriptors, and may not be clinically useful for planning treatment.
2. Concrete concepts are observable, measurable, limited by time and space, more exclusive, restricted by nature; concrete concepts constitute a specific category by naming a real thing or class of things and can be clinically useful for planning treatment.

Nomenclature: a system or set of terms or symbols; act or process of naming; a system of terms used in a particular science or discipline; compilation of accepted terms for describing phenomena.

Related factors: factors that appear to show some type of patterned relationship with the nursing diagnosis; may be described as antecedent to, associated with, related to, contributing to, or abetting

Taxonomy: type of classification; the theoretical study of systematic classifications including their bases, principles, procedures, and rules; the science of how to classify and identify

NANDA-APPROVED NURSING DIAGNOSTIC CATEGORIES*

This list represents the NANDA-approved nursing diagnostic categories for clinical use and testing (1988). Changes have been made in 15 labels for consistency.

PATTERN 1: EXCHANGING

1.1.2.1	Altered Nutrition: More Than body requirements
1.1.2.2	Altered Nutrition: Less Than body requirements

---

*These definitions are working definitions used in the development of Taxonomy I Revised - 1989 and are subject to change as work progresses.
*As published in the Summer 1988 NANDA Nursing Diagnosis newsletter.

1.1.2.3	Altered Nutrition: Potential for more than body requirements
1.2.1.1	Potential for Infection
1.2.2.1	Potential Altered Body Temperature
1.2.2.2	Hypothermia
1.2.2.3	Hyperthermia
1.2.2.4	Ineffective Thermoregulation
1.2.3.1	Dysreflexia
1.3.1.1	Constipation
1.3.1.1.1	Perceived Constipation
1.3.1.1.2	Colonic Constipation
1.3.1.2	Diarrhea
1.3.1.3	Bowel Incontinence
1.3.2	Altered Urinary Elimination
1.3.2.1.1	Stress Incontinence
1.3.2.1.2	Reflex Incontinence
1.3.2.1.3	Urge Incontinence
1.3.2.1.4	Functional Incontinence
1.3.2.1.5	Total Incontinence
1.3.2.2	Urinary Retention
1.4.1.1	Altered (Specify Type) Tissue Perfusion (Renal, Cerebral, Cardiopulmonary, Gastro-intestinal, Peripheral)
1.4.1.2.1	Fluid Volume Excess
1.4.1.2.2.1	Fluid Volume Deficit
1.4.1.2.2.2	Potential Fluid Volume Deficit
1.4.2.1	Decreased Cardiac Output
1.5.1.1	Impaired Gas Exchange
1.5.1.2	Ineffective Airway Clearance
1.5.1.3	Ineffective Breathing Pattern
1.6.1	Potential for Injury
1.6.1.1	Potential for Suffocation
1.6.1.2	Potential for Poisoning
1.6.1.3	Potential for Trauma
1.6.1.4	Potential for Aspiration
1.6.1.5	Potential for Disuse Syndrome
1.6.2.1	Impaired Tissue Integrity
1.6.2.1.1	Altered Oral Mucous Membrane
1.6.2.1.2.1	Impaired Skin Integrity
1.6.2.1.2.2	Potential Impaired Skin Integrity

PATTERN 2: COMMUNICATING

2.1.1.1	Impaired Verbal Communication

PATTERN 3: RELATING

3.1.1	Impaired Social Interaction
3.1.2	Social Isolation
3.2.1	Altered Role Performance
3.2.1.1.1	Altered Parenting
3.2.1.1.2	Potential Altered Parenting
3.2.1.2.1	Sexual Dysfunction
3.2.2	Altered Family Processes
3.2.3.1	Parental Role Conflict
3.3	Altered Sexuality Patterns

PATTERN 4: VALUING

4.1.1	Spiritual Distress (Distress of the Human Spirit)

PATTERN 5: CHOOSING

5.1.1.1	Ineffective Individual Coping
5.1.1.1.1	Impaired Adjustment
5.1.1.1.2	Defensive Coping
5.1.1.1.3	Ineffective Denial
5.1.2.1.1	Ineffective Family Coping: Disabling
5.1.2.1.2	Ineffective Family Coping: Compromised
5.1.2.2	Family Coping: Potential for Growth
5.2.1.1	Noncompliance (Specify)
5.3.1.1	Decisional Conflict (Specify)
5.4	Health-Seeking Behaviors (Specify)

PATTERN 6: MOVING

6.1.1.1	Impaired Physical Mobility
6.1.1.2	Activity Intolerance
6.1.1.2.1	Fatigue
6.1.1.3	Potential Activity Intolerance
6.2.1	Sleep Pattern Disturbance
6.3.1.1	Diversional Activity Deficit
6.4.1.1	Impaired Home Maintenance Management
6.4.2	Altered Health Maintenance
6.5.1	Feeding Self-Care Deficit
6.5.1.1	Impaired Swallowing
6.5.1.2	Ineffective Breastfeeding
6.5.2	Bathing/Hygiene Self-Care Deficit
6.5.3	Dressing/Grooming Self-Care Deficit
6.5.4	Toileting Self-Care Deficit
6.6	Altered Growth and Development

PATTERN 7: PERCEIVING

7.1.1	Body Image Disturbance
7.1.2	Self-Esteem Disturbance
7.1.2.1	Chronic Low Self-Esteem
7.1.2.2	Situational Low Self-Esteem
7.1.3	Personal Identity Disturbance
7.2	Sensory/Perceptual Alterations (Specify) (Visual, Auditory, Kinesthetic, Gustatory, Tactile, Olfactory)
7.2.1.1	Unilateral Neglect
7.3.1	Hopelessness
7.3.2	Powerlessness

PATTERN 8: KNOWING

8.1.1	Knowledge Deficit (Specify)
8.3	Altered Thought Processes

PATTERN 9: FEELING

9.1.1	Pain
9.1.1.1	Chronic Pain
9.2.1.1	Dysfunctional Grieving
9.2.1.2	Anticipatory Grieving
9.2.2	Potential for Violence: Self-Directed or Directed at Others
9.2.3	Post-Trauma Response
9.2.3.1	Rape-Trauma Syndrome
9.2.3.1.1	Rape-Trauma Syndrome: Compound Reaction
9.2.3.1.2	Rape-Trauma Syndrome: Silent Reaction
9.3.1	Anxiety
9.3.2	Fear

ACLS Guidelines

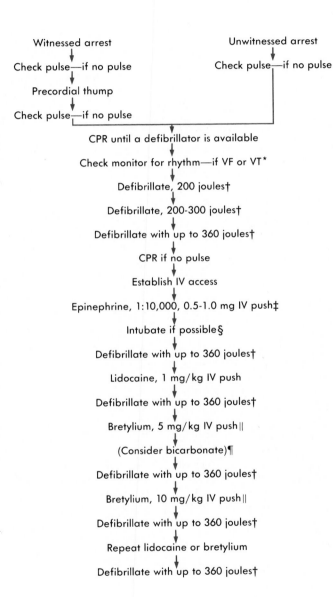

Witnessed arrest
↓
Check pulse—if no pulse
↓
Precordial thump
↓
Check pulse—if no pulse

Unwitnessed arrest
↓
Check pulse—if no pulse

CPR until a defibrillator is available
↓
Check monitor for rhythm—if VF or VT*
↓
Defibrillate, 200 joules†
↓
Defibrillate, 200-300 joules†
↓
Defibrillate with up to 360 joules†
↓
CPR if no pulse
↓
Establish IV access
↓
Epinephrine, 1:10,000, 0.5-1.0 mg IV push‡
↓
Intubate if possible§
↓
Defibrillate with up to 360 joules†
↓
Lidocaine, 1 mg/kg IV push
↓
Defibrillate with up to 360 joules†
↓
Bretylium, 5 mg/kg IV push‖
↓
(Consider bicarbonate)¶
↓
Defibrillate with up to 360 joules†
↓
Bretylium, 10 mg/kg IV push‖
↓
Defibrillate with up to 360 joules†
↓
Repeat lidocaine or bretylium
↓
Defibrillate with up to 360 joules†

Fig. B-1 Ventricular fibrillation (and pulseless ventricular tachycardia). This sequence was developed to assist in teaching how to treat a broad range of patients with ventricular fibrillation (VF) or pulseless ventricular tachycardia (VT). Some patients may require care not specified herein. This algorithm should not be construed as prohibiting such flexibility. Flow of algorithm presumes that VF is continuing. CPR indicates cardiopulmonary resuscitation.

*Pulseless VT should be treated identically to VF.

†Check pulse and rhythm after each shock. If VF recurs after transiently converting (rather than persists without converting), use whatever energy level has previously been successful for defibrillation.

‡Epinephrine should be repeated every 5 minutes.

§Intubation is preferable. If it can be accomplished simultaneously with other techniques, then the earlier the better. However, defibrillation and epinephrine are more important initially if the patient can be ventilated without intubation.

‖Some may prefer repeated doses of lidocaine, which may be given in 0.5-mg/kg boluses every 8 minutes to a total dose of 3 mg/kg.

¶Value of sodium bicarbonate is questionable during cardiac arrest, and it is not recommended for routine cardiac arrest sequence. Consideration of its use in a dose of 1 mEq/kg is appropriate at this point. Half of original dose may be repeated every 10 minutes if it is used. (Reproduced with permission from the American Heart Association: Textbook of advanced cardiac life support, 1989, The Association.)

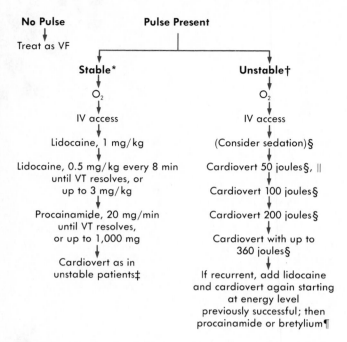

Treat as VF

Pulse Present

Stable*

O₂

IV access

Lidocaine, 1 mg/kg

Lidocaine, 0.5 mg/kg every 8 min
until VT resolves, or
up to 3 mg/kg

Procainamide, 20 mg/min
until VT resolves,
or up to 1,000 mg

Cardiovert as in
unstable patients‡

Unstable†

O₂

IV access

(Consider sedation)§

Cardiovert 50 joules§, ‖

Cardiovert 100 joules§

Cardiovert 200 joules§

Cardiovert with up to
360 joules§

If recurrent, add lidocaine
and cardiovert again starting
at energy level
previously successful; then
procainamide or bretylium¶

Fig. B-2 Sustained ventricular tachycardia (VT). This sequence was developed to assist in teaching how to treat a broad range of patients with sustained VT. Some patients may require care not specified herein. This algorithm should not be construed as prohibiting such flexibility. Flow of algorithm presumes that VT is continuing. VF indicates ventricular fibrillation.

*If patient becomes unstable (see footnote † for definition) at any time, move to "Unstable" arm of algorithm.

†Unstable indicates symptoms (e.g., chest pain or dyspnea), hypotension (systolic blood pressure <90 mm Hg) congestive heart failure, ischemia, or infarction.

‡Sedation should be considered for all patients, including those defined in footnote † as unstable, except those who are hemodynamically unstable (e.g., hypotensive, in pulmonary edema, or unconscious).

§If hypotension, pulmonary edema, or unconsciousness is present, unsynchronized cardioversion should be done to avoid delay associated with synchronization.

‖In the absence of hypotension, pulmonary edema, or unconsciousness, a precordial thump may be employed before cardioversion.

¶Once VT has resolved, begin intravenous (IV) infusion of antiarrhythmic agent that has aided resolution of VT. If hypotension, pulmonary edema, or unconsciousness is present, use lidocaine if cardioversion alone is unsuccessful, followed by bretylium. In all other patients, recommended order of therapy is lidocaine, procainamide, and then bretylium. (Reproduced with permission from the American Heart Association: Textbook of advanced cardiac life support, 1989, The Association.)

If rhythm is unclear and possibly ventricular
fibrillation, defibrillate as for VF. If asystole is present*

Continue CPR

Establish IV access

Epinephrine, 1:10,000, 0.5-1.0 mg IV push†

Intubate when possible‡

Atropine, 1.0 mg IV push (repeated in 5 min)

(Consider bicarbonate)§

Consider pacing

Fig. B-3 Asystole (cardiac standstill). This sequence was developed to assist in teaching how to treat a broad range of patients with asystole. Some patients may require care not specified herein. This algorithm should not be construed to prohibit such flexibility. Flow of algorithm presumes asystole is continuing. VF indicates ventricular fibrillation; IV, intravenous.

*Asystole should be confirmed in two leads.

†Epinephrine should be repeated every 5 minutes.

‡Intubation is preferable; if it can be accomplished simultaneously with other techniques, then the earlier the better. However, cardiopulmonary resuscitation (CPR) and use of epinephrine are more important initially if patient can be ventilated without intubation. (Endotracheal epinephrine may be used.)

§Value of sodium bicarbonate is questionable during cardiac arrest, and it is not recommended for the routine cardiac arrest sequence. Consideration of its use in a dose of 1 mEq/kg is appropriate at this point. Half of original dose may be repeated every 10 minutes if it is used. (Reproduced with permission from the American Heart Association: Textbook of advanced cardiac life support, 1989, The Association.)

Continue CPR

↓

Establish IV access

↓

Epinephrine, 1:10,000, 0.5-1.0 mg IV push*

↓

Intubate when possible†

↓

(Consider bicarbonate)‡

↓

Consider hypovolemia,
cardiac tamponade,
tension pneumothorax,
hypoxemia,
acidosis,
pulmonary embolism

Fig. B-4 Electromechanical dissociation. This sequence was developed to assist in teaching how to treat a broad range of patients with electromechanical dissociation. Some patients may require care not specified herein. This algorithm should not be construed to prohibit such flexibility. Flow of algorithm presumes that electromechanical dissociation is continuing. CPR indicates cardiopulmonary resuscitation; IV, intravenous.

*Epinephrine should be repeated every 5 minutes.

†Intubation is preferable. If it can be accomplished simultaneously with other techniques, then the earlier the better. However, epinephrine is more important initially if the patient can be ventilated without intubation.

‡Value of sodium bicarbonate is questionable during cardiac arrest, and it is not recommended for routine cardiac arrest sequence. Consideration of its use in a dose of 1 mEq/kg is appropriate at this point. Half of original dose may be repeated every 10 minutes if it is used. (Reproduced with permission from the American Heart Association: Textbook of advanced cardiac life support, 1989, The Association.)

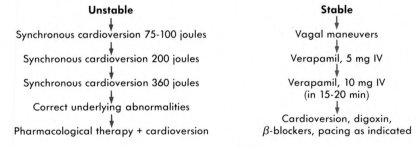

Unstable	**Stable**
↓	↓
Synchronous cardioversion 75-100 joules	Vagal maneuvers
↓	↓
Synchronous cardioversion 200 joules	Verapamil, 5 mg IV
↓	↓
Synchronous cardioversion 360 joules	Verapamil, 10 mg IV (in 15-20 min)
↓	↓
Correct underlying abnormalities	Cardioversion, digoxin, β-blockers, pacing as indicated
↓	
Pharmacological therapy + cardioversion	

If conversion occurs but PSVT recurs, repeated electrical cardioversion is *not* indicated. Sedation should be used as time permits.

Fig. B-5 Paroxysmal supraventricular tachycardia (PSVT). This sequence was developed to assist in teaching how to treat a broad range of patients with PSVT. Some patients may require care not specified herein. This algorithm should not be construed as prohibiting such flexibility. Flow of algorithm presumes PSVT is continuing. (Reproduced with permission from the American Heart Association: Textbook of advanced cardiac life support, 1989, The Association.)

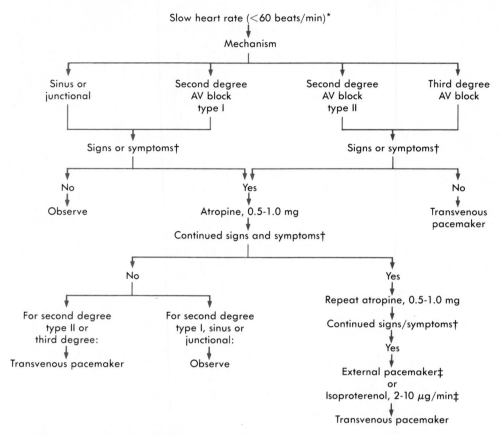

Fig. B-6 Bradycardia. This sequence was developed to assist in teaching how to treat a broad range of patients with bradycardia. Some patients may require care not specified herein. This algorithm should not be construed to prohibit such flexibility. AV indicates atrioventricular.

*A solitary chest thump or cough may stimulate cardiac electrical activity and result in improved cardiac output and may be used at this point.

†Hypotension (blood pressure <90 mm Hg), premature ventricular contractions, altered mental status or symptoms (e.g., chest pain or dyspnea), ischemia, or infarction.

‡Temporizing therapy. (Reproduced with permission from the American Heart Association: Textbook of advanced cardiac life support, 1989, The Association.)

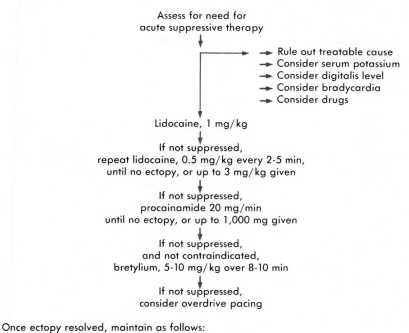

Once ectopy resolved, maintain as follows:
    After lidocaine, 1 mg/kg . . . lidocaine drip, 2 mg/min
    After lidocaine, 1-2 mg/kg . . . lidocaine drip, 3 mg/min
    After lidocaine, 2-3 mg/kg . . . lidocaine drip, 4 mg/min
    After procainamide . . . procainamide drip, 1-4 mg/min (check blood level)
    After bretylium . . . bretylium drip, 2 mg/min

Fig. B-7   Ventricular ectopy: acute suppressive therapy. This sequence was developed to assist in teaching how to treat a broad range of patients with ventricular ectopy. Some patients may require therapy not specified herein. This algorithm should not be construed as prohibiting such flexibility. (Reproduced from the American Heart Association: Textbook of advanced cardiac life support, 1989, The Association.)

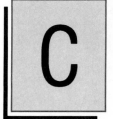

Physiologic Formulas for Critical Care

Mean (Systemic) Arterial Pressure (MAP)

$$\frac{\text{(Diastolic} \times 2) + \text{(Systolic} \times 1)}{3}$$

(Systemic)   (Systemic)

Systemic Vascular Resistance (SVR)

$$\frac{\text{MAP} - \text{RAP}}{\text{CO}} = \frac{\text{SVR in units}}{\text{Normal 10-18 units}}$$

$$\frac{\text{MAP} - \text{RAP}}{\text{CO}} \times 80 = \frac{\text{SVR in dynes/sec/cm}^{-5}}{\text{Normal 800-1400 dynes/sec/cm}^{-5}}$$

Systemic Vascular Resistance Index (SVRI)

$$\frac{\text{MAP} - \text{RAP}}{\text{CI}} \times 80 = \frac{\text{SVRI in dynes/sec/cm}^{-5}/\text{M}^2}{\text{Normal 2000-2400}}$$ dynes/sec/cm^{-5}/M^2

Pulmonary Vascular Resistance (PVR)

$$\frac{\text{PAP mean} - \text{PAW}}{\text{CO}} = \frac{\text{PVR in units}}{\text{Normal 1.2-3.0 units}}$$

$$\frac{\text{PAP mean} - \text{PAW}}{\text{CO}} \times 80$$
$$= \frac{\text{PVR in dynes/sec/cm}^{-5}}{\text{Normal 100-250 dynes/sec/cm}^{-5}}$$

MAP, mean arterial pressure; RAP, right atrial pressure; CO, cardiac output; CI, cardiac index; PAP mean, pulmonary artery mean pressure; PAW, pulmonary wedge pressure; PB, barometric pressure.

*pK = 6.1 is the dissociation constant of carbonic acid.

†PaCO$_2$ × .03 converts PaCO$_2$ from mm Hg to mEq/L.

‡1.25 is a constant used to take into account the normal respiratory quotient.

§47 is a constant used to correct for the normal water vapor pressure of humidified gas.

‖.003 is a constant used because 0.003 ml of oxygen will dissolve in each 100 ml of blood.

¶1.34 is a constant used because each gram of hemoglobin will carry 1.34 ml oxygen. Actually, if the hemoglobin is chemically pure (rare), each gram is capable of carrying 1.39 ml of oxygen. Since most hemoglobin has impurities, 1.34 is the accepted constant (see Chapter 17, reference #43).

Pulmonary Vascular Resistance Index (PVRI)

$$\frac{\text{PAP mean} - \text{PAW}}{\text{CI}} \times 80 = \text{PVRI in dynes/sec/cm}^{-5}/\text{M}^2$$

Henderson-Hasselbalch Equation (Blood pH)

$$pH = pK^* + \text{Log} \frac{\text{HCO}_3^- \text{ mEq/L (Base)}}{\text{PaCO}_2 \text{ mm Hg} \times .03† \text{(Acid)}}$$

$$pH = 6.1 = \text{Log} \frac{\text{HCO}_3^- \text{ mEq/L (Base)}}{\text{PaCO}_2 \text{ mEq/L (Acid)}}$$

Partial Pressure of Oxygen in the Alveolus (PaO$_2$, expressed in mm Hg)

$$\text{PaO}_2 = \text{PIO}_2 - (\text{PaCO}_2 \times 1.25)‡$$

Partial Pressure of Inspired Oxygen (PIO$_2$, expressed in mm Hg)

$$\text{PIO}_2 = \text{FIO}_2 \times (\text{PB} - 47)§$$

A-a Gradient (also known as A-a DO$_2$)

A-a gradient = PaO$_2$ − PaO$_2$ (expressed in mm Hg. Normal <10 mm Hg but normal increases with age and FIO$_2$.)

Calculation of the Oxygen Content (CaO$_2$)

Oxygen content is a measure of the total amount of oxygen carried in the blood; both the oxygen dissolved in plasma (PaO$_2$) and the oxygen bound to hemoglobin (SaO$_2$). Oxygen content is reported in ml/100 ml blood or as volume percent.

There are three steps in the CaO$_2$ calculation:

Step 1. Calculate the amount of oxygen dissolved in 100 ml of plasma—

$$\text{PaO}_2 \times .003‖ = \text{ml } O_2/100 \text{ ml plasma.}$$

Step 2. Calculate the amount of oxygen bound to hemoglobin—

$$\text{Hb} \times 1.34¶ \times \text{SaO}_2 = \text{ml of } O_2 \text{ bound to Hb.}$$

Step 3. Add the results of Steps 1 and 2 for the CaO$_2$.

Example: Patient A

PaO$_2$	100 mm Hg
SaO$_2$	.97
Hb	15 g%

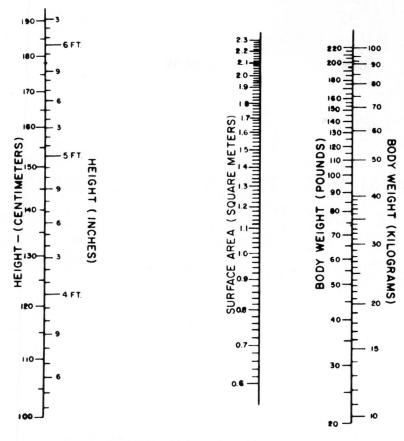

Fig. C-1 Body surface nomogram.

Step 1. $100 \times .003 = .3\ ml\ O_2$ in 100 ml plasma.
Step 2. $15\ g\% \times 1.34 \times .97 = 19.5$ ml O_2 bound to Hb.
Step 3. $.3 + 19.5 = 19.8\ vol\%\ CaO_2$.

Recommendations for Fluid Replacement Based on Body Surface Area (BSA)

1. Use body surface area nomogram to compute BSA (Fig. C-1).
2. For maintenance, consider administering 1500 ml/m² body surface per 24 hours.
3. For correction of a moderate fluid volume deficit and to continue maintenance, consider administering 2400 ml/m² of body surface area per 24 hours.
4. For correction of a severe fluid volume deficit and to continue maintenance, consider administering 3000 ml/m² of body surface area per 24 hours.

Remember that these are only general recommendations. Other specific clinical factors regarding a patient's condition (such as metabolic rate and organ dysfunction) need to be examined before the total required 24-hour fluid volume can be calculated.

Recommended fluid dosages for fluid replacement from Metheny NM and Snively WD: Nurses handbook of fluid balance, ed 4, Philadelphia, 1983, JB Lippincott Co.

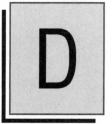

Therapeutic Touch in a High-Tech Environment

The use of touch as a form of caring for others is commonplace in nursing and yet the *therapeutic* value of touch is often either not recognized or simply discounted. In studying patients' perceptions of nurses' caring behaviors, Watson[14] found that patients most often rated nursing activities involving physical care and comfort as the ones more indicative of caring on the part of the nurse.

A rapidly growing number of nurses in the United States and 38 other countries are incorporating an intervention termed *therapeutic touch* into their practice. Therapeutic touch is a method of using one's hands to direct energies to help or heal. Therapeutic touch was first developed as a treatment modality for use by nurses in the early 1970s by Dolores Krieger, Ph.D., a physiologist and professor of nursing at New York University. Krieger's interest in therapeutic use of the hands was stimulated by her work with Dora Kunz, who derived the basic technique of therapeutic touch from the ancient practice of laying-on-of-hands.

CONCEPTUAL BASIS FOR THERAPEUTIC TOUCH

A basic assumption underlying the practice of Therapeutic Touch is the understanding of the human being as an energy field constantly interacting with other energy fields in the environment. This view of humans is also a core concept of *The Science of Unitary Human Beings,* developed by nurse-theorist Martha Rogers, a colleague of Kriegers.[13] Many of the concepts related to Rogers' conceptual model for nursing were incorporated by the Nurse Theorist group working with the North American Nursing Diagnosis Association (NANDA) in recommending the nine Human Response Patterns which now constitute NANDA's Taxonomy I Revised (see Chapter 1).

Another shared assumption of Rogers' and of therapeutic touch is that energies are interchanged in human interactions and modulated in a universal field which eventually permeates all matter. Through this perpetual energy exchange, all thoughts, emotions, and actions create changes that affect the energy fields of others.[2,16] Because energy is never destroyed, an unlimited amount is available when there is freedom of flow and synchronicity in the fields.[1] Blockage or disordered patterns of the energy flow in any field creates a negative influence.[16] The imbalance, then, is what may be experienced as mental or physical illness. In disease, the flow of energy is obstructed, disordered, and/or depleted.[10]

The nurse using therapeutic touch as an intervention has learned to attune to the universal energy field by making a conscious decision to help or heal. The nurse is then able to direct the life energy into patients and therefore enhance vitality.[10]

Nurses help patients assimilate the energy by releasing congestion and balancing areas where the energy flow has become disordered. Since the nurse is drawing on the universal energy field, she or he does not become drained of energy but is instead constantly replenished.[10]

The patient who is a recipient of therapeutic touch usually experiences a profound relaxation response during the treatment, and pain relief is a frequent component. The treatment itself generally lasts 10 to 15 minutes, although the nurse and patient may not be aware of the passage of time in the linear sense. The only known contraindication to using therapeutic touch is the patient's opposition to it, or if the patient's doubting that therapeutic touch may, in some way, be useful.

SCIENTIFIC BASIS FOR THERAPEUTIC TOUCH

In contrast to the laying-on-of-hands, therapeutic touch does not have a religious base, but rather a continually developing scientific research base. The research to date demonstrates that therapeutic touch is particularly effective in treating pain and anxiety, two very common nursing diagnoses in critical care. This research base is summarized in Table D-1. Although there is no significant difference in effect based on whether the therapeutic touch actually involves contact to the skin or is done by placing the hands 4 to 6 inches from the skin surface, there is a significant difference in outcome when using therapeutic touch versus casual touch or the touch of routine nursing care. This dif-

Table D-1 Research base for therapeutic touch

Author/year	Design	Variable studied	Subjects studied	Intervention used	Results
Krieger (1974)	Quasi-experimental	Hemoglobin	64 hospitalized adults	TT; routine care	Significant increase in TT group
Heidt (1979)	Experimental pre-post test	Anxiety	90 adult hospitalized cardiovascular patients	TT; casual touch; no touch	Significant decrease in TT group
Randolph (1979)	Experimental pre-post test	Physiological response to stressful stimuli	60 college students	Modified TT; modified MTT	No significant differences
Quinn (1982)	Experimental pre-post test	Anxiety	60 adult hospitalized cardiovascular patients	NCTT; MTT	Significant decrease in NCTT group
Fedoruk (1984)	Quasi-experimental repeated measures	Response to stress	17 neonates	NCTT; MTT	Significant decrease of stress on infant state
Connell-Meehan (1985)	Experimental pre-post test	Pain	108 postoperative adults	NCTT; MTT; medication	No significant differences between NCTT and MTT groups
Parkes (1985)	Experimental pre-post test	Anxiety	Gerontological hospitalized patients	NCTT; MTT; adapted MTT	No significant differences
Keller (1986)	Experimental pre-post test	Tension headache pain	60 adults	NCTT; MTT	Significant decrease in TT group

Adapted from Quinn JF: J Holistic Nurs 6(1):37, 1988.
TT, therapeutic touch; MTT, mimic therapeutic touch; NCTT, non-contact therapeutic touch.

ference is based on the mental/emotional state of the nurse giving the therapeutic touch treatment. Therapeutic touch used by a nurse who is free of distractions, focused on the individual, and consciously aware of wanting to help that individual is most effective in reducing anxiety and pain.

For the three studies in Table D-1, which show no significant differences in outcome after therapeutic touch treatment, Quinn points out that the findings may be more related to the nurse than the therapeutic touch treatment itself.[11] Specific factors may include such things as varying lengths of treatment times and varying skill levels of the nurses using the treatment. Overall, Quinn concludes that the designs of the therapeutic touch studies have become increasingly sophisticated, and a substantial foundation for future work in therapeutic touch research has been established.[11]

STEPS IN THERAPEUTIC TOUCH PROCESS

Therapeutic touch is a healing intervention that focuses on the individual as a whole. The process of therapeutic touch is itself a whole; however, for purposes of explication, six steps in this process will be identified and described.

Step I: Prepare the Patient

When feasible, a brief explanation of the process is provided, and verbal consent of the patient is obtained. The patient need not be fully responsive, however, to be a recipient of therapeutic touch, since the nurse will be working with the patient's energy field. Indeed, in the critical care setting, the patient will often be intubated, mechanically ventilated, and unresponsive while receiving therapeutic touch. In the outpatient setting, on the other hand, the patient may sit upright on a backless stool, thereby providing maximum access to the entire energy field.

Step II: Become Centered

In this step, the nurse becomes centered, which refers to quieting oneself and focusing inward, rather than on the distractions of the external environment. It is helpful at this point to focus thoughts on a desire or intent to help or heal the patient and to wish that the greatest good come for the patient as a result of the treatment. A sense of caring about the person with whom the nurse is working is often felt at this phase.

It is not easy to block out the stimulation of the all too noisy and active critical care unit. In the early stages of learning to use therapeutic touch, this phase takes more time. Relaxation tapes or meditation practice can assist one in developing the ability to become quickly centered in a moment or two, despite the external stimuli.

As the nurse is about to begin this step, the patient is instructed to think of being in a restful, quiet, and pleasant place. The patient is encouraged to continue with this image until the treatment is completed.

Step III: Assess the Patient/Energy Field

The focus of this step is to assess the patient's energy field for any imbalances or congestion of energy. This is a head-to-toe assessment that is accomplished by the nurse moving her or his hands in a slow to moderate pace down the energy field in the space from 4 to 6 inches away from the skin surface. With a patient lying supine in bed, the assessment is usually completed in less than 2 to 3 minutes. During this process, the nurse's hands will detect cues of imbalance by feeling sensations such as tingling, heat or cold, pressure, and/or a magnetic-type pulling. These cues assist the nurse in planning the type of energy modulation which will be done during the treatment phase in Step V.

Step IV: Smooth Out the Energy Field (Unruffle)

The energy field of the patient must first be free of old energy patterns of congestion and imbalance to prepare it for the next step of receiving new energy in a more healthful pattern. To accomplish this, the field is smoothed out or unruffled. In this step, the nurse's hands work from head to toe in a slow, rhythmic motion, each hand in a gentle synchrony with the other, moving over the field as if smoothing out wrinkles on a cloth. The patient's body may or may not be touched as unruffling proceeds.

Step V: Modulate or Repattern the Energy Field

In this step, the nurse's hands channel or direct the universal energy to areas of the body previously assessed as being out of balance. Focus is still maintained, however, on the person as a whole being, rather than allowing focus to narrow to only a part of the person. The appearance of this step is much like unruffling, or, the hands may, from time to time, become still over certain areas as the intention is mentally made to allow energy to flow to that area. The nurse attends to intuitive thoughts as her or his hands move either in the 4 to 6-inch space of surrounding the body, as in the assessment step, or actually touching the body. Since the research supports touch and non–touch therapeutic touch to be equally effective, it becomes the nurse's choice as to when and where each is used. Knowledge of the patient's preference in this matter, as well as respect for privacy, are important considerations during this step.

Step VI: Reassess and Complete the Treatment

Reassessment of the energy field is done at periodic intervals to ensure that imbalanced energy is becoming balanced in terms of the field feeling symmetrical from one side of the body to the other. In this manner, the treatment is completed. It is useful at the end of a therapeutic touch treatment to hold the patient's feet while thinking of the energy being pulled through the body and into the ground. This "grounding" maneuver eliminates the potential for leaving the patient feeling lightheaded, with too much energy in the head rather than flowing through the whole body.

The beginning therapeutic touch practitioner can find more details about this process in Krieger's book, *The Therapeutic Touch: How to Use Your Hands to Help or Heal,*[9] and Macrae's book, *Therapeutic Touch: A Practical Guide.*[10] To begin to experience the sensation of the energy field, the beginner may wish to practice exercises from Krieger's book. Additionally, each summer, classes are taught on the East and West coasts of the United States. Several schools of nursing throughout the country offer therapeutic touch in their curriculum. Continuing education classes are offered for the nursing community by school of nursing faculty or by other therapeutic touch practitioners.

SUMMARY

Although Therapeutic Touch may appear out of character in the "high-tech" environment of critical care, there is, in fact, a solid scientific basis for providing this therapeutic intervention. Critically ill patients may indeed be the ones most in need of "high touch" interventions by the critical care nurse.

REFERENCES

1. Bradley D: Energy fields: implications for nurses, J Holistic Nurs 5(1):32, 1987.
2. Dossey L: Space, time and medicine, Boulder, 1982, Shambhala.
3. Grad B: A telekinetic effect on plant growth, Int J Parapsychol 5:117, 1963.
4. Grad B: A telekinetic effect of plant growth II, Int J Parapsychol 6:473, 1964.
5. Grad B, Cadoret RJ, and Paul GI: An unorthodox method of wound healing in mice, Int J Parapsychol 3:5, 1961.
6. Heidt P: An investigation of the effects of therapeutic touch on anxiety of hospitalized patients (doctoral dissertation), New York, 1979, New York University.
7. Keller E and Bzdek VM: Effects of therapeutic touch on tension headache pain, Nurs Res 35(2):101, 1986.
8. Krieger D: The relationship of touch, with the intent to help or to heal, to subjects' in vivo hemoglobin values: a study in personalized interaction. In Proceedings of the Ninth American Nurses' Association Research Conference, New York, 1973, American Nurses' Association.
9. Krieger D: The therapeutic touch, Englewood Cliffs, NJ, 1979, Prentice Hall.
10. Macrae J: Therapeutic touch: a practical guide, New York, 1987, Alfred A Knopf.
11. Quinn JF: An investigation of the effect of therapeutic touch done without physical contact on state anxiety of hospitalized cardiovascular patients. Dissertation Abstracts International (University microfilms no. DA 82-26-788).
12. Quinn JF: Building a body of knowledge: research on therapeutic touch, J Holistic Nurs 6(1):37, 1988.
13. Rogers, M: An introduction to the theoretical basis of nursing, Philadelphia, 1970, FA Davis.
14. Watson J: Nursing: the philosophy and science of caring, Boston, 1979, Little, Brown & Co.
15. Watson J, and others: A model of caring: an alternative health care model for nursing practice and research. In Division of community health nursing practice (publ. NP-59), Kansas City, MO, 1979, American Nurses' Association.
16. Weber R: Philosophical foundations and frameworks for healing. In Brelli D and Heidt P, editors: Therapeutic touch, New York, 1981, Springer.

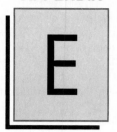

Universal Precautions for Prevention of Transmission of Human Immunodeficiency Virus, Hepatitis B Virus, and Other Bloodborne Pathogens in Health-Care Settings[*]

The purpose of this report is to clarify and supplement the Centers for Disease Control (CDC) publication entitled "Recommendations for Prevention of HIV Transmission in Health-Care Settings"[3].

In 1983, the CDC published a document entitled "Guideline for Isolation Precautions in Hospitals"[10] that contained a section entitled "Blood and Body Fluid Precautions." The recommendations in this section called for blood and body fluid precautions when a patient was known or suspected to be infected with bloodborne pathogens. In August 1987, the CDC published a document entitled "Recommendations for Prevention of HIV Transmission in Health-Care Setting."[3] In contrast to the 1983 document, the 1987 document recommended that blood and body fluid precautions be consistently used for all patients regardless of their bloodborne infection status. This extension of blood and body fluid precautions to *all* patients is referred to as "Universal Blood and Body Fluid Precautions" or "Universal Precautions." Under universal precautions, blood and certain body fluids of all patients are considered potentially infectious for human immunodeficiency virus (HIV), hepatitis B virus (HBV), and other bloodborne pathogens.

Universal precautions are intended to prevent parenteral, mucous membrane, and nonintact skin exposures of health-care workers to bloodborne pathogens. In addition, immunization with HBV vaccine is recommended as an important adjunct to universal precautions for health-care workers who have exposures to blood.[7,13]

Since the recommendations for universal precautions were published in August 1987, the CDC and the Food and Drug Administration (FDA) have received requests for clarification of the following issues: (1) body fluids to which universal precautions apply, (2) use of protective barriers, (3) use of gloves for phlebotomy, (4) selection of gloves for use while observing universal precautions, and (5) need for making changes in waste management programs as a result of adopting universal precautions.

BODY FLUIDS TO WHICH UNIVERSAL PRECAUTIONS APPLY

Universal precautions apply to blood and to other body fluids containing visible blood. Occupational transmission of HIV and HBV to health-care workers by blood has beeen documented.[5,7] *Blood is the single most important source of HIV, HBV, and other bloodborne pathogens in the occupational setting. Infection control efforts for HIV, HBV, and other bloodborne pathogens must focus on preventing exposures to blood as well as on delivery of HBV immunization.*

Universal precautions also apply to semen and vaginal secretions. Although both of these fluids have been implicated in the sexual transmission of HIV and HBV, they have not been implicated in occupational transmission from patient to health-care worker. This occurrence is not unexpected, because exposure to semen in the usual health-care setting is limited, and the routine practice of wearing gloves for performing vaginal examinations protects health-care workers from exposure to potentially infectious vaginal secretions.

Universal precautions also apply to tissues and to the following fluids: cerebrospinal fluid (CSF), synovial fluid,

[*]This appendix is modified from the Centers for Disease Control: Update: universal precautions for prevention of transmission of human immunodeficiency virus, hepatitis B virus, and other bloodborne pathogens in health-care settings, MMWR 37(24)377, 1988.

pleural fluid, peritoneal fluid, pericardial fluid, and amniotic fluid. The risk of transmission of HIV and HBV from these fluids is unknown; epidemiological studies in the health-care and community setting are currently inadequate to assess the potential risk to health-care workers from occupational exposures to them. However, HIV has been isolated from CSF, synovial, and amniotic fluid,[12,20,28] and HBsAg has been detected in synovial fluid, amniotic fluid, and peritoneal fluid.[1,17,21] One case of HIV transmission was reported after a percutaneous exposure to bloody pleural fluid obtained by needle aspiration.[22] Although aseptic procedures used to obtain these fluids for diagnostic or therapeutic purposes protect health-care workers from skin exposures, they cannot prevent penetrating injuries resulting from contaminated needles or other sharp instruments.

BODY FLUIDS TO WHICH UNIVERSAL PRECAUTIONS DO NOT APPLY

Universal precautions do not apply to feces, nasal secretions, sputum, sweat, tears, urine, and vomitus unless they contain visible blood. The risk of transmission of HIV and HBV from these fluids and materials is extremely low or nonexistent. In some of these fluids, HIV has been isolated and HBsAg has been demonstrated; however, epidemiological studies in the health-care and community setting have not implicated these fluids or materials in the transmission of HIV and HBV infections.[8,18] Some of the above fluids and excretions represent a potential source for nosocomial and community-acquired infections with other pathogens, and recommendations for preventing the transmission of nonbloodborne pathogens have been published.[10]

PRECAUTIONS FOR OTHER BODY FLUIDS IN SPECIAL SETTINGS

Human breast milk has been implicated in perinatal transmission of HIV, and HBsAg has been found in the milk of mothers infected with HBV.[17,18] However, occupational exposure to human breast milk has not been implicated in the transmission of HIV or HBV infection to health-care workers. This is mostly because the health-care worker does not have the same type of intensive exposure to breast milk as the nursing neonate. Although universal precautions do not apply to human breast milk, gloves may be worn by health-care workers in situations during which exposures to breast milk might be frequent, for example, in breast milk banking.

Saliva of some persons infected with HBV has been shown to contain HBV-DNA at concentrations 1/1,000 to 1/10,000 of that found in the infected person's serum.[15] HBsAg-positive saliva has been shown to be infectious when injected into experimental animals and in human bite exposures.[2,19,25] However, HBsAg-positive saliva has not been shown to be infectious when applied to oral mucous membranes in experimental primate studies[25] or through contamination of musical instruments or cardiopulmonary resuscitation dummies used by HBV carriers.[11,23] Epidemiological studies of nonsexual household contacts of HIV-infected patients, including several small series in which HIV transmission failed to occur after bites or after percutaneous

inoculation or contamination of cuts and open wounds with saliva from HIV-infected patients, suggest that the potential for salivary transmission of HIV is remote.[5,6,8,14,18] One case report from Germany has suggested the possibility of transmission of HIV in a household setting from an infected child to a sibling through a human bite.[27] The bite did not break the skin or result in bleeding. Because the date of seroconversion to HIV was not known for either child in this case, evidence for the role of saliva in the transmission of the virus is unclear.[27] Another case report suggested the possibility of transmission of HIV from husband to wife by contact with saliva during kissing.[24] However, follow-up studies did not confirm HIV infection in the wife.[6]

Universal precautions do not apply to saliva. General infection control practices already in existence—including the use of gloves for digital examination of mucous membranes and for endotracheal suctioning and handwashing after exposure to saliva—should further minimize the minute risk, if any, for salivary transmission of HIV and HBV.[3,26] Gloves need not be worn when feeding patients and when wiping saliva from skin.

Special precautions, however, are recommended for dentistry.[3] Occupationally acquired infection with HBV in dental workers has been documented,[7] and two possible cases of occupationally acquired HIV infection involving dentists have been reported.[5,16] During dental procedures, contamination of saliva with blood is predictable, trauma to health-care workers' hands is common, and blood spattering may occur. Infection control precautions for dentistry minimize the potential for nonintact skin and mucous membrane contact of dental health-care workers to blood-contaminated saliva of patients. In addition, the use of gloves for oral examinations and treatment in the dental setting may also protect the patient's oral mucous membranes from exposures to blood, which may occur from breaks in the skin of dental workers' hands.

USE OF PROTECTIVE BARRIERS

Protective barriers reduce the risk of exposure of the health-care worker's skin or mucous membranes to potentially infective materials. For universal precautions, protective barriers reduce the risk of exposure to blood, body fluids containing visible blood, and other fluids to which universal precautions apply. Examples of protective barriers include gloves, gowns, masks, and protective eyewear. Gloves should reduce the incidence of contamination of hands, but they cannot prevent penetrating injuries caused by needles or other sharp instruments. Masks and protective eyewear or face shields should reduce the incidence of contamination of mucous membranes of the mouth, nose, and eyes.

Universal precautions are intended to supplement rather than replace recommendations for routine infection control, such as handwashing and using gloves to prevent gross microbial contamination of hands.[9] Because specifying the types of barriers needed for every possible clinical situation is impractical, some judgment must be exercised.

The risk of nosocomial transmission of HIV, HBV, and

other bloodborne pathogens can be minimized if health-care workers use the following general guidelines.[*]

1. Take care to prevent injuries when using needles, scalpels, and other sharp instruments or devices; when handling sharp instruments after procedures; when cleaning used instruments; and when disposing of used needles. Do not recap used needles by hand or remove used needles from disposable syringes by hand. Do not bend, break, or otherwise manipulate used needles by hand. Place used disposable syringes and needles, scalpel blades, and other sharp items in puncture-resistant containers for disposal. Locate the puncture-resistant containers as close to the use area as is practical.

2. Use protective barriers to prevent exposure to blood, body fluids containing visible blood, and other fluids to which universal precautions apply. The type of protective barrier(s) should be appropriate for the procedure being performed and the type of exposure anticipated.

3. Immediately and thoroughly wash hands and other skin surfaces that are contaminated with blood, body fluids containing visible blood, or other body fluids to which universal precautions apply.

GLOVE USE FOR PHLEBOTOMY

Gloves should reduce the incidence of blood contamination of hands during phlebotomy (drawing blood samples), but they cannot prevent penetrating injuries caused by needles or other sharp instruments. The likelihood of hand contamination with blood containing HIV, HBV, or other bloodborne pathogens during phlebotomy depends on the following factors: (1) the skill and technique of the health-care worker, (2) the frequency with which the health-care worker performs the procedure (other factors being equal, the cumulative risk of blood exposure is higher for a health-care worker who performs more procedures), (3) whether the procedure occurs in a routine or emergency situation (during which blood contact may be more likely), and (4) the prevalence of infection with bloodborne pathogens in the patient population. The likelihood of infection after skin exposure to blood containing HIV or HBV will depend on the concentration of virus (viral concentration is much higher for hepatitis B than for HIV), the duration of contact, the presence of skin lesions on the hands of the health-care worker, and—for HBV—the immune status of the health-care worker. Although not accurately quantified, the risk of HIV infection following intact skin contact with infective blood is certainly much less than the 0.5% risk following percutaneous needlestick exposures.[5] In universal precautions, all blood is assumed to be potentially infective for bloodborne pathogens, but in certain settings (such as volunteer blood-donation centers) the prevalence of infection with some bloodborne pathogens (that is, HIV and HBV) is known to be very low. Some institutions have relaxed recommendations for using gloves for phlebotomy procedures by skilled phlebotomists in settings where the prevalence of bloodborne pathogens is known to be very low.

Institutions that do not require routine gloving for all phlebotomies should periodically reevaluate their policy. Gloves should always be available to health-care workers who wish to use them for phlebotomies. In addition, the following general guidelines apply.

1. Gloves should be used for performing phlebotomies when the health-care worker has cuts, scratches, or other breaks in her or his skin.

2. Gloves should be used in situations in which the health-care worker judges that hand contamination with blood may occur, for example, when performing phlebotomy on an uncooperative patient.

3. Gloves should be used when performing finger and/or heel sticks on infants and children.

4. Gloves should be used when persons are being trained in phlebotomy.

SELECTION OF GLOVES

The Center for Devices and Radiological Health, FDA, has responsibility for regulating the medical glove industry. Medical gloves include those marketed as sterile surgical or nonsterile examination gloves made of vinyl or latex. General purpose utility ("rubber") gloves are also used in the health-care setting, but they are not regulated by the FDA since they are not promoted for medical use. There are no reported differences in barrier effectiveness between intact latex and intact vinyl used to manufacture gloves. Thus, the type of gloves selected should be appropriate for the task being performed. The following general guidelines are recommended.

1. Use sterile gloves for procedures involving contact with normally sterile areas of the body.

2. Use examination gloves for procedures involving contact with mucous membranes, unless otherwise indicated, and for other patient care or diagnostic procedures that do not require the use of sterile gloves.

3. Change gloves between patient contacts.

4. Do not wash or disinfect surgical or examination gloves for reuse. Washing with surfactants may cause "wicking," that is, the enhanced penetration of liquids through undetected holes in the glove. Disinfecting agents may cause deterioration.

5. Use general-purpose utility gloves (such as rubber household gloves) for housekeeping chores involving potential blood contact and for instrument cleaning and decontamination procedures. Utility gloves may be decontaminated and reused but should be discarded if they are peeling, cracked, or discolored, or if they have punctures, tears, or other evidence of deterioration.

WASTE MANAGEMENT

Universal precautions are not intended to change waste management programs previously recommended by the CDC for health-care setting.[1] Policies for defining, collecting, storing, decontaminating, and disposing of infective

---

[*]The August 1987 publication should be consulted for general information and specific recommendations not addressed in this update.

waste are generally determined by institutions in accordance with state and local regulations. Information about waste management regulations in health-care settings may be obtained from state or local health departments or agencies responsible for waste management.

REFERENCES

1. Bond WW and others: Hepatitis B virus in peritoneal dialysis fluid: a potential hazard, Dial Transplant 11:592, 1982.
2. Cancio-Bello TP and others: An institutional outbreak of hepatitis B related to a human biting carrier, J Infect Dis 146:652, 1982.
3. Centers for Disease Control: Recommendations for prevention of HIV transmission in health-care settings, MMWR 36(2S), 1987.
4. Centers for Disease Control: 1988 agency summary statement for human immunodeficiency virus and report on laboratory-acquired infection with human immunodeficiency virus. MMWR 37(S4):1S, 1988.
5. Centers for Disease Control: Update: acquired immunodeficiency syndrome and human immunodeficiency virus infection among health-care workers. MMWR 37:299, 1988.
6. Curran JW and others: Epidemiology of HIV infection and AIDS in the United States, Science 239:610, 1988.
7. Department of Labor, Department of Health and Human Services: Joint advisory notice: protection against occupational exposure to hepatitis B virus (HBV) and human immunodeficiency virus (HIV), Washington, DC, 1987, US Department of Labor, US Department of Health and Human Services.
8. Friedland GH and others: Lack of transmission of HTLV-III/LAV infection to household contacts of patients with AIDS or AIDS-related complex with oral candidiasis, N Engl J Med 314:344, 1986.
9. Garner JS and Favero MS: Guideline for handwashing and hospital environmental control, Atlanta, 1985, US Department of Health and Human Services, Public Health Service, Centers for Disease Control, HHS publication no. 99-1117.
10. Garner JS and Simmons BP: Guideline for isolation precautions in hospitals, Infect control 4:245, 1983.
11. Glaser JB and Nadler JP: Hepatitis B virus in a cardiopulmonary resuscitation training course: risk of transmission from a surface antigen-positive participant, Arch Intern Med 145:1653, 1985.
12. Hollander H and Levy JA: Neurologic abnormalities and recovery of human immunodeficiency virus from cerebrospinal fluid, Ann Intern Med 106:692, 1987.
13. Immunization Practices Advisory Committee: Recommendations for protection against viral hepatitis, MMWR 34:313, 1985.
14. Jason JM and others: HTLV-III/LAV antibody and immune status of household contacts and sexual partners of persons with hemophilia, JAMA 255:212, 1986.
15. Jenison SA and others: Quantitative analysis of hepatitis B virus DNA in saliva and semen of chronically infected homosexual men, J Infect Dis 156:299, 1987.
16. Klein RS and others: Low occupational risk of human immunodeficiency virus infection among dental professionals, N Engl J Med 318:86, 1988.
17. Lee AKY, Ip HMH, and Wong VCW: Mechanisms of maternal-fetal transmission of hepatitis B virus, J Infect Dis 138:668, 1978.
18. Lifson AR: Do alternate modes for transmission of human immunodeficiency virus exist: a review, JAMA 259:1353, 1988.
19. MacQuarrie MB, Forghani B, and Wolochow DA: Hepatitis B transmitted by a human bite, JAMA 230:723, 1974.
20. Mundy DC and others: Human immunodeficiency virus isolated from amniotic fluid, Lancet 2:459, 1987.
21. Onion DK, Crumpacker CS, and Gilliland BC: Arthritis of hepatitis associated with Australia antigen, Ann Intern Med 75:29, 1971.
22. Oskenhendler E and others: HIV infection with seroconversion after a superficial needlestick injury to the finger [letter], N Engl J Med 315:582, 1986.
23. Osterholm MT and others: Lack of transmission of viral hepatitis type B after oral exposure to HBsAg-positive saliva, Br Med J 2:1263, 1979.
24. Salahuddin SZ and others: HTLV-III in symptom-free seronegative persons, Lancet 2:1418, 1984.
25. Scott RM and others: Experimental transmission of hepatitis B virus by semen and saliva, J Infect Dis 142:67, 1980.
26. Simmons BP and Wong ES: Guideline for prevention of nosocomial pneumonia, Atlanta, 1982, US Department of Health and Human Services, Public Health Service, Centers for Disease Control.
27. Wahn V and others: Horizontal transmission of HIV infection between two siblings [letter], Lancet 2:694, 1986.
28. Wirthrington RH and others: Isolation of human immunodeficiency virus from synovial fluid of a patient with reactive arthritis, Br Med J 294:484, 1987.

Index